AIDS

Papers from *Science*, 1982–1985

Edited by Ruth Kulstad

The American Association for the Advancement of Science

Library of Congress Cataloging-in-Publication Data
Main entry under title:

AIDS: Papers from Science, 1982–1985.

Includes index.
1. AIDS (Disease)—Addresses, essays, lectures.
I. Kulstad, Ruth. II. Science.
[DNLM: 1. Acquired Immunodeficiency Syndrome—collected works. WD 308 A2878]
RC607.A26A348   1986   616.97'92   85-28776
ISBN 0-87168-313-X
ISBN 0-87168-281-8 (pbk.)

This material originally appeared in *Science,* the official journal of the American Association for the Advancement of Science.

AAAS Publication No. 85-23

Printed in the United States of America

Other titles in this series of *Science* volumes include:

Biotechnology & Biological Frontiers
Edited by Philip H. Abelson

Neuroscience
Edited by Philip H. Abelson, Eleanore Butz, and Solomon H. Snyder

Astronomy & Astrophysics
Edited by Morton S. Roberts

Biotechnology & Biological Frontiers II (forthcoming)
Edited by Daniel E. Koshland, Jr.

Chemistry (forthcoming)
Edited by William Spindel and Robert M. Simon

Contents

Cases of AIDS in the United States
By Quarter-Year of Report to CDC

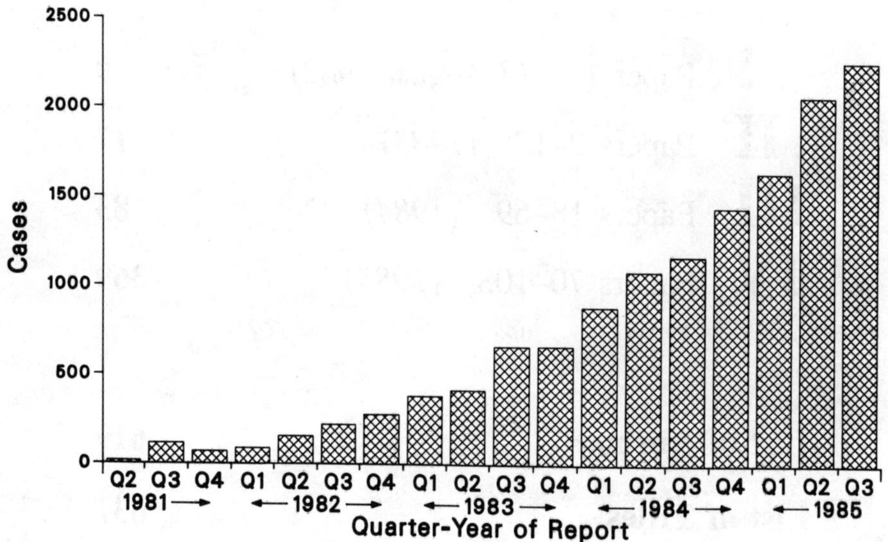

This graph shows cases of AIDS in the United States by quarter-year of report to the Centers for Disease Control. (Courtesy of W. Meade Morgan, CDC.)

Preface

The acquired immune deficiency syndrome (AIDS) is the top public health priority in the United States, and health officials all over the world are alarmed at the spread of this new disease. More funds for AIDS research are now becoming available, and increasing numbers of investigators are studying the disease. The rapid publication of the results of their work in many journals will continue to be an important part of the progress that is made in halting the epidemic. *Science* has already published some of the most frequently cited papers on AIDS, and a collection of them is useful now, both because of the experimental data they contain and because the papers provide a good source of references to related work in other journals. This volume joins other *Science* compendia on topics ranging from energy and food to biotechnology and neuroscience, all of which have helped disseminate essential information in important areas.

Included in this volume are research papers and a selection of news stories and letters that appeared in *Science* between August 1982 and September 1985. Not all the papers relate directly to AIDS research; some touch on aspects of the immune system that are not well understood, in AIDS or in other disorders, but are relevant because of the ideas they evoke. The news stories are by staff writers in the *Science* News and Comment and Research News departments. Many of them are by Dr. Jean Marx, who provided the first description of AIDS that *Science* published. Her stories give an explanation of what investigators are doing and why, and when arranged chronologically with the research papers, other news stories, and letters to the editor of *Science,* help give a picture of how far AIDS research has come and an indication of the directions in which it might go.

Thus the volume provides a brief history of the AIDS epidemic through September 1985, a history that also has sociologic interest. The research papers themselves reflect the interests and, perhaps, the beliefs of their authors, and indicate the state-of-the-art techniques applied to studies of the AIDS virus. The news stories focus on some of the problems associated with investigating a disease occurring predominantly—at least in the United States—in homosexual men, on the early reluctance of the federal government to provide adequate funds for research on AIDS, and on the problems that may be encountered in caring for huge numbers of sick and dying patients.

In the introduction to this volume, Dr. Myron Essex, chairman of the Department of Cancer Biology, Harvard University School of Public Health, provides an overview of research in AIDS to date. Dr. Essex, himself a leading AIDS researcher and senior author on several of the reports in the volume, has followed closely the expansion of the AIDS epidemic internationally; he was one of the first investigators to detect HTLV-related antibodies in AIDS patients and to find a disease similar to AIDS in monkeys. In the final paper in the volume, Dr. James Curran, chief of the AIDS Branch at the Centers for

Disease Control, provides an update—as of 30 August 1985—on the epidemiology of AIDS. Overall, it is apparent that the epidemic may still be at its beginning.

Since 1983, *Science*, like other journals, has made every effort to handle AIDS papers expeditiously. This would not have been possible without the help and cooperation of our outside reviewers, who are asked, at times, to drop what they are doing, criticize a manuscript, and convey their comments by telephone as well as in writing; of our authors, who must sometimes repeat experiments and make extensive revisions at the request of the reviewers and editors; and of members of the editorial, production, and support departments of *Science*, who must work together, and with the printer, at high speed while retaining their equanimity.

Ruth Kulstad
Science
October 1985

Introduction

October 1985

Introduction

October 1985

The Etiology of AIDS: Introduction and Overview

M. Essex

The acquired immune deficiency syndrome (AIDS) was first identified as a distinct clinical entity in 1981 by Gottlieb and his colleagues, who recognized that pneumocystis pneumonia was occurring at elevated rates in young homosexual males (*1*). The Centers for Disease Control soon proposed a working definition for the diagnosis of AIDS. Included in this definition were Kaposi's sarcoma (KS) and opportunistic infections with agents such as *Pneumocystis carinii* and *Mycobacterium avium*. Prior to the recognition of AIDS, these diseases were virtually unknown in young adults unless they occurred secondarily to some other process such as immunosuppression induced by cancer chemotherapy. The most obvious abnormality of the immune system seen in AIDS patients was a reversal in the ratio of helper to suppressor T lymphocytes, caused by an absolute reduction of T4 helper cells. The result is an impairment of both cell-mediated and humoral immune responses.

Numerous hypotheses were offered to explain the etiology of AIDS. Among them were the use of amyl nitrate or butyl nitrate "poppers," the effects on autoimmunity of repeated exposure to sperm, and an infectious agent. All of the hypotheses were influenced by observations that the greatest number of cases were in highly promiscuous homosexual males. Soon it became apparent that a similar or identical syndrome had begun at about the same time in distinctly different population groups, particularly intravenous drug abusers, hemophiliacs, recent immigrants from Haiti, and infants and blood transfusion recipients exposed to individuals from the other risk groups. Although some argued that the disease seen in different risk groups was not the same, upon further analysis it was apparent that the underlying immune lesions were very similar for the different risk groups, even though the spectrum of clinical presentation could vary.

With the realization that essentially the same disease had appeared for the first time in several different risk groups, the hypothesis that AIDS was caused by an infectious agent became more popular (*2*). There was still, however, considerable confusion about the types of infectious agents that should be considered. Viruses such as cytomegalovirus, Epstein-Barr virus, and hepatitis B were popular candidates at the earliest stages of the epidemic. This was partly because these agents were known to replicate to higher levels in male homosexuals or to have higher prevalence rates in this particular risk group (*3*).

During 1982 the possibility that AIDS might be caused by a member of the human T-lymphotropic virus (HTLV) family was discussed at professional meetings by Robert C. Gallo and myself. The first virus in this family had been discovered a few years earlier as the probable cause of adult T-cell leukemia (ATLL) (*4*), and was not included as a leading candidate for the cause of AIDS by most infectious disease epidemiologists. However, several characteristics of the HTLV's seemed particularly relevant to what was being observed in AIDS patients. For example, the HTLV's were the only viruses

4

known to preferentially infect T-helper lymphocytes (*5*), the target cells that become leukemic in ATLL. Once altered by HTLV, the T4 cells function in vitro as suppressor cells, even while maintaining the helper cell phenotype (*6*). HTLV was thought to be preferentially transmitted from males during sexual contact, from mother to child, and by blood transfusions (*7*).

Some skeptics found it hard to consider a retrovirus as a cause of immunosuppression. Yet, the T-lymphotropic feline leukemia viruses (FeLV) caused many more deaths in cats due to immunosuppression than to leukemia. And FeLV was known to suppress both the cell-mediated (*8*) and humoral (*9*) arms of the immune system, a situation similar to that seen in human AIDS. Furthermore, studies that were under way in Japan with HTLV-I indicated that persistently infected virus carriers had an elevated risk for the development of various infectious diseases less severe than AIDS (*10*). Some investigators suggested that a retrovirus should not be considered as a possible cause of AIDS because AIDS had not been recorded in Japan. But whatever agent caused this disease, it was very likely to be new because AIDS itself was a new disease. Thus, whether a cytomegalovirus or an HTLV was to be considered it would almost certainly have to represent a strain or type of agent that was different from those that had been in the human population for many years. What was not recognized at the time was how different the HTLV-III/LAV agent would be from other previously recognized T4 tropic HTLV's.

The first reports that provided experimental evidence for an association between an HTLV-type agent and AIDS were published in *Science* in May 1983 (*11-14*). This series of papers, from the laboratories of Gallo and Luc Montagnier, as well as my laboratory, provided evidence for the identification of a T-lymphotropic virus in several patients with AIDS or pre-AIDS, now called the AIDS related complex (ARC). Results from my laboratory indicated that about a third of the AIDS patients examined had antibodies that were cross- reactive with antigens of HTLV-I–infected T4 cells (*11*). Gallo and his colleagues reported the presence of HTLV antigens in T cells cultured from peripheral blood lymphocytes of two AIDS patients in France as well as the isolation of an HTLV from a patient in the United States (*12, 13*). The group at the Pasteur Institute reported finding HTLV-related antibodies in a patient with ARC who also yielded a virus that was cytopathic for cord blood lymphocytes (*14*). This virus would later be called the lymphadenopathy associated virus (LAV) by Montagnier and his colleagues.

During the ensuing months evidence began to accumulate that was compatible with an HTLV-type agent as a cause of AIDS. Elevated rates of antibodies cross-reactive with HTLV were also found in hemophiliacs, a group at high risk for development of AIDS (*15*). Recipients of blood transfusions were also reported among the various groups that developed AIDS (*16*), and we observed that transfusion-associated AIDS cases had usually received blood from a donor who was positive for HTLV antibodies (*17*). Yet retroviruses could only occasionally be isolated from AIDS or ARC patients, and antibodies could only be found in one-third to one-half of the patients, leaving many scientists skeptical that a retrovirus would be shown to cause AIDS.

What amounted to the proof that AIDS was caused by HTLV-III/LAV came when Gallo and his colleagues provided an overwhelming amount of evidence published in *Science* in May 1984 (*18-21*). The virus was isolated from 48 different donors, including 18 of 21 with ARC (*19*), and antibodies were detected in 88 percent of the AIDS patients (*21*). A cell line was described that could be used to grow large amounts of HTLV-III/LAV for biochemical studies and for antigen preparation (*18*). Several proteins specific for the virus were delineated (*20*), and an enzyme-linked immunosorbent assay (ELISA) and immunoblotting methods to be used for antibody screening were described (*21*).

At about the same time the cause of human AIDS was being revealed, several groups devoted attention to outbreaks of a similar disease in macaque monkeys. Large numbers of deaths from opportunistic infections, lymphoma, and retroperitoneal fibrosis had been recorded in several primate colonies (*22-25*). Because it was suggested that monkeys with this disease might provide an important model to study AIDS, the term simian AIDS or SAIDS was introduced. However, the spectrum of diseases involved in the SAIDS outbreak was variable, and the underlying cause was unclear. Initial suggestions that a monkey cytomegalovirus be considered soon gave way to the Mason Pfizer monkey retrovirus as a leading candidate (*26-28*). But by 1985 a new retrovirus that was antigenically similar to HTLV-III/LAV had also been detected in immunosuppressed monkeys (*29, 30*). This suggested that monkeys with an agent cross-reactive with HTLV-III/LAV could be used as a model for the pathogenesis of AIDS and for vaccine development.

The hypothesis that HTLV-I originated in Africa was raised by Gallo and his co-workers (*31*); Miyoshi and others had already obtained evidence that numerous species of Asian and African primates were infected with progenitor viruses designated STLV-I (*32*). In at least some instances, these, too, were associated with leukemia development (*33*). When clinical observations suggested that human AIDS (*34-36*), and thus HTLV-III/LAV, might also have originated in Africa, we decided to determine whether a virus related to HTLV-III/LAV might also exist in wild African monkeys. Such a virus, closely related to

both HTLV-III/LAV and STLV-III of macaques, was found infecting the majority of African Green monkeys, the species most prevalent in the region of central Africa where human AIDS was first reported (*37*). This suggested the possibility that HTLV-III/LAV entered the human population relatively recently from a primate source in Africa.

Analyses of the molecular structure and nucleotide sequence of HTLV-III/LAV and of the regulatory mechanisms utilized by the virus revealed several unexpected results. One unexpected finding was that HTLV-III/LAV was slightly larger than HTLV-I or HTLV-II and contained extra genes in the 3' end of the genome (*38-41*). It was also surprising to many investigators that HTLV-III/LAV had some homology with lentiviruses such as visna (*42*). The viral genome also had an unusual degree of genetic drift when one isolate was compared to another, and an unusual amount of extrachromosomal DNA (*43, 44*).

Earlier results with HTLV-I and HTLV-II indicated the presence of a previously unidentified gene, initially designated *x* or *lor*, and eventually labeled *tat* because the gene showed activity as a *trans*-activator of transcription (*45, 46*). The gene product of *tat*, designated p42, was believed to be involved in the immortalization of target lymphocytes (*47, 48*). In the case of HTLV-III, the same *tat* function was identified (*49*). In fact, the ability of the *tat* gene of HTLV-III to up-regulate transcription seemed about 1000-fold higher than that of SV40, and tenfold higher than that of HTLV-I.

For HTLV-III/LAV, the *env* glycoprotein gp120 represents the most immunogenic part of the virus (*50-53*). It is highly glycosylated, and considerably larger than the comparable external glycoproteins on most other retroviruses. It is thus the most appropriate antigen to use for antibody screening tests and in theory the molecule that would have to be used for

6

vaccine development. Although a considerable amount of genetic variation is seen within the *env* gene, several conserved regions are also present and presumably they can provide constant targets for the antibodies found in virus carrier individuals. The transmembrane protein gp41 also provides an important target for diagnostic antibodies, especially since it is difficult to obtain the delicate gp120 by concentrating virus from cell culture supernatant fluids.

At the time of this writing it has been just over 1 year since the evidence that HTLV-III/LAV causes AIDS was obtained by Gallo and his colleagues, and just over 2 years since retroviruses were first implicated in this disease by the Montagnier, Gallo, and Essex laboratories. During the ensuing time a very substantial amount of information has accumulated, providing extensive characterization of both the virus and the disease state, with much of the information published in *Science* and included in this volume. It has recently been recognized that the virus infects the central nervous system and causes brain lesions (*43*). Detailed studies on the immune defects, on drug treatment, and on vaccine development have just begun. Despite the present accumulation of knowledge we do not yet know how to cure the disease in the cases of AIDS already recorded or how to prevent disease development in the estimated one million asymptomatic Americans believed to be persistently infected with the virus (*54*). Although we do know much about how the virus is transmitted, the presence of the asymptomatic carrier state combined with the very long induction period suggests that several million more people may become infected before the epidemic peaks. One may hope that the next few years will represent a phase where the results of our research can be applied rapidly enough to control this highly unusual virus and its pathologic consequences.

October 1985

References

1. M.S. Gottlieb *et al.*, *N. Engl. J. Med.* **305**, 1425 (1981).
2. D.P. Francis, J.W. Curran, M. Essex, *J. Natl. Cancer Inst.* **71**, 1 (1983).
3. M.F. Rogers *et al.*, *Ann. Intern. Med.* **99**, 151 (1983).
4. B.J. Poiesz, F.W. Ruscetti, A.F. Gazdar, P.A. Bunn, J.E. Minna, R.C. Gallo, *Proc. Natl. Acad. Sci. U.S.A.* **77**, 7415 (1980).
5. M. Popovic *et al.*, *Science* **219**, 856 (1983).
6. Y. Yamada, *Blood* **61**, 192 (1983).
7. Y. Hinuma, *Gann* **28**, 211 (1982).
8. L.E. Perryman, E.A. Hoover, D.S. Yohn, *J. Natl. Cancer Inst.* **49**, 1357 (1972).
9. Z. Trainin, D. Wernicke, H. Ungar-Waron, M. Essex, *Science* **220**, 858 (1983).
10. M. Essex, M.F. McLane, N. Tachibana, D.P. Francis, T.H. Lee, in *Human T-Cell Leukemia/Lymphoma Virus*, R.C. Gallo, M. Essex, L. Groos, Eds. (Cold Spring Harbor Laboratory Press, Cold Spring Harbor, N.Y., 1984), p. 355.
11. M. Essex *et al.*, *Science* **220**, 859 (1983).
12. E.P. Gelman *et al.*, *ibid.*, p. 862.
13. R.C. Gallo *et al.*, *ibid.*, p. 865.
14. F. Barré-Sinoussi *et al.*, *ibid.*, p. 868.
15. M. Essex *et al.*, *ibid.* **221**, 1061 (1983).
16. J.W. Curran *et al.*, *N. Engl. J. Med.* **310**, 69 (1984).
17. H.W. Jaffee *et al.*, *Science* **223**, 1309 (1984).
18. M. Popovic, M.G. Sarngadharan, E. Read, R.C. Gallo, *ibid.* **224**, 497 (1984).
19. R.C. Gallo *et al.*, *ibid.*, p. 500.
20. J. Schüpbach, M. Popovic, R.V. Gilden, M.A. Gonda, M.G. Sarngadharan, R.C. Gallo, *ibid.*, p. 503.
21. M.G. Sarngadharan, M. Popovic, L. Bruch, J. Schüpbach, R.C. Gallo, *ibid.*, p. 506.
22. R.V. Henrickson *et al.*, *Lancet* **1983-I**, 388 (1983).
23. R.D. Hunt *et al.*, *Proc. Natl. Acad. Sci. U.S.A.* **80**, 5085 (1983).
24. N.L. Letvin *et al.*, *Lancet* **1983-II**, 599 (1983).
25. M. Gravell *et al.*, *Science* **223**, 74 (1984).
26. M.D. Daniel, N.W. King, N.L. Letvin, R.D. Hunt, P.K. Sehgal, R.C. Desrosiers, *ibid.*, p. 602.
27. P.A. Marx *et al.*, *ibid.*, p. 1083.
28. K. Stromberg *et al.*, *ibid.* **224**, 289 (1984).
29. P.J. Kanki *et al.*, *ibid.* **228**, 1199 (1985).
30. M.D. Daniel *et al.*, *ibid.* **228**, 1201 (1985).
31. R.C. Gallo, A. Sliski, F. Wong-Staal, *Lancet* **1983-II**, 962 (1983).
32. I. Miyoski, Y. Ohtsuki, M. Fujishita, S. Yoshimoto, I. Kubonishi, M. Minezawa, *Gann* **73**, 848 (1982).
33. T. Homma *et al.*, *Science* **225**, 716 (1984).
34. I.C. Bygbjerg, *Lancet* **1983-I**, 925 (1983).
35. J. Vandepitte, R. Verwilgen, P. Zachee, *ibid.*, p. 925.
36. N. Clumeck *et al.*, *N. Engl. J. Med.* **310**, 492 (1984).
37. P.J. Kanki, R. Kurth, W. Becker, G. Dreesman, M.T. McLane, M. Essex, *Lancet* **1985-I**, 1330 (1985).
38. L. Ratner *et al.*, *Nature (London)* **313**, 277 (1985).
39. S. Wain-Hobson, P. Sonigo, O. Danos, S. Cole, M. Alizon, *Cell* **40**, 9 (1985).
40. R. Sanchez-Pescador *et al.*, *Science* **227**, 484 (1985).
41. M.A. Muesing *et al.*, *Nature (London)* **313**, 480 (1985).
42. M.A. Gonda, F. Wong-Staal, R.C. Gallo, J.E. Clements, O. Narayan, R.V. Gilden, *Science* **227**, 173 (1985).
43. G.M. Shaw, B.H. Hahn, S.K. Arya, J.E. Groopman, R.C. Gallo, F. Wong-Staal, *ibid.* **226**, 1165 (1984).
44. B.H. Hahn, G.M. Shaw, S.K. Arya, M. Popovic, R.C. Gallo, F. Wong-Staal, *Nature (London)* **312**, 166 (1984).
45. W.A. Haseltine, J. Sodroski, R. Patarca, D. Briggs,

D. Perkins, F. Wong-Staal, *Science* **225**, 419 (1984).
46. J.G. Sodroski, C.A. Rosen, W.A. Haseltine, *ibid.*, p. 381.
47. T.H. Lee *et al.*, *ibid.* **226**, 57 (1984).
48. D.J. Slamon, K. Shimotohno, M.J. Cline, D.W. Golde, I.S.Y. Chen, *ibid.*, p. 61.
49. J. Sodroski *et al.*, *ibid.* **227**, 171 (1985).
50. L.W. Kitchen *et al.*, *Nature (London)* **312**, 367 (1984).
51. W.G. Robey *et al.*, *Science* **228**, 593 (1985).
52. F. Barin, M.F. McLane, J.S. Allan, T.H. Lee, J. Groopman, M. Essex, *ibid.*, p. 1094.
53. J. Allan *et al.*, *ibid.*, p. 1091.
54. J.W. Curran, W.M. Morgan, A.M. Hardy, H.W. Jaffee, W.W. Darrow, W.R. Dowdle, *ibid.* **229**, 1352 (1985).

August – December 1982

1.   New Disease Baffles Medical Community

Jean L. Marx

Within the past 4 years, a new disease of unknown cause and high virulence has afflicted more than 470 people, killing almost half of them. "It is a serious public health problem," says Harry Haverkos of the Centers for Disease Control (CDC), referring to what is known as acquired immunodeficiency syndrome (AIDS). "So far 184 people have died, which is more than the combined total of deaths attributed to toxic shock and the Philadelphia outbreak of Legionnaire's disease." Moreover, the toll continues to mount as 15 to 20 new cases are reported every week.

About one-third of the patients contract a hitherto rare form of cancer called Kaposi's sarcoma, although additional kinds of cancer are also turning up. The other major way in which the disease manifests itself is through infection by any of several pathogens. By far the most common is the protozoan *Pneumocystis carinii*, which causes a severe pneumonia. But the underlying problem is a defective immune system, which leaves the patients unable to resist the infections and, apparently, the cancer.

Not only is the disease a public health threat then, but analysis of the immune defect may have profound implications for research on cancer causation and the workings of the immune system. Michael Gottlieb of the University of California School of Medicine in Los Angeles describes it as "one of the most remarkable medical developments in 50 years. It may lead to important answers about immunoregulation and the origin of cancer."

Although other explanations have not been ruled out, most investigators currently think that the disease is caused by an infectious agent, possibly a new virus or a new variant of an existing virus. The spread of AIDS resembles that of hepatitis B virus.

Most of the patients—some 75 percent—are homosexual or bisexual men who are very active sexually. According to one study by the CDC, homosexuals who came down with AIDS averaged about 1100 sexual partners during their lifetime, whereas a control group of homosexual men averaged about 500.

The next biggest group of AIDS patients, some 12 percent, are users of intravenous drugs, such as heroin. Drug users, like sexually hyperactive homosexual males, have a high incidence of hepatitis B infections, which may be spread through sexual contact or by contaminated needles.

Hepatitis B is also transmitted through transfusion of whole blood or blood products. Recently, three individuals with hemophilia have come down with AIDS, an occurrence which is particularly disturbing because of the possibility that they acquired an infectious agent from the blood product they take to prevent bleeding. So far, however, there is no evidence linking ordinary blood transfusions to the immunodeficiency disease, Haverkos says. Hemophiliacs require two or three injections of clotting factor per week and the material is prepared from the blood of many individual donors, which means that hemophiliacs' total exposure to foreign substances is much greater than that of patients who receive transfusions of whole blood. The CDC has not been able to implicate any particular lot of clotting factor as a possible source of infection for these patients.

A third identifiable group of AIDS patients, who comprise 6 percent of the total, are Haitian immigrants to this country. At this time, no one knows how these individuals might have contracted the disease. They deny homosexual experience and, except for one patient, the use of intravenous drugs.

Finally, about 6 percent of AIDS patients do not fit into any of the three groups and have been classified as "other." Only 27 of the patients are women, and half of these use intravenous drugs.

Unusual cases of Kaposi's sarcoma began to attract notice a little over a year ago. For example, at about that time Alvin Friedman-Kien and Linda Laubenstein of New York University Medical Center acquired three young male homosexual patients with the cancer.

Kaposi's sarcoma had been very rare in this country. When it did occur it primarily affected elderly men—60 years of age or older—of Mediterranean origin or individuals whose immune systems were suppressed, either by cancer itself, cancer chemotherapy, or by drugs to prevent rejection of transplanted organs such as kidneys. But it was almost unheard of in young individuals who did not have these predisposing conditions. "Suddenly to see three cases of Kaposi's sarcoma in young men was most unexpected," Friedman-Kien remarks.

Similar cases soon began turning up, mostly in cities with large homosexual populations, including New York, Los Angeles, and San Francisco. The victims were male homosexuals of young or at most middle age. AIDS also began to be seen in intravenous drug users. "It is probably one of the first human cancers to be occurring in epidemic form," according to Friedman-Kien. (Burkitt's lymphoma in certain parts of Africa may be another.)

Moreover, the course of the sarcoma in these patients was much different from that in the older men. The latter usually have characteristic skin lesions on their legs. Their disease responds well to therapy and they rarely die from the cancer. But in the young patients the skin lesions were often located on the upper body, including the head and face. In addition, their internal organs were affected. Most of the patients respond poorly to therapy and death within 2 years is common.

The infections seen in AIDS patients, which first began to be noticed in about mid-1979, are also typical of those occurring in immunosuppressed individuals, but not in people who are generally healthy. The most common of these infections, which are called "opportunistic" because of their predilection for immunocompromised hosts, is *Pneumocystis* pneumonia. Roughly 60 percent of the AIDS patients, including some who also have the sarcoma, have *Pneumocystis* infections. Other infections, caused by viruses such as cytomegalovirus (CMV) and herpes simplex virus (HSV), by fungi such as *Candida* and *Cryptococcus*, by protozoans such as *Toxoplasma*, and by bacteria such as the tuberculosis bacillus, also occur.

The infections often have a relentlessly progressive course. Frederick Siegal of Mount Sinai School of Medicine says, "Infections that can be controlled with antimicrobials can be treated or suppressed, but eventually they recur or another infection overwhelms the patient." He estimates the long-term mortality of AIDS patients to be 65 percent.

The high incidence of Kaposi's sarcoma and the nature of the opportunistic infections in the patients suggested that their cellular immunity might be defective. As Siegal points out, "The organisms involved [in the infections] are mostly resisted by cellular immunity."

That the underlying defect affects cellular immunity has been borne out by several investigators. The patients' humoral immunity does not appear to be impaired; they have normal or elevated concentrations of antibodies in their blood.

The patients have low lymphocyte counts, often half or less than half of the normal lower limit of about 1500 lymphocytes per cubic millimeter of blood. In general, the antibody-secreting B lymphocytes are not much affected, but the T cells, the ones needed for cellular immunity, are both low in number and abnormal in composition. Gottlieb says, "In addition to the depletion of the total number of lymphocytes, certain subpopulations are more depleted than others."

In particular, the helper T cell subpopulation is greatly depleted or even missing, whereas the killer-suppressor T cell subpopulation is much less reduced. As might be expected from the names, helper T cells aid other immune cells to perform their functions and suppressor T cells inhibit them. Loss of the helpers, while the suppressor subpopulation remains more or less intact, could produce a profound suppression of cellular immunity, thus allowing the opportunistic infections to take hold.

The results also provide support for the controversial immune surveillance theory, which holds that immune cells help to protect against cancer by seeking out and destroying abnormal, cancerous cells before they can grow into a life-threatening tumor. In immunosuppressed patients, according to the theory, the cancer cells grow in the absence of the normal restraints. Precisely which immune cells might be important here is uncertain. In addition to the T cell abnormality, AIDS patients may have a reduced population of another type of immune cell, the natural killer, which has also been implicated in cancer cell surveillance.

According to Siegal, a shift in T cell subpopulations similar to that seen in AIDS patients, although less severe, occurs in many homosexual men. At this time, it is not known whether this is a subclinical manifestation of AIDS or is unrelated.

In addition, the CDC has received reports from physicians around the country of lymphadenopathy (enlarged lymph nodes) in homosexual men. By May of this year 57 patients had been reported. These individuals have enlarged lymph nodes in various locations throughout the body, and often experience fever, weight loss, fatigue, night sweats, diarrhea, and other symptoms of general malaise. Many of the patients with full-blown AIDS had similar symptoms in the months before they developed Kaposi's sarcoma or opportunistic infections. Moreover, profiles of the characteristics of the two groups—those with AIDS and those with the lymphadenopathy—are very similar. Thomas Spira of the CDC says, "The age distribution and other factors are virtually indistinguishable. . . . We don't know if the lymphadenopathy is a prodrome [premonitory symptom] or milder manifestation of the more severe disease, but our concern is that it is related." At least one of the lymphadenopathy patients has developed Kaposi's sarcoma.

The big question is what causes the immune defects of AIDS. For a time, health officials thought amyl nitrite and related vasodilator drugs might be involved. The drugs were used by practically all of the homosexual patients to intensify their sexual experiences. However, other patients among the intravenous drug users, Haitians, and hemophiliacs were not exposed to them. At most, the nitrites might have contributed to the homosexuals' immune deficiency without being its primary cause.

Most interest right now is focused on the possibility that an infectious agent causes AIDS. The resemblance of the population at risk to that at risk for hepatitis B suggests a viral pathogen, as does the discovery of the disease in hemophiliacs. In addition, David Auerbach and William Darrow of the CDC identified a cluster of nine AIDS cases in Los Angeles and Orange counties for whom they could establish sexual connections. This was out of a total of 19 cases at the time, although pertinent information could be obtained for only 13 of them. Auerbach says, "We estimate that it would be highly unlikely that these connections would occur at random. The finding speaks a little more strongly for some kind of infectious agent rather than some kind of toxic agent." One of the patients also had sexual contacts with AIDS patients in several other cities.

Gottlieb, for one, favors the idea that CMV plays an important role in AIDS. He suggests that it may be a major contributor to the development of Kaposi's sarcoma and may also help to produce the underlying immune defect. As he notes, the virus has been linked with Kaposi's sarcoma in other studies. It may be transmitted sexually, and homosexuals may have high rates of infection by CMV, up to 95 percent in some studies. Moreover, CMV is immunosuppressive, although the milder immunosuppression it causes has not been associated with Kaposi's sarcoma or opportunistic infections.

Nevertheless, there is a major problem with the idea that CMV, or any other known virus for that matter, causes AIDS. Neither homosexuality nor CMV is new, but the disease apparently is.

According to Haverkos, the earliest cases with the peculiar characteristics of the current disease that the CDC could identify began appearing in late 1978 and early 1979. The CDC came to this conclusion by examining tumor registries in several cities and their own records of requests for one of two major drugs used to treat *Pneumocystis* pneumonia. The CDC is the only source for this particular drug.

A new variant of CMV may have appeared a few years ago, but if it did, it has so far eluded detection. Many strains of CMV have been isolated from AIDS patients; the condition does not appear to be associated with any strain.

Another possibility is that the homosexual population at risk for AIDS experiences a more profound immunosuppression than members of the general population who might contract a viral infection, because they are exposed to many variants of CMV and other viruses. Spira favors the view that a new pathogen causes AIDS, but remarks, "As an alternate hypothesis, recurrent antigenic stimulation may cause a paralysis of the immune system." A similar explanation might apply to the hemophiliacs, who are exposed to many foreign antigens in the clotting factor preparations. The hypothesis also suffers from the problem of failing to explain how a new disease might have arisen, however.

Exposure to sperm from many sources may contribute to the immunodeficiency of homosexual men. Sperm are immunosuppressive if they enter the blood stream. Friedman-Kien, Laubenstein, and Pablo Rubinstein of the New York Blood Center and Bijan Safai's group at Memorial Sloan-Kettering Cancer Center have detected antibodies against sperm in the homosexual patients. These antibodies cross-react with T cells and could thus result in their depletion.

Neither Friedman-Kien nor Safai attributes AIDS solely to immunosuppression by sperm, however. Friedman-Kien says, "I don't think it is just the sperm; it may be a multiplicity of factors." A new virus, possibly carried by sperm, is a good possibility for one of the factors.

How the Haitians acquire AIDS, if they are not homosexuals or drug users, is one of the many puzzles of the disease. Nonetheless, their disease appears to be the same as that in the other groups. According to Spira and Margaret Fischl of Jackson Memorial Hospital in Miami, the Haitians with AIDS have a severe immune deficiency that closely resembles that of the other patients. "The syndrome we see in the Haitian group was strikingly similar to that in the gay community," Fischl explains.

Moreover, AIDS may be occurring in Haiti, too. B. Liautaud, a dermatologist in Port-au-Prince, recently reported 11 cases of Kaposi's sarcoma, a high number for such a small country. Fischl and Spira have begun immunological studies of some of these individuals to see if they have the same immunodeficiency as patients in this country.

Friedman-Kien and Safai point out that Haiti is a favorite vacation spot for many homosexual males. They might have carried the disease to or from that country. At present, no one knows if the syndrome being seen there began before or after AIDS in this country.

Although Kaposi's sarcoma is the most common cancer to be found in AIDS patients, it is not the only malignancy. This was not a surprise. Gottlieb remarks, "I would expect that we are going to see other cancers since these individuals are so profoundly immune deficient."

This expectation is rapidly being fulfilled. Friedman-Kien has now seen nine AIDS patients who have a cancer of the lymph system. In addition, three of the patients with Kaposi's sarcoma have also developed lymphomas.

According to John Ziegler of the Veterans Administration Hospital in San Francisco, Kaposi's sarcoma may be just one of a number of opportunistic tumors that may affect these immunosuppressed individuals. He and his colleagues have now found three individuals, young gay males with characteristics similar to those of the AIDS patients, who have a squamous carcinoma of the tongue. This cancer is rarely seen in young nonsmokers like these patients. One of the men was a lover of a patient with Kaposi's sarcoma. In addition, the San Francisco group has identified four AIDS patients who have a Burkitt's-like lymphoma.

Ziegler says, "The question arises— are these individuals susceptible to the cancers because of the activation of DNA viruses that are passed between the individuals?" All three of the cancers have been linked with members of the DNA-containing herpes virus family. Oral cancers, such as the squamous cell carcinoma, have been associated with HSV, Burkitt's lymphoma with Epstein-Barr virus (EBV), and, as already noted, Kaposi's sarcoma with CMV.

In fact, the Ziegler group has identified CMV DNA and proteins in sarcoma cells from AIDS patients, but not in normal cells from adjacent tissue. And they have found EBV in tumor cells from two of the lymphoma patients. Ziegler suggests that the immunosuppression of the patients may have allowed activation of the viruses, thus leading to the cancers. If his hypothesis is borne out, there would be another link for the chain of evidence supporting a causative role for the herpes viruses in cancer.

In addition to a possible role of the viruses in the etiologies of these cancers, there appears to be a genetic element influencing who gets the cancers, at least for Kaposi's sarcoma. According to Friedman-Kien, Laubenstein, and Rubinstein, there is an association between the sarcoma and a particular HLA antigen, the one designated DR5. The DR antigens, which are encoded by genes in the major histocompatibility complex, are thought to be involved in the regulation of immune responses. "Between 50 and 60 percent of the patients have HLA-DR5 in the classic as well as the homosexual variety of Kaposi's," says Friedman-Kien. "This indicates a genetic predisposition." Exactly how the DR5 antigen predisposes to Kaposi's sarcoma is not understood. Safai and Marilyn Pollack of Memorial Sloan-Kettering Cancer Center have similar findings.

In general, AIDS is providing researchers with a wealth of clues for investigating how the immune system works normally and how its malfunction can result in disease, including cancer. Meanwhile, a major effort is under way at CDC and elsewhere to pinpoint the agent or agents that cause the disease. "Identification of the cause and then prevention are the major goals," Gottlieb says.

January – December 1983

2. Spread of AIDS Sparks New Health Concern

Jean L. Marx

The relentless new disease called acquired immunodeficiency syndrome (AIDS) continues to spread. According to officials at the Centers for Disease Control (CDC), some 22 children, identified at medical centers in Newark, New York City, and San Francisco, are suspected of having the disorder. Most of the children were in close contact with parents or other adults who either have AIDS or are at high risk of contracting the disease.

Moreover, blood products have come under increased suspicion as vehicles for spreading AIDS. An infant who received several infusions of whole blood and blood products developed the condition. One of the donors, who had appeared well at the time he gave blood, eventually died of the disease. The CDC also reports the diagnosis of AIDS in four hemophiliacs, in addition to the three previously identified, confirming earlier suggestions that these individuals might be at high risk. "The problem in hemophiliacs is real," says the CDC's Harold Jaffe. "It isn't going to go away."

The latest reports support the hypothesis that AIDS is caused by an infectious agent, possibly a virus, that can be transmitted by close contact, including that between family members, or by blood products. The latter possibility raises a serious health issue about the safety of the blood products used by hemophiliacs and perhaps by the general public.

AIDS, which is thought to be a new disease, has a very poor prognosis. In the year and one-half since it was identified, 827 cases of AIDS have been reported to CDC, and 312 of the patients have died. Two or three new cases are reported to the CDC every day. Physicians treating the patients estimate that 65 percent will die within 2 years after the diagnosis, either of cancer, most often a hitherto rare type called Kaposi's sarcoma, or of any of several kinds of opportunistic infections, so-called because they strike individuals whose immune systems are defective. The underlying immune defect of AIDS affects the T lymphocytes, causing a profound suppression of the cellular arm of the immune system (*Science*, 13 August 1982).

The disease was first diagnosed in adults, principally in male homosexuals who had been extremely active sexually, users of intravenous drugs, and Haitians. The disease is apparently spread by sexual contact among homosexuals and by contaminated needles in the drug users. The reason for its prevalence in Haitians is unclear.

The mothers of several of the children who are now suspected of having AIDS are intravenous drug users; other mothers are Haitian. CDC officials hesitate to conclude unequivocally that the children have AIDS. Jaffe says, "We are having trouble sorting it out in children. We

20

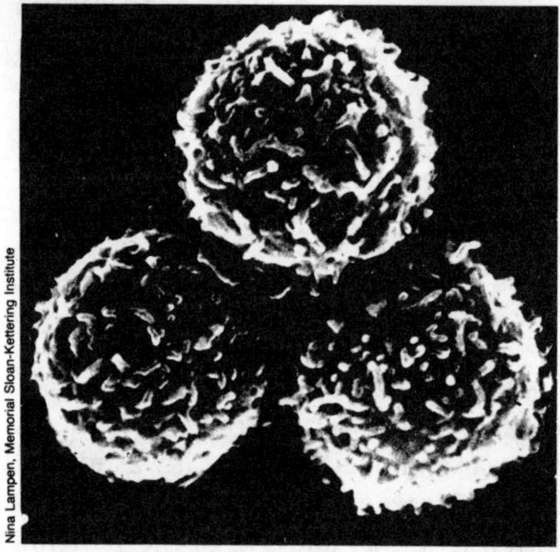

Normal blood lymphocytes.

don't have a single test for AIDS, and the children might have other types of immunodeficiencies. But their immune picture does not fit any of the well-described congenital immunodeficiencies."

The clinical picture presented by the children more closely resembles that of the adult AIDS patients. "If they were adults, it would be called AIDS," says James Oleske of St. Michael's Medical Center in Newark, where eight of the children have been identified. "These kids have immunological defects and infections that are characteristic of AIDS."

The most common life-threatening infection in the children, as in the adults, is a pneumonia caused by *Pneumocystis carinii*. Other infections, common in both the children and the adults, have been caused by viruses, including cytomegalovirus and herpes simplex virus, by yeast (*Candida*), and by *Mycobacterium avium-intracellulare*. So far none of the children have had cancer.

The principal immune defects of the children are also similar to those of adult patients. These include a marked decrease in the total number of T lymphocytes and a decrease in the ratio of helper T cells to suppressor T cells.

Arye Rubenstein of the Albert Einstein College of Medicine notes that the immune defects of the children are very different from those seen in congenital immunodeficiencies, in which the normal development of T or other immune cells is blocked with the result that the mature active cells are not formed. "The [AIDS] kids have mature T cells," Rubenstein explains, "but the proportion of helper and suppressor subsets is abnormal."

Ten of the most severely affected children have died, four of them infants who first became ill between 2 and 5 months of age. These children may have acquired AIDS while still in the womb, CDC officials suggest, or else very shortly after birth.

Two of the female children who died had the same mother, a prostitute and drug user who has AIDS symptoms herself. The woman's third daughter has some symptoms characteristic of AIDS, but has not suffered from life-threatening infections and is included in the less severely affected group of possible AIDS children. Clinicians are watching these children to see if their conditions worsen and become full-blown AIDS.

The presence of AIDS symptoms in three daughters of the same mother might suggest an inherited immune defect. However, they had different fathers and it is unlikely that all would inherit the disease unless the defective gene were dominant, which is not the case for the known congenital immunodeficiencies. Alternatively and more probably, the three children might have been exposed to an infectious agent for AIDS, although it is still possible that they might have inherited an increased susceptibility to that agent. Evidence for genetic susceptibility has been found in adult AIDS patients.

AIDS resembles hepatitis B in the groups affected, especially the male homosexuals and intravenous drugs users, and in the apparent mode of transmission through intimate contact and through blood products.

The evidence for transmission to hemophiliacs is now clear-cut, CDC officials say. Altogether there are seven confirmed cases in heterosexual male hemophiliacs, two of whom were less than 10 years old, plus one in a homosexual male.

No common lot of clotting factor, which might have been the source of an infectious agent, has been identified as being used by the patients. The seven patients received clotting factor preparation containing material from the blood of many individuals, which makes tracking down any AIDS patient among the donors very difficult.

The one AIDS case in which an AIDS victim has been identified among blood donors was that of an infant boy who was in the group of children studied by Arthur Ammann and his colleagues at the University of California Medical Center in San Francisco. The infant did not have any close contacts with AIDS victims. In the month after his birth, he had received numerous transfusions of whole blood and subfractions of blood, including packed cells and platelets, to treat Rh disease, which is caused by an incompatibility between the baby's blood type and his mother's. A total of 19 donors contributed the blood products. One of them, CDC investigators learned, was a man who developed AIDS some 8 months after he had donated blood. If the infant did contract AIDS because he was infected by an agent in the man's blood, the case has serious implications for the use of blood products. The agent must have been present and infectious for several months before it caused obvious symptoms.

The CDC is currently investigating the cases of two adult AIDS patients who do not have any of the common risk factors, but who did receive blood transfusions, to see if any of the donors might have developed AIDS.

Because of the serious nature of AIDS, its immediate threat to hemophiliacs who must have clotting factor, and its potential threat to a much wider population if it proves to be generally transmissible in blood products, Edward Brandt, assistant secretary for health in the U.S. Department of Health and Human Services, has called for an advisory committee to consider the current situation and determine what preventive steps ought to be taken regarding the collection of blood and its use. The committee meets on Tuesday, 4 January (2 weeks after this issue of *Science* went to press). The possibility that there may be a long latent period between the time of infection, by an as yet unidentified agent, and the emergence of AIDS symptoms will not make their task any easier.

3.   Health Officials Seek Ways to Halt AIDS

Jean L. Marx

On 4 January 1983 the Centers for Disease Control (CDC) convened a workshop at its Atlanta headquarters to assess the options for halting the spread of the new disease called acquired immunodeficiency syndrome or, more commonly, AIDS. The main topic of discussion was the possibility that the disease, which may kill up to 70 percent of the patients within 2 years of diagnosis, might be spread in blood and blood products.

The CDC recently reported that hemophiliacs are at high risk of contracting AIDS, which may be transmitted by an infectious agent in the blood clotting factor preparations that they take (*Science*, 7 January 1983). The Center's Bruce Evatt told the workshop that AIDS was the second leading cause of death for hemophiliacs in 1982, even though the disease was first discovered in hemophiliacs in the summer of that year. Eight hemophiliacs who had none of the other known risk factors died from AIDS, compared to some 40 who died of bleeding. James Curran, head of the CDC task force investigating AIDS, says, "The sense of urgency is greatest for hemophiliacs. The risk for others [who receive blood products] now appears small, but is unknown."

Suspicion has been cast on blood products in addition to clotting factor, however. An infant contracted AIDS after receiving red blood cells that had come from a man who developed the disease several months after he donated the blood. The CDC is also investigating the cases of two adults who developed AIDS after receiving blood transfusions during surgery. The two did not belong to any of the known high-risk groups, which include, in addition to hemophiliacs, homosexual and bisexual men who are extremely active sexually, users of intravenous drugs, and Haitians. In each case, investigators have identified a blood donor who has certain characteristics associated with AIDS, including a particular immune defect, although neither donor has actually developed the disease.

The CDC investigators have also identified several AIDS patients who donated blood. None of the recipients has contracted the condition, but there is still cause for worry. Thomas Spira of the CDC points out that there may be a long lag period, a year or more, between the time of exposure to the causative agent and the onset of AIDS. In other words, although there is currently no firm evidence linking ordinary blood transfusions to transmission of the disease, it is too early to rule out such a link.

The workshop participants easily reached agreement on some preventive measures that might check the spread of

AIDS. About 75 percent of the AIDS victims are homosexual or bisexual men in whom the disease is thought to be sexually transmitted. There was general agreement that homosexual men should avoid sexual contact with known or suspected AIDS patients, minimize the number of their sexual partners, and refrain from anonymous sexual contacts. Heterosexuals might follow the same suggestions because, according to Curran, there are indications that AIDS may also be transmitted by heterosexual sex and other forms of intimate personal contact, such as that between mother and child.

The seriousness of the threat of AIDS transmission by blood products and what, if anything, ought to be done in the current state of uncertainty remained thorny issues for the workshop participants. Not everyone agrees with the conclusion, accepted by CDC officials and many other investigators, that AIDS is caused by an infectious agent, presumably a virus, which could contaminate blood products. Louis Aledort, the medical director of the National Hemophilia Foundation, says, "I think it is too easily concluded that there is a transmissible agent. I can't rule it out but the data are not there yet." Aledort favors the idea that hemophiliacs, as well as homosexuals and intravenous drug users, because they are exposed to a great number of foreign antigens, experience a high degree of antigenic stimulation that effectively wears out their immune systems.

Nevertheless, because of the seriousness of AIDS, many participants were in favor of introducing measures to prevent persons who might be carrying an infectious agent from donating blood or plasma. The question is how to do this, especially in view of the long latent period of the disease and the possibility that many individuals who do not have full-blown AIDS may have a milder form or be asymptomatic carriers of an infectious agent.

Asking members of high-risk groups to voluntarily refrain from donating blood is one relatively uncontroversial approach, although it would probably not eliminate all potential carriers. Automatically excluding all members of high-risk groups is another, although this measure has the disadvantage of stigmatizing all homosexual males when only a fraction—those who are extremely sexually promiscuous—are likely to transmit an AIDS agent. Past and present users of intravenous drugs, who may be hepatitis carriers, and hemophiliacs are already excluded. Potential donors may also be screened for AIDS symptoms through a physical examination or a medical history.

Finally, the blood itself may be screened. Since the agent has not been identified, it would be necessary to use a "surrogate agent" as a marker for AIDS infectivity. The best candidate for this is an antibody to the core antigen of the hepatitis B virus. According to Spira, testing for this antibody in donated blood would detect about 90 percent of the donors who might transmit an AIDS agent, including persons with full-blown AIDS, those with the milder symptoms, and members of high-risk groups.

Some workshop participants favored requiring the test for all blood collection centers, but Aaron Kellner of the New York Blood Center dissented. "It is one thing to do these tests in the laboratory and another in the real world," he said. Kellner suggests that a few blood collection centers in the cities where AIDS is most prevalent—New York, San Francisco, and Los Angeles—undertake pilot studies to assess the feasibility and costs (including lost blood donations) of doing the antibody test.

The next step after the workshop is the preparation by CDC officials of a list of options for containing AIDS. This list will be submitted to Edward Brandt, assistant secretary for health in the U.S. Department of Health and Human Services, whose office will decide which options, if any, to implement.

Meanwhile, hemophiliacs who need clotting factor face an uneasy situation. Oscar Ratnoff, a hemophilia specialist from University Hospitals in Cleveland, proposes that they might minimize their risk of AIDS by using clotting factor cryoprecipitate instead of concentrate. A given lot of cryoprecipitate is made from material donated by one individual whereas each lot of concentrate contains material from an average of 5000 donors.

Cryoprecipitate may not be potent enough to control bleeding of some patients, however. The National Hemophilia Foundation recommends that new patients be given cryoprecipitate as long as possible, but that hemophiliacs who are already using the concentrate continue to do so. According to Dennis Donohue of the Bureau of Biologics of the Food and Drug Administration, an effort to prepare a safer clotting factor concentrate by removing or inactivating contaminating viruses is under way.

The biggest question of all still remains. What causes AIDS? Donald Armstrong of Memorial Sloan-Kettering Cancer Center expressed the hope that investigators not be distracted from answering that question. "I have no doubt that this is an infectious disease," he asserted. "I think we have to find the agent. A surrogate agent isn't good enough."

Research News

20 May 1983

4. Human T-Cell Leukemia Virus Linked to AIDS

Jean L. Marx

Five reports in the 20 May 1983 issue of *Science* suggest a possible link between the serious new disease, acquired immune deficiency syndrome (AIDS) and human T-cell leukemia virus (HTLV), which has been associated with a rare type of human cancer. Investigators at the Harvard University School of Public Health, the National Cancer Institute, and the Pasteur Institute have found evidence of HTLV infection in patients with AIDS or at high risk of developing the syndrome. The evidence includes isolation of the virus itself from a few patients, detection of the viral DNA in T cells from two cases, and also a much higher incidence of antibodies against HTLV in AIDS patients than in controls.

It is still too early to tell whether HTLV actually causes AIDS. The disease is characterized by immune suppression, which results in high susceptibility to opportunistic infections by agents that do not usually cause serious illnesses in healthy people but can prove devastating to individuals with defective immune responses. HTLV may be just another of these opportunistic pathogens, a consequence rather than a cause of AIDS. Max Essex of the Harvard group says, "I definitely do not want anyone to get the impression that we have proof of cause. What we do have is a good lead."

A good lead is much needed. Since AIDS first became manifest in 1981, more than 1350 cases have been reported to the Centers for Disease Control (CDC). The mortality rate may be 70 percent or higher, and the number of cases continues to grow by four to five per day. Epidemiological studies strongly suggest that AIDS is caused by an infectious agent, although other possibilities have not been conclusively ruled out. Efforts to identify the infectious agent have proved frustrating.

According to Robert Gallo of the National Cancer Institute (NCI), there are a number of reasons for taking a close look at HTLV as a possible cause of AIDS. First is the prevalence of HTLV in the Caribbean area and in Africa. The Caribbean area, especially Haiti, and equatorial Africa have been suggested as possible sources of the putative AIDS agent.

In the United States, Haitian immigrants constitute the third largest group of AIDS patients. The largest group consists of homosexual and bisexual men who have been extremely active sexually, and the second largest includes users of illegal intravenous drugs. Hemophiliacs are a fourth group with increased risk of AIDS.

AIDS has apparently spread among homosexuals by sexual contact and among drug users by contaminated needles. It is believed to have been transmitted to hemophiliacs by way of the blood clotting factor preparations that they must take. But the Haitians have always been a puzzle, because the vast majority deny both homosexual practices and drug use and they have not been exposed to clotting factor preparations. The identification of a causative virus in the Haitian population could help clear up this mystery.

Secondly, HTLV primarily infects T cells. As Gallo puts it, "HTLV is extraordinarily T-cell tropic." The primary AIDS defect also seems to be in the T lymphocytes, which are reduced in number in the patients and abnormal in composition. The helper T cells, which are needed to activate certain immune responses, including antibody production by the B lymphocytes, are very low in number, whereas the killer-suppressor cells are much less affected. The loss of helpers, while the activities of suppressor T cells remain more or less intact, could produce the profound suppression of the immune response that is characteristic of AIDS.

A third point of similarity is mode of transmission. As noted previously, AIDS spreads by intimate contact and through blood products. "Everything we know about HTLV suggests that intimate contact is needed for transmission," Gallo remarks. He points out that the viral envelope, which is required for infectivity, is very fragile. It tends to

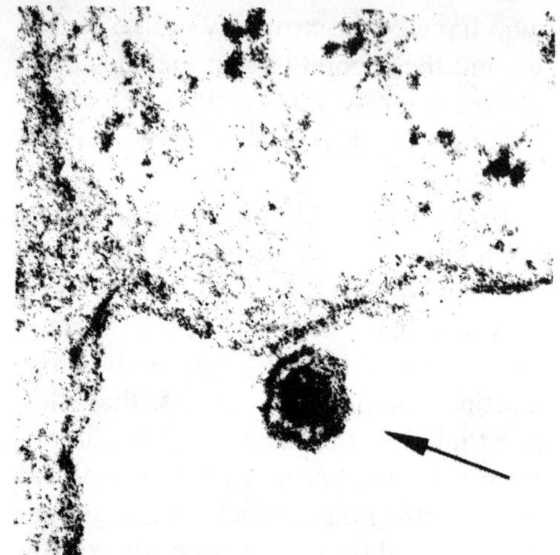

Human T-cell leukemia virus

come off when the virus buds from infected cells, thus rendering the particles incapable of infecting new cells. Gallo speculates that direct cell-to-cell contact may be required for the spread of HTLV.

Finally, there are precedents for a virus causing both a leukemia and immunosuppression. This is true for feline leukemia virus, which has been studied for many years in the Essex laboratory. "More cats are killed as a result of feline leukemia virus causing immunosuppression than by feline leukemia virus causing leukemia," Essex says.

The virus generally impairs T-cell responses in the animals. Previous attempts to demonstrate an effect on antibody production had failed, but the Essex group now finds that natural infection by feline leukemia virus suppresses the antibody response to an antigen that normally requires the cooperation of helper T cells to elicit antibody production. Feline leukemia virus also has a preference for infecting T cells and pro-

duces primarily T cell leukemias. The antibody response may be deficient, Essex speculates, because of a problem with the helper T cells.

Previous failures to demonstrate a viral effect on antibody production may be attributable to the differing responses of cats to naturally occurring and laboratory-induced infections. The natural infections are more effective at suppressing the immune response of cats than infections induced by such laboratory methods as directly injecting the virus.

HTLV is one of the retroviruses, which have RNA as their genetic material. In infected cells, the RNA is copied into DNA, which may then become integrated into the DNA genome of the host cell and bring about the cell's cancerous transformation. To determine whether AIDS patients showed signs of infection by HTLV the Gallo group looked for viral DNA in the patients' T cells.

They detected the viral DNA in the cells of two of 33 patients, but did not find it in T cells from any of 25 healthy homosexual males. They were able to isolate infectious HTLV particles from the T cells of one of the two individuals who were positive for viral DNA and also from two additional patients. This is from a total of about 20 patients whose T cells were used in attempts to isolate HTLV. In addition, a French group, under the direction of Luc Montagnier of the Pasteur Institute in Paris, has isolated a related virus from the T cells of a homosexual male with lymphadenopathy, a condition that may be a mild form of AIDS or a forerunner of the full-blown disease.

There is more than one type of HTLV. About 35 isolates of the virus have been made throughout the world. Roughly 25 of these have been characterized and most are of the type designated HTLV-I, which was originally isolated by the Gallo group. A second type of the virus, which is designated HTLV-II, has been isolated from the cells of a patient with hairy cell leukemia.

The NCI workers have characterized one of their three HTLV isolates from AIDS patients and it is HTLV-I. The virus isolated by the French group is neither HTLV-I nor -II, but represents a third variant of the virus. Although the members of the HTLV family are distinguished on the basis of structural variations in one of the internal proteins of the viral particle, they have other features in common, including their preference for infecting T cells and the rather unusual properties of their enzyme for copying RNA into DNA.

Gallo suggests that logistical problems might explain why viral DNA could be detected in the cells of so few AIDS patients. "If infection leads to a decline in the population of infected cells, you may not be able to find them by the time you get frank disease," he explains. In fact, the NCI workers could not detect integrated viral DNA in T cells from blood samples taken at a later date from the two patients who had earlier given positive results. The same problem might affect attempts to isolate the virus itself. Lymphocytes from the spleen or lymph nodes might be a better source of virus than the peripheral blood cells used for the NCI studies. The French workers isolated their virus from lymph node cells.

If HTLV does cause AIDS then there must be a way of maintaining the immunosuppressed state even after the virus is no longer detectable. The immune systems of the patients do not appear to recover.

Simply finding HTLV or the DNA in AIDS patients does not mean that the virus caused the disease. "From our data it could be an opportunistic infection," Gallo concedes. "But Essex's data argue that it is more than opportunistic."

Essex and his Harvard and CDC collaborators detected antibodies against membrane-associated antigens of HTLV in at least 25 percent of 75 AIDS and 23 lymphadenopathy patients. Another 10 percent or so would be positive if the investigators used a somewhat less stringent criterion for a positive antibody test.

In contrast, only one of 81 homosexual controls who had been matched for age, race, and place of residence with 36 of the AIDS patients had the antibodies. The one positive individual was a friend, but not a sex partner, of one of the patients. Only two of an additional 305 controls, including homosexuals who had visited a venereal disease clinic, healthy blood donors, kidney dialysis and chronic hepatitis patients, had the antibodies. "The message is that 25 to 40 percent of AIDS cases have the antibodies and 1 percent or less of control groups do," Essex says.

Other attempts to identify differences in viral exposures between AIDS patients and controls have not turned up such a large discrepancy between the two groups. Nevertheless, some 50 percent of the patients did not have the antibodies, either because the test was not sensitive enough to detect them or because their immune systems failed to make the antibodies—or because they had not been infected by HTLV.

Militating against the possibility that HTLV causes AIDS, Gallo says, is the relatively short period of time required for the immune deficiency disease to develop. CDC officials have reported the latency period of AIDS to be several months to a year. The T-cell leukemia caused by HTLV may require years, if not decades, to develop after infection by the virus.

Perhaps more disconcerting than the discrepancies in the latency periods of the two conditions is the apparent lack of AIDS in southern Japan, an area where the rate of HTLV infection is very high. Some 25 percent of the population there have antibodies against the virus, compared to 4 to 5 percent in Haiti and 1 percent in the United States.

Either AIDS exists in that part of Japan but has not been diagnosed, which seems unlikely especially in view of the publicity AIDS has received during the past year, or the Japanese may respond differently to the infection. Another possibility, Gallo points out, is that a change occurred in the HTLV family in Africa or Haiti that conferred a new capability for immune suppression on the virus. Comparison of the nucleotide sequences of the DNA of viral isolates from the various sources may help to clarify this issue.

Why some people might develop AIDS as a consequence of HTLV infection while others get leukemia is unclear. It might be an as yet undetermined difference in the infecting HTLV or in the host response to the infection. It might depend on the site at which the viral DNA integrates in the genome of infected cells.

In any event, there are now a number of approaches that may be taken to clarify the relation between HTLV and AIDS. A prospective study of high-risk individuals to see whether HTLV infection precedes or follows development of AIDS is a possibility. Another is to look at people who have other types of immune suppression, children with congenital immunodeficiency diseases or kidney transplant patients, for example, to see if they too have an increased number of HTLV infections.

If HTLV does eventually prove to be the cause of AIDS, then a specific test for the early diagnosis of the condition may be feasible. Especially desirable is an assay for the AIDS agent in blood. The possibility that the condition may be transmitted in blood products has naturally generated a great deal of concern. Ultimately a vaccine may be developed to protect high-risk individuals. But that all awaits firm proof of the cause of AIDS.

Report

20 May 1983

5. Suppression of the Humoral Antibody Response in Natural Retrovirus Infections

Ze'ev Trainin, Dorothee Wernicke, Hannah Ungar-Waron, and Max Essex

As a group, retroviruses often infect lymphoid tissues and many cause leukemias (*1*). Some, such as the feline leukemia virus (FeLV), cause many more deaths by predisposing the host to acute infections by other pathogens than by inducing leukemia (*2*). Cats infected with FeLV were previously shown to have prolonged homograft rejection responses (*3*), but, in the same study, no evidence was found that the humoral immune response was impaired. In the study reported here we found that the humoral response to the synthetic multichain polypeptide (L-tyrosine-L-glutamic acid)-poly-DL-alanine-poly-L-lysine, denoted (T,G)AL, was significantly depressed in healthy cats that were naturally infected with FeLV compared to uninfected controls. In cats that were persistently viremic with FeLV the major antibody response to (T,G)AL, normally seen at days 9 to 14 after immunization, was both delayed and greatly reduced.

Eight outbred adult cats that became persistently viremic with FeLV in their natural environment were studied. By means of indirect fixed-cell immunofluorescence (*4*), viremia was confirmed in each cat for a period of at least 6 months at the time of inoculation with antigen. The FeLV-infected cats were also judged to be clinically healthy, both before and during the course of the experi-

ments. Six uninfected healthy adult cats from similar environments were used as controls. Each animal was subcutaneously immunized with 1 mg of (T,G)AL in complete Freund's adjuvant. Blood was taken from the jugular vein at day 0, just before immunization, and subsequently every second day until day 11 and at intervals of several days thereafter for a total of about 110 days. The serum samples were tested for antibodies against (T,G)AL by means of an enzyme-linked immunoadsorbant assay (ELISA) as described by Ungar-Waron *et al.* (*5*).

The results are shown in Table 1 and Fig. 1. In the uninfected control group the first evidence of antibody production to (T,G)AL was detected between days 3 and 5. A major increase in antibody titer was detected at days 10 to 13 in the uninfected animals. The antibody titer increased rapidly to a very high level at about day 14, and then increased gradually to day 30 with individual end-point titers of 1:640 to 1:10,240 (Table 1). The antibody titers subsequently decreased at days 60 to 80.

Of the eight FeLV-infected cats, two showed a first peak of antibody response to (T,G)AL at day 3, which was similar to the peak seen in all six of the uninfected animals. No antibodies to (T,G)AL were found at days 3 to 5 in six of the

Table 1. Humoral antibody titers against (T,G)AL in FeLV-infected cats and uninfected control cats during the first month after immunization.

Cat number	Time after infection (days)					
	0	3 to 5	10 to 12	14 to 16	18 to 20	27 to 31
			Cats infected with FeLV			
1	< 10	< 10	< 10	10*	20	80
2	< 10	40	10	20	20	80
3	< 10	10			20	160
4	< 10	< 10	< 10	< 10	< 10	10
5	< 10	< 10	10	·40	80	640
6	< 10	< 10		160	320	320
7	< 10	< 10	< 10	< 10	< 10	< 10
8	< 10	< 10	< 10	< 10	< 10	< 10
Geometric mean		1.15	1.22	6.62	10.15	34.27
			Uninfected control cats			
9	< 10	10	1,280	2,560	5,120	10,240
10	< 10	10	320	640	2,560	5,120
11	< 10	10	2,560	5,120	5,120	2,560
12	< 10	10	40	80	160	1,280
13	< 10	20	20	160	80	640
14	< 10	10	10	40	640	640
Geometric mean		11.22	141.56	402.72	903.65	2,032.36

*Reciprocal of the highest twofold dilution of serum that gave a positive reaction (starting with an initial dilution of 1:10).

eight immunized FeLV-infected cats. A significant difference could be shown between the two groups at day 5 after immunization (Student's _t_-test). In five of eight FeLV-infected cats a low level of antibody production against (T,G)AL could be detected by days 14 to 20. Two of the eight infected cats did not respond to (T,G)AL at all, and a third showed a response that was only barely detectable by days 27 to 31. The range of peak titers for the other five FeLV-infected cats was 1:80 to 1:640 (Table 1). Only one of the eight infected animals developed a titer that was as high as any of the six uninfected cats by day 31, and the geometric mean antibody titers were approximately 60 to 120 times higher for the uninfected cats. The antibodies present at the first peak (days 3 to 5) were predominantly immunoglobulin M for both groups, whereas the second peak (after day 10) was primarily immunoglobulin G as determined with ELISA (5).

Cats that are naturally infected with FeLV have a greatly increased risk of developing bacterial, viral, and parasitic diseases such as septicemia, stomatitis, peritonitis, pneumonia, haemobartonellosis, and toxoplasmosis (2). Presumably, many of these infections, which are usually controlled in part by the humoral immune system, would be subclinical in the absence of immune suppression by FeLV. We observed a delay in the humoral immune response in six of eight FeLV-infected cats and a diminished peak in the antibody response in six of the eight infected animals. These results

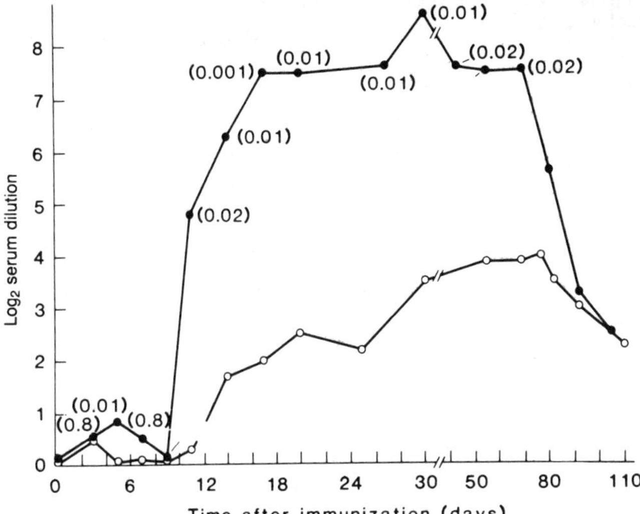

Fig. 1. Titer (geometric mean) of antibodies against the synthetic antigen (T,G)AL in (○) cats with natural, chronic infections of FeLV and (●) uninfected control cats. The numbers in parentheses represent the respective *P* values of the Student's *t*-test for the difference between the mean antibody titers for the two groups at each particular interval.

indicate that FeLV infection causes a severe immune impairment which is expressed as a delayed humoral response and by prolonged depressed concentrations of detectable antibodies in the serum.

The polypeptide (T,G)AL is known to be a T-cell–dependent antigen in rodents (6). One would expect it to evoke the same general class of response in cats. That most of the infected cats could, after a certain time, respond to the antigen allows us to speculate that the impairment lies in the T-helper cell function, and that once the B cells are triggered antibodies can be produced. A specific impairment of OKT-4 positive T-helper cells occurs in cells from humans infected with the adult T-cell leukemia virus (7).

Little is known about the way in which FeLV causes immunosuppression. Results by Mathes *et al.* implicated a virion structural protein of approximately 15,000 daltons (8). In earlier studies, infection with FeLV was associated with prolongation of allograft rejection (3),

thymic atrophy (9), depletion of paracortical lymphoid tissues (9), decreased response to T-cell mitogens (10), depressed peripheral blood lymphocyte counts (2), and diminished mobility of lymphocyte membrane capping (11). Despite these results, which appear to reflect both general impairment of lymphoid tissues and specific impairment of T-cell responses, earlier attempts to show that humoral immunity was depressed by FeLV infection were unsuccessful (3). Many of these studies were, however, conducted with cats that were inoculated in the laboratory with a particular strain of FeLV. Our results indicate that the humoral antibody response is diminished in cats that are naturally infected with FeLV.

References and Notes

1. N. Teich, J. Wyke, T. Mark, A. Bernstein, W. D. Hardy, Jr., in *RNA Tumor Viruses*, R. Weiss, N. Teich, H. Varmus, J. Coffin, Eds. (Cold Spring Harbor Press, Cold Spring Harbor, N.Y., 1982), p. 785.
2. M. Essex, W. D. Hardy, Jr., S. M. Cotter, R. M. Jakowski, A. Sliski, *Infect. Immun.* 11, 470 (1975); R. G. Olsen, L. E. Mathes, S. W. Nichols, in *Feline Leukemia*, R. G. Olsen, Ed.

(CRC Press, Boca Raton, Fla., 1981), p. 149; W. D. Hardy, Jr., P. W. Hess, E. G. MacEwen, A. J. McClelland, E. E. Zuckerman, M. Essex, S. M. Cotter, *Cancer Res.* **36**, 582 (1976); L. J. Anderson, O. Jarrett, H. M. Laird, *J. Natl. Cancer Inst.* **47**, 807 (1971); S. M. Cotter, W. D. Hardy, Jr., M. Essex, *J. Am. Vet. Med. Assoc.* **166**, 449 (1975).
3. L. E. Perryman, E. A. Hoover, D. S. Yohn, *J. Natl. Cancer Inst.* **49**, 1357 (1972).
4. W. D. Hardy, Jr., L. J. Old, P. W. Hess, M. Essex, S. M. Cotter, *Nature (London)* **244**, 266 (1973).
5. H. Ungar-Waron, I. Davidson, Z. Trainin, *J. Immunol. Methods* **53**, 175 (1982).
6. E. Mozes and J. Haimovich, *Nature (London)* **278**, 56 (1979).
7. M. Essex, *J. Natl. Cancer Inst.* **69**, 981 (1982).
8. L. E. Mathes, R. G. Olsen, L. C. Hebebrand, E. A. Hoover, J. P. Schaller, P. W. Adams, W. S. Nichols, *Cancer Res.* **39**, 950 (1979).
9. E. A. Hoover, L. E. Perryman, G. J. Kociba, *ibid.* **33**, 145 (1973); L. J. Anderson, O. Jarrett, H. M. Laird, *J. Natl. Cancer Inst.* **47**, 807 (1971).
10. G. L. Cockerell, E. A. Hoover, S. Krakowa, R. G. Olsen, D. S. Yohn, *ibid.* **57**, 1095 (1976).
11. J. E. Dunlap, W. S. Nichols, L. C. Hebebrand, L. E. Mathes, R. G. Olsen, *Cancer Res.* **39**, 956 (1979).
12. We thank M. F. McLane and R. Zuckerman for technical assistance, B. Willkie for providing antisera to cat immunoglobulins M and G, and D. Eardley and W. D. Hardy, Jr., for stimulating discussions. This work was supported by PHS grants CA-13885 and CA-18216.

7 February 1983; revised 11 April 1983

Report

20 May 1983

6.   Antibodies to Cell Membrane Antigens Associated with Human T-Cell Leukemia Virus in Patients with AIDS

M. Essex, M.F. McLane, T.H. Lee, L. Falk, C.W.S. Howe, J.I. Mullins, C. Cabradilla, and D.P. Francis

The human T-cell leukemia virus (HTLV), initially described in 1980 (*1*), was isolated from an American patient with mycosis fungoides, a form of T-cell lymphoma with extensive skin manifestations. Subsequently, the same virus was found in other individuals with lymphoid malignancies in this country and in various other geographical areas (*2–4*). Two regions of the world where both the virus and T-cell malignancies occur at increased rates are the Caribbean islands (*5–7*) and Southern Japan (*8–10*). In such areas from 4 to 37 percent of the healthy adults have antibodies to HTLV (*6, 7, 10, 11*). This contrasts with less than 1 percent of the healthy adults tested from selected regions of the continental United States, Western Europe, or Northern Japan who have such antibodies (*10–12*).

The acquired immune deficiency syndrome (AIDS) is a newly described disease that has recently been observed in several U.S. cities and in Haiti (*13–15*). The incidence of AIDS has been increasing dramatically. Although the disease was initially seen only in sexually active homosexual men, it has now been recognized in intravenous drug users, patients with hemophilia, Haitian immigrants, and heterosexual contacts of members of other high-risk groups (*15–17*). The syndrome, suspected to be of viral origin (*17*), is characterized by the development of Kaposi's sarcoma (KS), pneumonia caused by *Pneumocystis carinii* (PCP), and infections with various other opportunistic microorganisms. Such infections apparently develop because of an immune dysfunction that is characterized by lymphopenia with an imbalance of the normal ratio of T-helper cells to T-suppressor cells (*14, 16, 18*).

Patients with AIDS have increased titers of antibodies to cytomegalovirus and to the Epstein-Barr virus, and a higher prevalence of antibodies to hepatitis A virus and *Treponema pallidum* (*16*). The cytomegalovirus, which was previously considered as a potential cause of the African form of KS (*19*), has also been viewed as a candidate agent for a causative role in the form of KS seen in AIDS patients.

Since individuals with AIDS are probably at greater risk than the normal population for infection with many agents, including those transmitted by blood or by close contact, we decided to determine if they had increased rates of exposure to HTLV. Serum samples examined for antibodies were obtained from 75 patients with AIDS including 72 men (60 homosexual) and 3 women. These included 34 cases of KS, 30 cases of PCP, 11 cases that had both PCP and KS, and 23 homosexual men with lymphadenopathy (LAS), a syndrome that sometimes progresses to AIDS (*20*). These samples were examined, under code, along with samples from three control groups. The control groups were as follows. Group 1, 81 matched homosexual men including 9 friends of AIDS patients, 47 patients from a venereal disease (VD) clinic, and 25 patients of private physicians, all matched to 36 of the AIDS patients for age, race, sexual preference, and place

of residence. [For the selection of these cases and the controls, see (*16, 21*)]. Group 2, 118 unmatched homosexual male controls who visited a VD clinic in Chicago in 1978. This series of patients has been described before (*22*). Group 3, 137 first-time volunteer blood donors that gave blood in Philadelphia in 1977. The two last groups were collected before the recognition of AIDS. The samples were classified and coded at the Centers for Disease Control in Atlanta, and sent frozen to Boston for examination.

Several procedures have been used to survey serum samples for evidence of exposure to HTLV. These include radioimmunoassays for antibodies to p24, the major virion core protein (*6–8, 12*), and, with the use of HTLV-infected cells, indirect fixed-cell immunofluorescence (*9, 10, 23*) and indirect living-cell immunofluorescence (*8, 11*). We used the last procedure with two reference HTLV-infected cell cultures, Hut 102 (*1*) and MT 2 (*4*), and two HTLV-uninfected human lymphoid lines, 8402, a T-cell line (*24*), and NC37, a B-cell line that is negative for HTLV and positive for the Epstein-Barr virus genome and lacks surface immunoglobulin (*24*). Hut 102 is the prototype HTLV-infected T-cell culture established from an American patient and MT 2 is a standard HTLV-infected T-cell line established with virus from a Japanese patient. Both are of the OKT 4 phenotype (*3, 25*). When sufficient serum was available, selected samples were also checked by radioimmunoprecipitation with [^{35}S]methionine-labeled HTLV-infected cells or by the lactoperoxidase method with ^{125}I-labeled cells as previously described (*26, 27*).

When samples were judged to be positive on the basis of their ability to cause fluorescence on more than 50 percent of the target cells, 10 of 34 and 9 of 34 of the serum samples from KS patients were positive for the HTLV-associated cell membrane antigen (HTLV-MA) on Hut 102 cells and MT 2 cells, respectively (Tables 1 and 2). Also, 7 of 30 AIDS patients with PCP and 6 of 23 patients with LAS were positive on Hut 102. Overall, 19 of 75 AIDS patients were positive for HTLV-MA at the 50 percent level on Hut 102, compared to only 1 of 81 of the matched control samples, 0 of 118 unmatched homosexual samples, and 1 of 137 of the adult blood donor control samples (Table 2). Twenty-nine samples were tested from patients with chronic active hepatitis and 21 samples were tested from kidney dialysis pa-

tients. None of these 50 were positive. Of the 19 serum samples from AIDS patients that were positive for antibodies to HTLV-MA and reacted with 50 percent or more of the Hut 102 cells, all but two reacted with more than 60 percent of the cells and most reacted with more than 70 percent. This range in reactivity is very similar to that seen with positive reference sera obtained from Japanese patients with HTLV-related T-cell leukemia (*11*). The one matched control sample that was positive was from the limited series of nine samples collected as matched friends of AIDS patients. In all categories the results obtained when the MT 2 target cell was used were similar to the results obtained with the Hut 102

Table 1. Presence of antibodies to HTLV-MA in patients with AIDS, in patients with LAS, and in adult male homosexual controls. The Hut 102 and MT 2 cell lines were cultured as described earlier and used at peak phase of logarithmic growth (*1*, *8*). The cells (1×10^6 to 2×10^6) were washed twice in phosphate buffered saline (PBS) and exposed to 40 μl of a 1:4 dilution of previously centrifuged serum for 30 minutes at 37°C. Each preparation was then washed twice with PBS and reacted with 40 μl of a 1:20 dilution of fluorescein conjugated F(ab')$_2$ fragment of goat antiserum to human immunoglobulins (IgA + IgG + IgM) (Cappel, Cochranville, Pennsylvania). The samples were again incubated at 37°C for 30 minutes, washed twice with PBS, and examined by fluorescence microscopy. Serum samples were judged as positive if at least 50 percent (or 40 percent when indicated) of the cells showed specific fluorescence. All samples were coded and read in a double-blind manner. A positive and a negative reference human serum sample (*7*) was included in each test.

Category	Cells positive (> 50 percent)		Cells positive (< 40 percent)	
	Hut 102	MT 2	Hut 102	MT 2
AIDS patients				
KS patients	10/34 (29)*	9/34 (27)	14/34 (41)	11/34 (32)
PCP patients	7/30 (23)	6/30 (20)	10/30 (33)	7/30 (23)
Patients with both KS and PCP	2/11 (18)	3/11 (27)	3/11 (27)	4/11 (36)
LAS patients	6/23 (26)	6/23 (26)	7/23 (30)	7/23 (30)
Matched homosexual controls†				
Friends of patients	1/9 (11)	1/9 (11)	1/9 (11)	1/9 (11)
Patients from VD clinic	0/47 (0)	0/47 (0)	0/47 (0)	0/47 (0)
Private practice controls	0/25 (0)	0/25 (0)	0/25 (0)	0/25 (0)

* Number of individuals positive over the total number tested and percent positive.   † Matched to 36 of the AIDS patients.

Table 2. Presence of antibodies to HTLV-MA in patients with AIDS, in patients with LAS, in matched and unmatched healthy male homosexual controls, and in blood donors. The procedure used is described in the legend for Table 1.

Category	Greater than 50 percent of cells positive	
	Hut 102	MT 2
AIDS patients	19/75 (25)*	18/75 (24)
LAS patients	6/23 (26)	6/23 (26)
Matched homosexual controls†	1/81 (1)	1/81 (1)
Unmatched homosexual controls	0/118 (0)	0/118 (0)
Blood donors	1/137 (0.7)	2/137 (1.5)
Kidney dialysis patients	0/21 (0)	0/21 (0)
Chronic active hepatitis patients	0/29 (0)	0/29 (0)

*Number of individuals positive over total number tested and percent positive.   †All were matched to 36 of the AIDS patients.

target. Of the 27 samples in all categories that were positive at the 50 percent level on Hut 102 cells (Table 2), 19 of 27 or 70 percent were also positive at the 50 percent level on MT 2. No difference was observed in the proportion of antibody positive samples in the 36 matched AIDS cases compared to the 39 unmatched cases. Fourteen serum samples that were positive for antibodies to HTLV-MA were also tested for reactivity with 8402 and NC37 cells. All were negative on both targets.

Twenty positive serum samples from AIDS and LAS patients were available in sufficient quantities to carry out immunoprecipitation of solubilized [^{35}S]-methionine-labeled Hut 102 cells. Of these, 16 (75 percent) precipitated either p24, the major HTLV core protein, or p28, a polyprotein containing p24 (*1, 23, 28*), or both. Examples of these reactions are shown in Fig. 1. Most also precipitated p61, an HTLV-related glycoprotein that is detected at the surface of Hut 102 cells with positive reference sera obtained from Japanese T-cell lymphoma patients that react with HTLV-MA (*11*). In most cases, however, the reactivity

with the serum samples by immunoprecipitation was weak. Four samples from HTLV-MA antibody-negative AIDS patients were also tested by immunoprecipitation and each was negative for all known HTLV-related proteins detected by this technique.

The antigens that make up the HTLV-MA reactivity, which appears to be specific to HTLV-infected cells, include p61 and p28 (*30*). Whether p61 represents the product of a cell gene that is activated by HTLV or a direct product of the HTLV genome has not been established. One histocompatibility antigen, DR5, has been seen more often than expected in patients with KS (*30*). However, it seems very unlikely that HTLV-MA antibodies are directed to DR5 because the reference cells Hut 102 and MT 2 both lack this antigen (*3, 31*).

These results suggest that at least 25 percent of AIDS patients have evidence of exposure to HTLV or a closely related agent. Although another 10 percent or more could be considered weakly positive if a lower cutoff was used for the evaluation (Table 1), about half of the patients were clearly negative for

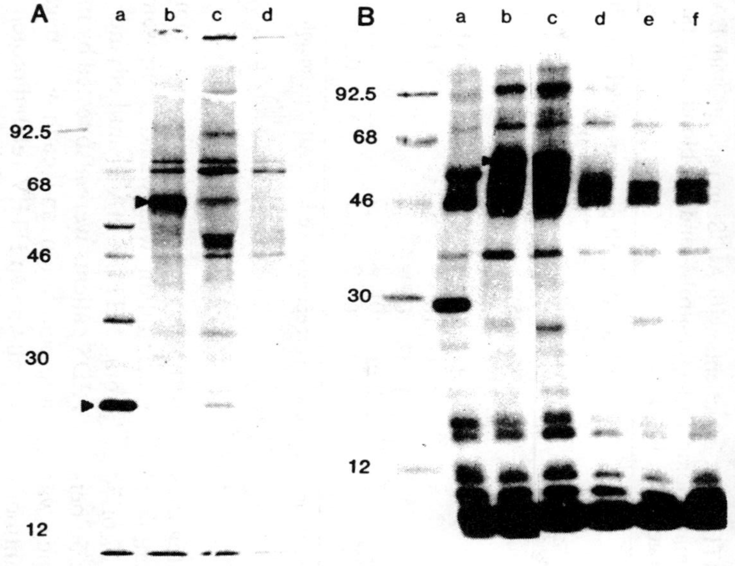

Fig. 1. Reactivity of serum samples from AIDS patients positive for antibodies to HTLV-MA as determined by sodium dodecyl sulfate (SDS)–polyacrylamide gel electrophoresis. (A) Hut 102 cells at their peak log phase of growth were harvested and exposed to [^{35}S]methionine [100 μCi/ml; specific activity 1050 Ci/mmole; New England Nuclear (NEN)], for 2 to 4 hours. A soluble cell lysate was obtained after disruption with RIPA buffer (0.15M NaCl, 0.05M tris-HCl, pH 7.2, 1 percent Triton X-100, 1 percent sodium deoxycholate, and 0.1 percent SDS) and centrifuged for 1 hour at 100,000g. The lysate supernatant was cleared once with 10 μl of reference negative control serum bound to Protein-A–Sepharose CL-4B (Protein-A beads) before portions were reacted with 10 μl of the following sera preabsorbed with Protein A beads: (a) reference goat antiserum to purified p24 of HTLV (5 μl) (8); (b) representative fluorescence-positive reference serum from a Japanese patient with adult T-cell leukemia (8); (c) serum from a representative individual with AIDS that was positive for antibodies to HTLV-MA by membrane immunofluorescence; (d) serum from a representative healthy homosexual control individual that was negative for HTLV-MA by membrane immunofluorescence. Immunoprecipitates were eluted in a sample buffer containing 0.1M Cleland's reagent, 2 percent SDS, 0.08M tris-HCl, pH 6.8, 10 percent glycerol, and 0.2 percent bromophenol blue by boiling at 100°C for 2 minutes. Samples were analyzed in a 12.5 percent acrylamide resolving gel with 3.5 percent stacking gel according to the discontinuous buffer system of Laemmli (38). The molecular weight markers, purchased from NEN, were ^{14}C-labeled phosphorylase b (92,500), bovine serum albumin (68,000), ovalbumin (46,000), carbonic anhydrase (30,000), and cytochrome c (12,000). (B) Surface-labeling was carried out by lactoperoxidase-catalyzed radioiodination. Three portions of 5×10^6 Hut 102 cells with greater than 99 percent viability were iodinated separately with 1 mCi of carrier-free Na^{125}I (NEN) in the presence of 50 μl of Enzymobeads (Bio-Rad) and 25 μl of 1 percent β-D-glucose. After the reaction was terminated, three portions of iodinated cells were pooled and the same procedures as those described in (A) were followed to prepare cell lysates. Portions of cell lysate, after being cleared once, were reacted with 10 μl of each of the following sera: (a) reference goat antiserum to purified p24 of HTLV (8); (b) representative serum positive for HTLV-MA by membrane immunofluorescence, from a Japanese patient with T-cell leukemia (8); (c) and (d) serum samples from two representative patients with AIDS that were positive for antibodies to HTLV-MA by membrane immunofluorescence [(d) was judged negative by immunoprecipitation]; and (e) and (f) serum samples from two representative healthy homosexual controls that were negative for antibodies to HTLV-MA by membrane immunofluorescence.

HTLV-MA antibodies. However, the prevalence rate for exposure to HTLV was at least 10- to 40-fold higher in AIDS patients compared with other homosexual controls, a situation that was not seen for other infectious agents evaluated in the same individuals (16).

Human T-cell leukemia virus is a lymphotropic retrovirus that preferentially infects T-helper cells (2, 32). Although most lymphoma cells of the type associated with HTLV are of the helper-cell phenotype, they actually show suppressor rather than helper activity when evaluated in vitro (33). Little or nothing is known about whether HTLV ever causes immunosuppression in healthy carriers. However, other naturally occurring retroviruses, such as the feline leukemia virus, cause thymic atrophy (34), lymphopenia (35), and profound immunosuppression (36).

The mechanisms by which HTLV is transmitted is unknown. Transmission by blood transfusion has been considered (37), but this could only account for a small proportion of the infections. The rate of infection in spouses of patients with T-cell lymphoma is elevated (7), suggesting that HTLV might be transmitted by sexual intercourse or other types of close contact. As mentioned above, two areas where HTLV infection is frequent are Southern Japan and the Caribbean. To our knowledge AIDS has not been reported in Japan. It has, however, been well documented in Haitians (17).

Our results indicate that homosexual patients with AIDS and LAS have increased risk for infection with HTLV or a related agent. Such individuals should be monitored to determine rates for development of lymphoma, especially those of T-cell origin. Our results also suggest that HTLV should, along with cytomegalovirus and other agents, be studied to determine what role, if any, it might play in the development of AIDS.

References and Notes

1. B. J. Poiesz, F. W. Ruscetti, A. F. Gazdar, P. A. Bunn, J. D. Minna, R. C. Gallo, *Proc. Natl. Acad. Sci. U.S.A.* **77**, 7415 (1980).
2. B. J. Poiesz, F. W. Ruscetti, M. S. Reitz, V. S. Kalyanaraman, R. C. Gallo, *Nature (London)* **294**, 268 (1981); V. S. Kalyanaraman, M. G. Sarngadharan, M. Robert-Guroff, I. Miyoshi, D. Blayney, D. Golde, R. C. Gallo, *Science* **218**, 571 (1982); M. Popovic, P. S. Sarin, M. Robert-Guroff, V. S. Kalyanaraman, D. Mann, J. Minowada, R. C. Gallo, *ibid.* **219**, 856 (1983); I. Miyoshi, I. Kubonishi, S. Yoshimoto, T. Akagi, Y. Ohtsuki, Y. Shiraishi, K. Nagata, Y. Hinuma, *Nature (London)* **294**, 770 (1981).
3. R. C. Gallo, D. Mann, S. Broder, F. W. Ruscetti, M. Maeda, V. S. Kalyanaraman, M. Robert-Guroff, M. S. Reitz, Jr., *Proc. Natl. Acad. Sci. U.S.A.* **79**, 5680 (1982).
4. M. Yoshida, I. Miyoshi, Y. Hinuma, *ibid.*, p. 2031.
5. D. Catovsky *et al.*, *Lancet* **1982-I**, 639 (1982).
6. W. A. Blattner *et al.*, *Int. J. Cancer* **30**, 257 (1982).
7. J. Schüpbach, V. S. Kalyanaraman, M. G. Sarngadharan, W. A. Blattner, R. C. Gallo, *Cancer Res.* **43**, 866 (1983).
8. M. Robert-Guroff, Y. Nakao, K. Notake, Y. Ito, A. Sliski, R. C. Gallo *Science* **215**, 975 (1982).
9. Y. Hinuma, K. Nagata, M. Hanaoka, M. Nakai, T. Matsumoto, K.-I. Kinoshita, S. Shirakawa, I. Miyoshi, *Proc. Natl. Acad. Sci. U.S.A.* **78**, 6476 (1981).
10. Y. Hinuma *et al.*, *Int. J. Cancer* **29**, 631 (1982).
11. N. Tachibana, M. F. McLane, T. H. Lee, C. Howe, V. S. Kalyanaraman, R. C. Gallo, M. Essex, in preparation.
12. R. C. Gallo *et al.*, *Cancer Res.*, in press.
13. A. E. Friedman-Kien, *J. Am. Acad. Dermatol.* **5**, 468 (1971).
14. M. S. Gottlieb, R. Schroff, H. M. Schanker, I. D. Weisman, P. T. Fan, R. A. Wolf, A. Saxon, *N. Engl. J. Med.* **305**, 248 (1982).
15. Centers for Disease Control Task Force on Kaposi's Sarcoma and Opportunistic Infections, *ibid.* **306**, 248 (1982).
16. M. F. Rogers *et al.*, Task Force on Acquired Immune Deficiency Syndrome, *Ann. Intern. Med.*, in press.
17. D. P. Francis, J. W. Curran, M. Essex, *J. Natl. Cancer Inst.* **71**, 1 (1983).
18. F. P. Siegal *et al.*, *N. Engl. J. Med.* **305**, 1439 (1981).
19. G. Giraldo *et al.*, *Int. J. Cancer* **15**, 839 (1975).
20. Centers for Disease Control Task Force on Kaposi's Sarcoma and Opportunistic Infections, *Morbid. Mortal. Weekly Rep.* **31**, 249 (1982).
21. H. W. Jaffee *et al.*, *Ann. Intern. Med.*, in press.
22. M. T. Schreeder *et al.*, *J. Infect. Dis.* **146**, 7 (1982).
23. N. Yamamoto and Y. Hinuma, *Int. J. Cancer* **30**, 289 (1982).
24. J. Azocar and M. Essex, *J. Natl. Cancer Inst.* **63**, 1179 (1979).
25. I. Miyoshi, S. Yoshimoto, I. Kubonishi, H. Taguchi, Y. Shiraishi, Y. Ohtsuki, T. Akagi,

Gann **72**, 997 (1981).
26. A. P. Chen, M. Essex, M. Kelliher, F. deNoronha, J. A. Shadduck, J. Y. Niederkorn, D. Albert, *Virology* **124**, 274 (1983).
27. J. J. Marchalonis, R. E. Cone, V. Santer, *Biochem. J.* **124**, 921 (1971).
28. V. S. Kalyanaraman, M. G. Sarngadharan, P. A. Bunn, J. D. Minna, R. C. Gallo, *Nature (London)* **294**, 217 (1981).
29. T. H. Lee, M. F. McLane, C. Howe, N. Tachibana, M. Essex, in preparation.
30. N. O'Hara and S. W. Chang, *Ann. Intern. Med.* **97**, 617 (1982).
31. D. L. Mann, M. Popovic, P. Sarin, C. Murray, B. F. Hanes, D. M. Strong, R. C. Gallo, W. A. Blattner, in preparation.
32. M. Essex, *J. Natl. Cancer Inst.* **69**, 981 (1982).
33. Y. Yamada, *Blood* **61**, 192 (1983).
34. E. A. Hoover, L. E. Perryman, G. J. Kociba, *Cancer Res.* **33**, 145 (1973).
35. M. Essex, W. W. Hardy, Jr., S. M. Cotter, R. M. Jakowski, A. Sliski, *Infect. Immun.* **11**, 470 (1975).
36. L. E. Perryman, E. A. Hoover, D. S. Yohn, *J. Natl. Cancer Inst.* **49**, 1357 (1972); Z. Trainin, D. Wernicke, H. Ungar-Waron, M. Essex, *Science* **220**, 858 (1983).
37. I. Miyoshi, M. Fujishita, H. Taquchi, Y. Ohtsuki, T. Akagi, Y. M. Morimoto, A. Nagasaki, *Lancet* **1982-I**, 683 (1982).
38. U. K. Laemmli, *Nature (London)* **227**, 680 (1970).

39. Supported by grant RD-173 from the American Cancer Society and NIH grants CA 18216, 2T32CA09031 and 5T32HL07523. C.W.S.H. is also a member of the Department of Hematology at Brigham-Women's Hospital. We thank R. Gallo for stimulating discussions, reference reagents, and the exchange of information prior to publication.

24 March 1983; revised 11 April 1983

Report

20 May 1983

7. Proviral DNA of a Retrovirus, Human T-Cell Leukemia Virus, in Two Patients with AIDS

Edward P. Gelmann, Mikulas Popovic, Douglas Blayney, Henry Masur, Gurdip Sidhu, Rosalyn E. Stahl, and Robert C. Gallo

Acquired immune deficiency syndrome (AIDS) is a new disease whose incidence in the United States has increased steadily since 1979 (*1*). The disorder was first noted in male homosexuals who presented with opportunistic infections, predominantly *Pneumocystis carinii* pneumonia (*2*), or with Kaposi's sarcoma (*3*). The syndrome has recently been found in other groups including intravenous drug users (*4*), Haitian immigrants to the United States (*5*), hemophiliacs (*6*), and inmates at a New York state prison (*7*). Although patients with AIDS usually come to medical attention because of Kaposi's sarcoma or opportunistic infections, the underlying disorder affects the patients' cell-mediated immunity (*8*). The T-cell dysfunction is often marked by an absence of delayed hypersensitivity, an absolute lymphopenia, and reversal of the usual ratio of phenotypic T-helper (OKT4$^+$) to T-suppressor (OKT8$^+$) cells whereby the latter come to predominate among circulating lymphocytes (*8*). Although the epidemiologic data suggest an infectious, possibly viral, etiology for AIDS, no agent has been linked etiologically to the disease. Many of the patients have chronic infection with cytomegalovirus (*9*) or hepatitis B virus, but the presence of these agents may be characteristic of the social history of the patients and may have preceded the disease or may represent infections permitted by the immune deficit.

We have been testing the hypothesis that AIDS is caused by a human retrovirus related to the human T-cell leukemia virus, HTLV (*10*). Retrovirus infection, known to cause leukemias, lymphomas, and solid tumors in several species of animals and T-cell malignancies in man, has also been shown to result in immune deficiency in some cats infected with feline leukemia virus (*11*). The target cell for the putative AIDS agent may be the T cell or a T-cell subset. Since HTLV is a T-cell tropic retrovirus (*12*), it can be linked hypothetically to other human T-cell disorders. The finding of AIDS in Haitians who may not have been exposed to other risk factors for the disease may be important since HTLV appears to be endemic in the West Indies (*13*). The search for evidence of retrovirus infection poses many problems. Several of the hallmarks of such infection, namely virus production, complete provirus integration into the host DNA, and antibody response to viral antigens have not been found in retrovirus-induced neoplasms. In a disease characterized by cellular depletion, as AIDS appears to be, it may be difficult to sample a patient's cells during the period of virus replication before the affected cell population becomes too small to detect. Since patients with AIDS show depressed antibody formation in response to some new stimuli (*14*), their antibody response to the putative infectious agent may also be depressed. In several patients with leukemia, the presence of HTLV was documented by finding the virus in cultured lymphocytes (*15*) or by identifying proviral sequences in fresh leukemic cells

(*16*), but serum antibodies to HTLV proteins were not detected. Conversely, antibodies to HTLV have been found in a small number of healthy people (*17*), especially in individuals who have been in close contact with HTLV positive patients (*18*).

A sensitive and perhaps more specific indicator of active retrovirus infection is the presence of the integrated proviral genome in the host cell chromosomal DNA. As part of their normal replicative cycle, retroviruses transcribe a DNA copy of their RNA genome. This copy is inserted colinearly into the host cell DNA and is then replicated during cell division and passed to daughter cells. This proviral DNA serves as a template for copies of new RNA genomes for virus production and may alter the expression of cellular genes near the chromosomal insertion site. We have tested fresh peripheral blood lymphocytes from AIDS patients for the presence of integrated HTLV provirus and now report that such viral sequences were present in two cases of AIDS.

The patients were diagnosed as having AIDS by the clinical presentation of opportunistic infection or Kaposi's sarcoma and by an immunologic profile as described above. Lymphocytes were isolated from 50 ml of peripheral blood by Ficoll-Hypaque gradient and immediately treated with sodium dodecyl sulfate and proteinase K, after which high-molecular-weight DNA was prepared by standard techniques. The DNA samples (5 μg) were treated with a restriction endonuclease, usually Eco RI, and analyzed by Southern blot hybridization (*19*) to radiolabeled cloned HTLV DNA (*20*). The viral probe, pCR$_{CH}$, represents 2.4 kb of the HTLV genome, predominantly the *env* region. Under stringent conditions of hybridization (see Fig. 1 legend),

40

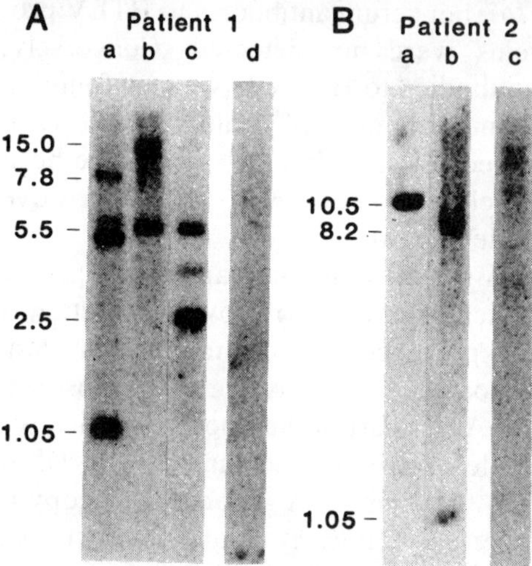

Fig. 1. Southern blot hybridization of the HTLV probe pCR$_{CH}$ to restriction enzyme–digested lymphocyte DNA from AIDS patients. Five micrograms of high-molecular-weight DNA were digested with the designated restriction enzyme under conditions described by the supplier. The DNA was subjected to electrophoresis on 0.8 percent agarose and blotted on nitrocellulose filters. The filters were heated in a vacuum at 80°C for 2 hours, and the DNA was then hybridized to ^{32}P-labeled pCR$_{CH}$ at 37°C in 0.45M NaCl, 50 percent formamide, and 10 percent dextran sulfate, overnight. The filters were washed in 0.15M NaCl at 60°C and autoradiographed overnight. (A) Patient 1. Digests of DNA from cultured T cells with (lane a) Bam HI, (lane b) Eco RI, and (lane c) Pst I. Lane d contains Eco RI–digested fresh peripheral blood lymphocyte DNA samples 4 months after the cells were taken for culture. (B) Patient 2. Digests of fresh peripheral blood lymphocyte DNA: (lane a) 5 μg of DNA digested with Eco RI; (lane b) 3 μg of DNA digested with Bam HI; (lane c) 5 μg of DNA, sampled 2 months after the DNA obtained for (lanes a and b), digested with Eco RI.

the probe hybridized only to DNA from virus-infected cells. In surveys of leukemic cell DNA for HTLV we have used Eco RI, which does not cleave the viral DNA, to excise a single restriction frag-

ment, usually larger than 10 kb, which contains the integrated provirus and can be detected by the pCR$_{CH}$ probe (*16*). Positive findings were confirmed by using the restriction enzyme Bam HI to cleave the sample DNA to yield a 1.05-kb fragment from proviral DNA which is also internal to the pCR$_{CH}$ fragment and is easily seen on a Southern blot when it is hybridized with that probe.

Patient 1 was a 32-year-old black male from New York City. He had intermittent fevers, lymphadenopathy, and *Pneumocystis carinii* pneumonia, and showed loss of weight. A blood count revealed the following: white cells, 4500 cell/mm^3; lymphocytes, 765 cell/mm^3; and an OKT4$^+$/OKT8$^+$ lymphocyte ratio of 0.2. Interviews with the patient and his family indicated that there was no history of malignancy. The patient's only travel outside the United States was for a year's military service in Vietnam; he was an admitted homosexual and denied that he had ever received a blood tranfusion or used intravenously administered illicit drugs.

When peripheral blood lymphocytes from this patient were cultured in the presence of human T-cell growth factor (TCGF) (*21*), a line of TCGF-dependent cells became established. These cells contained HTLV viral antigens, p19 (*22*) and p24 (*23*), produced reverse transcriptase activity in the culture fluid (*10*), showed the presence of type-C virus particles when thin sections were examined by electron microscopy, and contained integrated HTLV proviral DNA (*24*).

Figure 1 shows the results obtained by the Southern blot hybridization technique. The two bands of higher molecular weight cleaved by Eco RI in Fig. 1A (lane b) indicate the presence of two complete proviral copies. The 5.5-kb band represents a partial provirus. The extra proviral copies may have arisen in culture, since increased copies of provirus and defective viral genomes occur commonly when HTLV-infected T cells are passed in vitro for prolonged periods of time (25). Digestion with Bam HI gave the 1.05-kb internal fragment and Pst I cleaved a 2.5-kb internal fragment. This analysis did not reveal any differences between this HTLV isolate, HTLV-I$_{CR}$, and other HTLV-I isolates derived from malignant T cells (26).

Although this patient's fresh lymphocytes were not assayed for viral sequences at the time his cells were cultured, he did possess circulating antibodies to HTLV core proteins p24 and p19 (27). One year after he first became ill the patient developed a cerebral lymphoma (cell type undetermined). At that time no HTLV sequences could be found in his circulating lymphocytes (Fig. 1A, lane d).

Patient 2 was a 48-year-old black male resident of Philadelphia. He became ill with extensive perianal *Herpes simplex* and two nodular lesions of Kaposi's sarcoma. A blood count showed the following: white cells, 2400 cells/mm^3; total lymphocytes, 432 cell/mm^3; and an OKT4$^+$/OKT8$^+$ ratio of 0.1. From interviews with the patient and his family it was learned that he was homosexual, there was no history of malignancy, and that he had lived the first 12 years of his life in Alabama and then moved to Philadelphia. His only travel outside the United States had been to Canada, and he had never had a blood transfusion or used intravenously administered illicit drugs.

Fresh, uncultured, peripheral blood lymphocytes from this patient were analyzed by the Southern blot hybridization technique (Fig. 1B). A single-copy HTLV genome was seen in the Eco RI digestion. Digestion with Bam HI confirmed the presence of the viral genome by cleaving the internal 1.05-kb restriction fragment. To determine what fraction of the patient's peripheral blood lymphocytes were infected with HTLV, we compared the intensity of hybridization of the patient's DNA to dilutions of cloned viral DNA, that is, the CR$_{CH}$ insert, mixed with salmon sperm DNA as a carrier. The amount of cloned CR$_{CH}$ insert added to each lane was calculated to represent the density of viral copies per cell as shown in Fig. 2. By including on the Southern blot a known amount of lymphocyte DNA from patient 2 and comparing the autoradiographic intensity of the HTLV sequences in this DNA (arrow) with the intensity of the dilutions of this cloned insert, we were able to estimate that between 1/8 and 1/16 (about 10 percent) of the patient's peripheral lymphocytes contained HTLV provirus at the time of sampling. A second analysis of the patient's peripheral blood lymphocytes obtained 2 months after the first showed that the HTLV provirus could no longer be detected (Fig. 1B, lane c). At both times this patient had circulating antibodies to disrupted whole HTLV (28).

We also used the Southern blot technique to test DNA randomly sampled from peripheral blood lymphocytes of 31 other individuals with AIDS. No HTLV sequences were detected.

That the viral genome of HTLV was found to be integrated into peripheral blood lymphocyte DNA in 2 of 33 AIDS patients tested thus far may reflect an etiologic association that is detectable by our methods only in a small percentage

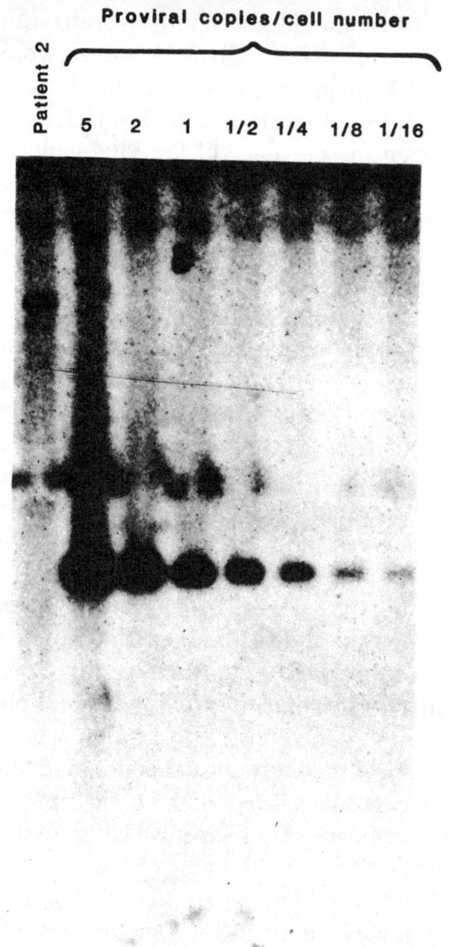

Fig. 2. Determination of the density of HTLV proviral copies in fresh peripheral blood lymphocytes of patient 2. Southern blot hybridization was performed as in Fig. 1. The first lane contains 3 µg of Eco RI–digested DNA from patient 2. The lanes to the right contain different amounts of the pCR$_{CH}$ cloned fragment added to 3 µg of salmon sperm DNA. The ratio of pCR$_{CH}$ insert to carrier salmon sperm DNA is calculated to represent the ratio of viral copy to cell number listed at the top of each lane.

of cases. Because of the depressed cell population numbers and the possible toxicity of the virus to the host cell it

may be necessary to develop alternative sampling techniques. A baseline for the presence of HTLV DNA sequences in the peripheral blood of healthy patients is unknown. We have thus far tested only 25 healthy homosexual males, none of whom had detectable virus. That both of the positive cases in our study are black is important since blacks may have a predisposition for HTLV expression; HTLV-induced lymphocytic malignancies appear to be endemic in the Caribbean basin area (*13*). A disproportionate number of the HTLV lymphomas studied in our laboratory occurred in blacks (*13*). The only large survey for nonleukemic HTLV-positive individuals in the United States was a screening of stored serum samples from patients attending a venereal disease clinic in the southeastern United States. Three percent of the samples, predominantly from black people, reacted positively with HTLV antigen (*29*).

Our results, if they do reflect an etiologic role for HTLV in AIDS, suggest a possible mechanism of disease induction. Restriction enzyme identification of two integration sites in one patient's cells and a single site in another implies a mono- or oligoclonal proliferation of infected cells. After exposure to the virus one or a few infected cells proliferated until they represented at least 10 percent of the circulating lymphocytes, a level enabling us to detect the sequence. HTLV is a T-cell tropic virus that apparently chiefly infects the OKT4$^+$ subset (*25*). The two patients with HTLV studied here had been ill for some months before we sampled their infected lymphocytes. Since OKT4$^+$ cells are markedly reduced in AIDS, it is less likely that these cells were infected with the virus. It seems more likely that the infected cells were suppressor T cells whose function was in some way altered by virus infection. Virus-induced proliferation of a T-suppressor clone may be an initiating step in AIDS. Studies of the HTLV integration sites in the DNA of these two patients, of the possible transmission of AIDS to animals, of transfusion recipients who contract AIDS, and of the genome of the HTLV isolated from AIDS patients compared to that of HTLV from T-cell neoplasias may shed further light on the involvement of HTLV in AIDS.

References and Notes

1. Center for Disease Control, Task Force on Kaposi's Sarcoma and Opportunistic Infections, *N. Engl. J. Med.* **306**, 248 (1982).
2. "*Pneumocystis* pneumonia—Los Angeles," *Morbid. Mortal. Weekly Rep.* **30**, 250 (1981); "Kaposi's sarcoma and *Pneumocystis* pneumonia among homsexual men—New York City and California," *ibid.*, p. 305.
3. A. E. Friedman-Kien *et al.*, *Ann. Int. Med.* **96**, 693 (1982).
4. K. Gold, L. Thomas, G. P. Garrett, *N. Engl. J. Med.* **307**, 498 (1982).
5. J. Vieira, E. Frank, T. J. Spira, S. H. Landesman, *ibid.* **308**, 125 (1983).
6. "*Pneumocystis carinii* pneumonia among persons with Hemophilia A," *Morbid. Mortal. Weekly Rep.* **31**, 365 (1982).
7. J. P. Hanrahan, G. P. Wormser, C. P. Maguire, L. J. DeLorenzo, G. Gravis, *N. Engl. J. Med.* **307**, 498 (1982).
8. M. Gottlieb, R. Schroff, H. M. Schanker, J. D. Weisman, P. T. Fan, R. C. Wolf, A. Saxon, *ibid.* **305**, 1425 (1981); H. Masur *et al.*, *ibid.*, p. 1431.
9. C. Urmacher, P. Myskowski, M. Ochoa, M. Kris, B. Safai, *Am. J. Med.* **72**, 569 (1982).
10. For brief reviews, see R. C. Gallo and F. Wong-Staal, *Blood* **60**, 545 (1982); R. C. Gallo and M. R. Reitz, *J. Natl. Cancer Inst.* **69**, 1209 (1982); B. J. Poiesz, F. W. Ruscetti, A. F. Gazdar, P. A. Bunn, J. D. Minna, R. C. Gallo, *Proc. Natl. Acad. Sci. U.S.A.* **77**, 7415 (1980); I. Miyoshi, I. Kubonishi, S. Yoshimoto, T. Akagi, Y. Ohtsuki, Y. Shiraishi, K. Nagata, Y. Hinuma, *Nature (London)* **294**, 770 (1981); B. J. Poiesz, F. W. Ruscetti, M. S. Reitz, V. S. Kalyanaraman, R. C. Gallo, *ibid.*, p. 268; B. F. Haynes, S. W. Miller, T. J. Perker, J. O. Moore, P. H. Dunn, D. P. Bolognesi, R. S. Metzger, *Proc. Natl. Acad. Sci. U.S.A.* **80**, 2054 (1983).
11. M. Essex, W. D. Hardy, S. M. Cotter, R. C. Jakowsku, A. Sliski, *Infect. Immun.* **11**, 470 (1975); Z. Trainin, D. Wernicke, H. Unger-Waron, M. Essex, *Science* **220**, 858 (1983).
12. R. C. Gallo, D. Mann, S. Broder, F. W. Ruscetti, M. Maeda, V. S. Kalyanaraman, M. Robert-Guroff, M. S. Reitz, *Proc. Natl. Acad. Sci. U.S.A.* **79**, 5630 (1982).
13. W. A. Blattner *et al.*, *Int. J. Cancer* **30**, 257 (1982).
14. C. Lane and A. Fauci, personal communication.
15. P. S. Sarin *et al.*, *Proc. Natl. Acad. Sci. U.S.A.*, in press.
16. F. Wong-Staal, B. Hahn, V. Manzari, S. Colombini, G. Franchini, E. P. Gelmann, R. C. Gallo, *Nature (London)*, in press.
17. L. E. Posner, M. Robert-Guroff, V. S. Kalyanaraman, B. J. Poiesz, F. W. Ruscetti, B. Fossieck, P. A. Bunn, J. D. Minna, R. C. Gallo, *J. Exp. Med.* **154**, 333 (1981).
18. M. Robert-Guroff *et al.*, *ibid.* **157**, 248 (1983).
19. E. M. Southern, *J. Mol. Biol.* **98**, 503 (1975).
20. V. Manzari, F. Wong-Staal, G. Franchini, S. Colombini, E. P. Gelmann, S. Oroszlan, S. Staal, R. C. Gallo, *Proc. Natl. Acad. Sci. U.S.A.* **80**, 1574 (1983).
21. B. J. Poiesz, F. W. Ruscetti, J. W. Mier, A. M. Woods, R. C. Gallo, *ibid.* **77**, 6815 (1980).
22. M. Robert-Guroff, K. Fahey, M. Maeda, Y. Nakao, Y. Ito, R. C. Gallo, *Virology* **122**, 297 (1982).
23. V. S. Kalyanaraman, M. G. Sarngadharan, B. J. Poiesz, F. W. Ruscetti, R. C. Gallo, *J. Virol.* **38**, 906 (1981).
24. M. Popovic *et al.*, in preparation.
25. E. P. Gelmann, F. Wong-Staal, P. Sarin, R. C. Gallo, unpublished observations.
26. M. Popovic, P. S. Sarin, M. Robert-Guroff, V. S. Kalyanaraman, D. Mann, J. Minowada, R. C. Gallo, *Science* **219**, 856 (1983).
27. M. Robert-Guroff *et al.*, unpublished data.
28. W. C. Saxinger and R. C. Gallo, in preparation.
29. C. Saxinger, M. Robert-Guroff, D. Blayney, W. Blattner, R. C. Gallo, unpublished observations.
30. We thank many collaborators who sent us clinical specimens for testing: A. Machur, A. Friedman-Kien, B. Safai, M. Lange, J. Gutterman, J. Groopman, N. Steigbigel, and I. Jaffrey. We also thank A. Fauci and C. Lane for immunological testing, A. LoMonico for technical assistance, E. Richardson for cell culturing, J. Ames for clinical coordination, and F. Wong-Staal and V. Manzari for helpful discussions.
* Present address: Medicine Branch, Building 10, Room 12N226, National Cancer Institute, Bethesda, Md. 20205.
† To whom reprint requests should be addressed.

3 March 1983; revised 18 April 1983

Report

20 May 1983

8. Isolation of Human T-Cell Leukemia Virus in Acquired Immune Deficiency Syndrome (AIDS)

Robert C. Gallo, Prem S. Sarin, E.P. Gelmann, Marjorie Robert-Guroff, Ersell Richardson, V.S. Kalyanaraman, Dean Mann, Gurdip D. Sidhu, Rosalyn E. Stahl, Susan Zolla-Pazner, Jacque Leibowitch, and Mikulas Popovic

Human T-cell leukemia-lymphoma virus, HTLV, was first discovered in and isolated from mature T cells associated with certain T-cell malignancies in adults in the United States (*1*). Since the isolation and characterization of the first two isolates, HTLV-I$_{CR}$ and HTLV-I$_{MB}$ (*1, 2*), several new isolates of HTLV were obtained in our laboratory from patients and in a few instances from clinically healthy individuals in the United States, Israel, the West Indies, and Japan (*3*). Recently, a new human retrovirus, called HTLV-II, was identified in (*4*) and isolated from (*5*) cultured cells from a patient with hairy cell leukemia; this isolate is related to but quite distinct from all other HTLV isolates. Independent detection and isolation of HTLV have now also been reported from Japan, Europe, and other laboratories in the United States (*6*). Detailed characterization of the HTLV isolates indicates that all but HTLV-II are very similar to each other (*3, 7*); none are endogenous in man (*2*); and all are readily distinguishable from the known animal retroviruses by nucleic acid hybridization (*8*), immunological assays of structural proteins (*9*), and reverse transcriptase (*10*). Specific antibodies to HTLV proteins have been found in serum samples from adults with mature T-cell leukemia (*11*), and the data from serological and epidemiological studies indicate that HTLV is endemic in certain regions of the world, particularly the Caribbean region and southern Japan (*12*). We are testing the possibility that HTLV is associated with the newly described acquired immune deficiency syndrome (AIDS) (*13*). This disease, which has been described with increasing frequency since the first case reports (*14, 15*), is suspected of being caused by a transmissible agent (*16*).

Patients with AIDS are now known to include male homosexuals (*13*), intravenous drug users (*17*), Haitian immigrants to the United States (*18*), and hemophiliacs (*19*). Clinical signs of the disease include opportunistic infections, predominantly *Pneumocystis carinii* pneumonia (*13*), and Kaposi's sarcoma (*20*) in previously healthy persons. Studies of cell-mediated immunity in patients with AIDS have demonstrated generalized impairment of T-lymphocyte functions, including lymphopenia, cutaneous anergy, and reduced helper T-lymphocyte (OKT4$^+$) subpopulations. This results in reversed ratios of helper to suppressor T-lymphocyte (OKT4$^+$/OKT8$^+$), poor lymphocyte responsiveness to mitogens, and, in some cases, decreased natural killer cell activity (*21*). The epidemiology of this syndrome—that is, the increasing incidence and clustering of cases, particularly in New York and California—suggests the involvement of a transmissible agent (*14, 15*). Patients with AIDS are often chronically infected with cytomegalovirus (*22*) or hepatitis B virus (*23*). Serum antibodies that react with membrane proteins from HTLV-infected cells have been found in many AIDS patients (*24*), and HTLV sequences have been found in DNA from two of 33 AIDS cases (*25*). Here we describe the isolation of HTLV from peripheral blood T lymphocytes from one U.S. patient with AIDS, and report briefly on the finding of HTLV antigens in T cells cultured from peripheral blood T lymphocytes of two cases of AIDS in France.

Peripheral blood T cells from the U.S. patient, EP, were grown in suspension culture in the presence of partially purified human T-cell growth factor (TCGF) (*26*) as described (*3, 26*). The morphology of the virus is shown in Fig. 1. Data on the identification of HTLV in the T cells are summarized in Table 1. The morphology was that of a type-C retrovirus, with the virus being indistinguishable from the earlier HTLV isolates. By using monoclonal antibodies and hyperimmune sera we determined that the T cells contained the HTLV core proteins p19 and p24, respectively. These results also showed that the new isolate belongs to the HTLV group.

We then transmitted the virus from the patient's peripheral blood lymphocytes into T cells from human umbilical cord blood (C183 cells). The donor (EP) cells were x-irradiated (6000 R) and then washed and cocultivated with recipient cord blood T cells of the opposite sex as described (*3*) (Table 1). Analyses of the sex chromosomes and HLA profiles (his-

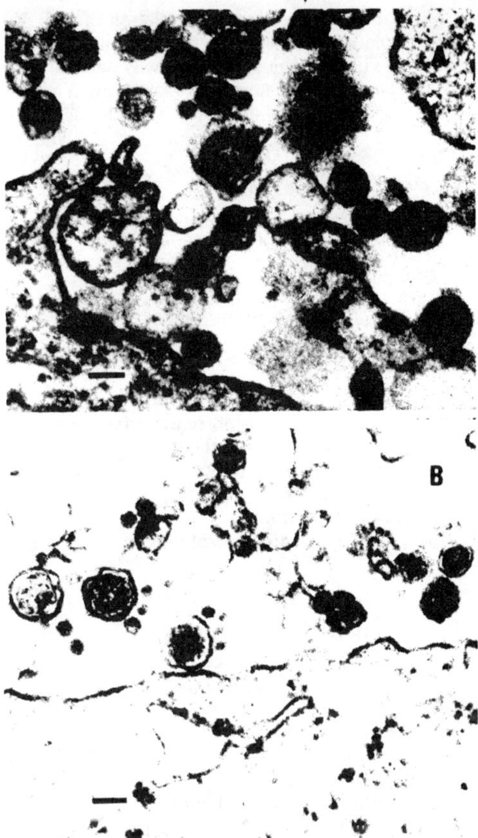

Fig. 1. Electron micrographs of (A) T cells from a patient (EP) with AIDS and (B) human umbilical cord blood T cells (C183/EP) cocultured with EP cells. Many mature type-C particles are visible in the extracellular space of both cell lines (scale bars, 100 nm).

tocompatibility antigens) distinguished the recipient cord blood cells from the EP cells. Subsequent cell sorter analysis with monoclonal antibodies showed that both the donor EP cells and the recipient C183 cells were infected with the virus (C183/EP cells) and that cells in both lines were mature T cells. They reacted with monoclonal antibodies to OKT3$^+$ (Pan T), OKT4$^+$ (helper-inducer), OKT8$^+$ (cytotoxic-suppressor), and 9.6$^+$

46

Table 1. Detection and isolation of HTLV in peripheral blood T cells of an AIDS patient and isolation of the virus by transmission into T cells from umbilical cord blood obtained from newborns. The T-cell line was derived from the peripheral blood of patient EP, a 32-year-old black male homosexual from New York City who had *Pneumocystis carinii* pneumonia with abnormal lymphocyte function characteristic of AIDS (*23*). N.D., not done; M, male; F, female.

Characteristics of the cultured T cells	Source of T cells		
	AIDS patient (EP)	Normal cord blood T cells (C183)	Cord blood (C183) T cells infected with HTLV$_{EP}$
HTLV expression*			
p24 (ng/mg)	40	0	500
p19 (percent positive cells)	9	0	37
Reverse transcriptase activity (pmole/ml extract)	81	0	21
Virus particles (electron microscopy)	+	N.D.	+
Sex chromosome†	M	F	F
Growth potential/morphology	Indefinite/uniform (few binucleated cells)	Limited/ uniform (normal)	Indefinite/polymorph (bi- and multinucleated cells)
TCGF requirements (units)‡	< 0.7	1	< 0.1
TCGF receptors (TAC) (percent/mean fluorescence units)§	77/475	20/150	42/1255
Transferrin receptors (5E9) (percent/mean fluorescence units)§	12/19	N.D.	28/1015
Lymphoid surface phenotype§			
Pan T (OKT3, 3A1, 9.6) (percent)	45 to 95	95	21 to 61
OKT4 (percent)	76	85	40
OKT8 (percent)	46	10	20
Histocompatibility antigen expression			
HLA-DR determinants (DA2, 3.1) (percent/mean fluorescence units)§	59/236	0	56/2363
Additional HLA antigens	Bw35, Bw62	0	Bw62, DR4, MB3, MT2

*The core protein p24 was detected by RIPA in cell extracts (*9*), and p19 was detected by IFA on fixed cells (*28*). Reverse transcriptase activity in culture fluids was assayed as described (*10*), and the activity expressed as picomoles of ^{3}H-labeled deoxythymidine monophosphate incorporated into trichloracetic acid–precipitable DNA per milliliter of 30 times concentrated culture fluid. †The HTLV$_{EP}$ isolate was transmitted into human cord blood T cells (C183) by cocultivation as described (*3*). Sex chromosomes and HLA antigens were used as markers for identification of HTLV-infected cells. Phytohemagglutinin-stimulated T cells (control) from cord blood were grown in the presence of TCGF and processed simultaneously with HTLV positive T cells. ‡Values for TCGF were determined by probit analysis; one unit of TCGF is defined as the amount necessary to give 50 percent of the maximum [^{3}H]thymidine incorporation by normal T cells (C183) in the presence of a standard TCGF preparation. §The binding of monoclonal antibodies reacting with TCGF and transferrin receptors, HLA-DR determinants as well as with lymphoid cell surface antigens using Pan T, helper-induced (OKT4), and suppressor-cytotoxic (OKT8) antibodies was determined by cytofluorometry with a fluorescence-activated cell sorter (FACS). The HLA profiles were determined as previously described (*2*) by comparing HTLV-infected C183/EP [HLA-A3, B27, B12 (Bw62), Cw2, DR4, MB3, MT2] to normal C183 cord blood T cells (HLA-A3, B27, B12, Cw2); in the case of EP, the HTLV positive T cells [HLA-A2, Aw30, B17, B18 (Bw35, Bw62), Cw5, DR2, MT1, MT2] were compared to B cells (HLA-A2, Aw30, B17, B18, Cw5, DR2, MT1, MT2) from the patient. The full identity in HLA profiles was found in both cases; however, as previously demonstrated (*2*), the expression of additional HLA antigens associated with HTLV infection was also detected.

(sheep red blood cell receptor). Both the EP and C183/EP cell lines had indefinite growth potential, cell surface alterations such as expression of inappropriate HLA antigens, and other properties similar to other HTLV-infected cord blood T cells (*27*).

We found HTLV antigens in both the EP and C183/EP cell lines by means of an indirect immunofluorescence assay (IFA) with a highly specific monoclonal antibody for p19 (*28*) and by a competition radioimmunoprecipitation assay (RIPA) for the major viral core protein p24 (*9*). Extracellular virus particles were visible in the electron microscope and verified by the finding of reverse transcriptase activity associated with extracellular particles in both cell lines (Fig. 1, A and B, and Table 1).

As shown in Fig. 2, the slopes of the competition curves in homologous RIPA's for p24 in cell extracts from both cell lines were very similar to those for p24 from isolates of the HTLV-I subgroup, indicating that the isolate from patient EP is closely related to the HTLV-I subgroup. By this assay the new isolate appears to be less closely related to the HTLV-II subgroup (*29*). We call this isolate HTLV-I$_{EP}$. Analysis of the nucleic acids of the HTLV isolated from EP also indicated its similarity to viruses of the HTLV-I subgroup (*29*).

The AIDS patients in France were female. One was a Haitian, the other was a Caucasian who had visited Haiti. Peripheral blood T cells from both patients were cultured with partially purified TCGF and, by means of hyperimmune sera and monoclonal antibodies, were shown to express HTLV antigen and the core proteins p19 and p24. Present data indicate that the virus can be transmitted to normal cord blood T lymphocytes by

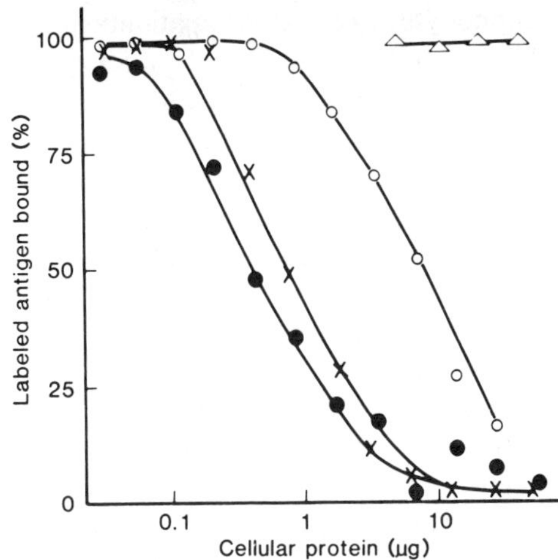

Fig. 2. Homologous competitive radioimmunoprecipitation assay of the major core protein p24 with cell extracts of established T-cell lines. Symbols: ○, cells from AIDS patient EP; ●, C183/EP cells (cord blood T cells infected with HTLV$_{EP}$); △, normal cord blood T cells; and X, positive control cells (from a patient with a mature T-cell malignancy known to release HTLV).

the cocultivation technique. We have not yet determined whether these isolates from France belong to subgroup I or II of HTLV or to a new subgroup.

Antibodies specifically reactive with internal structural proteins of HTLV have been found in the serum of AIDS patients more frequently than in the normal population, but less than in serum from patients with HTLV-positive T-cell leukemia (*30*). The evidence from immunological, epidemiological, and molecular biological studies (*31*) for an association between HTLV and certain adult T-cell leukemias and lymphomas is much stronger. The less consistent detection of the virus in AIDS patients may reflect a depletion in the number of available target T cells in their peripheral blood, a hypothesis supported by the results of serial analyses of DNA peripheral blood

48

lymphocytes of AIDS patients (25). These results showed that patients initially positive for HTLV sequences may be negative with subsequent repeated blood samples.

Since HTLV is endemic in southern Japan, the apparent lack of epidemic AIDS in this region may argue against a causative role for HTLV in AIDS. However, the absence of an AIDS epidemic in the area might also be explained by a recent genomic modification in some HTLV strains in other areas of the world. Alternatively, people in southern Japan may have greater resistance to the T-cell suppressive effect of the virus. There are, of course, many precedents for variations in the susceptibility of different populations to a microorganism.

Whether or not the etiological agent of AIDS is an HTLV, it is interesting to consider the possible routes of transmission of such an agent. Most findings suggest transmission by blood transfusion and by intravenous drug administration. However, the high incidence of AIDS in homosexuals who apparently have not received blood transfusions or used intravenously administered drugs suggests that the agent is also transmitted during sexual contact by sperm or saliva. It may therefore be possible to detect HTLV antigen in these secretions and to transmit the virus to cord blood by the coculturing method. Since HTLV can also infect marmoset and other primate T cells (32), should this virus be established as the causative agent of AIDS it may also be possible to develop an animal model of the disease.

References and Notes

1. B. J. Poiesz, F. W. Ruscetti, A. F. Gazdar, P. A. Bunn, J. D. Minna, R. C. Gallo, *Proc. Natl. Acad. Sci. U.S.A.* **77**, 7415 (1980); B. J. Poiesz, F. W. Ruscetti, M. S. Reitz, V. S. Kalyanaraman, R. C. Gallo, *Nature (London)* **294**, 268 (1981).
2. R. C. Gallo, D. Mann, S. Broder, F. W. Ruscetti, M. Maeda, V. S. Kalyanaraman, M. Robert-Guroff, M. S. Reitz, *Proc. Natl. Acad. Sci. U.S.A.* **79**, 5680 (1982).
3. M. Popovic, P. S. Sarin, M. Robert-Guroff, V. S. Kalyanaraman, D. Mann, J. Minowada, R. C. Gallo, *Science* **219**, 856 (1983).
4. V. S. Kalyanaraman, M. G. Sarngadharan, M. Robert-Guroff, I. Miyoshi, D. Blayney, D. Golde, R. C. Gallo, *ibid.* **218**, 571 (1982).
5. A. Saxons, R. H. Stevens, D. W. Golde, *Ann. Int. Med.* **88**, 323 (1978).
6. I. Miyoshi, I. Kuboniski, S. Yoshimoto, T. Akagi, Y. Outsuki, Y. Shiraishi, K. Nagata, Y. Hinuma, *Nature (London)* **294**, 770 (1981); M. Yoshida, I. Miyoshi, Y. Hinuma, *Proc. Natl. Acad. Sci. U.S.A.* **79**, 2031 (1982); B. F. Haynes, S. E. Miller, T. O. Moore, P. H. Dunn, D. P. Bolognesi, R. S. Metzgar, *ibid.* **80**, 2054 (1983); M. Greaves, in preparation.
7. M. Popovic *et al.*, *Nature (London)* **300**, 63 (1982); M. S. Reitz, M. Popovic, B. F. Haynes, M. Clark, R. C. Gallo, *Virology*, in press.
8. M. S. Reitz, B. J. Poiesz, F. W. Ruscetti, R. C. Gallo, *Proc. Natl. Acad. Sci. U.S.A.* **78**, 1887 (1981).
9. V. S. Kalyanaraman, M. G. Sarngadharan, B. J. Poiesz, F. W. Ruscetti, R. C. Gallo, *J. Virol.* **38**, 906 (1981).
10. H. M. Rho, B. J. Poiesz, F. W. Ruscetti, R. C. Gallo, *Virology* **112**, 355 (1981).
11. L. E. Posner *et al.*, *J. Exp. Med.* **154**, 333 (1981); V. S. Kalyanaraman, M. G. Sarngadharan, P. A. Bunn, J. D. Minna, R. C. Gallo, *Nature (London)* **294**, 271 (1981).
12. M. Robert-Guroff, Y. Nakao, K. Notake, Y. Ito, A. Sliski, R. C. Gallo, *Science* **215**, 975 (1982); V. S. Kalyanaraman, M. G. Sarngadharan, Y. Nakao, Y. Ito, T. Aoki, R. C. Gallo, *Proc. Natl. Acad. Sci. U.S.A.* **79**, 1653 (1982); W. A. Blattner *et al.*, *Int. J. Cancer* **30**, 257 (1982).
13. "*Pneumocystis* pneumonia—Los Angeles," *Morbid. Mortal. Weekly Rep.* **30**, 250 (1981); "Kaposi's sarcoma and *pneumocystis* pneumonia among homosexual men—New York City and California," *ibid.*, p. 305.
14. Centers for Disease Control, Task Force on Kaposi's Sarcoma and Opportunistic Infections, *N. Engl. J. Med.* **306**, 248 (1982).
15. J. P. Hanrahan, G. P. Wormser, C. P. Maguire, L. J. DeLorenzo, G. Gravis, *ibid.* **307**, 498 (1982).
16. M. F. Rogers *et al.*, Task Force on Acquired Immune Deficiency Syndrome, *Ann. Int. Med.*, in press; D. P. Francis, J. W. Curran, M. Essex, *J. Natl. Cancer Inst.*, in press.
17. K. Gold, L. Thomas, G. P. Garrett, *N. Engl. J. Med.* **307**, 498 (1982).
18. J. Vieira, E. Frank, T. J. Spira, S. H. Landesman, *ibid.* **308**, 125 (1983).
19. "*Pneumocystis carinii* pneumonia among persons with Hemophilia A," *Morbid. Mortal. Weekly Rep.* **31**, 365 (1982).
20. A. E. Friedman-Kien *et al.*, *Ann. Int. Med.* **96**, 693 (1982).
21. M. Gottlieb, R. Schroff, H. M. Schanker, J. D. Weisman, P. T. Fan, R. C. Wolf, A. Saxon, *N.*

Engl. J. Med. **305**, 1425 (1981); J. Masur *et al.*, *ibid.*, p. 1431.
22. C. Urmacher, P. Myskowski, M. Ochoa, M. Kris, B. Safai, *Am. J. Med.* **72**, 569 (1982).
23. D. R. Francis and J. E. Maynard, *Epidemiol. Rev.* **1**, 17 (1979).
24. M. Essex, M. F. McLane, T. H. Lee, L. Falk, C. W. S. Howe, J. I. Mullins, C. Cabradilla, D. P. Francis, *Science* **220**, 859 (1983).
25. E. P. Gelmann, M. Popovic, D. Blayney, H. Masur, G. Sidhu, R. E. Stahl, R. C. Gallo, *ibid.*, p. 862.
26. J. W. Mier and R. C. Gallo, *Proc. Natl. Acad. Sci. U.S.A.* **77**, 6134 (1980); B. J. Poiesz, F. W. Ruscetti, J. W. Mier, A. M. Woods, R. C. Gallo, *ibid.*, p. 6815.
27. M. Popovic, G. Lange-Wantizin, P. S. Sarin, D. Mann, R. C. Gallo, *ibid.*, in press.
28. M. Robert-Guroff, F. W. Ruscetti, L. E. Posner, B. J. Poiesz, R. C. Gallo, *J. Exp. Med.* **154**, 1957 (1981).
29. R. C. Gallo *et al.*, unpublished data.
30. C. Saxinger and M. Robert-Guroff, unpublished data.
31. F. Wong-Staal, B. Hahn, V. Manzari, S. Colombi, G. Franchini, E. P. Gelmann, R. C. Gallo, *Nature (London)*, in press; R. C. Gallo and M. R. Reitz, *J. Natl. Cancer Inst.* **69**, 1209 (1982).
32. L. Falk, unpublished data.
33. We thank E. Read for technical assistance, B. Kramarsky for electron microscopy, R. Ting for karyotyping, and A. Mazzuca for editorial assistance. Supported in part by Interagency Agreement Y01-CP-00502 with the Uniformed Services University for the Health Sciences.

19 April 1983

Report

20 May 1983

9. Isolation of a T-Lymphotropic Retrovirus from a Patient at Risk for Acquired Immune Deficiency Syndrome (AIDS)

F. Barré-Sinoussi, J.-C. Chermann, F. Rey, M.T. Nugeyre, S. Chamaret, J. Gruest, C. Dauguet, C. Axler-Blin, F. Brun-Vézinet, C. Rouzioux, W. Rozenbaum, and L. Montagnier

The acquired immune deficiency syndrome (AIDS) has recently been recognized in several countries (*1*). The disease has been reported mainly in homosexual males with multiple partners, and epidemiological studies suggest horizontal transmission by sexual routes (*2*) as well as by intravenous drug administration (*3*), and blood transfusion (*4*). The pronounced depression of cellular immunity that occurs in patients with AIDS and the quantitative modifications of subpopulations of their T lymphocytes (*5*) suggest that T cells or a subset of T cells might be a preferential target for the putative infectious agent. Alternatively, these modifications may result from subsequent infections. The depressed cellular immunity may result in serious opportunistic infections in AIDS patients, many of whom develop Kaposi's sarcoma (*1*). However, a picture of persistent multiple lymphadenopathies has also been described in homosexual males (*6*) and infants (*7*) who may or may not develop AIDS (*8*). The histological aspect of such lymph nodes is that of reactive hyperplasia. Such cases may correspond to an early or a milder form of the disease. We report here the isolation of a novel retrovirus from a lymph node of a homosexual patient with multiple lymphadenopathies. The virus appears to be a member of the human T-cell leukemia virus (HTLV) family (9).

The retrovirus was propagated in cultures of T lymphocytes from a healthy adult donor and from umbilical cord blood of newborn humans. Viral core proteins were not immunologically related to the p24 and p19 proteins of subgroup I of HTLV (9). However, serum of the patient reacted strongly with surface antigen (or antigens) present on HTLV-I–infected cells. Moreover, the ionic requirements of the viral reverse transcriptase were close to that of HTLV. Recently, a type-C retrovirus was also identified in T cells from a patient with hairy cell leukemia. Analysis of the proteins of this virus showed they were related to, but clearly different from, proteins of previous HTLV isolates (10). Moreover, recent studies of the nucleic acid sequences of this new virus show it is less than 10 percent homologous to the earlier HTLV isolates (11). This virus was called HTLV-II to distinguish it from all the earlier, highly related viruses termed HTLV-I. The new retrovirus reported here appears to also differ from HTLV-II. We tentatively conclude that this virus, as well as all previous HTLV isolates, belong to a family of T-lymphotropic retroviruses that are horizontally transmitted in humans and may be involved in several pathological syndromes, including AIDS.

The patient was a 33-year-old homosexual male who sought medical consultation in December 1982 for cervical lymphadenopathy and asthenia (patient 1). Examination showed axillary and inguinal lymphadenopathies. Neither fever nor recent loss of weight were noted. The patient had a history of several episodes of gonorrhea and had been treated for syphilis in September 1982. During interviews he indicated that he had had more than 50 sexual partners per year and had traveled to many countries, including North Africa, Greece, and India. His last trip to New York was in 1979.

Laboratory tests indicated positive serology (immunoglobulin G) for cytomegalovirus (CMV) and Epstein-Barr virus. Herpes simplex virus was detected in cells from his throat that were cultured on human and monkey cells. A biopsy of a cervical lymph node was performed. One sample served for histological examination, which revealed follicular hyperplasia without change of the general architecture of the lymph node. Immunohistological studies revealed, in paracortical areas, numerous T lymphocytes (OKT3$^+$). Typing of the whole cellular suspension indicated that 62 percent of the cells were T lymphocytes (OKT3$^+$), 44 percent were T-helper cells (OKT4$^+$), and 16 percent were suppressor cells (OKT8$^+$).

Cells of the same biopsied lymph node were put in culture medium with phytohemagglutinin (PHA), T-cell growth factor (TCGF), and antiserum to human α interferon (12). The reason for using this antiserum was to neutralize endogenous interferon which is secreted by cells chronically infected by viruses, including retroviruses. In the mouse system, we had previously shown that antiserum to interferon could increase retrovirus production by a factor of 10 to 50 (13). After 3 days, the culture was continued in the same medium without PHA. Samples were regularly taken for assay of reverse transcriptase and for examination in the electron microscope.

After 15 days of culture, a reverse transcriptase activity was detected in the culture supernatant by using the ionic conditions described for HTLV-I (*14*). Virus production continued for 15 days and decreased thereafter, in parallel with the decline of lymphocyte proliferation. Peripheral blood lymphocytes cultured in the same way were consistently negative for reverse transcriptase activity, even after 6 weeks. Cytomegalovirus could be detected, upon prolonged co-cultivation with MRC5 cells, in the original biopsy tissue, but not in the cultured T lymphocytes at any time of the culture.

Virus transmission was attempted with the use of a culture of T lymphocytes established from an adult healthy donor of the Blood Transfusion Center at the Pasteur Institute. On day 3, half of the culture was cocultivated with lymphocytes from the biopsy after centrifugation of the mixed cell suspensions. Reverse transcriptase activity could be detected in the supernatant on day 15 of the coculture but was not detectable on days 5 and 10. The reverse transcriptase had the same characteristics as that released by the patient's cells and the amount released remained stable for 15 to 20 days. Cells of the uninfected culture of the donor lymphocytes did not release reverse transcriptase activity during this period or up to 6 weeks when the culture was discontinued.

The cell-free supernatant of the infected coculture was used to infect 3-day-old cultures of T lymphocytes from two umbilical cords, LC1 and LC5, in the presence of Polybrene (2 μg/ml). After a lag period of 7 days, a relatively high titer of reverse transcriptase activity was detected in both of the cord lymphocyte cultures. Identical cultures, which had not been infected, remained negative. These

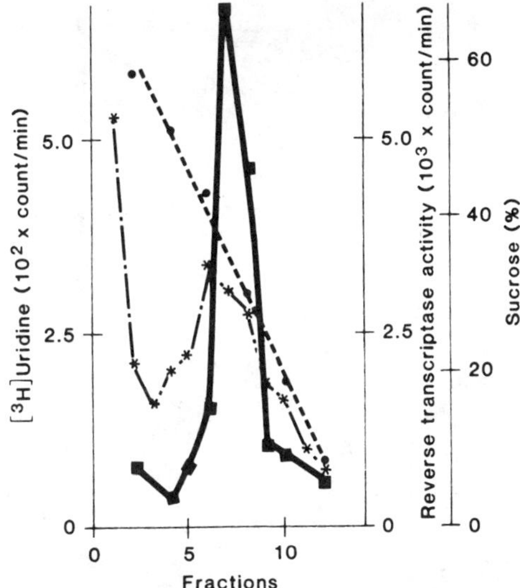

Fig. 1. Analysis of virus from patient 1 on sucrose gradients. Cord blood T lymphocytes infected with virus from patient 1 were labeled for 18 hours with [³H]uridine (28 Ci/ mmole, Amersham; 20 μCi/ml). Cell-free supernatant was ultracentrifuged for 1 hour at 50,000 rev/min. The pellet was resuspended in 200 μl of NTE buffer (10 mM tris, pH 7.4, 100 mM NaCl, and 1 mM EDTA) and was centrifuged over a 3-ml linear sucrose gradient (10 to 60 percent) at 55,000 rev/min for 90 minutes in an IEC type SB 498 rotor. Fractions (200 μl) were collected, and 30 μl samples of each fraction were assayed for DNA polymerase activity with 5 mM Mg^{2+} and poly(A) · oligo-(dT)$_{12-18}$ as template primer; a 20-μl portion of each fraction was precipitated with 10 percent trichloroacetic acid and then filtered on a 0.45-μm Millipore filter. The ³H-labeled acid precipitable material was measured in a Packard β counter.

two successive infections clearly show that the virus could be propagated on normal lymphocytes from either newborns or adults.

That this new isolate was a retrovirus was further indicated by its density in a sucrose gradient, which was 1.16, and by its labeling with [³H]uridine (Fig. 1). Electron microscopy of the infected umbilical cord lymphocytes showed charac-

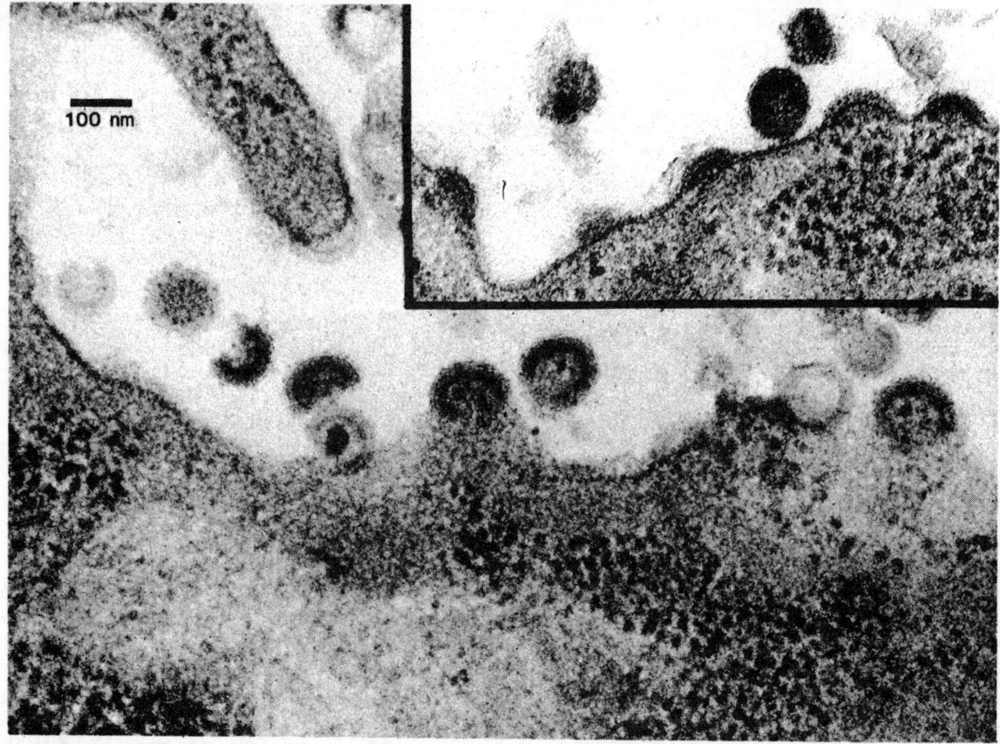

Fig. 2. Electron microscopy of thin sections of virus-producing cord lymphocytes. The inset shows various stages of particle budding at the cell surface.

teristic immature particles with dense crescent (C-type) budding at the plasma membrane (Fig. 2).

Virus-infected cells from the original biopsy as well as infected lymphocytes from the first and second viral passages were used to determine the optimal requirements for reverse transcriptase activity and the template specificity of the enzyme. The results were the same in all instances. The reverse transcriptase activity displayed a strong affinity for poly(adenylate · oligodeoxythymidylate) [poly(A) · oligo(dT)], and required Mg^{2+} with an optimal concentration (5 mM) slightly lower than that for HTLV (14) and an optimal pH of 7.8. The reaction was not inhibited by actinomycin D. This character, as well as the preferential

specificity for riboseadenylate · deoxythymidylate over deoxyadenylate · deoxythymidylate, distinguish the viral enzyme from DNA-dependent polymerases.

We then determined whether or not this isolate was indistinguishable from HTLV-I isolates. Human T-cell leukemia virus has been isolated from cultured T lymphocytes of patients with T lymphomas and T leukemias [for a review, see (9)]. The antibodies used were specific for the p19 and p24 core proteins of HTLV-I. A monoclonal antibody to p19 (15) and a polyclonal goat antibody to p24 (16) were used in an indirect fluorescence assay against infected cells from the biopsy of patient 1 and lymphocytes obtained from a healthy donor and in-

Table 1. Indirect immunofluorescence assay. Cells were washed with phosphate-buffered saline (PBS) and resuspended in the same buffer. Portions (5×10^4 cells) were spotted on slides, air-dried and fixed for 10 minutes at room temperature in acetone. Slides were stored at $-80°C$ until use. Twenty microliters of either monoclonal antibody to HTLV p19 (diluted 1/400 in PBS) or goat antibody to HTLV p24 (diluted 1/400 in PBS) or serum from patient 1 diluted 1/10 in PBS was applied to cells and incubated for 45 minutes at 37°C. The appropriate fluorescein-conjugated antiserum (antiserum to mouse, goat, or human immunoglobulin G) was diluted and applied to the fixed cells for 30 minutes at room temperature. Slides were then washed three times in PBS. Cells were stained with Evans blue solution for 15 minutes and then washed extensively with water before microscopic examination.

	Immunofluorescence (percent positive)		
Cell type	Antibody to p19	Antibody to p24	Serum from patient 1
Normal blood lymphocytes			
N 10916	−	−	−
LC$_1$	−	−	−
HTLV-producing cells			
C$_{91}$/PL	+ (90 to 100)	+ (90 to 100)	+ (90 to 100)
C$_{10}$/MJ$_2$	+ (90 to 100)	+ (90 to 100)	+ (90 to 100)
Virus-producing cells from			
Patient 1	−	−	+ (90 to 100)
LC$_1$/patient 1	−	−	± (0.5 to 2)
Patient 2	−	−	+ (90 to 100)

fected with the same virus. As shown in Table 1, the virus-producing cells did not react with either type of antibody, whereas two lines of cord lymphocytes chronically infected with HTLV (*17*) and used as controls showed strong surface fluorescence.

When serum from patient 1 was tested against infected lymphocytes from the biopsy the surface fluorescence was as intense as that of the control HTLV-producing lines. This suggests that serum of the patient contains antibodies that recognize a common antigen present on HTLV-I–producing cells and on the patient's lymphocytes. Similarly, cord lymphocytes infected with the virus from patient 1 did not react with antibodies to p19 or p24. Only a minor proportion of the cells (about 1 percent) reacted with the patient's serum. This may indicate that only this fraction of the cells was infected and produced virus. Alterna-

tively, the antigen recognized by the patient's serum may contain cellular determinants that show less expression in T lymphocytes of newborns.

We also cultured T lymphocytes from a lymph node of another patient (patient 2) who presented with multiple adenopathies and had been in close contact with an AIDS case. These lymphocytes did not produce viral reverse transcriptase; however, they reacted in the immunofluorescence assay with serum from patient 1. Moreover, serum from patient 2 reacted strongly with control HTLV-producing lines (not shown). In order to determine which viral antigen was recognized by antibodies present in the two patients' sera, several immunoprecipitation experiments were carried out. Cord lymphocytes infected with virus from patient 1 and uninfected controls were labeled with [^{35}S]methionine for 20 hours. Cells were lysed with detergents, and a cyto-

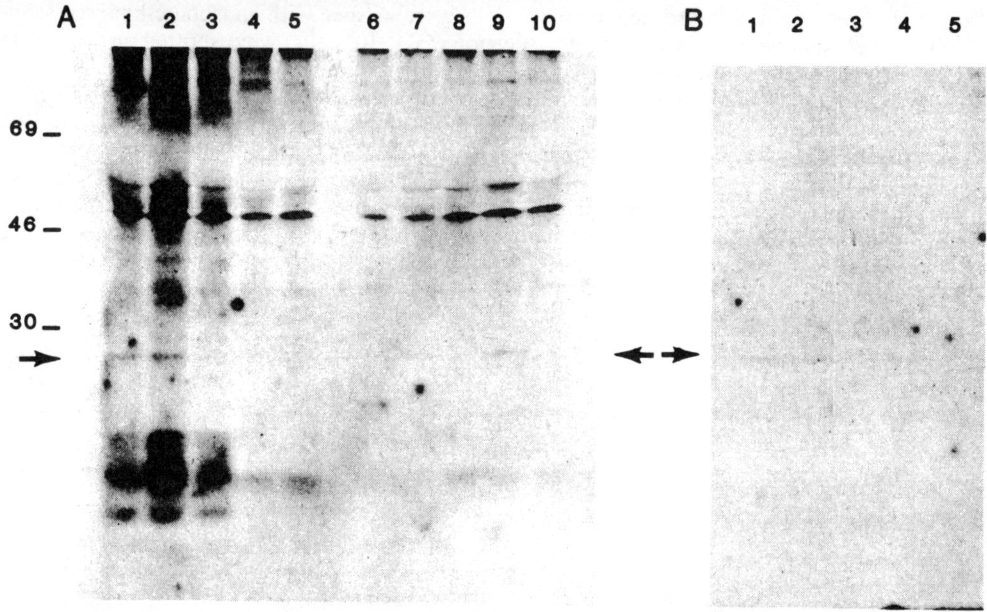

Fig. 3. Immunoprecipitation of ^{35}S-labeled viral proteins. Cord blood T-lymphocytes infected with virus from patient 1 were incubated overnight in culture medium containing one-fifth of the normal concentrations of methionine in minimum essential medium, [^{35}S]methionine (1500 Ci/mmole, Amersham; 50 μCi/ml), and 10 percent dialyzed fetal calf serum. The virus was purified by banding on a sucrose gradient as described in Fig. 1. Labeled cells were resuspended in 10 μl of saline and then lysed with 90 μl of RIPA buffer (18) containing aprotinin (500 U/ml; Zymofren, Specia) at 4°C for 15 minutes. The supernatant of a 10,000g centrifugation of the cell extract was used for immunoprecipitation. A similar extract was made from HTLV-producing C$_{91}$/PL cells (17). (A) Portions (20 μl) of cell extracts were mixed with 6 μl of serum, incubated for 2 hours at 37°C and overnight at +4°C. Then, 60 μl of a suspension of Protein A–Sepharose (10 mg/ml in RIPA buffer) were added. After 45 minutes of incubation at 4°C, immunocomplexes bound to Protein A–Sepharose were washed five times with RIPA buffer by centrifugation, heated for 3 minutes at 100°C in denaturing buffer and electrophoresed on 12.5 percent polyacrylamide-SDS slab gel (19). Lanes 1 to 5: Extract of LC$_1$ cells infected with virus from patient 1 and tested against 1, serum from patient 1; 2, serum from patient 2; 3, serum of a healthy donor; 4, goat antiserum to HTLV-Ip24; 5, normal goat serum. Lanes 6 to 10: C91/PL (HTLV-producing) cell extract tested with: 6, serum from patient 1; 7, serum from patient 2; serum of a healthy donor; 4, goat antiserum to HTLV-Ip24; 5, normal goat serum. (B) Portions (20 μl) of the band containing virus from patient 1 were treated with various antisera and processed as described for cell extracts. Lane 1, serum from patient 1; 2, serum from patient 2; 3, serum of a healthy donor; 4, serum of another healthy donor; 5, goat antiserum to HTLV-Ip24. Arrows indicate the p24–p25 protein. Molecular weights (in thousands) are indicated on the left.

plasmic S10 extract was made. Labeled virus released in the supernatant was banded in a sucrose gradient. Both materials were immunoprecipitated by antiserum to HTLV-1 p24, by serum from patients 1 and 2, and by serum samples from healthy donors. Immunocomplexes were analyzed by polyacrylamide gel electrophoresis under denaturing conditions. Figure 3 shows that a p25 protein present in the virus-infected cells from patient 1 and in LC1 cells infected with this virus, was specifically recognized by serum from patients 1 and 2 but not by antiserum to HTLV-1 p24 or serum of normal donors. Conversely, the p24 present in control HTLV-infected cell extracts was recognized by antibodies to HTLV but not by serum from patient 1. A weak band (lane 2, Fig. 3B) could hardly be seen with serum from patient 2, suggesting some similarities of the p25 protein from this patient's cells with HTLV-1 p24. When purified, labeled virus from patient 1 was analyzed under similar conditions, three major proteins could be seen: the p25 protein and proteins with molecular weights of 80,000 and 45,000. The 45K protein may be due to contamination of the virus by cellular actin which was present in immunoprecipitates of all the cell extracts (Fig. 3).

These results, together with the immunofluorescence data, indicate that the retrovirus from patient 1 contains a major p25 protein, similar in size to that of HTLV-I but different immunologically. The DNA sequences of these and other members of the HTLV family are being compared. All attempts to infect other cells such as a B-lymphoblastoid cell line (Raji), immature or pre-T cell lines (CEM, HSB$_2$), and normal fibroblasts (feline and mink lung cell lines) were unsuccessful.

The role of this virus in the etiology of AIDS remains to be determined. Patient 1 had circulating antibodies against the virus, and some of the latter persisted in lymphocytes of his lymph node (or nodes). The virus-producing lymphocytes seemed to have no increased growth potential in vitro compared to the uninfected cells. Therefore, the multiple lymphadenopathies may represent a host reaction against the persistent viral in-

fection rather than hyperproliferation of virus-infected lymphocytes. Other factors, such as repeated infection by the same virus or other bacterial and viral agents may, in some patients, overload this early defense mechanism and bring about an irreversible depletion of T cells involved in cellular immunity.

References and Notes

1. Centers for Disease Control, Task Force on Kaposi's Sarcoma and Opportunistic Infections, *N. Engl. J. Med.* **306**, 248 (1982).
2. M. Marmor *et al.*, *Lancet* **1982-II**, 1083 (1982); S. Fannin *et al.*, *Morbid. Mortal. Weekly Rep.* **31**, 305 (1982).
3. Centers for Disease Control, Task Force on Kaposi's Sarcoma and Opportunistic Infections, *Morbid. Mortal. Weekly Rep.* **31**, 507 (1982).
4. M. C. Poon *et al.*, *ibid.*, p. 644.
5. R. E. Stahl, A. Friedman-Kien, R. Dubin, M. Marmor, S. Zolla Parner, *Am. J. Med.* **73**, 171 (1982).
6. D. Mildvan *et al.*, *Morbid. Mortal. Weekly Rep.* **31**, 249 (1982).
7. R. O'Reilly *et al.*, *ibid.*, p. 665.
8. W. Rozenbaum *et al.*, *Lancet* **1982-II**, 572 (1982).
9. R. C. Gallo and M. S. Reitz, Jr., *J. Natl. Cancer Inst.* **69** (No. 6), 1209 (1982).
10. V. S. Kalyanaraman *et al.*, *Science* **218**, 571 (1982).
11. E. Gelmann, F. Wong-Staal, R. Gallo, personal communication.
12. The cells were grown in RPMI-1640 medium supplemented with antibiotics, $10^{-5}M$ β-mercaptoethanol, 10 percent fetal calf serum, 0.1 percent sheep antibody to human α interferon (neutralizing titer, 6 IU at 10^{-5}), and 5 percent TCGF, free of PHA.
13. F. Barré-Sinoussi *et al.*, *Ann. Microbiol. (Inst. Pasteur)* **130B**, 349 (1979).
14. B. J. Poiesz *et al.*, *Proc. Natl. Acad. Sci. U.S.A.* **77**, 7415 (1980).
15. M. Robert-Guroff *et al.*, *J. Exp. Med.* **154**, 1957 (1981).
16. V. S. Kalyanaraman *et al.*, *J. Virol.* **38**, 906 (1981).
17. M. Popovic, P. S. Sarin, M. Robert-Guroff, V. S. Kalyanaraman, D. Mann, J. Minowada, R. C. Gallo, *Science* **219**, 856 (1983).
18. R. E. Karess *et al.*, *Proc. Natl. Acad. Sci. U.S.A.* **76**, 3154 (1979).
19. U. K. Laemmli, *Nature (London)* **227**, 608 (1970).
20. We thank Dr. Fradellizi for gifts of T-cell growth factor, R. C. Gallo for providing antibodies to HTLV and for HTLV-producing cells, Mrs. Le François for preparation of the cord lymphocytes, M. Lavergne (Institut Pasteur, Production) for gifts of fluorescein-conjugated antisera, F. Huraud for performing some of the HTLV tests, and members of the French Working Group on AIDS for helpful discussion.

19 April 1983

10. AIDS Fears Spark Row Over Vaccine

David Dickson

Paris. Growing public concern in France about the spread of acquired immune deficiency syndrome (AIDS) is threatening the health of what appears, at least so far, to be an innocent victim—French efforts to promote foreign sales of a vaccine against hepatitis B. The vaccine is produced by the Institut Pasteur Production (IPP), a private company owned 51 percent by a subsidiary of the nationalized oil company Elf Acquitaine and 49 percent by the Institut Pasteur in Paris.

Last week, the president of IPP, Yves Garnier, filed suit against the Paris-based newspaper *Liberation* over a series of articles which appeared at the end of June raising questions about the safety of IPP's vaccine. The articles concentrated in particular on the company's use of American blood plasma, which is mixed with plasma from European sources, to produce the vaccine. They raised the possibility that, since AIDS is thought to be transmitted by some blood products, the vaccine could become a carrier for the disease.

While admitting that this theoretical possibility exists, IPP nevertheless maintains that each batch of its hepatitis B vaccine has been carefully checked for the presence of both viruses and retroviruses (and is now being double checked by government inspectors) and that no such problem has been discovered. The company claims the newspaper's articles have unnecessarily stirred up public concern about the safety of a vaccine which has been widely and safely used since

its introduction 2 years ago. It has expressed particular anger over a front page headline "Pasteur Institut Suffers from Gay Cancer," and is demanding 1 million francs (about $140,000) in damages.

French medical journalists have, in turn, accused the company of excessive secrecy over the procedures followed in the production of the vaccine. They point, for example, to the fact that the Ministry of Health was not initially informed about the use of the American plasma in the production of some batches of the vaccine, and that the company appears to be out of step with a recommendation from the Council of Europe concerning the prevention of AIDS, which suggests the avoidance, whenever possible, of "the import of blood products from countries where the payment of blood donors considerably increases the risk of contamination."

The controversy has come at a particularly sensitive time for IPP, since it is locked in intense competition for foreign sales, especially to Third World countries, with Merck Sharp & Dohme, whose hepatitis B vaccine is produced by a different process. Already several countries have decided in favor of the American vaccine.

Scientists at the Pasteur Institut are no less happy than IPP with the way the controversy has blown up in the French press, and in particular over the way that questions about their research have been raised by the action of what is, formally, a separate company.

Following the appearance of the *Liberation*

articles, the institute took the almost unprecedented step of calling a press conference to deny charges of impropriety, issuing a strongly worded warning against journalists spreading anxiety among the public "on the basis of fragmentary information," throwing discredit on research institutes and on French biological research "by questioning their methods and their integrity," and planting unfounded doubts about the quality of a vaccine, thereby threatening "the success of a French industry whose revenues go primarily to research."

The controversy is particularly ironic for scientists at Pasteur because some of them are deeply involved in identifying the possible causes of AIDS. In particular, the group headed by virologist Luc Montagnier earlier this year identified a retrovirus that had been isolated from the T cells of a homosexual male with the symptoms that often precede AIDS (*Science*, 20 May 1983).

At the time, the Pasteur discovery seemed to support a general hypothesis being developed in several U.S. laboratories that AIDS might be caused by the human T cell leukemia virus (HTLV), based on evidence of HTLV infection in patients who have either contracted or were at high risk for the syndrome. (There is, however, some debate over whether HTLV infection is a cause or a symptom of AIDS.) More recently, says Montagnier, other properties of the virus isolated by the Pasteur group indicate that it may not be as similar to the conventional HTLV virus as was originally thought—a finding which could lead to significant new developments in understanding the etiology of the syndrome.

France has also been at the forefront of attempts to understand the epidemiology of AIDS in Europe. Soon after the first reports from the U.S. Centers for Disease Control in 1981, an informal group of interested physicians and researchers in Paris rapidly started gathering data on its incidence in France (still relatively low, with about 60 known cases) and speculating about its possible pathology.

As formal recognition of the AIDS problem began to grow, a high level working group was established by the Ministry of Industry and Research to support more intensive studies, in particular of the epidemiology of the disease. Several major laboratories in France have now expressed an interest in participating in this research, while at the European level a meeting is being held in Denmark next month to coordinate approaches toward the detection and characterization of AIDS, the appropriate treatment for sufferers, and the research needed to study its epidemiological aspects.

As for research into the virus itself, the French researchers are now turning—for reasons of both time and the availability of facilities—to the U.S. National Cancer Institute for assistance in cloning the virus they have discovered so that its properties can be carefully studied.

Montagnier suggests this is a "very good example" of international collaboration in research, given the substantially higher level of resources currently available for such research in the United States. Phillipe Lazar, director-general of the National Institute of Health and Medical Research (INSERM), admitted last week that the "academicism" which tends to dominate the French approach to the support of research sometimes made it difficult to respond with "the intensity and the rapidity" that a particular problem—such as quickly determining the characteristics of a virus potentially associated with AIDS—might require.

11. Congress, NIH Open Coffers for AIDS

Gina Kolata

Fears about the spread of acquired immune deficiency syndrome, AIDS, an enigmatic disease that primarily afflicts homosexual men, have opened up a substantial source of new funds for biomedical research. Although there have been many complaints that the disease has been relatively neglected, this year alone the federal government will spend more on AIDS research than was spent over an 8-year period on Legionnaire's disease and toxic shock combined.

The chief source of this unprecedented spending spree is the Department of Health and Human Services, which is already devoting $14.5 million to AIDS research this year. Congress may add another $12 million in the 1983 supplemental appropriations bill still in conference. In addition, the department is supporting many scientists studying subjects directly related to AIDS, although they are not officially counted among the recipients of AIDS research grants. Several nongovernmental organizations have also begun to put money into the field.

The federal government is pouring money into AIDS research partly as a response to political pressures generated by fears that the disease may turn into a major epidemic. Furthermore, the homosexual community has become an important voting block in certain areas of the country and politicians have called for increased funds. The fears are heightened by the fact that although the chief route of transmission seems to be through sexual contact, it is not yet known how AIDS spreads. So far, the disease has afflicted some 1600 people and about 165 new cases are added in the United States each month. In addition, about 125 cases have so far been reported in other countries. The incubation period is estimated to be from 6 months to 3 years.

It is, however, extremely difficult to predict how many new cases of AIDS there are likely to be because conditions favoring the spread of AIDS are rapidly changing. For example, bathhouses frequented by homosexual men have reported a dramatic decline in business, as male homosexuals forgo the sexual promiscuity that used to be an integral part of life for many of them. In New York, epidemiologists had predicted that the number of new cases of AIDS would double over the past 6 months, but the rate of spread has held constant at two new cases per day. New York City health commissioner David Sencer attributes the slowdown of the AIDS epidemic in the city to changing practices among homosexuals.

But AIDS is not attracting a surge of research dollars just because it is a deadly disease. It is also scientifically exciting. Richard Krause, an infectious disease expert who is director of the National Institute of Allergy and Infectious Diseases, explains, "People have been interested in AIDS from the very beginning [about 2 years ago]. They are interested because it is clearly a severe abnormality of the immune system. We all expect that once we unravel the abnormality, we will learn a great deal about how the immune system works and we will learn how to correct the immunological deficiencies in these patients and in patients with immunological deficiencies that are unrelated to AIDS." AIDS, in fact, is so enormously intriguing to all sorts of scientists, from immunologists, to cancer researchers, to infectious disease experts, that despite all the research money available, there is simply not enough to finance everyone who wants to get into the field.

Since last October, the NIH has funded two batches of AIDS research applications and a third group of applications will be considered in August. Anne Thomas of the NIH notes that the institute routinely reviews applications by convening a committee of scientists to rate the various proposals. However, in the case of the AIDS proposals, she says, "We did try to cut down on the time of review by doing mail balloting. This is very unusual for us."

Not only were the NIH grants reviewed expeditiously but they frequently were for larger amounts than usual. The average NIH grant is for $120,000 per year. In contrast, R. Gordon Douglas of Cornell Medical Center received $243,271 for the first year of his 3-year grant to study the immunology and virology of AIDS patients. John Fahey of the University of California at Los Angeles was awarded $273,954 for the first year of a 3-year study of the use of chemotherapy and substances such as interferon to prevent and treat AIDS. Frederick Siegal of Mount Sinai Hospital in New York got $289,011 for the first year of his 3-year grant to study early defects in the immune systems of AIDS patients. Paul Volberding of the University of California at San Francisco was awarded $526,229 for the first year of his 5-year study of the immune systems of AIDS patients and apparently healthy persons at risk for AIDS. Arye Rubenstein of Yeshiva University received $506,685 for the first year of a 3-year study of infants born to mothers who were the sexual partners of AIDS patients. "I don't think people really are aware of the major awards that we've made," Thomas says.

In addition to these proposals, the NIH funds other research that is related to AIDS but comes through normal channels. This includes work on the human T cell leukemia virus, on infectious diseases that afflict AIDS patients, on immunodeficiencies, and on Kaposi's sarcoma. Then there are the scientists employed by NIH who are funded through the NIH intramural program. Many of these investigators have turned over their laboratories to AIDS research.

To further speed up the pace of AIDS research, NIH is starting a newsletter which will be disseminated to about 200 scientists starting in late July. The purpose of the newsletter is to keep the investigators informed of each others' results, especially negative ones. This way, they will be able to avoid fruitless approaches and experiments that do not work.

Not everyone, however, is happy with the level or style of NIH funding. Alvin Friedman-Kien of New York University, who is one of the discoverers of AIDS, believes NIH has moved too slowly in funding AIDS research. To get research funds, Friedman-Kien accepted the offer of a friend of an AIDS patient to organize an auction. It was held on 12 April at the Leo Castelli Gallery in Soho where the 400 people who attended each paid $50 admission. A total of $55,000 was raised.

David Purtilo of the University of Nebraska had a grant application turned down because it was not given a high enough rating to be funded. But he continues to do AIDS research. "We're basically borrowing money," he says. "A lot has been from my own pockets. I'm a pathologist so I make a fairly good salary. I've also dipped into department funds."

Concern about AIDS has generated other funding sources as well, including an AIDS Medical Foundation, chaired by Mathilde Krim of Sloan-Kettering Institute for Cancer Research. Krim was an early advocate of increased funding for interferon research. "We decided to put this foundation together because we feel a desperate need for money. Instead of a fluke, AIDS is a real medical problem and there has been no money," she contends. Asked about the recent NIH request for research proposals, Krim claimed that from the time a scientist writes a proposal until the time he gets funds "takes easily 18 months. We feel we can't wait. We have dying patients on our hands."

The AIDS Medical Foundation has put together a list of prospective individual donors and is soliciting $1000 from each. The foundation also hopes to get $500,000 from corporations and foundations. Frank Hoffey, vice chairman of the foundation, says, "The early donations are encouraging. The promises are even more encouraging—this includes the whole spectrum from private citizens to corporate donors."

Still another new source of funds is the Cancer Research Institute in New York, a nonprofit organization, established 30 years ago, that describes itself as "devoting all its resources to the immunological approach to cancer." The institute has put out a call for grant applications and plans to award a total of $350,000 in maximum grants of $70,000 each.

Homosexual organizations also have dipped into their pockets to fund AIDS research. For example, the AIDS/Kaposi's Sarcoma Research and Education Foundation, which is a San Francisco organization that has only been in existence for 1 year, has begun supporting research. "We've raised most of our money from the gay community," says Edward Power of the foundation. "But there are many, many more people applying for research money than we have money to give."

Report

2 September 1983

12. Cell-to-Cell Transfer of Interferon-Induced Antiproliferative Activity

Richard E. Lloyd, J. Edwin Blalock, and G. John Stanton

Interferons (IFN's) can induce a wide range of activities in cells and the mechanism for these responses is generally attributed to the direct interaction of IFN with membrane receptors on each target cell (*1*). Recently, IFN was shown to have an amplification system in which IFN-treated cells indirectly induce antiviral activity (*2–6*) in other cells. It was hypothesized that a secondary messenger molecule is transferred from the IFN-induced cell to the recipient cells which then express the antiviral activity of IFN (*7*). Here we show that the antiproliferative activity of IFN can also be transferred between cells.

For these experiments we used two cell systems in which the effect of IFN was transferred across the species preference barrier of IFN (to xenogeneic cells) and the recipient cells could be separated from the donor cells prior to the assay of antiproliferative activity. Figure 1A shows that cocultivation of mouse L1210 lymphoblastoid cells with human IFN-treated WISH cells resulted in the transfer of significant antiproliferative activity to the L1210 cells, as measured by reduced incorporation of [^{3}H]thymidine into cellular DNA. Both recombinant IFN-γ (*8, 9*) and partially purified IFN-α were able to induce an effective dose response. Likewise, mouse IFN-treated L cells transferred antiproliferative activity to human lymphoblastoid Daudi cells (Fig. 1B). In all cases, the amount of antiproliferative activity transferred followed asymptotic dose-response curves of similar magnitude. The reduction in growth rate was not due to the direct effect of IFN since donor cells were thoroughly washed before coculturing with recipient cells. Assay of supernatant fluids at the end of the 4-hour coculture period failed to detect carry-over of IFN unless more than 1000 IU had been used to induce the cells, in which case only 1 to 3 U/ml were detected. Also, the phylogenetic barrier of IFN was shown to be effective because direct treatment of L1210 cells with 100 IU of human IFNα or Daudi cells with 100 U of mouse IFN-α and -β resulted in no decrease in [^{3}H]thymidine incorporation (Fig. 1). In our system the incorporation of [^{3}H]thymidine into DNA was shown to be an accurate measure of cell growth, both in lymphoblastoid cells that were cocultured with IFN-treated cells or lymphoblastoid cells cultivated alone in dilutions of IFN (*10*). An assay of specific chromium release (*11*) suggested that nonspecific cellular cytotoxicity was not responsible for the observed reduction in cellular growth rate (*12*).

We also tested the ability of other human IFN's to induce antiproliferative transfer. When human IFN-β (specific activity 10^6 U per milligram of protein) or IFN-γ (specific activity 10^5 U/mg)

62

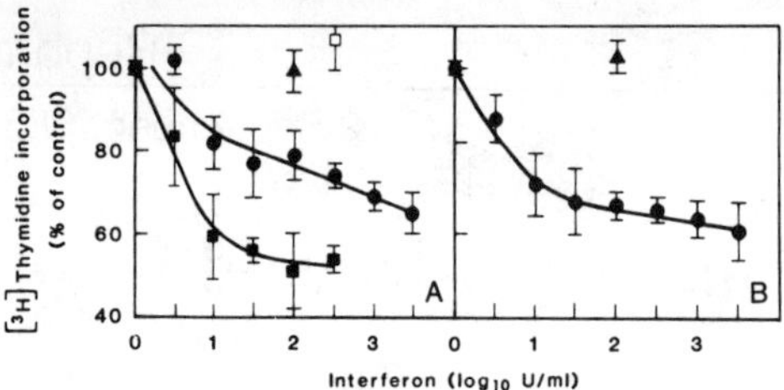

Fig. 1. Transfer of IFN-induced antiproliferative activity to lymphoblastoid cells. (A) Human amnion WISH cells (6×10^4 per well)
were plated into Costar 96-well microculture
plates in 0.1 ml (per well) of Eagle's minimum
essential medium (EMEM) supplemented
with 10 percent fetal calf serum (FCS), penicillin (100 U/ml), and streptomycin (100 µg/
ml). After overnight incubation, the cells were
treated for 4 hours with dilutions of human
IFN-α (specific activity 10^6 U per milligram of
protein) (●), recombinant human IFN-γ (specific activity 1.7×10^4 U per milligram of
protein) (■), or control supernatants for the
recombinant IFN (□), then were washed
three times with EMEM with 2 percent FCS.
L1210 cells in conditioned growth medium
(RPMI 1640 with 5 percent FCS and antibiotics) were added to each well (2×10^5 per
well) and the cells were cocultured for 4 hours
at 37°C in an atmosphere of 5 percent CO_2 (●,
■, □) or cultured alone with human IFN-α
(▲). The plastic nonadherent L1210 cells were
loosened from WISH cell monolayers by gentle agitation of the supernatant with a Titertek
multichannel micropipette and the suspended
cells were transferred to a new microculture
plate. The L1210 cells were exposed for 1
hour to 2µCi of [^{3}H]thymidine (Amersham)
before DNA was precipitated with acid and
collected on 25-µm glass-fiber filters (Gelman) for scintillation counting. Human IFN
was titrated on WISH cells (20) and mouse
IFN was titrated on L cells with a slightly
modified plaque reduction assay (21). (B) The
incorporation of [^{3}H]thymidine by human
Burkitt lymphoma Daudi cells (American
Type Culture Collection) after coculture with
L cells treated with virus-induced (22) mouse
IFN-α and -β. Procedures were as described
above, except Daudi cell growth medium was
RPMI 1640 with 12 percent FCS, and control
Daudi cells were cultured with mouse IFN-α
and -β (▲). The data represent the mean and
standard error of the mean for five experi-
ments (two experiments with recombinant
IFN), each performed in triplicate.

were used to induce the transfer of antiproliferative activity to L1210 cells, the
dose-response curves were similar in
shape and magnitude to those in Fig. 1
(data not shown).

Figure 2, A and B, shows the results of
two typical experiments in which antiviral activity was transferred to L1210 or
Daudi cells concurrently with antiproliferative activity. In both cell systems,
transfer of antiproliferative and antiviral
activity correlated well with the IFN
dose, and the results of many experiments showed that high antiproliferative
activity was transferred together with
high antiviral activity. This suggests that
these distinct biological activities may be
induced by a similar mechanism.

Figure 2C shows that antiproliferative
activity was rapidly transferred to Daudi
cells, that is, within 30 minutes of the
initiation of coculturing with donor cells.

By 2 hours the maximum activity had
been transferred and the activity was
stable through at least 14 hours of coculture conditions. These data agree with
previous reports concerning the time in
coculture necessary to transfer antiviral
activity between cells (7).

We have previously shown that the
transfer of antiviral activity is not mediated by soluble factors released by cells
and is dependent on cell contact (13). To
investigate whether soluble mediators induce antiproliferative activity, we treated WISH or L cells with IFN and
washed them as described in Fig. 1.
They were then incubated for 12 hours.
Then L1210 or Daudi cells, respectively,
were incubated for 6 hours in the supernatants from the WISH or L cells and
found to incorporate the same levels of
[^{3}H]thymidine as the controls. Interferon
was not detectable in the supernatants

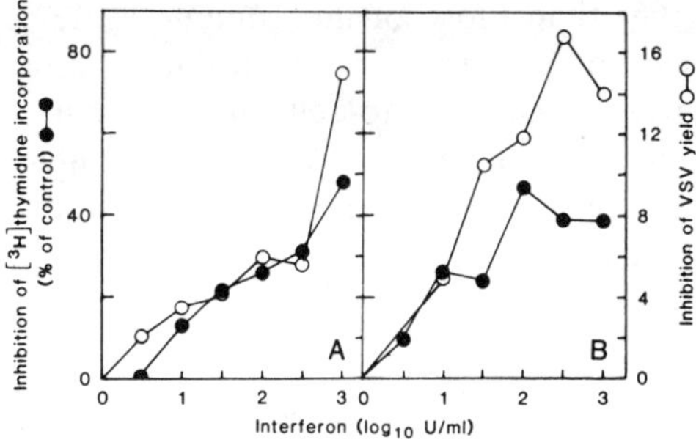

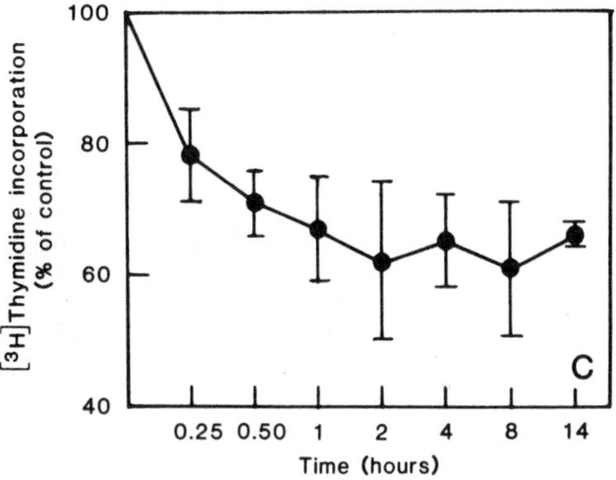

Fig. 2. Concurrent transfer of antiproliferative and antiviral activity and kinetics of transfer.

(A) Human IFN-α treated WISH cell monolayers were cocultured with L1210 cells for 4 hours and then antiproliferative activity was assessed in the L1210 cells as described in Fig. 1. After the L1210 cells were removed from coculture, antiviral activity was measured by challenging the L1210 cells with vesicular stomatitis virus (*VSV*) at a multiplicity of infection of 0.05. Virus yields were determined 18 hours later by a microplaque assay (*21*). (B) Mouse L cells treated with IFN-α and -β were cocultured with Daudi cells for 4 hours and then antiproliferative activity was assessed in the Daudi cells as described in Fig. 1. Antiviral activity was measured by challenging the Daudi cells with VSV as described above. (C) Kinetics of the transfer of antiproliferative activity from L cells to Daudi cells. L cells (1.5 × 10^6 per well) in 24-well Falcon dishes were treated overnight with 300 U of mouse IFN-α and -β, then washed three times and overlaid with a 1-ml suspension of Daudi cells (1.5 × 10^6 per milliliter) at time point 0. At the indicated times points, the Daudi cells were removed from the L cells and exposed to [^{3}H]thymidine as described in Fig. 1B. The data represent the mean and standard error of the mean of three experiments compared to control cocultured cells.

(data not shown). Thus, the transfer of antiproliferative activity is probably not mediated by the release of soluble factors but does appear to depend on some type of attachment or intimate contact between inducer and receptor cells, since the transfer of antiproliferative activity was prevented by gently rocking cocultures of IFN-treated L cells and Daudi cells.

The data suggest that the transfer of antiproliferative activity is specifically induced by treatment of homologous cells with IFN. Not only did recombinant IFN-γ effectively induce the transfer of antiproliferative activity in a dose-dependent manner (Fig. 1A), whereas control supernatants did not, but the other types of IFN tested thus far also induced antiproliferative transfer. Each

of these IFN's was prepared from different cell types, and four were highly purified (specific activity 10^5 to 10^6 U per milligram of protein). Another experiment showed that the transfer of antiproliferative activity from L cells to Daudi cells was abolished by prior treatment of the mouse IFN-γ with antiserum to IFN-γ (*14*) (data not shown).

We have also found that several other types of cells, including human leukocytes, are capable of participating in the transfer of antiproliferative activity. The levels of antiproliferative activity transferred are comparable to the direct effect of IFN on L1210 or Daudi cells both in our experiments (data not shown) and those of others (*15, 16*). The transfer of antiproliferative and antiviral activity appears to occur by the same or a similar mechanism. Although IFN is specifically required to induce the transfer of antiproliferative or antiviral activity, IFN is apparently not the direct effector molecule responsible for inhibiting proliferation in the recipient cells. The evidence is as follows: (i) antiproliferative activity can be effectively transferred between xenogeneic cells that do not respond to heterologous IFN, (ii) transfer will occur if IFN is removed before the cells are cocultured, and (iii) supernatants from IFN-induced cells do not induce antiproliferative activity in recipient cells. Thus the transfer appears to be mediated by a contact-dependent mechanism and the results support the hypothesis that antiviral activity is transferred by means of a secondary messenger, possibly through low-resistance membrane channels such as gap junctions (7).

Our results suggest a novel mechanism by which IFN may indirectly regulate cell growth. These cellular interactions could be an important host defense mechanism against neoplasias in tissues, especially where IFN diffusion is poor. Gresser *et al.* reported that a strain of L1210 cells cloned for IFN resistance was still responsive to IFN antitumor therapy in mice (*17*) and attributed these results to the effect of IFN on the host's immune response. The present findings, together with data indicating the probable transfer of antiviral activity in vivo (*18*), suggest that the antitumor effects on IFN-resistant cells may have been due, in part, to the transfer of antiproliferative activity from responding normal mouse cells. Similarly, the human IFN–induced inhibition of human tumor cells in nude mice, which was attributed to a direct effect of IFN only on the human tumor cells, could also have been due to the transfer of activity from mouse effector leukocytes (*19*). Such a defense mechanism suggests that cells

other than those of the immune system may play a role in controlling tumor growth where cell-to-cell contact occurs. This mechanism also provides a new system in which basic cell-to-cell communication may be investigated.

References and Notes

1. R. M. Friedman, *Science* **156**, 1760 (1967).
2. J. E. Blalock and S. Baron, *Nature (London)* **269**, 422 (1977).
3. J. E. Blalock and G. J. Stanton, *J. Gen. Virol.* **41**, 325 (1978).
4. J. E. Blalock, J. Georgiades, H. M. Johnson, *J. Immunol.* **122**, 1018 (1979).
5. T. K. Hughes, J. E. Blalock, S. Baron, *Arch. Virol.* **58**, 77 (1977).
6. J. E. Blalock, D. A. Weigent, M. P. Langford, G. J. Stanton, *Infect. Immun.* **29**, 356 (1980).
7. J. E. Blalock and S. Baron, *J. Gen. Virol.* **42**, 363 (1979).
8. Recombinant human IFN-γ was kindly supplied by W. Fiers, Laboratorium voor Moleculair Biologie, Gent, Belgium.
9. R. Devos, H. Cheroutre, Y. Taya, W. Degrave, H. V. Heuverswyn, W. Fiers, *Nucleic Acids Res.* **10**, 2487 (1982).
10. Intracellular thymidine from L1210 cells was measured by high-performance liquid chromatography (HPLC) on an ion-pair reversed-phase column (Serva Feinbiochemica). We used the protocol described for Fig. 1A, except the cell numbers were scaled up 15 times to be performed in 35-mm petri dishes (LUX). The WISH cells treated with 100 U of IFN-α transferred antiproliferative activity effectively and reduced [³H]thymidine incorporation into the DNA of the L1210 cells by 37 percent. However, HPLC analysis revealed no significant changes in the amount of intracellular thymidine from L1210 cells whether they had been cocultured with IFN-treated WISH cells, directly treated with human IFNα, or left untreated. The direct effects of IFN on cellular [³H]thymidine incorporation and cell growth also were compared. L1210 cells or Daudi cells in the log phase of growth were treated directly with dilutions of homologous mouse or human IFN for 48 hours and then cell counts and [³H]thymidine incorporation were determined. When number of cells and the incorporated radioactivity were plotted logarithmically against the units of IFN, parallel curves were obtained which suggested an accurate correlation between [³H]thymidine incorporation and cell growth..
11. D. A. Weigent, M. P. Langford, E. M. Smith, J. E. Blalock, G. J. Stanton, *Infect. Immun.* **32**, 508 (1981).
12. The specific chromium release assays showed that IFN-treated (1000 IU) WISH or L cells are not cytotoxic toward L1210 cells (3.7 percent specific ⁵¹CR release) or Daudi cells (3.3 percent specific ⁵¹CR release) even after 22 hours of cocultivation. Furthermore, routine microscopic examination of L1210 or Daudi cells after coculture with IFN-treated cells did not reveal significant cytotoxicity as determined by trypan blue dye uptake.
13. J. E. Blalock, *Infect. Immun.* **23**, 496 (1979).

14. L. C. Osbourne, J. A. Georgiades, H. M. Johnson, *Cell. Immunol.* **53**, 65 (1980).
15. M. Tovey, D. Brouty-Boyé, I. Gresser, *Proc. Natl. Acad. Sci. U.S.A.* **72**, 2265 (1975).
16. A. A. Creasey, J. C. Bartholomew, T. Merigan, *ibid.* 1471 (1980).
17. I. Gresser, C. Maury, D. Brouty-Boyé, *Nature (London)* **239**, 167 (1972).
18. S. Kohl, L. S. Loo, S. B. Greenberg, *J. Immunol.* **128**, 1107 (1982).
19. F. R. Balkwill, E. M. Moodie, V. Freedman, K. H. Fantes, *Int. J. Cancer* **30**, 231 (1982).
20. J. G. Tilles and M. Finland, *Appl. Microbiol.* **16**, 1706 (1968).
21. J. B. Campbell, T. Grunberger, M. A. Kochman, S. L. White, *Can. J. Microbiol.* **21**, 1247 (1975).
22. W. R. Fleischmann and E. H. Simon, *J. Gen. Virol.* **20**, 127 (1973).
23. Supported by the James W. McLaughlin Fellowship Fund and NIH grants EY 03348 and AM 30046.

25 February 1983

Report

9 September 1983

13. Antibodies to Human T-Cell Leukemia Virus Membrane Antigens (HTLV-MA) in Hemophiliacs

M. Essex, M.F. McLane, T.H. Lee, N. Tachibana, J.I. Mullins, J. Kreiss, C.K. Kasper, M.-C. Poon, A. Landay, S.F. Stein, D.P. Francis, C. Cabradilla, D.N. Lawrence, and B.L. Evatt

Hemophiliac patients, most of whom receive infusions of blood clotting preparations, become exposed to products from thousands of blood donors. Such hemophiliacs may also have abnormal T-lymphocyte profiles (*1*). Along with homosexual men with multiple partners, Haitians, and intravenous drug abusers, hemophiliacs represent one of the major risk groups for developing the acquired immunodeficiency syndrome (AIDS) (*2*).

Most researchers suspect that AIDS may be caused, at least in part, by an infectious agent (*3*). Such an agent would presumably be transmitted only with great difficulty, and in the case of intravenous drug abusers and hemophiliacs it could perhaps be transmitted by blood or blood products. Among the many candidate etiologic agents that have received

research attention is the human T-cell leukemia virus (HTLV) (*4*). We recently reported that AIDS patients have substantially increased rates of exposure to HTLV; this conclusion was based on our finding, by means of indirect membrane immunofluorescence (IMI) and radioimmunoprecipitation (RIP), an antibody to HTLV-infected cells in the blood of AIDS patients (*5*). Independently, Gallo and co-workers reported that HTLV had been isolated from one AIDS patient and proviral sequences had been found in two (*6*).

Using the same procedures that we described earlier (*5*), we examined serum samples from 172 hemophiliacs that were asymptomatic, two hemophiliacs with AIDS, and one with severe lymphadenopathy. Of the 172 asymptomatic hemophiliacs, 45 were from Atlanta, Georgia; 41 were from Birmingham, Alabama; 39 were from Los Angeles, California; and 47 were from New York City (see Table 1). Only one sample was examined from each individual. Except in the case of the New York hemophiliacs and the control blood donors, all the serum samples were collected in late 1982 or early 1983. Thirty-nine of the samples from New York hemophiliacs were collected in 1978 and 1979; the remaining eight samples were collected in 1976, 1977, or 1981. Also examined were serum samples from 47 healthy workers at the hospitals or laboratories where HTLV-producer cell cultures or tissue samples from patients were handled (the Harvard School of Public Health Laboratory, the Centers for Disease Control, the University of Buffalo, and the University of Alabama Medical Center). These last samples were collected in 1982 or 1983.

All samples were initially checked at a 1:4 serum dilution in a double-blind, coded way with the use of two standard reference HTLV-producer cell lines, Hut 102 and MT 2. The procedure used has been described (5, 7). All samples that reacted with Hut 102 or MT 2, or both, by IMI were subsequently screened on HTLV-negative T- and B-cell lines to confirm specificity, and those that specifically reacted with 40 percent or more of the Hut 102 or MT 2 cells were considered positive.

Overall, about 12 percent of the samples from asymptomatic hemophiliacs gave a positive reaction with at least 40 percent of the Hut 102 or MT 2 cells, and 8.7 percent reacted with at least 50 percent of the cells in one or both of the positive reference lines (Table 1). Samples from the Birmingham hemophiliacs showed the lowest proportion of positive reactions (4.9 percent); samples from the New York hemophiliacs showed the highest proportion of positive reactions (19 percent). Only two samples were available from hemophiliacs with AIDS, and one was positive for HTLV-MA antibody by IMI. Another sample from a 14-year-old hemophiliac with severe lymphadenopathy was also positive.

All ten of the samples from hemophiliacs in Atlanta and Los Angeles that gave a positive reaction by IMI, and six of the nine samples from New York hemophiliacs that gave a positive reaction, were available for testing by RIP of [^{35}S]methionine-labeled Hut 102 cells or [^{35}S]cysteine-labeled cells (Fig. 1). This procedure was also described previously (5). Eleven of the 16 showed either clear immunoprecipitation or weak precipitation of proteins that migrate in the same position as those regularly detected with reference sera to HTLV-related proteins. In particular, those antigens detected included glycoprotein 61 (gp61), which is the protein detected most frequently by human antibodies from HTLV-infected T-cell leukemia patients of Japanese origin or from AIDS patients (5, 8). Whether the gp61 is virus-encoded or an HTLV-activated cellular protein has not been resolved. It appears, however, to be distinct from the T-cell growth factor–receptor protein which migrates to a different position as detected by a reference monoclonal antibody (provided by T. Waldmann, National Cancer Institute).

Figure 1 illustrates the presence of antibodies to gp61 in representative hemophiliacs from Atlanta (lane f) and New York (lane g). The same reaction was seen with serum from a representative healthy Japanese individual

Table 1. Presence of antibodies to HTLV-MA in hemophiliacs and related controls. Each sample was tested at a 1:4 dilution on the reference cells (Hut 102 and MT 2) taken during the peak phase of logarithmic growth. The procedure followed was exactly as described earlier (5). Each test included positive and negative reference sera, and all samples were tested in a double-blind manner.

Category	Tested	> 50 percent cells positive using			> 40 percent cells positive using		
		Hut 102	MT 2	Either Hut 102 or MT 2	Hut 102	MT 2	Either Hut 102 or MT 2
Asymptomatic hemophiliacs							
Atlanta, Georgia	45	2 (4.4)*	3 (6.7)	3 (6.7)	3 (6.7)	4 (8.9)	5 (11)
Birmingham, Alabama	41	2 (4.9)	0	2 (4.9)	2 (4.9)	0	2 (4.9)
Los Angeles, California	39	1 (2.6)	2 (5.1)	3 (7.7)	4 (10)	5 (13)	5 (13)
New York, New York	47	5 (11)	7 (15)	7 (15)	5 (11)	9 (19)	9 (19)
Total	172	10 (5.8)	12 (7.0)	15 (8.7)	14 (8.1)	18 (10)	21 (12)
Healthy lab or hospital workers	47	0	0	0	0	0	0
Adult blood donors†	137	1 (0.7)	1 (0.7)	1 (0.7)	1 (0.7)	1 (0.7)	1 (0.7)
Chronic active hepatitis†	29	0	0	0	0	0	0
Hemodialysis†	21	0	0	0	0	0	0
Hemophiliacs with AIDS or severe lymphadenopathy‡	3	2 (67)	2 (67)	2 (67)	2 (67)	2 (67)	2 (67)

*Number and percentage positive shown in parentheses.   †From (5).   ‡Two had confirmed AIDS and one had lymphadenopathy.

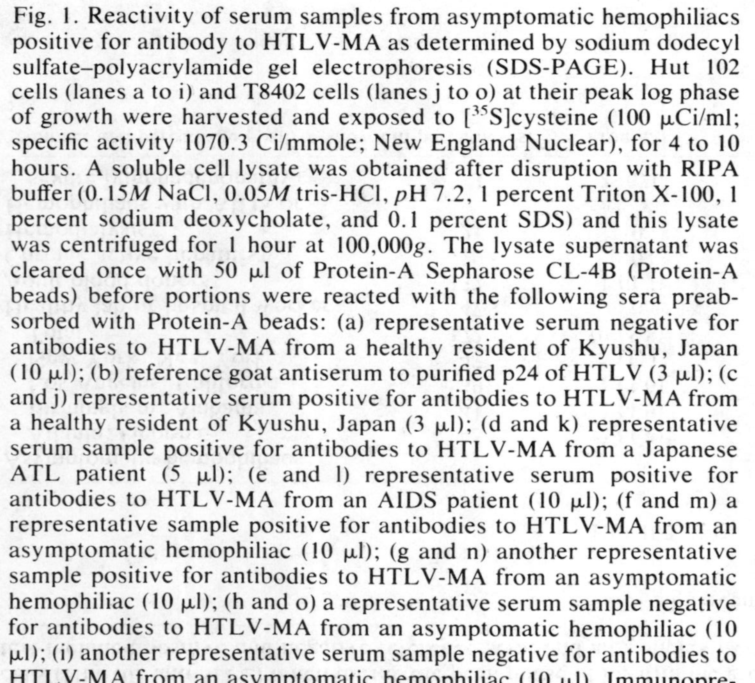

Fig. 1. Reactivity of serum samples from asymptomatic hemophiliacs positive for antibody to HTLV-MA as determined by sodium dodecyl sulfate–polyacrylamide gel electrophoresis (SDS-PAGE). Hut 102 cells (lanes a to i) and T8402 cells (lanes j to o) at their peak log phase of growth were harvested and exposed to [^{35}S]cysteine (100 μCi/ml; specific activity 1070.3 Ci/mmole; New England Nuclear), for 4 to 10 hours. A soluble cell lysate was obtained after disruption with RIPA buffer (0.15M NaCl, 0.05M tris-HCl, pH 7.2, 1 percent Triton X-100, 1 percent sodium deoxycholate, and 0.1 percent SDS) and this lysate was centrifuged for 1 hour at 100,000g. The lysate supernatant was cleared once with 50 μl of Protein-A Sepharose CL-4B (Protein-A beads) before portions were reacted with the following sera preabsorbed with Protein-A beads: (a) representative serum negative for antibodies to HTLV-MA from a healthy resident of Kyushu, Japan (10 μl); (b) reference goat antiserum to purified p24 of HTLV (3 μl); (c and j) representative serum positive for antibodies to HTLV-MA from a healthy resident of Kyushu, Japan (3 μl); (d and k) representative serum sample positive for antibodies to HTLV-MA from a Japanese ATL patient (5 μl); (e and l) representative serum positive for antibodies to HTLV-MA from an AIDS patient (10 μl); (f and m) a representative sample positive for antibodies to HTLV-MA from an asymptomatic hemophiliac (10 μl); (g and n) another representative sample positive for antibodies to HTLV-MA from an asymptomatic hemophiliac (10 μl); (h and o) a representative serum sample negative for antibodies to HTLV-MA from an asymptomatic hemophiliac (10 μl); (i) another representative serum sample negative for antibodies to HTLV-MA from an asymptomatic hemophiliac (10 μl). Immunoprecipitates were eluted in a sample buffer containing 0.1M Cleland's reagent, 2 percent SDS, 0.08M tris-HCl, pH 6.8, 10 percent glycerol, and 0.2 percent bromophenol blue by boiling at 100°C for 2 minutes. Samples were analyzed in a 12.5 percent acrylamide resolving gel with 3.5 percent stacking gel according to the discontinuous buffer system of Laemmli (11). The molecular weight markers, purchased from New England Nuclear, were ^{14}C-labeled phosphorylase b (92,500), bovine serum albumin (68,000), ovalbumin (46,000), carbonic anhydrase (30,000), and cytochrome c (12,000). Arrow indicates the 61,000-dalton glycoprotein.

from the HTLV-endemic region (lane c), serum from a representative Japanese patient with the HTLV-related adult T-cell leukemia (ATL) (lane d) (8), and with serum from a representative AIDS patient (lane e). All of the latter individuals also reacted in a positive manner by IMI. No precipitation of the gp61 was observed with sera from two hemophiliacs that reacted negatively by IMI (lanes h and i). Similarly, no reaction occurred with a serum from an IMI-negative healthy Japanese individual from the HTLV-endemic area (lane a). Neither the IMI-positive sera from hemophiliacs nor the IMI-positive sera from the Japanese individuals reacted with comparable proteins on T8402, an HTLV-uninfected human T-cell line (lanes j to o).

To demonstrate that the reactivity seen by RIP with the gp61 band was common to both the Japanese IMI-positive sera and the IMI-positive hemophiliac sera, we conducted adsorption studies (Fig. 2). The prior incubation of [^{35}S]methionine-labeled Hut 102 lysate with IMI-positive sera from either a Japanese ATL patient (lane d) or a healthy Japanese individual from the endemic area (lanes c and g) resulted in the loss of reactivity when the same lysate was subsequently exposed to IMI-positive hemophiliac sera. This reaction could not be blocked by incubating with IMI-negative sera from Japanese individuals (lane b); thus, the pattern of reactivity with sera from hemophiliacs was similar to that seen with IMI-positive sera from Japanese individuals or AIDS patients.

Although increased rates of exposure to HTLV are known to occur among Caribbean islanders and southern Japanese, hemophiliacs represent the first group in the continental U.S. population other than AIDS cases (5), homosexual males with lymphadenopathy (5), or selected groups of leukemia patients (7) that has elevated rates of exposure to HTLV. We did not detect any individuals that were HTLV-MA antibody–positive among 47 laboratory or hospital workers, 29 patients with chronic active hepatitis, or 21 patients on hemodialysis (Table 1). Among 137 healthy blood donors from Philadelphia in 1977, only one was positive. By the same procedure, Gallo *et al.* found only 4 of 538 normal U.S. blood donors to be positive (7).

Hemophiliacs represent one of the major risk groups for development of AIDS (2, 3, 10). They may receive blood elements from tens of thousands of donors in a relatively brief period of time and they frequently receive both blood and blood products (10). The likelihood that blood from healthy HTLV-carrier individuals may be present in the donor pool thus seems high. Although the current results are compatible with our earlier observations that AIDS patients have rates of exposure to HTLV above those seen in matched controls (5), they do not necessarily add evidence to a hypothesis that would etiologically associate HTLV and AIDS. For example, hemophiliacs may have abnormalities of the immune system prior to exposure to HTLV (1). The infusion of HTLV-carrier blood or blood products into a preconditioned host might then enhance the possibility of infection.

As a group, hemophiliacs probably have more frequent contact with major medical centers than the other subpopulations at risk for developing AIDS. Because of this, they may provide one of the most appropriate populations for prospective studies to determine if HTLV-exposed people have a relative increase in risk for disease development.

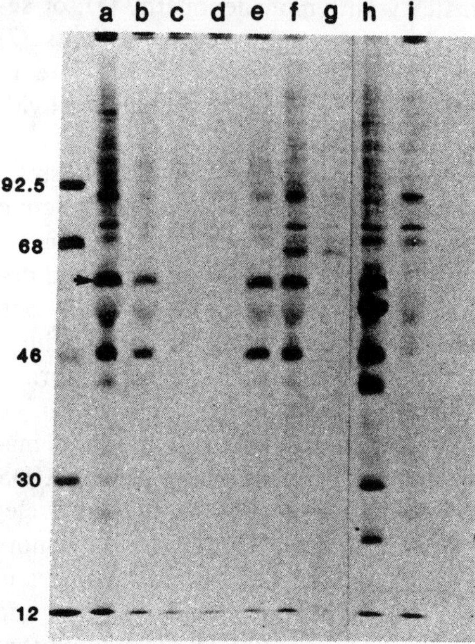

Fig. 2. Blocking of antibody reactivity to HTLV-related antigens present in serum samples of two representative asymptomatic hemophiliacs. Equal portions of cell lysate from Hut 102 cells, prepared by the same procedures as described in Fig. 1, except substituting the [^{35}S]cysteine with [^{35}S]methionine,

were first reacted with 10 µl of the following sera preabsorbed to Protein-A beads: (b) reference human serum negative for antibodies to HTLV-MA [same as sample (a) in Fig. 1]; (c) and (g) reference human serum positive for antibodies to HTLV-MA [same as sample (c) in Fig. 1]; (d) reference Japanese ATL serum sample [same as sample (d) in Fig. 1]; (e) reference goat antiserum to p24 [same as sample (b) in Fig. 1]; (a) and (f) phosphate-buffered saline only. After incubation for 90 minutes at 4°C, preabsorbed cell lysate was withdrawn from each tube and centrifuged at 100,000g for 15 minutes. The lysate supernatant was then reacted with 10 µl of the following sera preabsorbed to Protein-A beads: (a to e) a representative serum sample positive for antibodies to HTLV-MA from a hemophiliac [same as sample (f) in Fig. 1] and (f) and (g) another representative serum sample positive for antibodies to HTLV-MA from a hemophiliac [same as sample (g) in Fig. 1]. Lane (h) shows the reactivity of a reference human serum [same as sample (c) in Fig. 1] positive for antibodies to HTLV-MA which was used to preabsorb with cell lysate. Lane (i) shows the reactivity of a representative serum negative for antibodies to HTLV-MA from a hemophiliac [same as sample (h) in Fig. 1]. Immunoprecipitates were analyzed in the same way as described in Fig. 1. The arrow indicates the 61,000-dalton glycoprotein.

References and Notes

1. M. M. Lederman, O. D. Ratnoff, J. J. Scillian, P. K. Jones, B. Schacter, *N. Engl. J. Med.* **308**, 79 (1983); J. E. Menitove, R. H. Aster, J. I. Caspar, *ibid.*, p. 83; A. Landay, M.-C. Poon, T. Abo, S. Stagno, A. Lurie, M. D. Cooper, *J. Clin. Invest.* **71**, 1500 (1983).
2. K. C. Davis, C. R. Horsburgh, Jr., U. Hasiba, A. L. Schocket, C. H. Kirkpatrick, *Ann. Intern. Med.* **98**, 284 (1983); M.-C. Poon, A. Landay, E. F. Prasthofer, S. Stagno, *ibid.*, p. 287; J. L. Elliott, W. L. Hoppes, M. S. Platt, J. G. Thomas, J. P. Patel, A. Ganser, *ibid.*, p. 290.
3. D. P. Francis, J. W. Curran, M. Essex, *J. Natl. Cancer Inst.* **71**, 1 (1983).
4. B. J. Poiesz *et al.*, *Proc. Natl. Acad. Sci. U.S.A.* **77**, 7415 (1980).
5. M. Essex *et al.*, *Science* **220**, 859 (1983).
6. R. C. Gallo *et al.*, *ibid.*, p. 865; E. P. Gelmann *et al.*, *ibid.*, p. 862.
7. R. C. Gallo *et al.*, *Cancer Res.* **43**, 3892 (1983); M. G. Robert-Guroff *et al.*, *Science* **215**, 975 (1982).
8. T. H. Lee, C. Howe, M. F. McLane, N. Tachibana, M. Essex, *Leuk. Rev.* **1**, 294 (1983); N. Tachibana *et al.*, in preparation.
9. T. Uchiyama, J. Yodoi, K. Sagawa, K. Takatsuki, H. Uchino, *Blood* **50**, 481 (1977).
10. J. W. Curran, B. L. Evatt, D. N. Lawrence, *Ann. Intern. Med.* **98**, 401 (1983); G. C. White III and H. R. Lesesne, *ibid.*, p. 403.
11. U. K. Laemmli, *Nature (London)* **227**, 680 (1970).
12. Supported in part by grants RD-173 from the American Cancer Society and CA 18216 from the National Institutes of Health. T.H.L. is supported by Institutional Research Service Award 2-T32-CA09031. M.-C. Poon is now located at Foothill Hospital, Calgary, Alberta, Canada. We thank R. Gallo for the reference goat antiserum to HTLV p24.

15 August 1983

14.   Apes and AIDS

Constance Holden

In an effort to discover the cause of acquired immune deficiency syndrome (AIDS), the National Institute of Allergy and Infectious Diseases is awarding $933,000 to the University of Texas at Bastrop for a 3-year research project involving 11 chimpanzees that will be innoculated with tissues and fluids from AIDS victims.

But some animal welfare groups have registered objections to the research. Shirley McGreal of the International Primate Protection League is circulating petitions to stop the project, which she claims will subject the chimps to the "mental torture" of "solitary confinement." The Humane Society, according to anatomist John McArdle, also opposes the experiment. He says this is another example of scientists "jumping to the animal model immediately" when the purposes of the experiment would be served by in vitro and epidemiological studies. He speculates that AIDS may be stress-related because immune function is susceptible to stress, and claims that putting chimps in stressful circumstances would therefore defeat the purpose of the project.

Officials at the National Institutes of Health (NIH), which is supporting a good deal of AIDS research, say there is good reason to think AIDS is caused by an infectious agent, particularly since researchers have recently been successful in transmitting simian AIDS in macaques in whom the disease has occurred spontaneously. The project follows in the footsteps of past exercises in isolating infectious agents such as the hepatitis B virus, in which animals have been used to obtain samples throughout the course of the disease from its inception. Veterinarian David Johnson of the Division of Research Services says the chimps will be kept in cages in one room, not in solitary confinement.

The protests of the animal welfare people are part of a larger goal, which is to close down all seven of the NIH-funded regional primate centers (Bastrop is not one of them). NIH is not only out of sympathy with that but has formulated a National Chimpanzee Breeding Plan. Now that chimps can no longer be gotten from Africa, NIH wants to promote the establishment of a self-sustaining captive breeding population among the 1200 chimps kept by U.S. biomedical research institutions.

15.   Acquired Immune Deficiency Syndrome Abroad

Jean L. Marx

Epidemiologists have been tracking the spread of acquired immune deficiency syndrome (AIDS) in the hope of identifying the still elusive cause of this devastating disease. Participants at a recent meeting* presented data showing that AIDS, which was originally discovered in this country, is now widespread. It is found in Europe and in Canada, although not in the epidemic proportions seen here where there have been about 2700 cases and more than 1100 deaths. The disease is also present in Central Africa and in Haiti where the incidence is relatively high.

As of October of this year, 268 cases of AIDS had been reported in Europe, according to figures compiled by the World Health Organization and the Danish Cancer Society. The clinical symptoms closely resemble those observed in the United States. The patients suffer severe immunological deficiencies, leaving them prey to opportunistic infections and a hitherto rare form of cancer called Kaposi's sarcoma.

But, notes Jean Brunet of the French Ministry of Health, "There is an important difference between the American and European cases. One-quarter of the [European] cases were diagnosed in African patients." Eighteen of the 100 AIDS patients in France have links to Central Africa.

In addition, of the 40 cases in Belgium, "all are related in some way to Central Africa," according to Jan Desmyter of the Catholic University of Leuven (Louvain). They had either lived in the area themselves or had a sexual partner who had lived there. Zaire, the largest and most populous country in the region, has contributed the most cases.

The link to Central Africa is interesting because of what it may reveal about the origins of AIDS. The disease is thought to be a new one, at least in the United States where it was identified only in 1981. Where it originated is a big question because the answer may help epidemiologists identify the cause, which is generally, although not universally, thought to be an infectious agent, probably a virus.

Studies of AIDS in Central Africa are just beginning and the full extent of the problem there is unclear. "There are certainly cases in Africa," says Thomas Quinn of the National Institute of Allergy and Infectious Diseases, who recently returned from Zaire, "but it is premature to say how many cases there are. How long the disease has been there and the extent to which it has spread are questions we are working on now."

It is not yet known whether AIDS existed in Central Africa before it turned up here, but Kaposi's sarcoma has been

---

*Conference on Acquired Immune Deficiency Syndrome, which was sponsored by the New York Academy of Sciences and held in New York City on 14 to 17 November 1983.

occurring there for many years. AIDS patients, most of whom are young or middle-aged men in the United States, get an unusually virulent form of this cancer, which primarily affects the upper part of the body and frequently spreads to the lymph nodes and internal organs. They usually die within 2 to 3 years.

The more classical form of the sarcoma, which was originally described in the late 1800's by Moritz Kaposi, affects primarily elderly men of Mediterranean origin. This type occurs on the legs, does not spread rapidly to other organs, and responds well to treatment. In addition, the patients' immune responses remain more or less normal, in contrast to the marked immune suppression seen in AIDS patients.

Both the virulent and milder forms of Kaposi's sarcoma occur in Central Africa, Quinn says. The virulent cancer usually affects children and young adults but older individuals also develop this form occasionally. "These cases look very similar clinically to their counterparts with AIDS," Quinn says. "The question remains, is this virulent form AIDS?" The team with which Quinn is working has not yet completed the immunological studies needed to determine whether the patients have AIDS-like immunological deficiencies.

They are also interested in possible associations between viruses and the Central African patients. The current leading candidate for the cause of AIDS is human T-cell leukemia virus, although the case for this agent is in no way ironclad (*Science*, 20 May 1983). In addition, cytomegalovirus has been linked to Kaposi's sarcoma. However, it seems unlikely that this virus, which has been around much longer than AIDS, causes the disease unless a new mutated strain has arisen.

In the United States, the most common means by which AIDS spreads is sexual intercourse among homosexuals. The largest group of AIDS patients, more than 70 percent of the total, consists of homosexual and bisexual males who have had very large numbers of sex partners, a life-style that virtually guarantees the dissemination of infectious diseases. In Africa, AIDS does not appear to spread by homosexual contact, according to Quinn. Moreover, Desmyter says that 40 percent of the patients seen in Belgium are women.

Heterosexual sex may be a more likely form of transmission in the African patients. In the United States, women who lived with bisexual men or drug addicts, the second largest group of AIDS patients here, have contracted the disease. AIDS is transmitted among drug addicts by contaminated needles, a possible mode of transmission in Africa, too.

The third largest group of AIDS patients in the United States consists of Haitian immigrants. In Haiti itself, a country with a population of about 6 million, some 150 to 175 cases have now been identified, according to Jean-Michel Guerin of the Groupe de Recherches sur les Maladies Immunitaire en Haiti, in Port-au-Prince.

AIDS began turning up in Haiti at about the same time that the disease was identified here. Because that country is a favorite vacation spot for U.S. homosexuals, there have been suggestions that the disease may have originated in Haiti and been brought back to New York by returning homosexuals, a suggestion about which Haitian officials are understandably sensitive. There is at present no conclusive evidence for that theory, and the disease might have moved in the opposite direction. AIDS is not found in rural Haiti, Guerin notes. "It appears to us that the disease is an urban disease in a population that is in contact with tourists." The extent and nature of possible contacts between Haitians and Central Africans are currently unknown.

Haitian officials are also sensitive about suggestions that Haitians constitute a separate risk group simply because they are Haitians. Transmission among them is likely to occur by the standard routes, sexual contact and contaminated needles or blood products, Guerin says. The male patients, who constitute about

70 percent of the total in Haiti, rarely admit to homosexual practices, but these cannot be ruled out. "Homosexuality is a taboo subject in Haiti, and it is hard to get the information," Guerin explains.

A great many questions about AIDS, including the big one concerning the nature of the causative agent, remain unanswered. Nevertheless, the epidemiological studies are providing some interesting leads. As Quinn puts it, "The work in Zaire may give us some important clues about the course and spread of AIDS throughout the world."

Report

9 December 1983

16. Productive Infection and Cell-Free Transmission of Human T-Cell Leukemia Virus in a Nonlymphoid Cell Line

P. Clapham, K. Nagy, R. Cheingsong-Popov, M. Exley, and R.A. Weiss

Human T-cell leukemia virus (HTLV) is a C-type RNA tumor virus associated with a mature form of adult T-cell leukemia-lymphoma (ATLL). HTLV was first isolated and characterized from patients in the United States (*1*) and later in Japan (*2*), and in patients of West Indian origin (*3*) and in Israel (*4*). Human umbilical cord lymphocytes and peripheral blood lymphocytes cocultivated with HTLV-releasing lymphoma cells become infected and transformed in vitro (*4, 5*). Transformation of simian and rabbit peripheral blood T cells by HTLV has also been reported (*6*). Several of the T-cell lines transformed in vitro produce larger quantities of HTLV particles than the original tumor lines.

We have recently demonstrated that cocultivation of HTLV-producing cells with a variety of human and animal nonlymphoid cell types induces cell fusion, leading to the formation of large, multinucleated syncytia as a result of HTLV expression (*7*). These observations indicate that HTLV interacts with the surface of a number of cell types. Further studies with vesicular stomatitis virus (VSV) pseudotypes bearing the envelope glycoproteins of HTLV showed that there is a broad range of cells susceptible to pseudotype infection (*8*). Thus the expression of HTLV receptors is not restricted to lymphoid cells, because many cell types derived from diverse mammalian species are permissive for HTLV adsorption and penetration.

In this report we describe the productive infection of a nonlymphoid human cell line by American and Japanese strains of HTLV. Furthermore, we show that cell-free transmission of HTLV is achieved in this line.

Permissivity of HOS cells to HTLV replication. Five human and five animal cell lines known to have receptors for HTLV (*8*) were cocultivated with HTLV-producing C91/PL T cells. The human cells were 7605L embryonic lung fibroblasts, HOS osteogenic sarcoma cells, RD rhabdomyosarcoma cells, HeLa cervical carcinoma cells, and EJ bladder carcinoma cells. Animal cells were Vero African green monkey kidney cells, Fcf2th canine thymus murine sarcoma virus (MSV)–transformed S^+L^- cells, feline CCC MSV-transformed S^+L^- cells, CCL64 mink lung cells, and XC Rous sarcoma virus (RSV)–induced rat sarcoma cells. In the first set of experiments HTLV-producing cells were not x-irradiated but during serial passage the lymphoma cells were soon lost from the adherent cultures. The cells were maintained in Dulbecco-modified Eagle's medium with 5 to 10 percent fetal calf serum and were passaged for 5 months.

Although each of the ten cell types cocultivated with HTLV-producing cells was susceptible to HTLV penetration and eight were susceptible to HTLV-induced cell fusion, only one cell type, the HOS cell line (*9*), was permissive for HTLV replication. During the first 2 weeks of cocultivation, cell fusion oc-

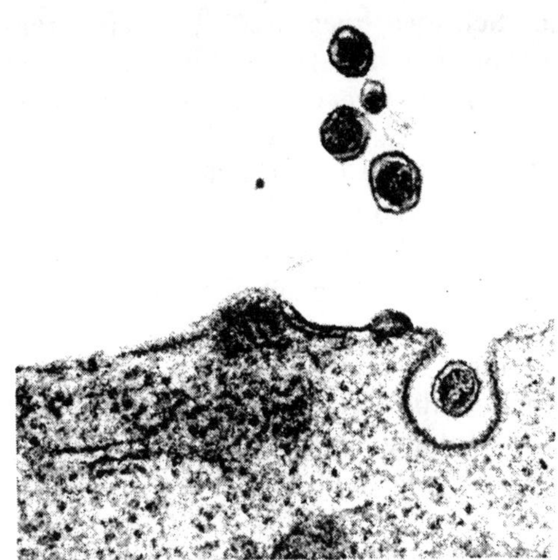

Fig. 1. Budding and mature virions resembling HTLV produced by HOS/PL cells. One particle is contained within a coated pit ($\times 105,000$).

curred among the HOS cells, but with the loss of C91/PL cells on passage, the syncytia disappeared. However, after 8 weeks' passage syncytia reappeared in the HOS cell monolayer indicating productive infection. By 10 weeks the cultures were full of syncytia, after which they gradually disappeared again. Virtually no syncytia could be seen by 12 weeks, although by this stage almost all cells expressed HTLV antigens. It appears that only the uninfected cells are sensitive to syncytium induction by HTLV. When all the cells express HTLV envelope antigens, the cell surface receptors become saturated and no further cell fusion takes place. The virus-infected subline was designated HOS/PL.

C-type particles with the morphology of HTLV were observed as budding and mature virions in electron micrographs of HOS/PL cultures (Fig. 1). No virus particles were evident in uninfected HOS cells. The relative amount of virus

76

particles was measured by reverse transcriptase assay (Table 1) in which there was a preference for Mn^{2+} cations. HTLV production by HOS/PL cells was slightly higher than C91/PL cells, the T-cell line used for cocultivation.

HOS cells were also cocultivated with MT2 cells, producing a Japanese strain of HTLV known as ATLV (2). After 3 months syncytia appeared and by 4 months the HOS/MT2 subline produced substantial amounts of viral antigens.

Immunological properties of HTLV produced by HOS/PL cells. When the fully infected HOS/PL cells were mixed with uninfected HOS or XC "indicator" cells, syncytia were induced in the indicator cells (Table 1). Syncytium induction was specifically inhibited in the presence of ATLL patients' sera, as described previously for HTLV-producing T cells (7), demonstrating HTLV membrane antigen specificity.

VSV particles bearing HTLV envelope glycoproteins can be produced by infecting HTLV-producing T cells with VSV (8). VSV(HTLV) pseudotypes were detected following infection of HOS/PL cells with VSV (Table 1). The plaque-forming activity of these pseudotypes was completely neutralized by serum (at a 1:250 dilution) from a patient with ATLL.

An indirect immunofluorescence assay for HTLV structural antigens was carried out with serum from an antibody-positive ATLL patient. Nearly 100 percent of HOS/PL cells expressed HTLV antigens (Fig. 2). Bright fluorescent regions in the cytoplasm and spots on the cell surface were observed as well as diffuse fluorescence around the nucleus. In addition, immunofluorescence revealed by monoclonal antibody to the HTLV core antigen p19 (10) was positive in HOS/PL cells (Table 1). No significant fluorescence was observed in uninfected HOS cells.

Table 1. Virus production, syncytium induction, pseudotype formation, and antigen expression by HOS/PL cells.

Cell line	Reverse trans-ciptase*	Syn-cytium induc-tion†	VSV (HTLV) pseudo-type titer‡	Percentage of cells immunofluorescent			
				HTLV antigens§		T-cell marker¶	IL-2 recep-tor ‖
				ATLL	p19		
C91/PL	16361	+++	3×10^3	87	89	72	85
HOS/PL	18890	++++	5×10^4	98	82	0	0
HOS	926	−	$< 10^1$	0	0	0	0

*Assay of viral RNA-directed DNA polymerase, expressed as the counts per minute of [³H]TMP incorporated during incubation for 60 minutes at 37°C (7).   †XC indicator cells were cocultivated with test cells for 18 hours and examined for syncytia (7). The results are expressed as the percentage of nuclei contained within syncytia: −, no syncytia; +++, 30 to 50 percent; ++++, > 50 percent.   ‡Plaque-forming units per milliliter of vesicular stomatitis virus (VSV) with envelope antigens specific to HTLV (8).   §Indirect immunofluorescence on fixed cells using serum from an antibody-positive ATLL patient (7) and monoclonal antibody to p19 (10).   ¶Indirect immunofluorescence with UCHT1 monoclonal antibody (12) on live cells.   ‖ Indirect immunofluorescence with anti-Tac monoclonal antibody (14) on live and fixed cells.

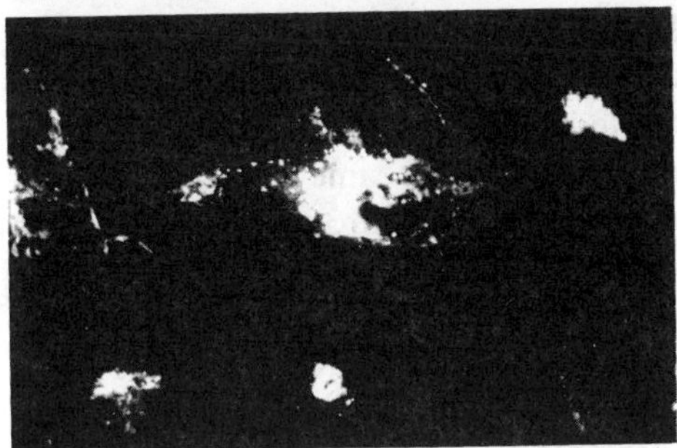

Fig. 2. Immunofluorescence of fixed HOS/PL cells treated with serum from a patient with ATLL and goat antiserum to human immunoglobulin G conjugated with fluorescein isothiocyanate.

HTLV-specific proteins synthesized by HOS/PL cells were also detected by radioimmunoprecipitation and gel electrophoresis (Fig. 3). Immunoprecipitation by monospecific antiserum to p24 (*11*) revealed the synthesis in HOS/PL cells of proteins with apparent molecular weights of 27,000, 37,000, and 57,000. With serum from an ATLL patient, further labeled proteins were precipitated, the major one being a broad band of 66,000 apparent molecular weight. All the major proteins present in C91/PL cells were also present in HOS/PL cells but with the exception of actin were not seen in uninfected HOS cells.

The results of the antibody-specific immunofluorescence, immunoprecipitation, syncytium inhibition, and pseudotype neutralization experiments show conclusively that the virus produced by HOS/PL cells is HTLV.

HOS cells lack T-cell markers and IL-2 receptors. HOS and HOS/PL cells were tested for expression of a surface antigen common to all T cells, recognized by UCHT1 monoclonal antibody (*12*). Neither cell type was positive for this antigen, providing additional evi-

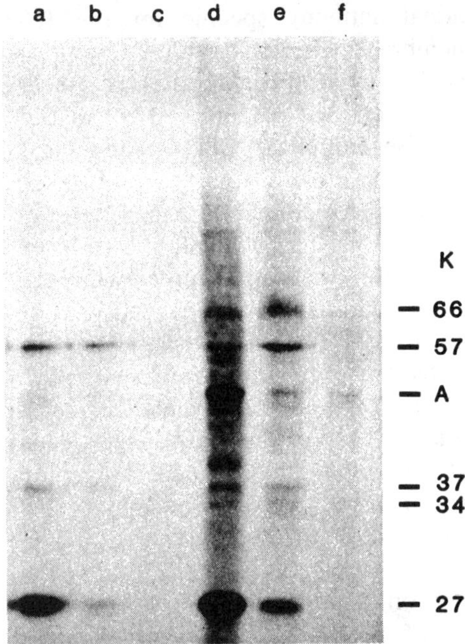

Fig. 3. Radiofluorograph of immunoprecipitation followed by polyacrylamide gel electrophoresis of [^{35}S]methionine-labeled proteins synthesized in HTLV-infected and uninfected cell lines. Lanes a, b, and c: precipitation of C91/PL, HOS/PL, and HOS lysates, respectively, by rabbit antiserum to p24 serum (*10*). Lanes d, e, and f: precipitation of C91/PL, HOS/PL, and HOS lysates, respectively, by human ATLL serum. HTLV-specific polypeptides with molecular weights of 27,000 (27K), 34K, 37K, 57K, and 66K are indicated. Defined proteins ranging from 21K to 85K (not shown) were used as molecular weight markers in the same gel. *A*, actin.

dence besides their morphology and reported origin (*9*) that HOS cells are not T cells.

T-cell growth factor, also known as interleukin-2 (IL-2), is a glycoprotein synthesized and secreted by certain T lymphocytes following activation with antigen or mitogen (*13*). IL-2 is required for proliferation and maintenance of mature T cells in long-term culture. Monoclonal antibody specific for the IL-2 membrane receptor (anti-Tac) suppresses IL-2–induced proliferation of T cells, and blocks the binding of IL-2 to cells (*14*). Several of the HTLV-producing T-lymphoma cells do not require exogenous IL-2 for proliferation in culture. All HTLV-transformed T-cell lines, however, express the IL-2 receptor which becomes preferentially associated with the virions of HTLV (*15*). It has been suggested that the IL-2 receptor may play a role in HTLV infection and transformation (*15*). We therefore investigated whether the expression of IL-2 receptors was involved in the infection of HOS cells by HTLV.

To detect the presence of IL-2 receptors on the membranes of HOS and HOS/PL cells, we performed indirect immunofluorescence with anti-Tac monoclonal antibody (Table 1). With this assay the presence of IL-2 receptors was detected in C91/PL T cells but neither in virus-producing HOS/PL nor in uninfected HOS cells, indicating that the IL-2 receptor is not necessary for HTLV replication and is not equivalent to the HTLV receptor.

HOS HTLV transforms T cells. To determine whether HTLV produced by HOS/PL cells is able to transform T lymphocytes, x-irradiated HOS/PL cells were cocultivated with phytohemagglutinin (PHA)-stimulated mixed human tonsil lymphocytes initially in the presence of IL-2. A transformed, HTLV-producing line of IL-2–independent T cells became established within 6 weeks. Thus the T-cell transforming property of HTLV was not lost upon passage through HOS cells.

Cell-free transmission of HOS HTLV. The infection of HOS cells was repeated and confirmed with x-irradiated (5000 R) HTLV-producing C91/PL and HOS/PL cells. When fresh HOS cells were cocultivated with x-irradiated HOS/PL cells, the HOS cells became infected and produced HTLV within 3 weeks, rather than 10 weeks that elapsed after cocultivation with C91/PL cells. Since the amount of virus released from HOS/PL and C91/PL cells was not markedly different as measured by reverse transcriptase (Table 1), this result suggests that HTLV produced by HOS/PL cells has become adapted for more efficient replication in this cell type.

It may be argued that cocultivation of HOS cells with HTLV-infected T cells allowed the transfer of chromosomes bearing HTLV proviruses into the HOS cells by cell fusion, even though the HOS cells did not bear T-cell markers. We therefore attempted to perform cell-free transmission of the HTLV. Clarified and filtered (0.2 μm) medium harvested from HOS/PL cell cultures was added to subconfluent cultures of HOS cells in the presence of DEAE-Dextran (25 μl/ml). After incubation for 1 hour at 37°C, growth medium was added and the cells were passaged twice a week. After 3 weeks the infected cells produced syncytia, and complete infection was established within 7 weeks.

On repeating cell-free infection of HOS cells, the appearance of HTLV antigens and syncytia was followed by immunofluorescent and cytological assays performed at 1, 3, 7, 14, 21, 28, and 35 days after infection. Syncytia first became evident 14 days after infection and by 21 days numerous syncytia were seen. HTLV antigens were first detectable by immunofluorescence 21 days after infection, increasing in cell number and intensity thereafter. It is likely that a very small proportion of cells are initially infected and that the virus progressively spreads through the culture during subsequent passage. However, we cannot rule out the possibility that the majority of cells become infected by the original inoculum but do not express viral antigens until several weeks later.

Discussion. HTLV has been successfully transmitted by cocultivation to other human, simian, and rabbit cells of lymphoid origin (*4–6*). Cell-free transmission of HTLV to human bone marrow cells has recently been observed (*16*). Here we show that HTLV is transmissible to nonlymphoid cells, by cocultivation with infected cells as well as by culture with filtered medium from such cells, and that virus-producing cell lines can be established. The uninfected HOS line and the HOS/PL and HOS/MT2 sublines proliferate in culture medium supplemented with fetal calf serum, without a requirement for specific growth factors. Bovine leukosis virus, which is distantly related to HTLV, can also be transmitted to nonlymphoid cells (*17*).

Because HTLV-transformed T cells represent cells derived from an unknown, minority T-cell subset in fresh lymphocyte cultures, there exist no control, uninfected cell lines directly comparable to the HTLV-infected cells. HOS, HOS/PL, and HOS/MT2 cells provide such a system, which is now being used in serological studies of ATLL and AIDS patients. This system enables us to distinguish in immunofluorescence studies between virus-specific and cell-specific antibodies in these patients' sera. HOS/PL cells are also useful as a source reagent for serological assays because they consistently produce high titers of HTLV antigens.

Experiments on the infection of HOS cells with HTLV-2 (*18*) and with HTLV-like viruses isolated from AIDS patients (*19*) and from nonhuman primates (*20*) should make possible detailed comparisons of the various HTLV strains.

References and Notes

1. B. J. Poiesz, F. W. Ruscetti, A. F. Gazdar, P. A. Bunn, J. D. Minna, R. C. Gallo, *Proc. Natl. Acad. Sci. U.S.A.* **77**, 7415 (1980); B. J. Poiesz, F. W. Ruscetti, M. S. Reitz, V. S. Kalyanaraman, R. C. Gallo, *Nature (London)* **294**, 268 (1981).
2. I. Miyoshi *et al., Nature (London)* **294**, 770 (1981); M. Yoshida, I. Miyoshi, Y. Hinuma, *Proc. Natl. Acad. Sci. U.S.A.* **79**, 2031 (1982).
3. D. Catovsky *et al., Lancet* **1982-I**, 639 (1982); F. A. Vyth-Dreese, J. E. De Vries, *ibid.* **1982-II**, 993 (1982); W. A. Blattner *et al., ibid.* **1983-II**, 61 (1983).
4. M. Popovic *et al., Science* **219**, 856 (1983).
5. I. Miyoshi, I. Kubonishi, S. Yoshimoto, Y. Shiraishi, *Gann* **72**, 978 (1981).
6. I. Miyoshi *et al., Lancet* **1982-II**, 1016 (1982); I. Miyoshi *et al., Gann* **74**, 1 (1983).
7. K. Nagy, P. Clapham, R. Cheingsong-Popov, R. A. Weiss, *Int. J. Cancer* **32**, 321 (1983).
8. K. Nagy, R. A. Weiss, P. Clapham, R. Cheingsong-Popov, in *Human T-Cell Leukemia-Lymphoma Viruses*, R. C. Gallo, M. Essex, L. Gross, Eds. (Cold Spring Harbor Laboratory, Cold Spring Harbor, N.Y., in press).
9. R. M. McAllister, M. B. Gardner, A. E. Greene, C. Brandt, W. W. Nichols, B. H. Landing, *Cancer* **27**, 397 (1971).
10. M. Robert-Guroff, F. W. Ruscetti, L. E. Posner, B. J. Poiesz, R. C. Gallo, *J. Exp. Med.* **154**, 1957 (1981).
11. V. S. Kalyanaraman, M. G. Sarngadharan, B. Poiesz, F. W. Ruscetti, R. C. Gallo, *J. Virol.* **38**, 906 (1981).
12. P. C. L. Beverley and R. E. Collard, *Eur. J. Immunol.* **11**, 329334 (1981).
13. K. A. Smith, *Immunol. Rev.* **51**, 337 (1980); F. W. Ruscetti and R. C. Gallo, *Blood* **57**, 379 (1981).
14. W. J. Leonard, J. M. Depper, T. Uchiyama, K. A. Smith, T. A. Waldmann, W. C. Green, *Nature (London)* **300**, 267 (1983).
15. Z. Lando *et al., Nature (London)* **305**, 733 (1983).
16. P. Markham and R. C. Gallo, personal communication.
17. M. J. van der Maaten, J. M. Miller, A. D. Boothe, *J. Natl. Cancer Inst.* **52**, 491 (1974); D. C. Graves and J. F. Ferrer, *Cancer Res.* **36**, 4152 (1976).
18. V. S. Kalyanaraman *et al., Science* **218**, 571 (1982).
19. R. C. Gallo *et al., Science* **220**, 865 (1983); F. Barré-Sinoussi *et al., ibid.*, p. 868.
20. I. Miyoshi *et al., Lancet* **1982-II**, 658 (1982).
21. We thank R. C. Gallo for providing C91/PL cells and ATLL patient's serum, I. Miyoshi for the MT2 cells, R. M. McAllister for the HOS cells, M. Robert Guroff for monospecific antibodies to HTLV, T. A. Waldmann for anti-Tac monoclo-

nal antibody, P. C. L. Beverley for UCHT1 T-cell monoclonal antibody, and J. Timar for preparing the electron micrograph. This study was supported by a joint grant from the Medical Research Council and the Cancer Research Campaign.

31 August 1983; accepted 26 October 1983

Letter to the Editor

16 December 1983

17. Retrovirus Terminology

Toshiki Watanabe, Motoharu Seiki, and Mitsuaki Yoshida

A human retrovirus, human T-cell leukemia virus (HTLV), was first isolated by Gallo and his colleagues in 1980 from a cell line established from a patient with cutaneous T-cell lymphoma (mycosis fungoides) (*1*). Subsequently, ATLV (adult T-cell leukemia virus) (*2, 3*) was isolated from the cell line MT-2, established by Miyoshi *et al.* (*4*), from Japanese patients with adult T-cell leukemia-lymphoma (ATL). This disease was discovered by Takatsuki and his colleagues (*5*) as a unique T-cell malignancy clustered in the southwest part of Japan. These two independent viral isolates were shown to be closely associated with ATL by epidemiological and molecular biological studies.

HTLV and ATLV were shown to be similar by immunological cross-reactivities (*6*) and nucleic acid hybridization (*7*). However, the data were not sufficient to prove the identity of these two viral isolates because the immunological cross-reactivities of the core proteins p19 and p24 reflected only part of the *gag* gene of the viral genomes and be-cause the viral complementary DNA preparations were not representative. Recently, we determined (*8*) the total nucleotide sequence of the ATLV genome cloned in λATK-1. On the basis of this structural information, we compared the provirus genomes of HTLV and ATLV integrated in the cell lines HUT-102 and MT-2, respectively, by Southern blotting analysis using five viral gene-specific probes. With every specific probe the expected viral fragments were identical for the HTLV and ATLV proviruses (*9*). These results clearly indicate that the locations of the gene-specific sequences and the cleavage sites of some restriction enzymes are identical in the proviral genomes integrated in HUT-102 and MT-2. Thus, we can conclude that HTLV and ATLV are the same, even if they differ in their base replacements, small insertions, or deletions. This conclusion indicates that the viral populations in the southwest of Japan and in the Caribbean have a common origin.

In view of these results we propose to use the term HTLV rather than ATLV, respecting the first isolate of this retrovirus. We will use the terminology "ATK strain of HTLV ($HTLV_{ATK}$)" for the ATLV previously cloned and reported as λATK-1, and whose total sequence was determined (8). At the conference on human T-cell leukemia viruses held at Cold Spring Harbor in September 1983, a letter proposing that the term HTLV be used for the retrovirus was signed by the following: W. A. Blattner, National Cancer Institute, Bethesda; D. Catovsky, Hammersmith Hospital, London; M. Essex, Harvard University School of Public Health; R. C. Gallo, National Cancer Institute, Bethesda; M. Greaves, Imperial Cancer Research Fund, London; Y. E. Ito, Kyoto University; I. Miyoshi, Kochi Medical School; K. Takatsuki, Kumamoto University Medical School; R. A. Weiss, Institute of Cancer Research, London; and M. Yoshida, Cancer Institute, Tokyo.

References

1. B. J. Poiesz *et al.*, *Proc. Natl. Acad. Sci. U.S.A.* **77**, 7415 (1980).
2. M. Yoshida, I. Miyoshi, Y. Hinuma, *ibid.* **79**, 2031 (1982).
3. Y. Hinuma *et al.*, *ibid.* **78**, 6476 (1981).
4. I. Miyoshi *et al.*, *Nature (London)* **294**, 770 (1981).
5. T. Uchiyama *et al.*, *Blood* **50**, 481 (1977).
6. V. S. Kalyanaraman *et al.*, *Proc. Natl. Acad. Sci. U.S.A.* **79**, 1653 (1982); J. Nagy *et al.*, *Int. J. Cancer* **32**, 321 (1983).
7. M. Popovic *et al.*, *Nature (London)* **300**, 63 (1982).
8. M. Seiki, S. Hattori, Y. Hirayama, M. Yoshida, *Proc. Natl. Acad. Sci. U.S.A.* **80**, 3618 (1983).
9. T. Watanabe *et al.*, *Virology*, in press.

January – December 1984

18. Transmission of Simian Acquired Immunodeficiency Syndrome (SAIDS) with Blood or Filtered Plasma

Maneth Gravell, William T. London, Sidney A. Houff, David L. Madden, Marinos C. Dalakas, John L. Sever, Kent G. Osborn, Donald H. Maul, Roy V. Henrickson, Preston A. Marx, Nicholas W. Lerche, Srinivasa Prahalada, and Murray B. Gardner

Many different infectious agents have been isolated from patients with acquired immunodeficiency syndrome (AIDS), but none of these has been clearly implicated as the cause of this disease. The difficulty of identifying the cause of AIDS has been compounded by the lack of a susceptible experimental animal. A spontaneous outbreak of a disease clinically and pathologically similar to AIDS in humans was recently described in rhesus monkeys (*Macaca mulatta*) housed in an outdoor corral at the California Primate Research Center of the University of California, Davis (CPRC) (*1*). Affected animals had symptoms similar to those of AIDS victims including profound immunosuppression, lymphadenopathy, splenomegaly, multiple opportunistic infections, persistent diarrhea, chronic wasting, and high mortality. Some animals also had cutaneous fibrosarcomas. A similar immunosuppressive disease was reported to occur in macaque monkeys housed at the New England Primate Research Center in Southborough, Massachusetts (*2*). An understanding of SAIDS is important so that methods can be developed to protect nonhuman primates from this devas-

tating disease. Such studies may also provide clues to the etiology and pathogenesis of AIDS in humans and serve as a useful model for investigation of prophylaxis and therapy.

We recently reported on the experimental transmission of SAIDS from two animals at the CPRC to four rhesus monkeys at the National Institutes of Health (NIH) that were negative for cytomegalovirus (CMV) antibody (*3*). Inocula for these studies were mixtures of unfiltered supernatant fluids from 10 percent homogenates of various organs with or without buffy coat cells from blood. In this report we narrow our focus on the cause of SAIDS by describing transmission of the syndrome to rhesus monkeys using whole blood or filtered plasma from diseased animals.

These studies were carried out at two geographically separated sites, NIH and CPRC, with inocula from different donor animals. The experiments were performed independently but the data were shared.

Four juvenile rhesus monkeys were each inoculated intravenously with 0.9 ml of heparinized whole blood from either of two moribund donor animals with experimentally transmitted SAIDS (Table 1). The clinical history and pathology of the donor animals were described previously (*3*). Monkeys 1 and 2, inoculated at NIH, were 8.5 and 8 months of age, respectively, and monkeys 3 and 4, inoculated at CPRC, were both 11 months of age. All four inoculated animals developed SAIDS; three of them became moribund and died 2 and 3 months after inoculation. Animal 1 remains alive with persistent generalized lymphadenopathy and splenomegaly 5 months after inoculation (Table 1).

In an attempt to characterize the SAIDS agent, plasma from two donor animals with advanced disease was filtered, sequentially, through two 0.45-μm Millipore filters to minimize the chance of filter failure. At CPRC, the integrity of the filters was further verified by retention of a mixture of *Staphylococcus aureus* and *Escherichia coli* by the same filter used to filter the SAIDS plasma. Confluent growth of the bacteria occurred on agar medium prior to filtration of the mixture, but no growth by either organism was seen after filtration.

Four juvenile rhesus monkeys were each inoculated with 3 ml of the filtered plasma from two animals with SAIDS (Table 1). Monkeys 5 and 6, inoculated at NIH, were negative for antibody to rhesus monkey CMV and were 11 and 8 months of age, respectively. At CPRC, animals 7 and 8, both 14 months of age, had antibody to rhesus monkey CMV. Two to four weeks after inoculation with filtered plasma, all four recipient animals developed SAIDS (Table 1). The disease progressed rapidly in three of the animals, leading to a moribund condition and death 5 to 9 weeks after inoculation. The fourth recipient (monkey 8) remains alive with persistent generalized lympha-

denopathy and splenomegaly 3 months after inoculation.

The postmortem findings in the six animals that died with SAIDS were similar (Table 1). The findings paralleled those seen in spontaneous (*1*) and experimental SAIDS (*3*). A characteristic feature was lymphoid depletion of the lymph node cortices, splenic white pulp, and thymic cortex. This was moderate to severe in four of the six cases as evidenced by loss of lymphocytes in both follicular (B cell) and paracortical and periarterial (T cell) zones of the lymph nodes and spleen, respectively. Immunoblasts were sparse and plasma cells virtually absent. In one animal (monkey 6) there was active follicular hyperplasia. The nodes showed sinus histiocytosis and erythrophagocytosis. In four animals examined, the bone marrows were abnormally hypercellular and showed an increase in erythroid and granulocytic precursors, occasional lymphoid nodules, and histiocytic proliferation. Other findings of note were enterocolitis (giardiasis, trichomoniasis, cryptosporidiosis) in five animals, cellulitis and focal suppurative lymphadenitis in two animals, and proliferative glomerulonephritis or interstitial nephritis in single animals. Cytomegalic cells with herpes-like intranuclear inclusions were seen disseminated throughout organs of monkey 5. In monkeys with spontaneous SAIDS, the virus associated with similar inclusion-bearing cells has been identified as monkey CMV by hybridization in situ (*4*).

Studies of the mitogenic responses of lymphocytes from animals in which SAIDS was induced by inoculation with whole blood (monkey 3) or filtered plasma (monkeys 7 and 8) were compared with those of uninoculated healthy con-

Table 1. Transmission of SAIDS with blood or filtered plasma.

Animal number and sex	Inoculum and donor numbers	Clinical and laboratory findings	Pathological findings
1 Female (B-923)*	Blood B-784	Lymphadenopathy, splenomegaly, transient lymphopenia	Alive 5 months after inoculation
2 Female (B-925)*	Blood B-784	Lymphadenopathy, splenomegaly, neutropenia, anemia, lymphopenia, weight loss, hypoproteinemia, diarrhea, dehydration, edema of the perineum and lower limbs	Died 10 weeks after inoculation. Moderate lymphoid depletion, glomerulonephritis, cellulitis, suppurative lymphadenitis, bone marrow hyperplasia
3 Female (20141)*	Blood B-883	Lymphadenopathy, splenomegaly, neutropenia, anemia, lymphopenia, weight loss, hypoproteinemia, thrombocytopenia	Died 9 weeks after inoculation. Moderate lymphoid depletion, enterocolitis, hypercellular bone marrow
4 Female (20335)*	Blood B-883	Same as monkey 3, plus diarrhea, but no thrombocytopenia	Died 11 weeks after inoculation. Moderate lymphoid depletion, enterocolitis, interstitial nephritis, bone marrow hyperplasia
5 Female (B-911)*	Filtered plasma B-784	Same as monkey 3, plus diarrhea and polymyostitis, but no thrombocytopenia	Died 5 weeks after inoculation. Moderate lymphoid depletion, disseminated inclusion-bearing cells, enterocolitis (giardiasis and trichomoniasis), lymph node abcess
6 Female (B-920)*	Filtered plasma B-784	Same as monkey 5, but no hypoproteinemia	Died 9 weeks after inoculation. Lymphoid follicular hyperplasia, paracortical depletion, sinus histiocytosis, enterocolitis (giardiasis and trichomoniasis)
7 Male (20383)*	Filtered plasma 20265	Same as monkey 3	Died 5 weeks after inoculation. Severe lymphoid depletion, enterocolitis, bone marrow hyperplasia
8 Male (20325)*	Filtered plasma 20265	Lymphadenopathy, splenomegaly, neutropenia	Alive 3 months after inoculation

*Number by which animal was identified in colony.

Table 2. Immunological data from rhesus monkeys with SAIDS. Immunoglobulin concentration (in milligrams per deciliter) from ten normal rhesus monkeys were as follows: IgM, 100 to 310; mean (standard deviation) 226 (68), median, 250; IgG, 560 to 1600; mean (S.D.) 976 (263), median, 950; IgA, 57 to 340; mean (S.D.) 234 (107), median 240.

Animal number	Disease stage	When tested	Mitogen stimulation index			Helper/ suppressor ratio (OKT$_4$/ OKT$_8$)	Immunoglobulin concentrations (mg/dl)		
			Con A	PHA	PWM		IgM	IgG	IgA
3 (20141)*	Late SAIDS	At death	9.6	9.3	45.1	2.7	< 35	< 283	< 57
7 (20383)*	Late SAIDS	At death	37.0	9.8	2.7	2.7	58	540	125
8 (20325)*	Early SAIDS	At 5 weeks	181.7	93.1	28.4	2.3	58	510	170
9 (19071)*	No SAIDS	Normal control	105.0	58.5	20.4	2.2			
10 (18995)*	No SAIDS	Normal control	262.7	119.2	25.5	3.1			

*Number by which animal was identified in colony.

trols matched for age and sex. Lymphocytes from SAIDS animals and controls were stimulated with phytohemagglutinin (PHA), concanavalin A (Con A), and pokeweed mitogen (PWM) by the standard procedures (3). Results of these studies showed that in the early stages of SAIDS, lymphocyte responses to these mitogens were not impaired. However, in animals with advanced disease, lymphocyte stimulation indices were significantly lower than those of controls, with the exception of the PWM response in monkey 3 (Table 2). Concentrations of immunoglobulins M, G, and A (IgM, IgG, and IgA), determined by radial immunodiffusion, were also very low in these animals (Table 2). Regardless of the time after inoculation and severity of disease, there was no evidence in animals with SAIDS of inversion of helper to suppressor T cell ratios determined with T_4 and T_8 monoclonal antibodies (Table 2). In this regard, the monkeys with SAIDS differed from humans with AIDS.

Numerous attempts were made to isolate viruses from the whole blood or filtered plasma that transmitted SAIDS. A variety of cell cultures were used including the continuous monkey kidney cell lines Vero and MA-104; low-passage Flow 7000 and W138 human fibroblasts, low-passage rhesus monkey kidney and lung fibroblast cells; and low-passage lung fibroblasts from the monkey *Erythrocebus patas*. No viral isolations were made from the blood or filtered plasma that caused SAIDS or from similar samples from recipient monkeys that developed SAIDS.

We previously reported that SAIDS could be experimentally transmitted to rhesus monkeys by inoculation with supernatant fluids from 10 percent homogenates (clarified by centrifugation at low speed) of organs from donor animals with SAIDS (3). Rhesus monkey CMV was isolated from the SAIDS-l inoculum used in those studies and from the urine of all four inoculated animals. However, SAIDS did not develop in rhesus monkeys intravenously inoculated with a high-passage laboratory strain of rhesus monkey CMV (283T) or with a recent isolate from a normal healthy animal, passed only three times in vitro (3). To determine whether a unique strain of CMV might be the cause of SAIDS, we inoculated two rhesus monkeys with an isolate of rhesus monkey CMV made from the SAIDS-l inoculum and passed four times in vitro in Flow 7000 human fibroblasts (3). These animals also did not develop SAIDS. In addition, rhesus monkeys with preexisting high titers of antibody to CMV have become infected naturally and experimentally with SAIDS. Rhesus monkey CMV was not isolated from the filtered plasma or whole blood used to transmit SAIDS, nor has it been isolated from CMV antibody negative animals receiving these inocula. These data suggest that rhesus monkey CMV is not the etiologic agent of SAIDS.

Since human T-cell leukemia virus (HTLV) has been associated with human AIDS (5), evidence was sought for the presence of a similar agent in SAIDS. Antibody to the p24 polypeptide of HTLV was not found by radioimmunoassay in infectious plasma from monkeys with SAIDS or in healthy rhesus monkeys housed with diseased monkeys and thus at risk of acquiring the immunodeficiency syndrome (6). Also, a significant reverse transcriptase activity was not detected in infectious plasma (6). However, these results only rule out a marked retroviremia and further studies with in vitro culture techniques are required (*6*). Type C retrovirus particles were not seen by electron microscopy in thin sections of lymph nodes or bone marrow or in cultured T cells of animals with SAIDS (*7*).

Although simian adenoviruses were not isolated from the filtered plasma or whole blood used to produce SAIDS, they have been isolated from many animals with SAIDS. Adenoviruses were isolated from all four experimentally inoculated monkeys (B-784, B-649, B-883, and B-884) from our previous study (*3*). The isolate from B-784 was typed as adenovirus type 11 (*8*). Filtered plasma from B-784 was the inoculum for monkeys 5 and 6 described in this report. An adenovirus was also isolated from the urine, feces, and kidney of monkeys 5 and 6 and also from the mesenteric node of monkey 6. Typing of these isolates has not been completed. Simian adenovirus type 23 was isolated from the feces of two rhesus monkeys that received urine from monkey B-784 (*7*). Adenovirus type 11 was also isolated from a healthy uninoculated normal control animal randomly selected from the CPRC colony, suggesting that these adenovirus isolates are opportunistic agents not etiologically linked to SAIDS.

The present studies demonstrate the experimental transmission of SAIDS with whole blood or filtered plasma. All recipients (eight of eight rhesus monkeys) developed signs of SAIDS within 2 to 4 weeks after inoculation, and (six of the eight recipients became moribund and died between 5 and 11 weeks after inoculation. We have also succeeded in transmitting SAIDS to two rhesus monkeys inoculated with pooled serum from diseased animals (data not shown). The transmission of SAIDS with infectious plasma that was passed through a 0.45-μm pore size filter provides evidence that the causative agent is small and probably a virus. These results are consistent with a recent report on transmission of a similar disease to macaque monkeys with cell-free material. However, in that study, a filtrate of lymphoma tissue was used as the inoculum (*2*). Efforts must now be focused on identifying and characterizing the etiologic agent of SAIDS. Such studies will contribute to the understanding and control of both SAIDS and human AIDS.

References and Notes

1. R. V. Henrickson *et al.*, *Lancet* **1983-I**, 388 (1983).
2. R. D. Hunt *et al.*, *Proc. Natl. Acad. Sci. U.S.A.* **80**, 5085 (1983); N. L. Letvin *et al.*, *Lancet* **1983-II**, 599 (1983).
3. W. T. London *et al.*, *Lancet* **1983-II**, 869 (1983).
4. M. Bryant, unpublished data.
5. M. Essex *et al.*, *Science* **220**, 859 (1983); E. P. Gelmann *et al.*, *ibid.*, p. 862; R. C. Gallo *et al.*, *ibid.*, p. 865; F. Barré-Sinoussi *et al.*, *ibid.*, p. 868.
6. L. Arthur and R. Gilden, personal communication.
7. R. Munn, personal communication.
8. R. L. Heberling, personal communication.
9. We thank R. Hamilton, R. Atkins, B. Curfman, and R. Brown of NIH and P. Moody, M. Bleviss, A. Spinner, R. Beards, and J. Tribble of CPRC for technical assistance. Supported in part by PHS grant RR00169 from the NIH Division of Research Resources.

4 October 1983; accepted 25 October 1983

Report

13 January 1984

19.   Gene for T-Cell Growth Factor: Location on Human Chromosome 4q and Feline Chromosome B1

Leonard J. Seigel, Mary E. Harper, Flossie Wong-Staal, Robert C. Gallo, William G. Nash, and Stephen J. O'Brien

T-cell growth factor (TCGF) was originally discovered as a component of conditioned medium from lectin-stimulated primary cultures of human lymphoid cells that permitted long-term proliferation in vitro (*1, 2*). Exploitation of this discovery led to the cloning of T-cell populations of defined function and specificity (*3*) and the use of TCGF to establish cell lines from certain mature T-cell tumors (*4*). These cells respond to TCGF without prior activation with lectin or antigen, apparently because of constitutive expression of the TCGF receptor (*5*). From these cell lines the retrovirus human T-cell leukemia virus (HTLV) was isolated (*6*). TCGF-dependent lymphocyte cultures of normal or leukemic individuals are invariably mature T cells as determined by the expression of an array of T-cell markers and the lack of any B cell or immature lymphoid determinants (*1*). Although normal lymphocyte cultures require the continuous presence of TCGF for growth, many of the HTLV-infected cell lines gradually become independent of exogenous TCGF (*2*), suggesting that they either produce their own TCGF or by-pass the normal TCGF–TCGF receptor system required for proliferation.

Homogeneously purified human TCGF is a single polypeptide with a molecular weight of 15,000 (*7*). Recently, almost identical molecular clones of the structural gene for human TCGF were derived from complementary DNA (cDNA) libraries of a leukemic T-cell line (Jurkat) (*8*) and from normal peripheral blood lymphocytes (*9*). Use of cloned TCGF sequences as probes suggested that human TCGF is encoded by a single cellular gene containing introns. We have used a molecular TCGF clone to map the gene in the normal human genome and in the genome of the HUT-102 B2 lymphoma cell line from which the original isolate of HTLV was obtained. HUT-102 B2 has become TCGF-independent and produces low levels of TCGF messenger RNA (mRNA) and biologically active TCGF (*2, 9*).

TCGF was mapped in normal cells with use of a panel of 43 somatic cell hybrids (rodent cells × normal human lymphocytes) (*10*). The human chromosome constitution was monitored by G-trypsin banding (*10, 11*), G-11 chromosome staining (*12*), and electrophoretic resolution of up to 36 isozyme markers previously mapped to each of the 23 human chromosomes (*13*). The TCGF gene was visualized as a 3.5 kilobase (kb) doublet-fragment in human DNA after digestion with Eco RI (Fig. 1a) and Southern hybridization analysis (*14*) with

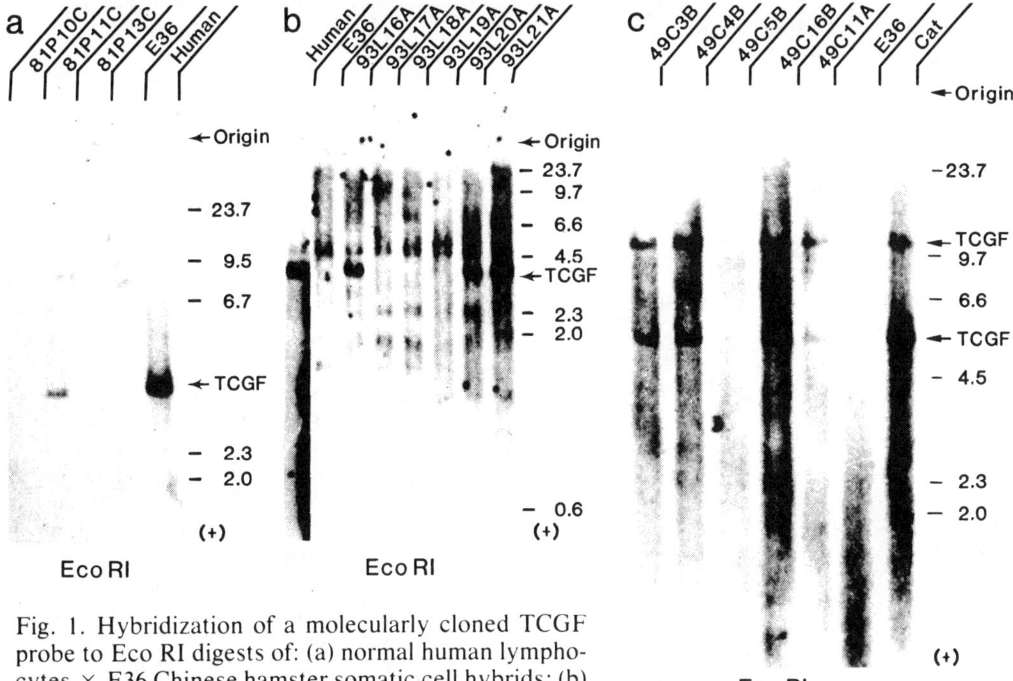

Fig. 1. Hybridization of a molecularly cloned TCGF probe to Eco RI digests of: (a) normal human lymphocytes × E36 Chinese hamster somatic cell hybrids; (b) HUT-102 B2 × E36 Chinese hamster cell hybrids; and (c) normal feline lymphocytes × E36 Chinese hamster cell hybrids. Restriction endonuclease-digested genomic DNA was subjected to electrophoresis on 0.7 percent agarose gels, transferred to nitrocellulose filters (*14*), and hybridized with a ^{32}P-labeled TCGF cDNA probe (*9*) in a solution containing 50 percent deionized formamide, 0.01 percent bovine serum albumin, 0.01 percent Ficoll, and 0.01 percent polyvinylpyrrolidone, a threefold (3×) concentration of SSC (1× SSC is 0.15M sodium chloride plus 0.015N sodium citrate), 20 mM sodium phosphate buffer, pH 6.5, and 10 percent dextran sulfate. After hybridization at 42°C for 24 to 48 hours, the filters were rinsed in 2× SSC, washed for 60 minutes in three changes of 0.2× SSC, and 0.1 percent sodium dodecyl sulfate at 50°C, rinsed in 0.2× SSC, and exposed to x ray film for 7 to 10 days at −70°C.

a nick-translated probe derived from a 1.1-kb molecular clone that includes the human TCGF locus (*9*). Under the stringent conditions used (see legend to Fig. 1), Eco RI digests of the rodent cell DNA produced no hybridization in this region of the filter. Thus, by Eco RI digestion of the hybrid panel (Fig. 1a), it was possible to determine which hybrids retained the human TCGF gene and the chromosome on which it resided. The presence of the TCGF fragment was 98 percent concordant with human chromosome 4 (HSA4)

and its included isozyme loci phosphoglucomutase 2 (*PGM2*) and peptidase S (*PEPS*) (Fig. 2a). The single discordant hybrid clone, 80H2C, had the genotype *HSA4*⁻, *PGM2*⁻; *PEPS*⁻; *TCGF*⁺. Because this hybrid did not contain any obvious rearranged human chromosomes, it may have contained a small transposition of HSA4 which was not apparent in the G-11 and G-trypsin analysis. Each of the remaining 22 human chromosomes showed high discordance (22 to 46 percent; Fig. 2a) with TCGF

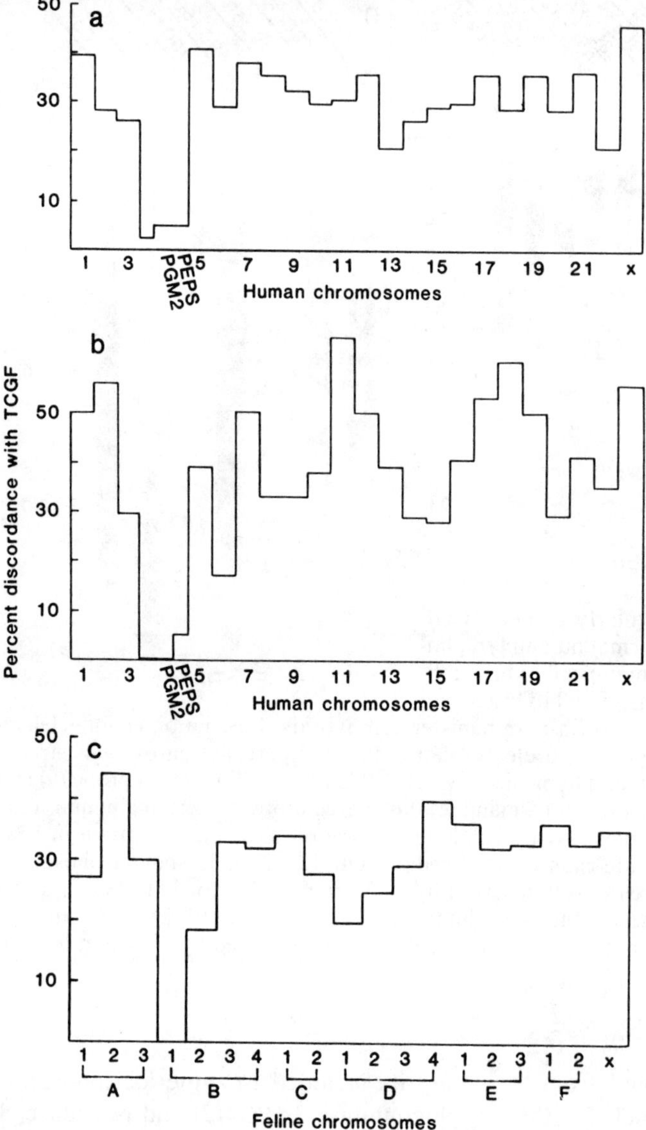

Fig. 2. Concordance of 23 human or 19 feline chromosomes and *TCGF* gene in three different panels of somatic cell hybrids (see text). Chromosome scores represent the consensus result of karyotypic and isoenzyme scores. Thirty-six isoenzyme systems diagnostic for each human chromosome were run on each human × rodent cell hybrid (*13*). Thirty-three isoenzyme systems diagnostic for feline chromosomes were run on each cat × rodent cell hybrid (*11, 13*). The details of isoenzyme analysis of human and feline cell hybrids has been described previously (*13*). The percentage discordance is presented for each chromosome with TCGF for: (a) 43 normal human lymphocyte × rodent somatic cell hybrids; (b) 18 HUT-102 B2 × rodent somatic cell hybrids; and (c) 37 cat × rodent somatic cell hybrids.

permitting the assignment of TCGF to human chromosome 4.

In situ hybridization of the TCGF cDNA clone to normal human chromosome preparations confirmed the assignment of TCGF to HSA4 and further identified the gene on the long arm. A nick-translated ^{3}H-labeled TCGF probe was hybridized at different concentrations between 10 and 100 ng/ml and then exposed autoradiographically for 4 to 27 days (*15*). In an analysis of 60 mitotic spreads, 33 percent of the metaphase spreads that could be scored exhibited label on the midportion of HSA4q. These labeled sites, each consisting of one to

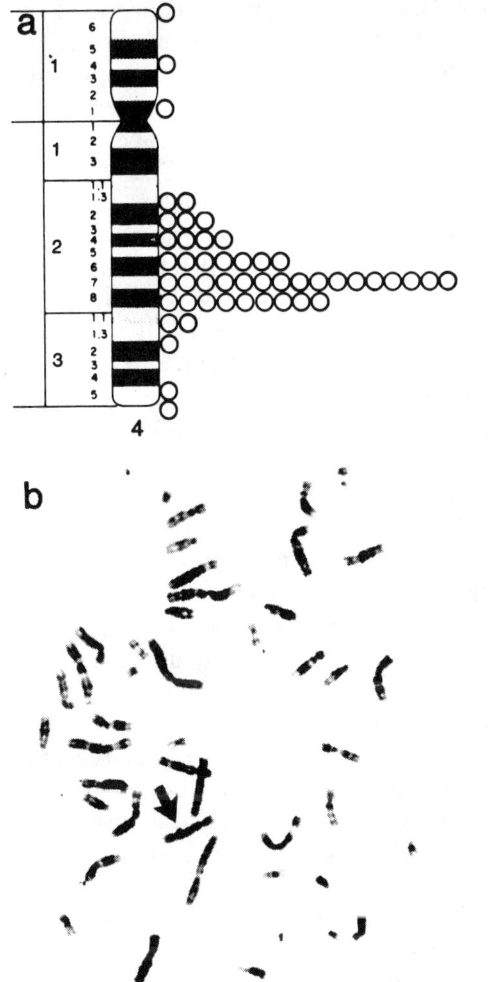

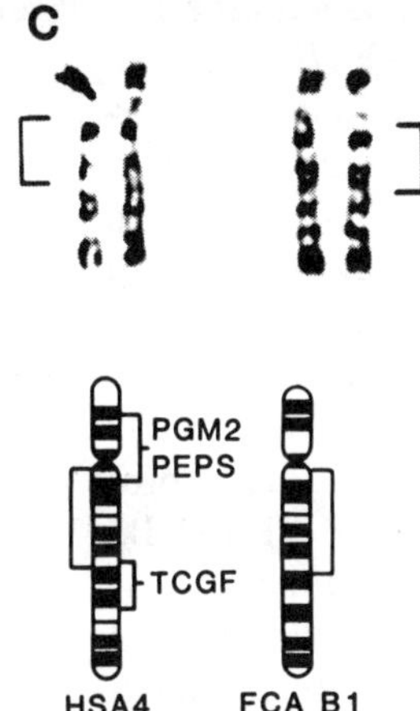

Fig. 3. Identification of the TCGF gene on chromosome 4. (a) Distribution of labeled sites on 47 No. 4 chromosomes after in situ hybridization of the TCGF probe. Of 49 total grains, 32 (65 percent) were clustered on segment q26–28. The probe was hybridized at 50 ng/ml and was then exposed autoradiographically for 27 days. (b) Human metaphase cell hybridized with TCGF probe at 100 ng/ml and exposed for 4 days, illustrating typical labeling of the midportion of the long arm of chromosome 4 (q27–28) (arrow). The TCGF probe was ^{3}H-labeled by nick translation to 3.7×10^7 counts per minute per microgram. (c) Giemsa-banded comparison of human chromosome 4 (*HSA4*) with chromosome B1 (*FCA B1*) of the domestic cat. The outside brackets indicate regions of banding homology. The selected chromosome examples shown are from early metaphase. A consensus schematic of these chromosome pairs is presented below to better illustrate the region of banding homology. Within the homologous region, negatively stained human band q23 contains slightly less chromosomal material than the homologous feline band. The regional portions of enzyme loci *PGM2*, *PEPS*, and *TCGF* are indicated for HSA4.

three grains, represented 20 percent (21 out of 107) of all labeled sites distributed throughout the 60 metaphase spreads. Compilation of grain positions from a large number ($N = 47$) of labeled No. 4 chromosomes indicated significant clustering of grains on segment q26–28 (65 percent) (Fig. 3a). These results are illustrated by the representative metaphase cell in Fig. 3b. Thus, on the basis of this significant labeling of a small segment on the long arm of chromosome 4, we con-

cluded that the TCGF gene was on HSA4q26–28.

The dependence of certain HTLV-producing human cell lymphoma lines on TCGF for proliferation in vitro prompted us to examine these and other human cells for the molecular and chromosomal integrity of the TCGF locus. Restriction enzyme digests (with six enzymes) of nine human cell lines, including the HTLV-infected lines HUT-102 (6) and MJ (16), all expressed the same patterns after Southern blot analysis with the 1.1-kb TCGF molecular probe (*17*). We observed no intraspecific human polymorphisms or any HTLV- or tumor-associated perturbations of the TCGF locus. To examine the chromosomal position of TCGF in an HTLV-associated tumor, we prepared and characterized a panel of 18 somatic cell hybrids between E36 Chinese hamster cells and HTLV-producing human lymphoma HUT-102 B2 with G-11 stain and isozyme markers as described above. TCGF was 100 percent concordant with HSA4 and the associated isozyme markers, *PGM2* and *PEPS*, and appreciably discordant (17 to 60 percent) with the remaining human chromosomes (Figs. 1b and 2b). These results confirm the assignment of *TCGF* to HSA4 and are consistent with the absence of chromosomal or molecular rearrangement of the TCGF locus in the etiology of the HUT-102 lymphoma.

A striking conservation of linkage homology between the genetic maps of the domestic cat and man was recently demonstrated (*11, 18*). When the linkage map of 31 homologous biochemical loci in both species was compared, only a few exceptions to linkage conservation were observed. We used the human TCGF clone and a panel of 37 cat × rodent somatic cell hybrids to map the feline chromosomal homolog of *TCGF*. The panel was expanded and analyzed with human TCGF by the same strategies that we used for the human analysis. The feline TCGF gene was visualized as a pair of fragments of 5.2 and 9.7 kb after digestion of cellular DNA with Eco RI and Southern blot analysis with the 1.1-kb TCGF clone being used as a probe (Fig. 1c). Homologous DNA segments from rodents did not appear in this region of the gels. The two fragments from

cat DNA were precisely concordant in 37 hybrids. The simplest interpretation of this observation is that an Eco RI site exists within the feline DNA sequence homologous to the TCGF probe.

The presence of feline TCGF was 100 percent concordant with feline chromosome B1 and highly discordant (30 to 60 percent) with the other 18 feline chromosomes (Fig. 2c), thereby permitting assignment of the feline TCGF gene to feline chromosome B1 (FCA B1). FCA B1 has previously been implicated as homologous to human chromosome 4 because both chromosomes contain the structural gene for the peptidase-S (*PEPS*) (*11, 18*). To extend this analysis, we sought to examine the possibility of cytological (G-banding) homology between these chromosomes. In Fig. 3c we show high-resolution banding of the feline chromosome B1, and of human chromosome 4 at a similar level of extension. The centromere proximal regions of the long arms of both chromosomes (FCA B1q and HSA4q12–24) displayed nearly identical banding. It is important to consider that the long arms of both human 4q and feline B1q are believed to be ancestral in that they do not contain the chromosome rearrangements that occurred after the divergence of the primate and carnivore orders (*18*). Because of the linkage cytological homologies reported here between the two chromosome arms, we propose that the proximal portions of HSA4q and FCA B1q be added to the five previously defined homologous chromosome segments between the primates and carnivores (*18*).

Our results indicate that human TCGF is encoded by a single locus on human chromosome 4q26–28. The only other lymphokine loci mapped to date in man are those of the interferon family: interferon, leukocyte type, HSA9 (*19*), and interferon, immune type, HSA12 (*20*). Other growth factors have not been chromosomally assigned, although a DNA sequence of human platelet–derived growth factor (PDGF) has recently been shown to be 90 percent homologous to the retroviral oncogene *sis* (*21*), which has been mapped to chromosome 22 (*22*). Presumably, the human homolog of *sis* codes for at least part of PDGF. Another oncogene, c-*raf* (*23*), has two homologous sequences in humans, one of which, c-*raf*-2, has been mapped to human chromosome 4 (*24*). The TCGF locus and c-*raf*-2 do not appear to be identical for two reasons. First, c-*raf*-2 is an apparent pseudogene which has termination signals in each reading frame (*25*). Second, the nucleotide sequences of *TCGF* (*14, 15*) and c-*raf*-2 (*25*) have been determined. A computer-assisted comparison of the two sequences using the ALIGN program (*26*) did not reveal any significant homology. In addition, c-*raf*-2 and *TCGF* are probably not closely linked since at least one of our hybrids, 80H9AC, has the genotype $HSA4^-$, $PGM2^-$, $PEPS^-$, raf-2^+, and $TCGF^-$. This hybrid has an unidentifiable rearranged human chromosome which apparently contains the *raf*-2 segment and none of the other HSA4 loci, including TCGF. The additional 15 human oncogene loci mapped to date are dispersed on other human chromosomes (*27*).

That growth factors may play a role in the onset of neoplasia has been an attractive hypothesis for some time. The near identity of a gene sequence of *PDGF* and v-*sis* has added credence to this hypothesis (*21*). A characteristic translocation involving chromosome 4 (q21) and chromosome 11 has been observed in some cases of acute leukemia (*28*). However, recent phenotypic studies suggesting that the t(4;11)-associated acute leukemia represents a proliferation of myeloid progenitor cells (*29*) as well as the identification of the TCGF gene on q26–28 make it difficult to implicate TCGF in the etiology of this disease. Nonetheless, the occurrence of *TCGF* on chromosome 4 adds an important aspect to the continuing genetic analysis of oncogenes, growth factors, and retroviruses that have been implicated as regulators of normal growth and development as well as in the etiology of neoplasia (*27*).

References and Notes

1. D. A. Morgan, F. W. Ruscetti, R. C. Gallo, *Science* **193**, 1007 (1976); F. W. Ruscetti, D. A. Morgan, R. C. Gallo, *J. Immunol.* **119**, 131 (1977); S. Gillis, M. M. Ferm, W. Ou, K. A. Smith, *ibid.* **120**, 2027 (1978); F. W. Ruscetti, J. W. Mier, R. C. Gallo, *J. Supramol. Struct.* **13**, 229 (1980).
2. J. E. Gootenberg, F. W. Ruscetti, J. W. Mier, A. Gazdar, R. C. Gallo, *J. Exp. Med.* **154**, 1403 (1981).
3. S. Gillis and K. A. Smith, *Nature (London)* **268**, 154 (1977); S. Gillis, P. E. Baker, F. W. Ruscetti, K. A. Smith, *J. Exp. Med.* **148**, 1093 (1978); J. Watson, *ibid.* **150**, 1510 (1979).
4. B. J. Poiesz, F. W. Ruscetti, J. W. Mier, A. M. Woods, R. C. Gallo, *Proc. Natl. Acad. Sci. U.S.A.* **77**, 6815 (1980); R. C. Gallo, B. J. Poiesz, F. W. Ruscetti, in *Modern Trends in Human Leukemia*, R. Neth, R. C. Gallo, T. Graft, K. Mannweiler, K. Winkler, Eds. (Springer-Verlag, Munich, 1981), vol. 5, pp. 502–514.
5. T. Waldmann *et al.*, *Clin. Res.* **31**, 547a (1983).
6. B. J. Poiesz, F. W. Ruscetti, A. F. Gazdar, P. A. Bunn, J. D. Minna, R. C. Gallo, *Proc. Natl. Acad. Sci. U.S.A.* **77**, 7415 (1980).
7. J. W. Mier and R. C. Gallo, *ibid.*, p. 6134.
8. T. Taniguchi, H. Matsui, T. Fujita, C. Takaoka, N. Kashima, R. Yoshimoto, J. Hamuro, *Nature (London)* **302**, 305 (1983).
9. S. Clark *et al.*, in preparation.
10. S. J. O'Brien, W. G. Nash, J. L. Goodwin, D. R. Lowry, E. H. Chang, *Nature (London)* **302**, 839 (1983); S. J. O'Brien, T. I. Bonner, M. Cohen, C. O'Connell, W. G. Nash, *ibid.* **303**, 74 (1983).
11. S. J. O'Brien and W. G. Nash, *Science* **216**, 257 (1982).
12. M. Bobro and J. Cross, *Nature (London)* **251**, 77 (1974).
13. S. J. O'Brien, J. M. Simonson, M. E. Eichelberger, in *Techniques in Somatic Cell Genetics*, J. Shay, Ed. (Plenum, New York, 1982); T. B. Shows and P. J. McAlpine, *Cytogenet. Cell Genet.* **32**, 221 (1982); H. Harris and P. A.

Hopkinson, in *Handbook of Enzyme Electrophoresis in Human Genetics* (North-Holland, Amsterdam, 1976).
14. E. M. Southern, *J. Mol. Biol.* **98**, 503 (1975).
15. M. E. Harper, G. Franchini, J. Love, M. I. Simon, R. C. Gallo, F. Wong-Staal, *Nature (London)* **304**, 169 (1983); M. E. Harper, A. Ullrich, G. F. Saunders, *Proc. Natl. Acad. Sci. U.S.A.* **78**, 4458 (1981); M. E. Harper and G. F. Saunders, *Chromosoma* **83**, 431 (1981).
16. M. Popovic *et al.*, *Science* **219**, 856 (1983).
17. The human cells examined included: HeLa, BeWo, 143B, A673, JAR, WiDR, VA-2 [S. J. O'Brien *et al.*, *In Vitro* **16**, 119 (1980)], HUT-102 B2 p105 (*16*), and MJ (*16*). The restriction endonucleases used were: Eco RI, Pst I, Hind I, Xba I, Hind III, and Sst I. The patterns for all the cells with each restriction enzyme were identical.
18. W. G. Nash and S. J. O'Brien, *Proc. Natl. Acad. Sci. U.S.A.* **79**, 6631 (1982).
19. D. Owerbach *et al.*, *ibid.* **78**, 3123 (1981).
20. S. L. Naylor, A. Y. Sakaguchi, T. B. Shows, M. L. Law, D. Goeddel, P. W. Gray, *J. Exp. Med.* **157**, 1020 (1983).
21. R. F. Doolittle *et al.*, *Science* **221**, 275 (1983); M. D. Waterfield *et al.*, *Nature (London)* **304**, 35 (1983).
22. R. Dalla-Favera, R. C. Gallo, A. Giallongo, C. M. Croce, *Science* **218**, 686 (1982); D. C. Swan, O. W. McBride, K. C. Robbins, D. A. Keithley, E. P. Reddy, S. A. Aaronson, *Proc. Natl. Acad.*

Sci. U.S.A. **79**, 4691 (1982).
23. U. R. Rapp *et al.*, *Proc. Natl. Acad. Sci. U.S.A.* **80**, 4218 (1983).
24. T. I. Bonner, S. J. O'Brien, W. G. Nash, U. R. Rapp, C. C. Morton, P. Leder, *Science* **223**, 71 (1984).
25. G. Mark and U. R. Rapp, personal communication.
26. M. O. Dayhoff and W. C. Barker, *Atlas of Protein Sequence and Structure 1965* (National Biochemical Research Foundation, Washington, D.C., 1978).
27. J. D. Rowley, *Nature (London)* **301**, 290 (1983); see S. J. O'Brien, Ed., *Genetic Maps* [(Cold Spring Harbor Laboratories, Cold Spring Harbor, N.Y., 1984), vol. 3], for complete reference.
28. M. Oshimura, A. I. Freeman, A. A. Sanberg, *Cancer (Brussels)* **40**, 1161 (1977); E. L. Prigogina *et al.*, *Hum. Genet.* **53**, 5 (1979); H. Van Den Berghe *et al.*, *ibid.* **46**, 173 (1979).
29. J. L. Parkin *et al.*, *Blood* **60**, 1321 (1982); M. Nagasaka *et al.*, *ibid.* **61**, 1174 (1983).
30. We thank J. Simonson, R. Bauer, M. Eichelberger, N. White, and J. Love for excellent technical assistance and R. Reeves for discussion and technical advice. We thank G. Mark for communication of the unpublished sequence of c-*raf*-2 and for assistance in the sequence comparisons.

14 September 1983; accepted 26 October 1983

Report

10 February 1984

20. A New Type D Retrovirus Isolated from Macaques with an Immunodeficiency Syndrome

Muthiah D. Daniel, Norval W. King, Norman L. Letvin, Ronald D. Hunt, Prabhat K. Sehgal, and Ronald C. Desrosiers

Endemic immunodeficiency diseases in colonies of macaque monkeys at the New England Regional Primate Research Center (NERPRC) and the California Primate Research Center at Davis have many similarities to the acquired immunodeficiency syndrome (AIDS) in humans (*1, 2*). Consistent immunologic abnormalities have been noted in affected macaques of the NERPRC colony. Proliferative responses of their peripheral blood lymphocytes to antigens and lectins are dramatically diminished (*1*). Furthermore, ratios of the T4 (helper/

inducer) to T8 (suppressor/cytotoxic) circulating T-lymphocytes of the macaques in the colony at greatest risk for developing this syndrome (*Macaca cyclopis*) are considerably less than those in other macaques (*1*). Peripheral blood smears from affected monkeys reveal an immature circulating mononuclear cell with vacuolated cytoplasm and prominent nucleoli (*1*).

We have transmitted spontaneously occurring lymphomas in rhesus monkeys to healthy monkeys by means of tumor cell suspensions (*3*). The recipient animals developed undifferentiated or poorly differentiated lymphomas or parenchymal lymphoproliferative abnormalities suggestive of early lesions of lymphoma. They also developed opportunistic infections with agents such as cytomegalovirus (CMV) and *Cryptosporidium* and showed evidence of an abnormal peripheral blood mononuclear cell morphologically similar to that seen in macaques with the immunodeficiency syndrome. These findings suggested a link between the transmissible lymphomas and the immunodeficiency syndrome in macaques. In fact, by inoculating previously healthy macaques with either tissue or a cell-free filtrate from a macaque lymphoma we were able to transmit the immunodeficiency syndrome (*4*). The recipients developed evidence of profound lymphocyte dysfunction or died with infections by opportunistic agents, including *Candida albicans*, *Cryptosporidium*, and CMV.

These studies implicated an infectious agent in the syndrome. Attempts to isolate a virus from macaques with this syndrome were made by using explant cultures of minced tissues (lymph nodes, spleens, and parenchymal tissues) and by cocultivation of cell suspensions, minced

tissues, and throat and rectal swabs with a battery of indicator cell lines. Viruses identified by these approaches included adenoviruses, simian virus 40 (SV40), CMV, paramyxoviruses including measles virus, and foamy viruses. Viruses were identified on the basis of reactivity in indirect immunofluorescence tests with specific antisera and by electron microscopy. None of these viruses, however, seemed likely to be etiologic in the macaque immunodeficiency syndrome.

We reasoned that since the presumed etiologic virus was causing immunosuppression, we might be able to isolate it by cocultivation of tissue from an infected animal with lymphoid cell lines. We used tissue from two 3-year-old *M. cyclopis* (Mc) in late stages of the immunodeficiency disease. One, Mc 184-80, was dehydrated and had lymphadenopathy (*5*). Peripheral blood mononuclear cells (PBM) from this animal showed no significant in vitro proliferative responses to pokeweed mitogen, concanavalin A, xenogeneic cells, or *Candida albicans* antigen. Lymph node biopsies 1 month before the animal's death revealed an effacement of nodal architecture with an absence of follicles and a depletion of lymphocytes. At necropsy, paramyxovirus inclusions were noted in periportal hepatocytes and CMV inclusions were seen in lymph nodes. Nodular aggregates of mature lymphocytes were seen in the bone marrow.

The second macaque, Mc 398-80, was dehydrated, cachetic, and had generalized lymphadenopathy (*5*). A lymph node biopsy 7 months before the animal's death revealed paracortical hyperplasia and sinus histiocytosis with erythrophagocytosis. CMV was isolated from oral swabs. Although PBM from this animal showed normal in vitro proliferative responses to lectins and antigens, a dramatic depletion of lymphocytes from lymph nodes was noted at necropsy. Furthermore, nodular infiltrates consisting of small, well-differentiated lymphocytes were noted in the kidneys. These unusual findings and the progression of morphological changes in lymph nodes are characteristic pathologic features of the macaque immunodeficiency syndrome (6).

Peripheral blood lymphocytes from Mc 398-80 and Mc 184-80 were cocultivated with Raji cells, a lymphoblastoid B cell line of human origin, and examined microscopically daily with the cell cultures being split at 3- to 4-day intervals. After 7 days, large unusual cells began to appear in the cultures (Fig. 1A). These cells varied in size, with some being as much as 20 times larger than normal Raji cells. Examination of these cells after fixing and staining with hematoxylin and eosin revealed that the smaller cells had one or sometimes two nuclei, whereas the large cells had multiple, closely packed nuclei, often two to four times larger than the nuclei of normal Raji cells (Fig. 1B). The cytoplasm was scant, granular, and usually vacuolated. No inclusion bodies were seen. Electron microscopic examination revealed numerous type D retrovirus particles in the large vacuolated cells (Fig. 1, C to E). Infected cells contained intracytoplasmic A particles that were budding with a complete nucleoid from the cell membrane. Mature particles had a central nucleoid and lacked surface spike projections on their envelope. These findings are characteristic of type D retroviruses.

The original selection of Raji cells for use in these cocultivations was fortuitous since 12 other B and T cell lines did not display the unusual cytopathic changes when infected with this agent.

Several control experiments showed that these results were not due to artifact. Virus was passed from infected cultures to uninfected Raji cells by means of supernatants from the cocultivations passed through a 0.2-μm filter; secondary infections again resulted in the large, bizarre cells. Mason-Pfizer monkey virus (MPMV), a type D retrovirus originally isolated from a mammary neoplasm in a rhesus monkey (*Macaca mulatta*), and squirrel monkey type D retrovirus (SMRV-D) produced the same type of cytopathic effect on Raji cells. Raji cell cultures from four separate laboratories have behaved similarly upon infection with type D retroviruses. Control Raji cell cultures examined by electron microscopy on three separate occasions did not show these virus particles, and the large cells shown in Fig. 1A were never seen in control cultures. The unusual cytopathic effect of this virus on Raji cells has allowed us to titer the virus by limiting dilution; virus titers in the supernatants of infected Raji cell cultures have been shown to exceed 10^6 infectious particles per milliliter.

The Raji cocultivation procedure thus provides an efficient, convenient means for isolating and growing type D retroviruses and does not appear to permit the growth of potential contaminating viruses such as foamy viruses, CMV, and SV40. Cocultivation of infected Raji cell supernatants with indicator monolayer cultures has not revealed the outgrowth of other virus types. We have also isolated type D retrovirus from macaque pharyngeal secretions and from supernatant fluids of lymph node and spleen monolayer cultures using the Raji cocultivation procedure.

The relation of these new virus isolates to MPMV was examined by cutting replicative intermediate DNA (Hirt supernatant DNA) from infected cells with restriction endonucleases and analyzing it by Southern blot hybridization (Fig. 2). Cells infected with D398 (the isolate from Mc 398-80) and D184 (the isolate from Mc 184-80) contained replicative intermediate DNA of about the same size as MPMV (approximately 8.2 kilobase pairs). Approximately ten times more Hirt supernatant DNA from D398

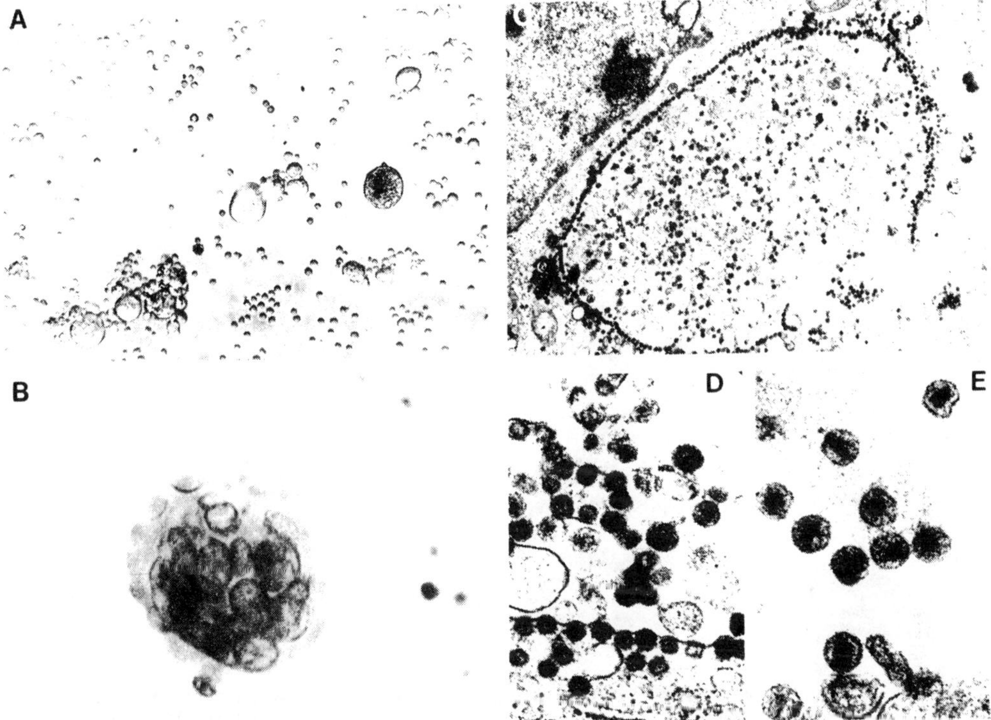

Fig. 1. Raji cells infected with retrovirus isolate from animal Mc 398-80. Approximately 5×10^5 peripheral mononuclear cells from Mc 398-80 were cocultivated with 10^7 Raji cells in 10 ml of RPMI 1640 medium containing 10 percent fetal calf serum. Peripheral mononuclear cells were prepared by Ficoll-Hypaque density gradient centrifugation. Cell cultures were split at 3- to 4-day intervals. For electron microscopy, cell pellets were fixed with 1 percent glutaraldehyde followed by osmium tetroxide and embedded in Epon 812. Thin sections were prepared with an ultramicrotome and stained with uranyl acetate and Sato's lead stain. (A) Large, unusual Raji cells 9 days after cocultivation (Leitz Diavert inverted light microscope, ×340). (B) Large multinucleated Raji cell after fixation and staining with hematoxylin and eosin (×1600). (C) Electron micrograph of a portion of one of the large Raji cells in which there are numerous viral particles aligned around and budding into a cytoplasmic vacuole (×12,000). (D) Higher magnification electron micrograph of a retrovirus-filled vacuole. Numerous cytoplasmic, 90-nm type A retrovirus particles are in the process of budding through the membrane of the vacuole to become enveloped 120-nm type D particles. The enveloped particles are devoid of surface spikes and have a centrally located nucleoid (×60,000). (E) Electron micrograph of a group of extracellular, enveloped viral particles with barrel-shaped nucleoids and blunt knobby surface projections on the envelope, morphologic features characteristic of mature type D retroviruses (×75,000).

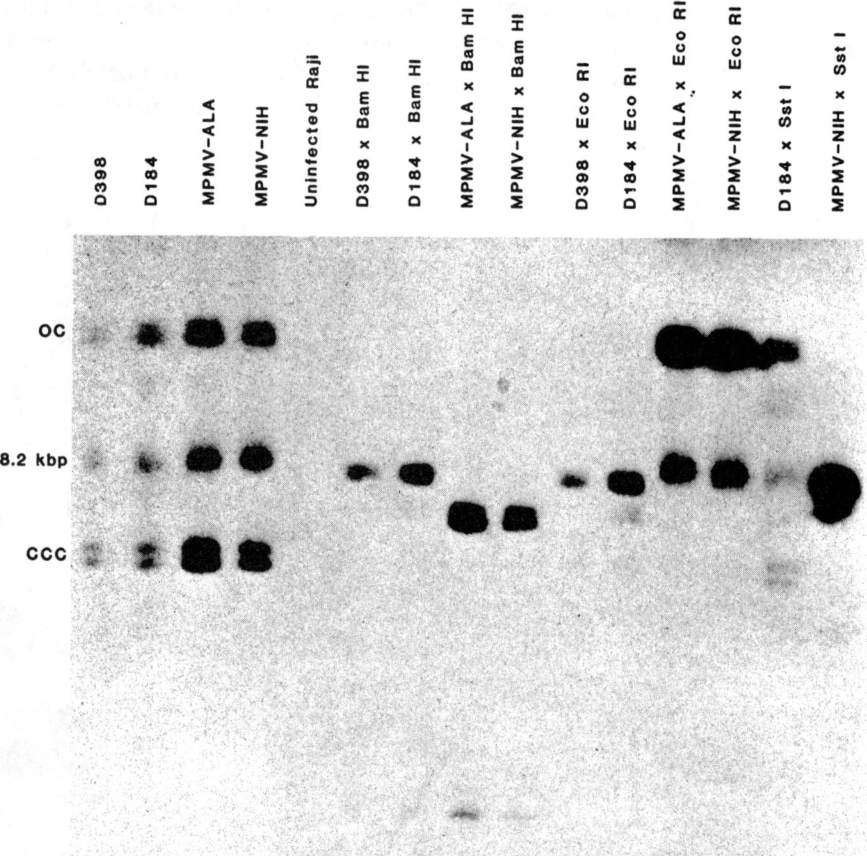

Fig. 2. Relatedness of type D retrovirus isolates to Mason-Pfizer virus by Southern blot hybridization. Raji cells (approximately 3×10^5 per milliliter) were infected with Mason-Pfizer monkey virus (*MPMV*) obtained from two sources (E. Hunter, University of Alabama, and Research Resources, National Institutes of Health), with type D retrovirus from Mc 398-80 (*D398*), and from Mc 184-80 (*D184*) at a multiplicity of infection of approximately 0.1. Virus titers were determined by limiting dilution on Raji cells. Seventy-two hours after infection, the cells were harvested and Hirt supernatant DNA was prepared (*13*). Portions of DNA, uncut or cut with the indicated restriction endonuclease, were subjected to electrophoresis through a 1.0 percent agarose gel and blotted to nitrocellulose by the procedure of Southern (*14*). Eight times more Hirt supernatant DNA from D398 and D184 than from MPMV infected cells was applied to the gel to give similar intensity in the autoradiogram. When equal volumes of the Hirt supernatant DNA's were subjected to electrophoresis in parallel slots, the ethidium bromide stain intensity of the mitochondrial DNA revealed equivalent yields (within 10 percent) from the four infected cultures as well as the uninfected control culture. A ^{32}P-labeled 2.5-kb fragment of MPMV DNA obtained from the cloned DNA pMP-6 (*7*) was hybridized with transferred DNA at 67°C in $4 \times$ SSC (0.6*M* sodium chloride plus 0.06*M* sodium citrate) and 0.1 percent sodium dodecyl sulfate, and the filter was rinsed extensively and placed onto film (*15*). The fragment was purified by electroelution from an agarose gel following digestion of pMP-6 DNA with Hind III. When equal amounts of Hirt supernatant DNA were applied to the gel, lanes containing MPMV DNA gave a much stronger signal (not shown). *CCC* and *OC* correspond, respectively, to the expected locations of covalently closed circular and open circular forms of retroviral DNA; the doublets at these positions probably represent molecules with one and two long terminal repeats.

and D184 infected cells than from MPMV infected cells was required to give approximately equal intensity in the autoradiogram when a ^{32}P-labeled MPMV DNA fragment was used as the hybridization probe. That D398 and D184 are indeed distinct from MPMV is reflected in differences in restriction endonuclease fragmentation patterns (Table 1). For example, while Eco RI and Bam HI cut D398 and D184 DNA once each, Bam HI cut MPMV DNA twice and Eco RI did not cut MPMV DNA at all (Fig. 2). When MPMV DNA was compared to D398 and D184 DNA with Pst I and Hpa II being used as the restriction enzymes, very different fragmentation patterns were observed. We have recently cloned the full length D398 Bam HI fragment into pBR322 and derived detailed restriction endonuclease maps. These maps were compared to MPMV maps (7). Although there were some similarities, especially with Hpa I and Hind III, most (> 50 percent) restriction endonuclease sites were not conserved. Thus these results demonstrate that D398 and D184 are distinct from but related to MPMV. Furthermore, the restriction endonucleases that have been used to date did not show any differences between the D398 and D184 isolates. Restriction endonuclease maps for cloned squirrel monkey type D retrovirus (SMRV-D) DNA (8) also clearly distinguish SMRV-D from D398 and D184 (Table 1).

We obtained additional type D retrovirus isolates from four of seven *M. cyclopis* with lymphadenopathy and neutropenia. Peripheral blood lymphocytes from 34 apparently healthy *M. cyclopis* yielded no type D retrovirus when cocultivated with Raji cells.

Since new type D retrovirus isolates

Table 1. Number of restriction endonuclease cleavage sites in replicative intermediate DNA from infected cells.

Restriction endonuclease	Source of replicative intermediate DNA			
	D398	D184	MPMV	SMRV-D*
Eco RI	1	1	0	1
Bam HI	1	1	2	3
Sst I	0	0	1	3
Kpn I	1	1	1	0

*Data from Chiu *et al.* (8) and Chiu and Aaronson (12).

were obtained from *M. cyclopis* with this immunodeficiency syndrome but not from apparently healthy *M. cyclopis*, one may speculate as to whether this virus is responsible for the endemic disease in our macaque colony. When Fine *et al.* (9) inoculated 68 newborn *M. mulatta* with MPMV, 41 of the monkeys died during the 35 weeks following inoculation with a disease spectrum that included lymphadenopathy, anemia, neutropenia, opportunistic infections, and failure to thrive. These clinical findings are strikingly similar to those in macaques with the immunodeficiency syndrome at NERPRC. Long-term study of experimentally infected juvenile macaques will be needed to determine definitively whether type D retroviruses are indeed the cause of the macaque immunodeficiency syndrome or whether they are opportunistic agents.

It is conceivable that the type D retroviruses of macaques represent an extended family of viruses. In this regard, we have found that endogenous DNA sequences from healthy macaque tissues contain large amounts of DNA homologous to MPMV DNA (10); similar results have been obtained in another laboratory

(*11*). A family of related type D retroviruses could conceivably cause a spectrum of immunodeficiency diseases in nonhuman primates.

References and Notes

1. N. L. Letvin *et al.*, *Proc. Natl. Acad. Sci. U.S.A.* **80**, 2718 (1983).
2. R. V. Henrickson *et al.*, *Lancet* **1983-I**, 388 (1983).
3. R. D. Hunt *et al.*, *Proc. Natl. Acad. Sci. U.S.A.* **80**, 5085 (1983).
4. N. L. Letvin *et al.*, *Lancet* **1983-II**, 599 (1983).
5. Hematologic data for Mc 184-80 were as follows: hemoglobin, 7.4 g/dl with microcytic hypochromic indices; a leukocyte count of $1.5 \times 10^3/\text{mm}^3$ with a differential count of 46 percent neutrophils, 6 percent band forms, 46 percent lymphocytes, and 2 percent monocytes. Hypoproteinemia was detected with total protein 3.3 g/dl, albumin 1.6 g/dl, and globulin 1.7 g/dl. The data for Mc 398-80 were: hemoglobin, 9.6 g/dl with microcytic hypochromic indices; a leukocyte count of $4.8 \times 10^3/\text{mm}^3$ with a differential count of 21 percent neutrophils, 5 percent band forms, 67 percent lymphocytes, 3 percent eosinophils, 2 percent monocytes, and 2 percent blast forms. Liver function tests were normal.
6. N. W. King, R. D. Hunt, N. L. Letvin, *Am. J. Pathol.* **113**, 382 (1983).
7. C. Barker, J. Wills, E. Hunter, in preparation.
8. I.-M. Chiu, P. R. Andersen, S. A. Aaronson, S. R. Tronick, *J. Virol.* **47**, 434 (1983).
9. D. L. Fine *et al.*, *J. Natl. Cancer Inst.* **54**, 651 (1975).
10. R. Desrosiers, in preparation.
11. E. Hunter, personal communication.
12. I.-M. Chiu and S. Aaronson, personal communication.
13. B. Hirt, *J. Mol. Biol.* **26**, 365 (1967).
14. E. M. Southern, *ibid.* **98**, 503 (1975).
15. R. C. Desrosiers, *J. Virol.* **39**, 497 (1981).
16. We thank E. Hunter and S. Aaronson for providing materials and information prior to publication and for helpful discussion, E. Gelmann for interest in this work, and A. Bakker, B. Price, W. Aldrich, and J. MacKey for technical assistance. This work was supported by grants RR00168 from NIH Division of Research Resources and R01-A1 20729 from USPHS.

1 November 1983; accepted 20 December 1983

Report

17 February 1984

21. Lymphokine Production by Cultured Human T Cells Transformed by Human T-Cell Leukemia-Lymphoma Virus-I

S.Z. Salahuddin, P.D. Markham, S.G. Lindner, J. Gootenberg, M. Popovic, H. Hemmi, P.S. Sarin, and R.C. Gallo

T cells play an important role in cell-mediated immunity both as effector cells and as modulators of cell proliferation and function. Many of these T-cell functions are mediated by soluble, biologically active molecules called lymphokines (*1*). These include among others: macrophage migration inhibitory factor (MIF) (*2*), leukocyte migration inhibitory factor (LIF) (*2*), leukocyte migration enhancing factor (MEF) (*2*), neutrophil migration-inhibitory factor (NIF-T) (*3*), macrophage activating factor (MAF) (*4*), differentiation inducing factor (DIF) (*5*), colony stimulatig factor (CSF) (*6*), eosinophil growth and maturation activity (eos. GMA) (*6*), interleukin 3 (IL-3) (*7*), fibroblast activating factor (FAF) (*8*), chemotactic factors (*1*), lymphotoxins (*9*), T-cell growth factor (TCGF) (*10*), B-cell growth factor (BCGF) (*11*), interferon (*12*), and other activities involved with helper and suppressor T-cell function. Some of these activities are well characterized while most essentially remain phenomenological observations not associated with distinct molecules. Progress in biological and biochemical characterization of many of these activities has been hampered by difficulties in obtaining sufficient amounts of active material. The most common sources have been mitogen-stimulated fresh peripheral blood mononuclear cells, some established leukemic T-cell lines (*13*), and hybrid cell lines established by fusion of activated fresh T cells with established T-cell lines (*14*). We and others have also described the production of some biological activities by T-cell lines established in cultures from patients positive for human T-cell leukemia virus (HTLV-I). For example, Gootenberg *et al.* (*15*) described the constitutive production of low levels of TCGF by the cell line HUT 102, and Le *et al.* (*16*) reported that a subclone of this cell line could liberate α- and γ-interferon. Also, cell line MO, established from a patient with a variant of hairy cell leukemia, was reported to liberate γ-interferon and CSF (*17*). MO was subsequently found to produce a subtype of HTLV-I, HTLV-II (*18*). In this report we extend these observations and describe a new approach to the routine production of several human lymphokines based on the development of T-cell lines immortalized in vitro by infection with HTLV-I (*19*).

The T-cell lines were established from patients with HTLV-positive T-cell malignancies (*15*) or from human umbilical cord blood and bone marrow T cells transformed in vitro by HTLV-I (*19*). All of them (Table 1), with the exception of UK, grew without exogenous TCGF. As previosly described (*19*), the HTLV-I–infected cell lines grew with a population doubling time of 40 to 60 hours and reached a saturation density of $1^{-3} \times 10^6$ cells per milliliter. Most of the cell lines [established adult T-cell leukemia-lymphoma donors and HTLV-I–transformed cord blood and adult bone marrow leukocytes] were reactive with monoclonal antibodies Leu 1 (T-cell specific), OKT 11 (E-rosette receptor specific, data not shown).

As shown in Table 2, T lymphocytes from leukemic donors and transformed cord blood were usually positive for the OKT 4/Leu 3a (helper/inducer) phenotype and negative for OKT 8/Leu 2a (cytotoxic/suppressor phenotype) (*19*). Some HTLV-I–transformed bone marrow T cells, however, were OKT 8/Leu 2a positive and OKT4/Leu 3a negative, and some expressed neither set of antigens. The HTLV-I–transformed lymphocytes usually had an atypical, granular-globular staining pattern for nonspecific esterase and acid phosphatase as has been reported for HTLV-I–transformed T lymphocytes. These cells lacked myeloid cytochemical markers, for example, myeloperoxidase and chloroacetate esterase, and B-lymphocyte markers, for example, surface immunoglobulin and Epstein-Barr virus nuclear antigens (*19*). All cell cultures contained HTLV-I–specific nucleic acids, expressed at least low levels of viral proteins (*19*), and with the exception of C43/UK, C63/CR FII, B1/MJ, and B2/CR FII released intact HTLV. The four nonproducer cell lines (Table 1) described here did not release HTLV detectable by banding in sucrose, electron microscopic observation, or by transmission to susceptible cells. However, these cells contained at least one copy per cell of HTLV proviral DNA and transcribed viral RNA, but levels of viral structural proteins were 10- to 100- fold lower than in virus-producing cells (*19, 20*).

Fluid from cell cultures was collected

Table 1. Characteristics of HTLV-I–transformed human T lymphocytes. T cells, initially established in suspension culture from peripheral blood of adult patients with T-cell leukemia-lymphoma, were lethally irradiated and used as a source of virus to infect umbilical cord blood T cells and adult bone marrow T cells by cocultivation procedure. Virus donor cells are represented by the initials of the donor leukemia patient. Other cell lines used are labeled C for cord blood or B for bone marrow followed by sample number in the numerator and the cell line used as a source of HTLV in the denominator. All cell lines shown except UK grew independently of added TCGF. Cell lines C43/UK, C63/CR FII, B2/CR FII, and B1/MJ were nonproductively infected by HTLV.

Culture desig-nation	Surface phenotype*					HTLV protein† p19,p24
	OKT3	OKT4/ Leu 3a	OKT8/ Leu 2a	OKT10	Leu 7	
Cultured leukemic T cells						
CR FII	0	100	0	0	0	90
MJ	40	90	0	0	4	90
UK	100	100	0	0	0	50
Transformed umbilical cord blood T cells						
C9/MJ-1	0	100	0	0	0	80
C9/MJ-2	18	90	0	0	0	85
C10/UK-1	0	80	0	0	0	80
C10/UK-2	45	35	4	10	0	90
CS/MJ	80	70	30	0	0	75
C91/PL	20	50	0	0	0	60
C43/UK	15	90	0	0	0	0
C63/CR FII	20	100	0	0	0	0
Transformed adult bone marrow T cells						
B1/MJ	0	0	0	0	0	0
B2a/MJ	40	20	2	8	4	80
B2b/MJ	30	12	4	10	4	65
B2/UK	80	3	45	4	4	80
B2/CR FII	0	90	0	0	0	0
B3a/MJ	10	15	7	5	0	70
B3b/MJ	5	100	16	4	0	30
B8b/C10UK	8	10	0	0	0	90
B9a/C10UK	23	5	40	5	3	45
B9/C10MJ	0	0	0	0	3	80
B9b/C10UK	15	0	36	10	4	90
B10/C10UK	35	5	45	40	6	8
B11/C10UK	40	8	38	10	5	25

*Cell type specific monoclonal antibodies were used to characterize live cells by an indirect immunofluorescence procedure (*19*). Numbers indicate the percentage of positive cells reacting with the indicated antibody. In addition, all cell cultures were negative for surface-bound immunoglobulins, Epstein-Barr virus nuclear antigen, OKT6 and OKM1, and positive for HLA-DR antigens (780 percent) and TCGF receptors (750 percent).   †Antibodies to purified HTLV structural proteins p24 and p19 were used in indirect immunofluorescence assays on fixed cells (*19*). Numbers indicated the percentage of positive cells.

Table 2. Lymphokines released by HTLV-I–transformed human T lymphocytes. The cultures were as described in the legend for Table 1. Serial dilutions of conditioned media, collected from cell lines 24 to 48 hours after a change of medium, were tested for the indicated activities and compared to standard positive control samples as described in the text. For MIF, a migration index of ≤ 0.8 indicates activity. Supernatant fluids from PPD-treated normal human mononuclear leukocytes were used as positive controls. For LIF and MEF, a migration index of ≤ 0.08 represents LIF and ≥ 1.2 MEF activity. For MAF, an activity of ≥ 20 percent was considered significant. Fluids from concanavalin A–treated human monocytes were used as a positive control with 40 to 50 percent cytotoxicity. For DIF, + indicates 500 to 1000 U/ml; + +, 1000 to 10,000 U/ml; + + +, > 10,000 U/ml; and −, < 500 U/ml. For CSF, values represent the number of colonies (≥ 50 cells per colony) per 10^5 fresh bone marrow cells seeded in 0.33 percent agarose. Eos. GMA, assessed as the ability of conditioned media to induce and support cell division and maturation of eosinophils from fresh bone marrow or umbilical cord blood. Symbols: +, maturation and one cell doubling; + +, maturation and two to four cell doublings in 2 weeks; + + +, maturation and more than four doublings in 2 weeks; −, no growth and negligible maturation. For FAF, + indicates that labeled thymidine incorporation in resting human fibroblast cells was about two times greater than with medium only; −, indicates an activity less than twice that of background. For interferon, the data are expressed as international units of interferon activity compared to a 5000 U/ml standard.

Culture designation	MIF (migration index)	LIF/MEF (migration index)	MAF (% cytotoxicity)	DIF (U/ml)	CSA (colonies/ 10^5 cells)	Eos. GMA	FAF	Interferon −PHA/+PHA (U/ml)
				Biological activities				
Cultured leukemic T cells								
CR FII	0.22	1.40	< 20	+	150	+ + +	+	14/0
MJ		0.75	< 20	+	50	+ + +	+	0/0
UK		0.62	< 20		5	+ + +	−	
Transformed umbilical cord blood T cells								
C9/MJ-1	0.55	0.70	< 20	+ +	40	+	+	0/0
C9/MJ-2		1.25	< 20	+ +	60		+	0/0
C10/UK-1			< 20	+ + +	125	+ + +	+	0/0
C10/MJ-2	0.62	1.05	31	+ + +	0	+ + +	+	0/0
C5/MJ	0.51	1.20	21	+	50		−	0/0
C91/PL	0.34	1.30	< 20	+	40		+	0
C43/UK	0.31	1.40	35	+ +	70	+ + +	−	0/0
C63/CR FII	0.67	1.70	36	+ + +	40	+ + +	+	0/0
Transformed adult bone marrow T cells								
B1/MJ	0.67	1.00	< 20	+ + +	25	+	+	0/600
B2a/MJ	0.38	0.60	26	+	60	+	+	0/0
B2b/MJ		0.55	72	+ +	60	+	+	524/3900
B2/UK			54	+	75	+	+	
B2/CR FII			< 20	+ + +	30	+ + +	+	832/416
B3a/MJ	0.51		73	+	50	+	+	39/0
B3b/MJ				+	0			0/0
B8b/C10UK		0.75	67	+ +	65	+ +	+	39/0
B9a/C10UK	0.40	1.70	< 20	+ +	75	−	−	212/316
B9/C10MJ			< 20	+	100			0/0
B9b/C10UK		0.70			56	+	−	4400/4062
B10/C10UK	0.56	0.70	< 20	+	95	+	+	1400/4054
B11/C10UK			< 20	+	60		+	274/2400

24 to 48 hours after a complete media change, and was clarified by low-speed centrifugation and filtration (0.22 μm). Serial dilutions were tested for biological activity by established procedures. All media and reagents were screened for endotoxin activity and only endotoxin-free materials were tested. As positive controls we used conditioned media from normal human peripheral blood mononuclear leukocytes stimulated with mitogen. In addition to the HTLV-transformed T-cell lines listed in Table 2, fluids from other sources were tested and found negative for the activities described in this report. For example, the media and fetal calf serum used for growing all the cell cultures, conditioned media from a "pre–T-cell" line established from a leukemic patient [Molt 4 (21)], B-cell lines from normal donors (22), and long-term myeloid and monocytic cell cultures (23) were tested. Some of the monocytic cells did liberate lymphocyte activating factor (LAF), prostaglandin E, lysozyme, and CSF (data not shown).

MIF, defined as the ability to inhibit the migration of fresh human macrophages, was tested by a microcapillary procedure (2, 24, 25). The area (in square centimeters) of migration of treated versus untreated adult peripheral blood macrophages (25) was expressed as a migration index. Cell culture fluids from normal human mononuclear leukocytes treated with purified protein derivative (PPD) were used as positive controls for MIF. Compared to untreated macrophages with a migration index ranging from 0.80 to 1.20, macrophages treated with conditioned media from several cell lines had a reduced migration index, that is, ≤ 0.80 (Table 2).

LIF, defined as a factor involved in restricting granulocyte migration from the site of an inflammatory response,

and MEF, a factor that enhances this migration, were assayed in the same way as MIF (24). The responder cells were mature granulocytes prepared from adult peripheral blood by differential centrifugation in Ficoll-Hypaque. Fluids from several cell lines either restricted leukocyte migration (migration index of ≤ 0.80, defined as LIF activity) or stimulated leukocyte migration (migration index of ≥ 1.20, or less defined as MEF activity).

MAF, a factor that nonspecifically activates macrophages for extracellular killing, was tested by a procedure described by Fidler *et al.* (26). Monocyte-macrophages, prepared as for the MIF assay, were first "activated" by incubation for 24 hours either with conditioned medium from the HTLV-I–transformed T-cell lines or with MAF-positive supernatant fluids collected from concanavalin A–treated human peripheral blood monocytes. Both resulted in a 40 to 50 percent level of cytotoxicity. The activated cells were then added to radiolabeled melanoma cell line A376 and, after an additional 72 hours of incubation, the cytolytic effect was determined by measuring the residual radioactivity in the melanoma cells. MAF activity is expressed as the percentage of cytotoxicity compared to that obtained with nonactivated cells. Approximately one-half of the cell lines tested released a significant amount (≥ 20 percent) of activity (Table 2).

DIF, a factor released by activated lymphocytes that induces the morphological and functional maturation of human myeloid leukemia cells (5), was assayed by incubation of the promyelocytic cell line HL-60 (27) for 4 days in the presence of 10 n*M* retinoic acid (5) and increasing concentrations of test cell fluids. Differentiation of HL-60 was determined by the increased number of cells able to reduce nitroblue tetrazolium or to phagocytize yeast (28). Media from all cell lines assayed induced HL60 maturation and contained DIF ranging from 500 to 2000 U/ml (Table 2).

CSF, a family of factors able to support the growth and maturation of monocytes and granulocytes in semisolid medium (6, 23, 29), was assayed by incubating fresh bone marrow leukocytes in 0.3 percent agarose containing various concentrations of test fluids. Many of the cell lines released CSF at levels comparable to or higher than positive control samples from a human trophoblast cell line (30) (Table 2). The type of cells forming the colonies were granulocytic or monocytic as determined by Wright-Giemsa staining of colonies picked from the agarose plates or by staining in situ (31) (data not shown).

Eos. GMA, a factor that supports the maturation and cell division of fresh eosinophils in vitro (6), was assayed by incubation of conditioned media from T-cell lines with fresh bone marrow or cord blood mononuclear leukocytes. In positive samples the usually small population of recognizable eosinophils was rapidly expanded by a combination of limited cell replication and maturation of immature cells (Table 2). The resulting cell population was > 90 percent eosino- as confirmed by Luxol fast blue staining and electron microscopic examination for characteristic granuoles (data not shown).

FAF, a product of human peripheral blood lymphocytes that stimulates the active proliferation of quiescent fibroblasts (8), was assayed by testing the ability to stimulate [^{3}H]thymidine uptake in resting cells from fibroblast cell line CCD1SK in an assay described by Schmidt *et al.* (32). Conditioned media

from many of the cell lines were positive in this assay (Table 2). This biological activity is similar to that described for platelet-derived growth factor (PDGF) (33). By means of immunopurification techniques with hyperimmune sera against purified human PDGF, cell lysates from all of the HTLV-I–transformed cell lines tested contained material related to PDGF (34).

Interferon, which belongs to a family of glycoproteins liberated by lymphocytes, exhibits a potent effect on virus replication and cell growth. Interferon was assayed by a plaque-reduction technique in which we used vesticular stomatitis virus (VSV) with monolayers of the human cell line WISH as a target (35). Test samples collected from the cell line were induced, or not induced, by exposure to phytohemagglutinin-P (PHA-P; 5 µg/ml for 24 hours) and incubated with target cells for 24 hours before infection with VSV. Interferon activity, measured by comparison to an international standard (5000 U/ml), was not detected in fluids from induced or uninduced cells established from T-cell leukemia-lymphoma patients or from HTLV-transformed cord blood T cells (Table 2). However, several HTLV-transformed bone marrow cell lines produced substantial levels of interferon, often without PHA-P induction. This activity was destroyed (≥ 80 percent) by treatment at *p*H 2 for 24 hours, suggesting that the activity was caused by γ-interferon (12, 35) (data not shown). Whether or not all HTLV-I-positive cells liberate γ-interferon needs further investigation. All cell lines examined, including some found negative for interferon production in the biological assay, transcribe detectable levels of polyadenylate-containing RNA recognized by cloned γ-interferon complementary DNA assayed by Northern

108

blot procedures (*36*).

TCGF (also known as interleukin-2) is liberated by activated T lymphocytes and participates in the regulation of T-cell growth (*10, 37*). Cell culture fluids concentrated 20 times and eluates from intact T cells treated at low *p*H (*15*) were examined for TCGF activity by a thymidine uptake procedure (*37*). TCGF was detected at low levels in conditioned media or bound to the cell membrane of some cell lines established from adult T-cell leukemia-lymphoma patients, for example, CR and MJ. However, with the exception of membrane-bound TCGF detected on C9/MJ-1, no activity was associated with any of the other HTLV-I–transformed cord blood or bone marrow T cells (data not shown).

In addition to the factors described in Table 2, tests for other biological activities were performed. For example, IL-3, an activity liberated by mitogen-activated lymphocytes which supports the growth of immature hemotopoietic cells in vitro, was produced by many of the cell lines (*38*). Also BCGF, assayed by a thymidine uptake procedure (*39*), was produced by some cell lines (data not shown).

Several biologically active molecules produced by monocytic cells [lymphocyte activating factor (LAF), prostaglandin E, and lysozyme] were also assayed. Prostaglandin E and lysozyme, assayed by radioimmunoassay and a radial diffusion procedure (*23*) were not detected. However, a low level of LAF, assayed with fresh thymocytes from C3H/HEJ mice as indicator cells (*40*), was detected in some of the cell lines tested (*41*).

The biological activities described herein were detected in unconcentrated tissue culture fluids from most of the HTLV-positive T-cell lines studied and, in contrast to nonactivated T cells from normal donors (*1*), they were constitutively produced in most instances. No attempt was made to optimize the expression or recovery of the activities and it is likely that higher levels of activity could be obtained with proper manipulation. The role HTLV plays in the induction of lymphokine synthesis is unclear. It is not known, for example, whether the lymphokines described would normally be produced by the subsets of T cells infected by HTLV-I or whether infection by HTLV-I induces their synthesis. It is clear that a productive HTLV infection is not necessary since transformed cells not producing virus, for example C43/UK, C63/CR FII, B2/CR FII, and B1/MJ, also produce the lymphokines. These HTLV-transformed nonproducer T-cell lines will be of particular value in the study of these lymphokines since they reduce the potential biohazard caused by the presence of HTLV.

The ability to establish immortalized T-cell lines by infection with HTLV should prove useful for studies of the biological activities detected, some of which are otherwise difficult to obtain in large quantities. The HTLV-transformed T cells should also provide sources of messenger RNA for the genetic cloning of the biological factors.

References and Notes

1. J. W. Hadden, J. R. Sadlik, A. H. Warfel, *The Lymphokines, Biochemistry and Biological Activity*, J. W. Hadden and W. E. Steward, II, Eds. (Humana Press, Clifton, N.J., 1981), p. 73; J. P. Dumonde, *Nature (London)* **244**, 38 (1969).
2. R. E. Rocklin, *J. Immunol.* **116**, 816 (1976).
3. R. H. Weisbart, R. Billing, D. Golde, *J. Lab. Clin. Med.* **93** (No. 4), 622 (1979).
4. R. B. Herberman *et al.*, *Immunol. Rev.* **44**, 43 (1979).
5. I. L. Olsson, T. Olofsson, N. Maaritzon, *J. Natl. Cancer Inst.* **67**, 1225 (1981); I. L. Olsson, T. R. Breitman, R. C. Gallo, *Cancer Res.* **42**, 3298 (1982); T. R. Breitman, B. R. Keene, H. Heimmi, *Cancer Survey*, E. Rozengurt and M. B. Spoon, Eds. (Oxford Univ. Press, London, in press).

6. R. E. Stanley, *Proc. Natl. Acad. Sci. U.S.A.* **76**, 2969 (1979); J. T. Prival, M. Paran, R. C. Gallo, A. M. Wu, *J. Natl. Cancer Inst.* **53**, 1583 (1974); C. Tarella, F. W. Ruscetti, B. J. Poiesz, A. Woods, R. C. Gallo, *Blood* **59**, 1330 (1982).
7. J. N. Ihle, L. Pepersack, L. Rebar, *J. Immunol.* **126**, 2184 (1981).
8. S. M. Wahl and C. L. Gately, *ibid.* **130**, 1226 (1983).
9. B. W. Papermaster, M. E. Smith, J. E. McEntire, in *The Lymphokines, Biochemistry and Biological Activity*, J. W. Hadden and W. E. Stewart II, Eds. (Humana Press, Clifton, N.J., 1981), p. 149.
10. D. A. Morgan, F. W. Ruscetti, R. C. Gallo, *Science* **193**, 1007 (1976).
11. M. Howard *et al.*, *J. Exp. Med.* **155**, 914 (1982).
12. J. E. Blalock, J. A. Georgiades, M. P. Langford, H. M. Johnson, *Cell. Immunol.* **49**, 390 (1980).
13. D. W. Golde, S. G. Quan, M. J. Cline, *Blood* **57**, 1068 (1978); L. Chess, R. E. Rocklin, R. P. McDermott, J. R. David, S. F. Schlossman, *J. Immunol.* **115**, 315 (1975).
14. T. L. Ratliff, D. L. Thomasson, R. E. McCool, W. J. Catalona, *Cell. Immunol.* **68**, 311 (1982); J. Le *et al.*, *J. Immunol.* **130**, 1231 (1983).
15. J. E. Gootenberg, F. W. Ruscetti, R. C. Gallo, *J. Immunol.* **129**, 1499 (1982).
16. J. Le, W. Pronsky, D. Henriksen, J. Vilcek, *Cell. Immunol.* **72**, 157 (1982).
17. I. Nathan, J. E. Gropman, S. G. Quan, N. Bersch, D. W. Golde, *Nature (London)* **292**, 842 (1981).
18. V. S. Kalyanaraman, M. G. Sarngadharan, B. J. Poiesz, F. W. Ruscetti, R. C. Gallo, *J. Virol.* **38**, 906 (1981).
19. B. J. Poiesz, F. W. Ruscetti, M. S. Reitz, V. S. Kalyanaraman, R. C. Gallo, *Nature (London)* **294**, 268 (1981); M. Popovic *et al.*, *Science* **219**, 856 (1983); P. D. Markham *et al.*, *Int. J. Cancer* **31**, 413 (1983); S. Z. Salahuddin *et al.*, *Virology*, **129**, 51 (1983).
20. S. Z. Salahuddin *et al.*, unpublished data.
21. B. I. S. Srivastava and J. Minowada, *Biochem. Biophys. Res. Commun.* **51**, 529 (1973).
22. P. D. Markham, F. Ruscetti, Z. Salahuddin, R. E. Gallagher, R. C. Gallo, *Int. J. Cancer* **23**, 148 (1979).
23. S. Z. Salahuddin *et al.*, *Blood* **58**, 931 (1981); S. Z. Salahuddin, P. D. Markham, R. C. Gallo, *J. Exp. Med.* **155**, 1842 (1982).
24. B. A. Maurer *et al.*, *Immunopharmacology* **1**, 57 (1978).
25. E. S. Klanerman, A. J. Schroit, W. E. Folger, I. J. Fidler, *J. Clin. Invest.*, in press.
26. I. J. Fidler, *J. Natl. Cancer Inst.* **55**, 1159 (1975).
27. S. J. Collins, R. C. Gallo, R. E. Gallagher, *Nature (London)* **270**, 347 (1977).
28. T. R. Breitman, S. E. Selnic, S. J. Collins, *Proc. Natl. Acad. Sci. U.S.A.* **77**, 2936 (1980).
29. T. R. Bradley and D. Metcalf, *Aust. J. Expt. Biol. Med. Sci.* **77**, 6134 (1966); D. H. Pluznik and L. Sachs, *J. Cell. Comp. Physiol.* **66**, 319 (1966).
30. F. W. Ruscetti, J. Y. Chou, R. C. Gallo, *Blood* **59**, 86 (1982).
31. J. Lidbeck and J. C. Marson, *Exp. Hematol.* **7**, 166 (1979).
32. J. A. Schmidt, S. B. Mizel, D. Cohen, I. Green, *J. Immunol.* **128**, 2177 (1982).
33. H. N. Antoniades, *Proc. Natl. Acad. Sci. U.S.A.* **78**, 7314 (1981).
34. S. Z. Salahuddin, T. Pantazis, P. D. Markham, H. N. Antoniades, R. C. Gallo, unpublished data.
35. R. D. Arbirt, P. Leary, M. J. Levin, *Infect. Immun.* **35**, 383 (1982).
36. S. Avya and R. C. Gallo, unpublished data.
37. J. W. Mier and R. C. Gallo, *Proc. Natl. Acad. Sci. U.S.A.* **77**, 6134 (1980).
38. J. Ihle, S. Z. Salahuddin, P. D. Markham, R. C. Gallo, unpublished data.
39. A. Maizel *et al.*, *Proc. Natl. Acad. Sci. U.S.A.* **79**, 5998 (1982).
40. I. Grey, R. K. Gershon, B. H. Waksman, *J. Exp. Med.* **136**, 128 (1972).
41. G. Cannon, S. Z. Salahuddin, P. D. Markham, R. C. Gallo, unpublished data.
42. We thank I. J. Fidler for certain of the MAF assays, G. Cannon (Litton Bionetics) for the MIF, LIF/MEF, MAF, and FAF assays, and A. Patel, S. Roberson, B. Read, and A. Fladager for technical assistance. S.G.L. was supported by grant 344/1-1 from the Deutsche Forschungsgemeinschaff.

14 October 1983; accepted 14 December 1983

22.   Simian AIDS: Isolation of a Type D Retrovirus and Transmission of the Disease

Preston A. Marx, Donald H. Maul, Kent G. Osborn, Nicholas W. Lerche, Peggy Moody, Linda J. Lowenstine, Roy V. Henrickson, Larry O. Arthur, Raymond V. Gilden, Maneth Gravell, William T. London, John L. Sever, Jay A. Levy, Robert J. Munn, and Murray B. Gardner

The simian acquired immunodeficiency syndrome (SAIDS), which occurs endemically in colonies of macaque monkeys in the United States (*1, 2*), resembles the acquired immunodeficiency syndrome (AIDS) in humans in overall clinical manifestations, pathology, and immune deficiency. However, in the simian form of the disease, the ratio of helper to suppressor T cells is not reversed, nor is there a high incidence of *Pneumocystis carinii* pneumonia in affected monkeys. By means of a filterable agent present in tissue extracts and plasma of sick monkeys, SAIDS has been transmitted to healthy monkeys (*2, 3*). Here we report the isolation of a new type D retrovirus resembling Mason-Pfizer monkey virus (MPMV) from the blood of two rhesus monkeys (*Macaca mulatta*) with SAIDS. The virus was grown in tissue culture, and tissue culture fluids were used to transmit SAIDS to juvenile rhesus monkeys.

In a study of some of the biophysical properties of the then unidentified etiologic agent, we obtained plasma from an infected monkey (RM-20265) and mixed it in the cold (for 20 minutes) with an equal volume of ether to destroy the infectivity of ether-sensitive agents. Un-

treated plasma and ether-treated plasma were each inoculated into juvenile rhesus monkeys. After 6 months, the two animals that received ether-treated plasma remained healthy whereas the four animals that received untreated plasma developed SAIDS as defined previously (*1, 4*). Plasma from a rhesus monkey with SAIDS was subjected to ultracentrifugation, and the pellet, after being suspended in phosphate-buffered saline, was centrifuged to equilibrium in a 20 to 60 percent linear sucrose gradient. The gradient was divided into six fractions, and each fraction was inoculated intravenously into rhesus monkeys. Only the lightest two fractions (1.14 to 1.18 g/ml average density) transmitted SAIDS to recipient monkeys. These data indicated that the SAIDS agent had the physical properties of an enveloped virus.

The studies that led to the isolation of the SAIDS agent are summarized in Fig. 1. RM-18610 was a 3-year-old female with spontaneously occurring SAIDS (*5*). A mixture of tissue homogenates from RM-18610 was inoculated into RM-B883, who developed SAIDS 4 months later. A heparinized blood sample from RM-B883 was inoculated intravenously into two 12-month-old monkeys (RM-

Fig. 1. Schematic diagram of the SAIDS transmission studies which led to the isolation of a type D retrovirus and production of disease. Symbols: **, alive with overt clinical SAIDS; ***, dead from SAIDS. Dates are shown for the different steps of the studies. Numbers prefixed by RM- are identification numbers for rhesus monkeys. The monkeys were colony-bred and maintained in facilities accredited by the American Association for the Accreditation of Laboratory Animal Care. RM-18610 was a 3-year-old female. The other monkeys are also female and range in age from 1 to 2 years. To initiate the culture C1132, we exposed confluent primary rhesus monkey kidney cells (Rh-MK: M.A. Bioproducts, Walkersville, Maryland) to whole blood for 18 hours, then washed the cells free of blood and maintained them with minimum essential medium (Gibco) containing 10 percent fetal calf serum, 100 mM glutamine, and

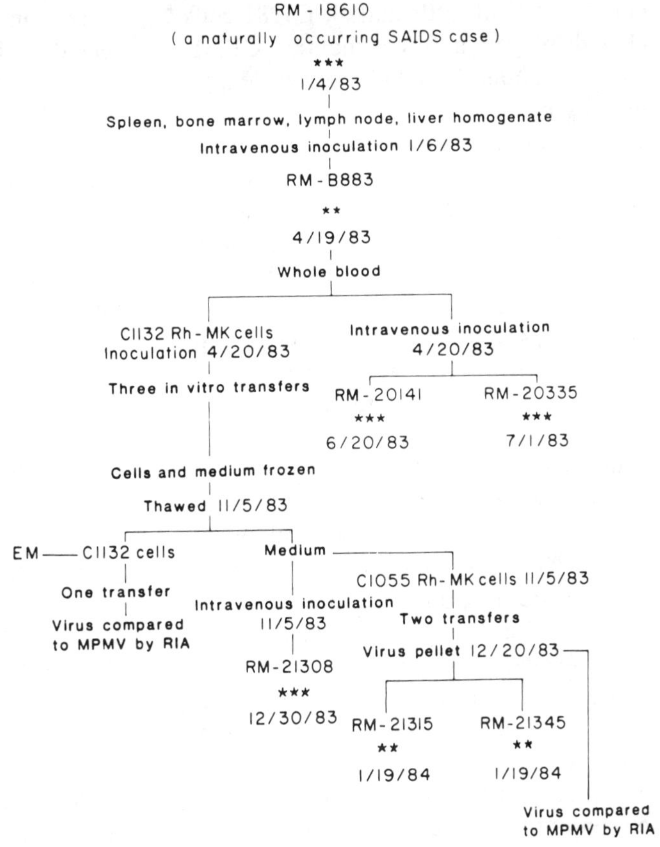

100 U of penicillin and 100 µg of streptomycin per milliliter. C1055 was initiated by treating subconfluent primary Rh-MK cells with Polybrene (5 µg/ml) for 24 hours and then inoculating the cultures with tissue culture fluid from C1132 (*EM*, electron microscopy).

20141, RM-20335) and into primary rhesus monkey kidney (Rh-MK) cells (culture C1132). RM-20141 and RM-20335 had an accelerated course of the disease and were moribund from SAIDS by 60 and 65 days after inoculation. Their symptoms were typical, and included generalized lymphadenopathy, splenomegaly, neutropenia, diarrhea, weight loss, and lymphoid depletion (*1–5*).

Cultures C1132 and C1281 (the latter being inoculated with blood from a different SAIDS case, RM-20265) were selected for further study because the blood used to infect these cultures had produced SAIDS in juvenile rhesus monkeys (*3*). Cells from the two cultures were passaged three times and a portion was prepared for electron microscopy and for hemadsorption assays. Some cells were stored in liquid nitrogen and their culture media were frozen at −70°C. C1132 cells displayed no cytopathic effect, but a few syncytia were noted. The culture was negative in the hemadsorption assay against the red cells of eight species (rhesus monkey, human, chicken, rabbit, guinea pig,

112

goose, rat, and rattlesnake). C1281 cells also displayed a few syncytia. C1281, and subsequently C1132, when examined by electron microscopy, had particles resembling type D retroviruses ranging in size from 110 to 130 nm (Fig. 2). Occasional budding particles, characteristic precursors of type D virions, were seen (6, 7). Uninfected Rh-MK cells showed no virus particles.

For transmission studies in vivo (Fig. 1), 4.0 ml of frozen medium from C1132 was thawed and inoculated intravenously into RM-21308, an 18-month-old female. This animal developed neutropenia, generalized lymphadenopathy, and splenomegaly after 16 days and by 30 days after inoculation had a decreased lymphocyte response to the mitogens concanavalin A, phytohemagglutinin, and pokeweed mitogen. At 52 days, the moribund animal was killed. Lymphoid tissue sections showed lymphoid depletion typical of SAIDS (1, 4). Two juvenile monkeys inoculated with comparable amounts of uninfected Rh-MK culture fluids still remain healthy 5 months after inoculation.

To confirm this observation, we subjected medium from C1132 to ultracentrifugation (50,000g) and, resuspended the pellet in fresh culture medium. Portions of this suspension were inoculated onto fresh Rh-MK cells (C1055). After two passages, 120 ml of the C1055 medium was subjected to ultracentrifugation, the pellet was resuspended in culture medium, and portions of the suspension were inoculated intravenously, without freezing, into two juvenile females (RM-21315 and RM-21345). These monkeys developed, by 16 days after inoculation, generalized lymphadenopathy, splenomegaly, and neutropenia, and their peripheral lymphocytes showed a decreased mitogenic response. Lymph nodes biopsied on days 16 and 23 showed changes typical of SAIDS. These two animals are still alive with SAIDS 8 weeks after inoculation.

No sex differences in susceptibility to SAIDS have been observed (1–5). In the present studies, two juvenile male monkeys (1 to 2 years old) inoculated with culture fluids from C1055 have developed the early signs of SAIDS 4 weeks

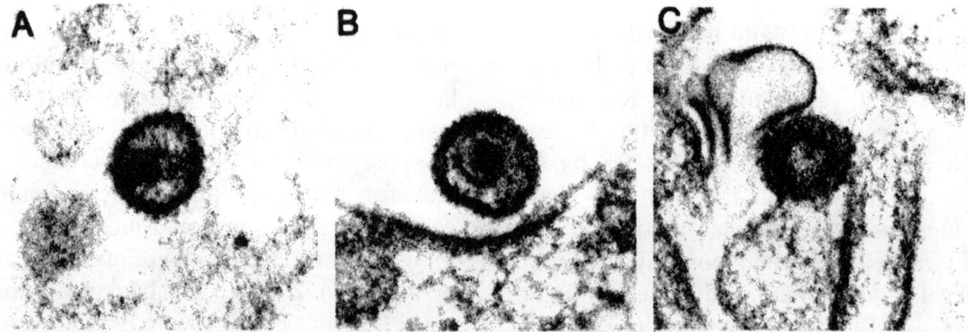

Fig. 2. (A and B) Transmission electron microscopy of thin sections of (A) C1132 cells and (B) C1281 cells stained with uranyl acetate and lead citrate. Cells were trypsinized, centrifuged, and fixed in Karnovsky's solution (18). (A) A virion is shown with the cylindrical core characteristic of type D retroviruses (7). (B) a similar particle is shown sectioned perpendicular to the virion in (A). (C) C1132 cells containing a budding virion with a ring-shaped core characteristic of type D retroviruses. (×100,000)

after inoculation (generalized lymphadenopathy and splenomegaly).

The tissue culture fluids used in the SAIDS transmission experiments were assayed for antigens of MPMV, a type D retrovirus originally isolated from a rhesus monkey with a spontaneously occurring breast tumor (7). Viral pellets prepared by ultracentrifugation showed complete competition in a homologous radioimmunoassay (RIA) for the MPMV core antigen p27 (Fig. 3A). The slopes of the competition curves were similar to the slope of the MPMV standard indicating a close antigenic relationship to MPMV p27. The endogenous type D virus of langur monkeys (*Presbytis* species) (PO-1-Lu) also competed in the assay. This result was not surprising since PO-1-Lu is genetically related to MPMV (7). In contrast, pellets prepared from C1132 and C1055 did not compete in a homologous RIA for the MPMV envelope glycoprotein gp70 (Fig. 3B), even when viral antigen concentrates were 250-fold more than necessary for detectable competition. Mouse mammary tumor virus, Rauscher murine leukemia virus, and human T-cell leukemia virus type 1 (HTLV-1) did not compete in either assay. Thus the gp70 in the culture fluids may be antigenically different from MPMV gp70 or may have been sheared during ultracentrifugation. This latter explanation seems unlikely since pelleted virus was highly infectious for rhesus monkeys and Rh-MK cells, and the infectious agent sedimented as an enveloped virus in a sucrose gradient.

Pellets prepared by ultracentrifugation of medium from C1055 were found to be negative in an RIA broadly reactive for type C viruses. In this assay we used antiserum (8) prepared in goats by sequential immunization with purified core proteins of several type C retroviruses. The radiolabeled antigen in the assay

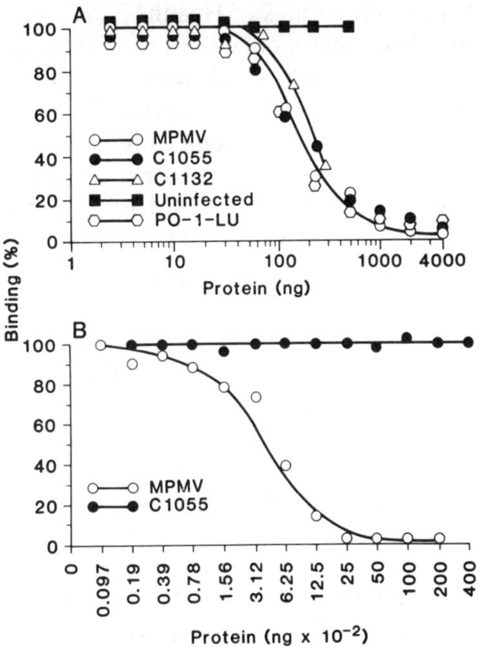

Fig. 3. Homologous RIA for (A) MPMV p27 and (B) MPMV gp70. Pellets obtained by ultracentrifugation of cultures were disrupted by 1 hour of incubation in 0.01M tris-HC1, pH 7.8, 0.1M NaCl, 0.001M EDTA, 0.1 percent Triton X-100 and 0.05 percent sodium desoxycholate, and then tested in twofold serial dilutions for ability to compete with ^{125}I-labeled viral proteins for binding limiting amounts of antisera. Antisera and unlabeled antigen were incubated for 1 hour at 37°C, and then ^{125}I-labeled antigen was added (20,000 count/min). After incubation for 1 hour at 37°C and overnight at 4°C, antigen-antibody complexes were precipitated by addition of 20 μl of *Staphylococcus aureus* (10 percent) and centrifugation at 2500g for 30 minutes. Radioactivity in the pellets was determined in a gamma counter. All the results were normalized to 100 percent binding in the absence of competing antigens.

was the p28 core protein of the endogenous primate type C virus (CPC-1). The viral pellets were also negative when tested in an RIA for the HTLV-1 core antigen p24. These results suggest that type C viruses are not present in C1055.

Studies were also conducted at the

National Institutes of Health. Pooled serum from two monkeys (RM-20414 and RM-20322) with spontaneously occurring SAIDS at the California Primate Research Center was sent to NIH where it was inoculated into two male rhesus monkeys, RM-B991 and RM-B992, both of which developed SAIDS. Pooled filtrates of serum (0.45 μm pore size) from these monkeys were inoculated into RM-E17. When RM-E17 developed advanced SAIDS, 1.0 ml of serum was collected and used to inoculate primary bone marrow cells (5×10^7 cells per 75-cm^2 vessel) obtained from a normal rhesus monkey. Cultures were maintained at 37°C in enriched McCoy 5a medium containing 0.1 μM hydrocortisone and 25 percent fetal calf serum. After five serial passages, high reverse transcriptase activity was detected in fluids collected from adherent fibroblast cells of the bone marrow cell culture. After four additional passages of the infected fibroblasts, a virus was purified from the culture fluids by isopycnic banding in a neutral sucrose gradient. The fraction occurring in the ultraviolet absorption peak at 1.15 g/ml was inoculated into two rhesus monkeys (RM-E427 and RM-B959). Both animals developed SAIDS after 5 weeks and died at 8 weeks. Type D retrovirus was seen by electron microscopy in the fraction occurring at 1.15 g/ml, and the reverse transcriptase activity associated with this band showed a preference for Mg^{2+} when tested with polyriboadenylate · oligodeoxyribothymidylate$_{12 \text{ to } 18}$ and polyribocytidlyate · oligodeoxyriboguanylate$_{12 \text{ to } 18}$ (9). These are all characteristics of type D retroviruses.

Thus a type D retrovirus that is partially related to MPMV appears to be the etiologic agent of SAIDS in the macaques at the California Primate Research Center. This virus contains the core protein but not a detectable envelope glycoprotein of MPMV and has been repeatedly isolated from cells inoculated with blood from monkeys with SAIDS. Its etiologic role in SAIDS must be further confirmed by neutralization with appropriate antisera and with molecular and biologically cloned isolates. A similar virus grown in Raji cells has been obtained from macaques with SAIDS at the New England Regional Primate Center (10), although successful induction of SAIDS with virus grown in Raji cells was not reported. The restriction endonuclease cleavage pattern of our retrovirus isolate appears to be identical to that of the New England isolate (10, 11).

The association of this type of retrovirus with SAIDS is not unexpected. After the initial isolation of MPMV (7), early passage virus was inoculated into newborn rhesus monkeys and, although no tumors occurred, almost all animals developed a syndrome very similar to SAIDS (12). However, later in vitro passages of MPMV were nonpathogenic for newborn rhesus monkeys (12). Our review of the histopathology of one such monkey dying in 1972 showed lymphoid depletion typical of SAIDS. A mixture of type C and type D retroviruses was also recently isolated from a pigtailed macaque (*Macaca nemestrina*) with enzootic retroperitoneal fibrosis at the University of Washington Primate Center (13). This isolate was lost during cultivation in vitro and is not available for comparison with the SAIDS retrovirus (13).

These results focus further attention on the role of retroviruses in the etiology of human AIDS (14). They also indicate that the blood stream is a source of the SAIDS virus. However, in contrast to the murine (15) and feline (16) models of retrovirus-induced immunosuppression, the amount of virus in SAIDS plasma and tissue is very low ($\leq 10^4$ particles per milliliter), (*17*) and the virus is a type D rather than type C retrovirus. This simian model should prove useful for determining how an infectious retrovirus causes depletion of lymphoid cells and for the development of measures for controlling SAIDS in primates.

References and Notes

1. R. V. Henrickson *et al.*, *Lancet* **1983-I**, 388 (1983).
2. R. D. Hunt *et al.*, *Proc. Natl. Acad. Sci. U.S.A.* **80**, 5085 (1983); N. L. Letvin *et al.*, *Lancet* **1983-II**, 599 (1983).
3. M. Gravell *et al.*, *Science* **223**, 74 (1984).
4. K. G. Osborn *et al.*, *Am. J. Pathol.* **114**, 94 (1984).
5. W. T. London *et al.*, *Lancet* **1983-II**, 869 (1983).
6. M. A. Gonda *et al.*, *Arch. Virol.* **56**, 297 (1978).
7. D. Fine and G. Schochetman, *Cancer Res.* **38**, 3123 (1978).
8. R. V. Gilden, *Adv. Cancer Res.* **22**, 157 (1975).
9. M. Gravell, in preparation.
10. M. D. Daniel *et al.*, *Science* **223**, 602 (1984).
11. E. Hunter, personal communication.
12. D. L. Fine *et al.*, *J. Natl. Cancer Inst.* **54**, 651 (1975); D. Fine, personal communication.
13. E. Hefti, *Virology* **127**, 309 (1983); S. Panem, personal communication.
14. M. Essex *et al.*, *Science* **220**, 859 (1983); E. P. Gelmann *et al.*, *ibid.*, p. 862; R. C. Gallo *et al.*, *ibid.*, p. 865; F. Barré-Sinoussi *et al.*, *ibid.*, p. 868.
15. H. Friedman and W. S. Ceglowski, in *Progress in Immunology*, B. Amos, Ed. (Academic Press, New York, 1971), pp. 815–829.
16. M. Essex, *Am. J. Vet. Res.* **34**, 809 (1973).
17. P. Marx, in preparation.
18. M. J. Karnovsky, *J. Cell Biol.* **27**, 137A (1965).
19. We thank M. Bryant, R. Cardiff, D. Fine, E. Hunter, and C. Barker for discussions; R. Cork, J. Katilus, B. Bencken, J. Bess, A. Spinner, R. Beards, J. Tribble, J. Lund, and M. Bleviss for technical assistance; L. Click and A. Dean for manuscript preparation; C. Sarason for artwork; and the Federal Express Corporation for overnight delivery. Supported by grants RR00169, AI20573-01, contract N01-CO-23910, and Interagency Agreement from Blood Division, NHLBI with Division of Research Resources, NIH, and by special appropriation from the state of California.

20 January 1984; accepted 13 February 1984

Report

9 March 1984

23. T-Cell Growth Factor Gene: Lack of Expression in Human T-Cell Leukemia-Lymphoma Virus-Infected Cells

Suresh K. Arya, Flossie Wong-Staal, and Robert C. Gallo

T-cell growth factor (TCGF, interleukin 2) is required for the continuous proliferation of specifically activated mature T lymphocytes (*1*). Similarly, some neoplastic mature T cells require TCGF for their growth in vitro, although in some cases without the requirement of prior antigen and lectin activation (*2*). This is apparently because at least some of these cells already possess TCGF receptors (*3*). Some mature T cells infected with human T-cell leukemia-lymphoma virus (HTLV) require TCGF for growth early in culture. Subsequently, many of the HTLV-infected cell lines become independent of exogenously added TCGF (*4*). Some of these cell lines constitutively produce and respond to their own TCGF (*3*), while other cell lines do not elaborate detectable extracellular TCGF (*5*). The question thus arises whether the latter cell lines are truly independent of TCGF or produce small quantities of TCGF, sufficient for growth but undetectable by conventional assay procedures. Moreover, it is possible that these HTLV-infected cells produce TCGF that is not externalized and that would not be detected in extracellular medium. A more direct answer to this question could be obtained from a study of TCGF messenger RNA (mRNA) in these cells. This is now possible because a human TCGF complementary DNA (cDNA) sequence has been molecularly cloned (*6, 7*), providing a sensitive probe for evaluating the expression of the TCGF gene. We have previously demonstrated that the production of TCGF is regulated at the transcriptional level (*7*). Therefore, if these cell lines synthesize TCGF, whether externalized or not, they would be expected to contain TCGF mRNA. Here we show that several of the TCGF-independent cell lines do not contain detectable TCGF mRNA, suggesting that the immortalization of mature T cells by HTLV may sometimes be by mechanisms that bypass the TCGF-TCGF receptor system.

The TCGF gene recently cloned from a normal human lymphocyte cDNA library (*7*) was identical to the clone from the human lymphoma Jurkat cell line (*6*) and contained the complete coding sequence for TCGF, in addition to 5′ and 3′ untranslated sequences. We have shown that this gene is transcribed into an 11S to 12S mRNA in all human TCGF-producing cells (*7*). To determine if such an mRNA species was also present in HTLV-infected cells, we analyzed polyadenylate [poly(A)]-containing RNA from these cells by the Northern blot procedure, using cloned TCGF DNA as a probe (Fig. 1). The cell lines examined included those derived from HTLV-positive T-cell malignancies (HUT 102, MO, MI, and MJ), those obtained by HTLV infection of normal human cord blood and bone marrow cells in vitro (C5/MJ, C10/MJ, B2/UK, and MT-2), and an uninfected mature neoplastic T-cell line (HUT 78) (see legend to Fig. 1). The Jurkat cell line, which produces abundant TCGF upon stimulation with phytohemagglutinin (PHA) and 12-*O*-tetradecanoylphorbol-13-acetate (TPA) (*7, 8*), served as a positive control.

As expected, 11S to 12S TCGF mRNA was readily detected in stimulated Jurkat cells. A similar mRNA species was also detected in HTLV-infected HUT 102 and MO cells, and also in HUT 78 cells. We estimate (*9*) that Jurkat, MO, and HUT 102 cells, respectively, contain about 40 to 50, 5 to 10, and less than 5 copies of TCGF mRNA per cell. None of the other HTLV-infected cells contained detectable TCGF mRNA. Since TPA in combination with PHA increases the level of TCGF mRNA in some cells (*7*), a number of HTLV-infected cells were also examined after treatment with TPA and PHA. This treatment did not cause the induction of TCGF mRNA in cells that were previously negative (Fig. 1). It was possible that some of these cells synthesized TCGF mRNA that was only distantly related to our cloned TCGF sequence. Such an mRNA could possibly arise from the use of an alternative splicing mechanism or possible polymorphism of the TCGF gene. This was tested by lowering the stringency of hybridization and hybrid detection. Instead of the 50 percent formamide used under standard conditions (see legend to Fig. 1), 40 percent formamide was used. This is equivalent to reducing the temperature at which hybridization was performed by

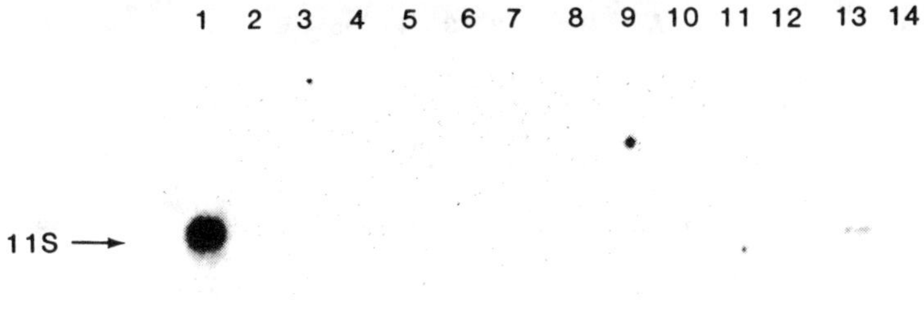

Fig. 1. Expression of TCGF gene in HTLV-infected cells. Poly(A)-selected RNA, size-separated by agarose gel electrophoresis, was hybridized with labeled cloned TCGF DNA.

11S →

Lanes 1 to 14 are for RNA from: 1, PHA plus TPA-stimulated Jurkat cells; 2, TCGF-independent HUT 78 cells; 3, TCGF-independent HUT 102 cells; 4, another preparation of TCGF-independent HUT 102 cells; 5, TCGF-independent C5/MJ cells; 6, TCGF-dependent C5/MJ cells; 7, TCGF-independent C10/MJ cells; 8, TCGF-independent C10/MJ cells treated with TPA-PHA; 9, TCGF-independent B2/UK cells; 10, TCGF-independent B2/UK cells treated with TPA-PHA; 11, TCGF-independent MT-2 cells; 12, TCGF-dependent MI cells; 13, TCGF-independent MO cells; and 14, TCGF-independent Molt 4 cells (immature T). Poly(A)-selected RNA was obtained as described (15). After denaturation at 65°C in 50 percent formamide, RNA (10 μg per lane) was subjected to electrophoresis in 1 percent agarose slab gel containing 6 percent formaldehyde and transferred to a Zeta Probe membrane (Bio-Rad Laboratories) by electroelution (7). Hybridization with ^{32}P-labeled nick-translated cloned TCGF DNA was performed at 37°C for 16 hours in a mixture containing 50 percent formamide, five times standard sodium chloride and sodium citrate (SSC, 0.15M NaCl and 0.015M sodium citrate, pH 7), 0.05M sodium phosphate buffer (pH 7), five times PM (0.02 percent each of bovine serum albumin, polyvinylpyrrolidone, and Ficoll 400), yeast RNA (200 μg/ml), denatured DNA (20 μg/ml), 0.1 percent sodium dodecyl sulfate (SDS), and 10 percent dextran sulfate. The membrane was subsequently washed repeatedly with SSC and 0.1 percent SDS at 65°C, air dried, and exposed to a Kodak XAR film with the use of intensifying screens. Where indicated, cells were treated with TPA (10 ng/ml) and PHA (1 μg/ml) for 20 hours.

about 7°C. In addition, the filters were washed at 45°C instead of 65°C as under standard conditions. While TCGF mRNA was readily detected in cell lines that gave positive results under standard conditions, such mRNA was not detected in negative cell lines even under reduced strirgency conditions (data not shown).

To ensure that the integrity of RNA was maintained during the hybridization procedure, we used two additional probes spanning the 12S to 18S mRNA range: namely, cloned γ-interferon (γ-IFN) DNA and a cloned sequence designated JD15. The latter cloned DNA was obtained from a Jurkat cDNA library and is specifically expressed in stimulated lymphocytes (10). As shown in Fig. 2, the γ-IFN probe detected a specific 12S to 13S mRNA species in C5/MJ, C10/MJ,

B2/UK, and MI cells, and the level of this mRNA was increased by treatment with PHA and TPA. Further, all the HTLV-infected cell lines contained varying amounts of 17S to 18S mRNA corresponding to cloned JD15 DNA. Thus, the lack of detectable TCGF mRNA in some HTLV-infected cells was not due to the degradation of RNA. It is interesting that there was a reverse correlation between the synthesis of TCGF and γ-IFN mRNA in these cells. Though TCGF may stimulate γ-IFN production by normal peripheral blood lymphocytes (11), γ-IFN mRNA was synthesized in these HTLV-infected cells without the concomitant synthesis of TCGF mRNA. Conversely, Jurkat cells stimulated with PHA and TPA synthesized TCGF mRNA in the absence of γ-IFN mRNA (Figs. 1 and 2). As expected,

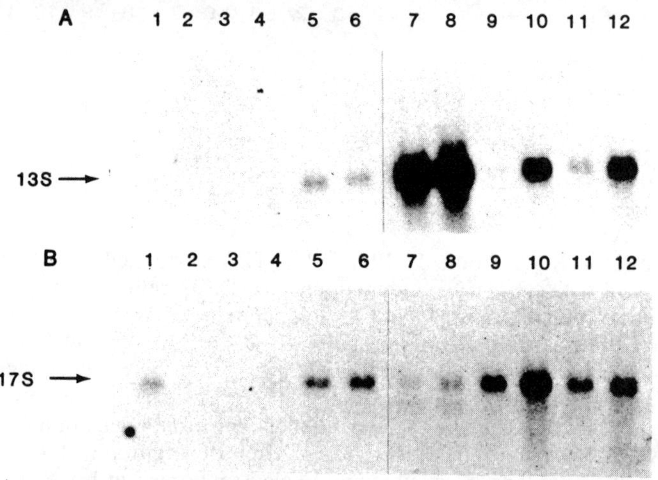

Fig. 2. Expression of (A) γ-interferon gene and (B) JD15 gene in HTLV-infected cells. Analysis was performed as described in the legend to Fig. 1. Lanes 1 to 12 contain the same RNA's as in lanes 1 to 12 of Fig. 1.

PHA-stimulated normal lymphocytes synthesized both TCGF and γ-IFN mRNA's (data not shown).

Two primary HTLV-infected neoplastic cell lines (HUT 102 and MO) contained TCGF mRNA; the level in HUT 102 was barely detectable. These cells are known to produce low levels of TCGF (3) and it has been postulated that the continued abnormal proliferation of these transformed cells may be due to the concomitant presence of cells bearing TCGF receptors and cells producing TCGF (12). Two other primary HTLV-infected cell lines (MI and MJ), whether dependent or independent of added TCGF for growth, did not contain detectable TCGF mRNA. The cell lines infected with HTLV in vitro, such as C5/MJ, C10/MJ, B2/UK, and MT-2, which grow independently of added TCGF (4, 13), also did not contain detectable levels of TCGF mRNA. The lack of detectable TCGF mRNA in these cells was not due to the poor quality of RNA preparations or other artifacts. It was also not due to a selective loss of this mRNA during poly(A) selection, since total unselected RNA gave the same results as poly(A)-selected RNA (data not shown). Thus, these cells appeared to be truly independent of TCGF for growth. Since the procedure used here can detect one or a few copies of TCGF mRNA per cell (9), the results rule out an autostimulation mechanism in which each cell produces and responds to its own TCGF (12). Some of these cell lines have been examined by in situ hybridization. Of hundreds of cells examined, not a single cell displaying a specific hybridization signal with the TCGF probe was detected (14). Thus, no cell in the population appeared to express TCGF mRNA, suggesting that a parastimulation mechanism, in which a few cells in a population produce sufficient TCGF to sustain the growth of the population, was also not evident.

These results suggest that TCGF production is not always needed for the growth of HTLV-infected T cells. Since all cells possess TCGF receptors (3), it is possible that changes in or influences on

TCGF receptors are sufficient for continued T-cell growth without the need for any growth factor. Alternatively, it is possible that a protein not related to TCGF produced by normal lymphocytes stimulates proliferation of some neoplastic T cells. If this is the case, this protein must also be significantly different from the TCGF released by such neoplastic T cells as Jurkat, since the normal and Jurkat TCGF gene and mRNA are identical (7). In either case, cells transformed by HTLV may use other mechanisms to regulate control.

References and Notes

1. D. A. Morgan, F. W. Ruscetti, R. C. Gallo, *Science* 193, 1007 (1980); K. A. Smith, S. Gillis, P. E. Baker, D. McKenzie, F. Ruscetti, *Ann. N.Y. Acad. Sci.* 332, 423 (1979); J. W. Mier and R. C. Gallo, *Proc. Natl. Acad. Sci. U.S.A.* 77, 6134 (1980); B. M. Stadler, S. F. Dougherty, J. J. Farrar, J. J. Oppenheim, *J. Immunol.* 127, 1491 (1981).
2. B. J. Poiesz, F. W. Ruscetti, J. W. Mier, A. M. Woods, R. C. Gallo, *Proc. Natl. Acad. Sci. U.S.A.* 77, 6815 (1980); F. W. Ruscetti and R. C. Gallo, *Blood* 57, 379 (1981).
3. J. E. Gootenberg, F. W. Ruscetti, J. W. Mier, A. Gazdar, R.C. Gallo, *J. Exp. Med.* 154, 1403 (1981); R. J. Robb, *Immunobiology* 161, 21 (1982); T. A. Waldmann *et al.*, *Clin. Res.* 31, 547A (1983).
4. M. Popovic *et al.*, *Science* 219, 856 (1983); P. D. Markham *et al.*, *Int. J. Cancer* 31, 413 (1983).
5. J. Gootenberg, M. Popovic, P. Markham, R. C. Gallo, unpublished results.
6. T. Tanigushi, H. Matsui, T. Fujita, C. Takaoka, N. Kashima, R. Yoshimoto, J. Hamuro, *Nature (London)* 302, 305 (1983).
7. S. C. Clark, S. K. Arya, F. Wong-Staal, *Proc. Natl. Acad. Sci. U.S.A.*, in press.
8. S. Gillis and J. Watson, *J. Exp. Med.* 152, 1709 (1980).
9. E. H. Westin *et al.*, *Proc. Natl. Acad. Sci. U.S.A.* 79, 2490 (1982).
10. S. K. Arya, unpublished results.
11. T. Kasahara, J. J. Hooks, S. F. Dougherty, J. J. Oppenheim, *J. Immunol.* 130, 1784 (1983).
12. R. C. Gallo, *Blood Cells* 7, 313 (1981).
13. I. Miyoshi, I. Kubonishi, S. Yoshimoto, *Nature (London)* 294, 770 (1981).
14. C. C. Trainor and M. S. Reitz, personal communication.
15. S. K. Arya, *Nature (London)* 284, 71 (1980); *Int. J. Biochem.* 14, 19 (1982).
16. We thank S. C. Clark of Genetics Institute, Boston, for MO RNA and γ-IFN probe.

25 November 1983; accepted 29 December 1983

Report

16 March 1984

24. Novel Viral Sequences Related to Human T-Cell Leukemia Virus in T Cells of a Seropositive Baboon

Hong-Guang Guo, Flossie Wong-Staal, and Robert C. Gallo

Human T-cell leukemia virus (HTLV) is a family of related T-cell tropic retroviruses associated with a specific subtype of mature T-cell malignancy in man (1). Two subgroups of HTLV have been identified thus far. Members of the first subgroup, HTLV-I, are highly related to each other, if not identical. These include the initial isolates of the virus in the United States (2, 3) as well as additional isolates from patients in this country (4, 5), Israel (4), South America (4), Japan (4, 6), and the Caribbean (4). Members of the second subgroup, HTLV-II, are only distantly related to HTLV-I as determined by serological cross-reactivities of their proteins (7) and molecular hybridization studies with cloned viral genomes (8, 9). Only two HTLV-II isolates have been obtained,

120

the first from a patient with a T-cell variant of hairy cell leukemia, and the second from a patient with acquired immunodeficiency syndrome (AIDS) (*10*). Recently, antibodies against HTLV antigens have been found in several Old World monkey species, including Japanese and Chinese macaques, African green monkeys, and baboons (*11–13*). It has been proposed that HTLV can be spread between macaques and humans in Japan (*11*). However, we have evidence that macaques are also seropositive in regions of Japan where HTLV is not endemic in the human population (*13*), suggesting independent entries of the virus into man and other primates. We have analyzed DNA from a T-cell line established from a baboon that was seropositive for HTLV antigens. We found the viral sequences to be related to but distinct from HTLV-I and HTLV-II.

A T-lymphocyte cell line (991-ICC) was established from peripheral leukocytes of a baboon (*Papio cynocephalus*) that is seropositive for HTLV antigens by the enzyme-linked immunosorbent assay (ELISA). The baboon was a recipient of cellular material (bone marrow, lymph node, spleen, and peripheral blood) from a leukemic baboon from Sukumi, U.S.S.R., as part of a U.S.–U.S.S.R. joint virology study during 1973–1975 (*14*). The cell line releases typical type-C particles and extracellular reverse transcriptase, and reacts positively with a monoclonal antibody against the 19,000 dalton core protein (p19) of HTLV as well as a hyperimmune antibody against HTLV p24 (*15*).

High molecular weight DNA from 991-ICC was examined for the presence of HTLV-related sequences by Southern blot hybridization (Fig. 1). DNA from cell lines infected with HTLV-I (lane 1) and HTLV-II (lane 3) were used as posi-

tive controls and uninfected human cells were used as a negative control. DNA from many primates, including baboons, lacks sequences closely related to HTLV (data not shown). The restriction endonuclease Sst I cuts in the long terminal repeat (LTR) of many HTLV-I isolates and in the LTR, as well as internally in HTLV-II. When it was used to cut 991-ICC DNA a single band of 8.5 kb was produced that hybridized to the cloned HTLV-I genome. A similar size band was observed in the DNA of HTLV-I infected cells, corresponding to a complete genome with one LTR. This result indicates that like HTLV-I, the provirus in 991-ICC is only cut in the LTR by Sst I. However, Bam HI, which yields a characteristic internal band in all known HTLV-I isolates and two internal bands of 5.0 kb and 3.5 kb in HTLV-II, did not give discernible discrete bands in 991-ICC DNA, suggesting that Bam HI may cut not at all or once in the provirus of 991-ICC and that the infected cell population is polyclonal. Pst I, which gives three internal bands of 2.4, 1.6, and 1.3 kb with HTLV-I genomes, generated four detectable bands of 1.7, 1.5, 1.3, and 0.9 kb from 991-ICC DNA. The multiple high molecular weight bands are probably junction fragments. Thus these experiments indicate that the provirus in 991-ICC is distinct from HTLV-I and HTLV-II. Hybridization to an HTLV-II probe revealed specific bands in HTLV-I and HTLV-II DNA but not in 991-ICC (Fig. 2), indicating the baboon provirus is more related to HTLV-I than to HTLV-II.

To determine whether the provirus in 991-ICC is homologous to only a restricted portion of HTLV-I, we used the complete clone as well as subclones containing only *pol* or *env*-pX sequences of HTLV-I. pX is a region at the 3′ end of

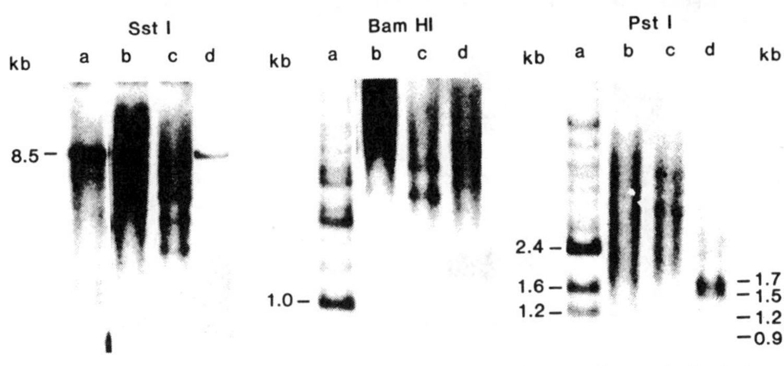

Fig. 1. The distinction between the provirus in 991-ICC and HTLV-I and HTLV-II. DNA from CH, an HTLV-I infected cell line (lane a), normal human thymus (lane b), MO, an HTLV-II infected cell line (lane c), and 991-ICC (lane d) were digested with the enzymes Sst I, Bam HI, and Pst I as shown, subjected to electrophoresis in 0.8 percent agarose gels, and transferred to nitrocellulose filters (20). Hybridization was carried out with ^{32}P-labeled DNA representing the complete HTLV-I genome that has been purified away from the vector on agarose gels. After incubation at 37°C for 20 hours in a solution containing triple-strength standard saline citrate, 50 percent formamide, 20 percent dextran sulfate, and 5× Denhardt's solution [0.1 percent bovine serum albumin, Ficoll, polyvinylpyrrolidone] and ^{32}P-labeled HTLV DNA (2 × 10^6 count/min), the filters were washed with two changes of double-strength SSC and 0.1 percent sodium dodecyl sulfate (SDS) at room temperature for 10 minutes each and at 65°C for another 10 minutes. Autoradiography was for 20 to 48 hours.

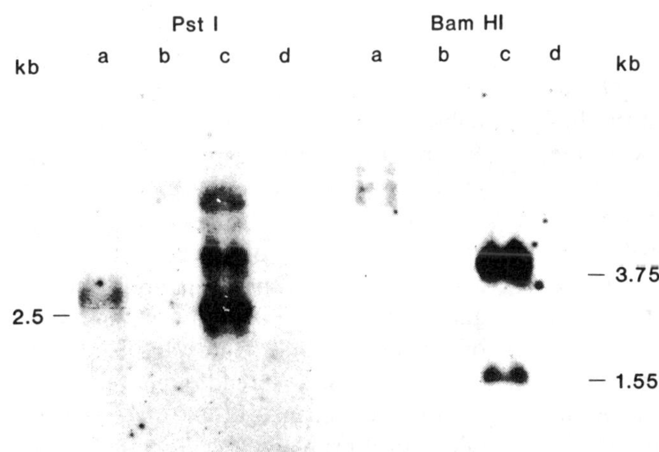

Fig. 2. Lack of detectable homology of 991-ICC provirus to HTLV-II. Duplicate filters, prepared as described in legend to Fig. 1, were hybridized to a subclone of HTLV-II corresponding to 2.5 kb of 3' sequences. As in Fig. 1, lanes a to d are, respectively, CH (HTLV-I), normal thymus, MO (HTLV-II), and 991-ICC.

the HTLV genome that has open reading frames for several small peptides (16). With the Pst I digestion, we were able to detect strong hybridization using all three probes (Fig. 3A) and we can assign the 1.7-kb band in the *pol* region, the 1.5-kb band overlapping the *pol* and *env* regions, and the 0.9-kb band in the *env* region. The 1.2-kb band detected by the total HTLV-I genome is probably located in the *gag* region for which a subclone is not available. All the hybridizable bands withstand stringent washing conditions of 0.5× SSC (standard saline citrate) and 65°C (Fig. 3B), suggesting that they are closely related to HTLV-I over

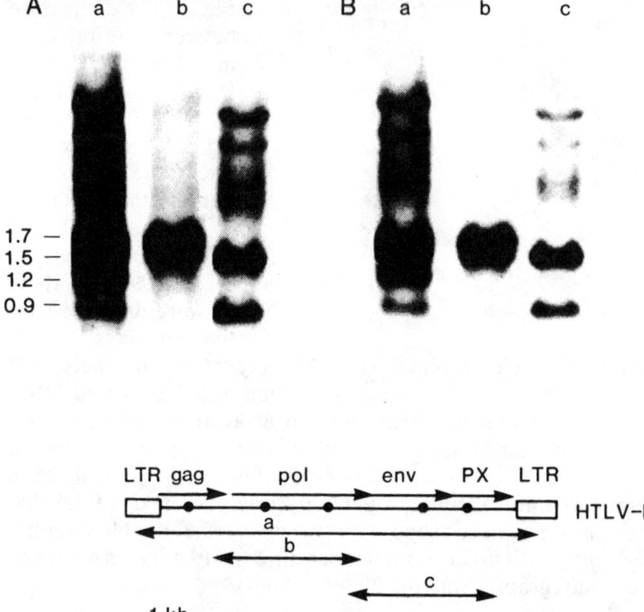

Fig. 3. Hybridization of specific HTLV-I probes to the 991-ICC provirus. 991-ICC DNA was digested with Pst I and blot hybridized to the entire HTLV-I genome (probe a), HTLV-I *pol* sequences (probe b), and *env*-pX sequences (probe c). The filters were washed in (A) double-strength SSC and 0.1 percent SDS at room temperature, and (B) 0.5× SSC and 0.1 percent SDS at 65°C.

the entire genome. The relatively weak hybridization signal of 991-ICC DNA to the HTLV-I probe compared to the homologous control (see Fig. 1) may be due to infection of only a small percentage of the 991-ICC cells. In fact, immunofluorescence analysis of these cells with antibodies against HTLV antigens showed that less than 10 percent of the cells express viral antigens (*15*).

The provirus that we have identified in cultured T lymphocytes from a baboon, although related to HTLV-I, is clearly distinct from all known HTLV-I isolates. Serological surveys have demonstrated clusters of HTLV carriers in southwestern Japan, the Caribbean basin, parts of South America, southeastern United States, and Africa. In the United States, healthy carriers of the virus are unusual and are found mainly in rural black populations. Although the survey of primates for a related virus has been less extensive, several Old World monkey species,

including Japanese and Chinese macaques and African green monkeys and baboons, have been seropositive (*15*). In Japan, the distribution of virus in primates is much wider than in the human population (*15*). These observations suggest that the entry of virus into primates and man occurred independently and argues against a present-day transmission of virus between primates and man. Because of the widespread infection of Africans and because of the presence of Old World primates, including baboons, in Africa, we proposed that the origin of HTLV in the Caribbean, the United States, and South America was from entry of infected Africans to the Americas (*17*). Further, HTLV may have been brought to Japan by the 16th century Portuguese seamen who also had contact with Africa (*17*). Isolates of HTLV-I from patients in the United States, Japan, the Caribbean, and South America are closely related, if not identical, by restriction enzyme mapping (*8, 18*). Our present data suggest that the virus found in one baboon is related to but distinct from HTLV-I. Yamamoto *et al.* (*19*) have found that HTLV and a virus from an African green monkey contain identical core antigens but distinguishable envelope proteins. We also have evidence that more than one virus variant occurs in Old World monkeys (not shown), suggesting that infection of primates may have occurred much earlier than infection of man. Like HTLV, the primate viruses are T-cell tropic. We propose to name these viruses PTLV for primate T-lymphotropic viruses. Whether PTLV are involved in leukemogenesis in primates remains to be determined.

References and Notes

1. R. C. Gallo *et al.*, *Cancer Res.* **43**, 3892 (1983).
2. B. J. Poiesz *et al.*, *Proc. Natl. Acad. Sci. U.S.A.* **77**, 7415 (1980).
3. B. J. Poiesz, F. W. Ruscetti, M. S. Reitz, V. S. Kalyanaraman, R. C. Gallo, *Nature (London)* **294**, 268 (1981).
4. M. Popovic *et al.*, *Science* **219**, 856 (1983).
5. B. F. Haynes *et al.*, *Proc. Natl. Acad. Sci. U.S.A.* **80**, 2054 (1983).
6. I. Miyoshi *et al.*, *Nature (London)* **294**, 770 (1981).
7. V. S. Kalyanaraman *et al.*, *Science* **218**, 571 (1982).
8. F. Wong-Staal *et al.*, *Nature (London)* **302**, 626 (1983).
9. E. P. Gelmann, G. Franchini, V. Manzari, F. Wong-Staal, R. C. Gallo, *Proc. Natl. Acad. Sci. U.S.A.*, in press.
10. M. Popovic *et al.*, unpublished data.
11. I. Miyoshi *et al.*, *Lancet* **1982-II**, 658 (1982).
12. N. Yamamoto *et al.*, *ibid.* **1983-I**, 240 (1983).
13. C. Saxinger *et al.*, in preparation.
14. B. A. Lapin, in *Nonhuman Primates and Medical Research* (Academic Press, New York, 1973), p. 213.
15. C. Saxinger *et al.*, in *Human T-Cell Leukemia Viruses*, R. C. Gallo, M. Essex, L. Gross, Eds. (Cold Spring Harbor Laboratory, Cold Spring Harbor, N.Y., in press).
16. M. Seiki, S. Hattori, Y. Hirayama, M. Yoshida, *Proc. Natl. Acad. Sci. U.S.A.* **80**, 3618 (1983).
17. R. C. Gallo, A. Sliski, F. Wong-Staal, *Lancet* **1983-II**, 962 (1983).
18. B. Hahn *et al.*, unpublished data.
19. N. Yamamoto *et al.*, in preparation.
20. E. M. Southern, *J. Mol. Biol.* **98**, 503 (1975).
21. We thank M. Reitz, C. Saxinger, and S. Josephs, Tumor Cell Biology, NCI, for helpful discussions; N. Yamamoto of the Institute of Virus Research, Kyoto, Japan, for unpublished data; and T. Soltis for secretarial assistance.

9 November 1983; accepted 19 December 1983

Report

23 March 1984

25. Transformation and Cytopathogenic Effect in an Immune Human T-Cell Clone Infected by HTLV-I

Hiroaki Mitsuya, Hong-Guang Guo, Mary Megson, Cecelia Trainor, Marvin S. Reitz, Jr., and Samuel Broder

The human type-C retrovirus known as human T-cell leukemia-lymphoma virus (HTLV) was first isolated from neoplastic cells derived from black patients in the United States with adult T-cell malignancies (*1, 2*). It has been suggested that HTLV and bovine leukemia virus (BLV) have a common ancestry (*3*). Most of the HTLV isolates studied are very similar to one another (*4, 5*) and belong to the subgroup HTLV-I, a family of acquired viruses with T-cell tropism (6). In coculture, cells producing HTLV can infect other cells and transform them (7, 8). This transformation reduces or eliminates the normal requirement for T-cell growth factor (TCGF) or interleukin-2.

Despite recent advances, much remains to be learned about the relation between HTLV infection and immune function. Populations in which HTLV is endemic can be found in the West Indies and southern Japan, where the virus is associated with the development of a T-cell leukemia or lymphoma, often made up of neoplastic cells with suppressor immunoregulatory function (9, 10). Other regions of the world where HTLV is endemic include the southeastern United States, parts of South America, and portions of Africa (11).

In the endemic areas of Japan and the Caribbean, 6 percent (and in selected districts up to 37 percent) of adults are asymptomatic carriers of the virus (12). In the United States, HTLV infection is linked to fulminant T-cell lymphoproliferative disorders in adults, complicated by hypercalcemia and opportunistic infections (11).

The full spectrum of diseases associated with HTLV is not known. There are data supporting the hypotheses that certain patients with the recently defined acquired immunodeficiency syndrome (AIDS) either have an increased risk of infection with viruses in the HTLV family or developed the disease as a result of infection with a strain of HTLV (13). Studies with outbred cats indicate that there is a clear precedent for the latter possibility in that feline leukemia virus (FeLV) can mediate an infectious form of immunodeficiency (14). Indeed, such an immunodeficiency involves an increased risk of bacterial, viral, and parasitic infections and it is commonly encountered in veterinary practice. However, the factors that govern whether the retrovirus will cause a neoplasm, an immunodeficiency, or both, are not defined.

We have investigated populations of HTLV-specific, cytotoxic T cells that were derived from a patient (M.J.) whose HTLV-bearing lymphoma was in remission (15). We now report a human T-cell clone that has been infected and transformed by the HTLV that itself had served as its target antigen. The clone initially had potent specific cytotoxic activity that waned with time in culture, and it spontaneously proliferated in the absence of TCGF. The spontaneous proliferation of the clone was profoundly and specifically inhibited by exposure to autologous HTLV-bearing tumor cells. The genome of the clone contained one copy of an HTLV provirus.

We generated cultures of immune T cells from the peripheral blood of patient M.J. after his neoplasm was in remission (15). These uncloned, starting T-cell populations required TCGF for propagation in vitro. Such T cells mediated specific cellular immune reactions in vitro against HTLV-I, including proliferation in response to cultured HTLV-I–bearing tumor cells and a form of HTLV-specific cytotoxicity restricted by products of the major histocompatibility complex (MHC). In the current studies, immune T cells were exposed to infectious HTLV and cloned. Cloning of the immune T cells was undertaken by limiting dilution (0.5 cells per well) in round-bottom microtiter wells containing lectin-free TCGF and a feeder-layer of irradiated mononuclear cells obtained from the patient in remission. The wells also contained a lethally irradiated population of HTLV-producing autologous tumor cells. Within 21 days, one microtiter well was noted to contain a very rapidly growing population of cells (designated clone K7). These cells expressed the same surface markers of mature cytotoxic T cells (OKT-3$^+$, -4$^-$, -8$^+$, DR$^+$, and Tac$^+$) that characterized the uncloned, starting T cells. They also expressed the patient's HLA phenotype: A1, B8, B27, Cw6, Cw7, DR3, and DR7. (These phenotypic properties remained stable throughout the course of these studies.) The K7 cells proliferated in the absence of TCGF (although the rate of replication could be increased by exogenous TCGF). The cells were propagated in the absence of MJ-tumor cells for further study.

The immune cytotoxic effector function of the noncloned, starting population and clone K7 is illustrated in Fig. 1,

A and B. Shortly after cloning, K7 cells mediated substantial cytotoxic activity against autologous HTLV-bearing tumor cells and other histocompatible cells infected with HTLV. Clone K7 was cytotoxic only for cells that were infected with HTLV, and then only when histocompatible target cells were used. However, with time in culture, clone K7 progressively lost cytotoxic activity (Fig. 1C). It was not possible to restore the cytotoxic activity by recloning the cells. Clone K7 spontaneously proliferated in the absence of TCGF, and phytohemagglutinin (PHA), a polyclonal T-cell mitogen, did not affect the spontaneous proliferation of clone K7 (Fig. 2A).

The capacity to recognize an antigen and respond by proliferating in the absence of exogenous TCGF is one of the hallmarks of immune T cells. The uncloned, starting population of immune T

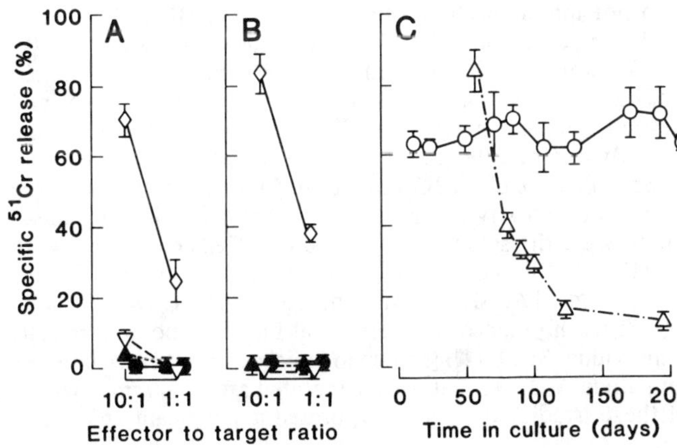

Fig. 1. Functional properties of clone K7. (A) Cytotoxic effector activity of the parent cultured T-cell line (MJ-CTL). (B) Initial cytotoxic effector activity of clone K7 cells derived from MJ-CTL. Standard 4-hour ^{51}Cr-release assays were used to assess the specific cytotoxic activity of cultured T cells as previously described (15). The release of radioactivity (R) into the surrounding medium by target cells labeled with ^{51}Cr is an index of cell destruction. The percentage specific release of ^{51}Cr was determined by the following formula: $\{[(R_{test}) - (R_s)]/[(R_{max}) - (R_s)]\} \times 100$, where R_{test} is the ^{51}Cr released in the assay, R_s is the spontaneous release, and R_{max} is the maximum release of radioactivity. MJ-CTL and clone K7 cells were tested on day 62 in culture. Target cells were HTLV-bearing autologous tumor cell line, MJ-tumor ($\diamond$); HTLV-bearing tumor cell line from an unrelated donor, HUT-102-B2 ($\blacktriangle$); Epstein-Barr virus–transformed autologous B cells ($\bullet$); and an erythroid line, K562 ($\triangledown$). (C) Progressive loss of cytotoxic activity of clone K7. In each ^{51}Cr release assay, the cytotoxicity of the parent cultured T-cell line, MJ-CTL ($\bigcirc$) and clone K7 ($\triangle$) against autologous HTLV-bearing tumor cells (MJ-tumor cells), was determined. The ratio of effector to target cells for each determination was 10 to 1. Cloning took place on day 35 in culture.

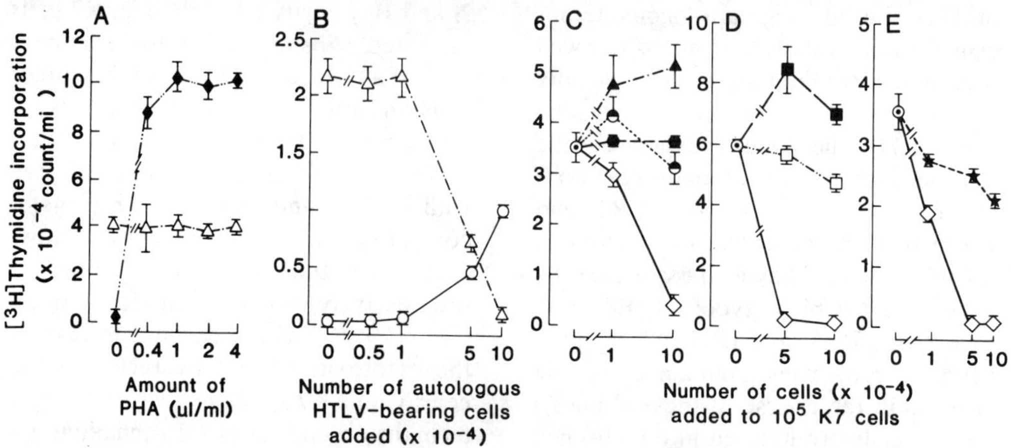

Fig. 2 (A and B). Altered properties of clone K7. (A) Loss of proliferative response to the nonspecific mitogen phytohemagglutinin-M (PHA-M). Clone K7 cells (△) (10^5) and peripheral blood mononuclear cells from a normal individual (◆) were cultured for 3 days with various amounts of PHA-M (Gibco) in the absence of exogenous TCGF in 200 μl of RPMI 1640 medium supplemented with 10 percent heat-inactivated fetal calf serum, 4 mM L-glutamine, and penicillin (50 unit/ml) and streptomycin (50 μg/ml) at 37°C in humidified air containing 5 percent CO_2. In the final 5 hours of culture the cells were exposed to 0.5 μCi of [^{3}H]thymidine. They were then harvested onto glass fibers and assessed for the incorporation of isotope as an indicator of proliferation. The results are expressed as the mean counts per minute ± one standard deviation for triplicate determinations. Clone K7 proliferates spontaneously and the proliferative rate is not affected by PHA; this provides a control showing that nonspecific stimuli at the surface membrane do not inhibit proliferation of the clone. (B) Inhibition of proliferation upon exposure of clone K7 to autologous HTLV-bearing cells. Clone K7 cells (10^5) (△) and the parent line, MJ-CTL (○), were cocultured with various numbers of irradiated autologous HTLV-bearing cells (MJ-tumor cells) for 3 days, exposed to [^{3}H]thymidine, and harvested as described above. The spontaneous proliferation of clone K7 was inhibited by the addition of irradiated MJ-tumor cells. By contrast the parent line was stimulated to proliferate under the same conditions. (C to E) Specificity of clone K7 inhibition. Clone K7 cells (10^5) were cultured in the presence or absence (⊙) of a variety of irradiated (12,000 rad) cells for 3 days. Assays of [^{3}H]thymidine incorporation were the same as in (A) and (B). Cells cocultured with clone K7 cells were MJ-tumor (◇); HUT-102-B2 (▲), Epstein-Barr virus–transformed B cells from patient M.J. (●), and a normal individual M.M. (⊖) who shared A1, B8, Cw6, DR3, and DR7 with patient M.J. [shown in (C)]; freshly harvested peripheral blood mononuclear cells from patient M.J. (□) and a normal individual M.M. (■) [shown in panel (D)]; and PHA-induced TCGF-dependent T-cell blasts from patient M.J. (★) that were generated after his tumor was in remission [shown in (E)]. None of these irradiated cells incorporated a significant amount of [^{3}H]thymidine when cultured alone.

cells from patient M.J. proliferated specifically in response to irradiated, autologous HTLV-bearing tumor cells (MJ-tumor cells) (Fig. 2B). However, under the same conditions, exposure of K7 to autologous HTLV-bearing tumor cells caused an inhibition of proliferation and cell death in a dose-dependent fashion.

The addition of TCGF to the K7 cells at the time of initial exposure to irradiated MJ-tumor cells did not prevent the inhibitory effects (data not shown). Neither HTLV-infected nor -uninfected cells from unrelated individuals could bring about these inhibitory effects. Similarly, a variety of autologous cells obtained from the patient after his neoplasm was in remission (including fresh peripheral blood mononuclear cells, Epstein-Barr virus–transformed B cells, and PHA-induced T-cell blasts) did not cause these inhibitory effects (Fig. 2, C to E). Comparably treated MJ-tumor cells had no inhibitory effects on the proliferation of MOLT-4 (an HTLV-negative T-cell line), HUT-102-B2 (an HTLV-positive T-cell line), or PHA-stimulated T cells from an unrelated normal individual in control coculture experiments. A monoclonal antibody to the p19 group-specific antigen (*gag*) protein of HTLV-I did not appreciably affect the responses of K7 cells discussed above.

However, in preliminary experiments we observed that the inhibitory effect exerted by MJ-tumor cells on clone K7 could be partially abrogated by the addition of irradiated syngeneic (but not allogeneic) peripheral blood mononuclear cells taken from patient M.J. in remission.

We then determined whether K7 cells were infected with HTLV. K7 cell DNA was digested with the restriction endonuclease Eco RI, which does not cleave within the proviral DNA. The resultant Southern blot contains a single proviral fragment (Fig. 3), indicating that there is only one copy of HTLV and that the K7 cell population is monoclonal with respect to the HTLV integration site. This

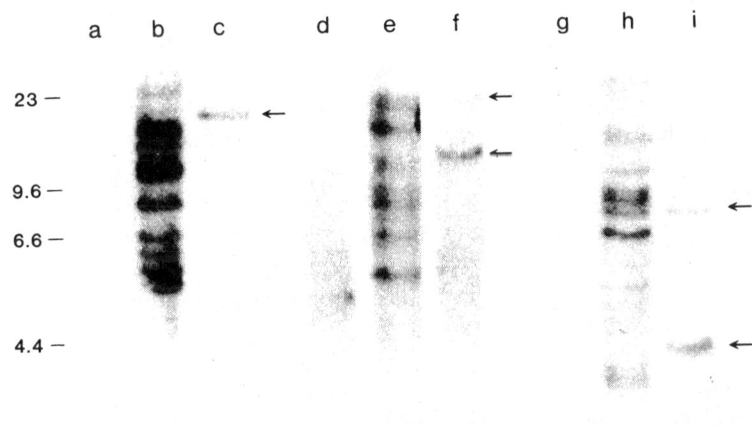

Fig. 3. HTLV Proviral sequences in clone K7 DNA. The DNA was digested with Eco RI (lanes a to c), Sst I (lanes d to f), or Pvu II (lanes g to i) and analyzed by the Southern blotting technique with an HTLV LTR (R-U5) probe. The DNA was from an uninfected cord blood B-cell line (lanes a, d, and g), HTLV-bearing tumor cells from patient M.J. (lanes b, e, and h), or clone K7 (lanes c, f, and i). Arrows show the provirus-containing K7 DNA fragment (or fragments), and the lines on the left-hand side show the position of the Hind III fragments of λ phage DNA as a marker. High molecular weight DNA was digested with Pronase–sodium dodecyl sulfate and extracted with organic solvents essentially as described (*16*). For Southern blots. 25 to 30 μg of DNA was digested for 16 hours at 37°C with 60 units of the indicated enzyme and a buffer as specified by the manufacturer. Restriction endonuclease digests were subjected to electrophoresis overnight at 40 V in 0.5 percent agarose, transferred to nitrocellulose, and analyzed by hybridization to a nick-translated ^{32}P-labeled excised insert containing the R-U5 region of the LTR sequences of HTLV-I$_{CR}$ cloned in plasmid PBR-322 (*17*). Filters were washed extensively in 0.075M NaCl, 7.5 mM sodium citrate (pH 7) at 65°C. Sst I was from Bethesda Research Laboratories, Gaithersburg, Maryland, and Eco RI and Pvu II were from Boehringer Mannheim, Indianapolis, Indiana.

128

provides an independent indicator of a monoclonal origin for the K7 cell population. This contrasts with the multiple integration sites observed in MJ-tumor cells (the long-term line of autologous HTLV-bearing tumor cells), a pattern commonly observed in cultured HTLV-producing tumor cells (*16*). Digestion with the restriction endonuclease Sst I, which cleaves the HTLV-I$_{MJ}$ provirus once internally, results in two fragments labeled by an HTLV probe for a long terminal repeat (LTR) (Fig. 3). This implies that there are LTR sequences at both the 5' end and the 3' end of the provirus. The restriction endonuclease Pvu II cuts several times within the HTLV provirus. Pvu II digests of K7-cell DNA give two fragments that label with the LTR probe and are, therefore, proviral-host DNA junction fragments. This confirms that the proviral population is integrated in the same site in all the K7 cells and that the provirus indeed has LTR sequences at both the 5' and 3' ends. In addition, in each of the Pvu II and Sst I digests, the size of at least one of the junction fragments differs from any of the junction fragments in MJ-tumor cell DNA (Fig. 3), indicating that the cell lineage of clone K7 is different from that of the neoplastic cells from the same patient. Digestion with Sma I gives a characteristic 4.3-kb fragment labeled with a probe consisting of the Cla I–Hind III fragment of HTLV clone λCR-1 (*17*), indicating that the 3' half of the virus is present (data not shown). Southern blots with other enzymes and a complete HTLV proviral probe, λ23-3 (*18*), suggest that there are no gross deletions or rearrangements of the HTLV provirus. In spite of the apparently complete HTLV provirus, virus expression was restricted during the course of these studies. There was no detectable expression of the *gag* proteins p19 or p24 during the first 275 days after cloning [about 30 passages] (not shown). During this time, viral RNA was not detectably expressed in the majority of the K7 cells as determined by in situ hybridization to fixed K7 cells. A few cells (10 to 20 percent) appeared to express low levels of viral RNA. Since the same cells were negative for viral *gag* proteins, it appears that either the RNA did not include functional *gag* messenger RNA or it was not translated at detectable levels. However, we do not yet know the reasons for the observed restriction of HTLV expression in K7 cells (*19*).

To our knowledge, clone K7 is the first example of a functional cytotoxic T cell transformed by a human retrovirus. Perhaps the current results can be viewed in the context of the receptor-mediated leukemogenesis theory, which to date has been predicated on data from studies of retrovirus-associated lymphomas of rodents (*20*). The theory proposes that antigen-specific lymphocytes can be a target for infection by an oncogenic retrovirus, a point that has not been fully resolved in animals (*21*). According to this theory, retrovirus-induced lymphomas can be the progeny of normal cells that bear antigen-specific T-cell receptors for engaging viral envelope antigens. Binding of a retrovirus to these cells is postulated to provide both a portal of infection and a continuous mitogenic signal. Such events could have played a role in the emergence of the human T-cell clone K7 in the current studies, although the receptor-mediated leukemogenesis theory per se would not explain the inhibitory effects of exogenous HTLV after the clone emerged.

The mechanisms for the specific inhibition of this clone by its antigen HTLV are not known. Normal human T-cell clones that are specific for discrete peptides of influenza A virus can be rendered unresponsive to antigen by incubation with high concentrations of the appropriate peptide (*22*). This state of specific unresponsiveness is defined by a failure to mount a proliferative response to antigen in vitro and is perhaps akin to certain forms of immunologic tolerance. Perhaps clone K7 represents HTLV-induced transformation and expansion of a T cell that had already been programmed for such unresponsiveness. In this context, K7 cells might serve as an in vitro model for immunologic tolerance based on a mechanism of clonal deletion. Alternatively, the insertion of HTLV (or a mutant strain of the virus) into a critical domain within the genome could induce or predispose reactive T cells to somatic errors that cause them to recognize exogenous viral antigens as a negative signal. These are topics for future research that could have implications in understanding the relation between retroviruses in T-cell neoplasms and acquired immunodeficiency disease states.

References and Notes

1. B. J. Poiesz, F. W. Ruscetti, A. F. Gazdar, P. A. Bunn, J. D. Minna, R. G. Gallo, *Proc. Natl. Acad. Sci. U.S.A.* **77**, 7415 (1980).
2. B. J. Poiesz, F. W. Ruscetti, M. S. Reitz, V. S. Kalyanaraman, R. C. Gallo, *Nature (London)* **294**, 268 (1981).
3. R. C. Gallo, A. Sliski, F. Wong-Staal, *Lancet* **1983-II**, 962 (1983).
4. Y. Hinuma *et al., Proc. Natl. Acad. Sci. U.S.A.* **78**, 6476 (1981).
5. M. Popovic *et al., Nature (London)* **300**, 63 (1982).
6. R. C. Gallo *et al., Proc. Natl. Acad. Sci. U.S.A.* **79**, 5680 (1982).
7. M. Popovic, P. S. Sarin, M. Robert-Guroff, V. S. Kalyznaraman, D. Mann, J. Minowada, R. C. Gallo, *Science* **219**, 856 (1983).
8. M. Popovic, G. Lange-Wantzin, P. S. Sarin, D. Mann, R. C. Gallo, *Proc. Natl. Acad. Sci. U.S.A.* **80**, 5402 (1983).
9. T. Uchiyama, K. Sagawa, K. Takatsuki, H. Uchino, *Clin. Immunol. Immunopathol.* **10**, 24 (1978).
10. T. Hattori, T. Uchiyama, T. Toibana, K. Takatsuki, H. Uchino, *Blood* **58**, 645 (1981).
11. P. A. Bunn, Jr., *et al., N. Engl. J. Med.* **309**, 257 (1983); R. C. Gallo, unpublished data.
12. Y. Hinuma *et al., Int. J. Cancer* **29**, 631 (1982).
13. R. C. Gallo *et al., Science* **220**, 865 (1983); E. P. Gelmann *et al., ibid.*, p. 862; M. Essex *et al.*, p. 859; *ibid.* **221**, 1061 (1983).
14. M. Essex, W. D. Hardy, Jr., S. M. Cotter, R. M. Jakowski, A. Sliski, *Infect. Immun.* **11**, 470 (1975); W. D. Hardy, Jr., *et al., Cancer Res.* **36**, 582 (1976); S. M. Cotter, W. D. Hardy, Jr., M. Essex, *J. Am. Vet. Med. Assoc.* **166**, 449 (1975); Z. Trainin, D. Wernicke, H. Unger-Waron, M. Essex, *Science* **220**, 858 (1983).
15. H. Mitsuya *et al., J. Exp. Med.* **158**, 994 (1983). Patient M.J. is a 54-year-old white male with circulating antibodies against internal structural proteins of HTLV. In 1977 he was diagnosed as having cutaneous T-cell lymphoma, and he eventually became a complete responder to a regimen of chemotherapy, whole-body electron beam irradiation, and topically applied nitrogen mustard. The patient's disease was in clinical remission when these studies were initiated in January 1983.
16. F. Wong-Staal *et al., Nature (London)* **302**, 626 (1983).
17. V. Manzari *et al., Proc. Natl. Acad. Sci. U.S.A.* **80**, 1574 (1983).
18. M. F. Clarke, E. P. Gelmann, M. S. Reitz, Jr., *Nature (London)* **305**, 60 (1983).
19. After approximately 1 year in culture (50 passages), some K7 cells were found to express p19 and p24 proteins as well as virus particles, confirming the presence of a complete provirus and indicating that the restriction of HTLV expression was a reversible phenomenon.
20. I. C. Weissman and M. S. McGrath, *Curr. Top. Microbiol. Immunol.* **98**, 103 (1982).
21. J. N. Ihle and J. C. Lee, *ibid.*, p. 85.
22. J. R. Lamb, B. J. Skidmore, N. Green, J. M. Chiller, M. Feldmann, *J. Exp. Med.* **157**, 1434 (1983).
23. We thank R. C. Gallo for helpful advice.

7 December 1983; accepted 21 February 1984

26. Transfusion-Associated AIDS: Serologic Evidence of Human T-Cell Leukemia Virus Infection of Donors

H.W. Jaffe, D.P. Francis, M.F. McLane, C. Cabradilla, J.W. Curran, B.W. Kilbourne, D.N. Lawrence, H.W. Haverkos, T.J. Spira, R.Y. Dodd, J. Gold, D. Armstrong, A. Ley, J. Groopman, J. Mullins, T.H. Lee, and M. Essex

The acquired immunodeficiency syndrome (AIDS) is a recently recognized human disease whose incidence in the United States has been rapidly increasing (*1, 2*). Patients with AIDS suffer from at least one type of malignancy, Kaposi's sarcoma, and various life-threatening opportunistic infections, the most common of which is *Pneumocystis carinii* pneumonia. The disease is characterized by diverse immunologic abnormalities, including lymphocyte dysfunction and depletion of the T-helper subpopulation of lymphocytes (*3*).

Although the etiology of AIDS is unknown, epidemiologic observations suggest that it is caused by an infectious agent transmitted sexually and, less commonly, through parenteral exposure to blood or blood products (*4*). In the United States, about 94 percent of patients reported to have AIDS belong to one or more of the following groups: homosexual or bisexual men, abusers of intravenous drugs, persons born in Haiti, and persons with hemophilia (*2*). Another 1 percent of AIDS patients do not belong to any of these groups but received transfusions of blood or blood components within 5 years before the onset of their illness. These cases are classified as transfusion-associated AIDS and have been described in detail elsewhere (*5, 6*).

Among the agents studied as a possible cause of AIDS are retroviruses, including the human T-cell leukemia virus (HTLV) (*7*). Compared with control individuals, AIDS patients have a higher prevalence of antibodies directed against membrane antigens of HTLV-infected cells (HTLV-MA) as measured by indirect membrane immunofluorescence and radioimmunoprecipitation techniques (*8*). In studies in which serum from Japanese T-cell leukemia patients and asymptomatic carriers was used, the major antigens detected by antisera to HTLV-MA have been defined (*9*). They include two glycoproteins, designated gp 61 and gp 45, that are encoded by the *env* gene of HTLV (*9*). The prevalence of antibodies to HTLV-MA is also increased in homosexual men with chronic, generalized lymphadenopathy (*8*), an illness that has been associated with AIDS (*10*). Human T-cell leukemia virus has been isolated from the lymphocytes of AIDS patients, both American (*11*) and Japanese (*12*), and DNA sequences that hybridized with a cloned HTLV DNA probe were detected in two other patients (*13*). A retrovirus thought to be related to HTLV has also been isolated from a lymph node of a French homosexual man with chronic lymphadenopathy (*14*). Whether these findings reflect an etiologic role for a retrovirus in AIDS or are simply a consequence of these viruses infecting AIDS patients opportunistically is unknown.

In an attempt to evaluate further the serologic relationship of HTLV or a related virus to AIDS, we have studied patients with transfusion-associated AIDS and the persons who donated blood or blood components to these patients. As of 1 January 1984, the Centers for Disease Control (CDC) had received reports of 32 adults with transfusion-associated AIDS. An additional patient (patient 5), a 69-year-old man with Kaposi's sarcoma, whose age exceeds the limit of 60 years specified for Kaposi's sarcoma patients in the CDC surveillance definition for AIDS (*4*), is included in this report because his abnormal immunologic studies and rapidly fatal clinical course suggest that he did, in fact, have AIDS. For 12 of these 33 cases, donor investigations have been completed. An investigation is considered complete when all available donors (i) have been interviewed regarding risk factors for AIDS, (ii) have been examined for physical findings suggestive of AIDS, and (iii) have provided a blood sample.

Several classes of serum were obtained to serve as controls. These included 298 randomly selected specimens collected during 1979 and 1980 from volunteer blood donors in Philadelphia, Pennsylvania (100 specimens), Madison, Wisconsin (99 specimens), and Tucson, Arizona (99 specimens). Also included for comparison were 81 previously tested serum samples collected in 1981 from

homosexual men matched by age, race, and residence to a sample of AIDS patients (*8, 15*) and 45 samples obtained in 1982 from homosexual men in Ithaca, New York.

Serum specimens from patients with transfusion-associated AIDS, donors to these patients, and control subjects were coded and sent frozen to Boston to test for antibodies to HTLV-MA by a method that has been described (*8, 16*). Briefly, a 1:4 dilution of serum was added to two HTLV-I-infected cell lines, Hut 102 and MT 2; the cells were washed; and a fluorescein-conjugated $F(ab')_2$ fragment of goat antibody to human immunoglobulins G, A, and M was added. The cells were washed again, and the proportion of cells having fluorescence was determined for each cell line. Samples with 40 percent or more of the cells having fluorescence on either cell line were considered positive. Positive samples were tested on uninfected lymphoid cell lines to exclude nonspecificity. A negative and a positive control serum sample were included in each coded test.

Of the 12 patients with transfusion-associated AIDS, 11 had *Pneumocystis carinii* pneumonia and one had Kaposi's sarcoma (Table 1). Only one of the 12 patients had an onset of illness before April 1982. For the ten patients who received transfusions on only one occasion, the interval between receipt of blood or blood components and onset of illness ranged from 13 to 40 months (mean, 24.6 months; median, 22.5 months).

Antibodies to HTLV-MA were detected in three of eight patients for whom serum samples were available (Table 1). Thus, the proportion (37.5 percent) of transfusion-associated AIDS patients who had detectable antibodies to HTLV-

Table 1. Illness, transfusion history, and presence of antibodies to HTLV-MA in patients with transfusion-associated AIDS. PCP is *Pneumocystis carinii* pneumonia; KS is Kaposi's sarcoma; and NA indicates that no specimen was available for testing.

Pa-tient	Diag-nosis	Antibodies to HTLV-MA	Month of		Time from transfusion to illness onset (months)
			AIDS onset	Transfusion	
1	PCP	+	June 1981	November 1977	44
				April 1980*	15
2	PCP	−	April 1982	February 1979	39
				July 1979*	34
				June 1981*	11
3	PCP	NA	April 1982	January 1981	16
4	PCP	+	May 1982	February 1980	28
5	KS	NA	September 1982	May 1981	17
6	PCP	NA	October 1982	December 1979	35
7	PCP	−	November 1982	August 1979	40
8	PCP	−	December 1982	March 1980	34
9	PCP	−	January 1983	August 1981	18
10	PCP	+	January 1983	November 1980	27
11	PCP	NA	January 1983	January 1982	13
12	PCP	−	February 1983	September 1981	18

*Date of receipt of blood from a high-risk donor.

MA was very similar to the proportion (36 percent) of seropositive individuals among previously reported patients with AIDS not associated with transfusion (8).

The number of donors to the 12 patients described in Table 1 ranged from 2 to 34 (mean, 13.1; median, 6) (Table 2). Of the total of 157 donors, 117 (74.5 percent) were evaluated. The overall prevalence of antibodies to HTLV-MA was significantly higher in the donors to AIDS patients (9 of 117; 7.7 percent) than in random blood donors (1 of 298; 0.3 percent) ($P < 0.0001$; Fisher's exact test) (Table 3). Among the 12 sets of donors to AIDS patients, 9 sets included one donor with antibodies to HTLV-MA.

As reported earlier, most patients with transfusion-associated AIDS had received blood from one or more "high-risk" donors within 5 years before the onset of symptoms in the patient (6). A donor was considered to be at high risk if he or she had AIDS, was a member of a group with increased risk for AIDS, or had an abnormally low ratio of T-helper to T-suppressor lymphocytes (< 1.00) ascertained as described (15). Donors not meeting these criteria were considered "other" donors. Among the 12 sets of donors to the AIDS patients described in this report, 11 included a high-risk donor; two such donors were found for patient 3 (Table 2). Eight of the 12 high-risk donors belonged to known AIDS risk groups. Although none of the high-risk donors had illnesses that met the surveillance definition for AIDS, 4 of the 12 had generalized lymphadenopathy when examined at the time they were interviewed (19 to 51 months after they had donated blood).

Among the nine donors who showed positive results for antibodies to HTLV-

Table 2. Prevalance of antibodies to HTLV-MA in blood donors to patients with transfusion-associated AIDS. T_H/T_S is the ratio of T-helper to T-suppressor lymphocytes.

Patient	Donors (No.)	Donors evaluated (No.)	AIDS risk group	Generalized lymphadenopathy	T_H/T_S	Antibodies to HTLV-MA	Other donors (ratio of antibody-positive to total donors)
1	3	3	None	Yes	0.6 (0.7)*	+	0/2
2	28	18	Homosexual man	Yes	0.8 (1.3)	+	0/17
3	20	13	Intravenous drug user	No	1.5 (1.8)	+	0/11
			None	No	0.9 (0.9)	−	
4	6	6	Homosexual man	No	0.5	+	0/5
5	3	1	Homosexual man	No	0.4 (0.7)	+	0/0
6	2	2	Homosexual man	Yes	0.7	−	0/1
7	4	4	Homosexual man who used intravenous drugs	Yes	1.7	+	0/3
8	4	2	None	No	0.6	−	0/1
9	6	3	Homosexual man	No	0.7	−	0/2
10	16	11	None	No	0.3	−	1/10
11	31	28	No high-risk donor identified				1/28
12	34	26	Homosexual man	No	0.6	−	1/25

*The value in parentheses is the result of testing a follow-up specimen (normal ratio, ≥ 1.0).

Table 3. Prevalence of antibodies to HTLV-MA in blood donors to patients with transfusion-associated AIDS, random blood donors, and healthy homosexual men.

Category	Number tested	Antibody positive	
		Number	Percent
Blood donors to AIDS patients			
High-risk donors	12	6	50.0
Other donors	105	3	2.9
Total	117	9	7.7
Random blood donors			
Philadelphia	100	0	
Madison	99	0	
Tucson	99	1	1.0
Total	298	1	0.3
Healthy homosexual men			
Matched with AIDS patients	81	1	1.2*
Unmatched	45	0	
Total	126	1	0.8

*Result previously published (8).

MA, six were classified as high-risk donors (Table 2). These high-risk donors were significantly more likely to have had detectable antibodies to HTLV-MA (6 of 12; 50 percent) than the other donors to these patients (3 of 105; 2.9 percent) ($P < 0.0001$; Fisher's exact test) (Table 3).

The six antibody-positive high-risk donors were the only seropositive persons in their donor sets (Table 2). Five of the six belonged to known AIDS risk groups; the one exception denied belonging to such groups but had generalized lymphadenopathy and a low ratio of T-helper to T-suppressor lymphocytes. Three of the four high-risk donors with generalized lymphadenopathy had detectable antibodies to HTLV-MA.

Of the three antibody-positive "other" donors, two belonged to donor sets that included a seronegative high-risk donor; the third had donated blood to patient 11, for whom no high-risk donor was identified (Table 2). No risk factor for AIDS could be found in these donors, and they had neither signs nor symptoms of AIDS. None had received transfusions within the previous 5 years. These three donors were a 33-year-old married white man, a 22-year-old unmarried white woman, and a 40-year-old married white man.

We have shown that blood donors to patients with transfusion-associated AIDS had a significantly higher prevalence of antibodies to HTLV-MA than a control group of blood donors, and 9 of 12 donor sets studied had at least one seropositive donor. Furthermore, among the donors to the AIDS patients, those identified as possible sources of AIDS transmission on the basis of epidemiologic and immunologic criteria were significantly more likely to be antibody positive than other donors to these patients. The high prevalence of antibodies to HTLV-MA in homosexual male donors was unexpected, since these antibodies were rare in homosexual controls (Table 3) (8). This difference contrasts with that expected for other viruses such as Epstein-Barr virus, cytomegalovirus, hepatitis B virus, and other agents, where the background prevalence in homosexual controls is very high (15). An unusually high prevalence of antibodies to HTLV-MA in AIDS patients (36 percent), homosexual men with chronic lymphadenopathy (30 percent), and patients with hemophilia (5 to 19 percent), a group at increased risk for AIDS, has been reported (8, 16).

The meaning of the higher prevalence of positive results for antibodies to HTLV-MA in certain people who donated blood to AIDS patients is not yet clear. One hypothesis is that this test is measuring antibody to HTLV or a serologically related virus and that this virus is the etiologic agent of AIDS. The donors, although they remain either asymptomatic or develop chronic lymphadenopathy, might transmit the virus though their donated blood to recipients who, after incubation periods of up to 40 months, develop AIDS. Several investigators have suggested that HTLV, apart from any association with the AIDS disease spectrum, may be transmitted through transfusion of blood from asymptomatic carriers of the virus (*17*). This hypothesis is also consistent with the pathogenic pattern of illness associated with another retrovirus, feline leukemia virus, which can be transmitted to cats by blood and can, after a long latency period, produce manifestations ranging from asymptomatic seroconversion to lymphoid malignancy and fatal opportunistic infection (*18*).

An alternative hypothesis is that certain donors have antibody to HTLV-MA or a serologically related virus, but this virus is not the cause of AIDS. The high-risk donors may have been predisposed to infection with this virus because of their individual practices or because both AIDS patients and the high-risk donors have a particular form of immune suppression, caused by another agent, that makes these individuals especially susceptible to retroviral infection. Immune dysfunction might also have led to a reactivation of latent retroviral infection and, hence, to antibody expression. However, neither apparently healthy homosexual men nor renal-transplant recipients, a patient group with drug-induced immune dysfunction, have an increased prevalence of antibodies to HTLV-MA (Table 3) (*19*). Nonetheless, the occurrence of AIDS in the recipients

may have been the result of infection with another, as yet undetected, agent present in the blood of either the high-risk donors or other donors.

Neither hypothesis explains the antibody-positive "other" donors who appear to be outside the groups so far identified as being at risk for AIDS. Further work is required to understand fully the relationship between positive results for antibodies to HTLV-MA and AIDS.

At the present time, no test exists that will specifically screen out blood capable of transmitting AIDS. However, the study of individuals who have donated blood to patients with transfusion-associated AIDS offers an opportunity to examine the transmission of this disease and to evaluate potential "screening tests." Furthermore, study of these donors may help to elucidate the possible role of retroviruses or other viruses in AIDS.

References and Notes

1. Centers for Disease Control Task Force on Kaposi's Sarcoma and Opportunistic Infections, *N. Engl. J. Med.* **306**, 248 (1982).
2. "Update: Acquired immunodeficiency syndrome (AIDS)—United States," *Morbid. Mortal. Weekly Rep.* **32**, 688 (1984).
3. M. S. Gottlieb *et al.*, *N. Engl. J. Med.* **305**, 1425 (1981); H. C. Lane, H. Masur, L. C. Edgar, G. Whalen, A. H. Rook, A. S. Fauci, *ibid.* **309**, 453 (1983).
4. H. W. Jaffe, D. J. Bregman, R. M. Selik, *J. Infect. Dis.* **148**, 339 (1983).
5. J. R. Jett, J. N. Kuritsky, J. A. Katzmann, J. A. Homburger, *Ann. Intern. Med.* **99**, 621 (1983).
6. J. W. Curran *et al.*, *N. Engl. J. Med.* **310**, 69 (1984).
7. B. J. Poiesz, F. W. Ruscetti, A. F. Gazdar, P. A. Bunn, J. D. Minna, R. C. Gallo, *Proc. Natl. Acad. Sci. U.S.A.* **77**, 7415 (1980).
8. M. Essex *et al.*, *Science* **220**, 859 (1983).
9. T. H. Lee, J. E. Coligan, T. Homma, M. F. McLane, M. Tachibana, M. Essex, *Proc. Natl. Acad. Sci. U.S.A.*, in press.
10. C. E. Metroka *et al.*, *Ann. Intern. Med.* **99**, 585 (1983).
11. R. C. Gallo *et al.*, *Science* **220**, 865 (1983); R. C. Gallo, personal communication.
12. I. Miyoshi *et al.*, *Lancet* **1983-II**, 275 (1983).
13. E. P. Gelmann *et al.*, *Science* **220**, 862 (1983).

14. F. Barré-Sinoussi *et al.*, *ibid.*, p. 868.
15. M. F. Rogers *et al.*, *Ann. Intern. Med.* **99**, 151 (1983).
16. M. Essex *et al.*, *Science* **221**, 1061 (1983).
17. I. Miyoshi *et al.*, *Lancet* **1982-I**, 683 (1982); W. C. Saxinger and R. C. Gallo, *ibid.*, p. 1072; K. Okochi, H. Sato, Y. Hinuma, *Vox Sang.*, in press.
18. W. D. Hardy, Jr., in *The Virology, Immunology, and Epidemiology of the Feline Leukemia Virus*, W. D. Hardy, Jr., M. Essex, A. J. McClelland, Eds. (Elsevier/North-Holland, New York, 1980), pp. 33–78.
19. In an unpublished study by M. Essex and M. Hirsch (Massachusetts General Hospital), 2 of 93 kidney transplant patients had antibodies to HTLV-MA when their sera were tested with previously described methods (*8, 16*). In another unpublished study by M. Essex, J. Bailey, and T. Guthrie (Medical College of Georgia), none of 17 patients with systemic lupus erythematosus, a disease of immunoregulatory dysfunction, had positive results for the antibodies.
20. We thank the many physicians, blood banks, and health departments that assisted in the investigations described in this report.

27 February 1984; accepted 6 March 1984

Report

20 April 1984

27. Characterization of Exogenous Type D Retrovirus from a Fibroma of a Macaque with Simian AIDS and Fibromatosis

Kurt Stromberg, Raoul E. Benveniste, Larry O. Arthur, Harvey Rabin, W. Ellis Giddens, Jr., Hans D. Ochs, William R. Morton, and Che-Chung Tsai

Human acquired immunodeficiency syndrome (AIDS) is characterized pathologically by lymphoid depletion, depressed cellular and humoral immune functions, opportunistic infections, and unusual neoplasms, particularly Kaposi's sarcoma and, less frequently, lymphomas (*1*). An acquired immunodeficiency syndrome similar in certain respects to human AIDS has been observed in macaques at the New England (*2*) and California (*3*) Regional Primate Research Centers (RPRC). The simian AIDS (SAIDS) at the New England RPRC occurs primarily in *Macaca cyclopis* in which some of the affected animals died with lymphoproliferative lesions (*2*). SAIDS in the California facility is epidemic in *M. mulatta* and two cases of cutaneous fibrosarcomas have been reported in rhesus monkeys (*4*). At the RPRC at the University of Washington, various macaques, primarily *M. nemestrina* but also *M. mulatta*, *M. fuscata*, and *M. fascicularis*, show an immunodeficiency syndrome characterized by persistent diarrhea, progressive weight loss, anemia, lymphocytopenia, unusual chronic infections (noma and cryptosporidiosis), and a peculiar fibromatous tumor termed retroperitoneal fibromatosis (RF) (*5, 6*). Histologically, there is marked thymic atrophy, follicular and paracortical atrophy of lymph nodes, and variable myeloid and lymphoid hyperplasia in bone marrow. Neither RF nor immunodeficiency has been observed among colony-born or feral baboons housed at the Washington RPRC. Retroperitoneal fibromatosis, which is characterized by an aggressive proliferation of highly vascular fibrous tissue, often remains localized to the peritoneum. However, in over one-fourth of the cases it progresses to involve the entire abdominal cavity, inguinal canal, and thoracic cavity. A cutaneous form has been recognized in a small number of RF-affected animals and resembles the cutaneous fibrosarcomas seen in the California colony (3). Immunohistochemical studies have shown factor VIII–related antigen in endothelial and scattered fibroblast-like cells throughout the RF lesions (6), similar to that described for Kaposi's sarcoma (7). Thus, in its progressive form, SAIDS at the RPRC in Washington includes the triad of lymphoid depletion, opportunistic infections, and an unusual neoplasm (RF).

We have investigated the immune status of monkeys with RF. In an experiment involving four *M. nemestrina* monkeys with biopsy-confirmed lesions of RF and three age- and sex-matched controls, peripheral blood mononuclear cells were cultured in the presence of optimal concentrations of phytohemagglutinin (PHA), concanavalin A (Con A), or pokeweed mitogen (PWM) (8). Results for the RF-affected animals were expressed as the percentage of the average net [^{3}H]thymidine incorporation by lymphoid cells of the three controls. The results showed that responses of lymphoid cells of RF animals were 2 to 12 percent of the control value for PHA, 1 to 13 percent of the control value for Con A, and 5 to 66 percent of the control

value for PWM. Antibody responses to the T-cell–dependent antigen bacteriophage ϕX174 (9) were measured in two rhesus monkeys with biopsy-confirmed RF and two age- and sex-matched controls. Control monkeys showed a typical primary immunoglobulin M (IgM) response and a brisk and amplified secondary response consisting mainly of immunoglobulin G (IgG) antibody. In contrast, RF-affected animals had a markedly depressed primary response (both animals less than 1 percent of controls) and failed to amplify and switch from IgM to IgG during the secondary response. Similarly depressed immune responses have been observed in homosexual men with lymphadenopathy and reversed ratios of helper to suppressor lymphocytes (10).

To examine the etiology of SAIDS at the Washington RPRC, RF tissue from an immunodeficient rhesus monkey was cocultivated with heterologous mammalian cells known to support the replication of a wide variety of primate viruses (11). After only 2 weeks, a Mg^{2+}-dependent reverse transcriptase activity was detected in the conditioned medium from a dog thymus cell line (FCf2Th). Electron microscopic examination of the virus (Fig. 1) revealed typical (12) type D retroviral particles, indistinguishable from Mason-Pfizer monkey virus (MPMV), in which intracytoplasmic type A particles were common (Fig. 1A), and budding occurred by envelopment of preformed A particles (Fig. 1B). Budding of virions with incomplete nucleoids was also observed (Fig. 1C) and, characteristic of MPMV, nucleoids of the mature virions were cone shaped (Fig. 1D).

This isolate, designated SAIDS-D/Washington, can be grown to high titers in mammalian cell lines of human, canine, rhesus, bat, and mink origin (13).

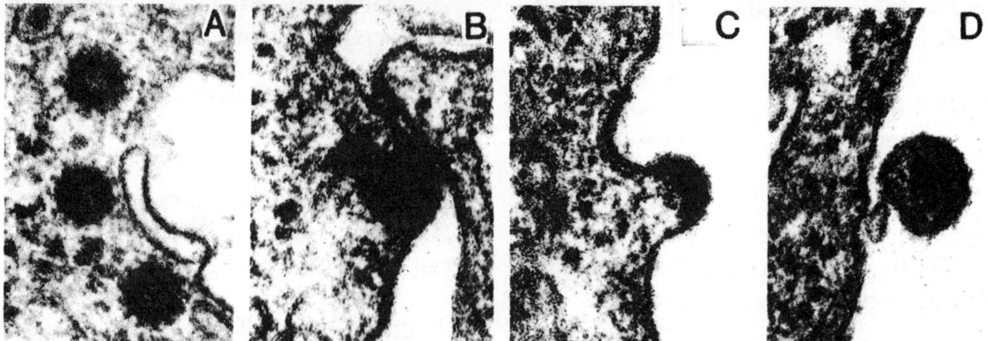

Fig. 1. Morphology of the SAIDS-D viral isolate grown in canine FCf2Th cells. (A) Intracytoplasmic type A particles; (B) budding by envelopment of preformed A particles; (C) budding virions with incomplete nucleoids; and (D) cone or barrel-shaped nucleoids of the "mature" virions. The specimens were prepared as previously described (*12*). (×105,000)

These cells that support SAIDS-D virus growth remained fibroblastic and no cytopathic effect or morphological evidence of transformation was observed. However, after infection of several cell lines chosen for their flat morphology and ability to be transformed, foci of proliferating or otherwise abnormal cells were observed in mouse NIH 3T3 cells (*13*).

The antigenic relatedness of SAIDS-D virus to other type D viruses was determined in specific radioimmunoassays (RIA) for the major core protein (p27) and the major envelope glycoprotein (gp70) purified from MPMV. Other type D viruses used as competitors were the endogenous virus of langurs (PO-1-Lu) and the endogenous virus of squirrel monkeys (SMRV). As shown in Fig. 2A, lysed virus pellets of SAIDS-D, MPMV, and PO-1-Lu effectively competed in the MPMV p27 assay. The extent of competition and similarity of the slopes of the competition curves indicate close immunological relatedness of the core proteins of these three viruses. SMRV type D virus, as well as type C retroviruses, did not compete in the MPMV p27 assay.

Figure 2B shows that the envelope protein of SAIDS-D appears immunologically distinct from MPMV since, like PO-1-Lu and SMRV, it did not compete in the MPMV gp70 assay. SAIDS-D virus was also found to be negative in a broadly specific RIA for type C virus core antigens as well as in an RIA for human T-cell leukemia virus core antigen (*14*).

To further characterize the SAIDS-D virus from *M. mulatta*, we compared the nucleic acid sequence homology and thermal stability between this isolate and other known primate retroviruses. A retrovirus previously described from the spleen of a *M. nemestrina* with RF (*15*) was not related to MPMV and consisted of a mixture of type C and type D viruses. This isolate was lost during cultivation (*16*) and is thus not available to compare with SAIDS-D virus. Table 1 shows the results obtained after hybridization of a radioactively labeled DNA transcript of SAIDS-D virus to the cellular DNA extracted from tissues of various primate species or from virus-infected cells. The DNA hybrids were digested with S_1 nuclease at low stringency (*17*). Liquid hybridization under these conditions reveals more initial information about overall quantitative nucleic acid homologies than can be obtained by comparison of limited restriction endo-

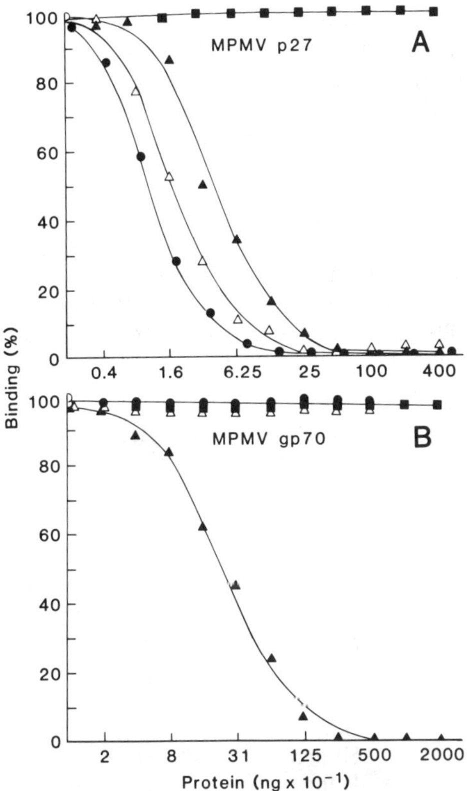

Fig. 2. Competitive RIA for the MPMV major core protein (p27) and envelope glycoprotein (gp70). Detergent-disrupted viruses were tested for their ability to compete with the binding of ^{125}I-labeled viral proteins to limiting amounts of antisera (24). All results are normalized to 100 percent binding in the absence of competing antigens. The reagents used were (A) antibody to MPMV p27: ^{125}I-labeled MPMV p27; (B) antibody to MPMV gp70: ^{125}I-labeled MPMV gp70. Viruses include MPMV (▲), SAIDS-D virus (●), PO-1-Lu (△), and SMRV (■). Other retroviruses that were negative in both assays (data not shown) were mouse mammary tumor virus, Rauscher murine leukemia virus, an endogenous type C virus of stump-tailed macaques, and human T-cell leukemia virus.

nuclease digests. The SAIDS-D isolate is distinct from all other primate retroviruses, but is partially related (36 to 38 percent) to MPMV and the endogenous langur virus. No homology was detected to the DNA of the New World type D isolate from squirrel monkeys. Previous hybridization experiments have shown that MPMV and langur endogenous virus are partially related (22 to 33 percent homology) (18). In reciprocal experiments not shown here, ^{3}H-labeled DNA transcripts prepared from MPMV and langur virus each hybridize approximately 30 percent to the cellular DNA of SAIDS-D–infected cells.

The thermal stability of nucleic acid hybrids can also be used as an index of the degree of base-pair mismatching between DNA strands. As shown in Table 1, the hybrids formed between SAIDS-D viral DNA transcripts and the cellular DNA of MPMV- or langur virus-infected cells dissociate at approximately 12°C lower than the homologous hybrid. Although there may be regions of the SAIDS-D viral genome that are not well represented in our DNA transcripts, the low degree of nucleic acid sequence homology between SAIDS-D virus and the other Old World monkey type D viruses is probably due to an accumulation of base-pair mutations rather than to a recombinational event involving a major portion of the Mason-Pfizer genome.

The cellular DNA of several primate species was tested for nucleic acid sequence homology to the SAIDS-D virus. Table 1 shows that the highest degree of homology was obtained with DNA from the Colobinae subfamily of Old World monkeys, in particular langur DNA (51 percent). The cellular DNA from all Old World monkeys belonging to the subfamily Cercopithecinae (including several macaque species) hybridize 33 to 38 percent to the viral probe. A pig-tailed macaque with RF revealed the presence of SAIDS-D viral sequences in the tumor tissue as shown by the high final extent of hybridization obtained. Spleen cellular DNA from the same animal hybridized 48 percent to the viral probe. This level of hybridization is greater than that observed in normal pig-tailed macaque DNA, and may reflect a low level of

Table 1. Nucleic acid homology and thermal stability between SAIDS-D/Washington viral DNA and the cellular DNA from various species. A ^{3}H-labeled DNA transcript of the SAIDS-D virus grown in the canine cell line FCf2Th was synthesized from detergent-disrupted virus and purified over alkaline sucrose gradients (*18*). ^{3}H-Labeled DNA viral probes consisting of > 13S DNA were hybridized to the various cellular DNA's. The percentage hybridization is the saturating normalized value obtained after digestion of the hybrids with nuclease S_1 (*17*). The actual final extent of hybridization to DNA extracted from the SAIDS-D virus–infected cell line varied from 80 to 94 percent; the remainder of the probe hybridized to dog cellular DNA. All hybridizations were carried out to a C_0t value of 3×10^4; the standard deviation of the values varied from ±2.6 to ±4.1 percent, based on five separate hybridization experiments with four cellular DNA samples and viral DNA probes. The T_m is the temperature at which 50 percent of the DNA hybrids dissociated. The various primate viral isolates were grown in canine (FCf2Th), human (A549), and bat (Tb1Lu) cell lines. C_0t is defined as moles of nucleotide per liter times seconds.

Species	Virus	Source of cellular DNA	Hybridization (%)	T_m (°C)
Cell lines				
Rhesus monkey (*M. mulatta*)	SAIDS-D	Canine	100	93.4
Rhesus monkey (*M. mulatta*)	MPMV	Human	38	81.5
Langur (*P. obscura*)	PO-1-Lu	Bat	36	82.0
Squirrel monkey (*S. sciureus*)	SMRV	Canine	2	
Stump-tailed macaque (*M. arctoides*)	M109	Human	7	
Baboon (*P. papio*)	M7	Canine	8	
Owl monkey (*A. trivirgatus*)	OMC-1	Bat	1	
Gibbon (*H. lar*)	M144	Human	6	
Woolly monkey (*Lagothrix* spp.)	SSV	Human	6	
Tissue				
Pig-tailed macaque* (*M. nemestrina*)		RF	92	91.6
Pig-tailed macaque* (*M. nemestrina*)		Spleen	48	
Pig-tailed macaque (*M. nemestrina*)		Liver	35	
Rhesus monkey (*M. mulatta*)		Liver	34	
Lion-tailed macaque (*M. silenus*)		Spleen	33	
African green (*C. sabaeus*)		Spleen	38	
Langur (*P. obscura*)		Testes	51	
Colobus (*C. guereza*)		Liver	42	
Gibbon (*H. lar*)		Spleen	2	
Human (*H. sapiens*)		Spleen	1	
Howler monkey (*Alouatta* spp.)		Spleen	3	
Mouse (*Mus caroli*)		Liver	2	
Dog (*C. familiaris*)		Liver	6	
Cow (*B. taurus*)		Thymus	1	

*Spleen and retroperitoneal fibroma cellular DNA were obtained from a pig-tailed macaque (animal T82050) with RF and its associated immunodeficiency.

SAIDS-D viral sequences present in the spleen of this particular monkey. Thus, SAIDS-D virus from *M. mulatta* is present in the fibromatous tissue and spleen of a second macaque species, *M. nemestrina*, from the same primate colony. Moreover, we have recently obtained multiple viral isolates from different tissues of diseased animals of this species (*13*).

The Old World monkeys of Africa and Eurasia are divided into two distinct subfamilies. The Cercopithecinae include baboon, macaque, African green, patas, and related species belonging to eight genera, while the Colobinae include *Colobus* from Africa and five genera of Southeast Asian monkeys including *Presbytis* (langurs). Previous studies showed that DNA probes prepared from the langur type D virus hybridize to other primate DNA's with the final extent of hybridization and the thermal stability of the hybrids formed correlating with the phylogenetic distance of the primates from langur (*18*). A portion of the MPMV genome can also be detected in the cellular DNA's of all Old World monkeys, particularly in those of the Colobinae subfamily (*18, 19*). The high degree of hybridization of SAIDS-D/ Washington viral DNA to langur DNA suggests that this virus, like MPMV, may also have arisen from an endogenous langur virus. The sequence divergence of MPMV and SAIDS-D viruses may reflect the rapid evolution of infectious viruses relative to the genetically transmitted endogenous viral gene sequences.

A type D retrovirus related to MPMV has been isolated from *M. cyclopis* at the New England RPRC (*20*), and another type D virus has been isolated from the blood of rhesus monkeys with SAIDS at the California RPRC. This latter group has also induced SAIDS using tissue culture fluids containing type D retrovirus (*21*). The differences between these two isolates and the one described here from the Washington RPRC remain to be determined. It is possible that this class of type D retroviruses is infectious in macaques and produces the disease spectrum that is defined as simian AIDS.

The gibbon class of type C viruses, which is tumorigenic in primates (*22*), is believed to have been derived by transspecies infection of these apes with endogenous viruses from various species of Southeast Asian rodents, such as *Mus caroli* or *Mus cervicolor* (*23*). It thus appears that MPMV, SAIDS-D viruses, and the gibbon class of infectious primate viruses may have been acquired by infections from the endogenous viruses of other mammalian species that cohabit the same geographic area. Southeast Asia, where both macaques and langurs reside, may thus be a reservoir for the SAIDS-D viruses.

References and Notes

1. C. M. Reichert, T. J. O'Leary, D. L. Levens, C. R. Simrell, A. M. Macher, *Am. J. Pathol.* **112**, 357 (1983).
2. N. L. Letvin *et al., Proc. Natl. Acad. Sci. U.S.A.* **80**, 2718 (1983).
3. R. V. Henrickson *et al., Lancet* **1983-I**, 388 (1983); K. G. Osborn *et al., Am. J. Pathol.* **114**, 94 (1984).
4. W. T. London *et al., Lancet* **1983-II**, 869 (1983).
5. W. E. Giddens *et al., Lab. Invest.* **40**, 294 (1979); W. E. Giddens, Jr., W. R. Morton, E. Hefti, S. Panem, H. Ochs, *Viral and Immunological Disease in Nonhuman Primates* (Liss, New York, 1983).
6. C. C. Tsai, G. A. Blakley, H. Uno, B. Frohna, T. F. C. S. Warner, *Lab. Invest.* **50**, 61 (1984); T. F. C. S. Warner, H. Uno, C. C. Tsai, W. E. Giddens, Jr., *ibid.*, p. 65.
7. W. H. Burgdorf, K. Mukai, J. Rosai, *Am. J. Clin. Pathol.* **75**, 167 (1981); M. Nadji, A. R. Morales, J. Ziegles-Weissman, N. S. Penneys, *Arch. Pathol. Lab. Med.* **105**, 274 (1981).
8. H. D. Ochs *et al., Blood* **55**, 243 (1980); A. K. Junker *et al., Pediatr. Res.*, in press.
9. H. D. Ochs, S. D. Davis, R. J. Wedgwood, *J. Clin. Invest.* **50**, 2559 (1971).
10. M. S. Gottlieb *et al., N. Engl. J. Med.* **305**, 1425 (1981); H. C. Lane, H. Masur, G. Whalen, A. H. Rood, A. S. Fauci, *ibid.* **309**, 453 (1983).

11. R. E. Benveniste, M. M. Lieber, D. M. Livingston, C. J. Sherr, G. J. Todaro, *Nature (London)* **248**, 17 (1974).
12. B. Kramarsky, N. H. Sarkar, D. H. Moore, *Proc. Natl. Acad. Sci. U.S.A.* **68**, 1603 (1971); M. A. Gonda, D. L. Fine, M. Gregg, *Arch. Virol.* **56**, 297 (1977).
13. R. E. Benveniste *et al.*, in preparation.
14. V. S. Kalyanaraman, M. G. Sarngadharan, B. Poiesz, F. W. Ruscetti, R. C. Gallo, *J. Virol.* **38**, 906 (1981).
15. E. Hefti, J. Ip, W. E. Giddens, Jr., S. Panem, *Virology* **127**, 309 (1983).
16. S. Panem, personal communication.
17. R. E. Benveniste *et al.*, *Biochem. Biophys. Res. Commun.* **81**, 1363 (1978).
18. R. E. Benveniste and G. J. Todaro, *Proc. Natl. Acad. Sci. U.S.A.* **74**, 4557 (1977).
19. W. Drohan, D. Colcher, G. Schochetman, J. Schlom, *J. Virol.* **23**, 36 (1977).
20. M. D. Daniel *et al.*, *Science* **223**, 602 (1984).
21. P. A. Marx *et al.*, *ibid.*, p. 1083.
22. T. G. Kawakami *et al.*, *Nature (London) New Biol.* **235**, 170 (1972); T. G. Kawakami, G. V. Kollias, Jr., C. Holmberg, *Int. J. Cancer* **25**, 641 (1980).
23. M. M. Lieber *et al.*, *Proc. Natl. Acad. Sci. U.S.A.* **72**, 2315 (1975).
24. L. O. Arthur, B. W. Altrock, G. Schochetman, *Virology* **110**, 270 (1981).
25. Supported in part with federal funds from the Department of Health and Human Services under contracts N01-CO-23910 with Program Resources, Inc., and N01-CO-23909 with Litton Bionetics, Inc.; and NIH grants RR00166 and RR01203 from the Division of Research Resources. We thank B. Kramarsky for electron microscopy, W. B. Knott, R. W. Hill, T. C. Shaffer, and S. A. Vargo for technical assistance, and D.A. Huffer for clerical assistance.

10 February 1984; accepted 12 March 1984

28. Rectal Insemination Modifies Immune Responses in Rabbits

Jon M. Richards, J. Michael Bedford, and Steven S. Witkin

Antibodies to spermatozoa and to circulating immune complexes (CIC's) are present in apparently healthy homosexual men (*1, 2*) and at increased concentrations in homosexuals with lymphadenopathy or acquired immunodeficiency syndrome (AIDS) (*2, 3*). The etiology of AIDS is not clear; however, the fact that a large proportion of AIDS cases have been found in highly sexually active homosexual men suggests that the syndrome may have some relation to circulating antibodies evoked as a result of semen deposition in the alimentary canal. Human seminal fluid apparently contains components that potentially can suppress the immune response (*4, 5*),

and syngeneic mouse spermatozoa injected intravenously are reported to be immunosuppressive as determined by mixed lymphocyte culture (*6*).

We used rabbits to ascertain whether CIC's or antibodies to sperm can result from rectal insemination and whether this affects the ability to mount an immune response. Rabbit ejaculates collected with an artificial vagina were pooled and examined with a microscope for motile sperm, which were counted. Healthy males were restrained and 1 ml of fresh semen (containing about 10^8 sperm) was deposited in the rectum to a depth of 5 cm at weekly intervals with a No. 7 French rubber catheter. To ensure that this had not traumatized the rectal mucosa, feces passed after the procedure were examined and found to be heme-negative. Rabbits treated by depositing 1 ml of saline in the same manner on the same schedule were used as controls.

Blood was drawn into heparinized tubes at weekly intervals for immunological analyses. The total red and white cell counts, differential white cell count, and total concentrations of immunoglobulin G (IgG), immunoglobulin M (IgM), and immunoglobulin A (IgA) in the serum were not affected by these treatments. Nor was the ability of concanavalin A, phytohemagglutinin, and rabbit spermatozoa to induce proliferation of the peripheral blood lymphocytes (PBL's) reduced. However, after an 8-week period of weekly rectal inseminations there was a significant ($P < 0.01$, Student's t-test) increase in CIC's and in IgG and IgA reactive with rabbit sperm (Fig. 1); no changes were seen in the control rabbits. Antibodies to seminal fluid antigens were not detected.

Rectal insemination for longer periods (up to 8 months) did not bring about a further increase in CIC's or antibodies to sperm. However, levels of IgG reactive with normal rabbit PBL's, apparent by 2 to 4 months, increased throughout the 8-month period. Serum samples obtained from each rabbit before treatment and at the end of treatment were assayed for IgG that reacted with normal rabbit PBL's. Immunoglobulin G reactive with PBL's in semen-treated rabbits doubled on average, whereas saline-treated controls showed no such change ($P < 0.01$, Student's t-test) (Table 1).

In addition to producing IgG reactive with PBL's, semen-treated rabbits produced IgG reactive with asialo GM1 (7). This neutral glycolipid is not present on

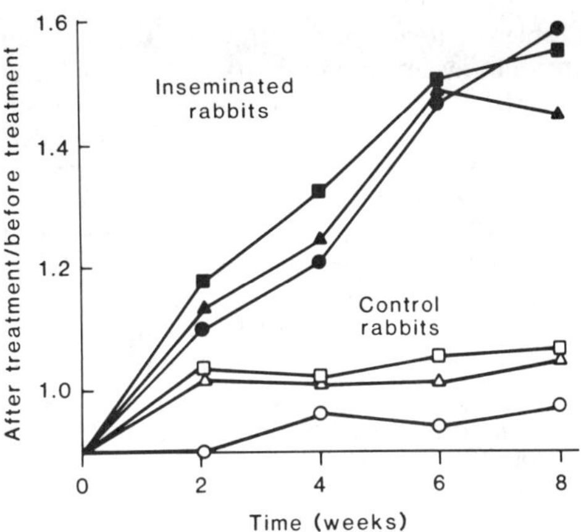

Fig. 1. Appearance of CIC's and sperm-reactive IgG and IgA after rectal insemination. Plasma from five inseminated rabbits and five controls were assayed for CIC's by a Raji cell ELISA (16) and for IgG and IgA by an ELISA with rabbit sperm bound to wells of a microtiter plate (1). Each value is the mean of at least three determinations that varied less than 10 percent. Symbols: (●, ○) IgG, (▲, △) IgA, and (■, □) CIC's.

B cells (8) but occurs on the surface of murine natural killer and peripheral T cells and on rabbit and human sperm (7). Previous studies have shown that injection of antibody to asialo GM1 into mice (9) or rats (10) decreases natural killer cell function in these animals and that 36 percent of homosexuals with AIDS have antibody to asialo GM1 in their serum (7).

We also studied the responsiveness of semen-treated animals to T cell–dependent antigens—in this case keyhole limpet hemocyanin (KLH) and sheep red blood cells (SRBC's). Since the means for assessing natural killer cell function in rabbits have not yet been developed and since mitogen-induced lymphocyte proliferation appeared to be unaffected after rectal insemination, immune function in the experimental males was assessed by evaluating the immune re-

144

Table 1. Reactivity of IgG in serum from rectally inseminated rabbits with normal rabbit PBL's. The last serum sample from each rabbit and the sample obtained before treatment began were analyzed for IgG reactive with normal rabbit PBL's. The PBL's were prepared (15) and 5×10^4 cells were fixed with glutaraldehyde to the wells of microtiter plates. Wells were washed with phosphate-buffered saline (PBS) and Tween and incubated for 2 hours with 1:10 dilutions of test serum. IgG bound to the rabbit lymphocytes was then measured by incubating wells with 1:200 dilutions of alkaline phosphatase–conjugated swine antibodies to rabbit IgG (gamma chain–specific) for 90 minutes, washing wells with PBS-Tween, and adding 0.2 ml of p-nitrophenylphosphate (1 mg/ml) in 10 percent diethanolamine (pH 9.8). After 30 minutes the optical density at 405 nm was determined. Each value is the mean of at least three determinations that varied less than 10 percent.

Treatment	IgG (before treatment/ after treatment)	Treatment	IgG (before treatment/ after treatment)
Semen	3.4	Saline	0.9
Semen	1.1	Saline	1.1
Semen	2.0	Saline	1.2
Semen	2.8	Saline	0.7
Semen	1.7		
Mean	2.2		0.98

sponse to these T cell–dependent antigens. Rabbits were immunized intravenously with KLH or SRBC's for 4 to 5 days and antibody responses were determined daily by measuring hemagglutination of KLH-coated or uncoated SRBC's (11) and by measuring KLH- or SRBC-specific IgG, IgM, and IgA with the enzyme-linked immunosorbent assay (ELISA) (12). Table 2 summarizes the hemagglutination results of SRBC-immunized normal and treated rabbits. Hemagglutination in serum from rectally

Table 2. Hemagglutination response to SRBC's by rabbits receiving rectal semen. Rabbits were given 2 ml of 10 percent SRBC's in 0.9 percent NaCl every day for 4 days. Before each injection and every day after the injections were discontinued, 3 ml of blood was collected for analysis of the SRBC hemagglutination titer (11).

Treatment	Day of peak titer	Peak titer
Saline	7	1:2048
Saline	6	1:2048
Saline	5	1:2048
Semen	6	1:64
Semen	6	1:2048
Semen	6	1:64
Semen	9	1:64

inseminated animals was significantly lower than that in serum from controls ($P < 0.01$), and IgM, IgG, and IgA titers were similarly diminished. Table 3 shows the outcome of a 5-day intravenous KLH immunization. A reduction in each antibody isotype was associated with animals receiving rectal semen. The differences in IgG, IgA, and IgM binding were all significant at $P < 0.01$, $P < 0.02$, and $P < 0.01$, respectively.

In conclusion, rectal insemination of homologous semen into rabbits had several consequences. Sperm in the rectum evoked the formation of antibodies to sperm despite the presence of seminal plasma, which has been held to be immunosuppressive (5). Furthermore, as judged by representative serial sections of tissue taken at autopsy, this response occurred in the absence of insemination-associated trauma to the gut lining or perianal area, possible elements in the etiology of the sperm antibody response seen in homosexual men ($1, 2$). While the rectally inseminated rabbits did not de-

Table 3. Peak production of antibody to KLH in rabbits. Polystyrene microtiter plates were incubated with KLH (10 µg/ml) in carbonate buffer (*p*H 9.8) overnight at 4°C. The plates were washed in PBS-Tween and 0.1 ml of a 1:10,000 dilution of rabbit serum was added to each well. After being incubated at room temperature, the plates were washed with PBS-Tween and incubated with alkaline phosphatase–conjugated swine antibody to rabbit IgM, IgG, or IgA (heavy chain–specific) for 90 minutes. After a final wash with PBS-Tween, 0.2 ml of *p*-nitrophenylphosphate (1 mg/ml) in 10 percent diethanolamine (*p*H 9.8) was added to each well. The optical density at 405 nm was determined at 30 minutes and wells that had been reacted with normal rabbit serum were used as blank reference wells. Each value is the mean (and standard deviation) of at least three determinations for each of four rabbits.

Anti-body	Optical density at 405 nm	
	Normal rabbits	Semen-treated rabbits
IgM	1.643 (0.216)	0.732 (0.110)
IgG	1.511 (0.124)	0.976 (0.201)
IgA	0.410 (0.116)	0.165 (0.086)

velop the opportunistic infections typically seen in AIDS patients, their reduced responsiveness to T cell–dependent antigens suggests a possible link in this respect. The basis of this effect is not yet known. We have found no significant difference in the rate of clearance of ^{51}Cr-labeled SRBC's in antigen-naïve inseminated and control rabbits, indicating that macrophage interaction with the antigen was not impaired after rectal insemination. Moreover, it is unlikely that the reduced humoral response was due to net lymphocyte depletion, since total PBL counts did not change. However, the appearance of CIC's and antibodies to asialo GM1 in the serum of rectally inseminated rabbits and the fact that serum from the rectally inseminated rabbits inhibited mitogen-induced proliferation of control PBL's in vitro (*13*) raises two possibilities. The first is that CIC's can interfere with immune function (*14*). They have been associated with a number of pathological states (*14*), including AIDS (*1, 2*). Second, the presence of IgG reactive with asialo GM1 in the serum of rectally inseminated rabbits may also be a factor in the decreased immune response. When presented in association with sperm-surface allogeneic histocompatibility antigens, this surface antigen may evoke an autoimmune response leading to the appearance of antibodies reactive with subsets of the T lymphocyte or natural killer cell populations. CIC's or cross-reactive antibodies could foster a degree of suppression by interfering directly with lymphocyte functions or by inducing alterations in the production of soluble mediators of the immune response.

References and Notes

1. S. S. Witkin and J. Sonnabend, *Fertil. Steril.* **39**, 337 (1983).
2. S. S. Witkin *et al.*, *AIDS Res.* **1**, 31 (1983).
3. J. Sonnabend, S. S. Witkin, D. T. Purtilo, *J. Am. Med. Assoc.* **249**, 2370 (1983).
4. S. S. Witkin, J. M. Richards, A. Bongiovanni, G. Zelikovsky, *Am. J. Reprod. Immunol.* **3**, 23 (1983).
5. D. Stites, C. Lammel, G. Brooks, in *Immunobiology of Neisseria gonorrhoeae*, G. Brooks *et al.*, Eds. (American Society for Microbiology, Washington, D.C., 1978), pp. 344–345.
6. U. Hurtenbach and G. Shearer, *J. Exp. Med.* **155**, 1719 (1982).
7. S. S. Witkin, J. Sonnabend, J. Richards, D. Purtilo, *Clin. Exp. Immunol.* **54**, 346 (1983).
8. K. Stein, G. Schwarting, D. Marcus, *J. Immunol.* **120**, 676 (1978).
9. M. Kasai *et al.*, *Nature (London)* **291**, 334 (1981).
10. T. Barlozzari, C. Reynolds, R. Herberman, *J. Immunol.* **131**, 1024 (1983).
11. J. S. Garvey, N. Cremer, D. Sussdorf, *Methods in Immunology* (Benjamin, Reading, Pa., ed. 3, 1977), pp. 356–360.
12. A. Voller, D. Bidwell, A. Bartlett, in *Manual of Clinical Immunology*, N. Rose and H. Friedman, Eds. (American Society for Microbiology, Washington, D.C., 1980), pp. 359–371.
13. S. S. Witkin, J. M. Richards, A. M., Bongiovanni, I. R. Yu, *Ann. N.Y. Acad. Sci.*, in press.

14. A. Theofilopoulos and F. Dixon, *Adv. Immunol.* **28**, 89 (1979).
15. M. Kunz, J. Innes, M. Wecksler, *J. Exp. Med.* **143**, 1042 (1976).
16. S. S. Witkin *et al.*, *J. Clin. Lab. Immunol.* **10**, 193 (1983).
17. The excellent technical assistance of A. M.

Bongiovanni and I. R. Yu is gratefully acknowledged. These studies were supported by grants HD16587 and CA 35018 from the National Institutes of Health and by the Rockefeller Foundation and the AIDS Medical Foundation.

3 January 1984; accepted 7 February 1984

29. Strong New Candidate for AIDS Agent

Jean L. Marx

In the 3 years since AIDS (acquired immune deficiency syndrome) was first identified, the cause of the disease has been intensely sought and often just as intensely debated. Most investigators expected that an infectious agent, probably a virus, would turn out to cause AIDS, but this was by no means a universal view. The 4 May 1984 issue of *Science* contains four reports from Robert Gallo of the National Cancer Institute and his many collaborators that appear to settle the matter.

According to these workers, a newly discovered subgroup of the human T-cell leukemia virus family, designated HTLV-III, is closely linked to the disease. The virus itself has been isolated from more than one-third of patients with full-blown AIDS and from nearly 90 percent of individuals with symptoms indicating that they may have an early form of the disease. Antibodies to HTLV-III have been found in 90 to 100 percent of AIDS patients, a finding that indicates that they have been infected with the agent. "I think that Dr. Gallo has identified the cause of AIDS," says Jerome Groopman of New England Dea-

coness Hospital and Harvard Medical School, "and I am a very cautious, skeptical person who has been involved with AIDS from the start."

In addition, Luc Montagnier of the Pasteur Institute in Paris and his colleagues have also been finding a virus in patients with AIDS and early AIDS. The Pasteur virus may be the same as HTLV-III, although this has not yet been definitively established.

Identification of the AIDS agent has enormous clinical implications. At the very least, it should be possible to develop a specific assay to identify blood that might be contaminated with the virus. The 10,000 to 15,000 hemophiliacs in this country are at high risk of developing the disease because the clotting factor preparations they must take to prevent uncontrollable bleeding are usually prepared from blood contributed by thousands of donors. According to figures compiled by ·the Centers for Disease Control in Atlanta, nearly 30 hemophiliacs have developed AIDS.

People who receive whole blood are at much lower risk, but the potential number of people who might be exposed is very large. Some 4 million people are transfused every year. So far, 46 people with no other risk factors have developed AIDS, apparently as a result of transfusions. A means of testing for the AIDS agent would do much to allay fears of contracting a dread disease as a result of a needed medical treatment.

The identification should also help to define the natural history and clinical course of the disease. At present the definition of AIDS is descriptive. It involves, among other things, a finding of severe immune depression, with depletion of helper T cells in particular, in patients for whom no other causes of an immune deficiency, such as cancer or organ transplantation, can be identified. They must also have either life-threatening opportunistic infections or Kaposi's sarcoma, a cancer that was rare and found only in older men of Mediterranean ancestry before it began turning up in AIDS patients. Full-blown AIDS has a high mortality rate. About 1750 of the more than 4000 victims have died.

But this severe form of AIDS may represent just the tip of the iceberg. Many additional individuals show such symptoms as lymphadenopathy (a condition characterized by swollen lymph nodes, fever, and malaise) and depressed helper T-cell counts without having the devastating illness characteristic of the full-blown disease. These people may be classified as having early AIDS (pre-AIDS as it is sometimes called). About 10 percent eventually develop the more serious symptoms, but at present there is no way to predict whose condition will worsen. Without a definitive test for AIDS it is difficult to tell whether their symptoms are related to AIDS at all. A number of viral infections cause a transient immune suppression that resembles that seen in AIDS.

The test for the HTLV-III antibodies may help to clear up some of these uncertainties. "It is tremendously exciting. To really have the possibility of a diagnostic test is a breakthrough," Groopman says. In some cases the result may alleviate the fears of a high-risk individual who has been having symptoms of AIDS. Groopman cites the case of a homosexual male who showed evidence of immune abnormalities although HTLV-III antibodies could not be detected in his blood. He turned out to have a case of mononucleosis from which he is now recovering.

In contrast, individuals who learn that they have a positive antibody test will hardly be comforted. The ambiguous symptoms make it difficult to differentiate between a mild case and one that will progress. However, as Bijan Safai of Memorial Sloan-Kettering Cancer Center points out, earlier detection of AIDS may have clinical benefits. "If you treat early, you may be able to reverse the immune deficiency."

But there is another problem. An individual who displays no or only mild AIDS symptoms is still capable of harboring the agent and may transmit it to others. Since sexual intercourse both of the heterosexual and homosexual varieties is a major pathway of transmission, an individual who learns that he or she shows signs of infection will face a major dilemma, to say the least.

There may be an enormous demand for the test. Virtually every blood bank will have to examine all donated blood. The high-risk groups in this country include some 15,000 hemophiliacs, an unknown number of users of illicit intravenous drugs, and about half a million Haitians. In addition, there are perhaps 20 million homosexual males, although this figure is only an estimate at best.

However, only an unknown percentage of these are highly promiscuous and therefore at high risk.

Identification of the AIDS agent also opens the way to a vaccine to protect high-risk persons against the disease. "The data in these four reports make a very good case that this virus is associated with the disease," notes Vincent DeVita, director of NCI. "Attempts to develop a vaccine would be the next step." One thing that will have to be learned is whether antibodies to HTLV-III can protect against the development of AIDS. Vaccine testing may begin in 2 to 3 years, according to officials of the Department of Health and Human Services.

HTLV first turned up a few years ago when Gallo's group and that of Yorio Hinuma of Kyoto University in Japan independently isolated a virus from leukemia cells of patients with malignancies affecting the T lymphocytes, which play a major role in immune responses. This virus, now designated HTLV-I, is currently the best candidate for a human cancer virus. The Gallo group also identified a second, much more rare HTLV variant, designated HTLV-II, which is also associated with T-cell malignancies.

The first reports linking HTLV's to AIDS began to appear about a year ago (*Science*, 20 May 1983). The Gallo group found either infectious HTLV particles or DNA related to the HTLV genome in T cells from a few AIDS patients. At the same time investigators from the Pasteur Institute in Paris also reported the isolation of an HTLV-like virus from an individual with signs of early AIDS. The Paris isolate, which has not yet been fully characterized, appeared different from HTLV-I and -II. In addition, Max Essex of the Harvard University School of Public Health found antibodies against HTLV-I in about 30 percent of patients with AIDS or early AIDS.

Although these findings were considered intriguing and "a good lead," they did not constitute definitive proof of HTLV involvement in AIDS. For one thing, most of the patients did not show evidence of HTLV infection. For another, a hallmark of AIDS is high susceptibility to infection by opportunistic pathogens that can take advantage of the patient's compromised immune system. The HTLV infections might also be opportunistic—that is, consequences rather than causes of AIDS.

Nevertheless, all during this research Gallo and his colleagues were tantalized by indications of a viral presence in cells from many additional AIDS patients. The indications included electron micrographs showing what appeared to be viral particles, the presence of reverse transcriptase (an enzyme that copies RNA into DNA and is a component of viruses such as HTLV that have RNA as their genetic material), and the ability to infect fresh human lymphocytes by culturing them with the AIDS cells. Infected cells always died, however. "We couldn't characterize these isolates because, unlike the leukemic cells, we couldn't get T cells from AIDS patients to grow," Gallo explains. The investigators were able to tell that the isolates were neither HTLV-I nor -II because they were not detected by monoclonal antibodies against those strains.

The turning point came about 10 months ago. Mikulas Popovic of the Gallo laboratory identified cloned cell lines, derived from human lymphoid leukemia cells, that would continue to grow after infection with the uncharacterized virus. "We were able to mass-produce the virus for the first time," Gallo notes. They at last had enough material to determine the properties of the virus and compare it with HTLV-I and -II. Moreover, they could develop analytic reagents for characterizing all their isolates, which now total 51.

The newly identified virus has RNA for its genetic material, like the other HTLV's, and also resembles them in size and shape. Its reverse transcriptase has a molecular weight of about 100,000 and requires magnesium ions for its activity, additional points of resemblance to HTLV-I and -II. There are significant differences, however. Jörg Schüpbach of the NCI laboratory has found that the proteins of the newly isolated virus, now called HTLV-III, are similar to those of the other HTLV's, especially HTLV-II, but they are not identical. In addition, Suresh Arya and Flossie Wong-Staal have found that the viral nucleic acids, although showing homology throughout the genome, are different.

The most significant difference between HTLV-III and the other two variants, at least with respect to their potential pathogenicity, involves their effects on cells. According to Gallo, when cultured cells are infected with HTLV-I or -II, a few cells undergo cancerous transformation. This is consistent with the association of these two viruses with the T-cell malignancies. In contrast, HTLV-III does not appear to transform cells in that way, although it does have cell-killing effects.

All three HTLV's specifically infect T cells of the class that includes the helper cells, which, as their name suggests, help other immune cells to carry out their functions. The immune deficiencies of AIDS patients are largely, if not entirely, caused by a severe depletion of helper T cells—such as might be produced by a virus that specifically kills them.

In any event, the Gallo group has now isolated HTLV-III from roughly 85 percent of 21 individuals with early AIDS symptoms and from about 35 percent of patients with the full-blown disease (26 of 72). The latter figure may be lower than it is in actuality. When the investigators calculated the percentage, they used the total of all the AIDS samples sent to them, even though some had deteriorated to the point where they were of questionable value for analysis. In addition, it may be more difficult to detect virus-infected cells in patients with advanced AIDS because the susceptible cell population is so severely depleted in them.

The Gallo group did not detect the virus in blood samples from 115 heterosexual donors. Only 1 of 22 homosexual males who appeared healthy when their blood samples were taken carried the virus. That individual subsequently developed AIDS.

In addition, as described in their 4 May 1984 *Science* report, M. G. Sarngadharan of Litton Bionetics, Inc., in Kensington, Maryland; Gallo; and their colleagues found antibodies to HTLV-III in nearly 90 percent of AIDS patients (43 of 49) and in about 80 percent of 14 homosexual men with the milder, early symptoms. They also detected the antibodies in 7 of 17 homosexual men with no clinical AIDS symptoms. At least two of these were long-term sex partners of AIDS victims, and all the men were clinic patients, which means that they may not be representative of the total homosexual population.

Only 1 of 186 other controls was positive for the antibodies. The controls included a number of patients with conditions in which the function of the immune system is disrupted. This makes it unlikely that the antibodies are associated with nonspecific immune defects instead of HTLV-III infection.

In another study that was just completed, with the use of an improved method for detecting the HTLV-III antibodies, 100 percent of the AIDS patients were positive. Groopman, who supplied samples for this study, says, "The assay picked out 100 percent of the AIDS and lymphadenopathy syndrome [pre-AIDS] patients. There were no false positives and no false negatives. I can tell you it was remarkable." The study was conducted under double-blind conditions. The investigators did not know which samples were which until the antibody analyses were completed and the code was broken on 10 April.

The antibodies detected in the blood of the AIDS patients are directed primarily against the major protein forming the outer envelope of the HTLV-III particle. These antibodies are apparently capable of cross-reacting to some extent with the envelope protein of HTLV-I, which probably explains why roughly one-third of AIDS patients were positive in the earlier study by the Essex group. The antigen actually detected by the Essex assay is a membrane protein, which has a molecular weight of roughly 60,000 and is found on the surfaces of cells infected with HTLV-I. Recent work by the Essex and Gallo groups has shown that this is the precursor of the 46,000-dalton envelope protein of HTLV-1.

Meanwhile, the Pasteur workers have now made nearly a dozen isolates of their virus, which they call lymphadenopathy-associated virus (LAV), from AIDS and pre-AIDS patients. Using samples supplied by the CDC, they have also detected antibodies to LAV in blood from about 90 percent of U.S. AIDS and pre-AIDS patients.

LAV, like the HTLV's, has RNA as its genetic material. It appears to infect the same subpopulation of T cells as the HTLV's. The presumption is that LAV will turn out to be the same as HTLV-III. Gallo plans to collaborate with the Pasteur group to determine whether that is the case. Gallo notes, incidentally, that HTLV-III does not appear to be closely related to the virus that has recently been identified as the cause of an AIDS-like disease of monkeys.

According to Gallo, the nucleic acid studies of HTLV-III suggest that the virus may not be new, as has been speculated. AIDS was just identified in 1981. The nucleic acid data show that the HTLV-III RNA is similar throughout the genome to the RNA's of HTLV-I and -II. "It looks as though there is some kind of common ancestor," Gallo says. "It has probably existed for a long time." The possibility remains, however, that HTLV-III underwent some recent subtle change.

Gallo speculates that the HTLV's originated in Africa. HTLV-I has been detected in Old World monkeys, but not in New World monkeys. AIDS may have emerged only recently as a result of population shifts from rural areas of Africa to the cities where there would be greater chances of contact with foreign visitors who could have carried the agent to new locales, such as the United States or Haiti, which also has a relatively high incidence of the disease. Alternatively, the virus might have been exported directly by an emigrating African. Many of the AIDS cases identified in Europe have links to Central Africa and the condition has been found there as well.

Traditionally, final proof that a particular agent causes a disease usually involves showing that Koch's postulates can be met. One of the postulates requires that the host be injected with the agent to see whether the disease develops. With an illness as deadly as AIDS this will never be possible with human subjects. But showing that HTLV-III can be used to produce an effective vaccine would go a long way to removing whatever doubts might remain about whether it is the AIDS agent.

Report

4 May 1984

30. Detection, Isolation, and Continuous Production of Cytopathic Retroviruses (HTLV-III) from Patients with AIDS and Pre-AIDS

Mikulas Popovic, M.G. Sarngadharan, Elizabeth Read, and Robert C. Gallo

Epidemiologic data suggest that the acquired immunodeficiency syndrome (AIDS) is caused by an infectious agent that is horizontally transmitted by intimate contact or blood products (*1–3*). Though the disease is manifested by opportunistic infections, predominantly *Pneumocystis carinii* pneumonia (*4*), and by Kaposi's sarcoma (*5*), the underlying disorder affects the patient's cell-mediated immunity (*6*), resulting in absolute lymphopenia and reduced subpopulations of helper T lymphocytes (OKT4$^+$). Moreover, before a complete clinical manifestation of the disease occurs, its prodrome, pre-AIDS, is frequently characterized by unexplained chronic lymphadenopathy or leukopenia involving helper T lymphocytes (*5, 6*). This leads to the severe immune deficiency of the patient and suggests that a specific subset of T cells could be a primary target for an infectious agent. Although patients with AIDS or pre-AIDS are often chronically infected with cytomegalovi-

rus (*7*) or hepatitis B virus (*8*), for various reasons these appear to be opportunistic or coincidental infections. We have proposed that AIDS may be caused by a virus from the family of human T-cell lymphotropic retroviruses (HTLV) (*9*) that includes two major, well-characterized subgroups of human retroviruses, called human T-cell leukemia-lymphoma viruses, HTLV-I (*9–12*) and HTLV-II (*9, 11, 13*). The most common isolate, HTLV-I, is obtained mainly from patients with mature T-cell malignancies (*9, 12*). Seroepidemiological studies, the biological effects of the virus in vitro, and nucleic acid hybridization data indicate that HTLV-I is etiologically associated with the T-cell malignancy of adults that is endemic in certain areas of the south of Japan (*14*), the Caribbean (*15*), and Africa (*16*). HTLV-II was first isolated from a patient with a T-cell variant of hairy cell leukemia (*13*). To date, this is the only reported isolate of HTLV-II from a patient with a neoplastic disease. Virus isolation and seroepidemiological data show that both HTLV-I and HTLV-II can sometimes be found in patients with AIDS (*17*).

That a retrovirus of the HTLV family might be an etiological agent of AIDS was suggested by the findings (i) that another retrovirus, feline leukemia virus, causes immune deficiency in cats (*18*); and that (ii) retroviruses of the HTLV family are T-cell tropic (*12, 19*); (iii) preferentially infect helper T cells (OKT4$^+$) (*12, 19*); (iv) have cytopathic effects on various human and mammalian cells, as demonstrated by their induction of cell syncytia formation (*20*); (v) can alter some T-cell functions (*21*); (vi) can in some cases selectively kill T cells (*22*); and (viii) may be transmitted by intimate contact and blood products (*9*). Also consistent with an HTLV etiology were the results of Essex and Lee and their colleagues showing the presence of antibodies to cell membrane antigens of HTLV-infected cells in serum samples from more than 40 percent of patients with AIDS (*23*). This antigen has since been defined as part of the envelope of HTLV (*24*). The more frequent detection in AIDS patients of antibodies to a membrane protein rather than to HTLV-I internal structural core proteins (*25*), together with the low incidence of isolations of HTLV-I or HTLV-II from AIDS patients, also suggested that a new variant of HTLV might be present.

The original detection and isolation of HTLV-I were made possible by the discovery of T-cell growth factor (TCGF) (*26*), also called interleukin 2 (IL-2), which stimulates the growth of different subsets of normal and neoplastic mature T cells (*27*), and by the development of sensitive assays for reverse transcriptase (RT), an enzyme characteristic of retro-

viruses (*28*). The procedures used previously for the transmission and continuous production of HTLV-I and -II were first worked out in mammalian cells transformed by avian sarcoma virus (*29*). These methods involved cocultivation of the transformed cells with cells permissive for the particular virus strain. Normal human T cells in cocultivation experiments preferentially yielded HTLV of both subgroups. Some of these viruses showed an immortalizing (transforming) capability for certain target T cells (*9, 12*). We thought that HTLV variants that have cytopathic effects on their target cells but do not immortalize them might be more important in the cause of AIDS. In fact, such variants were frequently but only transiently detected when normal T cells were used as targets in cocultivation or cell-free transmission experiments. This transience was our main obstacle to the isolation of these cytopathic variants of HTLV from patients with AIDS or pre-AIDS. We subsequently found a cell line that is highly susceptible to and permissive for cytopathic variants of HTLV. This cell line can grow permanently after infection with the virus. We report here the establishment and characterization of this new immortalized T-cell population and its use in the isolation and continuous high-level production of HTLV variants from patients with AIDS and pre-AIDS.

Several neoplastic human cell lines established in vitro were assayed for susceptibility to infection with HTLV-I and -II and with many of the more cytopathic retroviruses isolated from AIDS patients (*30*). One neoplastic aneuploid T-cell line, derived from an adult with lymphoid leukemia, was found to be susceptible to infection with the new cytopathic virus isolates. This cell line, termed HT, has produced HTLV-variants in sufficient quantities to permit the development of specific immunologic reagents and nucleic acid probes that can be used to characterize new isolates and compare them with HTLV-I and HTLV-II (*30*). These cytopathic variants differ from HTLV-I and -II not only in their biological effects but also in several immunological assays and in their morphology (*31*). They nevertheless have many properties similar to HTLV-I and -II. For example, they are T4 lymphotropic, they have a similar RT (*30*), they cross-react with several structural proteins in heterologous radioimmune assays with serum from AIDS patients and with antisera to the virus raised in animals (*31*), and they induce syncytia. These new HTLV isolates are collectively designated HTLV-III, although it is not yet proved that they are identical.

The cell line HT was tested for HTLV before being infected in vitro and was negative by all criteria including lack of proviral sequences (*32*). Continuous production of HTLV-III was obtained after repeated exposure of parental HT cells (3×10^6 cells pretreated with polybrene) to concentrated culture fluids harvested from short-term cultures of T cells (grown with TCGF) obtained from patients with AIDS or pre-AIDS. The concentrated fluids were first shown to contain particle-associated RT. When cell proliferation declined, usually 10 to 20 days after exposure to the culture fluids, the fresh (uninfected) HT cells were added to the cultures. Culture fluids from the infected parental cell line were positive for particulate RT activity, and about 20 percent of the infected cell population was positive in an indirect immune fluorescence assay in which we used serum from a hemophilia patient with pre-AIDS (patient E.T.). Serum from E.T. also contained antibodies to proteins of disrupted HTLV-III (*33*) but did not react with cells infected with HTLV-I or HTLV-II.

The parental T-cell population was extensively cloned in order to select the most permissive clones that would preserve high rates of growth and virus production (for example, see clones 4 and 9 in Table 1). A total of 51 single-cell clones were obtained by both capillary (*34*) and limited dilution (*35*) techniques using irradiated mononuclear cells from peripheral blood of a healthy donor as a feeder. The clones were infected with HTLV-III by exposure to concentrated virus (2×10^6 cells of each clone and 0.1 ml of virus). Then cell growth and morphology, expression of cellular viral antigens, and RT activity in culture fluids were assessed 6 and 14 days after infection. Results for eight of these clones are shown in Table 1. Although all of these clones were susceptible to and permissive for the virus, there were considerable differences in their ability to proliferate after infection. For example, the cell number decreased by 10 to 90 percent from the initial cell count within 6 days after infection. The percentage of T cells positive for viral antigens ranged from 10 to 80 percent, as determined by immune fluorescence assays with serum from patient E.T. and with antiserum from rabbits infected repeatedly with disrupted HTLV-III. At 14 days after infection, the total cell number and the proportion of HTLV-III positive cells had increased in all eight clones. The virus positive cultures consistently showed a high proportion of round giant cells containing numerous nuclei (Fig. 1a). These cells resemble those induced by HTLV-I and -II (*9*) except that the

154

nuclei exhibit a characteristic ring formation. Electron microscopic examinations showed that the cells released considerable amounts of virus (Fig. 1b).

Both virus production and cell viability of the infected clone H4 (H4/HTLV-III) were monitored for several months. Although virus production fluctuated (Fig. 2a), culture fluids harvested and assayed at approximately 14-day inter-

Table 1. Response of cloned T-cell populations to infection with HTLV-III. Single-cell clones were isolated as described (*34, 35*) from a long-term cultured aneuploid HT cell line exhibiting mature T-cell phenotype [OKT3$^+$ (62 percent), OKT4$^+$ (39 percent), and OKT8$^-$] as determined by cytofluorometry with a fluorescence-activated cell sorter. The cultures are routinely maintained in RPMI 1640 medium containing 20 percent fetal calf serum (FCS) and antibiotics. The terminal cell density of the parental cell culture, seeded at a concentration of 2×10^5 cells per milliliter of culture media, was in the range of 10^6 to 1.5×10^6 cells per milliliter after 5 days of culture.

Characteristics after infection	Clones*							
	H3	H4	H6	H9	H17	H31	H35	H38
Total cell number ($\times 10^6$)								
At 6 days	1	1.5	1.5	0.3	0.4	0.3	0.5	1.8
At 14 days	2.2	7.3	7.5	10	4.7	5.0	4.5	3.2
Multinucleated cells (%)*								
At 6 days	24	42	32	7	13	14	30	45
At 14 days	45	48	45	30	22	45	60	60
Immunofluorescence positive cells (%)†								
At 6 days								
Rabbit antiserum to HTLV-III	55	56	32	32	39	21	10	87
Patient serum (E.T.)	56	29	21	ND	ND	ND	ND	73
At 14 days								
Rabbit antiserum to HTLV-III	50	74	60	97	71	40	20	80
Patient serum	45	47	56	78	61	43	22	89
Reverse transcriptase activity ($\times 10^4$ cpm/ml)‡								
At 6 days	2.4	1.8	2.1	4.1	2.6	1.4	1.7	2.5
At 14 days	16.2	18.1	16.1	20.2	17.1	13.4	15.1	18.2

*Cell smears were prepared from cultures 6 and 14 days after infection and stained with Wright-Giemsa. Cells with more than five nuclei were considered to be multinucleated. Cloned cells from uninfected cultures also contained some multinucleated giant cells; however, the arrangement of the multiple nuclei in a characteristic ring formation (see Fig. 1a) was lacking and the number of these cells was much less (0.7 to 10 percent). †Cells were washed with phosphate-buffered saline (PBS) and resuspended in the same buffer at concentration 10^6 cells per milliliter. Approximately 50 µl of cell suspension was spotted on a slide, air dried, and fixed in acetone for 10 minutes at room temperature. Slides were stored at −20°C until use. Twenty microliters of either rabbit antiserum to HTLV-III (diluted 1:2000 in PBS) or serum from the patient (E.T.) diluted 1:8 in PBS was applied to cells and incubated for 50 minutes at 37°C. The fluorescein-conjugated antiserum to rabbit or human immunoglobulin G was diluted and applied to the fixed cells for 30 minutes at room temperature. Slides were then washed extensively before microscopic examinations. The uninfected parental cell line as well as the clones were consistently negative in these assays. ND, not done. ‡Virus particles were precipitated from cell-free supernatant as follows: 0.3 ml of $4M$ NaCl and 3.6 ml of 30 percent (weight to volume) polyethylene glycol (Carbowax 6000) were added to 8 ml of harvested culture fluids and the suspension was placed on ice overnight. The suspension was centrifuged in a Sorvall RC-3 centrifuge at 2000 rev/min at 4°C for 30 minutes. The precipitate was resuspended in 300 µl of 50 percent (by volume) glycerol (25 mM tris-HCl, pH 7.5, 5 mM dithiothreitol, 150 mM KCl, and 0.025 percent Triton X-100). Virus particles were disrupted by addition of 100 µl of 0.9 percent Triton X-100 in 1.5M KCl. Reverse transcriptase assays were performed as previously described (*10, 28*) (see comments to Fig. 2b) and expressed in counts per minute per milliliter of culture medium.

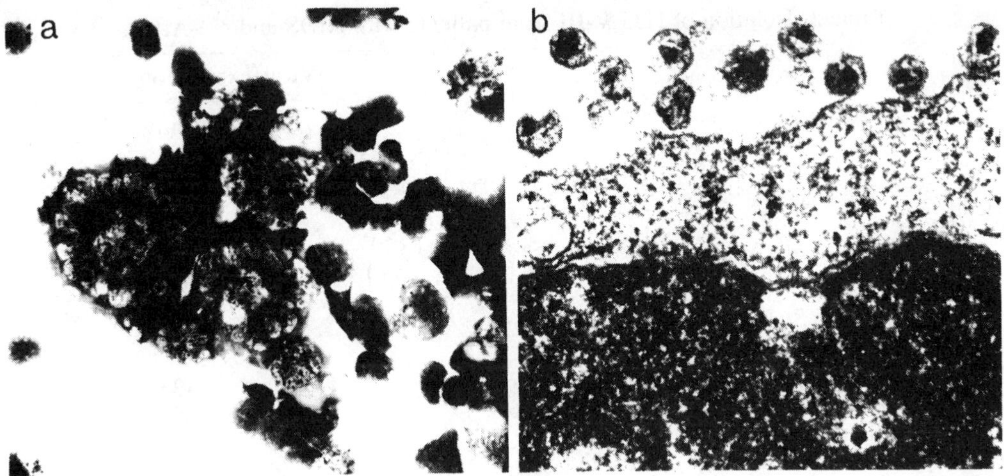

Fig. 1. Light and electron microscopic examination of clone H4/HTLV-III. (a) H4/HTLV-III cells were characterized by the presence of large multinucleated cells that showed, with Giemsa-Wright staining, a characteristic arrangement of their nuclei (×350). (b) Electron micrograph of the cells showing the presence of extracellular viral particles (×60,000).

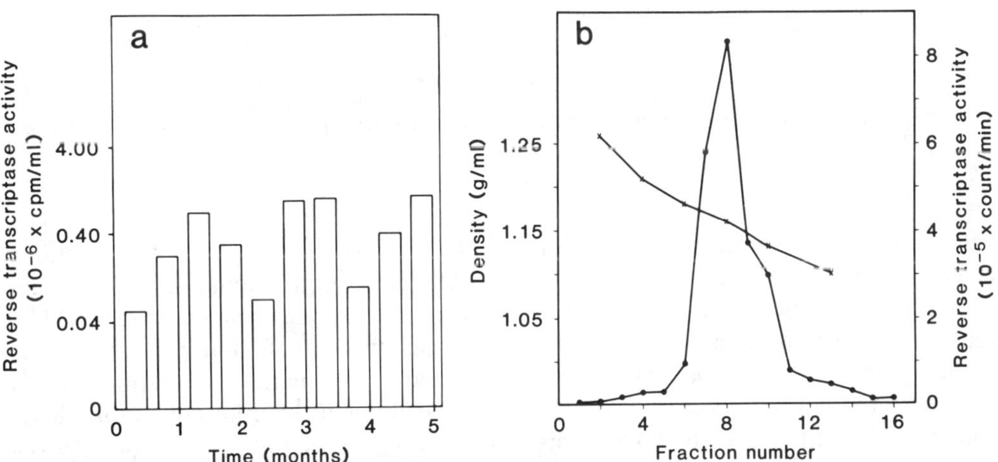

Fig. 2. (a) Continuous HTLV-III production from H4/HTLV-III in long-term culture was characterized by fluctuation in the amount of released virus as assessed by RT activity in the culture fluid (for details, see Table 1 and Fig. 2b). Viability of the infected cells was in the range of 60 to 90 percent. (b) Sucrose density gradient banding of HTLV-III showed the highest particulate RT activity at a density of 1.16 g/ml. A cell-free virus concentrate from a culture of H4/HTLV-III was layered on a 20 to 60 percent (by weight) sucrose gradient in 10 mM tris-HCl (pH 7.4) containing 0.1M NaCl and 1 mM EDTA and centrifuged overnight at 35,000 rev/min in a Spinco SW47 rotor. Fractions of 0.7 ml were collected from the bottom of the gradient and portions were assayed for RT ($\bullet$) with (dT)$_{15}$ · (A)$_n$ being used as the primer template and Mg^{2+} as the divalent cation according to the methods described earlier (*10, 28*). Density of sucrose (X) was determined by refractive index measurements.

Table 2. Isolation of HTLV-III from patients with AIDS and pre-AIDS.

Pa-tient*	Diagnosis	Origin	RT Activity ($\times 10^4$ cpm)	Virus expression†		Elec-tron micros-copy
				Percent positive cells in immune fluorescence assay		
				Rabbit anti-serum	Serum from E.T.	
R.F.	AIDS (heterosexual)	Haiti	0.25	80	33	ND
S.N.	Hemophiliac (lymphadenopathy)	United States	6.3	10	ND	+
B.K.	AIDS (homosexual)	United States	0.24	44	5	+
L.S.	AIDS (homosexual)	United States	0.13	64	19	+
W.T.	Hemophiliac (lymphadenopathy)	United States	3.2	69	ND	ND

*Cocultivation with H4 recipient T-cell clone was performed with fresh mononuclear cells from peripheral blood of patients R.F. and S.N., respectively. For patients B.K. and L.S. cocultivation was performed with T cells grown in the presence of exogenous TCGF (10 percent by volume) for 10 days. The ratio of recipient to donor (patients') cells was 1:5. The mixed cultures were maintained in RPMI 1640 medium (containing 20 percent FCS and antibiotics) in the absence of exogenous TCGF. H9 cells were also infected by exposing the cells to concentrated culture fluids harvested from T-cell cultures of patient W.T. The cultures were grown in the presence of exogenous TCGF for 2 weeks before the culture fluids were harvested and concentrated. Cells of H9 clones were treated with polybrene (2 µg/ml) for 20 minutes and 2×10^6 cells were exposed for 1 hour to 0.5 ml of 100-fold concentrated culture fluids positive for particulate RT activity.   †HTLV-III virus expression in cells infected by the coculture and cell-free methods was assayed approximately 1 month after cultivation in vitro. Note a considerable fluctuation in HTLV-III expression. For details of the RT and indirect immune fluorescence assays see Table 1.

vals consistently showed particulate RT activity which has been followed for over 5 months. The viability of the cells ranged from 65 to 85 percent and the doubling time of the cell population was approximately 30 to 40 hours (data not shown). Thus the data show that this permanently growing T-cell population can continuously produce HTLV-III.

The yield of virus from H4/HTLV-III cells was assessed by purification of concentrated culture fluids through a sucrose density gradient and assays of particulate RT activity in each fraction collected from the gradient. As shown in Fig. 2b, the highest RT activity was found at a density of 1.16 g/ml, which is similar to other retroviruses. The highest RT activity was found in the fractions with the largest amount of virus, as determined by electron microscopy. The actual number of viral particles determined by this method was estimated (36) to be about 10^{11} per liter of culture fluid.

We have used clones H4 and H9 for the long-term propagation of HTLV-III from patients with AIDS and pre-AIDS. HTLV-III was isolated from four patients by the cocultivation method and from one patient by cell-free infection of these T-cell clones (Table 2). The transmission was monitored by RT activity, electron microscopic examinations, and expression of viral protein. When the H4 cells thus infected were fixed with acetone and tested with rabbit antiserum to

HTLV-III and with serum from patient E.T., the percentage of positive cells was between 5 and 80 percent. HTLV-III has also been isolated in our laboratory from a total of 48 patients by the more conventional methods for isolation of HTLV (*30*). Some of these isolates have now successfully been transmitted to the HT clones for production and detailed analyses.

A few T-lymphocyte retroviruses that differed from HTLV-I and -II but were associated with lymphadenopathy syndrome were detected earlier (*37, 38*). One such virus, called LAV, was reported to be unrelated to HTLV-I or -II (*38*). Moreover, serum samples from 37.5 percent of patients with AIDS were found to react with it (*38*). In contrast, HTLV-III is related to HTLV-I and -II (*31, 39*) and, by all criteria, this new virus belongs to the HTLV family of retroviruses. In addition, more than 85 percent of serum samples from AIDS patients are reactive with proteins of HTLV-III (*33*). These findings suggest that HTLV-III and LAV may be different. However, it is possible that this is due to insufficient characterization of LAV because the virus has not yet been transmitted to a permanently growing cell line for true isolation and therefore has been difficult to obtain in quantity.

The transient expression of cytopathic variants of HTLV in cells from AIDS patients and the previous lack of a cell system that could maintain growth and still be susceptible to and permissive for the virus represented a major obstacle in detection, isolation, and elucidation of the precise causative agent of AIDS. The establishment of T-cell populations that continuously grow and produce virus after infection opens the way to the routine detection of cytopathic variants of HTLV in AIDS patients and provides

the first opportunity for detailed immunological (*31, 33*) and molecular analyses of these viruses.

References and Notes

1. Centers for Disease Control Task Force on Kaposi's Sarcoma and Opportunistic Infections, *N. Engl. J. Med.* **306**, 248 (1982).
2. J. P. Hanranhan, G. P. Wormser, C. P. Maquire, L. J. DeLorenzo, G. Davis, *ibid.* **307**, 498 (1982).
3. J. W. Curran *et al.*, *ibid.* **310**, 69 (1984).
4. "Pneumocystis pneumonia—Los Angeles," *Morbid. Mortal. Weekly Rep.* **30**, 250 (1981).
5. "Kaposi's sarcoma and pneumocystis pneumonia among homosexual men—New York City and California," *ibid.*, p. 305; A. E. Friedman-Klein *et al.*, *Ann. Int. Med.* **96**, 693 (1982).
6. M. Gottlieb *et al.*, *N. Engl. J. Med.* **305**, 1425 (1981); J. Masur *et al.*, *ibid.*, p. 1431.
7. C. Urmacher, P. Myskowski, M. Ochoa, M. Kris, B. Safai, *Am. J. Med.* **72**, 569 (1982).
8. D. R. Francis and J. E. Maynard, *Epidemiol. Rev.* **1**, 17 (1979); N. Clumeck *et al.*, *N. Engl. J. Med.* **310**, 492 (1984).
9. R. C. Gallo, in *Cancer Surveys*, L. M. Franks, L. M. Wyke, R. A. Weiss, Eds. (Oxford Univ. Press, Oxford, in press).
10. B. J. Poiesz *et al.*, *Proc. Natl. Acad. Sci. U.S.A.* **77**, 7415 (1980); M. Yoshida, I. Miyoshi, Y. Hinuma, *ibid.* **79**, 2031 (1982).
11. M. S. Reitz, M. Popovic, B. F. Haynes, S. C. Clark, R. C. Gallo, *Virology* **26**, 688 (1983).
12. M. Popovic *et al.*, *Science* **219**, 856 (1983).
13. V. S. Kalyanaraman *et al.*, *ibid.* **218**, 571 (1982).
14. Y. Hinuma *et al.*, *Proc. Natl. Acad. Sci. U.S.A.* **78**, 6476 (1981); M. Robert-Guroff *et al.*, *Science* **215**, 975 (1982); V. S. Kalyanaraman *et al.*, *Proc. Natl. Acad. Sci. U.S.A.* **79**, 1653 (1982).
15. W. A. Blattner *et al.*, *Int. J. Cancer* **30**, 257 (1982).
16. W. C. Saxinger *et al.*, in *Human T-Cell Leukemia Viruses*, R. C. Gallo, M. Essex, L. Gross, Eds. (Cold Spring Harbor Press, Cold Spring Harbor, N.Y., in press).
17. R. C. Gallo *et al.*, *Science* **220**, 865 (1983); E. P. Gelmann *et al.*, *ibid.*, p. 862; M. Popovic *et al.*, in preparation.
18. M. Essex, W. D. Hardy, Jr., S. M. Cotter, R. M. Jakowski, A. Sliski, *Infect. Immun.* **11**, 470 (1975); W. D. Hardy, Jr., *et al.*, *Cancer Res.* **36**, 582 (1976); L. J. Anderson, O. Jarret, H. M. Laird, *J. Natl. Cancer Inst.* **47**, 807 (1971).
19. R. C. Gallo *et al.*, *Cancer Res.* **43**, 3892 (1983); F. Wong-Staal *et al.*, *Nature (London)* **302**, 626 (1983).
20. K. Nagy, P. Clapham, R. Cheinsong-Popov, R. A. Weiss, *Int. J. Cancer* **32**, 321 (1983).
21. M. Popovic *et al.*, in preparation.
22. H. Mitsuya, H. G. Guo, M. Megson, C. D. Trainor, M. S. Reitz, S. Broder, *Science* **223**, 1293 (1984).
23. M. Essex *et al.*, *ibid.* **220**, 859 (1983).
24. J. Schüpbach, M. G. Sarngadharan, R. C. Gallo, *ibid.*, in press; T. H. Lee *et al.*, *Proc. Natl. Acad. Sci. U.S.A.*, in press.
25. M. Robert-Guroff *et al.*, in preparation.
26. D. A. Morgan, F. W. Ruscetti, R. C. Gallo, *Science* **193**, 1007 (1976).

158

27. F. W. Ruscetti, D. A. Morgan, R. C. Gallo, *J. Immunol.* **119**, 131 (1977); B. J. Poiesz, F. W. Ruscetti, J. W. Mier, A. M. Woods, R. C. Gallo, *Proc. Natl. Acad. Sci. U.S.A.* **77**, 6134 (1980).
28. R. C. Gallo, F. W. Ruscetti, R. E. Gallagher, in *Hematopoietic Mechanisms*, B. Clarkson, P. A. Marks, J. Till, Eds. (Cold Spring Harbor Press, Cold Spring Harbor, N.Y., 1978), vol. 5, p. 671.
29. J. Svoboda, *Natl. Cancer Inst. Monogr.* **17**, 277 (1964); J. Svoboda and R. Dourmashkin, *J. Gen. Virol.* **4**, 523 (1969); M. Popovic, J. Svoboda, J. Suni, A. Vaheri, L. Ponten, *Int. J. Cancer* **19**, 834 (1977); M. Popovic, J. Svoboda, F. L. Kisselyov, K. Polakova, *Folia Biol.* **26**, 244 (1980).
30. R. C. Gallo *et al.*, *Science* **224**, 500 (1984).
31. J. Schüpbach, M. Popovic, R. V. Gilden, M. A. Gonda, M. G. Sarngadharan, R. C. Gallo, *ibid.* **224**, 503 (1984).
32. G. Shaw and F. Wong-Staal, unpublished data.
33. M. G. Sarngadharan, M. Popovic, L. Bruch, J. Schüpbach, R. C. Gallo, *Science* **224**, 506 (1984).
34. M. Popovic, M. Grofova, N. Valentova, D. Simkovic, *Neoplasma* **18**, 257 (1971).
35. H. F. Bach, B. J. Alter, B. M. Widmer, M. S. Segall, D. Dunlap, *Immunol. Rev.* **54**, 5 (1981).
36. J. H. Monroe and P. M. Brandt, *Appl. Microbiol.* **20**, 259 (1970).
37. F. Barré-Sinoussi *et al.*, *Science* **220**, 868 (1983).
38. L. Montagnier *et al.*, in *Human T-Cell Leukemia Viruses*, R. C. Gallo, M. Essex, L. Gross, Eds. (Cold Spring Harbor Press, Cold Spring Harbor, N.Y., in press).
39. S. Arya *et al.*, in preparation.
40. We thank B. Kramarsky for help in electron microscopic examination of HTLV-III infected cells, E. Richardson and R. Zicht for technical help, and A. Mazzuca for her editorial assistance.

30 March 1984; accepted 19 April 1984

Report

4 May 1984

31. Frequent Detection and Isolation of Cytopathic Retroviruses (HTLV-III) from Patients with AIDS and at Risk for AIDS

Robert C. Gallo, Syed Z. Salahuddin, Mikulas Popovic, Gene M. Shearer, Mark Kaplan, Barton F. Haynes, Thomas J. Palker, Robert Redfield, James Oleske, Bijan Safai, Gilbert White, Paul Foster, and Phillip D. Markham

The acquired immunodeficiency syndrome known as AIDS was initially recognized as a separate disease entity in 1981 (*1*). Groups reported to be at risk for AIDS include homosexual or bisexual males (about 70 percent of reported cases), intravenous drug users (about 17 percent of cases), and Haitian immigrants to the United States (about 5 percent of cases). Also at risk are heterosexual contacts of members of the highest risk group, hemophiliacs treated with blood products pooled from donors, recipients of multiple blood transfusions, and infants born of parents belonging to the high-risk groups (*2*). AIDS is diagnosed as a severe, unexplained, immune deficiency that usually involves a reduction in the number of helper T lymphocytes and is accompanied by multiple opportunistic infections or malignancies. A number of other clinical manifestations, when occurring in members of a group at risk for AIDS, are identified as its prodrome (pre-AIDS). These include unexplained chronic lymphadenopathy or leukopenia involving a reduction in the number of helper T lymphocytes (1, 2). The increasing incidence of this disease, the types of patients affected, and other epidemiological data suggest the existence of an infectious etiologic agent that can be transmitted by intimate contact or by whole blood or separated blood components (2). As indicated by Popovic et al. (3), we and others have suggested that specific human T-lymphotropic retroviruses (HTLV) cause AIDS (4, 5). Many properties of HTLV are consistent with this idea (6).

An association of members of the HTLV family with T lymphocytes from some AIDS or pre-AIDS patients was reported previously. For example, the first subgroup of HTLV to be characterized, HTLV-I, was isolated recently from T cells from about 10 percent of AIDS patients, and a virus related to HTLV-II was isolated from one AIDS patient (4). Another HTLV isolate was obtained from the lymph nodes of a patient with lymphadenopathy and at risk for AIDS (7). This isolate has been difficult to grow in quantities sufficient to permit its characterization. HTLV proviral DNA was detected in T lymphocytes from two additional AIDS patients (8) and HTLV-related antigens were found in another two patients (4). Studies in which disrupted HTLV-I or the purified structural proteins (p24 or p19) were used to detect antibodies in serum samples from patients with AIDS and pre-AIDS indicated that 10 to 15 percent of the patients had been exposed to HTLV-I (9). Essex and his co-workers, using HTLV-infected T-lymphocyte cultures to detect antibody in serum samples, found that about 35 percent of patients with AIDS and pre-AIDS had been exposed to HTLV (5). Further studies suggested that at least some of the antigens detected in this system were products of the genome of a member of the HTLV family (10), but it was not known whether the antibodies were specifically against HTLV-I, HTLV-II, or a virus of a different subgroup.

With the availability of large quantities of HTLV-III (3), it became possible to develop specific immunological reagents that would facilitate its characterization. HTLV-III was found to share many properties with other HTLV isolates (6), but it was morphologically, biologically, and antigenically distinguishable (3, 11). Here we describe the detection and isolation of HTLV-III from a large number of patients with AIDS and pre-AIDS.

For these studies we used cell culture conditions previously developed in our laboratory for the establishment of T lymphocytes in culture and for the detection and isolation of HTLV-I and HTLV-II from leukemic donors (12). Evidence for the presence of HTLV-III included: (i) viral reverse transcriptase (RT) activity (12) in supernatant fluids; (ii) transmission of virus by coculturing T cells with irradiated donor cells or with cell-free fluids (3, 13); (iii) observation of virus by electron microscopy (12, 13); and (iv) the expression of viral antigens in indirect immune fluorescence assays using serum from a patient positive for antibodies to HTLV-III as described (5, 11), or antisera prepared against purified, whole disrupted HTLV-III (11). Cells and supernatant fluids were also monitored for the expression of HTLV-I and HTLV-II by using antibodies to the viral structural proteins p19 and p24 and by indirect immune fluorescence and radioimmunoprecipitation procedures (14).

As summarized in Table 1, we found HTLV-III in 18 of 21 samples from patients with pre-AIDS, from three of four clinically normal mothers of juvenile

Table 1. Detection and isolation of HTLV-III from patients with AIDS and pre-AIDS. Peripheral blood leukocytes were banded in Ficoll-Hypaque, incubated in growth medium (RPMI 1640, 20 percent fetal bovine serum, and 0.29 mg of glutamine per milliliter) containing phytohemagglutinin (PHA-P; 5 μg/ml) for 48 hours at 37°C in a 5 percent CO_2 atmosphere. They were then refed with growth medium containing 10 percent purified T-cell growth factor (TCGF). Cells and conditioned media from these lymphocytes were assayed for the presence of HTLV-III. Samples exhibiting more than one of the following were considered positive: repeated detection of a Mg^{2+}-dependent reverse transcriptase activity in supernatant fluids; virus observed by electron microscopy; intracellular expression of virus-related antigens detected with antibodies from seropositive donors or with rabbit antiserum to HTLV-III; or transmission of particles, detected by RT assays or by electron microscopic observation, to fresh human cord blood, bone marrow, or peripheral blood T lymphocytes. All isolates are distinguishable from HTLV-I or HTLV-II by several criteria and are classified as HTLV-III on the basis of similar morphological features observed by electron microscopy (Fig. 1); similar cytopathic effects (3); antigenic cross-reactivity (11); and nucleic acid analysis (16).

Diagnosis*	Number positive for HTLV-III	Number tested	Percent positive
Pre-AIDS	18	21	85.7
Clinically normal mothers of juvenile AIDS patients	3	4	75.0
Juvenile AIDS	3	8	37.5
Adult AIDS with Kaposi's sarcoma	13	43	30.2
Adult AIDS with opportunistic infections	10	21	47.6
Clinically normal homosexual donors	1	22	4.5
Clinically normal heterosexual donors	0	115	0

*With the exception of the normal heterosexual donors and some of the clinically normal mothers of juvenile AIDS patients, all others belong to one of the groups of people identified as being at risk for AIDS (homosexual males, intravenous drug users, Haitian immigrants, heterosexual contacts of members of a group at risk, hemophiliacs treated with pooled blood products, recipients of multiple blood transfusions, and infants born of parents belonging to other groups at risk). Pre-AIDS includes patients with unexplained chronic lymphadenopathy and leukopenia, with an inverted T4 (helper)/T8 (suppressor) lymphocyte ratio. The clinically normal, nonpromiscuous, homosexual subjects are from Washington, D.C., and are believed to be at moderate risk. The clinically normal heterosexual donors include both male and female subjects believed not to be at risk for AIDS.

AIDS patients, three of eight juvenile AIDS patients, 13 of 43 of adult AIDS patients with Kaposi's sarcoma, and 10 of 21 adult AIDS patients with opportunistic infections. Virus was detected in only one of 22 samples from clinically normal, nonpromiscuous homosexual males believed to be at only moderate risk for AIDS. It is interesting, however, that 6 months after these tests were conducted the one positive normal homosexual subject developed AIDS. In no instance, 0 of 115, was virus detected in or isolated from cells of the normal volunteers. Samples from 15 of these were tested under rigorously controlled conditions, which included addition of antibody to α-interferon.

Primary cells from patients usually produce virus for 2 to 3 weeks (Fig. 1). After this time the production of virus declines even though the culture may contain actively replicating cells that can be maintained for long periods in the

Fig. 1. Reverse transcriptase activity from lymphocytes established in cell culture from a patient with pre-AIDS. Viable cell number and Mg^{2+}-dependent RT activity were determined by established procedures (*13*). Symbols: ○, viable cell number in 1.5 ml of growth medium; ●, RT in 5 μl of fivefold concentrated conditioned medium sampled at the indicated time. A sudden vertical drop in the dashed curve indicates the time of subculturing of cells to the indicated cell number. Arrow indicates the time of addition of rabbit antiserum to α-interferon to a portion of the cultured cells (also see legend to Table 1).

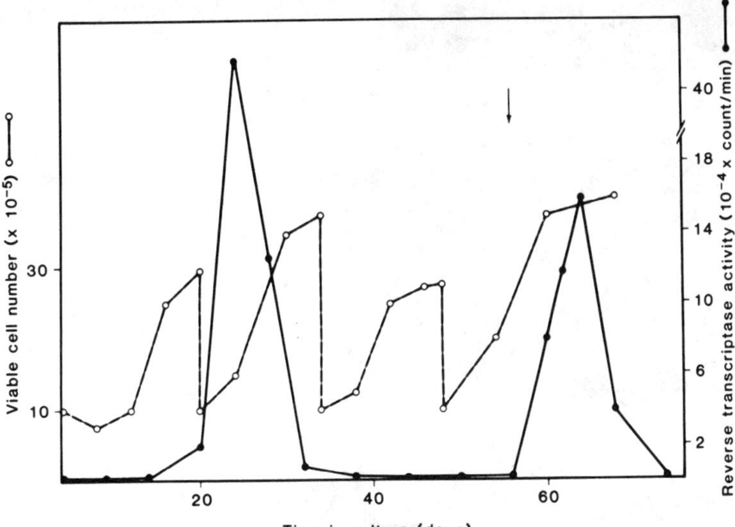

presence of added T-cell growth factor (TCGF). In some instances virus release can be reinitiated by the addition of antibody to α-interferon (Fig. 1). The HTLV-III–producing cell cultures were characterized by established immunological procedures (*13*). They were predominantly T lymphocytes (E rosette receptor–positive, OKT3$^+$ and Leu1$^+$) with a helper-inducer phenotype (OKT4$^+$ and Leu3$^+$).

The fairly uniform morphological appearance of HTLV-III is shown in Fig. 2. The diameter of the virus is 100 to 120 nm, and it is produced in high numbers from infected cells by budding from the cell membrane. A possibly unique feature of this virus is the cylindrical shaped core observed in many mature virions.

The incidence of virus isolation reported here probably underestimates its true incidence since many tissue specimens were not received or handled under what we now recognize as optimal conditions (*15*). This is particularly so for the samples received from late-stage AIDS patients. Such samples usually contain many dying cells and very few viable T4 lymphocytes. However, a high proportion of patients with AIDS and pre-AIDS have circulating antibody to HTLV-III (*11*).

The HTLV-III produced by cultured T cells from patients with AIDS and pre-AIDS is highly infectious and can be readily transmitted to fresh umbilical cord blood and adult peripheral blood or bone marrow lymphocytes. The production of HTLV-III by these cells is transient, often declining to undetectable levels by 2 to 3 weeks after infection (data not shown). The transmission of HTLV-III to an established T-cell line (*3*), however, now makes possible its production in large quantities for detailed analyses and for development of

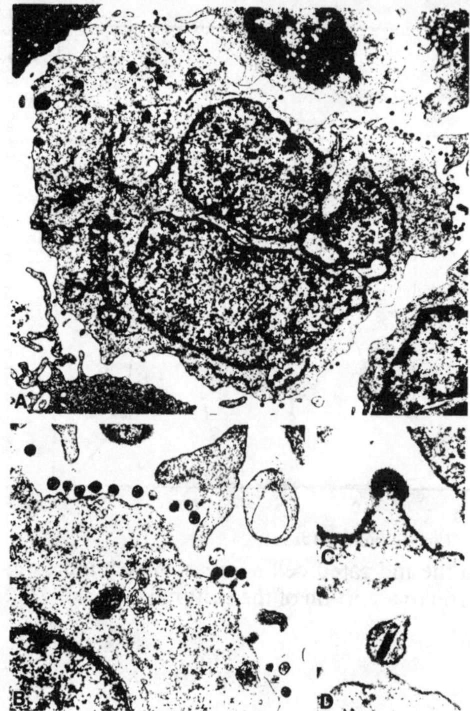

Fig. 2. Transmission electron micrographs of fixed, sectioned lymphocytes from a patient with pre-AIDS. (A) ×10,000; (B) ×30,000; (C and D) ×100,000.

reagents for its detection (*3, 11*).

That the viruses we have named HTLV-III belong to the HTLV family is indicated by their T cell tropism, Mg^{2+}-dependent RT of high molecular weight, antigenic cross-reactivity with HTLV-I and -II (*11*), cytopathic effects on T lymphocytes (*3*), and their morphological appearance in the electron micrograph. HTLV-III also contains some structural proteins similar in size to those of other members of the HTLV family (*11*).

These studies of HTLV-III isolates from patients with AIDS and pre-AIDS and from some healthy individuals at risk for AIDS provide strong evidence of a causative involvement of the virus in AIDS.

References and Notes

1. M. S. Gottlieb *et al.*, *N. Eng. J. Med.* **305**, 1425 (1981); H. Masur *et al.*, *ibid.*, p. 1431; F. P. Siegal *et al.*, *ibid.*, p. 1439.
2. Centers for Disease Control, *Morbid. Mortal. Week. Rpt.* **32**, 688 (1984); J. W. Curran *et al.*, *N. Eng. J. Med.* **310**, 69 (1984); G. B. Scott, B. E. Buck, J. G. Letterman, F. L. Bloom, W. P. Parks, *ibid.*, p. 76; J. Oleske *et al.*, *J. Am. Med. Assoc.* **249**, 2345 (1983).
3. M. Popovic *et al.*, *Science* **224**, 497 (1984).
4. R. C. Gallo *et al.*, *ibid.* **220**, 865 (1983); M. Popovic and R. C. Gallo, in preparation.
5. M. Essex *et al.*, *Science* **220**, 859 (1983); M. Essex *et al.*, in *Human T-Cell Leukemia Viruses*, R. C. Gallo, M. Essex, L. Gross, Eds. (Cold Spring Harbor Press, Cold Spring Harbor, N.Y., in press).
6. R. C. Gallo *et al.*, *Cancer Res.* **43**, 3892 (1983); in *Cancer Surveys*, L. M. Franks *et al.*, Eds. (Oxford Univ. Press, Oxford, in press).
7. F. Barré-Sinoussi *et al.*, *Science* **220**, 868 (1983).
8. E. P. Gelmann *et al.*, *ibid.*, p. 862.
9. M. Robert-Guroff *et al.*, in *Human T-Cell Leukemia Viruses*, R. C. Gallo, M. Essex, L. Gross, Eds. (Cold Spring Harbor Press, Cold Spring Harbor, N.Y., in press).
10. T. H. Lee *et al.*, personal communication; J. Schüpbach, M. G. Sarngadharan, R. C. Gallo, in preparation.
11. M. G. Sarngadharan, M. Popovic, L. Bruch, J. Schüpbach, R. C. Gallo, *Science* **224**, 506 (1984); J. Schüpbach *et al.*, *ibid.*, p. 503.
12. B. J. Poiesz *et al.*, *Proc. Natl. Acad. Sci. U.S.A.* **77**, 7415 (1980); B. J. Poiesz, F. W. Ruscetti, M. S. Reitz, V. S. Kalyanaraman, R. C. Gallo, *Nature (London)* **294**, 268 (1981); V. S. Kalyanaraman *et al.*, *Science* **218**, 571 (1982).
13. P. D. Markham *et al.*, *Int. J. Cancer* **31**, 413 (1983); P. D. Markham, S. Z. Salahuddin, B. Macchi, M. Robert-Guroff, R. C. Gallo, *ibid.* **35**, 13 (1984); S. Z. Salahuddin *et al.*, *Virology* **129**, 51 (1983).
14. M. Robert-Guroff and R. C. Gallo, *Blut* **47**, 1 (1983); V. S. Kalyanaraman, M. G. Sarngadharan, B. J. Poiesz, F. W. Ruscetti, R. C. Gallo, *J. Virol.* **81**, 906 (1981); C. Saxinger and R. C. Gallo, *Lab. Invest.* **49**, 371 (1983).
15. For virus isolation, samples of freshly drawn, heparinized peripheral blood or bone marrow, yielding a minimum of 10^7 viable cells (greater than 90 percent), are needed. These samples must contain the cells of interest, namely, OKT4⁺ T cells, which are frequently depleted in AIDS patients.
16. S. Arya *et al.*, in preparation.
17. We thank M. Gonda for electron microscopy and A. Patel, S. Roberson, A. Fladager, and E. Reid for technical assistance. We are also indebted to many clinical collaborators who provided patient materials.

30 March 1984; accepted 19 April 1984

32. Serological Analysis of a Subgroup of Human T-Lymphotropic Retroviruses (HTLV-III) Associated with AIDS

Jörg Schüpbach, Mikulas Popovic, Raymond V. Gilden, Matthew A. Gonda, M.G. Sarngadharan, and Robert C. Gallo

Members of the family of human lymphotropic retroviruses (HTLV) have the following features in common: a pronounced tropism for OKT4$^+$ lymphocytes (*1*), a reverse transcriptase (RT) with a high molecular weight (100,000) and a preference for Mg^{2+} as the divalent cation for optimal enzymatic activity (*2, 3*), and the capacity to inhibit T cell function (*4*) or, in some cases, kill T cells (*5*). Many HTLV also have the capacity to transform infected T cells (*1*). The two major subgroups that have been characterized (*6*) are HTLV-I, which is causatively linked to certain adult T-cell malignancies (*7*), and HTLV-II, which was first identified in a patient with hairy cell leukemia (*8*).

Viruses of the HTLV family have been detected in some patients with the acquired immunodeficiency syndrome (AIDS) (*9*) or with pre-AIDS, a condition frequently progressing to AIDS (*10*). A high proportion of patients with AIDS or pre-AIDS, as well as a significant number of hemophiliacs, have antibodies in their serum that recognize a cell surface glycoprotein (gp61) that is present on certain human T cells infected with HTLV-I (*11*). Gp61 and p65, a slightly larger protein that is a homolog of gp61 and occurs in another cell line producing HTLV-I, were subsequently shown to be related to the HTLV viral glycoprotein (*12, 13*). Studies of blood transfusion recipients who later developed AIDS and of their blood donors have revealed the presence, in the blood of the donors, of antibodies to a retrovirus of the HTLV family (*14*). These findings suggest an involvement of viruses of the HTLV family in the cause of AIDS and pre-AIDS. An involvement of HTLV-I alone appeared doubtful, however, because antibody titers to gp61 of HTLV-I in these patients are generally very low and antibodies to the structural proteins of HTLV, notably p24 and p19 (*15*), are not detectable in most AIDS patients (*16*). Instead, it seemed likely that another member of the HTLV family might be involved in the etiology of AIDS. Here we describe our studies of a group of cytopathic viruses (collectively designated HTLV-III) isolated from patients with AIDS or pre-AIDS. Isolation of these viruses was achieved by means of a novel system permitting the continuous growth of T-cell clones infected with the cytopathic types of HTLV found in these disorders (*17*). We show that antigens associated with human cells infected by HTLV-III are specifically recognized by antibodies in serum from AIDS and pre-AIDS patients, and present a preliminary biochemical and immunological analysis of these antigens.

Lysates of two immortalized and infected human T-cell clones, H4/HTLV-III and H17/HTLV-III (*17*), were tested with samples of human serum in a strip radioimmunoassay (RIA) based on the Western blot technique (*18*). The sera were from patients with AIDS or pre-AIDS, from contacts of such patients, and from homo- or heterosexual male controls. Sera from the same patients were also tested by the enzyme-linked immunosorbent assay (ELISA) with purified HTLV-III as part of a larger, systematic serologic study of the prevalence of antibodies to HTLV-III in AIDS and pre-AIDS patients (*19*).

Representative results are shown in Fig. 1. Sera from patients with AIDS or pre-AIDS, and from some homosexuals and heroin-addicts, recognized a number of specific antigens not detected by sera from heterosexual subjects. The most prominent reactions were with antigens of the following molecular weights: 65,000, 60,000, 55,000, 41,000, and 24,000. Antigens with molecular weights of approximately 88,000, 80,000, 39,000, 32,000, 28,000, and 21,000 gave less prominent reactions. The reaction with the antigen of 55,000 (p55) only occurred in sera that also recognized p24, suggesting a relationship between the two antigens.

The specificity of these reactions was studied by comparing lysates of H4/HTLV-III and H17/HTLV-III with lysates of the same cell clones, H4 and H17, before viral infection (Fig. 2A). No antigen from the uninfected clones reacted with the sera, with the exception of a protein with a molecular weight of 80,000 in H17 which bound antibodies from all of the human serum samples tested (see Fig. 1B) but not from rabbit or goat serum. Antigens newly expressed after viral infection and recognized by the human serum used for this analysis included p65, p55, p41, p39, p32, and p24. A large protein with a molecular weight of approximately 130,000 and a protein of 48,000 were also detected. With this serum, p55 consistently appeared as a doublet of bands of similar intensity. With normal human serum, none of the antigens was detected (not shown). These results show clearly that the antigens detected after virus infection are either virus-coded proteins or cellular antigens specifically induced by the infection.

The antigens of H4/HTLV-III were also compared with antigens from virus purified from the culture fluids of H4/HTLV-III (Fig. 2B). Extensive accumulation of p24 and p41 [see (*20*)] occurred in the virus preparation (Fig. 2B, panels I and II). Protein stains showed that these molecules are the major components of the virus preparation (*19*). P24 and p41 may therefore be considered viral structural proteins. Furthermore, an antigen with a molecular weight of approximately 110,000 was detected in the virus preparation but was below limit of detection in the cells. Also, p39 [see (*20*)] was present in the virus preparation. It is interesting that p24 in the virus preparation consistently appeared as a doublet (p24/p23), whereas in the cells it appeared as p24 alone. The significance of this is under investigation. P55 was not detected in the virus; however, the intensity of the p55 band in the cells (Fig. 2B,

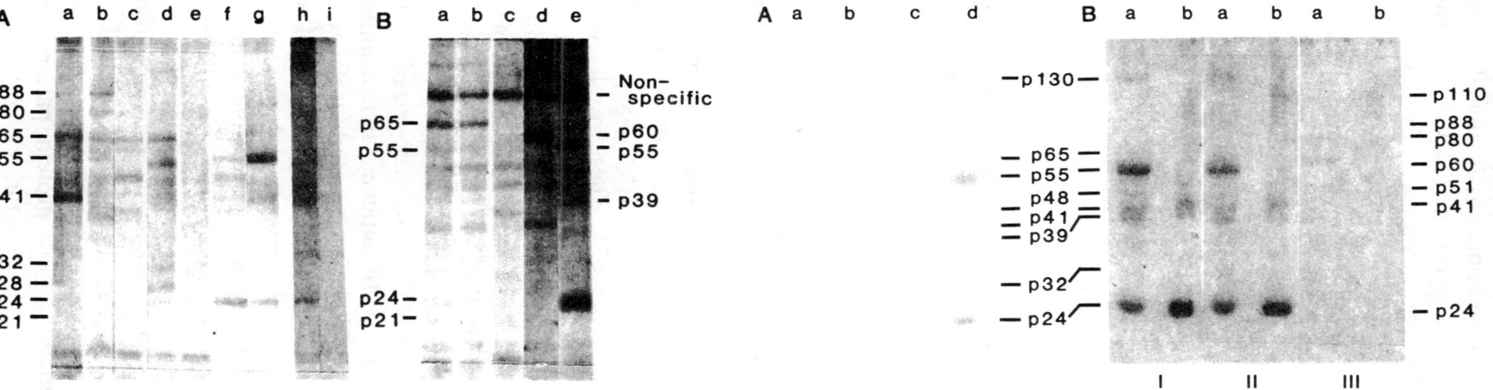

Fig. 1 (left). Serologic detection of antigens in HTLV-III producer cell clones. Strip RIA were performed with human serum as described elsewhere in detail (21). Briefly, lysates of HTLV-III producer cell clones were subjected to electrophoresis under reducing conditions on preparative sodium dodecyl sulfate (SDS)–polyacrylamide slab gels, and electroblotted to nitrocellulose sheets (18). The sheets were cut into strips. These were incubated with human serum diluted 1:100. After three thorough washings, bound antibodies of immunoglobulin G (IgG) and immunoglobulin M (IgM) classes were made visible with radiolabeled, affinity-purified goat antiserum to human IgG and IgM (H-chain specific) and autoradiography. (A) Analysis with H4/HTLV-III cells. (Lanes a, d, and g) U.S. patients with AIDS; (lane b) a French heterosexual male who developed AIDS after receiving a blood transfusion in Haiti (24); (lane c) an AIDS patient from Switzerland; (lane e) a normal heterosexual control; (lane f) a French pre-AIDS patient (24); (lane h) a Swiss heterosexual drug addict; (lane i) a normal homosexual control. (B) Analysis with H17/HTLV-III cells. (Lane a) An infant with AIDS whose mother is a prostitute; sera from both are highly positive for antibodies to the HTLV membrane antigen (11, 25) and in our ELISA with disrupted HTLV-III (19); (lane b) same serum as in (A), lane d; (lane c) normal heterosexual control; (lane d) another Swiss AIDS patient; (lane e) a Swiss heterosexual male intravenous drug abuser with generalized lymphadenopathy and thrombocytopenic purpura (pre-AIDS).   Fig. 2 (right). (A) Specificity of the antigens recognized. Lysates of cloned cells before and after infection with HTLV-III were analyzed by the Western blot technique (18) with a 1:500 dilution of the serum shown in Fig. 1B, lane e. (Lane a) The H17 clone before and (lane b) the same clone after infection (H17/HTLV-III); (lane c) the H4 clone before and (lane d) the same clone after infection (H4/HTLV-III). All reactive antigens are virus-related with the exception of that with a molecular weight of 80,000 in H17 cells; this antigen binds antibodies from all human sera investigated. Normal human serum did not bind to any of the virus-related bands (not shown). (B) Comparison of antigens in (lanes a) cells and (lanes b) virus. Lysates of H4/HTLV-III (250 μg per lane) or virus purified from the cell culture fluids (19) (5 μg per lane) were analyzed with 1:500 dilutions of human sera. (Panel I) Same serum as in Fig. 2A; (panel II) serum of a Swiss male homosexual with fatigue and generalized lymphadenopathy (pre-AIDS); (panel III) serum from same AIDS patient as in Fig. 1B, lane d. An antigen with a molecular weight of 110,000 and p41, p39, and p24 are enriched in the virus preparation [see (20)]. The serum in panel III recognized a subset of the antigens recognized by the sera used in panels I and II.

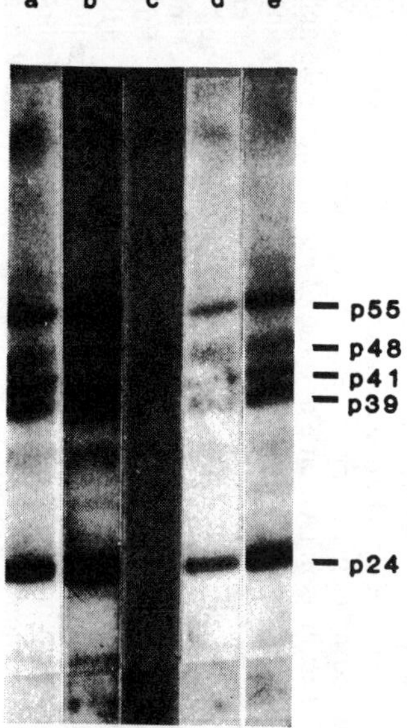

Fig. 3. Relation between HTLV-III and HTLV-II. Serum of an AIDS patient at a dilution of 1:500 was tested in a competition RIA on strips (20) prepared with H4/HTLV-III cells. (Lane a) The human serum was added directly to the strip (uncompeted control); (lanes b to e) the serum was first absorbed for 3 hours at 37°C with 1 mg of cellular extract. In (b) the absorption was with uninfected H4 cells (not producing virus); in (c) the absorption was with H4/HTLV-III cells producing HTLV-III (positive control); in (d) the absorption was with C3/44 cells (26) producing HTLV-II; in (e) the absorption was with HUT 102 cells producing HTLV-I (2).

lanes a) appeared to correlate with the intensity of p24/p23 in the virus preparation (Fig. 2B, lanes b), thus again suggesting a relation between these antigens. The p55 is probably a precursor of p24, since a group-specific antigen of similar size (Pr 54^{gag}) in HTLV-I–infected cells is the precursor of p24 and the other gag-coded proteins (21). Occasionally an additional set of antigens was recognized by a serum (Fig. 2B, panel III) but their relation to the antigens described above is unclear.

Thus we have shown that viral or virus-induced antigens in cloned human T cells infected with HTLV-III are specifically recognized by antibodies in the serum of patients with AIDS or pre-AIDS. The detection of p65 by many of the serum samples is of special interest. We have tested these sera on strips prepared from lysates of cells producing HTLV-I or -II. Some of these cells produce a p65 that has been shown (13) to be coded for by the env gene of HTLV-I and to be the homolog of the gp61 described by others (11, 12). Many of the sera recognizing p65 in HTLV-III–infected cells also recognized, though somewhat faintly, p65 in cells producing HTLV-I or -II, and some of them also recognized gag-related antigens (data not shown).

In addition, the reaction of some human sera with virus-related antigens of HTLV-III–infected cells could be partially inhibited by large amounts of extracts of cells producing HTLV-II (Fig. 3). When a human serum not recognizing p65 was used, the antigens for which there was competition included p55, p48, p41, p39, and p24. These results were confirmed by the demonstration that a rabbit antiserum raised against purified HTLV-III showed some reactivity with antigens of HTLV-II and, to a lesser extent, with HTLV-I. In contrast, antiserum to HTLV-II recognized both HTLV-I and -III antigens, and an antiserum to HTLV-I reacted well with HTLV-II, but only faintly with HTLV-III (22). Moreover, nucleotide sequences of HTLV-III have been found to be related to HTLV-I and -II (23). Although the morphology of HTLV-III particles appears to be somewhat different from the morphology of HTLV-I and -II (Fig. 4), and although some differences are also found in the protein patterns of purified virus preparations (19), these immunological and nucleic acid data

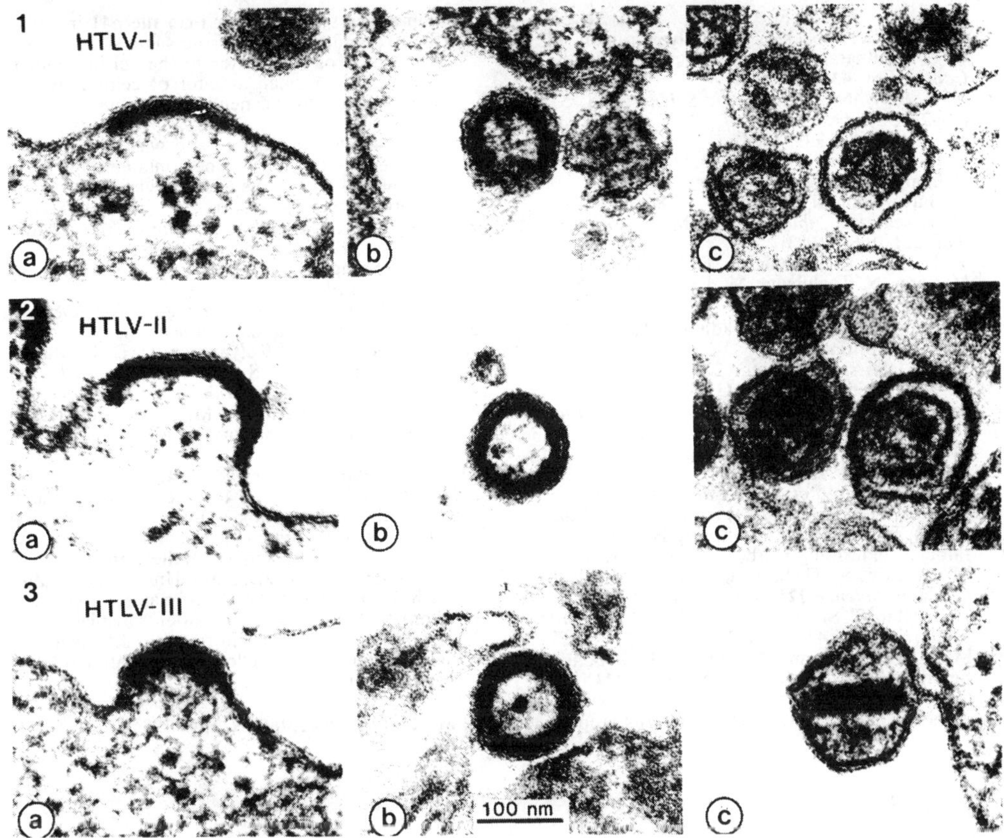

Fig. 4. Electron microscopy of thin sections of cells producing HTLV-I, -II, and -III. (Top) HUT 102 cells producing HTLV-I (*2*). (Middle) Cells from an AIDS patient (J.P.) producing HTLV-II (*24*). (Bottom) Cells from a patient [described in (*27*)] with pre-AIDS, producing HTLV-III. (Panels a) Virus particles budding from the cell membrane. (Panels b) Free particles have separated from the membrane. (Panels c) Free particles sectioned in a different plane. Note the dense, cylindrical core region of HTLV-III.

clearly indicate that HTLV-III is a true member of the HTLV family and that it is more closely related to HTLV-II than to HTLV-I.

References and Notes

1. M. Popovic, P. S. Sarin, M. Robert-Guroff, V. S. Kalyanaraman, D. Mann, J. Minowada, R. C. Gallo, *Science* **219**, 856 (1983); P. D. Markham, S. Z. Salahuddin, V. S. Kalyanaraman, M. Popovic, P. Sarin, R. C. Gallo, *Int. J. Cancer* **31**, 413 (1983); S. Z. Salahuddin, P. D. Markham, F. Wong-Staal, G. Franchini, V. S. Kalyanaraman, R. C. Gallo, *Virology* **129**, 51 (1983).
2. B. J. Poiesz, F. W. Ruscetti, A. F. Gazdar, P. A. Bunn, J. D. Minna, R. C. Gallo, *Proc. Natl. Acad. Sci. U.S.A.* **77**, 7415 (1980).
3. H. M. Rho, B. Poiesz, F. W. Ruscetti, R. C. Gallo, *Virology* **112**, 355 (1981); M. Seiki, S. Hattori, Y. Hirayama, M. Yoshida, *Proc. Natl. Acad. Sci. U.S.A.* **80**, 3618 (1983).
4. M. Popovic *et al.*, in preparation.
5. H. Mitsuya, H. G. Guo, M. Megson, C. O. Trainor, M. S. Reitz, S. Broder, *Science* **223**, 1293 (1984).
6. For a brief review, see M. G. Sarngadharan *et al.*, in *Human Carcinogenesis*, C. C. Harris and H. H. Autrup, Eds. (Academic Press, New York, 1983), p. 679.
7. V. S. Kalyanaraman, M. G. Sarngadharan, Y. Nakao, Y. Ito, T. Aoki, R. C. Gallo, *Proc. Natl. Acad. Sci. U.S.A.* **79**, 1653 (1982); M. Robert-Guroff, Y. Nakao, K. Notake, Y. Ito, A. H. Sliski, R. C. Gallo, *Science* **215**, 925 (1982); Y. Hinuma *et al.*, *Int. J. Cancer* **29**, 631 (1982); W. A. Blattner *et al.*, *ibid.* **30**, 257 (1982); J. Schüpbach, V. S. Kalyanaraman, M. G. Sarngad-

haran, Y. Nakao, R. C. Gallo, *ibid.* **32**, 583 (1983); J. Schüpbach, V. S. Kalyanaraman, M. G. Sarngadharan, W. A. Blattner, R. C. Gallo, *Cancer Res.* **43**, 886 (1983).

8. V. S. Kalyanaraman *et al.*, *Science* **218**, 571 (1982); E. P. Gelmann *et al.*, *Proc. Natl. Acad. Sci. U.S.A.* **81**, 993 (1984).
9. R. C. Gallo *et al.*, *Science* **220**, 865 (1983); E. P. Gelmann *et al.*, *ibid.*, p. 862.
10. F. Barré-Sinoussi *et al.*, *ibid.*, p. 868.
11. M. Essex *et al.*, *ibid.*, p. 859; M. Essex *et al.*, *ibid.* **221**, 1061 (1983).
12. T. H. Lee, J. E. Coligan, T. Homma, M. F. McLane, N. Tachibana, M. Essex, *Proc. Natl. Acad. Sci. U.S.A.*, in press.
13. J. Schüpbach, M. G. Sarngadharan, R. C. Gallo, *Science*, in press.
14. H. W. Jaffe *et al.*, *Science* **223**, 1309 (1984).
15. V. S. Kalyanaraman, M. G. Sarngadharan, P. A. Bunn, J. D. Minna, R. C. Gallo, *Nature (London)* **294**, 271 (1981); V. S. Kalyanaraman, M. Jarvis-Morar, M. G. Sarngadharan, R. C. Gallo, *Virology* **132**, 61 (1984).
16. M. Robert-Guroff *et al.*, in *Cancer Cells,* vol. 3, *Human T-Cell Leukemia Viruses,* R. C. Gallo and M. Essex, Eds. (Cold Spring Harbor Laboratory, Cold Spring Harbor, N.Y., in press).
17. M. Popovic, M. G. Sarngadharan, E. Read, R. C. Gallo, *Science* **224**, 497 (1984).
18. H. Towbin, T. Staehelin, J. Gordon, *Proc. Natl. Acad. Sci. U.S.A.* **76**, 4350 (1979).
19. M. G. Sarngadharan, M. Popovic, L. Bruch, J. Schüpbach, R. C. Gallo, *Science* **224**, 506 (1984).
20. Although in Fig. 2B the p41 in the virus prepara-tion appears to be larger than the p41 in cells, the two molecules are of the same size. During application of the lysates to the gel in another experiment, a small amount of cellular lysate was spilled into the neighboring lanes and the cellular p41 moved with the same velocity as the viral p41. A connecting band was thus formed between the p41 in the lane containing the cells and the p41 in the lane with the virus. The same situation occurred with p39 in cells and virus.
21. J. Schüpbach, V. S. Kalyanaraman, M. G. Sarngadharan, R. C. Gallo, in preparation.
22. M. G. Sarngadharan *et al.*, in preparation.
23. S. Arya *et al.*, in preparation.
24. J. B. Brunet *et al.*, *Lancet* **1983-I**, 700 (1983).
25. M. Essex, personal communication.
26. M. Popovic, V. S. Kalyanaraman, D. L. Mann, E. Richardson, P. S. Sarin, R. C. Gallo, in *Cancer Cells,* vol. 3, *Human T-Cell Leukemia Viruses,* R. C. Gallo and M. Essex, Eds. (Cold Spring Harbor Laboratory, Cold Spring Harbor, N.Y., in press).
27. R. C. Gallo *et al.*, *Science* **224**, 500 (1984).
28. We thank J. Ahmad for technical assistance and R. Lüthy and M. Vogt, Division of Infectious Diseases, Department of Medicine, University Hospital, Zurich, and O. Haller, Institute for Immunology and Virology, University of Zurich, Zurich, Switzerland, for making some sera from AIDS and pre-AIDS patients available and for providing clinical information. J.S. is a Fogarty International Fellow of the National Cancer Institute.

30 March 1984; accepted 19 April 1984

Report

4 May 1984

33. Antibodies Reactive with Human T-Lymphotropic Retroviruses (HTLV-III) in the Serum of Patients with AIDS

M.G. Sarngadharan, Mikulas Popovic, Lilian Bruch, Jörg Schüpbach, and Robert C. Gallo

The incidence of the acquired immunodeficiency syndrome (AIDS) in homosexual men with multiple sexual partners, intravenous drug abusers, hemophiliacs, blood transfusion recipients, and close heterosexual contacts of members of these high-risk groups (*1–7*) strongly suggests that the disease spreads by the transmission of an infectious agent (*8, 9*). The agent's primary targets within the body appear to be specific subpopulations of T cells. The severe immune deficiency of AIDS patients results from an unusually low proportion of helper T lymphocytes (OKT4$^+$) and a resulting lack of many helper functions, including production of antibodies by B cells (*1, 3*).

Retrovirus infections are known to lead to depressed immune functions in animal systems. For example, in cats, a major result of infection with feline leukemia virus (FeLV) is loss of normal immune function. More FeLV-infected cats die from consequences of this immune dysfunction than from the leukemia itself (*10*). FeLV provides an example of a single T-cell tropic retrovirus that causes both target cell proliferation (leukemia) and depletion (immunosuppression). By analogy, a human retrovirus with a tropism for T cells should be considered a serious candidate in the etiology of human AIDS. Two subgroups of a family of human T-lymphotropic retroviruses (HTLV) have been isolated and characterized (*11*). The first, HTLV-I, was isolated from a black American with an aggressive form of T-cell lymphoma (*12*) and has been etiologically linked to the pathogenesis of adult T-cell leukemia-lymphoma (ATL) (*13–15*). Infection with HTLV-I in vitro can alter T-cell function (*16*) and, in some cases, lead to T-cell death (*17*). HTLV-II was isolated from a patient with a T-cell variant of hairy cell leukemia (*18*).

Although there are distinct differences between HTLV-I and HTLV-II, they have the following common features: a tropism for OKT4$^+$ lymphocytes (*19*); a Mg^{2+}-dependent reverse transcriptase (RT) of high molecular weight (100,000) (*20*); some antigenic cross-reactivity in their proteins (*18*); a novel set of nucleotide sequences called pX at the 3′ end of the viral genome; a limited amount of nucleic acid homology in their genomes (*21*); and similar morphology. Both HTLV-I and HTLV-II have been isolated from cultured T cells of patients with AIDS (*22, 23*). Another retrovirus was isolated from a homosexual patient with chronic generalized lymphadenopathy (*24*), a syndrome that often precedes AIDS and is therefore referred to as pre-AIDS. Proviral DNA of HTLV-I was detected in the cellular DNA of two AIDS patients (*25*), and serum samples from some patients were shown to react with antigens of HTLV-I (*26*). A larger proportion of the sera reacted with a cell membrane antigen specific to HTLV-I–infected cells (*27*). This antigen has since been identified as a precursor of the envelope glycoprotein, gp46, of HTLV-I (*28, 29*). However, the correlation between AIDS and serum antibodies to HTLV-I protein (including the cell membrane antigen, p61) is weak.

These results are consistent with the idea that the primary cause of AIDS is another member of the HTLV family with limited cross-reactivities with the known HTLV subgroups. Sera with high titers of antibodies to the AIDS-specific virus might show a detectable reaction with antigens of HTLV-I and HTLV-II, whereas the reaction of sera with low titers might be too weak to recognize in such a cross-reactive system. Our attempts to isolate other retroviruses from AIDS patients resulted in the identification of a number of HTLV isolates that are similar to each other but are distinguishable from HTLV-I and HTLV-II. These new isolates are designated HTLV-III and are described in the accompanying reports (*30–32*). Here we describe the use of HTLV-III in an immunological screening of serum samples from patients with AIDS and pre-AIDS and from individuals at increased risk for AIDS.

The virus was purified from supernatants of cell cultures supporting the continuous production of HTLV-III (*30*). The virus showed a difference in the makeup of its protein components as revealed by sodium dodecyl sulfate (SDS)–polyacrylamide gel electrophoresis of a sucrose density banded preparation (Fig. 1, lane 2). Like HTLV-I (lane 1), and unlike common mammalian retroviruses (for example, Rauscher murine leukemia virus, lane 3), HTLV-III (lane 2) has a major group-specific antigen (*gag* protein) with a molecular weight of 24,000 (p24). It has a reverse transcriptase with a molecular weight of about 100,000, another protein with a molecular weight of 41,000 (presumably the envelope glycoprotein), and shows a tropism for OKT4$^+$ lymphocytes. However, it lacks the band separating at a molecular weight of 19,000 (p19). Instead, it has a smaller band that is missing in HTLV-I. Immunological studies presented in an accompanying report (*32*) also indicate that HTLV-III is antigenically different from HTLV-I and -II, but that it also shares a variety of antigenic determinants with them, especially with HTLV-II. This relatedness has also been confirmed by comparison of nucleotide sequences of the three types of HTLV (*33*).

Serum samples were obtained from patients with clinically documented AIDS, Kaposi's sarcoma, sexual contacts of AIDS patients, intravenous drug abusers, homosexual men, and heterosexual subjects. These sera were tested for their reactivity to HTLV-III by means of the enzyme-linked immunosorbent assay (ELISA) (*34*). Lysates of sucrose density banded HTLV-III were coated on 96-well microtiter plates. The test sera were diluted with normal goat serum, added to the wells, and allowed to react for 2 hours or overnight at room temperature. The primary immune complex formed with the antibodies in the human sera was detected by adding peroxidase-labeled goat antiserum to human immunoglobulins and assaying for a colored peroxidase reaction product (*34*). The results are presented in Table 1. Of 49 clinically diagnosed AIDS patients, 43 (88 percent) showed serum reactivity in

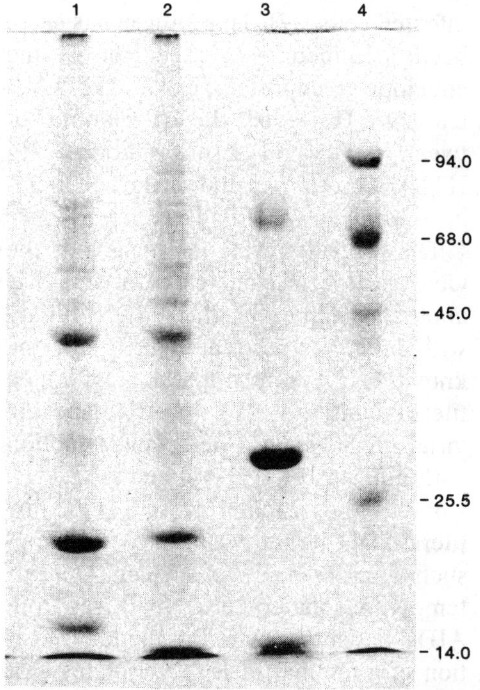

Fig. 1. Comparison of the SDS–polyacrylamide gel profile of HTLV-III with profiles of HTLV-I and Rauscher murine leukemia virus (R-MuLV). Lane 1, HTLV-I; lane 2, HTLV-III; lane 3, R-MuLV; lane 4, molecular weight standards: phosphorylase b (94,000), bovine serum albumin (68,000), ovalbumin (45,000), chymotrypsinogen (25,500), and lysozyme (14,000).

Table 1. Antibodies to HTLV-III in serum samples from patients with AIDS and pre-AIDS and from control subjects. Wells of 96-well Immulon plates were coated overnight with a lysate of density-banded HTLV-III (*30*) at 0.5 μg protein per well in 100 μl 50 m*M* sodium bicarbonate buffer, *p*H 9.6. The wells were washed with water and incubated for 20 minutes with 100 μl of 5 percent bovine serum albumin in phosphate buffered saline (PBS). The wells were washed again in water, and then 100 μl of 20 percent normal goat serum in PBS were added to each well, followed by 5 or 10 μl of the test sera. These were allowed to react for 2 hours at room temperature. The wells were washed three times with 0.05 percent Tween-20 in PBS and incubated for 1 hour at room temperature with peroxidase-labeled goat antiserum to human immunoglobulin G at a dilution of 1:2000 in 1 percent normal goat serum in PBS. The wells were successively washed four times with 0.05 percent Tween-20 in PBS and four times with PBS and reacted with 100 μl of the substrate mixture containing 0.05 percent orthophenylene diamine and 0.005 percent hydrogen peroxide in phosphate-citrate buffer, *p*H 5.0. The reactions were stopped by the addition of 50 μl of 4*N* H_2SO_4, and the color yield was measured with a Dynatech ELISA reader. Assays were done in duplicate and absorbance reading greater than three times the average of four normal negative control readings was taken as positive.

Subject	Number positive for antibodies to HTLV-III	Number tested	Percent positive
Patients with AIDS	43	49	87.8
Patients with pre-AIDS	11	14	78.6
Intravenous drug users	3	5	60
Homosexual men	6	17	
Sexual contact of AIDS patient	1	1	
Persistent fatigue	1	1	
Other	4	15	26.6
Other controls	1	186	0.5
Normal subjects	1	164	0.6
Patients with hepatitis B virus infection	0	3	
Patient with rheumatoid arthritis	0	1	
Patients with systemic lupus erythematosus	0	6	
Patients with acute mononucleosis	0	4	
Patients with lymphatic leukemias	0	8	

this assay. Two of the subjects whose serum reacted positively with the HTLV preparation had developed AIDS after receiving blood transfusions, one in Haiti and the other in Aruba. Of 14 homosexual men with pre-AIDS, 11 (79 percent) were positive. Of 17 homosexual men with no clinical symptoms of AIDS, seven were positive. At least one of these was known to be a long-time sexual partner of a patient with clinically diagnosed AIDS. Another had persistent fatigue and possibly other early symptoms of AIDS. Because these 17 men had been seeking medical assistance, they are not a representative sample of the homosexual population, and the high incidence of HTLV-III–specific antibodies in their sera may not reflect the true incidence in the homosexual population. One of the three intravenous drug abusers that were positive for serum antibodies to HTLV-III was also a homosexual. Serum samples from only one of 186 control subjects reacted positively in this test. These control subjects included three with hepatitis B virus infection, one with rheumatoid arthritis, six with systemic lupus erythematosus, four with acute mononucleosis, and eight with various forms of lymphatic leukemias and lymphomas, some of whom were positive for HTLV-I. The rest were normal donors of unknown sexual preference including laboratory workers ranging in age from 22 to 50.

To understand the molecular nature of the antigens recognized by ELISA, we conducted the following experiment. A lysate of HTLV-III was fractionated by SDS–polyacrylamide gel electrophoresis and transferred to a nitrocellulose sheet by the electrophoretic blotting (Western) technique of Towbin *et al.* (*35*). The nitrocellulose sheet was cut into 0.5-cm strips and reacted with samples of the human sera. Antigen-antibody complexes formed were detected by autoradiography after incubation of the strips with ^{125}I-labeled goat antibody to human immunoglobulin. Figure 2 shows that the antigen most prominently and commonly detected among all of the sera from AIDS patient had a molecular weight of 41,000 (p41). This corresponds to one of the major proteins of the virus (Fig. 1)

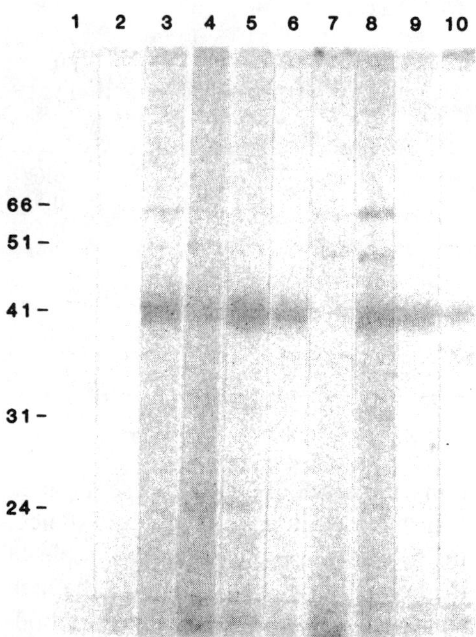

Fig. 2. Identification of HTLV-III antigens recognized by sera of AIDS patients. HTLV-III was lysed and fractionated by electrophoresis on a 12 percent polyacrylamide slab gel in the presence of SDS. The protein bands on the gel were electrophoretically transferred to a nitrocellulose sheet according to the procedure of Towbin *et al.* (*35*). Strip solid-phase radioimmunoassays were then performed as described (*36*). The sheet was incubated at 37°C for 2 hours with 5 percent bovine serum albumin in 10 mM tris-HCl, pH 7.5 containing 0.9 percent NaCl and cut into 0.5-cm strips. Each strip was incubated for 2 hours at 37°C and 2 hours at room temperature in a screw cap tube containing 2.5 ml of buffer-1 (20 mM tris-HCl, pH 7.5, 1 mM EDTA, 0.2M NaCl, 0.3 percent Triton X-100, and 2 mg of bovine serum albumin and 0.2 mg of human Fab per milliliter). Test sera (25 μl) were then added to individual tubes containing the strips and incubation was continued for 1 hour at room temperature and overnight in the cold. The strips were washed three times with a solution containing 0.5 percent sodium deoxycholate, 0.1M NaCl, 0.5 percent Triton X-100, 1 mM phenylmethylsulfonyl fluoride, and 10 mM sodium phosphate, pH 7.5. The strips were incubated for 1 hour at room temperature with 2.4 ml of buffer-1 and 0.1 ml of normal goat serum. Affinity-purified and ^{125}I-labeled goat antiserum to human immunoglobulin (μ chain and Fc fragment) (1.25 × 10^6 count/min) were added to the reaction mixture and the incubation was continued for 30 minutes at room temperature. The strips were washed as described, dried, mounted, and exposed to x-ray film. Strip 1, adult T-cell leukemia; strip 2, normal donor; strip 3, mother of a child with AIDS; strips 4 and 6 to 10, AIDS patients; and strip 5, patient with pre-AIDS.

and is presumably the envelope protein. Strip 7 shows the result obtained with serum from an AIDS patient that reacted negatively in the ELISA but in this more sensitive strip assay it gave a low, but definitely positive, result. Reactivity to p24 of the virus was generally very weak and was clear only in two cases (strips 4 and 5). This may be a reflection of the relative titer toward different antigens. One would expect the highest antibody titer against the envelope of the infecting agent, especially if the infection causes a pronounced immune deficiency and decreased capacity to make antibodies in response to subsequent antigenic challenge. Additional reactivities against antigens with molecular weights of 66,000 and 51,000 were seen in some sera. In strip 8 the serum reacted with an additional antigen that has a molecular weight of 31,000. These additional antigens appear to be related to those detected by sera from the same patients in HTLV-III–producing cells (*33*). Strips 1 and 2 show that sera from a patient with ATL who was positive for HTLV-I and from a normal subject do not react with the antigens of HTLV-III.

Of particular interest is the finding that among the serum samples that reacted positively with HTLV-III two were from young children (ages 7 months and 2 years). These children were free of known opportunistic infections including cytomegalovirus, Epstein-Barr virus, *Pneumocystis carinii*, and fungus. The mother of one of them was positive in both tests described here. The children presumably acquired the infection in utero, by their mother's milk, or by another route.

Among the positive serum samples from AIDS patients there appears to be a wide variation in antibody titer to HTLV-III. Generally, the titers in sera from patients with advanced AIDS are significantly lower than those in sera from newly diagnosed patients and patients with pre-AIDS. This is consistent with the idea that HTLV-III infection causes an initial lymphoid proliferation but eventually causes death of the target lymphocytes (OKT4$^+$) leading to the abnormal T4$^+$/T8$^+$ ratios and loss of helper T-cell functions including antibody production by B cells. Therefore, the low or negative result in the ELISA of sera from some cases of advanced AIDS may be a consequence of the natural course of the disease. To prove this it will be necessary to study antibody titers in sera obtained at intervals from subjects at risk for the disease. The serum of one AIDS patient showed a low positive titer, but serum from his homosexual partner with no symptoms of AIDS had a significantly higher antibody titer. It is interesting that the serum of one AIDS patient that was negative in the ELISA did show a definite but low positive reaction with p41 in the more sensitive Western blot assay (Fig. 2, strip 7). The ELISA with purified p41 might prove to be even more sensitive. It is significant that although HTLV proviral sequences were clearly detected in DNA from cell samples obtained from two AIDS patients early in the course of their disease, these sequences could not be detected in cells obtained after 1 year in one case and 2 months in the second case (*25*). It is conceivable that the subset of T lymphocytes that forms the target of the provirus had been depleted before the second samples were obtained in each case.

In conclusion, we have shown a high incidence of specific antibodies to HTLV-III in patients with AIDS and pre-AIDS. Among the antibody-positive cases reported here a few are of particular importance with respect to the transmission of the disease. For example, the mother of the baby with AIDS was positive for HTLV-III as was a long-term sexual partner of a homosexual with AIDS. Recipients of blood products originating from individuals at risk for AIDS were also positive for HTLV-III and, as described in an accompanying report (*31*), the virus has been isolated from several children with AIDS as well as from their mothers. The data presented here and in the accompanying reports (*30–32*) suggest that HTLV-III is the primary cause of AIDS.

References and Notes

1. M. S. Gottlieb, R. Schroff, H. M. Schanker, I. D. Weisman, P. T. Fan, R. A. Wolf, A. Saxon, *N. Engl. J. Med.* **305**, 1425 (1981).
2. H. Masur, M. A. Michelis, J. B. Greene, *ibid.*, p. 1431.
3. F. P. Siegal *et al.*, *ibid.*, p. 1439.
4. M. Poon, A. Landay, E. F. Prasthofer, S. Stagno, *Ann. Int. Med.* **98**, 287 (1983).
5. *Mortal. Morbid. Weekly Rep.* **31**, 697 (1983).
6. B. Moll, E. E. Emerson, C. B. Small, G. H. Friedland, R. S. Klein, I. Spigland, *Clin. Immunol. Immunopathol.* **25**, 417 (1982).
7. J. W. Curran, D. N. Lawrence, H. Jaffe, J. E. Kaplan, L. D. Zyla, M. Chamberland, R. Weinstein, K.-J. Lui, L. B. Schonberger, T. J. Spira, W. J. Alexander, G. Swinger, A. Ammann, S. Solomon, D. Auerback, R. Stoneberger, J. M. Mason, H. W. Haverkos, B. L. Evatt, *N. Engl. J. Med.* **310**, 69 (1984).
8. Centers for Disease Control, Task Force on Kaposi's Sarcoma and Opportunistic Infections, *ibid.* **306**, 248 (1982).
9. J. P. Hanrahan, G. P. Wormser, C. P. Maguire, L. J. De Lorenzo, G. Davis, *ibid.* **307**, 498 (1982).
10. M. Essex, W. D. Hardy, Jr., S. M. Cotter, R. M. Jakowski, A. Sliski, *Infect. Immun.* **11**, 470 (1975); W. D. Hardy, Jr., P. W. Hess, E. G. MacEwen, A. J. McClelland, E. E. Zuckerman, M. Essex, S. M. Cotter, *Cancer Res.* **36**, 582 (1976); L. J. Anderson, O. Jarrett, H. M. Laird, *J. Natl. Cancer Inst.* **47**, 807 (1971).
11. R. C. Gallo, in *Cancer Surveys*, L. M. Franks *et al.*, Eds. (Oxford Univ. Press, Oxford, in press).
12. B. J. Poiesz, F. W. Ruscetti, A. F. Gazdar, P. A. Bunn, J. D. Minna, R. C. Gallo, *Proc. Natl. Acad. Sci. U.S.A.* **77**, 7415 (1980).
13. V. S. Kalyanaraman, M. G. Sarngadharan, Y. Nakao, Y. Ito, T. Aoki, R. C. Gallo, *ibid.* **79**, 1653 (1982).
14. W. A. Blattner, V. S. Kalyanaraman, M. Robert-Guroff, T. A. Lister, D. A. G. Galton, P. Sarin, M. H. Crawford, D. Catovsky, M. Greaves, R. C. Gallo, *Int. J. Cancer* **30**, 257 (1982).
15. R. C. Gallo *et al.*, *Cancer Res.* **43**, 3892 (1983).
16. M. Popovic, N. Flomberg, D. Volkman, D. Mann, A. S. Fauci, B. DuPont, R. C. Gallo, in preparation.
17. H. Mitsuya, H. G. Guo, M. Megson, C. D. Trainor, M. S. Reitz, S. Broder, *Science* **223**, 1293 (1984).
18. V. S. Kalyanaraman, M. G. Sarngadharan, M. Robert-Guroff, I. Miyoshi, D. Blayney, D. Golde, R. C. Gallo, *ibid.* **218**, 571 (1982).
19. M. Popovic, unpublished observation.
20. H. M. Rho, B. J. Poiesz, F. W. Ruscetti, R. C. Gallo, *Virology* **112**, 355 (1981).
21. E. P. Gelmann, G. Franchini, V. Manzari, F. Wong-Staal, R. C. Gallo, *Proc. Natl. Acad. Sci. U.S.A.* **81**, 993 (1984).
22. R. C. Gallo *et al.*, *Science* **220**, 865 (1983).
23. M. Popovic *et al.*, in preparation.
24. F. Barré-Sinoussi *et al.*, *Science* **220**, 868 (1983).
25. E. P. Gelmann, M. Popovic, D. Blayney, H. Mazur, G. Sidhu, R. E. Stahl, R. C. Gallo, *ibid.* p. 862.
26. M. Robert-Guroff *et al.*, unpublished results.
27. M. Essex, M. F. McLane, T. H. Lee, L. Falk, C. W. S. Howe, J. I. Mullins, C. Cabradilla, D. P. Francis, *Science* **220**, 859 (1983).
28. J. Schüpbach, M. G. Sarngadharan, R. C. Gallo, *ibid.*, in press.
29. T. H. Lee, J. E. Coligan, T. Homma, M. F. McLane, M. Tochipana, M. Essex, *Proc. Natl. Acad. Sci. U.S.A.*, in press.
30. M. Popovic, M. G. Sarngadharan, E. Read, R. C. Gallo, *Science* **224**, 497 (1984).
31. R. C. Gallo *et al.*, *ibid.*, p. 500.
32. J. Schüpbach, M. Popovic, R. V. Gilden, M. A. Donda, M. G. Sarngadharan, R. C. Gallo, *ibid.* p. 503.
33. S. Arya *et al.*, in preparation.
34. C. Saxinger and R. C. Gallo. *Lab. Invest.* **49**, 371 (1983).
35. H. Towbin, T. Staehelin, J. Gordon, *Proc. Natl. Acad. Sci. U.S.A.* **76**, 4350 (1979).
36. J. Schüpbach, V. S. Kalyanaraman, M. G. Sarngadharan, R. C. Gallo, in preparation.
37. We thank K. L. Arnett for technical assistance and R. Lüthy and M. Vogt, Division of Infectious Diseases, Department of Medicine, University Hospital, Zurich, and O. Haller, Institute for Immunology and Virology, University of Zurich, Zurich, Switzerland, for providing us with sera from AIDS and pre-AIDS patients and for clinical information. J.S. is a Fogarty International Fellow of the National Cancer Institute.

30 March 1984; accepted 19 April 1984

Report

11 May 1984

34.   Antigens on HTLV-Infected Cells Recognized by Leukemia and AIDS Sera Are Related to HTLV Viral Glycoprotein

Jörg Schüpbach, M.G. Sarngadharan, and R.C. Gallo

Human T-cell leukemia-lymphoma viruses (HTLV) are a family of exogenous T-lymphotropic type C retroviruses strongly associated with adult T-cell leukemia (ATL) (*1*). Recently, additional attention has been given to these viruses as a result of the demonstration that a high proportion of patients with acquired immunodeficiency syndrome (AIDS) have antibodies that react with antigens on the surface of HTLV-producing transformed human T cells, such as the Hut 102 (*2*) and the MT 2 (*3*) cell lines (*4*). In some cases, HTLV was isolated from these patients or was shown to be integrated in the cellular genome (*5, 6*). In particular, one of the surface antigens, which is also widely recognized by antibodies from ATL patients (*7*), appears to be gp 61, a glycoprotein of molecular size 61,000 daltons (*4*). Whether this antigen is of viral or cellular origin is, however, still unknown. If it is cellular in origin, its expression might be induced by HTLV infection. However, another etiological agent yet to be identified might induce the same cellular protein. Therefore, it is unclear whether the antibodies indicate a direct involvement of HTLV in AIDS, and it has become imperative to define the origin of these antigens.

Using an HTLV-transformed virus-producing cell line we call G-25/MI (*6*), we found an antigen of 63,000 to 67,000 daltons (p65) which, like gp 61 in Hut 102 cells (*4, 7*), reacted strongly with sera from both ATL patients and healthy carriers of HTLV but did not react with sera from seronegative normals, as shown by a strip radioimmunoassay (RIA) based on the "Western blot" technique (*8*) (Fig. 1A). The G-25/MI cell line was established from the leukemic T cells of a black ATL patient from the Caribbean (*6*) and produces HTLV of type I. Although all of the sera from ATL patients or seropositive normals also detected the viral *gag*-related antigens p24 or p19 (or both) (*9, 10*), the recognition of p65 was much stronger in many sera. An antigen of 54,000 daltons was previously identified as the precursor of the viral *gag* proteins Pr54^{gag} (*11*). Moreover, antigens of about 41,000 and 80,000 daltons are detected by sera from some ATL patients or carriers but not by sera from normals.

A comparison of the intensities of the bands in Fig. 1A suggested that p65 is not related to *gag*. This was confirmed by the failure of large amounts of purified p24 (*9*) and p19 (*10*) to compete with p65 and by the failure of antibodies to

176

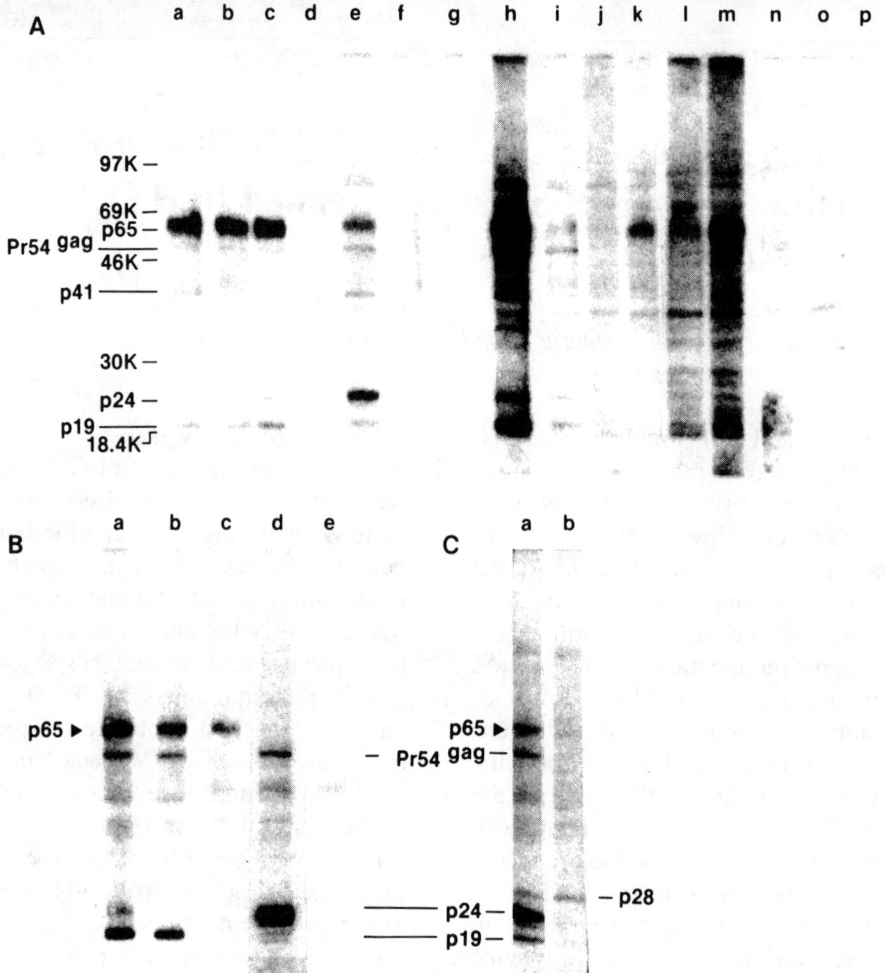

Fig. 1. (A) Recognition of p65 in HTLV-producer cells. Sera from patients with HTLV-positive
ATL (lanes a to g), HTLV carriers (lanes h to m), and uninfected controls (lanes n to p) were
analyzed in a strip RIA based on the Western blot technique (8), as described elsewhere (11).
Briefly, lysates of G-25/MI cells were subjected to electrophoresis under reducing conditions on
a preparative sodium dodecyl sulfate (SDS)–polyacrylamide slab gel (17) and transferred
electrophoretically to a nitrocellulose sheet (8). Strips cut from the sheet were reacted with
human test serum at a dilution of 1:500. Bound antibodies were made visible with radiolabeled
goat immunoglobulin G directed against human immunoglobulin. (B) Unrelatedness of p65 to
gag. Serum h [lane h in (A)] was diluted 1:1000 and used in strip RIA either without competing
material (lane a) or after being incubated for 3 hours at 37°C with 30 μg of purified HTLV p24
(lane b) or p19 (lane c). No competition with p65 was found. Furthermore, p65 was not
detected by an affinity-purified goat antibody to p24 (lane d) or by a monoclonal antibody to p19
(lane e). (C) Localization of p65 cross-reactive antigen on the cell surface. A human serum
diluted 1:500 was used either without competing material (lane a) or after being incubated for 3
hours at 37°C with 5 × 10^7 glutaraldehyde-fixed (18) G-25/MI cells (lane b). Antibodies to p65
and gag-related proteins were specifically absorbed by the cell surfaces, whereas antibodies to
an antigen of 28,000 daltons not present on the cell surface and not related to gag (12) remained
unaffected.

p24 and p19 to bind to p65 (Fig. 1B). A competition RIA on G-25/MI cell strips, with glutaraldehyde-fixed G-25/MI cells as the competing agent, showed that p65, or a cross-reactive antigen, is located on the cell surface (Fig. 1C). The surface of the fixed cells, which cannot be penetrated by antibodies, selectively absorbed antibodies to p65 and to some *gag*-related antigens, while leaving others uninfluenced, among them antibodies to a non-membrane antigen of 28,000 daltons (*12, 13*), thus ascertaining that the competition is not based on nonspecific absorption.

Competition strip RIA's with cellular and viral extracts (Table 1) revealed that antigens that cross-react with p65 are found in all tested human cell lines producing HTLV-I, such as Hut 102 (*2*), MT 2 (*3*), and G-11/MJ (*6*) (Table 1). The cell line G-11/MJ, a T-cell line producing HTLV-I, was initiated from a patient with cutaneous T-cell lymphoma (*6*). In comparison to G-25/MI, the competition with p65 by these cell lines was weak. No competition was found with phytohemagglutinin-activated normal human T cells or with JM, a human T-cell line not infected by HTLV (*14*). In comparison with the HTLV-producing cells, the viruses purified from them competed much better, with the exception of the G-25/MI virus that predominantly consists of particles lacking the envelope, as judged from the banding pattern in sucrose gradient centrifugation (data not shown). Antigens that cross-react with p65 are thus enriched in the virus preparations. An HTLV-transformed nonproducer cell line, NIH 82-15B, which had been established from human bone marrow by co-cultivation with G-11/MJ cells, did not compete with p65, whereas a virus-pro-

Table 1. Competition of p65 and *gag*-related antigens by various cellular and viral extracts. Competition RIA's were done on G-25/MI cell strips as described in Fig. 1. Symbols indicate that competition was $+++$, complete; $++$, strong; $+$, marginal; or $-$, absent.

Competing agent	Competition with	
	p65	*gag* antigens
Cells (50 μg of protein)		
G-25/MI	$+++$	$+++$
JM (Jurkat)	$-$	$-$
Normal human T cells	$-$	$-$
MT 2	$+$	$+++$
Hut 102	$+$	$+++$
G-11/MJ	$+$	$+++$
Purified viruses (10 μg of protein)		
G-25/MI	$-$	$+++$
MT 2	$++$	$+++$
Hut 102	$++$	$+++$
G-11/MJ	$++$	$+++$
Virus-producer and nonproducer cells (500 μg)		
G-11/MJ	$+++$	$+++$
NIH82/C2 (HTLV-producer)	$+++$	$+++$
NIH82/15B (HTLV-infected but nonproducer)	$-$	$-$

ducer cell line, NIH 82-C2, established from cord blood by cocultivation with the same G-11/MJ cells, competed well. The presence of p65 is thus associated with the expression of viral structural proteins.

To determine the nature of the p65–cross-reactive antigen (or antigens) in viruses, we made use of the observation that the G-25/MI virus absorbed all *gag*-related antibodies from serum h (lane h in Fig. 1A) while leaving antibodies to p65 uninfluenced (see Table 1). This absorbed serum was used to detect the antigens related to p65 on strips made from G-11/MJ virus, which was a good competitor for p65 (Table 1). The unabsorbed serum (lane b in Fig. 2A) detected p19, p24, and antigens of 32,000, 36,000, and 54,000 daltons, all of which are *gag*-related (*11*). In addition, two fainter bands of 46,000 and 51,000 daltons were detected, but no band of 65,000 daltons. The preabsorbed serum (lane c in Fig. 2A) detected two bands only, p46 and p51. Neither of these antigens was reactive with normal human serum (lane a in Fig. 2A). Thus, at least one of them had to account for the competition with p65 G-25/MI cell strips.

Table 1 also shows the presence of material that cross-reacts with p65 in MT 2 cells and MT 2 virus. A glycoprotein extract made from MT 2 cell culture fluids by adsorption to and elution from lentil lectin–agarose completely blocked the detection of p65 on G-25/MI cell strips (Fig. 2B). The glycoprotein responsible for the competition was shown to have a molecular size of 46,000 daltons by the technique used above. Unabsorbed serum incubated with strips made from the glycoprotein extract (Fig. 2C) strongly reacted with an antigen of 46,000 daltons (gp 46) and faintly with

antigens of 24,000 and 28,000 daltons (lane b in Fig. 2C), the latter two of them reactive with antibody to p24 (not shown). When incubated with G-25/MI virus, the serum reacted with gp 46 only (lane c in Fig. 2C), which is therefore responsible for the competition with p65. Experiments with the viruses purified from four different cells—G-11/MJ, NIH82-C2, Hut 102, and MT 2—showed that all of them have a strongly reactive gp46 (Fig. 2D).

Experiments analogous to those described in Fig. 2 were also done with strips made from Hut 102 cells. The serum rendered unreactive to *gag* still recognized a band comparable in intensity to p65 but somewhat smaller (not shown). This antigen, called p61 or gp61, is a cell surface glycoprotein unrelated to *gag* and the principal target of antibodies from patients with ATL and AIDS (*4, 7*). Our data show that p61 of Hut 102 and p65 of G-25/MI cells are homologous proteins.

In conclusion, we have established a relationship of homology between surface antigens of 61,000 and 65,000 daltons present in human T cells producing HTLV-I, but absent in HTLV-I–transformed nonproducer cells. Cross-reactive antigens are enriched in viruses purified from these cells. Taken together, the findings strongly suggest a viral origin of these antigens, though not definitely excluding the possibility that the presence of viral protein in the cell might lead to the expression of a cellular p65, which then copurifies with the virus. However, this theoretical possibility is rendered unlikely by the demonstration that the cross-reactive antigen in virus is not p65, but a glycoprotein of 46,000 daltons that contains all of the highly immunogenic determinants of p65 (Fig. 2B). These

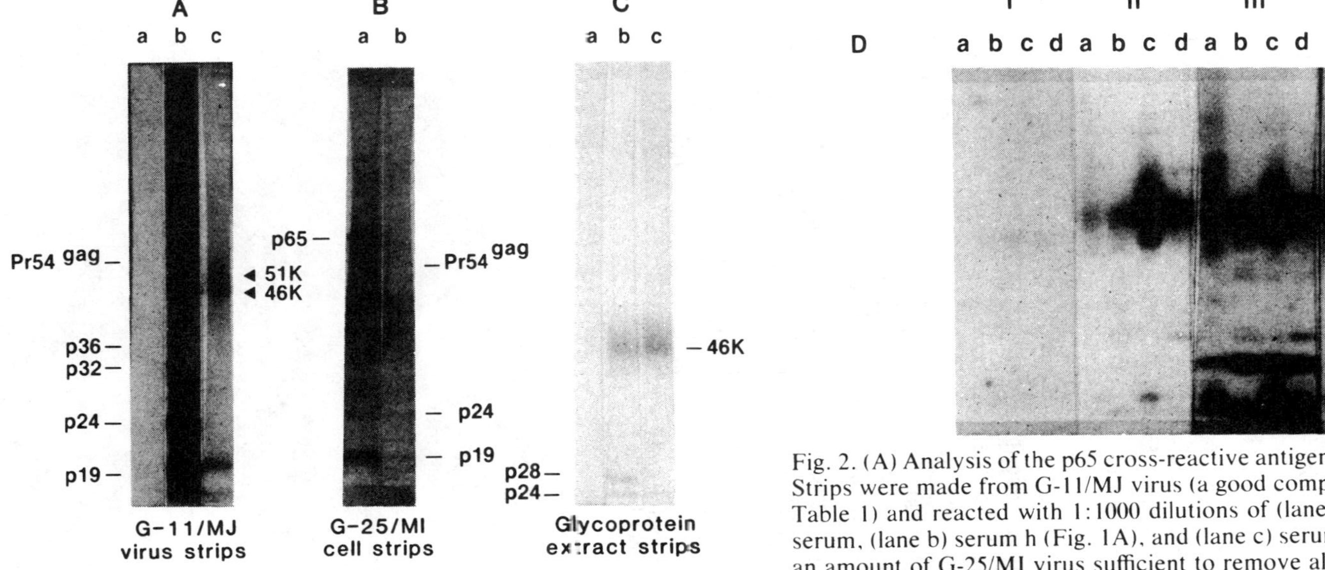

Fig. 2. (A) Analysis of the p65 cross-reactive antigens present in virus. Strips were made from G-11/MJ virus (a good competitor for p65; see Table 1) and reacted with 1:1000 dilutions of (lane a) normal human serum, (lane b) serum h (Fig. 1A), and (lane c) serum h absorbed with an amount of G-25/MI virus sufficient to remove all reactivity to *gag* while leaving the reactivity to p65 intact. This absorption removed all but the reactivities to p46 and p51, one of which thus had to account for the cross-reactivity to p65. (B) Competition with p65 by a glycoprotein extract. Strips made from G-25/MI cells were reacted with a 1:1000 dilution of serum h (Fig. 1A) either without competing material (lane a) or absorbed with 100 μl of a glycoprotein extract made from the cell culture fluids of MT 2 cells (lane b). This extract completely blocked the antibodies to p65. (C) Analysis of the p65 cross-reactive antigens in the MT 2 glycoprotein extract. Strips were made from the glycoprotein extract used in (B) and reacted with 1:1000 dilutions of (lane a) normal human serum, (lane b) serum h of Fig. 1A, and (lane c) serum h incubated with the G-25/MI virus to make it "monospecific" for p65. The only antigen not affected by this absorption is a glycoprotein of 46,000 daltons, thus responsible for the cross-reactivity with p65. (D) gp46 is a consistent component of purified viruses. Virus from the HTLV-I producer cell lines (lanes a) G-11/MJ, (lanes b) NIH 82-C2, (lanes c) Hut 102, and (lanes d) MT 2 was subjected to electrophoresis on an SDS–polyacrylamide gel and analyzed by Western blot with human sera diluted 1:1000. (I) Normal human serum; (II to IV) sera from ATL patients (III is serum e and IV is serum a of Fig. 1A).

findings are typical for the products of the envelope gene (*env*) of animal retroviruses (*15*). The *env* gene codes for a glycosylated precursor, which is then cleaved into the larger, highly immunogenic, main envelope glycoprotein and the smaller transmembrane glycoprotein, which is less immunogenic. Therefore, p65 and p61 probably represent the viral envelope precursor, which is readily detected in the cellular extracts because of the immunogenic envelope glycoprotein it contains. In the virus, the envelope glycoprotein may not be detected at the high serum dilution used. Alternatively, p65 or p61 may represent the major *env* glycoprotein, and the gp46 found in the virus may be a breakdown product of p65 and p61, as suggested for glycoproteins of 45,000 daltons often found in animal retrovirus preparations (*16*). In either case, the interpretation indicates a viral origin of p65 and p61.

References and Notes

1. For recent reviews, see R. C. Gallo and M. Essex, Eds., *Cancer Cells*, vol. 3, *Human T-cell Leukemia Viruses* (Cold Spring Harbor Laboratories, Cold Spring Harbor, N.Y., in press).
2. B. J. Poiesz, F. W. Ruscetti, A. F. Gazdar, P. A. Bunn, J. D. Minna, R. C. Gallo, *Proc. Natl. Acad. Sci. U.S.A.* **77**, 7415 (1980).
3. I. Miyoshi, I. Kubonishi, S. Yoshimoto, Y. Shiraishi, *Gann* **72**, 978 (1981).
4. M. Essex *et al.*, *Science* **220**, 859 (1983).
5. R. C. Gallo *et al.*, *ibid.*, p. 865; E. P. Gelmann *et al.*, *ibid.*, p. 862.
6. M. Popovic *et al.*, *ibid.* **219**, 856 (1983).
7. M. Essex *et al.*, *ibid.* **221**, 1061 (1983).
8. H. Towbin, T. Staehelin, J. Gordon, *Proc. Natl. Acad. Sci. U.S.A.* **76**, 4350 (1979).
9. V. S. Kalyanaraman, M. G. Sarngadharan, P. A. Bunn, J. D. Minna, R. C. Gallo, *Nature (London)* **294**, 271 (1981).
10. V. S. Kalyanaraman, M. Jarvis-Morar, M. G. Sarngadharan, R. C. Gallo, *Virology*, in press.
11. J. Schüpbach *et al.*, in preparation.
12. This 28,000-dalton protein was also found in another HTLV-infected cell line, G-11/MJ, and is, in contrast to a *gag*-related p28 of Hut 102 (*4*) and MT 2 (*13*) cells, unrelated to *gag* (*11*), and not part of the cell membrane, as shown by competition RIA.
13. N. Yamamoto and Y. Hinuma, *Int. J. Cancer* **30**, 289 (1982).
14. U. Schneider, H.-U. Schwenk, G. Bornkamm, *ibid.* **19**, 621 (1977).
15. For a review, see J. R. Stephenson, in *Molecular Biology of RNA Tumor Viruses*, J. R. Stephenson, Ed. (Academic Press, New York, 1980), p. 245.
16. J. H. Elder, J. W. Gautsch, F. C. Jensen, R. A. Lerner, J. W. Hartley, J. W. Rowe, *Proc. Natl. Acad. Sci. U.S.A.* **74**, 4676 (1977); H. Marquardt, R. V. Gilden, S. Oroszlan, *Biochemistry* **16**, 710 (1977); M. J. Krantz, M. Strand, J. T. August, *J. Virol.* **22**, 804 (1977).
17. U. K. Laemmli, *Nature (London)* **227**, 680 (1970).
18. J. Schüpbach *et al.*, *Blood* **62**, 616 (1983).
19. J.S. is a Fogarty International Fellow of the National Cancer Institute and also supported by the Swiss National Science Foundation.

12 December 1983; accepted 12 March 1984

35. The Interleukin-2 T-Cell System: A New Cell Growth Model

Doreen A. Cantrell and Kendall A. Smith

Mitosis of T lymphocytes results from the interaction of the T-lymphocytotrophic hormone interleukin-2 (IL-2) with specific membrane receptors (*1–4*). As a result of the availability of homogeneous IL-2 (*5*), the capability to examine IL-2 receptors quantitatively (*4–6*) and qualitatively (*7–11*), and the ability to synchronize IL-2 receptor-positive (receptor$^+$) T cells (*10*), it was possible to formulate new approaches to the determinants of T-cell cycle progression. Consequently, the basis for variable cell cycle transit times of individual cells among genetically homogeneous populations, a perplexing observation fundamental to the mechanisms that control cell proliferation, could finally be clarified. The results from several types of experiments indicate that T-cell cycle progression is predictable and depends on a critical threshold of interactions between IL-2 and the receptor that determines the quantal response, namely, cell division. Since IL-2 receptor density is heterogeneous and follows a log-normal distribution among T-cell populations, the cell cycle times of individual cells reflect the logarithmic-normal distribution of the IL-2 receptors.

Numerous experiments with many cell types (*12–23*) reveal that, within a cell population, the cell cycle times follow a normal distribution when examined as a function of the division rate (the rate-normal distribution) (*16, 17*). Kinetic studies of the cell cycle with either asynchronously proliferating populations or synchronized cell populations indicate that most of the variability in transit times occurs in the prereplicative phase (G_0-G_1) of the cell cycle since the replicative phases (S, G_2, M) remain relatively constant (*23*). Also, duration of the cell cycle is not genetically determined, nor is it passed on at division, since the correlations of cell cycle times for mother-daughter cells are generally poor (*23–26*). However, cycle times of sister cells do show a positive correlation, an indication that sibling cells inherit some property that contributes to similar cell cycle transit times for the next cycle, which then disappears by the subsequent cell cycle (*23–26*). Consequently, there is no selection for more rapidly growing cells, and cell populations retain the same rate-normal distribution of cell cycle times over many generations.

These and similar observations have led to the presentation of two basic models to explain the variability of cell cycle times. (i) The earlier deterministic model, proposed 20 years ago by Koch and Schaechter (*27*), is based on the assumptions that cells initiating their cycle are functionally different and that cell cycle variability arises from the cumulative effects of many small differences. (ii) The probabilistic model, originally proposed by Burns and Tannock (*28*) and extended by Smith and Martin and co-workers (*18, 20, 24–26, 28–30*), is based on the assumptions that cells initiating their cycle are functionally identical and that the transition of cells from an indeterminate resting phase to a determinant proliferative phase is regulated by a single Poissonian event, quite independent of other events or properties. While both models provide explanations for many of the observed data, in each instance there are discrepancies that point toward the presence of hidden variables operative in cell division kinetics. Accordingly, to achieve a better understanding of cell cycle control mechanisms, it appeared desirable to proceed beyond mathematical analysis of studies of cell populations and to correlate kinetic studies of cell growth with quantitative measurements of the critical factors known to promote DNA duplication and cellular division.

Recent advances in the dissection of the molecular mechanisms that regulate T-lymphocyte mitosis have permitted an analysis of the variables that determine the heterogeneity of interdivision times observed within proliferating T-cell populations. Such studies have become possible because IL-2 can now be purified to homogeneity by monoclonal antibody affinity adsorption (*5*). Furthermore, the development of a radiolabeled IL-2 binding assay made possible the quantitative measurement of IL-2 receptors (*4, 6*), and a recently described monoclonal antibody reactive with IL-2 receptors (anti-Tac) (*7–9*) made possible a qualitative assessment of IL-2 receptors within T-cell populations (*10, 11*). These re-

agents have been used to show that the initiation of T-cell cycle progression depends on immunostimulatory signals such as antigens, mitogenic lectins, or T-cell–specific monoclonal antibodies, whereas the transition from G_1 into the replicative phases of the cell cycle is mediated by IL-2 alone (*3, 4, 10, 11*).

The relevance of the IL-2 receptor hormone system to T-cell cycle progression is attested by experiments showing that the IL-2 receptor interaction is obligatory for DNA synthesis and mitosis; that is, monoclonal antibodies reactive with IL-2 (*5*), or the IL-2 receptor (*9*), inhibit T-cell proliferation by preventing IL-2 receptor binding. Moreover, the IL-2 membrane binding sites satisfy the criteria for authentic hormone receptors (such as high affinity, saturability, and ligand and target cell specificity), and the concentrations of IL-2 that bind to IL-2 receptors coincide precisely with those that promote T-cell proliferation (*4, 6*). Thus, as would be predicted from the interaction of a single ligand and a single class of high affinity receptors, at equilibrium the rate of T-cell proliferation is directly dependent on the concentration of IL-2 available to the cells (*4*).

A characteristic of the IL-2 hormone-receptor mechanism, which permits the synchronization of IL-2 receptor$^+$ cells, stems from the finding that, unlike those of all known hormone receptor systems, IL-2 receptors are not continuously expressed by T cells. Rather, receptor expression occurs only after appropriate immune stimulation and is thus transient (*10*). When cells are exposed to antigen or lectin, IL-2 receptors accumulate asynchronously among the individual cells within a population. Once a critical density of IL-2 receptors is reached, cell cycle progression ensues provided that an adequate concentration of IL-2 is present. If the initial immunostimulatory activating signal is removed, the number of IL-2 receptors progressively declines regardless of the maintenance of an adequate IL-2 concentration. In parallel, the proliferative rate of the cell population also declines, finally resulting in the reaccumulation of all of the cells within the population into the G_0-G_1 phase of the cell cycle. Of significance for our studies is that the reintroduction of the initial activating signal results in an acquisition of IL-2 receptors so accelerated that maximum receptor levels now occur within 18 to 24 hours. However, cell cycle progression resumes only when IL-2 is provided. Thus, a T-cell population can be synchronized into the G_0-G_1 phase of the cell cycle and can be stimulated to express maximal levels of IL-2 receptors. The kinetics of IL-2–dependent cell cycle progression can then be followed and analyzed in relationship to IL-2 receptor concentration and distribution among the cells within the population.

Heterogeneous Distribution of IL-2 Receptors

When the IL-2 receptor distribution of a T-cell population is analyzed by flow microfluorometry with anti-Tac, and the data are plotted on a linear scale, a skewed distribution pattern is obtained (Fig. 1A). However, if the data are plotted on a logarithmic scale, the receptor density follows a normal distribution with only a slight skewing toward a frequency of cells with a higher receptor concentration (Fig. 1B). The heterogeneous distribution of receptors within T-

cell populations could not be explained by receptor variation with the recognizable phases of the cell cycle, since identical receptor distribution patterns were observed with G_0-G_1 synchronized cells. Moreover, clonal variation of receptor density could not account for these observations, as identical patterns were consistently observed with cloned murine (data not shown) and human T-cell populations (*11*).

The log-normal distribution of IL-2 receptors within a T-cell population is strikingly reminiscent of the rate-normal distribution of cell cycle times. Because of the similarity of these distributions and because the IL-2-receptor interaction is obligatory for T-cell cycle progression, the possibility was considered that cell cycle variability is determined by the intrapopulation heterogeneity of IL-2 receptor density per cell. Should this supposition be correct, IL-2 receptor[+] cell populations would be heterogeneous with regard to their responsiveness to IL-2. Accordingly, to examine the functional implications of heterogeneous IL-2 receptor expression, the initial experimental approach was to establish whether conditions that limit IL-2 receptor interactions modify cell cycle progression, particularly with respect to the proportion of cells triggered.

IL-2 Concentration and Exposure Time Determine Cell Cycle Progression

Since the proportion of occupied receptors is dependent on the IL-2 concentration, and since the distribution of IL-2 receptors among the cells within a population follows a log-normal pattern, the absolute number of occupied receptors should vary according to the receptor

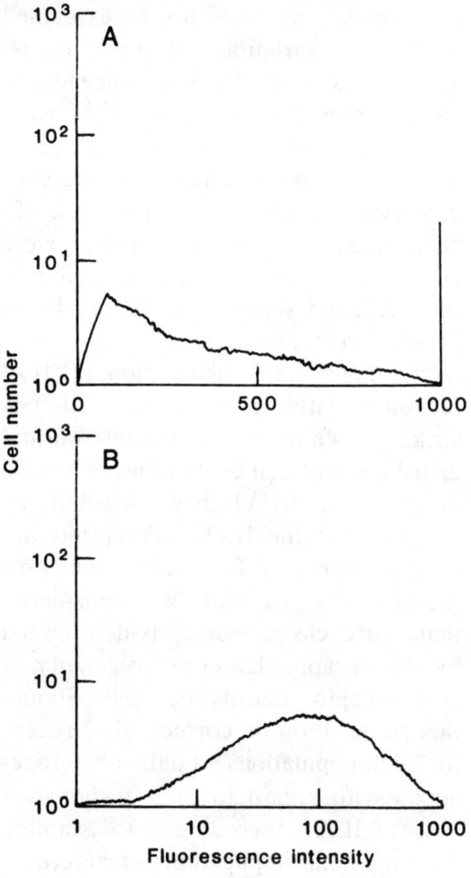

Fig. 1. Fluorescence of anti-Tac reactivity. Human peripheral blood mononuclear cells (PBM) isolated by Ficoll-Hypaque discontinuous gradient centrifugation were cultured (10^6 cells per milliliter) in RPMI 1640 medium supplemented with heat-inactivated fetal calf serum (10 percent) (RPMI 1640/10 percent fetal calf serum). Cells were stimulated with phytohemagglutinin (PHA) (1 µg/ml) for 72 hours to ensure expression of the IL-2 receptor. For analysis of anti-Tac reactivity, samples (10^6 cells) were incubated (1 hour, 4°C) with saturating concentrations of biotinylated anti-Tac (20 µg/ml) and fluorescein or Texas red–conjugated avidin (1 hour, 4°C). Anti-Tac reactivity was determined on an Orthocytofluorograph (System 50H, Orthodiagnostic System, Inc.) for analysis of linear plots of fluorescence intensity (A) and on an Epics 5 cell sorter (Coulter Electronics) for analysis of logarithmic plots of fluorescence intensity (B). The percentage anti-Tac$^+$ cells, estimated against a background of nonspecific labeling with normal mouse immunoglobulin (1 to 3 percent), was 84 percent (A) and 87 percent (B). For each plot 10,000 cells were collected.

density of each cell. Thus, if the number of occupied receptors is critical, a G_0-G_1 synchronized cell population with a heterogeneous IL-2 receptor profile would be expected to enter the proliferative phases of the cell cycle asynchronously, as a function of the IL-2 concentration. As a test for this assumption, phytohemagglutinin (PHA)-stimulated human peripheral blood mononuclear cells (PBM) were harvested from culture after 10 days of IL-2–dependent growth. The cells were again stimulated with PHA to ensure maximal receptor expression, cultured without IL-2 for 3 days to allow the accumulation of the cell population in the G_0-G_1 phase of the cell cycle, and

then exposed to various concentrations of IL-2. The entrance of the cells into the S phase of the cell cycle was monitored by incorporation of tritiated thymidine ($[^3H]TdR$) and by cytofluorometric analysis of propidium iodide (PI)–DNA binding. As anticipated, the proportion of cells that entered the cell cycle varied with time, depending on the IL-2 concentration (Fig. 2A). Within the population, the asynchronous entry of cells into S phase is reflected by the gradual increase in $[^3H]TdR$ incorporation at each IL-2 concentration and by the PI profile of the cells, which 24 hours after exposure to IL-2 is consistent with that of a population in asynchronous growth,

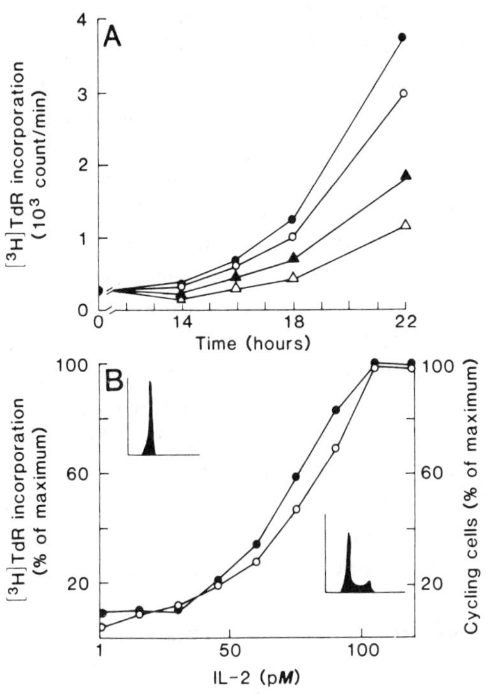

Fig. 2. IL-2 concentration-dependent T-cell cycle progression. (A) PHA-stimulated (72 hours) human PBM were harvested from IL-2–dependent proliferative growth after 10 days of culture, restimulated with PHA (1 μg/ml, 2 hours) to ensure maximal IL-2 receptor expression and cultured without IL-2 for 72 hours to allow for the reaccumulation of the cell population into G_0 or G_1. The synchronized cells were cultured (5×10^4 cells per milliliter) in a humidified atmosphere (5 percent CO_2 in air) in microtiter wells (0.2 ml per well) with the following concentrations of immunoaffinity-purified IL-2 (5): (●) 500 pM, (○) 100 pM, (▲) 50 pM, (△) 25 pM. Tritiated thymidine ([³H]TdR (Schwarz/Mann; specific activity, 2.0 μCi/ml) incorporation was monitored during 1-hour intervals (as indicated) by precipitation onto glass fiber filter paper and subsequent liquid scintillation counting. Symbols represent the mean of quadruplicate cultures. The standard errors of the mean in all cultures were < 5 percent. (B) Incorporation of [³H]TdR (●) and the percentage cycling cells (○) from a second experiment performed as described in (A) 24 hours after the addition of IL-2. The data are expressed as percent of maximum [³H]TdR incorporation ($50,526 \pm 536$ count/min per 10^5 cells). The percentage cycling cells was determined by labeling 10^6 cells with propidium iodide (50 μg/ml in 1.12 percent sodium citrate, 0.05 percent Nonidet P-40, and ribonuclease, 100 Kunitz unit/ml) and subsequent analysis for cellular DNA content (Orthocytofluorograph). The relative number of cells in the cycling phases of the cell cycle (S, G_2, and M) was estimated by the Quick Estimate method of cell cycle analysis provided with the Ortho 2150 Data Handler System. (Inset, upper left) Linear plot of DNA content for cells cultured without IL-2. (Inset lower right) Linear plot of DNA content for cells cultured with the maximum IL-2 concentration (250 pM). Identical data were obtained from three additional experiments.

comprised of cells exhibiting G_1, S, G_2, and M content of DNA. The IL-2 concentration-dependent effect is discerned by examining a single time interval after the addition of IL-2 (Fig. 2B). A typical sigmoid log-dose response curve resulted when the response of the cell population was monitored either by [³H]TdR incorporation or by PI analysis of the proportion of cells in the replicative phases of the cell cycle. The coincidence of the curves obtained by the different monitoring techniques also affirms the

validity of the interpretation that [³H]TdR incorporation, measured over short intervals, reflects the proportion of cells within the population that are in the replicative phase of the cell cycle.

The capability to synchronize the cell population into G_0-G_1 while simultaneously ensuring maximal IL-2 receptor expression by lectin stimulation also permitted an analysis of the effect of altering the IL-2 receptor exposure time on cell cycle progression. Although IL-2 receptor binding reaches equilibrium within 15 minutes, the results of the previous series of experiments led us to anticipate that the duration of IL-2 receptor interaction could be an important determinant of cell cycle progression. When a G_0-G_1 IL-2 receptor[+] population was exposed to 250 pM IL-2, a receptor-saturating concentration, for varying intervals, a 3-hour exposure was insufficient to trigger detectable DNA synthesis over the ensuing 26 hours (Fig. 3, inset). In four additional experiments, it was found that a minimum of 5 to 6 hours of IL-2 exposure was essential for triggering detectable cell cycle progression; moreover, exposure times in excess of 6 hours resulted in a progressively greater proportion of cells within the population entering the S phase. In the experiment shown in Fig. 3 (inset), exposure times of 6, 11, and 26 hours resulted in increasingly greater incorporation of [^{3}H]TdR at each interval studied.

If the cell cycle progression were determined by the extent of IL-2 receptor interactions, the IL-2 concentration would also be expected to influence the duration of exposure necessary to promote cell cycle progression. In fact, at 26 hours, 20 percent of the maximal [^{3}H]TdR incorporation occurred when 10 pM IL-2 was present for the entire 26-hour culture period, whereas 60 pM and 100 pM IL-2 were necessary to promote a similar effect when the IL-2 cellular exposure times were limited to 11 or 6 hours, respectively (Fig. 3). Therefore, both IL-2 concentration and the duration of IL-2 cellular interaction are critical determinants of cell cycle progression. There appears to be an interplay between these two variables, such that the proportion of cells responsive to suboptimal concentrations of IL-2 can be increased by lengthening the exposure period.

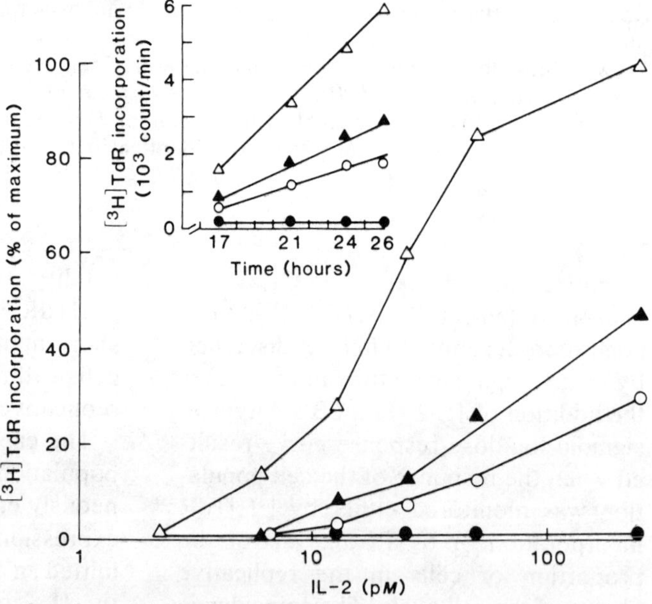

Fig. 3. The effect of varying the IL-2 exposure period on the proliferative response of G_0 or G_1 IL-2 receptor[+] T cells. IL-2 receptor[+] cells were synchronized (legend to Fig. 2) and exposed to IL-2 concentrations for different time intervals. IL-2 was then removed by washing, and the subsequent progression of the population into the S phase of the cell cycle was monitored by [^{3}H]TdR incorporation (1-hour intervals). The data represent the percent maximum [^{3}H]TdR incorporation after 26 hours of culture plotted as a function of IL-2 concentration after a 3-hour (●), 6-hour (○), 11-hour (▲), and 26-hour (△) exposure to IL-2. The inset shows the [^{3}H]TdR incorporation of each population (that is, 3-, 6-, 11-, and 26-hour exposure periods) in response to an IL-2 receptor saturating IL-2 concentration (250 pM) monitored at the times indicated.

IL-2 Receptor Concentration Determines Cell Cycle Progression

The above observations suggested that the absolute number of IL-2 receptor interactions occurring during G_1 was important in the initiation of the biological response. Moreover, as conditions that limit IL-2 receptor interactions modify the proportion of cells that enter the proliferative phases of the cell cycle, the observations were consistent with an underlying heterogeneity within the cell population with regard to the capacity to respond to a given concentration of IL-2. A possible explanation for this differential responsiveness is afforded by the observation that IL-2 receptor density is also heterogeneous and distributed log-normally within the cell population. Therefore it could be anticipated that, when the IL-2 concentration or exposure period is reduced, only cells with relatively high IL-2 receptor levels would be triggered to initiate DNA synthesis. Moreover, under conditions of saturating levels of IL-2, cells with a high IL-2 receptor density would exit from G_1 before cells with relatively low IL-2 receptor densities. Thus, synchronized T-cell populations that differ with respect to IL-2 receptor levels would be expected to enter the S phase of the cell cycle after varying periods of G_1.

In 16 experiments with cell populations that differed with respect to the mean IL-2 receptor density, the duration of G_1 ranged between 10 and 28 hours (mean duration = 18.5 ± 1.0 standard error of the mean) and varied inversely with the number of IL-2 receptors. Moreover, when cells from the same population were examined sequentially (Fig. 4), similar data were obtained. Human PBM cells were cultured for 3 days with lectin, washed and placed in lectin-

free and IL-2–free medium. After 8 days more than 95 percent of the cells had accumulated in G_0 or G_1, although the population still expressed relatively high levels of IL-2 receptors (anti-Tac mean fluorescence intensity, 270). The remainder of the cells were harvested from

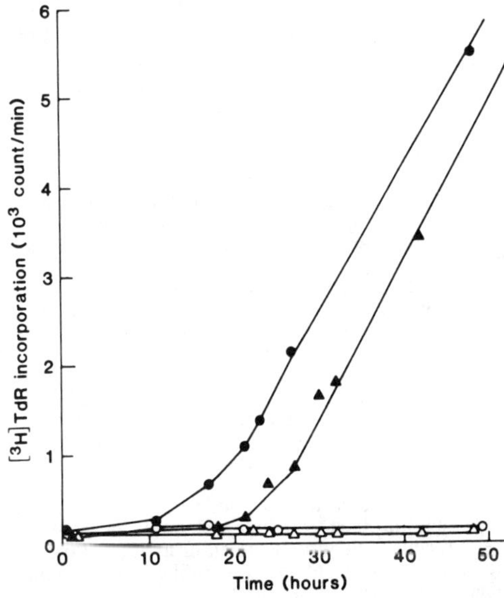

Fig. 4. The effect of IL-2 receptor density on T-cell cycle progression. Human PBM cells were cultured (1×10^6 cells per milliliter) for 72 hours with phytohemagglutinin (PHA) (1 μg/ml), washed, and placed into culture without PHA or IL-2. At day 8 (●) and day 11 (▲), the cells were washed and cultured with a receptor-saturating concentration (250 pM) of IL-2. Open symbols indicate cultures without IL-2 addition. Incorporation of [^{3}H]TdR was monitored as indicated at 1-hour intervals. Before the addition of IL-2, portions of each cell population were analyzed for IL-2 receptor expression with flow microfluorometry and anti-Tac (see legend to Fig. 1). A comparison of fluorescence intensity was made by means of the mean channel number for different plots (range 1 to 1000). The mean anti-Tac fluorescence intensity for the cells harvested after 8 days of culture was 270 and that for cells harvested after 11 days was 85. The mean fluorescence obtained with control immunoglobulin was 25 and 5, respectively.

188

Table 1. The proliferative response of IL-2 receptor[+] cell subpopulations separated on the basis of IL-2 receptor density.

Experiment	Culture (hours)	[³H]TdR incorporation*		
		Unseparated	IL-2 receptors	
			Low	High
1	38	10,461	6,555	12,571
2	40	30,852	13,160	39,122
3	40	38,064	4,248	51,344
4	48	19,824	5,556	36,754
5	31	26,120	10,760	59,600

*Synchronized IL-2 receptor[+] cells (cultured as described in the legend to Fig. 2) were labeled with anti-Tac (ascites 1:5000, 1 hour, 4°C), and fluorescein isothiocyanate (FITC)–conjugated rabbit antiserum to mouse immunoglobulin (1:20, 1 hour, 4°C). Viable cells were selected for high or low anti-Tac reactivity by means of a cell-sorting facility available with the Orthocytofluorograph. The mean fluorescence intensities of the unseparated cells, low IL-2 receptor subset and high IL-2 receptor subset were 375 ± 44, 162 ± 33, and 605 ± 34 (mean ± standard error of the mean), respectively. After the cells were sorted, unbound anti-Tac was removed from the cells by washing, and the separated and unseparated G_0 or G_1 cell populations were placed into culture in the presence of affinity-purified IL-2 (250 pM). At the indicated times [³H]TdR incorporation was determined during a 1-hour period. Data shown represent the mean number of counts per minute per 10^5 cells of quadruplicate cultures. The standard error of the mean of the quadruplicate determinations was <5 percent of the mean.

culture after 11 days, at which time the IL-2 receptor density of the population had decreased approximately threefold (anti-Tac mean fluorescence intensity, 85). On addition of 500 pM IL-2, the cell population with the higher IL-2 receptor density entered the S phase of the cell cycle 10 hours earlier than the population with lower IL-2 receptor density (Fig. 4).

Cell sorting experiments permitted a direct approach to the issue of the relevance of IL-2 receptor density and cell cycle progression (Table 1). Synchronized IL-2-receptor[+] cells were separated into subsets on the basis of low or high anti-Tac fluorescence intensity,

washed, and placed into culture with 500 pM IL-2. Entrance into the S phase of the cell cycle in each population was monitored at various intervals by [³H]TdR incorporation. The data from the longest interval studied (31 to 48 hours) indicate that the subsets with a high density of IL-2 receptors contained a greater proportion of cells within the S phase of the cell cycle. In a representative experiment, unseparated (Fig. 5A) and separated (Fig. 5, B and C) cell populations were examined at intervals after exposure to a receptor-saturating concentration of IL-2 (250 pM) (Fig. 5D). In the high density IL-2 receptor population the proportion of cells in the S phase of the cell cycle was greater than that in the low density IL-2 receptor subset; also, the higher density population appeared to account for most of the [³H]TdR incorporation of the unseparated population. In addition, as would be anticipated from the experiments with unseparated cell populations, the response of the separated cell populations was dependent on IL-2 concentration (Fig. 5E). At limiting IL-2 concentrations (10 to 20 pM), only the high IL-2 receptor density cells could be detected in the S phase of the cell cycle. Thus, the log-normal distribution of cellular IL-2 receptor density within a T-cell population is responsible for the normal sigmoid shape of the IL-2 log dose-response curve.

Conclusions

Our study shows that (i) synchronized T cells differ with respect to IL-2 receptor density and (ii) analysis of the key elements that control T-cell growth in relation to IL-2 receptor expression provides an explanation for cell cycle asynchrony within T-cell populations. IL-2–directed T-cell mitosis is a quantal response determined by a critical threshold of signals generated by the interaction between IL-2 and the IL-2 receptor. Thus, T-cell cycle progression is predict-

able, provided that the variables of IL-2 concentration, IL-2 receptor density, and the duration of the IL-2 receptor interactions are known.

To arrive at this interpretation, it was first necessary to identify that the IL-2

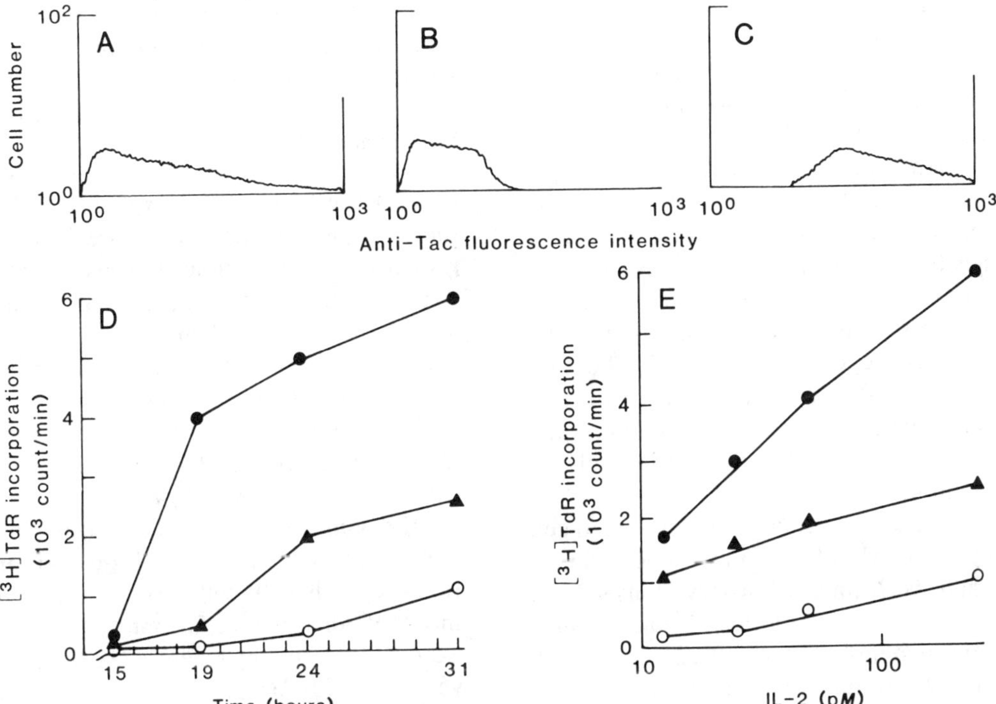

Fig. 5. The proliferative response of IL-2 receptor$^+$ cell subpopulations separated on the basis of IL-2 receptor density. Synchronized IL-2 receptor$^+$ cells (Fig. 2 legend) were labeled with anti-Tac (1:5000 dilution of ascites, 1 hour, 4°C) and rabbit FITC-conjugated antiserum to mouse immunoglobulin (1:20 dilution, 1 hour, 4°C). Viable cells were selected for low or high anti-Tac reactivity (Orthocytofluorograph). Analysis of anti-Tac reactivity of the unseparated cells (A), low anti-Tac reactive subset (B), and high anti-Tac reactive subset (C) is shown in the upper panels. The percentage anti-Tac$^+$ cells in the unseparated population was 97 percent (background labeling with control immunoglobulin, 1 to 3 percent). The mean fluorescence intensity plots shown in (A), (B), and (C) was 344, 158, and 646, respectively. After the cells were sorted, anti-Tac was removed from the cell suspensions by washing, and the separated and unseparated G_0 or G_1 cells were placed into culture in the presence of immunoaffinity-purified IL-2 (0 to 250 pM). Residual cell-bound anti-Tac did not prevent IL-2–mediated proliferation: although anti-Tac can block IL-2 receptor binding, antibodies must be present continuously at high concentrations (50 μg/ml; $3.3 \times 10^{-7}M$) to inhibit IL-2–dependent proliferation. (D) [^{3}H]TdR incorporation in response to receptor saturating concentrations of IL-2 (250 pM) of unseparated cells (▲), low anti-Tac reactive cells (○), and high anti-Tac reactive cells (●). (E) [^{3}H]TdR incorporation of unseparated (▲), low (○), and high (●) IL-2 receptor$^+$ cells, plotted as a function of IL-2 concentration after 31 hours of culture.

receptor interaction is the key event that signals T-cell cycle progression. In addition to the coincidence of the IL-2 binding and biological response curves (*4, 6*), this conclusion rests on the finding that prevention of the IL-2 receptor interaction completely abrogates T-cell proliferation (*5, 9*). However, the observation that IL-2 receptor density has a log-normal distribution within asynchronous, synchronized, and cloned T-cell populations provided new insight as to a cellular characteristic essential for growth, one which could underlie variability of cell cycle times. Review of the many reports where cell cycle variability has been investigated indicates that previous workers were hampered by a lack of knowledge of the variables that determine cell cycle progression in the systems under study. Moreover, so long as these variables remained hidden, they could not be analyzed quantitatively or qualitatively.

Thus an important issue relating to cell cycle variability is now amenable to analysis. Numerous observations in both prokaryotic (*12, 17, 20, 31*) and eukaryotic systems (*14–17, 19–22, 24–26, 29, 30, 32–34*) indicate that cell populations in exponential growth retain the same distribution of generation times over many cycles and that there is no selection for more rapidly growing cells. Consequently, there can be no strong mother-daughter correlation with respect to cell cycle transit times. In the T-cell system this leads to the prediction of a lack of a mother-daughter correlation with respect to IL-2 receptor number. Consistent with this prediction, when monoclonal antibodies to anti-Tac or IL-2 were used to detect receptor bound IL-2, cloned lines of murine and human T-cell populations showed the same heterogeneous log-normal distribution of IL-2 receptor expression as observed in polyclonal T-cell populations. These findings can be accounted for only if deterministic differences in IL-2 receptor levels are created at each cell division and modified in each cycle. Moreover, in addition to the inexact partitioning of membrane receptors between the daughter cells, the cellular components responsible for IL-2 receptor synthesis and degradation would also be expected to be distributed unequally. Thus, the importance of these findings resides not only in the logic of the explanation for the lack of selection for more rapidly growing cells over time, but also in the experimental directions provided by the knowledge that the elements in question are the IL-2 receptors and the determinants of IL-2 receptor expression.

The salient information derived from these studies relates to the probability that these concepts can be extrapolated to other cell systems. It is indeed striking that the growth characteristics found for IL-2–dependent T cells are identical to those of all other cells that have been examined, including bacteria (*12, 17, 20*), yeasts (*12, 32, 33*), protozoa (*14, 23*), and all mammalian cells (*15, 16, 19–26, 29, 30, 34*). Accordingly, it could be postulated that the mechanisms operative to signal DNA duplication and cell division are common to all living forms and that the specificity of cell cycle progression, especially in multicellular organisms, is conferred by cell-specific ligands and receptors. With the identification of the variables determining T-cell growth, it should now be possible to proceed beyond the IL-2 receptor interaction to begin to unravel the biochemical and molecular reactions that are critical for cell division. In addition, both normal

(*35*) and neoplastic (*36*) IL-2 receptor[+] cell populations are available for study. Thus, future experiments designed to understand the intracellular reactions triggered by the IL-2 receptor interaction may yet provide the means for discriminating between the mechanisms underlying normal and neoplastic cell growth.

References and Notes

1. D. A. Morgan, F. W. Ruscetti, R. C. Gallo, *Science* **193**, 1007 (1976).
2. S. Gillis and K. A. Smith, *Nature (London)* **268**, 154 (1977).
3. K. A. Smith, *Immunol. Rev.* **51**, 337 (1980).
4. ______, in *Genetics of the Immune Response*, E. Moller and G. Moller, Eds. (Plenum, New York, 1983), p. 151.
5. K. A. Smith, M. F. Favata, S. Oroszlan, *J. Immunol.* **131**, 1808 (1983).
6. R. J. Robb, A. Munck, K. A. Smith, *J. Exp. Med.* **154**, 1455 (1981).
7. T. Uchiyama, S. Broder, T. A. Waldmann, *J. Immunol.* **126**, 1393 (1981).
8. T. Uchiyama, D. L. Nelson, T. A. Fleisher, T. A. Waldmann, *ibid.*, p. 1398.
9. W. J. Leonard *et al.*, *Nature (London)* **300**, 267 (1982).
10. D. A. Cantrell and K. A. Smith, *J. Exp. Med.* **158**, 1895 (1983).
11. S. C. Meuer *et al.*, *Proc. Natl. Acad. Sci. U.S.A.* **81**, 1509 (1984).
12. C. D. Kelly and O. Rahn, *J. Bacteriol.* **2**, 147 (1932).
13. V. W. Burns, *J. Cell Comp. Physiol.* **47**, 537 (1956).
14. J. R. Cook and B. Cook, *Exp. Cell Res.* **28**, 524 (1962).
15. K. B. Dawson, H. Madoc-Jones, E. O. Field, *ibid.* **38**, 75 (1965).
16. J. F. Sisken and L. Morasca, *J. Cell Biol.* **25**, 179 (1965).
17. H. E. Kubitshek, *Cell Tissue Kinet.* **4**, 113 (1971).
18. J. A. Smith and L. Martin, *Proc. Natl. Acad. Sci. U.S.A.* **70**, 1263 (1973).
19. H. Miyamoto, E. Zeuthen, L. Rasmussen, *J. Cell Sci.* **13**, 879 (1973).
20. R. Shields, *Nature (London)* **293**, 755 (1978).
21. R. F. Brooks, D. C. Bennett, J. A. Smith, *Cell* **19**, 493 (1980).
22. P. S. Rabinovitch, *Proc. Natl. Acad. Sci. U.S.A.* **80**, 2951 (1983).
23. A. B. Pardee, B.-Z. Shilo, A. L. Koch, in *Hormones and Cell Culture*, G. H. Sato and R. Ross, Eds. (Cold Spring Harbor Laboratory, Cold Spring Harbor, N.Y., 1979), p. 373.
24. P. D. Minor and J. A. Smith, *Nature (London)* **248**, 241 (1974).
25. R. Shields and J. A. Smith, *J. Cell Physiol.* **91**, 345 (1977).
26. R. Shields, *Nature (London)* **267**, 704 (1977).
27. A. L. Koch and M. Schaechter, *J. Gen. Microbiol.* **29**, 435 (1962).
28. F. J. Burns and I. F. Tannock, *Cell Tissue Kinet.* **3**, 321 (1970).
29. R. F. Brooks, *Cell* **12**, 311 (1977).
30. R. Shields, R. F. Brooks, P. N. Riddle, D. F. Capellaro, D. Delia, *Cell* **15**, 469 (1978).
31. J. L. Spudich and D. E. Koshland, *Nature (London)* **262**, 467 (1976).
32. B. Shilo, V. Shilo, G. Simchen, *ibid.* **264**, 767 (1976).
33. L. H. Hartwell and W. Unger, *J. Cell Biol.* **75**, 422 (1977).
34. D. F. Peterson and E. C. Anderson, *Nature (London)* **203**, 642 (1964).
35. K. A. Smith and F. W. Ruscetti, *Adv. Immunol.* **31**, 137 (1981).
36. T. Hattori, T. Uchiyama, T. Toibana, K. Takatsuki, H. Uchino, *Blood* **58**, 645 (1981).
37. We thank Drs. T. Uchiyama and T. Waldmann for the monoclonal antibody (anti-Tac), Dr. M. Landy for editorial comments, and R. Miller for assistance with the cytofluorographic analysis. Supported in part by NIH grants CA-17643, CA-17323, CA-23108, and CA-26273 and by American Cancer Society grant CH-167.

12 December 1983; accepted 17 February 1984

Report

6 July 1984

36. Selective Tropism of Lymphadenopathy Associated Virus (LAV) for Helper-Inducer T Lymphocytes

David Klatzmann, Françoise Barré-Sinoussi, Marie Thérèse Nugeyre, Charles Dauguet, Etienne Vilmer, Claude Griscelli Françoise Brun-Vézinet, Christine Rouzioux, Jean Claude Gluckman, Jean-Claude Chermann, and Luc Montagnier

Epidemiological data indicate that the acquired immunodeficiency syndrome (AIDS) is caused by an infectious agent, probably a virus (*1–3*). Since a qualitative and quantitative defect of the helper-inducer T cell subset (T4$^+$) is the major immunological abnormality of this disease (*4, 5*), one would expect such a causative agent to express a tropism for T4$^+$ lymphocytes, resulting in alteration of their function.

We recently discovered a new group of human retroviruses that differ from human T-cell leukemia virus (HTLV-I) (*6–10*). The first member of this group was isolated from a nonimmunodepressed homosexual patient with persistent lymphadenopathy, a syndrome considered to be related to AIDS (*11, 12*). This virus has tentatively been named lymphadenopathy associated virus (LAV). Similar viruses were found in patients with frank AIDS, including the only hemophiliac patient with AIDS reported in France (*7*). Specific antibodies against LAV have been detected in approximately 70 percent of patients with persistent lymphadenopathy and 40 percent of AIDS patients studied (*8, 13*). We have now investigated whether the tro-pism of LAV is selective for the T4$^+$ subset in vivo as well as in vitro.

The studies in vivo were conducted with the help of an asymptomatic virus carrier, patient E.L., and his brother, patient D.L. Both patients have B hemophilia (*7*). Patient D.L. recently developed AIDS as assessed by successive opportunistic infections accompanied by a profound alteration of immune functions in vivo and in vitro. By means of techniques already described (*6–8*), a retrovirus similar to LAV was isolated repeatedly from his peripheral blood lymphocytes (PBL). This virus differs from HTLV-I (*9, 14, 15*). When examined by an immunofluorescence technique with antibodies to the structural proteins p24 or p19 of HTLV-I, fixed LAV-producing cells (*6*) were negative. Similarly, [^{35}S]methionine-labeled p25 of LAV was not precipitated by the antibodies to HTLV-I. Moreover, no antibody to HTLV-producing cell lines (C10/MJ, C91/PL) could be detected in the patient's serum by immunofluorescence, nor to HTLV p24 by the commercial enzyme-linked immunosorbent assay (ELISA; Biotech) or by a radioimmunoassay with a monoclonal antibody to p24 (*7*). No antibodies against LAV or HTLV could be detected in serum samples from parents of the patients, but E.L., like his brother, had circulating antibodies against LAV. However, apart from having hemophilia, E.L. was healthy and displayed normal immune functions. Nevertheless, LAV was isolated three times at monthly intervals from his PBL. The fact that no difference could be found between the viruses isolated from the brothers by serological and morphological studies, as well as the similar history of factor IX transfusion, strongly suggests that the viruses have a common origin (*7*). Since, contrary to AIDS patients, E.L. had normal numbers of helper-inducer lymphocytes, sufficient quantities of these cells could be purified and cultured to find out whether the virus displayed a selective tropism in vivo for any given blood cell population.

Preliminary experiments indicated that LAV can be propagated only in human T lymphocytes in vitro. We were unable to detect productive virus infection, as determined by reverse transcriptase (RT) activity, after in vitro infection of normal B lymphocytes, lymphoma cell lines (RAJI and MOLT4), or monocytes (*16*).

Peripheral blood lymphocytes of E.L. were fractionated into monocytes, B lymphocytes, and T lymphocytes. Helper-inducer ($T4^+$) and suppressor-cytotoxic ($T8^+$) fractions were then obtained by cellular affinity chromatography. This technique does not modify interleukin-2 (IL-2) production or proliferative or cytotoxic lymphocyte functions (*17*, and data not shown). Cells were then cultured as described (*6, 8*) in the presence of phytohemagglutinin (PHA) followed by IL-2. Reverse transcriptase was then sequentially measured in each culture

supernatant. When $T4^+$ or $T8^+$ lymphocytes from normal individuals are maintained under the same culture conditions, the baseline of RT remains negative. By comparison, a spontaneous increase of RT occurred as early as day 3 of culture in the $T4^+$ fraction from patient E.L. and reached a peak value of 700×10^3 count/min on day 10. It declined rapidly thereafter to less than 200×10^3 count/min on day 18 and remained low until the end of the culture period on day 45 (Fig. 1). During the same period, this activity was always below 4×10^3 count/min in the $T8^+$ culture, until day 60. Such a low degree of RT, compared to $T8^+$ cultures from normal noninfected lymphocytes ($< 2 \times 10^3$ count/min), probably reflects the small number of $T4^+$ contaminating cells. Moreover, when $T8^+$ lymphocytes were cocultivated with cord blood lymphocytes, in order to amplify the low virus production (*10*), no RT activity was detectable (data not shown).

Examination with the electron microscope revealed mature virus particles characterized by a small eccentric core, as well as virus budding at the cell surfaces, in the $T4^+$ but not in the $T8^+$ fraction (Fig. 2). These aspects were similar to those seen in the unfractionated T lymphocytes (*6–8*).

At the beginning of the culture, each cellular fraction was enriched to more than 95 percent and contained less than 2 percent of cells of the opposite phenotype. This phenotype remained unchanged throughout the period of culture in the $T8^+$ fraction with always less than 5 percent of contaminating cells. In contrast, a progressive disappearance of the markers identified by the monoclonal antibodies OKT3 and OKT4 was observed in the $T4^+$ cell fraction. Thus, the

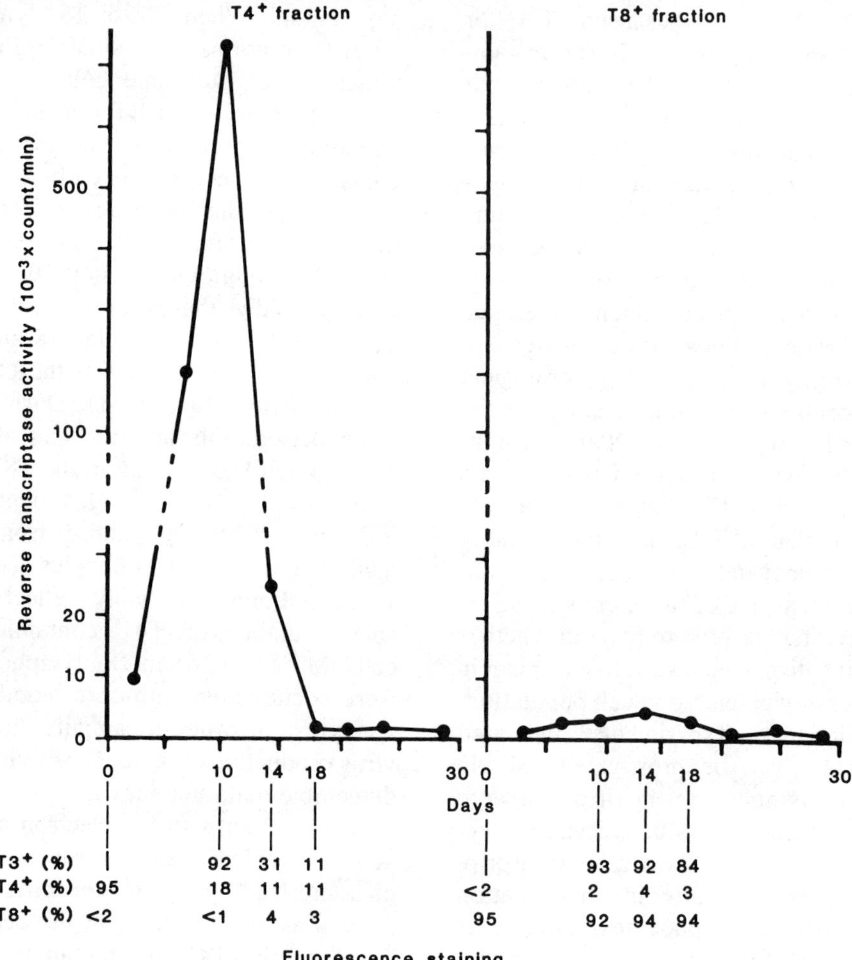

Fig. 1. Virus production and phenotype of cultured lymphocyte subsets. T4⁺ and T8⁺ fractions were purified by cellular affinity chromatography. A suspension of enriched T lymphocytes was obtained after depletion of monocytes by plastic-adherence, and by rosetting with aminoethyl-isothiouranium-treated sheep erythrocytes followed by centrifugation on a Ficoll-Hypaque gradient. The suspension usually contained 95 percent of T lymphocytes, the contaminating cells being mainly B lymphocytes. Approximately 6×10^7 T-enriched lymphocytes were incubated for 15 minutes at room temperature with 40 µl of OKT8 antibody (Ortho Diagnostic System) in 2 ml of RPMI 1640 medium supplemented with 5 percent autologous serum and 1 percent antibiotics. After two washes, cells were resuspended in 1 ml of medium and placed in a plastic column (Pharmacia K9/15) containing 5 ml of Sepharose 6-MB gel coupled with the 7S fraction of a goat antiserum to mouse immunoglobulin (Nordic). This gel (Pharmacia) was prepared following the manufacturer's specifications with 10 mg of proteins for 1 ml of gel. The antibody-labeled T lymphocytes were incubated in the gel for 15 minutes at room temperature. The T8⁻ population was recovered by washing the column with 30 ml of medium at a rate of 1 ml per minute. The T8⁺ fraction was then eluted by gentle mechanical agitation and washing with medium that had been warmed to 37°C. The efficiency of this method was checked by indirect immunofluorescence staining (4). All these procedures were performed under sterile conditions and the cell viability was excellent, as judged by trypan blue exclusion. Reverse transcriptase activity in culture was determined every 3 to 4 days, at the time of medium change (6). The cell suspension phenotypes were determined on days 0, 10, 14, and 18 after infection.

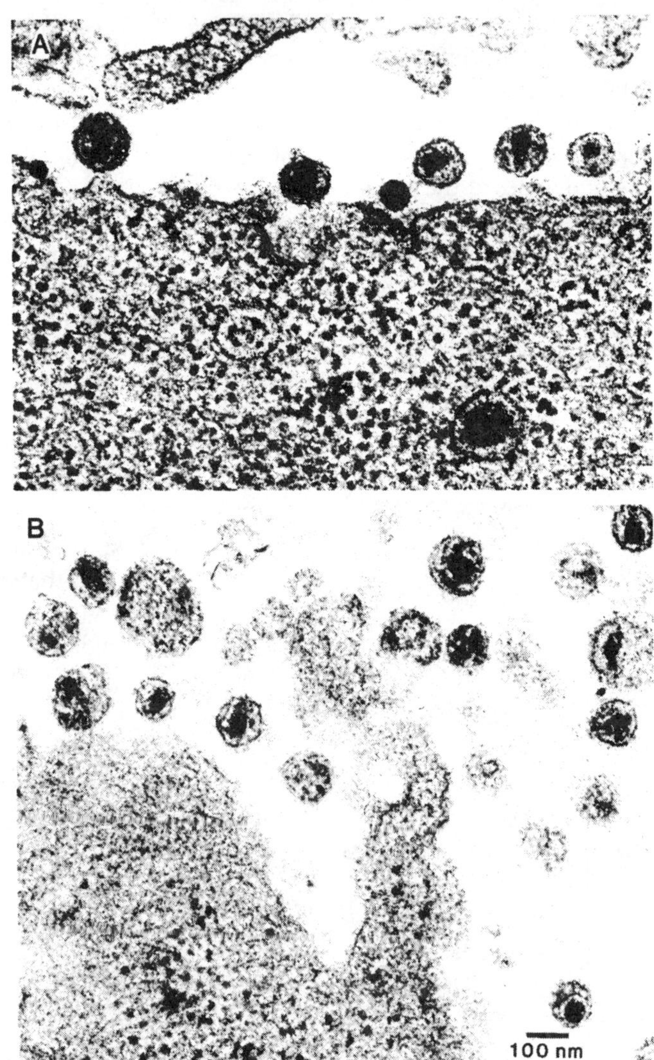

Fig. 2. Electron microscopy of viral particles in ultrathin section. (A) Portion of a T4 lymphocyte from a healthy donor, which had been infected by the virus isolated from patient E.L. Note the numerous mature particles with eccentric dense core in the external space. These particles are morphologically similar to D particles such as those found in Mason-Pfizer virus or the virus recently isolated from simian AIDS (27, 28). However, no antigenic relatedness was found between the p25 of the human virus and the p27 of Mason-Pfizer virus (29). (B) Portion of a T4 lymphocyte from patient E.L. at the time of virus production. Note the abundant mature virions around a piece of altered cytoplasm.

level of T4 expressing cells dropped to less than 20 percent as early as on day 6, when RT was already at 200×10^3 count/min. However, at that time, such cells continued to express OKT3 antigen, but half of them already showed an unusual weak and thin staining of the cell membrane compared to the normal patchy staining of the other half. Later on, percentages decreased to about 10 percent of $T3^+$ and $T4^+$ cells, whereas $T8^+$ cells never exceeded 4 percent in this fraction (Fig. 1). Since the disappearance of T4 antigens was not accompanied by the appearance of the T8 antigen, this phenomenon could not be related to a switch between these two membrane antigens. Such a switch has been observed only during culture of cloned cells, but not in bulk culture of either $T4^+$ or $T8^+$ purified cells (18, 19). Furthermore, the kinetics of the disappearance of T3 and T4 markers at the cell membrane was related to the kinetics of

196

virus production and could also be observed during infection of normal lymphocytes in vitro. This intriguing phenomenon may be due to virus-induced modulation of the expression of the T3-T4 molecules at the cell membrane, or by steric hindrance of the antibody binding site. Modifications in the expression of other membrane markers are currently under study.

After fixation (6), each cell fraction was also examined by indirect immunofluorescence with serum samples from the patient himself, his brother, his parents, or patients from whom similar viruses had been isolated. Both T4$^+$ and T8$^+$ fractions were strictly negative when tested with serum from the parents or other normal individuals with no antibodies against LAV. In contrast, when serum samples from E.L., D.L., or other patients were tested (all containing antibodies to LAV), a positive specific staining was observed in the T4$^+$ fraction and never in the T8$^+$ one. However, even at the peak of virus production, the percentage of stained cells in the T4$^+$ fraction only reached 10 percent. We suggest that the low percentage of T4$^+$ cells expressing viral antigens is due to the fact that only a fraction of T4$^+$ lymphocytes is susceptible to virus infection, indicating a heterogeneity in the T4$^+$ subset. It is also possible that the majority of the cells were infected but only a few were virus producers. The availability of molecular or immunological probes will be useful in discriminating between these possibilities.

Since virus production by infected cells is dependent on their proliferation (8), we verified that both fractions were able to proliferate under our culture conditions. Indeed, cell growth was followed every 3 or 4 days by counting these cells before they were systematically readjusted to 1×10^6 per milliliter. Proliferation of T8$^+$ cells was always greater than that of T4$^+$ lymphocytes as confirmed by [^{3}H]thymidine incorporation (Fig. 3). Thus, the absence of virus production in the T8$^+$ fraction could not be related to lower proliferation. Furthermore, in this experiment, as in others in which normal lymphocytes were infected in vitro by LAV, an early decrease of the T4$^+$ lymphocyte multiplication was noted at the same time that virus was being produced. The appear-

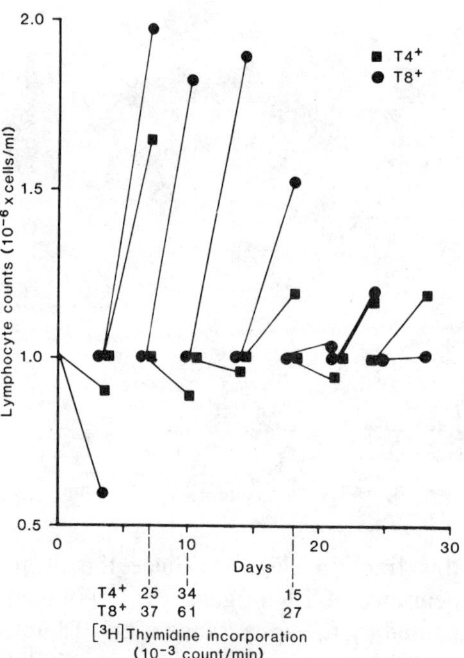

Fig. 3. Cell growth as followed by cell counting and [^{3}H]thymidine incorporation. Every 3 to 4 days, at the time of medium change, cells were counted and adjusted at 10^6 per milliliter. On days 7, 10, and 18, portions of cell suspension were labeled with [^{3}H]thymidine for 12 hours and material precipitated in trichloroacetic acid was counted in a liquid scintillation spectrometer.

ance of giant cells was also observed, indicating a cytopathic effect of the virus (Fig. 4).

To confirm these findings in vivo, we also investigated which lymphocyte populations from normal individuals were sensitive to infection by LAV or related retroviruses in vitro. We obtained PBL

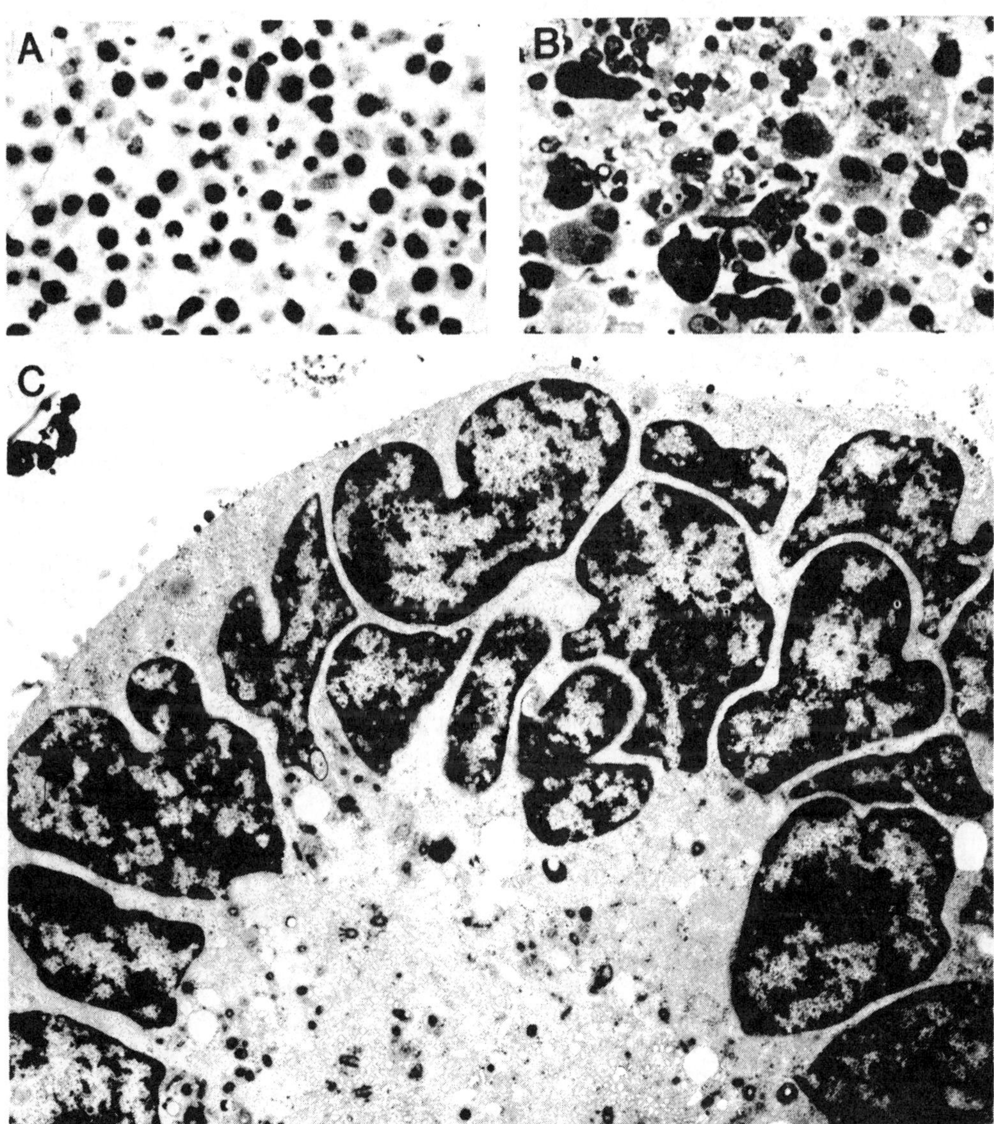

Fig. 4. (A and B) Light microscope picture of thin sections of cultured T4$^+$ lymphocytes from a healthy donor. Staining by toluidine blue. (A) Uninfected culture. (B) LAV-infected culture at the peak of virus production. Note the enlarged and giant cells. (C) Electron microscopy picture of a giant cell of (B). Note the numerous nuclei arising by cell fusion and the viral particles at the cell surface ($\times$8000).

from healthy Caucasian volunteers who had no antibodies against retroviruses and separated them into T, T4$^+$, and T8$^+$ fractions. Half of each fraction was separately infected with virus-containing cell-free supernatant. Reverse transcriptase was sequentially measured in each infected and uninfected culture. In three different experiments, using LAV-1 or virus isolated from E.L., we found that infected T4$^+$ lymphocytes displayed virus production, as assessed by an increase in RT which reached 30×10^3 to 100×10^3 count/min at the peak value and by electron microscopy. On the contrary, uninfected cultures of T4$^+$ or T8$^+$ cells as well as infected T8$^+$ fractions expressed less than 2×10^3 count/min throughout the culture period. When the T4$^+$ and T8$^+$ fractions were mixed, RT production was similar to that of the original unfractionated population, demonstrating that the technique used to separate the T cell subsets did not interfere with virus production (data not shown). Immunofluorescence staining showed no modification of the surface phenotype of the uninfected T4$^+$ or T8$^+$ cultured cells. In contrast, in the infected T4$^+$ fractions, a decrease of T4 and T3 markers was observed, but only when a high level of RT was produced in the culture.

It seems clear that the virus can be produced in vivo only by the T4$^+$ cells of the healthy carrier and that this selective tropism for T4$^+$ lymphocytes is identical to that observed after the in vitro infection of lymphocytes of healthy blood donors. It remains to be determined whether this phenomenon is due to a lack of recognition of specific receptors at the cell membrane of T8$^+$ cells or to a lack of expression of the proviral DNA. Data published by Gallo and co-workers (*10*) have suggested that HTLV shows a similar tropism in transformed cell lines derived from leukemic patients or immortalized after infection in vitro. In both situations, most cell lines were T4$^+$, but some others have been described as being T4$^+$ and T8$^+$ or T4$^-$ and T8$^-$ (*10, 14, 15, 20*) or even B cells (*21*). Tropism for T4 cells has also been suggested for a new HTLV isolate which resembles LAV, called HTLV-III (*22*).

That LAV was found in a "healthy" carrier whose brother had AIDS does not provide evidence against its causal role in the disease. First, the incubation period after virus infection may vary from one individual to another. Indeed, 3 months after these experiments were carried out, E.L.'s T4$^+$ lymphocytes decreased although he still showed no clinical symptoms (*23*). Second, individual variations in susceptibility (genetic background or natural history) to virus infection are well documented in man and mice (*24–26*) and, with respect to AIDS, are suggested by epidemiological data on regular sexual partners of AIDS patients. Third, since LAV infection of T4$^+$ cells impairs their proliferative capacity and causes cytopathogenic effects, the present results support the hypothesis that LAV is involved in AIDS and point to its possible interference with T-cell differentiation.

References and Notes

1. E. Dournon *et al.*, *Lancet* **1983-I**, 1040 (1983).
2. J. B. Brunet *et al.*, in *Epidemic Kaposi's Sarcoma and Opportunistic Infections in Homosexual Men: Expression of Acquired Immunoregulatory Disorder*, A. E. Friedman Kein, Ed. (Masson, New York, in press).
3. Centers for Disease Control, *Mortal. Morbid. Weekly Rep.* **31**, 305 (1982).
4. D. Klatzmann *et al.*, *Ann. N.Y. Acad. Sci.*, in press.
5. R. W. Schroff *et al.*, *Clin. Immunol. Immunopathol.* **27**, 300 (1983).
6. F. Barré-Sinoussi *et al.*, *Science* **220**, 868 (1983).
7. For the clinical details of these patients, see E. Vilmer *et al.*, *Lancet* **1984-I**, 753 (1984).
8. L. Montagnier *et al.*, in *Human T-Cell Leukemia Lymphoma Viruses*, R. C. Gallo, M. E.

Essex, L. Gross, Eds. (Cold Spring Harbor Laboratory, Cold Spring Harbor, N.Y., in press).
9. B. J. Poiesz *et al.*, *Proc. Natl. Acad. Sci. U.S.A.* **77**, 7415 (1980).
10. M. Popovic *et al.*, *Science* **219**, 856 (1983).
11. C. E. Metroka *et al.*, *Ann. Int. Med.* **99**, 585.
12. H. Kornfeld *et al.*, *N. Engl. J. Med.* **307**, 729 (1982).
13. F. Brun-Vézinet *et al.*, *Lancet*, in press.
14. P. D. Markham *et al.*, *Int. J. Cancer* **31**, 413 (1983).
15. M. Popovic *et al.*, *Proc. Natl. Acad. Sci. U.S.A.* **80**, 5402 (1983).
16. J.-C. Chermann *et al.*, *Antibiot. Chemother.* **32**, in press.
17. S. Chouaib *et al.*, *J. Immunol.* **132**, 1851 (1984).
18. G. F. Burns *et al.*, *Cell. Immunol.* **71**, 12 (1982).
19. D. Zagury *et al.*, *Int. J. Cancer* **31**, 705 (1983).
20. F. W. Ruscetti *et al.*, *ibid.*, p. 171.
21. N. Yamamoto *et al.*, *Nature (London)* **299**, 367 (1982).
22. M. Popovic *et al.*, *Science* **224**, 497 (1984); R. C. Gallo *et al.*, *ibid.*, p. 500.
23. E.L.'s lymphocyte phenotypes and functions were determined in August 1983 and January and February 1984. No lymphopenia was observed and the responses to mitogenic or allogenic stimulation were normal. The percentages of T-cell subsets were, respectively: T3: 70, T4: 33, T8: 27 in August 1983; T3: 52, T4: 5, T8: 52 in January 1984; T3: 65, T4: 14, T8: 50 in February 1984. The fractionation experiment reported here was performed in September 1983.
24. J. L. Virelizier *et al.*, *Arch. Virol.* **50**, 279 (1976).
25. F. B. Bang *et al.*, *Proc. Natl. Acad. Sci. U.S.A.* **46**, 1065 (1960).
26. D. T. Purtillo *et al.*, *Lancet* **1976-I**, 882 (1976).
27. M. D. Daniel *et al.*, *Science* **223**, 602 (1984).
28. P. A. Marx *et al.*, *ibid.*, p. 1083.
29. L. Montagnier *et al.*, *Ann. Virol. (Inst. Pasteur)*, **135E**, 119 (1984).

30. We thank C. Gazengel for providing the patient's sera, F. Chapuis, F. Rey, C. Axler, J. Gruest, and S. Chamaret for technical assistance, and E. Martin for typing the manuscript. We are indebted to G. Janossy (Royal Free Hospital, London) for information about the cellular affinity chromatography technique. This work was supported by grants from the Ministère de l'Industrie et de la Recherche (contracts 82 L 13.13., 83 C 14.11. and 83 C 14.14), Centre National de la Recherche Scientifique (CNRS), and Ligue Nationale contre le Cancer. F. Barré-Sinoussi, J. C. Chermann, and L. Montagnier are also members of the research team No. 147 of CNRS.

1 May 1984; accepted 29 May 1984

Report

6 July 1984

37. Adaptation of Lymphadenopathy Associated Virus (LAV) to Replication in EBV-Transformed B Lymphoblastoid Cell Lines

L. Montagnier, J. Gruest, S. Chamaret, C. Dauguet, C. Axler, D. Guétard, M.T. Nugeyre, F. Barré-Sinoussi, J.-C Chermann, J.B. Brunet, D. Klatzmann, and J.C. Gluckman

Lymphadenopathy associated virus (LAV) is a human T-cell lymphotropic retrovirus that was first isolated from the cells of a lymph node of a homosexual man with lymphadenopathy syndrome (LAS) (*1*). Similar isolates were made from several patients with the acquired immunodeficiency syndrome (AIDS), including a B hemophiliac (*2, 3*), a Zairian woman (*2*), a Zairian couple (*4*), and a Haitian man (*2*).

All viral isolates have in common a major, antigenically related protein with a molecular weight of 25,000 (p25), a Mg^{2+}-dependent reverse transcriptase (RT), mature virions with a morphology similar to that of equine infectious anemia virus (EIAV), and D type particles. The p25 of LAV is immunoprecipitated by serum from horses infected with EIAV, suggesting antigenic similarity with the core protein of this virus (5). In contrast, the p25 of LAV and LAV-related viruses is not antigenically related to the p24 of human T-cell leukemia virus type I (HTLV-I), the core proteins of Mason-Pfizer virus (5) or similar viruses isolated from simian AIDS (6), or to other known animal retroviruses (5). An important biological feature of members of the LAV family is their specific tropism for activated $T4^+$ (helper) lymphocytes, in which they induce a cytopathic effect without giving rise to immortalized lines (1, 2, 7). Initially, we found that LAV could not be grown in B lymphocytes, Raji cells, MOLT/4, or in several established fibroblastic lines (1).

We report here the successful adaptation of LAV to persistent infection of several lymphoblastoid cell lines obtained by the transformation of B lymphocytes with Epstein-Barr virus (EBV) as well as in one Burkitt lymphoma cell line. Thus, it is now possible to grow LAV on a large scale in permanent cell lines. The growth of LAV in EBV-transformed cells may have important implications for the pathogenic role of such viruses in AIDS and other diseases.

The first LAV isolate was initially propagated in cord blood lymphocytes and then in lymphocytes from several adult donors whose sera contained no antibody against LAV and whose lymphocytes did not spontaneously release LAV after activation (1). Blood from one particular donor, F.R., was used for the present experiments because of the high and regular yields of LAV obtained from his T lymphocytes upon infection. In these cultures, however, LAV produc-

tion was transient and was regularly followed by a decline of virus production and cell death.

Because LAV can induce T-cell fusion (2, 7) and because EBV is known to have fusion activity in B cells (8), we performed co-infection experiments of unfractionated lymphocytes (B and T) with both viruses. It was hoped that stable hybrids of LAV-infected T cells and of EBV-transformed B cells would be formed and that such hybrids would be able to continuously produce LAV.

Several regimens were tried. The one that gave rise to continuous productive infection of LAV was the following. Whole lymphocytes of F.R. were first stimulated for 24 hours with Protein A and then infected (9) with an EBV strain, M81, derived from a nasopharyngeal carcinoma (10). Five days later, half of this culture was infected with LAV as described (1) and then divided in two subcultures: one was cultured in medium lacking T-cell growth factor (TCGF; interleukin-2), the other in medium containing TCGF. As expected, the TCGF-fed culture produced LAV as detected by a peak of RT activity appearing between day 12 (day 6 after LAV infection) and day 21 in the supernatant. In contrast, the cells cultured in the absence of TCGF did not yield any detectable RT. This shows that at that time LAV was produced only by activated T cells maintained in TCGF, and not by B cells. On day 19, at the time of decline of LAV production, a subculture of the TCGF-fed cells received fresh T cells from the same donor; these T cells had been activated for 3 days with phytohemagglutinin (PHA) in order to provide new targets for the virus. Six days later (day 25), a new peak of RT appeared, but contrary to the first infection, it was not transient. It was followed by continuous but fluctuating production (Fig. 1) that subsequently increased to high amounts, greater than 100,000 count/min per milliliter of supernatant.

At the time of the second LAV infection, large cells transformed by EBV could be readily seen in this culture, as well as in the control culture not infected with LAV, indicating that immortalization of B cells by EBV had already occurred. The immortalized B-cell line was termed FR8. Continuous LAV production could thus be accounted for by a prolonged survival of infected T cells in the presence of the EBV-transformed lymphoblastoid line, or alternatively by B cells of the newly established lymphoblastoid line, or by T-B cell hybrids. To distinguish between these possibilities, the control, uninfected culture of EBV-transformed cells, which had not received TCGF, was exposed to infected cells from the same LAV passage as those used at the beginning of the experiment. The culture was thereafter maintained in the absence of TCGF. It was expected that, under these conditions, the T cells would rapidly decline. Indeed, we determined, by using the monoclonal antibody OKT3 (Ortho), that no T3$^+$ cell remained in the culture by day 49 and that the culture was composed only of B cells as determined by the presence of surface membrane immunoglobulins. LAV production began in this culture without any lag period (Fig. 2a). This experiment clearly established that the virus could grow on B lymphocytes but only after they had been transformed by EBV. This new property of LAV was probably acquired during passage in vitro before the co-infection experiment, since an earlier passage of LAV, from July 1983, could not grow in the FR8 lymphoblastoid line.

Sequence comparison of proviral

DNA's will help our understanding of the molecular basis of this change in tropism. Recent work on animal retroviruses suggests that the long terminal

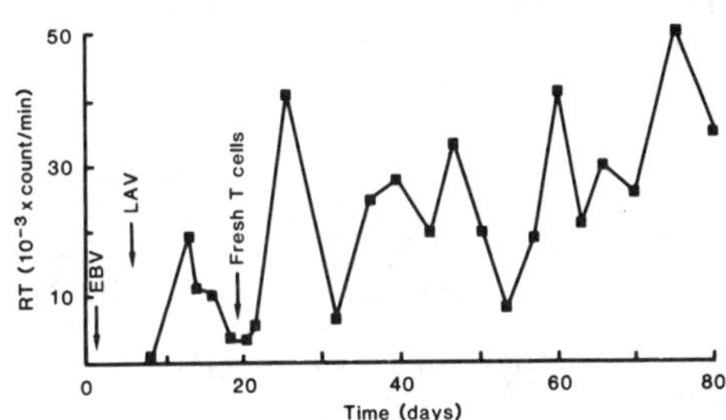

Fig. 1. EBV and LAV co-infection of lymphocytes from a blood donor (F.R.). The culture medium (RPMI 1640 with 10 percent fetal calf serum) included TCGF, antiserum to interferon α, and Polybrene, as described (1). Production of LAV was determined by assaying RT activity in 1-ml portions of pelleted virus (1).

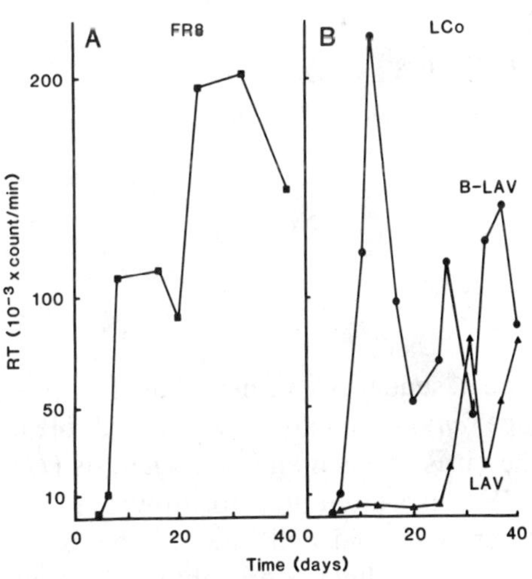

Fig. 2. (A) Virus production by the established FR8 lymphoblastoid line. The cells were infected with LAV at time zero as described (1). (B) Virus production by the LCo lymphoblastoid line after infection by LAV and B-LAV. Same medium as in Fig. 1, except that TCGF was omitted.

202

Table 1. Susceptibility and resistance to LAV and B-LAV infection of some established human lymphoid cell lines. Symbols: + +, viral-associated RT production more than 100,000 count/min per milliliter of supernatant (weekly average, two harvests a week); +, RT production between 10,000 and 100,000 count/min. No RT activity could be detected in the supernatant of any of the cell lines before infection with LAV.

Cell line	Presence of EBV genome	Retrovirus growth	
		LAV	B-LAV
Origin: B lymphocytes from adult donor			
FR8	Yes	+ +	+ +
BAR	Yes	+	+ +
BRA	Yes	–	–
DIER	Yes	–	–
Origin: B lymphocytes from umbilical cord blood			
LCo	Yes	+	+ +
LC1	Yes	–	–
Origin: Burkitt lymphoma			
Daudi	Yes	–	–
Namalwa	Yes	–	–
Raji	Yes	–	–
Chev	Yes	–	–
BJAB	No	–	+
BJAB/B95/8	Yes	–	+ +
Origin: T lymphoma			
MOLT/4	No	–	–
Origin: Myeloid leukemia			
HL60	No	–	–

repeat sequences rather than the envelope (*env*) gene may play a crucial role in the virus tropism and pathogenesis (*11*).

We also attempted to grow LAV on other lymphoid cell lines of the B lineage. Such lines were obtained in our laboratory by in vitro transformation of unfractionated lymphocytes from adult blood donors or umbilical cord blood with the M81 or the B95/8 strains of EBV. Only one other line from an adult

donor and one from umbilical cord blood could be productively infected by the virus (Table 1), after a lag period of 3 weeks. This selective infectibility, observed in three of the cell lines, suggests that LAV tropism may be restricted by a polymorphism expressed at the transformed B-cell membrane. Whether this polymorphism is related to HLA class I or class II determinants or to the expression of other membrane molecules is not known. It was interesting that the virus derived from the FR8 lymphoblastoid line could grow in the same lines with higher RT activity and with a shorter lag period (Fig. 2b). This suggests that after its passage in FR8 cells, LAV underwent a secondary adaptation to B cells. This adapted strain was termed B-LAV.

Several established lines from Burkitt lymphoma were also tested for their susceptibility to LAV and B-LAV infection. The BJAB (EBV negative) line could be infected by B-LAV, but not by LAV (Fig. 3). There was a 30-day lag period between exposure to infected cells and virus production. Upon its transformation in vitro by the B95/8 strain of EBV, BJAB could also be productively infected with B-LAV. This infected line showed the same lag (Table 1) and then produced four times as much virus as the original EBV negative BJAB line. Other B lymphoma lines did not show evidence of virus production, as assayed by RT activity at intervals for more than 2 months after infection. Negative results were also obtained with the T lymphoma line MOLT/4 and the HL60 myeloid line.

It was important to check whether or not the virus produced by the B-cell line retained the characteristics of the original LAV. The virus produced by LCo, a cell line derived from umbilical cord lym-

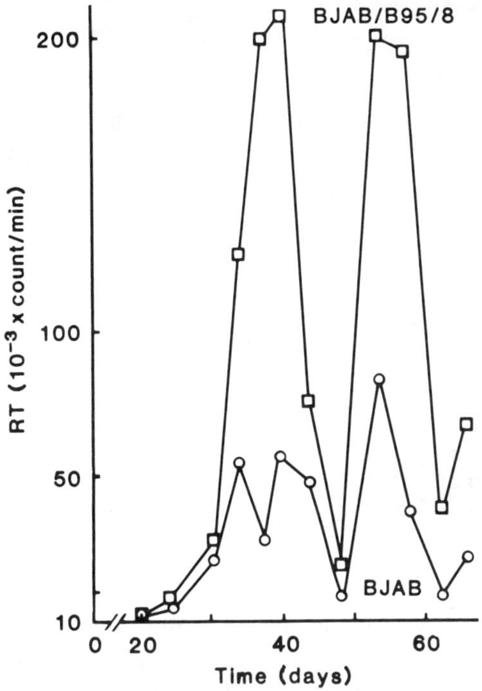

Fig. 3. Infection of the BJAB Burkitt lymphoma cell line and of its EBV-transformed derivative (BJAB/B95/8) with B-LAV. Same culture conditions as in Fig. 2

was immunoprecipitated by the same sera. No differences between the two strains could be found with regard to the ionic requirements of their RT (*1*, *12*) and their ultrastructural morphology (Fig. 5) [see (*1*, *5*)]. The virus produced by FR8, but not that produced by LCo, had a slightly higher density in sucrose gradi-

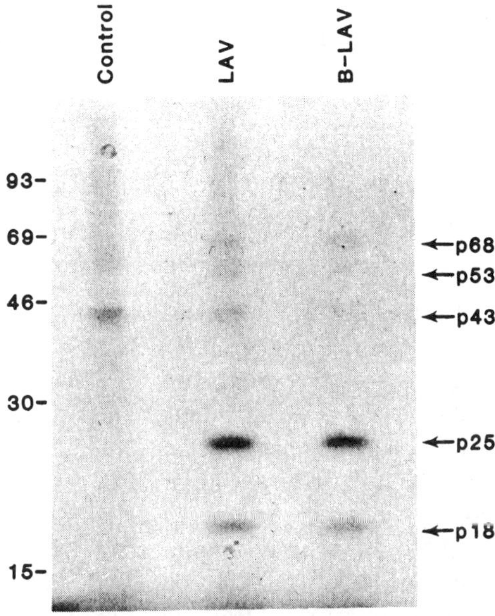

Fig. 4. Major proteins of LAV and B-LAV. LCo cells infected with LAV or B-LAV were labeled for 4 hours in RPMI 1640 medium lacking amino acids but containing 10 percent fetal calf serum in the presence of a mixture of ^{14}C-labeled amino acids (C.E.A., 40 to 50 mCi/mmol, 20 μCi/ml). The supernatant was centrifuged at 10,000*g* for 20 minutes and then at 45,000*g* for 20 minutes in a SW55 Beckman rotor. The viral pellet was resuspended in NTE buffer (*5*) and centrifuged to equilibrium in a Nycodenz gradient as described (*5*). Fractions of the virus-containing band were pooled and recentrifuged, and the pellet was dissolved in denaturing buffer, heated for 3 minutes at 100°C as described (*1*), and subjected to electrophoresis. The control is the supernatant of an uninfected LCo culture, processed exactly as described for the infected cultures.

phocytes, was metabolically labeled with [^{35}S]methionine or ^{14}C-labeled amino acids and purified on a Nycodenz gradient (*5*). Figure 4 shows the results of a comparison of polyacrylamide gel electrophoresis under denaturing conditions between B-LAV proteins and LAV proteins. The patterns were identical, showing a prominent p25, a p18, a low molecular weight protein at the bottom of the gel (p12), and three proteins of high molecular weight (43,000, 53,000, 68,000). The band at 43,000 may include a component of cellular origin, since it was also found in a similar preparation made from the control uninfected cells.

The p25 of B-LAV showed the same antigenicity as the p25 of LAV, since it

204

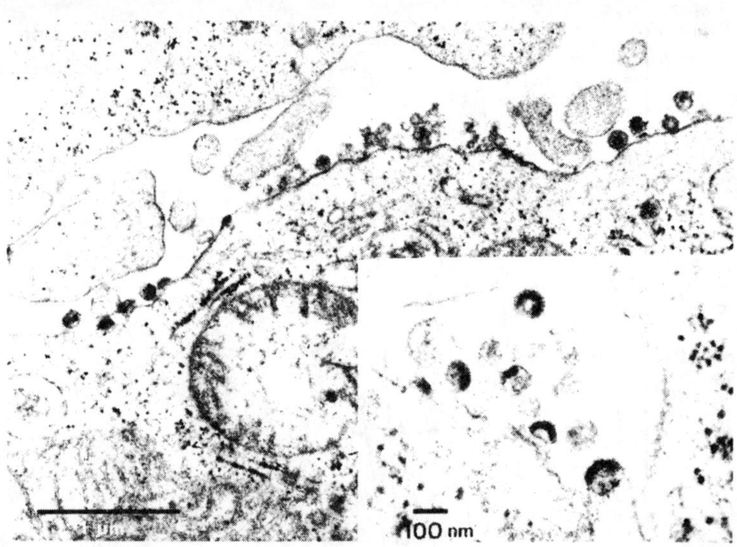

Fig. 5. Electron microscopic examination of a section of an LCo lymphoblastoid cell infected with B-LAV. Note the three typical aspects of LAV: budding particles, immature free particles with a dense crescent, and mature virions with dense eccentric core.

ent than LAV (1.18 instead of 1.17).

In addition, like LAV, B-LAV retained a selective tropism for the helper-inducer (T4$^+$) T-cell population of lymphocytes from normal donors infected in vitro (2). Peripheral blood lymphocytes of normal volunteers were fractionated into monocytes, B lymphocytes, and T lymphocytes. The T4$^+$ and T8$^+$ (suppressor/cytotoxic) fractions were obtained by cellular affinity chromatography. Cells were then cultured in the presence of PHA followed by TCGF. Each fraction was separately infected with virus-containing, cell-free supernatant, and RT was sequentially measured in each infected and uninfected culture. Only T4$^+$ lymphocytes displayed virus production with LAV as well as with B-LAV, under these conditions. Thus far it has not been possible to grow B-LAV in short-term cultures of B cells from F.R., either before or after stimulation of the cells with B-cell mitogens such as Protein A. It is not known whether the virus could grow in long-term cultures such as those maintained in the presence of B-cell growth factor (13). Studies of EBV antigen expression did not reveal any significant change in the FR8 and LCo lines after infection with the retrovirus. Both were 100 percent positive for the EBV nuclear antigen (EBNA). Early antigen (EA) expression could be detected in 0.1 percent of LCo cells and 3.5 percent of FR8 cells. No LCo cells were positive for viral capsid antigens (VCA), but 1.5 percent of FR8 cells had VCA. A search for the presence of EBV antigens (EA and VCA) in purified B-LAV preparations yielded negative results. The tests used included immunoprecipitation with polyclonal antibodies against EA and VCA and two monoclonal antibodies to the 52K and 85K components of EA (14). The role of EBV in the growth of LAV in B cells is not crucial since an EBV negative Burkitt lymphoma line could be infected by B-LAV. However, LAV production was four times higher in the same line supertransformed by the B95/8 strain of EBV, suggesting that

EBV could enhance LAV production. A similar enhancing effect by EBV on animal retrovirus expression was recently described for another BL line, RAMOS (*15*).

Such interaction between a human retrovirus and a herpesvirus may have some bearing on human pathology. It is possible that the adaptation of LAV to B lymphoid cells occurs in some situations in vivo. For example, during a late stage of AIDS, LAV could disseminate through EBV-infected B lymphocytes as well as through the $T4^+$ cell population. LAV-induced depression of the T lymphocyte mediated control over EBV infected B lymphocytes (*16*) could result in an expansion of the latter cells, which would constitute in turn a reservoir for LAV production. This phenomenon may also contribute to the increased frequency of B-cell lymphomas that has been reported in AIDS (*17*).

Our finding is of practical importance because LAV can now be produced continuously by some permanent cell lines growing in suspension without noticeable cytopathic effects.

Another laboratory has recently described the growth of HTLV type III in a T leukemia cell line (*18*). These independent findings will facilitate comparison between viral isolates, particularly between HTLV-III and LAV, and the development of reagents for serological tests.

References and Notes

1. F. Barré-Sinoussi *et al.*, *Science* **220**, 868 (1983).
2. L. Montagnier *et al.*, in *Human T Cell Leukemia Lymphoma Viruses*, R. C. Gallo, M. E. Essex, L. Gross, Eds. (Cold Spring Harbor Laboratory, Cold Spring Harbor, N.Y., in press).
3. E. Vilmer *et al.*, *Lancet* **1984-I**, 753 (1984).
4. A. Ellrodt *et al.*, *Lancet*, in press.
5. L. Montagnier *et al.*, *Ann. Virol. (Inst. Pasteur)* **135E**, 119 (1984).
6. L. Montagnier *et al.*, unpublished data.
7. D. Klatzmann *et al.*, *Science* **225**, 59 (1984).
8. G. J. Bayliss and H. Wolf, *Nature (London)* **287**, 164 (1980).
9. The conditions used for EBV infection were as follows: 10^7 cells were exposed to 3 ml of crude supernatant from EBV-producing marmoset cells for 1 hour at 37°C and, after centrifugation, were suspended in culture medium at a concentration of 10^6 per milliliter.
10. C. Desgranges *et al.*, *Biomedicine* **25**, 349 (1976).
11. J. Lenz *et al.*, *Nature (London)* **308**, 467 (1984); I. S. Y. Chen, J. McLaughlin, D. W. Golden, *ibid.* **309**, 276 (1984).
12. M. A. Rey *et al.*, *Biochem. Biophys. Res. Commun.*, in press.
13. T. Leanderson *et al.*, *Proc. Natl. Acad. Sci. U.S.A.* **79**, 7455 (1982).
14. G. R. Pearson *et al.*, *J. Virol.* **47**, 193 (1983).
15. R. D. Lasky and F. A. Troy, *Proc. Natl. Acad. Sci. U.S.A.* **81**, 33 (1984).
16. E. Klein *et al.*, *Cancer Res.* **41**, 4210 (1981).
17. Center for Disease Control, *Mortal. Morbid. Weekly Rep.* **31**, 277 (1982).
18. M. Popovic *et al.*, *Science* **224**, 497 (1984).
19. We thank F. Rey and C. Barreau for technical assistance. This work was supported by grants 83/L14-19 and 83 C 14-11 of the French Ministry of Research and Industry. Members of the Viral Oncology Unit are also members of Research Team 147 of the Centre National de la Recherche Scientifique.

14 May 1984; accepted 8 June 1984

Report

6 July 1984

38. Immunoregulatory Lymphokines of T Hybridomas from AIDS Patients: Constitutive and Inducible Suppressor Factors

Jeffrey Laurence and Lloyd Mayer

Patients with the acquired immunodeficiency syndrome (AIDS) have a marked but selective abnormality of immunoregulation, manifest by susceptibility to opportunistic infections and malignancies characteristic of certain genetic and iatrogenic immune deficiencies (*1*). We have previously shown that supernatants from lectin-free cultures of peripheral blood mononuclear cells (PBMC) obtained from homosexual males with AIDS or its prodromes can inhibit spontaneous and pokeweed mitogen (PWM)–induced B lymphocyte differentiation into plasmacytes, and T-cell blastogenic responses to antigen (*2*). These soluble suppressor factors (SSF) are the product of the interaction of T lymphocytes with adherent cells. T cells or T-cell factors from certain AIDS patients, but not from healthy homosexual or heterosexual controls or from heterosexual individuals with Epstein-Barr virus (EBV) or cytomegalovirus mononucleosis, can collaborate with normal adherent cells in the formation of SSF (*2, 3*). This system provides a model with which to examine cell subsets participating in the induction and expression of immunoregulatory defects in AIDS. The availability of functional T-cell hybrids derived from such patients would facilitate investigation of T lymphokine–mediated inhibitory phenomena, and permit direct comparisons with products isolated in other disorders linked to cell- or factor-mediated immunosuppression.

Human T-cell hybridomas secreting molecules able to interfere with T cell–directed polyclonal immunoglobulin (Ig) synthesis independent of T-lymphocyte mitogenesis (*4*), or with antibody production directly at the level of the B cell (*5*), have been described by others. In those studies the investigators used PBMC from healthy individuals enriched for activated suppressor T cells by exposure to concanavalin A (Con A) in vitro (*5*) or unstimulated T cells from patients with common variable hypogammaglobulinemia (*4, 6*). We have now immortalized peripheral T lymphocytes obtained from a homosexual male with unexplained generalized lymphadenopathy, persistent fever, malaise, and high titers of SSF-AIDS [see patient Sel. in (*2*)] by fusion with KE37.3.2, a hypoxanthine-guanine phosphoribosyl transferase–deficient mutant of the human T acute lymphoblastic leukemia line KE37, first isolated in our laboratory (*7*). Fusion products were selected in aminopterin and further identified as hybrids by demonstration of shared HLA class I allodeterminants between patient Sel. (HLA-A1,w29/B51,w35/cw4) and KE37.3.2

(HLA-A11,30/B35,44/cw4). These "SK" hybrids retained the membrane antigen profile of the parent line as detected by indirect immunofluorescence: 75 percent Leu-3a$^+$ (helper-inducer T lymphocyte subset); 0 percent Leu-2a$^+$ (suppressor-cytotoxic T subset); 0 percent Leu-4$^+$ (mature pan-T cell marker); >95 percent OKT10$^+$; and 0 percent HLA-DR$^+$ (detected with a murine monoclonal reagent, VG2). Neither the hybrid lines nor KE37.3.2 expressed human T-cell leukemia virus (HTLV) type I or type II products as determined by indirect intracellular immunofluorescence staining with a monoclonal antibody directed against the HTLV core protein p19. However, patient Sel. had serum antibody to LAV, an AIDS-associated retrovirus (8), as detected by an enzyme-linked immunosorbent assay (ELISA) for an antibody to the internal antigen p25 (9).

Figure 1 shows activities in the supernatants of initially uncloned cells in growth positive wells. Activities were determined by the ability of the supernatants to affect PWM-induced polyclonal Ig production by normal indicator PBMC in a reverse hemolytic plaque-forming cell (PFC) assay. Supernatant from KE37.3.2 had no effect in this system. Nine of 22 SK hybrid supernatants gave significant (>25 percent) constitutive inhibition of PFC; 2 of 22 showed enhancement (>25 percent); and 11 of 22 revealed no activity. Selected supernatants were reassessed after 48 hours of incubation with normal peripheral blood monocytes, isolated by Percoll gradient centrifugation or serial plastic adherence, and depleted of E-rosette$^+$ and surface Ig$^+$ cells (10). Two samples, SK8 and SK10, which formerly revealed no significant suppression, now evinced marked inhibition of Ig synthesis (Fig. 1). In no

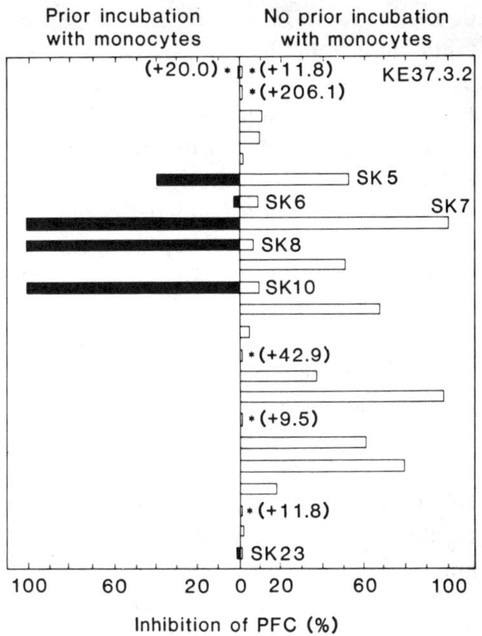

Fig. 1. Effect of T hybridoma factors on PWM-induced Ig production. Supernatants were harvested after 24 hours from cultures of 1×10^6 T hybrids maintained in 1 ml of RPMI 1640 medium containing 10 percent fetal bovine serum (medium) at 37°C in a 5 percent humidified CO_2 atmosphere. They were added, at a 1:9 final dilution (volume/volume), to 3×10^5 normal PBMC per microwell in 0.3 ml of medium, together with a 1:150 dilution of PWM. The contents of duplicate wells were harvested on day 6 of culture, and PFC determined by a reverse hemolytic plaque assay (2, 3). Some supernatants were reexamined after 48 hours of incubation at a 1:2 dilution in medium with 1.5×10^5 monocytes per milliliter, prepared as previously outlined (10). Data are expressed as the percent inhibition of PFC in the absence of factors.

instance did prior incubation of hybrid supernatants with monocytes remove constitutive SSF activity.

In agreement with the effector profile of SSF-AIDS elaborated by T lymphocyte–adherent cell interactions in patients with AIDS or its prodromes (2, 3), selected constitutive (SK7) and "induced" (SK8/monocyte) hybrid supernatants were noncytotoxic, as determined by supravital dye exclusion in 6-day PWM-stimulated indicator cultures. With normal target PBMC of divergent HLA-DR allotypes, SSF function proved not to be genetically constrained. Indomethacin (1 to 10 μg/ml), sheep antibody to human α-interferon (Interferon Sciences, Inc.; 1 to 10 units per culture), and a murine monoclonal antibody to human γ-interferon (1 to 10 units per culture) did not perturb SSF activity. In addition, SK7 and SK8/monocyte factors had no influence on a cytopathic effect–inhibition assay for γ-interferon, conducted with vesicular stomatitis virus and WISH cells (*11*).

Dilution curves for SK7 and SK8 supernatants, before and after exposure to monocytes, are given in Fig. 2A. Titers of hybridoma SSF are equivalent to or greater than those obtained with the patient's unstimulated PBMC (titer 1:1000). Figure 2B shows the kinetics of SSF activity. Corresponding to the spontaneous SSF-AIDS product (*2, 3*), SK7 and SK8/monocyte factors depressed PWM-induced Ig formation only if introduced within the first 48 hours of culture initiation. This supports the contention that the SSF is noncytotoxic, and that it is able to disrupt differentiation of B cells to plasmacytes during the critical period at which regulatory cell helper activity is maximal (*12*).

The cellular site of action of SSF was further examined by using B cell–enriched indicator populations activated with EBV; such populations act as helper T cell–independent polyclonal mitogens. Supernatants from SK7, SK8, and SK8/monocyte cultures did not block polyclonal PFC after EBV induction of allogeneic B cells. In contrast, supernatants from PBMC derived from normal and pre-AIDS patients, when activated with Con A, were capable of depressing such synthesis (data not shown). Restriction of SSF activity to the T lymphocyte was supported by absorption protocols. Purified populations of normal E-rosette[+] T cells, or non-T cells (B lymphocytes plus adherent cells) were incubated with SK7, SK8, or SK8/monocyte supernatants for 4 hours at 37°C. SSF activity in the SK7 and SK8/monocyte mixtures was diminished by prior incubation with T lymphocytes, whereas its activity did not change after absorption with the other immune cell subsets (Table 1). These absorptions do not definitively establish the presence of specific receptors for SSF-AIDS on T cells. To further address this question, we are attempting to radioactively label purified SSF-AIDS. This experiment does indicate that simple release of a preformed monokine under the influence of SK8 factor is unlikely, because 4 hours of incubation of SK8 supernatant with non-T cells proved inadequate to generate suppressor-effector factor (Table 1), which appears at about 12 hours of incubation and is maximal at 48 to 72 hours.

Lectin-free supernatants from patients with AIDS or its prodromes also inhibit antigen-induced T-cell proliferation (*2, 3*) and the blastogenic activity of normal T lymphocytes in response to various mitogens (*13*). Both SK7 and SK8/monocyte molecules were capable of depressing tetanus toxoid–mediated T-cell mitogenesis of PBMC from presensitized normal individuals (*2, 3*), as well as T-cell responses to optimal concentrations of Con A, PWM, and phytohemagglutinin [75 percent inhibition at a 1:100 dilution (volume to volume)].

The physicochemical properties of

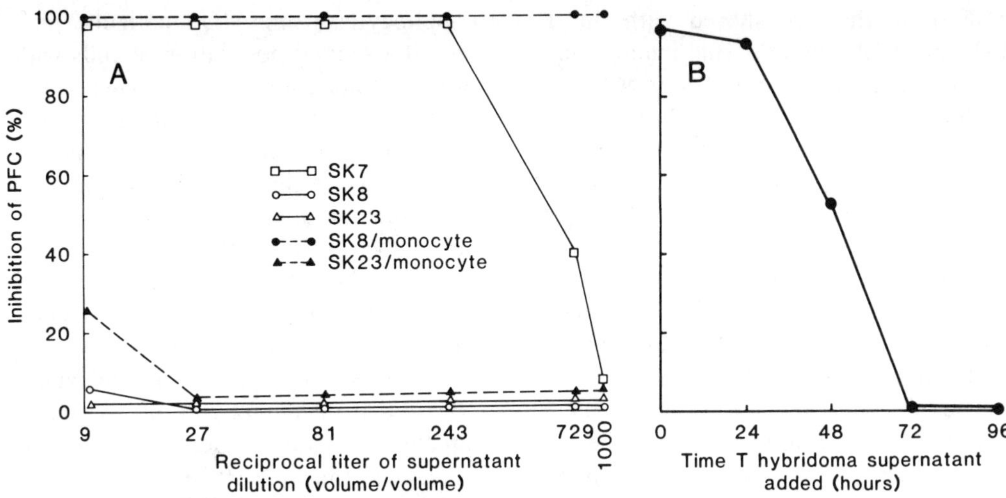

Fig. 2. (A) Dose-response curves for T hybridoma factors. The effects of varying dilutions of T hybrid supernatants, before and after incubation with monocytes, are illustrated. Data are expressed as the percent inhibition of PFC in 6-day PWM-induced indicator cultures. The dilution of SK8/monocyte factor capable of inhibiting PFC by 50 percent varied between 1:750 and 1:1500, depending on the target culture used. (B) Kinetics of T hybridoma factor suppression of T cell–dependent polyclonal Ig synthesis. In this representative experiment, T hybrid supernatants were added at a 1:9 final dilution (volume/volume) to PWM-induced indicator cultures at varying times after culture initiation. The contents of each culture were harvested on day 6 and evaluated in a reverse hemolytic plaque assay, with results expressed as in (A).

Table 1. Effect of absorption of T hybridoma factors with immune cell subpopulations on suppressor-effector activity. Supernatants generated as noted in the legend to Fig. 1 were used as sources of factor. They were reacted with adherent cell-depleted E-rosette$^+$ T cells, or non-T cells (B plus adherent cell) subsets, prepared as described (2, 10). 2×10^7 cells were incubated with 1 ml of factor at 37°C for 4 hours with constant rocking. Supernatants were collected by centrifugation and then added at a 1:9 final dilution to PWM-induced indicator cultures. Duplicate microwells were harvested on day 6 and the number of PFC determined in a reverse hemolytic plaque assay. KE37.3.2 supernatants were unaffected by these prior absorptions.

Supernatant added	Prior absorption with	Polyclonal Ig synthesis (PFC per 10^6 B cells)	Inhibition of PFC (%)
Medium		9975	
Medium/monocyte		9310	6.7
SK7		0	100.0
SK7	Non-T cells	0	100.0
SK7	T cells	7382	26.0
SK8		6650	33.3
SK8	Non-T cells	7980	20.0
SK8	T cells	7714	22.7
SK8/monocyte		0	100.0
SK8/monocyte	Non-T cells	0	100.0
SK8/monocyte	T cells	3990	60.0

SSF-AIDS that are shared with the T hybrid factor include partial inactivation upon heating for 60 minutes at 56°C, or with addition of $3 \times 10^{-5}M$ 2-mercaptoethanol on initiation of PWM-induced target cultures. Both products were resistant to 50 mM L-rhamnose and 50 mM n-acetyl-D-glucosamine, two carbohydrates reported to reverse the inhibitory effects of suppressor factors produced by Con A–activated PBMC and acting, respectively, on Ig production at the B-cell level (14) or on mitogen- and antigen-induced T-cell proliferation (15). The apparent size of SSF was determined by molecular sieve chromatography on Sephadex S-200. A major peak of suppressor activity for PWM-induced PFC was detected at approximately 47,000 daltons, migrating between ovalbumin (45,000) and albumin (67,000).

The exact mechanism of SSF effector function is obscure. As both SSF-AIDS and the T hybrid products must be present during the initial 48 hours of the PWM-induced PFC system, the period during which maximal helper factor activity is observed (16), SSF may block lymphokine synthesis, secretion, or receptor function. Supernatant from SK7 had no effect on the synthesis of interleukin-2 by a clone of the Jurkat human T-cell leukemia line, on the utilization of this lymphokine by an interleukin-2–dependent T-cell clone, or on peroxide-mediated macrophage cytotoxicity (17). The immunosuppressive effect is not directly related to LAV virion production because at least the constitutive hybridoma does not express virus by reverse transcriptase assay (9).

Data with SK8 support a two-step mechanism for the generation of the suppressor-effector molecules. It appears that certain T hybrid clones, such as T lymphocytes from AIDS patients, may recruit a second population of cells with the characteristics of monocytes in the inhibition of T cell–dependent immune responses. The afferent limb of suppressor activity in human diseases and in experimental animal systems may involve several pathways linked by T cell–monocyte collaborations. Production of nonspecific inhibitory factors by T cells from mice (18) and man (19) with systemic mycoses is dependent on substances liberated from monocytes of normal or infected individuals. Certain retroviruses, such as murine sarcoma virus, stimulate infected non-T cells to secrete potent soluble suppressors of lectin-mediated thymocyte proliferation and antibody synthesis (20). Induction of these factors is independent of virus particle production (21). Pierce and co-workers have recovered soluble immune response suppressor (SIRS) from several murine T hybridomas, and have demonstrated the feasibility of utilizing a continuous macrophage cell line to process or generate SIRS under the direction of T lymphokines (22, 23). At least two SIRS-like products have been identified in man (14, 15), one of which has been produced by a continuous T-cell line (15). SSF-AIDS and its related T hybrid products are distinguishable from these substances by the restriction of activity to T cell–dependent processes and the lack of susceptibility to specific sugars.

The question of long-term stability of our T hybridomas requires continued assessment. Repetitive recloning with selection of suitable clones, together with the maintenance of frozen stocks of cells, minimizes the problem of functional loss related to chromosomal attrition or other phenomena. SK7 and SK8 have remained in continuous culture, with two subclonings, for 10 months, with persistence of activity. (SK10 no longer expresses an active lymphokine, despite repetitive cloning.) These T hybrids may thus be exploited as potentially unlimited sources of immunoregulatory molecules. Correlations between the presence of SSF-AIDS in individuals with unexplained lymphadenopathy and fever, circulating antibody to LAV (24), and the subsequent development of AIDS (2, 3, 24) have been uncovered. The production of SSF by LAV-infected T4$^+$ cells, either alone or in collaboration with monocytes, would be analogous to the activation and release of helper and inducer lymphokines by normal cells infected with HTLV-I (25). We also attempted to detect SSF-AIDS in the sera of individuals with AIDS or its prodromes. No direct relation between the elaboration of this factor in vitro and the capacity of a given serum sample to depress T cell–dependent immune reactivities could be identified. This may be secondary to the binding of such molecules to T lymphocytes or other cellular receptors, with consequent depletion from the circulation, or to the simultaneous presence of helper or other factors which effectively block SSF detection in whole serum. Indeed, although inhibition of T-cell mitogenesis in vitro by serum from AIDS patients has been reported (26), such activity was not found by another group (27), and certain normal sera express inhibitory substances (28). However, SK7, SK8, and SK8/monocyte supernatants do have the capacity to induce an immunodeficiency state in vivo. Marked suppression of antigen-specific IgM antibody production was noted in BALB/c mice administered these factors intraperitoneally (29). If reproduced in vivo for other types of

immune response known to be defective in AIDS, this may serve as a useful animal model for the disorder. In addition, by comparison with a variety of T lymphokines now being tested clinically in an attempt to augment immunologic function of patients with AIDS and other immune deficiencies (30), our hybrid factors may be of therapeutic significance in the management of disorders requiring immunosuppression. Several groups have achieved in vitro the translation of murine antigen-specific (31) and SIRS (32) T hybridoma suppressor factors, and we have tentatively isolated SSF-AIDS activity from a rabbit reticulocyte lysate system using messenger RNA's derived from SK7 and SK8.

References and Notes

1. A. S. Fauci, *Ann. Intern. Med.* **100**, 92 (1984); M. S. Gottlieb, *ibid.* **99**, 208 (1983); J. Laurence, in *Sexuality: New Perspectives*, Z. DeFries, R. C. Friedman, R. Corn, Eds. (Greenwood, New York, in press).
2. J. Laurence, A. B. Gottlieb, H. G. Kunkel, *J. Clin. Invest.* **72**, 2071 (1983).
3. ________, *Ann. N.Y. Acad. Sci.*, in press.
4. C. Grillot-Courvalin, K. Dellagi, A. Chevalier, J. C. Brouet, *J. Immunol.* **129**, 1008 (1982); C. Grillot-Courvalin, J. C. Brouet, *Nature (London)* **292**, 844 (1982).
5. W. C. Greene, T. A. Fleisher, D. L. Nelson, T. A. Waldmann, *J. Immunol.* **129**, 1986 (1982).
6. J. M. Depper, W. J. Leonard, R. M. Black, T. A. Waldmann, W. C. Greene, *Clin. Res.* **30**, 346A (1982).
7. L. Mayer, S. M. Fu, H. G. Kunkel, *J. Exp. Med.* **156**, 1860 (1982).
8. F. Barré-Sinoussi *et al.*, *Science* **220**, 868 (1983).
9. J.-C. Chermann and L. Montagnier, personal communication.
10. M. K. Crow and H. G. Kunkel, *Clin. Exp. Immunol.* **49**, 338 (1982).
11. H. W. Murray, B. Y. Rubin, H. Masur, R. B. Roberts, *N. Engl. J. Med.* **310**, 883 (1984); B. Y. Rubin *et al.*, *J. Immunol.* **130**, 1019 (1983).
12. L. Mayer, S. M. Fu, H. G. Kunkel, *Immunol. Rev.*, in press.
13. H. S. Panitch, *Ann. N.Y. Acad. Sci.*, in press.
14. T. A. Fleisher, W. C. Greene, R. M. Blaese, T. A. Waldmann, *J. Immunol.* **126**, 1192 (1981).
15. W. C. Greene, T. A. Fleisher, T. A. Waldmann, *ibid.*, p. 1185.
16. C. J. Heijnen, F. Uytdetlang, C. H. Pot, R. E. Balleux, *ibid.*, p. 497.
17. Experiments performed by M. Suthanthiran and H. Murray, Cornell Medical College.

212

18. G. S. Deepe, Jr., S. R. Watson, W. E. Bullock, *J. Immunol.* **132**, 2064 (1984).
19. J. D. Stobo, *ibid.* **119**, 918 (1977).
20. J. B. Mizel *et al.*, *Proc. Natl. Acad. Sci. U.S.A.* **77**, 2205 (1980).
21. C. J. Ciancialo *et al.*, *Fed. Proc. Fed. Am. Soc. Exp. Biol.* **38**, 1364A (1979).
22. T. M. Aune and C. W. Pierce, *J. Immunol.* **127**, 368 (1981).
23. ______, *Proc. Natl. Acad. Sci. U.S.A.* **78**, 5099 (1981).
24. J. Laurence *et al.*, in preparation.
25. S. Z. Salahuddin, P. D. Markham, S. G. Lindner, J. Gootenberg, M. Popovic, H. Hemmi, P. S. Sarin, R. C. Gallo, *Science* **223**, 703 (1984).
26. S. Cunningham-Rundles, M. A. Michelis, H. Masur, *J. Clin. Immunol.* **3**, 156 (1983).
27. R. W. Schroff, M. S. Gottlieb, H. E. Prince, L. L. Chai, J. L. Fahey, *Clin. Immunol. Immunopathol.* **27**, 300 (1983).
28. S.-K. Oh *et al.*, *ibid.* **31**, 430 (1984).
29. J. Laurence, in preparation.
30. N. Flomenberg *et al.*, *J. Immunol.* **130**, 2644 (1983); A. A. Gottlieb *et al.*, *Clin. Res.* **32**, 504A (1984); H. C. Lane *et al.*, *ibid.*, p. 351A; M. Suthanthiran *et al.*, *ibid.*, p. 359A.
31. M. Taniguchi, T. Tokuhisa, M. Kanno, T. Honjo, in *T Cell Hybridomas*, H. V. Boehmer *et al.*, Eds. (Springer-Verlag, Berlin, 1982), pp. 33–41; D. R. Webb *et al.*, *ibid.*, pp. 53–59.
32. I. Nowowiejski, T. M. Aune, C. W. Pierce, D. R. Webb, *J. Immunol.* **132**, 556 (1984).

33. We thank Shu Man Fu for the monoclonal antibody VG2, P. Markham and R. C. Gallo for the p19, and B. Rubin for the antibody to γ-interferon. P. Crow, Rockefeller University, isolated monocyte subpopulations; M. Fotino, Tissue Typing Laboratory, New York Blood Center, performed the HLA-DR determinations; M. Grebenau, Rockefeller University, assisted with the column chromatography; and B. Rubin, New York Blood Center, conducted biologic assays for interferon. We thank A. Lorraine Hoy, W. Mann, and C. Thompson for technical expertise and P. Bolton for secretarial help. Supported by a grant from the New York Affiliate of the American Heart Association, the New York Community Trust, and by NIH grant CA 35018-01. J.L. is a Clinician-Scientist of the American Heart Association and an Academic Fellow of the William S. Paley Foundation.

1 May 1984; accepted 29 May 1984

Report

6 July 1984

39. Lymphadenopathy Associated Virus Infection of a Blood Donor–Recipient Pair with Acquired Immunodeficiency Syndrome

P.M. Feorino, V.S. Kalyanaraman, H.W. Haverkos, C.D. Cabradilla, D.T. Warfield, H.W. Jaffe, A.K. Harrison, M.S. Gottlieb, D. Goldfinger, J.-C. Chermann, F. Barré-Sinoussi, T.J. Spira, J.S. McDougal, J.W. Curran, L. Montagnier, F.A. Murphy, and D.P. Francis

Human retroviruses have been implicated as etiologic agents of the acquired immunodeficiency syndrome (AIDS). Evidence to support this causal association includes (i) the detection in blood from patients with AIDS and lymphadenopathy syndrome (LAS) of antibodies to membrane antigens of human T-cell lymphotropic virus, HTLV (*1*); (ii) the isolation in France from lymphocytes from a homosexual man with lymphadenopathy of a retrovirus called lymphadenopathy associated virus (LAV) (*2*); (iii) the detection of antibodies to membrane antigens of HTLV in serum from donors who gave blood to patients who subsequently developed transfusion-associated AIDS (3); and (iv) the documentation of infection in patients with AIDS, AIDS-related diseases, and their contacts by a retrovirus called HTLV-III (4). We now report the isolation and characterization of a retrovirus from blood from three AIDS patients and compare its antigenic relatedness to HTLV-I, HTLV-II, and LAV.

Whole blood for virus isolation and serologic testing was collected from a blood donor–recipient pair, each member of which had developed AIDS. The blood recipient was a 38-year-old woman who was well until she developed uterine bleeding necessitating surgery. With surgery she received 2 units of packed red blood cells obtained from two separate donors. Two weeks after surgery she developed a mononucleosis-like syndrome, which gradually disappeared. Two months after surgery one of the two blood donors to this woman was identified as a 24-year-old homosexual man who had been hospitalized with oral thrush and *Pneumocystis carinii* pneumonia. His ratio of T-helper to T-suppressor cells at that time was 0.02. The second blood donor to this woman was a healthy man with no risk factors for AIDS.

After the donor's history became known, the cellular immune status of the recipient was tested. She was found to have lymphopenia and a decreased ratio of T-helper to T-suppressor cells 7 months after surgery. Thirteen months after surgery she was hospitalized with *Pneumocystis carinii* pneumonia; her ratio of T-helper to T-suppressor cells was 0.46. She had no other known risk factors for AIDS and denied intravenous drug use, sexual contact with any members of groups with an increased incidence of AIDS, and other exposures to blood or blood products within the preceding 5 years.

The blood specimens used in this study were drawn 12 months after the onset of AIDS symptoms in the blood donor and 1 month after the onset of AIDS symptoms in the recipient. Blood was obtained from a third AIDS patient 20 months after the onset of symptoms; this patient was a homosexual man who had had generalized lymphadenopathy for 20 months before the onset of multiple severe opportunistic infections. He was not epidemiologically connected to the blood donor–recipient pair.

Two virus isolation techniques were used on specimens from these patients: (i) passage of cell-free supernatant fluids from primary patient lymphocyte cultures and (ii) cocultivation of patient lymphocytes with normal fetal cord blood lymphocytes. In both techniques lymphocytes were separated from fresh whole blood on Ficoll-Hypaque gradients and placed into culture with phytohemagglutinin (PHA). For cocultivation, fetal cord blood lymphocytes were added weekly to the patient's PHA-stimulated primary lymphocyte cultures to which interleukin-2 had been added. For the cell-free transmission assays, supernatant fluids were removed from the patient's PHA-stimulated primary lymphocyte cultures and added to cultures of fetal cord blood lymphocytes. Lymphocyte cultures were monitored for virus replication with immunofluorescence and particulate reverse transcriptase assays. When evidence of infection was noted by these methods, cells were examined by electron microscopy.

Antibody to LAV p25 was assayed with an immunoprecipitation method (5). LAV (from the Institut Pasteur, Paris) was purified from supernatant fluids of infected primary lymphocyte cultures (*6*). Supernatant fluids were harvested at the time of peak reverse transcriptase activity and centrifuged at 100,000*g* for 60 minutes. The pellet was solubilized, centrifuged through a 30 percent sucrose cushion, and subjected to phosphocellulose chromatography. The purified p25 was labeled with ^{125}I (*7*). Serum that precipitated at least 15 percent of the ^{125}I label after the addition of gluteraldehyde-fixed *Staphylococcus aureus* Protein A was considered positive.

Both the AIDS patient who donated blood and the patient who received his blood had antibodies to LAV, as assayed by radioimmunoprecipitation. In addition, virus was isolated from both patients' peripheral lymphocytes. Cell-free supernatant fluids from primary lymphocyte cultures from both patients were

found to be infectious when passaged into cultures of PHA-stimulated fetal cord blood lymphocytes. Significant elevations in particulate viral reverse transcriptase activity were observed after 4 days (Fig. 1). The reverse transcriptase activity was maximal when Mg^{2+} was used as the primary cation and when poly A/oligo dT was used as the template-primer. Little or no activity was found when Mn^{2+} was used as the cation or when poly dA/oligo dT was used as the primer. No reverse transcriptase activity was found in parallel uninoculated cultures of the same fetal cord blood lymphocytes.

When the inoculated cord blood lymphocyte cultures were examined by immunofluorescence with fluorescein isothiocyanate–conjugated human globulin fraction of antibody to LAV, antigen was distributed focally in the cytoplasm and

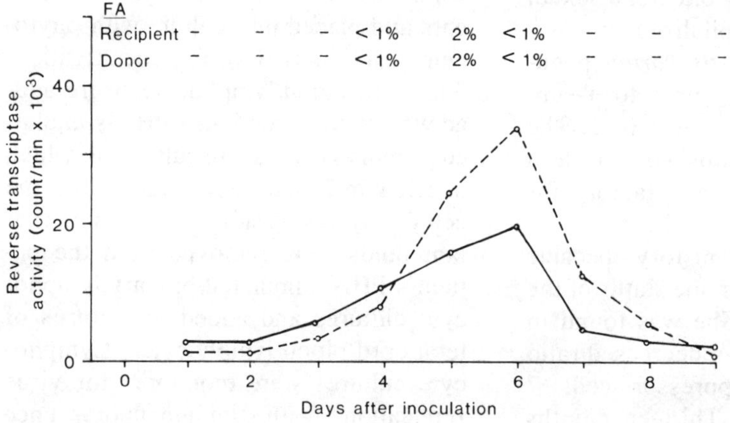

Fig. 1. Reverse transcriptase assays and immunofluorescence showing the dynamics of virus replication in fetal cord blood lymphocytes inoculated from material obtained from a blood donor and the recipient of his blood, both of whom developed AIDS. Supernatant fluids were removed from a 3-day donor cell culture and the 6-day recipient cell culture and after centrifugation (1000*g* for 15 minutes). Ten milliliters of each was inoculated onto human fetal cord blood lymphocyte cultures that had been treated with PHA for 3 days. Interleukin-2, antiserum to interferon (1:1000), and Polybrene (0.2 μg/ml) were added to the cultures. Samples of the cultured cells were examined daily by immunofluorescence (Fig. 2). Specimens of supernatant fluid were prepared daily for reverse transcriptase assay by centrifugation at 500*g* for 15 minutes. Supernatants were then pelleted (100,000*g* for 30 minutes) and assayed for particulate reverse transcriptase by using a template primer of $(A)_n$ $(dt)_{12-18}$ or $(dA)_n$ $(dT)_{12-18}$ in 7.5 m*M* Mg^{2+} or 0.1 m*M* Mn^{2+}.

as a rim beneath the plasma membrane of infected cells (Fig. 2). The proportion of cells with detectable antigen (about 2 percent) was maximal 1 day before maximum reverse transcriptase activity. As reverse transcriptase activity declined and the cells underwent cytopathic change, the immunofluorescence pattern became more diffuse throughout the cytoplasm and eventually was associated with cell debris.

The serum of the epidemiologically unrelated homosexual AIDS patient was negative for antibody to LAV p25. However, cells infected with material from his blood exhibited the same patterns of reverse transcriptase and immunofluorescence as found for the other patients.

Retrovirus particles were seen by electron microscopy in all cultures derived by cocultivation or infection with cell-free supernatant fluids from all three AIDS patients (Fig. 3). These particles budded from the plasma membranes of infected cells without involvement of any preformed intracytoplasmic structure. Nascent budding particles and immature particles had lucent centers; mature particles had small eccentric dense cores and usually an irregular shape. These virus particles were indistinguishable from those depicted in the original characterization of LAV (2, 6) but were different from the typical morphology of HTLV-I and -II.

Competitive radioimmunoassays were used to compare the major core proteins of the viruses isolated from the three AIDS patients with the analogous proteins of other human retroviruses. Virus from all three patients was separated by ultracentrifugation from lymphocyte culture supernatant fluids. These virus preparations were used as competitive antigens in homologous radioimmunoas-

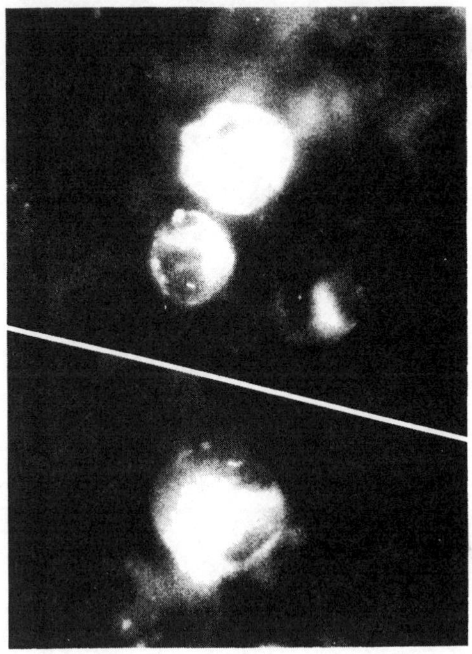

Fig. 2. Infected cultured lymphocytes from a blood donor (top) and the recipient of his blood (bottom) treated with one of two fluorescein isothiocyanate conjugates prepared from the immunoglobulin G fraction of the serum of two individuals with high titers of antibody to LAV. When used at a dilution of 1:100, both conjugates were unreactive on cells infected with HTLV-I, HTLV-II, herpes simplex virus types 1 and 2, cytomegalovirus, Epstein-Barr virus, and adenovirus (group reactivity). Cultured lymphocytes from the patients reacted with the conjugates to a dilution of 1:400.

says for HTLV-I p24, HTLV-II p24, and LAV p25 (Fig. 4). The three isolates from the AIDS patients did not compete in the homologous HTLV-I p24 or HTLV-II p24 assays. In contrast, each of the three isolates competed in the homologous LAV p25 assay. The quantitative pattern of this competition, as reflected by the shape and slope of the curves, indicates that their major core proteins were identical.

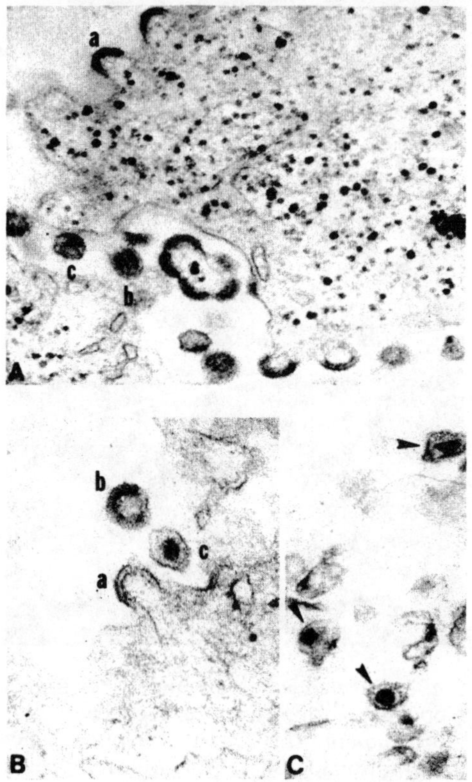

Fig. 3. Retrovirus particles in cocultivated lymphocytes from a blood donor–recipient pair, both of whom developed AIDS. (A) Donor lymphocyte culture with budding (*a*), immature (*b*), and mature (*c*) virus particles. (B) Recipient lymphocyte culture with virus particles in the morphogenic stages. (C) Recipient lymphocyte culture with mature virus particles having dense, eccentric, and bar-shaped nucleoids similar to those described for LAV. Lymphocytes from the blood donor and recipient were separated by Ficoll-Hypaque gradient centrifugation and placed in RPMI 1640 medium supplemented with 10 percent fetal calf serum, PHA (final concentration, 1:500), and antibiotics. On day 2 one lymphocyte culture from each patient was cocultivated with fresh human fetal cord lymphocyte cells (1×10^7) in 5 percent interleukin-2. Additional fresh fetal cord lymphocytes were added to the culture on days 10 and 17. Four days after the last addition of fetal cord lymphocytes, cultures were prepared by standard methods for thin-section electron microscopy.

The ultimate proof that LAV or any other virus is the cause of AIDS requires studies that cumulatively fulfill the modern equivalent of Koch's postulates. That is, an indicator (virus, viral protein, or viral nucleic acid) of a specific viral infection must be found in all or nearly all patients with AIDS or with signs or symptoms that frequently precede AIDS; antibody to the same virus must be shown to develop in constant temporal association with the development of AIDS; and transmission of the same virus to a previously uninfected experimental animal or to a human must be demonstrated with subsequent development of the disease. Progress toward fulfilling the first two postulates has been substantial; the findings reported here contribute to fulfillment of the third. The isolation of the same retrovirus from both a blood donor and the recipient of that donor's blood, a person with no other known source of infection, and the subsequent development of AIDS in this recipient suggests that this virus is the etiologic agent of AIDS. Isolating LAV from other AIDS patients and identifying LAV-specific antibodies in the serum of AIDS patients, including the donor-recipient pair reported here, but not in serum from persons in groups with low AIDS incidence (*4, 8*), provide further evidence for such an etiologic association.

An etiologic association between HTLV-III and AIDS was reported recently (*4*). The most likely explanation for the parallel evidence for HTLV-III and LAV being the cause of AIDS is that the two viruses are the same.

References and Notes

1. M. Essex *et al.*, *Science* **220**, 859 (1983).
2. F. Barré-Sinoussi *et al.*, *ibid.*, p. 868.
3. H. W. Jaffe *et al.*, *ibid.* **223**, 1309 (1984).

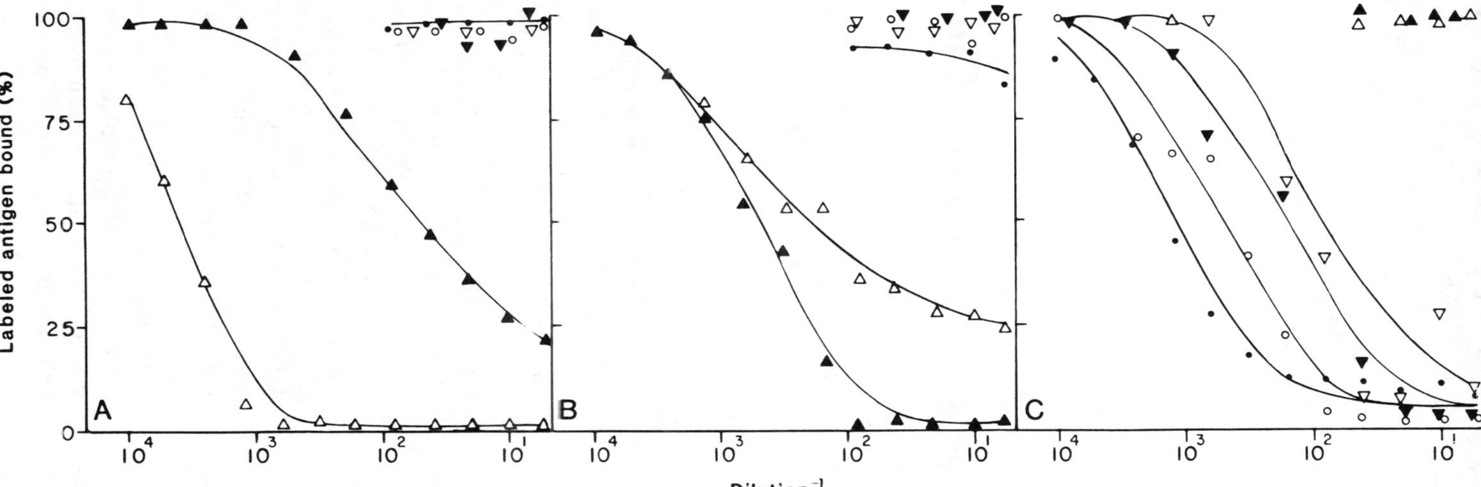

Fig. 4. Homologous competition radioimmunoassay of HTLV-I p24, HTLV-II p24, and LAV p25. Competition radioimmunoassays were carried out with ^{125}I-labeled HTLV-I p24, HTLV-II p24, LAV p25 and limiting dilution of hyperimmune rabbit antibody to HTLV-I (1:2000) or serum from patients M.O. (HTLV-II) (1:2000) and B.R.U. (LAV) (1:600) (2). Serial dilutions (100 μl) of solubilized virus (initial concentrate, 10 μg) in buffer 1 (20 mM Na$_2$HPO$_4$; pH 7.6), 200 mM NaCl, 1 mM EDTA, 0.3 percent Triton X-100, 0.1 mM phenylmethylsulfonyl fluoride, and bovine serum albumin (2 mg/ml) were incubated with the appropriate serum for 1 hour at 37°C. Labeled HTLV-I p24, HTLV-II p24, or LAV p25 (8000 count/min in 50 μl of buffer 1) was then added and the mixture was further incubated at 37°C for 2 hours and at 4°C overnight. A 20-fold excess of goat antiserum to rabbit immunoglobulin G or goat antiserum to human immunoglobulin G was then added and the volume was made up to 1 ml in buffer 1. The samples were further incubated at 37°C for 1 hour and at 4°C for 2 hours and then centrifuged at 2500 revolutions per minute for 20 minutes. The supernatants were aspirated and the radioactivity in the sediment was determined in a gamma counter. (A) Competition radioimmunoassay with rabbit antiserum to HTLV-I and ^{125}I-labeled HTLV-I p24. (B) Competition radioimmunoassay with serum from M.O. and ^{125}I-labeled HTLV-II p24. (C) Competition radioimmunoassay with serum from B.R.U. and ^{125}I-labeled LAV p25. Virus extracts used for competition were as follows: (●) LAV; (△) HTLV-I; (▲) HTLV-II; (○) supernatant (homosexual man, LAV/CDC-151); (▼) supernatant (blood donor, LAV/CDC-228); and (▽) supernatant (blood recipient, LAV/CDC-230).

4. P. Popovic, M. G. Sarngadharan, E. Read, R. C. Gallo, *ibid.* **224**, 497 (1984); R. C. Gallo *et al.*, *ibid.*, p. 500; J. Schüpbach *et al.*, *ibid.*, p. 224; M. G. Sarngadharan *et al.*, *ibid.*, p. 506.
5. V. S. Kalyanaraman *et al.*, *Nature (London)* **294**, 271 (1981).
6. L. Montagnier *et al.*, in *Human T-Cell Leukemia Viruses*, R. C. Gallo, M. Essex, L. Gross, Eds. (Cold Spring Harbor Laboratory, Cold Spring Harbor, N.Y., 1984).
7. F. C. Greenwood, W. M. Hunter, J. S. Glover, *Biochem. J.* **89**, 114 (1963).
8. V. S. Kalyanaraman *et al.*, *Science,* in press.
9. We thank J. V. Bennett and W. R. Dowdle for their advice, D. Golde for the M.O. (HTLV-II) serum, R. Dubois for the supply of clinical material, and T. Scott for manuscript preparation.

27 April 1984; accepted 31 May 1984

---

40. Antibodies to the Core Protein of Lymphadenopathy-Associated Virus (LAV) in Patients with AIDS

V.S. Kalyanaraman, C.D. Cabradilla, J.P. Getchell, R. Narayanan, E.H. Braff, J.-C Chermann, F. Barré-Sinoussi, L. Montagnier, T.J. Spira, J. Kaplan, D. Fishbein, H.W. Jaffe, J.W. Curran, and D.P. Francis

One of the first indications that a human retrovirus might have a role in the etiology of AIDS was the finding of an increased prevalence, in patients with AIDS and lymphadenopathy syndrome (LAS), of antibodies to membrane antigens of human T-cell leukemia virus type I (HTLV-I) infected lymphocytes (*1*). HTLV-I had been frequently isolated from patients with mature T-cell malignancies and is etiologically associated with adult T-cell malignancy endemic in southern Japan, the Caribbean islands, and Africa (*2, 3*). However, the rarity of HTLV-I isolates from AIDS and LAS patients and the low titer of antibodies to HTLV membrane antigens, together with the low prevalence of antibodies to virion core protein antigens of HTLV-I

(*4*), suggested that cross-reacting antibodies to a related retrovirus was responsible for the initial observations. At the same time, a T-lymphotrophic retrovirus, subsequently termed lymphadenopathy-associated virus (LAV), was described (*5*). This cytopathic retrovirus was isolated from a homosexual man with lymphadenopathy. That this virus is linked to AIDS is suggested by (i) the presence of antibody to the virus in AIDS and LAS patients (*6*), (ii) the repeated isolation of the virus from AIDS and LAS patients (*6*), and (iii) the isolation of the virus from a blood donor–recipient pair of AIDS patients (*7*). Another T-lymphotrophic retrovirus, termed HTLV-III, has been isolated repeatedly in similar circumstances and antibodies to this virus have also been found in a high proportion of AIDS and LAS patients (8). Although comparative studies of LAV and HTLV-III have not been reported, it is possible that the two viruses are the same.

We have developed a highly sensitive radioimmunoprecipitation assay that is specific for the major core protein, p25, of LAV. We used this assay, together with similar assays for antibodies to the core proteins (p24) of HTLV-I and HTLV-II, to determine antibody prevalence in groups of patients with AIDS on LAS, homosexual men, laboratory workers, and blood donors.

LAV was propagated in primary cultures of blood lymphocytes (5). At the time of peak reverse transcriptase (RT) activity, supernatant fluids were harvested from infected lymphocyte cultures by low-speed centrifugation, and virus was pelleted by ultracentrifugation (100,000g for 2 hours). Virus-containing pellets were resuspended, centrifuged through a 30 percent sucrose cushion, disrupted with detergent, and subjected to phosphocellulose chromatography (9). HTLV-I p24 and HTLV-II p24 were similarly purified by phosphocellulose chromatography as described (9). The purified products were iodinated and examined by polyacrylamide gel electrophoresis (Fig. 1): the HTLV-I p24, HTLV-II p24, and LAV p25 were purified to apparent homogeneity. The immunoprecipitation of ^{125}I-labeled antigen by serum samples from patients was initially carried out at a 1:25 dilution. Samples were considered positive when at least 15 percent of the label was precipitated after the addition of fixed staphylococcal Protein A cells. Titers of several positive sera ranged from 1:50 to over 1:10,000. The specificity of the

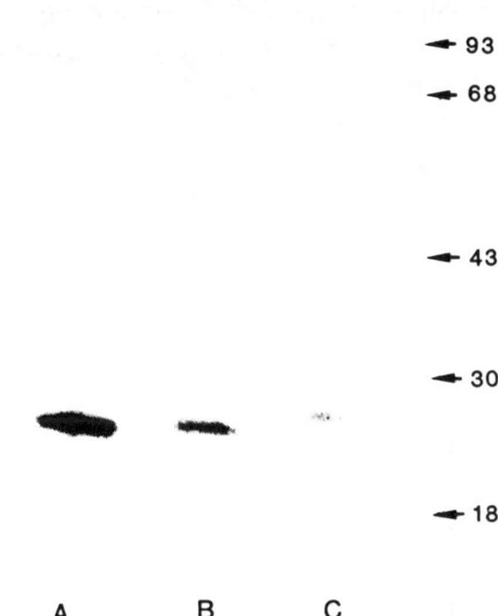

Fig. 1. Sodium dodecyl sulfate–polyacrylamide gel electrophoresis of ^{125}I-labeled core proteins of (lane A) HTLV-I, (lane B) HTLV-II, and (lane C) LAV. HTLV-I p24 was purified from HTLV-I as described (9). By the same techniques, HTLV-II p24 was purified from a cell line (MC) developed in our laboratory. This cell line, which contains the complete integrated genome of HTLV-II, produces large quantities of virus. LAV was purified from supernatant fluids of primary lymphocyte cultures as described (5). Virus pellets were prepared from supernatant fluids obtained at the time of peak reverse transcriptase activity. The resuspended pellets were concentrated by centrifugation through a 30 percent sucrose cushion and then subjected to phosphocellulose chromatography. The product of this purification procedure was examined for homogeneity by electrophoresis on polyacrylamide gel.

LAV p25 radioimmunoprecipitation assay was examined by a competitive radioimmunoassay (Fig. 2). Although unlabeled p25 from LAV competed well for homologous antibody (from patient B.R.U.), other retroviruses did not. The noncompeting viruses included HTLV-I, HTLV-II, Mason-Pfizer monkey virus, simian sarcoma virus, baboon endogenous virus, Rauscher murine leukemia virus, mouse mammary tumor virus, and equine infectious anemia virus.

Serum from AIDS patients was obtained either as part of various studies

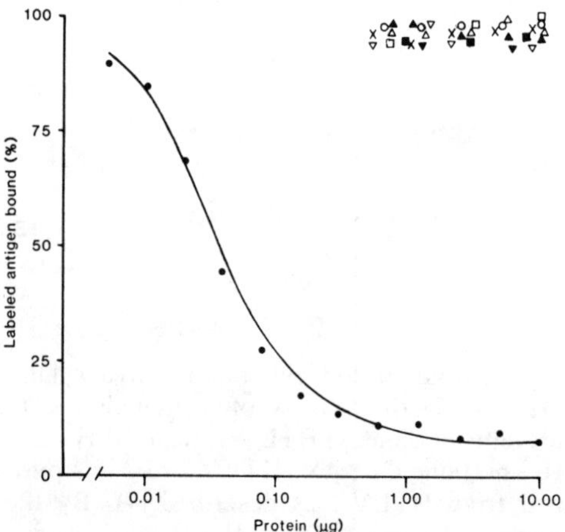

Fig. 2. Competitive RIA of the p25 of LAV and analogous core proteins of other retroviruses. The RIA's were carried out with ^{125}I-labeled LAV p25 and a limiting dilution of human serum positive for antibodies to LAV (B.R.U.). Serial dilutions (100 μl) of solubilized virus in buffer 1 [20 mM Na$_2$HPO$_4$ (pH 7.6), 200 mM NaCl, 1 mM EDTA. 0.3 percent Triton X-100, 0.1 mM phenylmethylsulfonyl fluoride, and bovine serum albumin (2 mg/ml)] were incubated with the appropriate serum for 1 hour at 37°C. Labeled LAV p25 (8000 count/min in 50 μl of buffer 1) was then added, and the mixture was further incubated at 37°C for 2 hours and at 4°C overnight. A 20-fold excess of goat antiserum to human immunoglobulin G was then added, and the volume made up to 1 ml in buffer 1. The samples were further incubated at 37°C for 1 hour and at 4°C for 2 hours and then centrifuged at 2500 rev/min for 5 minutes. The supernatant fluids were aspirated, and the radioactivity in the sediment was determined in a gamma counter. Virus extracts used for competition were as follows: ●, LAV; ▽, HTLV-I; ▼, HTLV-II; □, Mason-Pfizer monkey virus; X, simian sarcoma virus; and ○, equine infectious anemia virus; ■, baboon endogenous virus.

sponsored by the Centers for Disease Control (CDC) or as individual specimens submitted directly to CDC. Serum from LAS patients was obtained as part of an ongoing prospective study of this syndrome among homosexual men in Atlanta. Serum from CDC employees who worked in laboratories and other areas was obtained in 1983 and 1984; some of the laboratory workers were exposed to materials from AIDS patients. Serum samples were also collected from homosexual men, 18 years of age or older, who sought medical care at the San Francisco City Clinic. These samples were routinely collected from 1978 as part of ongoing studies of hepatitis B virus infection in homosexual men (10); specimens from 1984 were obtained, according to the same protocol, as part of a hepatitis B vaccine study (11). Serum from blood donors (provided by the National Red Cross) was chosen at random from samples obtained in 1980 and 1981. The donors were located in Tucson, Arizona; Madison, Wisconsin; and Philadelphia, Pennsylvania.

Specific antibody to the core protein of LAV p25 was present in serum from 41 percent of the AIDS patients and from 72 percent of the LAS patients (Table 1). In contrast, no antibody was detected in serum from the CDC employees or from the blood donors.

When we compared serum samples drawn in 1978 and 1984 from groups of homosexual men in San Francisco, we found a marked increase in antibody prevalence. In 1978, one of 100 homosexual men had antibody, and in 1984, 12 (24 percent) of 50 had antibody. Although the samples were collected and selected without known bias, to rule out confounding variables we are following the 1978 serum collection protocol exactly for the 1984 collection.

Table 1. Prevalence of antibodies to LAV p25 and the p24 of HTLV-I and HTLV-II in serum from AIDS and LAS patients and from control groups. Purified core proteins were labeled with ^{125}I and used as target antigens. Labeled antigen was added to serum samples and those samples that precipitated at least 15 percent of the label after the addition of staphylococcal Protein A were considered positive. N.D., not done.

Group	LAV p25			HTLV-I and HTLV-II p24		
	Number positive	Number tested	Percentage	Number positive	Number tested	Percentage
AIDS patients	51	125	41	7	125	5
LAS patients	81	113	72	0	113	
Controls						
Homosexual men						
1978	1	100	1	0	100	
1980	12	50	24	0	50	
Blood donors	0	189		0	N.D.	
Laboratory workers	0	70		0	70	

Table 2. Prevalence of antibodies to LAV p25 in serum from AIDS patients. All groups of AIDS patients are represented except hemophiliacs.

Group	Number positive	Number tested	Percentage
Homosexuals	42	100	42
Intravenous drug users	5	16	31
Haitians	2	5	40
Others	2	4	51
Total	51	125	41
Homosexuals by disease manifestation			
Kaposi's sarcoma	22	35	63
Opportunistic infection	29	90	33
Total	51	125	41

The prevalence of antibodies to LAV p25 varied only slightly among different groups of AIDS patients (Table 2). There was considerable variation, however, among AIDS patients with different disease manifestations. Patients with Kaposi's sarcoma alone had a significantly higher antibody prevalence [22 (63 percent) of 35] compared with patients who had only opportunistic infections [29 (34 percent) of 90] ($P = <0.005$, Student's t-test). These results are consistent with the observation that Kaposi's sarcoma patients are less immunodeficient than patients with opportunistic infections and support the contention that seropositivity decreases with disease progression.

Assays for antibodies to the p24's of HTLV-I and HTLV-II were conducted in parallel with the assays for LAV p25 antibody. The specificity of tests with these antigens has been described (*12*). Seven of the 125 AIDS patients had antibodies that precipitated the p24's of both HTLV-I and HTLV-II (Table 1). This concordance might be expected since the p24's of the two viruses are known to be cross-reactive (*12*). However, three of the same seven sera also precipitated the p25 of LAV—an unexpected result. Since neither HTLV-I p24 nor HTLV-II p24 competed in our LAV p25 competitive radioimmunoassay (RIA) (Fig. 2), and since p25 of LAV did not compete in complementary assays with homologous HTLV-I and HTLV-II p24 systems (*7*), this result must be explained otherwise. Some AIDS patients may have been infected with more than one virus, resulting in broadened specificity of antibody response. Other AIDS patients, infected with only one virus, may have developed a broader, more cross-reactive antibody against shared epitopes than has been found in the reference human and animal sera used in the development of the RIA. Support for possible shared common antigenic determinants among HTLV-I, HTLV-II, and LAV may come from nucleic acid hybridization studies in which varying degrees of homology between HTLV-I, HTLV-II, and LAV have been demonstrated (*13*). These studies indicate that LAV is more closely related to HTLV-II than to HTLV-I. LAV and HTLV-II cross-hybridize over most of their genomes, whereas LAV and HTLV-I cross-hybridize primarily in their *env* genes. This relationship may also account for the finding of antibodies in AIDS and LAS patients that react with those HTLV-I–encoded *env* gene products that are expressed on the plasma membranes of infected cells (*1*).

Thus we have shown that a high proportion of serum samples from patients with AIDS and LAS and from people at risk for AIDS has detectable antibodies to the major core protein of LAV. These antibodies also react specifically with LAV p25. Since other known type C and type D retroviruses do not cross-react in the competition RIA with ^{125}I-labeled p25 of LAV, these antibodies are not directed toward heterophile antigens that are commonly found in human serum (*14, 15*). The presence of antibody to LAV p25 in only 42 percent of the serum samples from AIDS patients may be due to the fact that these patients are highly immunosuppressed and have progressively lost the ability to make high-titer antibodies (*16, 17*). Another possible, but less likely, explanation may be that more than one virus is involved in the etiology of AIDS. A better indicator of LAV infection in these patients may be the presence of antibodies to the envelope glycoprotein of LAV. The antibody titers to the envelope glycoprotein may persist during the late stage of the disease while antibody to the core protein may decline to less than detectable levels. This has indeed been shown in the case of antibodies to the major core protein p24 and the presumptive envelope protein of HTLV-III (*8*).

Since we also find antibodies to LAV p25 in apparently normal homosexuals, the results of the study on the distribution of antibodies to LAV have to be interpreted with caution. For example, in the case of adult T-cell leukemia (ATL) in Japan, there is a clear etiological relation between the disease and HTLV-I (*15*). Even though nearly 25 percent of the population in the endemic area have antibodies to HTLV-I, only a minor percentage of the population gets ATL. Thus, as with ATL in Japan, other cofactors in addition to viruses may be involved in the causation of AIDS.

Note added in proof: A specific ELISA test with total LAV proteins detects LAV-specific antibodies in 95 percent of LAS patients and 70 to 95 percent of AIDS depending on the risk group and the stage of the disease.

References and Notes

1. M. Essex *et al.*, *Science* **220**, 859 (1983).
2. R. C. Gallo *et al.*, *Cancer Res.* **43**, 3892 (1983).
3. V. Hinuma *et al.*, *Proc. Natl. Acad. Sci. U.S.A.* **78**, 6476 (1981).
4. M. Robert-Guroff *et al.*, *Lancet*, in press.
5. F. Barré-Sinoussi *et al.*, *Science* **220**, 868 (1983).
6. L. Montagnier *et al.*, in *The Cancer Cell 3*, R. C. Gallo and M. Essex, Eds. (Cold Spring Harbor Laboratory, Cold Spring Harbor, N.Y., in press).
7. P. M. Feorino *et al.*, *Science* **225**, 69 (1984).
8. M. Popovic *et al.*, *ibid.* **224**, 497 (1984); R. C. Gallo *et al.*, *ibid.*, p. 500; J. Schüpbach *et al.*, *ibid.*, p. 503; M. G. Sarngadharan *et al.*, *ibid.*, p. 506.
9. V. S. Kalyanaraman *et al.*, *J. Virol.* **38**, 906 (1981).
10. M. T. Schreeder *et al.*, *J. Infect. Dis.* **146**, 7 (1982).
11. D. P. Francis *et al.*, *Ann. Intern. Med.* **97**, 362 (1982).
12. V. S. Kalyanaraman *et al.*, *Science* **218**, 571 (1982).
13. R. Narayanan *et al.*, in preparation.
14. V. S. Kalyanaraman *et al.*, *Nature (London)* **294**, 271 (1981).
15. V. S. Kalyanaraman *et al.*, *Proc. Natl. Acad. Sci. U.S.A.* **79**, 1653 (1982).
16. H. C. Lane *et al.*, *N. Engl. J. Med.* **309**, 453 (1983).
17. E. Vilmer *et al.*, *Lancet* **1984-I**, 753 (1984); C. Cabradilla *et al.*, in preparation.
18. We thank the many investigators at CDC, health departments, and hospitals who provided us with patient sera for testing. We also thank P. O'Malley of the San Francisco City Clinic, R. Dodd of the National Red Cross, and W. R. Dowdle, J. V. Bennett, and S. Hadler of CDC for help and cooperation.

4 May 1984; accepted 8 June 1984

Research News

27 July 1984

41. How the HTLV's Might Cause Cancer

Jean L. Marx

Two of the human T cell leukemia viruses, HTLV-I and -II, cause human blood cell malignancies, producing leukemias or lymphomas of T cells. Since the first identification of an HTLV about 5 years ago, the manner in which the viruses might cause the malignant transformation of cells has remained a mystery. New results from William Haseltine of Harvard Medical School and the Harvard School of Public Health and his colleagues, which are reported in the 27 July 1984 issue of *Science*, provide the first clues to the mechanism by which the viruses may transform cells. "It is the first thing that has come up concretely that might explain how the viruses cause leukemias," says Myron Essex of the Harvard School of Public Health.

The results are important not only because they open up potential approaches to the prevention and cure of the T-cell malignancies caused by the viruses, but also because they may provide new insights into the regulation of growth and other activities in cells that have a central role in controlling immune responses. In addition, the two viruses have a close relative, HTLV-III, which has been implicated as a likely cause of acquired immune deficiency syndrome (AIDS), and the work may help in understanding this devastating disease.

The model being proposed to explain transformation by HTLV-I and -II represents a new kind of transforming mechanism for a tumor virus of the retrovirus group. (Retroviruses have RNA genomes.) It postulates the production by the viruses of a protein that stimulates both their replication and that of their host cells.

Retroviruses, including the HTLV's, contain long terminal repeating sequences (LTR's) at the ends of their genomes. The LTR's carry regulatory segments, known as promoters and enhancers, which activate transcription of the viral genes into messenger RNA, the first step of protein synthesis. What Haseltine, with Joseph Sodroski and Craig Rosen, who are also at Harvard, has shown is that T cells that have been infected with HTLV-I or -II produce a factor, presumably a protein encoded by the viral genomes themselves, that increases transcription from the viral promoter in the LTR.

The results indicate that the factor can facilitate transcription from the viral promoter wherever this is located in the genome. This type of regulation is called *trans* regulation in molecular biology jargon. "It's nice because you don't need specific integration sites," Sodroski explains. "No matter where the virus goes it can make the factor."

The new findings may help to explain some of the peculiarities of transformation by the two HTLV's. Up until now retroviruses have been thought to transform cells by one of two general mechanisms. The transforming potential of the acute or rapidly acting retroviruses is encoded in specific viral genes, called

oncogenes, which are derived from cellular DNA sequences that became incorporated in the viral genomes during the course of infection. These oncogenes can cause transformation when reintroduced by the viruses into cells, both in living animals and in culture.

The chronic or slow-acting retroviruses, which generally cause leukemias, do not carry oncogenes but may transform by inserting an LTR near one of the cellular oncogene counterparts, thus eliciting its abnormal activation. These viruses do not transform cultured cells.

The HTLV's fit neither of the two models. They do not carry any of the two dozen or so known oncogenes. Moreover, none of their DNA sequences appear to be related to cellular sequences, making it unlikely that they carry any oncogene as these are commonly understood. In spite of the absence of an oncogene, however, HTLV-I and -II do transform cultured cells. It is also unlikely that they act by LTR insertion because the HTLV genome may integrate anywhere in the genome of transformed cells.

A regulatory factor that stimulates transcription from a viral promoter should increase replication of the virus. Haseltine, Sodroski, and Rosen propose that, in the case of HTLV-I and -II infected cells, the factor may also increase transcription of cellular genes, such as those that turn on cell division, and that this is what leads to the uncontrolled growth and other abnormalities of transformed cells. Work from Robert Gallo's laboratory at the National Cancer Institute, where the first HTLV was discovered, has shown that expression of some cellular genes, including that for the receptor for T-cell growth factor, is increased in cells transformed by the viruses. "It's opened up a new way of thinking about how a virus like this might transform a cell," says Dani Bolognesi of Duke University School of Medicine of the Harvard group's suggestion.

In contrast to the malignancies, AIDS is caused by T-cell death, not proliferation. If HTLV-III also produces a *trans*-acting regulatory factor, Haseltine, Sodroski, and Rosen suggest, it may act either to turn off genes that stimulate growth or to turn on those that cause cells to stop dividing.

There are precedents, incidentally, although not from the retroviruses, for transforming-virus production of a *trans*-acting regulatory factor that activates expression of both viral and cellular genes. Researchers from several laboratories have evidence that DNA-containing viruses, including adenovirus and SV40, act in this way.

The likely location in the HTLV genome of the gene coding for the *trans*-acting regulatory factor is in a region that was identified by Mitsuaki Yoshida and his colleagues at the Cancer Institute in Tokyo, Japan, as having four open reading frames and thus the potential of coding for four proteins. This region lies between the genes coding for the viral structural proteins and the 3' (right-hand) LTR, a region where retroviral oncogenes may be located, although, as already mentioned, the HTLV's do not carry any known oncogenes. The slowly transforming retroviruses do not contain a comparable stretch of RNA.

Haseltine and his colleagues have now compared the sequences of this region, which is roughly 1600 base pairs long, from HTLV-I and -II. They find the first 600 base pairs to be very different in the two viruses, whereas the last 1000 are very highly conserved. More than 80 percent of the amino acids in the proteins encoded by the conserved regions should be identical. "No other open reading frame has such a high degree of conservation," Haseltine says. "We predict that it will encode a protein that will affect transcription."

Essex and Tun-Hou Lee, also at the Harvard School of Public Health, have identified in HTLV-I transformed cell lines a viral protein with a molecular weight of 42,000, about the right size for a protein encoded by the long open reading frame. In one transformed line, which originated in Gallo's laboratory, it is the only viral protein made. This line is just as effective in stimulating transcription from the HTLV-I LTR as lines that make infectious viral particles. The Haseltine and Essex groups have shown that the 42-kilodalton protein is not related to the viral polymerase or structural proteins and that it is at least partly derived from the conserved reading frame. "So it proves that the long open reading frame is used," Haseltine says.

The HTLV's may not be the only RNA-transforming viruses that operate by *trans* regulation of gene transcription. Bovine leukemia virus induces a disease very similar to the leukemia associated with HTLV-I. The sequence of the bovine virus has recently been determined by Arsene Burny of the University of Brussels. It, too, contains a long open reading frame just inside the 3' LTR. The amino acid sequence of the protein encoded by this region is different from that of the comparable HTLV protein, but they both have similar arrangements of hydrophobic and hydrophilic regions.

If the proposed mechanism for transformation by the HTLV's is correct, then the way might be open to finding means of preventing or treating the cancers caused by the agents. For example, a vaccine might be derived from a virus modified so that it no longer produces the transcription-stimulating protein. For therapy, it might be possible to attach a lethal gene to an LTR that has been altered so that it works only in tumor cells that were transformed by HTLV-I or -II. That gene, if introduced into cells, would be transcribed in—and kill—only the tumor cells. At the very least, the new results on the HTLV's should open new lines of inquiry.

Research Article

27 July 1984

42. *Trans*-Acting Transcriptional Activation of the Long Terminal Repeat of Human T Lymphotropic Viruses in Infected Cells

Joseph G. Sodroski, Craig A. Rosen, and William A. Haseltine

The human T lymphotropic viruses (HTLV), a family of exogenous human retroviruses (*1*), are distinguished by the different diseases with which they are associated and by their structural features (*2*). HTLV-I is the etiologic agent of clinically aggressive adult T-cell leukemia-lymphoma (*1, 3*). HTLV-II is an infrequent isolate originally derived from a patient with a clinically benign T-cell cell variant of hairy cell leukemia (*2*). Recently, a new group of HTLV, HTLV-III, was isolated from patients with the acquired immune deficiency syndrome (AIDS) (*4*).

We wished to characterize the differences between the genomes of HTLV-I and HTLV-II that might account for their different disease associations. Experience with murine leukemia viruses indicated that transcriptional differ-ences mediated by the viral long terminal repeats (LTR's) are major determinants of virulence (*5*). The LTR regions of HTLV-I and -II diverge markedly in sequence (*2*). To determine whether these structural differences have functional significance, we investigated the ability of the LTR sequences of HTLV-I and -II to act as transcriptional elements.

Construction of HTLV-CAT recombinant plasmids. The transcriptional control elements of animal retroviral LTR's are contained within the U3 region (*6*). The LTR U3-R boundary, defined by the RNA transcriptional start site, has been determined for HTLV-I and -II (*2*). For our studies, we inserted the entire U3 and R regions of HTLV-I and -II at a site 5' to the chloramphenicol acetyltransferase (CAT) gene (pU3R-I and pU3R-II) (Fig. 1) (*7*). A third plasmid that contains

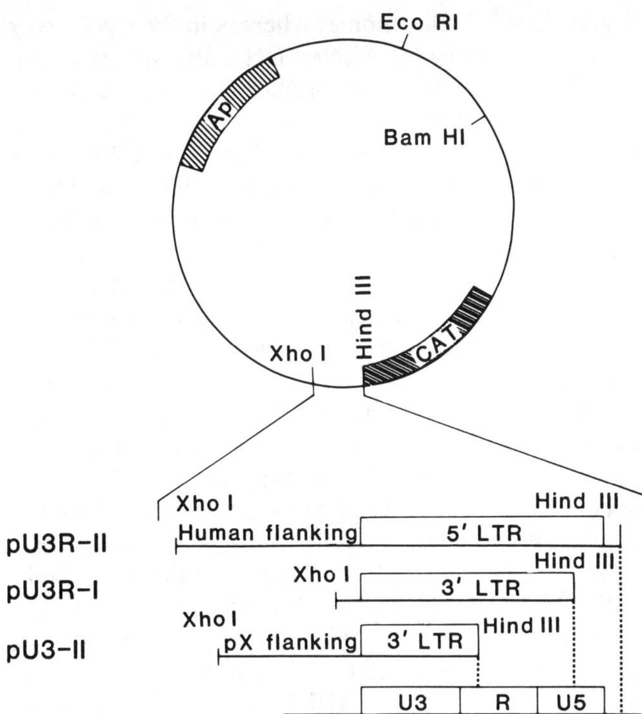

Fig. 1. Construction of recombinant plasmids. The diagram depicts the region of the HTLV LTR's placed 5' to the CAT gene (Ap, ampicillin resistance gene). pSV2CAT contains the SV40 early promoter region 5' to CAT (7). The recipient vector contains a Hind III–Xho I fragment of pSVIXCAT, a variant of pSV2CAT lacking the SV40 72-base pair enhancer region. Digestion with Hind III–Xho I removes the SV40 promoter region, allowing HTLV sequences to be placed 5' to CAT. HTLV LTR sequences were inserted into this vector by using natural restriction enzyme sites or by converting convenient sites to Hind III and Xho I sites with synthetic linkers. The sites used for cloning were as follows: (i) pU3R-I: pCR1, a defective proviral clone containing the HTLV-I 3' LTR (35), was digested with Rsa I and Mbo I, resulting in a fragment containing the U3, R, and 105 bp of the U5 region. (ii) pU3R-II: The complete 5' LTR from MO15A, a complete HTLV-II proviral clone (2), was cleaved with Bgl II (in the 5' cellular flanking sequence) and Eco RI, located 25 bp 3' to the terminus of the LTR. (iii) pU3-II: MO1A, a 3' HTLV-II LTR clone (2), was cleaved with Xho I (in the envelope gene) and Bam HI (47 bp downstream from the cap site). All recombinant DNA techniques were performed according to enzyme manufacturer's specifications. Plasmid DNA's were purified by centrifugation in CsCl$_2$ gradients prior to transfection.

only the U3 and a small portion of the R region of HTLV-II was also constructed, pU3-II (Fig. 1). Other plasmids used for comparative purposes contain either the entire SV40 enhancer-promoter region (pSV2CAT), the promoter of SV40 without the 72-base repeat regions that comprise the SV40 enhancer (pSVIXCAT), or the entire LTR of Rous sarcoma virus located 5' to the CAT gene (pRSVCAT) (7).

To test the transcriptional activity of the inserted HTLV sequences, we introduced the plasmid DNA into cells via transfection using either the calcium phosphate or DEAE-dextran methods (8). For each experiment the CAT activity directed by the plasmids that contained HTLV sequences was normalized to that of plasmids that contain the SV40 enhancer-promoter elements, known to function in a wide variety of cell types (7, 9). Levels of CAT enzymatic activity at 48 hours after transfection correlate closely with CAT-related messenger RNA (mRNA) levels, even when such messages differ in their 5' start sites, thereby providing a measure of the abili-

228

ty of the sequences 5' to the CAT gene to promote transcription (*7, 9*).

Expression of the CAT gene in fibroblast and epithelial cell lines. We tested the ability of the LTR sequences of HTLV-I and -II to act as transcriptional elements in fibroblasts and epithelial cells of murine, simian, and human origin. The data are summarized in Table 1 and Fig. 2.

In murine fibroblasts (NIH 3T3) (*10*), the activity of plasmids that contained the LTR sequences of HTLV-I was comparable to that of pSV2CAT and much higher than that produced by the plasmid that contained the SV40 promoter sequence alone. The HTLV-I sequences also yielded significant CAT activity upon transfection of simian (CV-1) cells (*11*), although this was lower than that observed for the pSV2CAT plasmid. The LTR sequences of HTLV-II directed no appreciable levels of CAT activity in either of these cell lines. These experiments suggest that the LTR sequences of HTLV-I function as efficient transcriptional elements in cells of different species, whereas the HTLV-II LTR sequences do not.

Upon transfection of pU3R-I into human epithelial and fibroblast cells [HeLa (*12*) and M1 (*13*)] the level of CAT activity was greater than that observed upon transfection of the same cells with pSV2CAT. Negligible CAT activity was observed upon transfection of these cells with pU3R-II or pU3-II. Thus, HTLV-I LTR sequences appear to function as transcriptional control elements in human cells that are not the natural targets for HTLV infection, whereas the HTLV-II LTR sequences do not.

In retrovirus-infected cells, LTR-mediated gene expression occurs from a provirus stably integrated into the host cell genome, whereas in the CAT assay, the transfected DNA directing transcription occurs primarily in an extrachromosomal state (*14*). To determine if the results obtained from the CAT assays are relevant to an understanding of HTLV LTR function in the integrated provirus, the HTLV LTR sequences used to direct CAT expression were positioned upstream of the neomycin phosphotransferase (*neo*) gene (*15*). These plasmids were transfected into murine and human cell lines and stably transfected colonies were selected in the presence of the neomycin analog G-418. The numbers of G-418–resistant colonies in NIH 3T3 cells transfected with pU3R-I-neo and pSV2neo were equal. In HeLa cells, pU3R-I-neo yielded about twice as many colonies as did pSV2neo. In both these cell lines, the neo plasmid directed by HTLV-II LTR failed to yield any G-418–resistant colonies. We conclude that the levels of CAT activity correlate well with the function of the LTR in the integrated state.

Expression in human lymphoid cells. In naturally acquired HTLV infections, most of the infected cells are of the T-cell lineage (*16*). However, some HTLV-producing cells expressing B-cell markers have been isolated (*17*). To determine the function of the HTLV LTR sequences within lymphocytes, we transfected cell lines of lymphoid origin with the plasmids described above. The cell lines used were: HUT 78, an OKT4$^+$ (helper-inducer) human T-cell line derived from an HTLV-negative patient with Sézary syndrome (this cell line lacks HTLV-I or HTLV-II proviral sequences) (*18*); and NC37, a B-cell line established from a normal donor and immortalized with Epstein-Barr virus (*18*).

Table 1. Relative CAT activity in transfected cells. The percent conversion of chloramphenicol to its acetylated forms in HTLV-CAT recombinant transfected cells was normalized against the percent conversion in similar cells transfected with pSV2CAT. To arrive at the values shown, we divided the slope of the time course from the CAT assays of the HTLV-CAT transfected cells by the slope of the pSV2CAT time course. Thus the values represent the percent acetylation per hour relative to that directed by pSV2CAT. The numbers represent the average of a minimum of three independent experiments with a variation no greater than ±20 percent between experiments. N.D., not done.

Cell line	Description	pSV2CAT	pU3R-I	pU3-II	pU3R-II	pRSVCAT
CV-1	Simian fibroblast cell line	1.0	0.2	<0.01	<0.01	N.D.
NIH 3T3	Murine fibroblast cell line	1.0	0.9	<0.01	<0.01	N.D.
M1	SV40-transformed human fibroblasts	1.0	2.2	<0.01	<0.01	N.D.
HeLa	Human cervical carcinoma line	1.0	2.2	<0.01	<0.01	1.6
NC37	Human B-lymphocyte line immortalized by Epstein-Barr virus	1.0	4.5	<0.01	<0.01	N.D.
HUT 78	HTLV-negative human T-lymphocyte line	1.0	4.5	<0.01	<0.01	2.1
C81-66-45	HTLV-I–immortalized nonproducer	1.0	74	<0.01	<0.01	N.D.
HUT 102	HTLV-I producer T-lymphocyte line	1.0	28	1.4	1.7	N.D.
MT2	HTLV-1 producer T-lymphocyte line	1.0	180	N.D.	5.5	2.4
C3-44	HTLV-II producer T-lymphocyte line	1.0	140	40	95	N.D.
HOS	Human osteosarcoma cell line	1.0	0.7	<0.01	<0.01	N.D.
HOS/PL	HTLV-I–infected HOS cell line	1.0	75	<0.01	<0.01	1.0

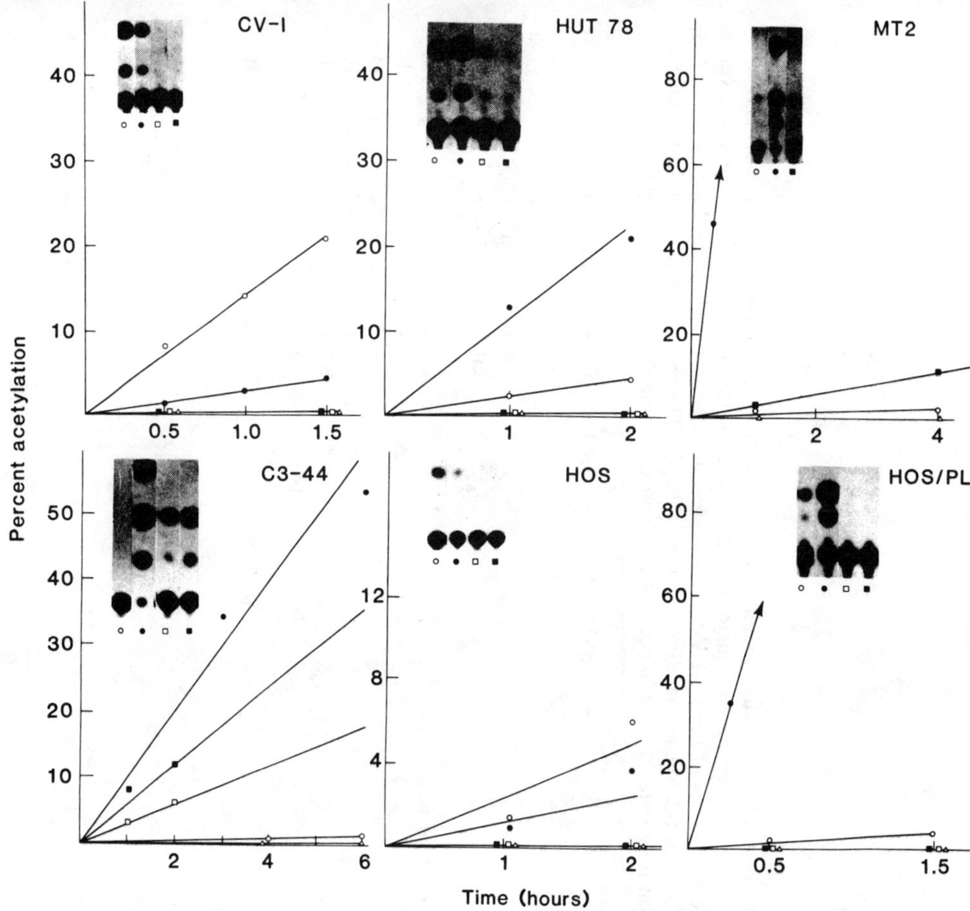

Fig. 2. Transient expression of the CAT gene directed by the HTLV LTR transcriptional elements. NIH 3T3 and CV-1 cells were transfected by a modification of the calcium phosphate coprecipitation technique (*8*). Approximately 1×10^6 cells were seeded on 100-mm dishes 24 hours prior to addition of the CaPO$_4$-DNA precipitate. One milliliter of the precipitate containing 5 to 10 μg of DNA was added to the medium, and the cells were incubated 4 hours at 37°C and then exposed to glycerol for 3 minutes. CV-1 cells were exposed to 10 percent dimethyl sulfoxide 24 hours after transfection. All other cell lines were transfected by a modification of the DEAE-dextran technique (*8*). Twenty-four hours before transfection adherent cells were seeded at a density of 1×10^6 cells per 10-cm^2 dish. Immediately prior to transfection cells were trypsinized, washed, and transfected in suspension with 5 to 8 μg of DNA, an amount shown to be less than saturating. Lymphocyte lines were transfected at a density of 1×10^6 to 5×10^6 cells per milliliter with 5 to 10 μg of DNA. Cells were harvested 48 hours after transfection, and cellular extracts were prepared by freeze-thawing three times. After a brief centrifugation to remove cell debris, extracts were analyzed for CAT activity as described (*7*) except that acetyl coenzyme A was present at 24 m*M*. Percent conversion of chloramphenicol to the acetylated forms was determined by ascending thin-layer chromatography and liquid scintillation counting of the spots cut from the plate. The graphs depict typical CAT assays over the time course indicated. Arrowheads indicate other data points that could not be accommodated in the graph. All experiments were performed a minimum of three times, and the slopes of the curves differ by no more than 20 percent from experiment to experiment. Symbols represent CAT activity directed by the plasmids: ●, pU3R-I; ○, pSV2CAT; □, pU3-II; and ■, pU3R-II; and △, pSVIXCAT. Insets show actual autoradiograms of a CAT assay and represent conversions obtained from one time period within the linear range of the assay.

The LTR sequences of HTLV-I directed the synthesis of significant amounts of the CAT gene product in the human T and B cells (Fig. 2 and Table 1). The ratio of pU3R-I activity to pSV2CAT activity was approximately twice as high as this ratio in fibroblasts and epithelial cell lines. These findings demonstrate that factors specific for the cell type modulate the activity of the HTLV-I LTR.

To our surprise, transfection of the HUT 78 or NC37 cells with plasmids containing HTLV-II LTR sequences resulted in no appreciable CAT activity. Thus, there are substantial differences in the cellular requirements for the function of HTLV-I and HTLV-II LTR sequences. Some human lymphoid cells apparently lack factors required for the efficient function of the HTLV-II LTR.

Expression in HTLV-infected cells. The inactivity of the HTLV-II LTR in the lymphoid cell lines suggested that factors specific to the HTLV target cell might be required for efficient expression of the CAT gene under control of the HTLV LTR's. For this reason we transfected HTLV-producing cell lines derived from infected individuals, or cell lines established by cocultivation of primary human lymphocytes with HTLV producer cell lines. The cell lines used include: HUT 102, an HTLV-I–producing OKT4⁺ T-lymphocyte line established from a patient with an HTLV-associated adult T-cell leukemia-lymphoma (mycosis fungoides) (*18*); MT2, an HTLV-I–producing cell line established by immortalization of primary T lymphocytes after cocultivation with an HTLV producer cell line (*19*); and C81-66-45, a subclone of C63/CR$_{II}$-4, derived by fusion of primary umbilical cord blood cells with an HTLV-I–producing cell line established from an adult T-cell

leukemia-lymphoma patient (this cell line does not produce virus but expresses a limited number of viral proteins) (*20*).

The results obtained upon transfection of these cell lines with pU3R-I were remarkable and unexpected. The level of CAT activity was 25- to 180-fold higher than that obtained with pSV2CAT.

Normalization of CAT activities for DNA uptake indicates that the increased ratio of CAT activity directed by the pU3R-I plasmid in infected cells represents a real increase and not only a relative increase compared to the activity in uninfected cells. Since the transfected DNA that expresses the CAT activity is mostly extrachromosomal, these results suggest that *trans*-acting factors in HTLV-infected cells stimulate the expression of genes directed by the HTLV-I LTR. Although low, the CAT activity directed by pU3R-II and pU3-II was substantially higher in most of the cells that contained HTLV-I proviruses than it was in uninfected cells.

Lymphocytes infected with HTLV exhibit changes characteristic of T cells activated by exposure to mitogenic or antigenic stimuli (*21*). To examine whether T-cell activation alone might permit increased expression of genes under the control of the HTLV LTR sequences, we transfected the HTLV-CAT and control plasmids into an HTLV-negative immature human T-cell line, Jurkat, both in the presence and absence of the T-cell mitogen phytohemagglutinin (PHA) (*18*). The Jurkat cell line displays many of the responses typical of activated T cells when treated with PHA (*18*). No effect of PHA stimulation on the relative levels of CAT activity directed by any of the plasmids was observed (data not shown). We conclude that mitogenic activation of T cells is probably insufficient to account for the stimulation of CAT activity in infected cells transfected with the HTLV-CAT plasmids.

Activity of the HTLV-II LTR. To determine if the HTLV-II LTR sequences could function in a cell line producing type II virus, the plasmids were transfected into the C3-44 cell line. C3-44 is an HTLV-II–producing cell line established by immortalization of primary lymphocytes following cocultivation with cells derived from an HTLV-II–infected individual (*18*). In this cell line, the level of CAT activity produced by both pU3R-II and pU3-II was approximately 40 times that of the same cells transfected with pSV2CAT DNA. Evidently, in the proper cellular environment, the HTLV-II LTR can function as an efficient transcriptional element.

The CAT activity of the plasmid containing the HTLV-I LTR sequence was also high, approximately 135 times that of pSV2CAT in C3-44 cells. The ratio of CAT activity directed by the plasmids containing the HTLV-I and -II sequences was 25:1 in HTLV-I–infected cells, and only 3:1 in HTLV-II–infected cells. This suggests the presence of *trans*-acting factors, that is, factors that can regulate the transcriptional activity of DNA molecules other than those that encode them. The *trans*-acting factors in HTLV-I–infected cells appear to differ from those of HTLV-II–infected cells in the ability to act on HTLV LTR sequences of different types. The high CAT activity in HTLV-infected cells might thus be a consequence of viral infection rather than of the specific type of cell infected.

A test for viral-associated trans-*acting factors.* To test the possibility that the high CAT production in cells containing HTLV proviruses could be attributed to the virus infection, we examined the ability of the plasmids containing the HTLV LTR sequences to function in uninfected (HOS) and HTLV-I–infected (HOS/PL) human osteogenic sarcoma cells (*22*). The HOS/PL cells were derived in vitro by cocultivation of HOS cells with HTLV-I–producing lymphocytes and do not express T-cell markers (*22*). The data of Table 1 and Fig. 2 show that the CAT activity induced by pU3R-I in the HOS/PL cells was more than 90 times that in uninfected cells. Neither HOS nor HOS/PL cells transfected with the plasmids containing HTLV-II LTR sequences expressed significant CAT activity.

We therefore conclude that *trans*-acting factors in HTLV-infected cells, either encoded directly by the virus or induced by viral infection, augment gene expression directed by the HTLV LTR sequences. This effect is not observed upon transfection of these plasmids into murine T lymphocytes infected with nonacute murine leukemia viruses (*23*). The expression of the *neo* gene directed by the HTLV-II LTR as reported by Chen *et al.* (*24*) is probably due to *trans*-acting factors present in the HTLV-II–infected recipient cells and not only due to tissue type-specific elements as they suggest.

Trans-*activation of transcription.* To determine if the *trans*-acting stimulation of CAT expression reflects increased transcription, RNA was isolated from transfected HOS and HOS/PL cells and analyzed by Northern blotting (*25*) with a probe derived from the CAT coding region (Fig. 3). No discrete transcripts of the expected size (1.6 to 1.7 kilobases) were detected in either HOS or HOS/PL cells transfected with pU3-II. Low but approximately equal amounts of CAT RNA were detected in HOS and HOS/PL cells transfected with pSV2CAT, consistent with the nearly equal amounts of DNA uptake and CAT activity seen in these matched cell types (see Fig. 2). With pU3R-I, however, the amount of CAT RNA in HOS/PL cells was markedly increased relative to that in HOS cells transfected in parallel. This increase probably occurred at the level of RNA transcription initiation. It could be argued that differences in the 5′ structure of CAT RNA affect the stability of the message in HTLV-infected cells. We think this is unlikely because *trans*-activation in HTLV-II–infected cells occurs with plasmids pU3R-I, pU3R-II, and pU3-II, which differ substantially in R region sequence and, therefore, in the leader sequence of the CAT transcripts. Moreover, we find that a plasmid containing a sequence rearrangement 5′ of the pU3R-I promoter (TATA box), but that leaves the known RNA transcriptional start site (2) unaltered, directs the same level of CAT activity in both uninfected and HTLV-infected cells (26). Thus, the *trans*-acting stimulation of HTLV LTR-directed gene expression must affect sequences distant from those present in the CAT transcripts, showing that the *trans*-activation is mediated at the level of initiation of RNA transcription.

Discussion

The phenomenon of *trans*-activation distinguishes HTLV from other non-acute transforming retroviruses. The ability of HTLV-I and -II to immortalize primary lymphocytes in vitro, the apparent absence of preferential integration sites in HTLV-induced tumors, and the

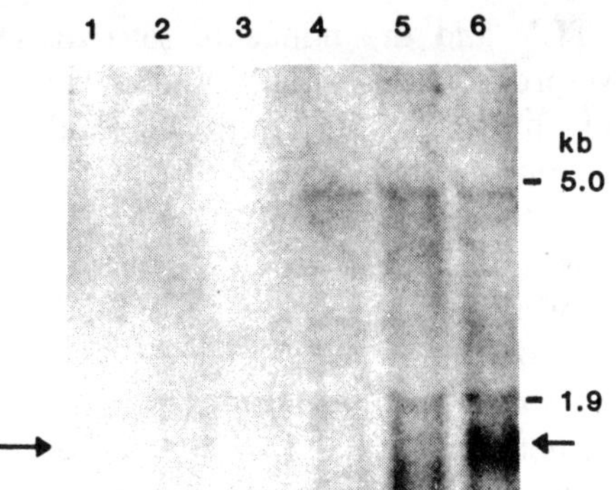

Fig. 3. Northern blot analysis of CAT messages in transfected cells. Approximately 2 × 10⁶ HOS or HOS/PL cells were transfected with 5 μg of pU3R-I, pU3-II, or pSV2CAT DNA by using calcium phosphate–DNA coprecipitation. Forty-eight hours after transfection, RNA was isolated. Fifty micrograms of total cellular RNA was sized on a denaturing gel, transferred to nitrocellulose, and hybridized to a nick-translated probe made from the Hind III–Bam HI CAT fragment as described (25). Nonspecific hybridization serves to identify the positions of the 28*S* and 18*S* ribosomal bands. Lanes 1 to 3 represent RNA from HOS cells, and lanes 4 to 6 from HOS/PL cells. Cells were transfected with pU3-II DNA (lanes 1 and 4), pSV2CAT DNA (lanes 2 and 5), or pU3R-I DNA (lanes 3 and 6). Arrows indicate the expected position of CAT messages with appropriate start and termination sites. Since the message sizes differ only minimally between the plasmids, comparison of hybridization signals between adjacent bands is appropriate. After Northern transfer, the nitrocellulose filter was stained with methylene blue to ensure equal transfer between lanes.

absence of chronic viremia also distinguish these viruses from most others (*19–21, 27–29*). The genome of HTLV also differs from the genomes of non-acute retroviruses by the presence of a long, 1600-base sequence located between the 3′ end of the envelope gene and the LTR (*30*).

To explain the differences in the structure and biological activity between

HTLV and the nonacute retroviruses, we propose that an HTLV-encoded protein mediates transcriptional regulation in *trans*, either directly via interaction with the HTLV LTR or indirectly via induction of cellular genes that effect the transcription of genes under HTLV LTR control.

Trans-acting transcriptional regulatory elements might alter the expression not only of viral genes but also cellular genes. One possibility is that in T cells, HTLV-I and -II regulate cellular genes that control proliferation, whereas HTLV-III regulates genes that terminate cell growth. In this regard, we note that the receptor for T-cell growth factor (interleukin-2), the HT3 gene product, and the JD-15 product are regularly expressed at high levels in lymphocytes infected with HTLV-I or -II (*18*). The specificity of HTLV transformation for the OKT4$^+$ (helper-inducer) subset of T lymphocytes may result from a restricted ability of the *trans*-acting transcriptional element to regulate growth control in specific differentiated T-cell subpopulations. Expression of a viral protein that mediates the biological effects of HTLV infection provides a natural explanation for the ability of HTLV-I and -II to transform cells in vitro and for the absence of preferential integration sites in tumor cells. We call this hypothesis the *trans*-acting transcriptional regulation hypothesis. The transforming proteins of some DNA tumor viruses, notably adenovirus and SV40, also activate expression of viral and cellular genes in *trans* (*31, 32*).

What might the identity of the virus-induced *trans*-acting product be? We note that the level of CAT activity directed by the HTLV-I LTR in the C81-66-45 line is comparable to the high activity in HTLV producer cells. Since the C81-66-45 line produces no virus, yet contains a 42-kilodalton viral protein precipitable by human antiserum to HTLV (*33*) the production of this protein may be sufficient to maintain the *trans*-activation phenomenon. In a separate study, we have shown that the region located between the envelope gene and the 3' LTR of both HTLV-I and HTLV-II can encode a polypeptide of about this size (*34*). This coding region includes sequences that are highly conserved (approximately 75 percent identical) in the two virus types, but the immediate flanking sequences are almost entirely divergent. The predicted amino acid sequences of these proteins are 77 percent identical. A subgenomic spliced 2.2-kilobase mRNA species that contains the 3' sequences, but not the *gag, pol*, or *env* genes, has been detected in HTLV-producing cells and in some fresh HTLV-associated tumors (*35, 36*). It is possible that this region encodes the 42-kilodalton protein seen in the C81-66-45 line, and that this protein mediates the *trans*-acting transcriptional effects of HTLV infection.

The T-cell malignancies associated with HTLV-I and HTLV-II infection differ in their clinical aggressiveness (*1, 2*). Here we have demonstrated marked differences in the ability of the HTLV-I and HTLV-II LTR sequences to direct CAT expression in a range of differentiated cell types. The number and type of cells infected by these different groups of HTLV may vary as a consequence of differences in LTR promoter strength, host cell range, or response to *trans*-acting transcriptional factors. The level of a viral protein effecting lymphocyte transformation may vary in a critical target cell as a result of differences in

LTR function. Further work to identify the HTLV-associated *trans*-acting factor, as well as its target sequences in the viral and host cell genome, should provide insight into the mechanism of transformation by this family of retroviruses.

References and Notes

1. B. J. Poiesz *et al.*, *Proc. Natl. Acad. Sci. U.S.A.* **77**, 7415 (1980); V. S. Kalyanaraman, M. Sarngadharan, P. Bunn, J. Minna, R. C. Gallo, *Nature (London)* **294**, 271 (1981); M. Robert-Guroff, F. Ruscetti, L. Posner, B. Poiesz, R. C. Gallo, *J. Exp. Med.* **154**, 1957 (1981); M. Yoshida, I. Miyoshi, Y. Hinuma, *Proc. Natl. Acad. Sci. U.S.A.* **79**, 2031 (1982).
2. V. S. Kalyanaraman *et al.*, *Science* **218**, 571 (1982); I. S. Y. Chen, J. McLaughlin, J. C. Gasson, S. C. Clark, D. S. Golde, *Nature (London)* **305**, 502 (1983); E. P. Gelmann, G. Franchini, V. Manzari, F. Wong-Staal, R. C. Gallo, *Proc. Natl. Acad. Sci. U.S.A.* **81**, 993 (1984); G. M. Shaw *et al.*, *ibid.*, in press; K. Shimotohno, D. W. Golde, M. Miwa, T. Sugimura, I. S. Y. Chen, *ibid.* **81**, 1079 (1984); J. G. Sodroski *et al.*, *ibid.*, in press; M. Seiki, S. Hattori, M. Yoshida, *ibid.* **79**, 6899 (1982).
3. M. Popovic *et al.*, *Nature (London)* **300**, 63 (1982).
4. M. Popovic, M. G. Sarngadharan, E. Read, R. C. Gallo, *Science* **224**, 497 (1984); R. C. Gallo *et al.*, *ibid.*, p. 500; J. Schüpbach *et al.*, *ibid.*, p. 503; M. Sarngadharan, M. Popovic, L. Bruch, J. Schüpbach, R. C. Gallo, *ibid.*, p. 506.
5. P. A. Chatis, C. A. Holland, J. W. Hartley, W. P. Rowe, N. Hopkins, *Proc. Natl. Acad. Sci. U.S.A.* **80**, 4408 (1983); L. DesGroseillers, E. Rassart, P. Jolicoeur, *ibid.*, p. 4203; J. Lenz *et al.*, *Nature (London)* **308**, 467 (1984); D. Celander and W. A. Haseltine, in preparation; C. Rosen, M. Cloyd, J. Lenz, W. A. Haseltine, in preparation.
6. H. M. Temin, *Cell* **27**, 1 (1981); *ibid.* **28**, 3 (1982).
7. C. M. Gorman, L. F. Moffat, B. H. Howard, *Mol. Cell Biol.* **2**, 1044 (1982); C. M. Gorman, G. T. Merlino, M. C. Willingham, I. Pastan, B. Howard, *Proc. Natl. Acad. Sci. U.S.A.* **79**, 6777 (1982).
8. F. L. Graham and A. J. van der Eb, *J. Virol.* **52**, 456 (1973); C. Queen and D. Baltimore, *Cell* **33**, 729 (1983).
9. M. D. Walker, T. Edlund, A. M. Boulet, W. J. Rutter, *Nature (London)* **306**, 557 (1983).
10. G. J. Todaro and H. Green, *J. Cell Biol.* **17**, 299 (1963).
11. F. C. Jensen *et al.*, *Proc. Natl. Acad. Sci. U.S.A.* **53**, 53 (1964).
12. G. O. Gey, W. D. Coffman, M. T. Kubicek, *Cancer Res.* **12**, 264 (1952).
13. B. Royer-Pokora, W. D. Peterson, W. A. Haseltine, *Exp. Cell Res.* **151**, 408 (1984).
14. B. Howard, M. Estes, J. Pagano, *Biochim. Biophys. Acta* **228**, 105 (1971); A. Loyter, G. A. Scangos, F. H. Ruddle, *Proc. Natl. Acad. Sci. U.S.A.* **79**, 422 (1982).
15. P. J. Southern and P. Berg, *Mol. Appl. Genet.* **1**, 227 (1982).
16. R. C. Gallo *et al.*, *Proc. Natl. Acad. Sci. U.S.A.* **79**, 5680 (1982).
17. N. Yamamoto, T. Matsumoto, Y. Koyanagi, Y. Tanaka, Y. Hinuma, *Nature (London)* **299**, 367 (1982); S. Z. Salahuddin and R. C. Gallo, personal communication.
18. V. Manzari *et al.*, *Proc. Natl. Acad. Sci. U.S.A.* **80**, 11 (1983); M. Popovic *et al.*, in preparation.
19. I. Miyoshi *et al.*, *Nature (London)* **294**, 770 (1981).
20. S. Z. Salahuddin *et al.*, *Virology* **129**, 51 (1983); B. Hahn *et al.*, *Nature (London)* **303**, 253 (1983).
21. M. Popovic, G. Lange-Wantzin, P. S. Sarin, D. Mann, R. C. Gallo, *Proc. Natl. Acad. Sci. U.S.A.* **80**, 5402 (1983).
22. P. Clapham, K. Nagy, R. Cheingsong-Popov, M. Exley, R. W. Weiss, *Science* **222**, 1125 (1983).
23. J. G. Sodroski *et al.*, unpublished data.
24. I. S. Y. Chen, J. McLaughlin, D. W. Golde, *Nature (London)* **309**, 276 (1984).
25. P. S. Thomas, *Proc. Natl. Acad. Sci. U.S.A.* **77**, 5201 (1980).
26. C. A. Rosen, J. G. Sodroski, W. A. Haseltine, in preparation.
27. B. Hahn, V. Manzari, S. Colombini, G. Franchini, R. C. Gallo, F. Wong-Staal, *Nature (London)* **305**, 340 (1983).
28. R. C. Gallo and F. Wong-Staal, *Blood* **60**, 545 (1982).
29. N. Yamamoto, M. Okada, Y. Koyanagi, M. Kannagi, Y. Hinuma, *Science* **217**, 737 (1982).
30. M. Seiki, S. Hattori, Y. Hirayama, M. Yoshida, *Proc. Natl. Acad. Sci. U.S.A.* **80**, 3618 (1983).
31. J. Brady, J. B. Bolen, M. Radonovich, N. Salzman, G. Khoury, *ibid.* **81**, 2040 (1984).
32. N. Jones and T. Shenk, *ibid.* **76**, 3665 (1979); J. R. Nevins, *Cell* **26**, 213 (1981); A. Berk, F. Lee, T. Harrison, J. Williams, P. A. Sharp, *ibid.* **17**, 935 (1979); R. B. Gaynor, D. Hillman, A. Berk, *Proc. Natl. Acad. Sci. U.S.A.* **81**, 1193 (1984).
33. T. H. Lee and M. Essex, personal communication.
34. W. A. Haseltine *et al.*, *Science* **225**, 419 (1984).
35. V. Manzari *et al.*, *Proc. Natl. Acad. Sci. U.S.A.* **80**, 1574 (1983).
36. G. Franchini, F. Wong-Staal, R. C. Gallo, in preparation.
37. We thank R. C. Gallo, F. Wong-Staal, S. Z. Salahuddin, D. Celander, R. Weiss, C. Gorman, B. Howard, and M. Essex for helpful discussions and materials. Supported by a Director's Grant from the American Cancer Society. J.G.S. and C.A.R. were supported by postdoctoral fellowships from the National Institutes of Health.

18 May 1984; accepted 21 June 1984

Report

27 July 1984

43.   Structure of 3′ Terminal Region of Type II Human T Lymphotropic Virus: Evidence for New Coding Region

William A. Haseltine, Joseph Sodroski, Roberto Patarca, Debra Briggs, Dennis Perkins, and Flossie Wong-Staal

The human T lymphotropic viruses (HTLV) are a family of retroviruses that are associated with T-cell abnormalities (*1*). Isolates known as HTLV-I are associated with an aggressive form of adult T-cell leukemia or lymphoma (*1*). An infrequent isolate known as HTLV-II was first identified in a patient with a T-cell variant of hairy cell leukemia (*2*). Recently, some viruses collectively called HTLV-III were isolated from patients with the acquired immune deficiency syndrome (*3*).

The genomes of HTLV-I and -II differ from those of the nonacute retroviruses, which encode only the *gag*, *pol*, and *env* genes, in that they have an additional sequence that is approximately 1600 nucleotides long. This sequence is located between the 3′ end of the *env* gene and the 5′ end of the U3 region of the proviral long terminal repeat (LTR) (*4*).

Although this sequence occupies a position similar to the *src* gene in Rous sarcoma virus, it is not homologous to conserved mammalian genes and therefore differs from the oncogenes of transforming retroviruses (*4*). There is some evidence that this region contains a functional gene. Heteroduplex analysis of HTLV-I and -II reveals a conserved sequence about 1000 nucleotides long near the 3′ terminus of the genome (*5*). Spliced messenger RNA (mRNA) species that contain sequences that are unique to the 5′ end of the viral genome (U5 LTR sequences) and a portion of the 3′ sequence are observed in HTLV-infected cells and in some fresh tumor cells (*6*). Seiki *et al.* (*4*) note that several open reading frames occur within the 3′ sequence of HTLV-I.

To obtain a clearer understanding of the potential role of the 3′ region of HTLV, we determined the primary nucleotide sequence of the region located between the 3′ end of the *env* gene and the LTR of a cloned HTLV-II provirus, MO15A (*7*).

The nucleotide sequence of 1557 bases of the 3′ terminal region of HTLV-II is presented in Fig. 1. This sequence can be divided into two regions. One region, 546 nucleotides long, is located at the 5′ end of the sequence and has either no or very little similarity to the corresponding sequences in HTLV-I. For this reason we call this sequence the nonconserved region (NCR). A second region, 1011 nucleotides long, comprises the 3′ portion of this sequence. This sequence is very similar to that of HTLV-I and is identical at 765 of 1011 nucleotides (76 percent identity).

A new gene? The perimeters of the 1011 nucleotide sequence of the HTLV-II genome correspond precisely with a single long open reading frame capable of encoding a polypeptide 337 amino acids long. A corresponding sequence of HTLV-I also encompasses a single long open reading frame capable of encoding a polypeptide 357 amino acids long. We call the nucleotide sequence containing these long open reading frames the LOR region (nucleotides 566 to 1557 in HTLV-II) (Fig. 1).

The predicted amino acid sequences of both polypeptides are presented in Fig. 1. The potential proteins encoded by the LOR regions of HTLV-I and -II are of approximately the same length and are identical in 259 of 337 of the amino acids (77 percent identity). The degree of similarity of these two proteins is even more striking if conservative amino acid substitutions are considered (89 percent similar). The distribution of hydrophilic and hydrophobic regions of these proteins is remarkably similar (Fig. 2).

We also note the existence of a splice acceptor consensus sequence located at the 5′ end of the open reading frame (Fig. 1). Although no methionine codon occurs at the 5′ end of the open reading frames of HTLV-I and -II, a fusion protein synthesized from a spliced mRNA can be envisioned. Several other splice acceptor sequences occur within this reading frame from which smaller fusion proteins might also be made.

These observations suggest that the 3′ terminal region of HTLV contains a new gene that encodes a protein with a molecular weight of at least 38,000. Such a protein could be translated from the 2.2-kb spliced mRNA species containing LOR sequences found in HTLV-infected cells (6). A protein of molecular weight 38,000 to 42,000 in HTLV-I–infected cell lines has been noted that is recognized by the serum of persons infected with HTLV-I, but not by serum from control subjects (8).

Several other open reading frames exist in the region between the *env* gene and the LTR of both HTLV-I and -II. Seiki *et al.* (4) have identified four such regions, pX I to pX IV. The pX IV region corresponds to the carboxyl terminus of the peptide that could be encoded by the LOR region. No region of predicted protein similarity could be found in HTLV-II that corresponds to pX I or pX III. A further argument against the functional importance of pX I is that an 11-nucleotide deletion that destroys the pX I open reading frame occurs in an HTLV-Ic isolate with apparently complete biological activity (9). Another open reading frame in the LOR region of HTLV-II (nucleotides 530 to 1325) includes a region exhibiting 65 percent amino acid homology to pX II. The significance of this similarity is not clear, because the pX II peptide is much shorter than the corresponding peptide in HTLV-II (87 compared to 265 amino acids). Sequence similarity here could arise as a result of conservation of the LOR protein in the other open reading frame.

We have also reported (8) that *trans*-acting factors, either directly encoded by HTLV or induced by HTLV infection, substantially augment gene expression directed by HTLV LTR sequences. The phenomenon of *trans*-activation distinguishes HTLV from other retroviruses. The unusual structure of the 3′ terminus of HTLV also distinguishes these from most other retroviruses. For this reason, we suggest that the protein encoded by the LOR region may mediate transcriptional changes observed in HTLV-infected cells. In this regard, we note that transcription directed by the HTLV-I

```
HTLV-II  ACCTGCTAGCTTCTGCAGCAAATCCCCATGGTTCGTCCCCCACCATTGACCCATCCACAGTCCTCTATACCAGATGAGTCGCCCCCGATGTTCCAGCCCG  100
HTLV-I   ACCAAGCACGCAATTATTGCAACCACATCGCCTCCAGCCTCCCCTGCCAATAATTAACCTCTCCCATCAAATCCTCCTTCTCCTGCAGCAACTTCCTCCT

         GACTCGAACTGAATAATTGCCTCAAATAGTTCCTCTAACCCCCGCTCACATTCCTCCCATAGGACCTTCTTTTCCCCTTCAAGGAAATCCACATAACCCT  200
         TTCAGCCTCCAAGGACTCCACCTCGCCTTCCAACTGTCTAGTCTAGCCATCAATCCCCAACTCCTGCATTTTTTCTTTCCTAGCACTATGCTGTTTCGCC

         GAAGCAAGTCACAAAACCCATCAAAACCAAGGAGTCCTATACACTCCAACTGCTGATGCCTTTCTTCCCTCTCCCGGCGCTTTTGATCCTTTTCCCGCGG  300
         TTCTCAGCCCCTTGTCTCCACTTGCGCTCACGGCGCTCCTGCTCTTCCTGCTTCCTCCTAGCGACGTCAGCGGCCTTCTTCTCCGCCCGCCTCCTGCGCC

         CGCTCCTTTCTGCGCCGCTCCCGCTCCTCACGCTCCTGCAGAAGTTTTAAGATCTCCCGCTGCTCCTCCGCCAACAGTCTCCGACGAGAGTCTCGCACCT  400
         GTGCCTTCTCCTCTTCCTTCCTTTTCAAATACTCAGCGGTCTGCTTTTCCTCCTCTTTCTCCCGCTCTTTTTTTCGCTTCCTCTTCTCCTCAGCCCGTCG

         GCTCGCTGACCGATCCCGACCCCAGAGGGCGGACCTTTTTGCTGTGTCCTTCTCGGTTCCTCTCCAGGGGGAGGCACACCAGATGTGAGACTCGCCTCTCCCT  500
         CTGCCGATCACGATGCGTTTCCCCGCGAGGTGGCGGCTTTCTCCCCTGGAGGGCCCCGTCGCAGCCGGCCGCGGGCTTTCCTCTTCTAAGGATAGCAAACCG

         GGTCTCCTAACGGCAATCTCCTAAAATAGTCTAAAAAATCACACA..................................................  545
         TCAAGCACAGCTTCCTCCTCCTCCTTGTCCTTTAACTCTTCCTCCAAGGATAATAGCCCGTCCACCCAATTCCTCCACCAGCAGGTCCTCCGGGCATGAC
```

Splice
acceptor

```
         ....................TAATTACAATCCTGTCTCCTCTCAGCCCATTTCCTAGGATTTGGACAGAGCCTCCTATATGGATACCC  613
                            L Q [S C L L S A H F] L [G F G Q S L L Y G Y P]
                                [P C L L S A H F] P [G F G Q S L L F G Y P]
         ACAGGCAAGCATCGAAACAGCCCTGCAGATACAAAGTTAACCATGCTTATTATCAGCCCACTTCCCAGGGTTTGGACAGAGTCTTCTTTTCGGATACCC

         CGTCTACGTGTTTGGCAATTGTGTACAGGCCGATTGGTGTCCCGTCTCAGGTGGTCTATGTTCCACCCGCCTACATCGACATGCCCTCCTGGCCACCTG  713
         [V Y V F G N] [C V Q A D W C P V S G G L C S T R L H R H A L L A T C]
         [V Y V F G D] [C V Q G D W C P I S G G L C S A R L H R H A L L A T C]
         AGTCTACGTGTTTGGAGACTGTGTACAAGGCGACTGGTGCCCCATCTCTGGGGGACTATGTTCGGCCCGCCTACATCGTCACGCCCTACTGGCCACCTG

         TCCAGAGCACCAACTCACATGGGACCCCATCGATGGACGCGGTTGTCAGCTCTCCTCTCCAATACCTTATCCCTCGCCTCCCCTCCTTCCCCACCCAGAG  813
         [P E H Q L T W D P I D G R V V S] [S P L Q Y L I P R L P S F F P T Q R]
         [P E H Q I T W D P I D G R V I G] [S A L Q F L I P R L P S F P T Q R]
         TCCAGAGCATCAGATCACCTGGGACCCCATCGATGGACGCGTTATCGGCTCAGCTCTACAGTTCCTTATCCCTCGACTCCCCTCCTTCCCCACCCAGAG

         AACCTCAAGGACCCTCAAGGTCCTTACCCCTCCCACCACTCCTGTCTCCCCCAAGGTTCCACCTGCCTTCTTTCAATCAATGCGAAAGCACACCCCCTA  913
         [T S R] [T L K V L T P P T T P V S] [P K V P P A F F] [Q S M R K H T P Y]
         [T S K] [T L K V L T P P I T H T T P N I P P S F L] [Q A M R K Y S P F]
         AACCTCTAAGACCCTCAAGGTCCTTACCCCGCCAATCACTCATCAACCCCCAACATTCCACCCTCCTTCCTCCAGGCCATGCCGCAAATACTCCCCCTT

         CCGAAATGGATGCCTGGAACCAACCCTCGGGGATCAGCTCCCCTCCCTCGCCTTCCCCGAACCTGGCCTCCGTCCCCAAAACATCTACACCACTGGGC  1013
         [R N G C L E P T L G D Q L P S L A F P] E [P G L R P Q N I Y T T W G]
         [R N G Y M E P T L G Q H L P T L S F P] D [P G L R P Q N L Y T L W G]
         CCGAAATGGATACATGGAACCCACCCTTGGGCAGCACCTCCCAACCCTGTCTTTTCCAGACCCGGACTCCGGCCACAAAACCTGTACCCCTCTGGGG

         AAAAACCGTAGTATGCCTATACCTATACCAGCTTTCCCCACCCATGACATGGCCACTTATACCCCATGTCATATTCTGCCACCCCAGACAATTAGGAGC  1113
         [K T V V C L] [Y L Y Q L S P P] M [T W P L I P H V I F C H P R Q L G A]
         [G S V V C M] [Y L Y Q L S P P I] [T W P L L P H V I F C H P G Q L G A]
         AGGCTCCGTTGTCTGCATGTACCTCTACCAGCTTTCCCCCCCCATCACCTGGCCCCTCCTGCCCCACGTGATTTTTTGCCACCCCGGCCAGCTCGGGGG

         CTTCCTCACCAAGGTGCCTCTAAAACGATTAGAAGAACTTCTATACAAAATGTTCCTACACACAGGGGCAGTCATAGTCCTCCCGGAGGACGACCTACC  1213
         [F L T K V P L] [K R L E E L L Y K M F] [L H T G A V I V L P E D] D L P
         [F L T N V P Y] [K R I E E L L Y K I S] [L T T G A L I I L P E D] C L P
         CTTCCTCACCAATGTTCCCTACAAGCGAATAGAAGAACTCCTCTATAAAATTTCCCTCACCACAGGGGCCCTAATAATTCTACCCGAAGACTGTTTGCC

         CACCACAATGTTCCAACCCGTGAGGGCTCCCTGTATCCAGACTGCCTGGTGTACAGGACTTCTCCCCTATCACTCCATCTTAACAACCCCAGGTCTAAT  1313
         [T T M] [F Q P V R A P C] [I Q T A W] C T [G L L P Y H S] [I L T T P G L I]
         [T T L] [F Q P A R A P V] [T L T A W] Q N [G L L P F H S] T [L T T P G L I]
         CACCACCCTTTTCCAGCCTGCTAGGGCACCCGTCACGCTAACAGCCTGGCAAAACGGCCTCCTTCCGTTCCACTCAACCCTCACCACTCCAGGCCTTAT

         ATGGACCTTCAATGACGGCTCACCAATGATTTCCGGCCCTTGCCCCAAAGCAGGGCAGCCATCTTTAGTAGTTCAGTCCTCCCTATTAATCTTCGAAAA  1413
         [W T F N D G S P M I S G P C P K] A [G Q P S L V V Q S S L L I F E K]
         [W T F T D G T P M I S G P C P K] D [G Q P S L V L Q S S S F I F H K]
         TTGGACATTTACCGATGGCACGCCTATGATTTCCGGGCCCTGCCCTAAAGATGGCCAGCCATCTTTCGTACTACAGTCCTCCTCCTTTATATTTCACAA

         ATTCCAAACCAAAGCCTTCCATCCCTCCTATCTACTCTCTCATCAGCTTATACAATACTCCTCCTTTCATAACCTTCACCTTCTATTCGATGAATACAC  1513
         [F Q T K A F H P S Y L L S H Q L I Q Y S S F H N L H L L F D E Y T]
         [F Q T K A Y H P S F L L S H G L I Q Y S S F H S L H L L F E E Y T]
         ATTTCAAACCAAGGCCTACCACCCCTCATTTCTACTCTCACACGGCCTCATACAGTACTCTTCCTTTCATAGTTTACATCTCCTGTTTGAAGAATACAC

         CAACATCCCTGTCTCTATTTTATTTAATAAAGAAGAGGCGGATGACAATGGCGACTAG.............................  1557
         [N I P V S I L F N K E E A D D N] G D .
         [N I P I S L L F N E K E A D D N] D H E P Q I S P G G L E P P S E K
         CAACATCCCCATTTCTCTACTTTTTAACGAAAAAGAGGCAGATGACAATGACCATGAGCCCCAAATATCCCCCGGGGGCTTAGAGCCTCCCAGTGAAAA
```

5' end of
LTR

```
         ......................
         H F R E T E V .
         ACATTTCCGAGAAACAGAAGTCTGA
```

LTR is activated to high levels in a cell line, C81-66, that expresses the 42,000-dalton HTLV-I–associated protein but not HTLV *gag*, *pol*, or *env* products (*8*). We further suggest that the HTLV LOR product mediates both the *trans*-activating and transforming effects of HTLV infection. We note that *trans*-acting transcriptional activities have been associated with the transforming genes of other tumor viruses, notably adenovirus and SV40 (*10, 11*). The existence of a potential transforming function within the HTLV genome may explain the ability of the virus to transform cells in vitro, as well as the absence of specific integration sites in tumor cells and the absence of chronic viremia in target tissues (*12–14*). Such a transforming function would differ from that of other retroviruses because, unlike the oncogenes, the sequence that encodes the putative transforming gene will not anneal to the highly conserved cellular sequences (*4*).

Comparison with the bovine leukemia virus genome. We noticed that the 3′ genome of another retrovirus, bovine leukemia virus (BLV), also contains an LOR frame located 3′ to the envelope glycoprotein gene that could encode a protein of a size similar to that of HTLV (*15, 16*) (Fig. 2). There is evidence for the existence of a subgenomic spliced mRNA species that contains the 3′ open reading frame but not the *gag*, *pol*, and *env* gene sequences in BLV-producing cell lines (*17*).

Although the similarity in structure of the HTLV and BLV proteins is insufficient to indicate that they have a common functional role, the overall similarity in genomic structure, including the location of a 5′ NCR and 3′ LOR frame, and the previously described similarity in protein antigenicity of the two viruses (*1, 14*) suggests that they are functionally similar. Moreover, there is a similarity in the distribution of hydrophobic and hydrophilic regions of the HTLV and BLV polypeptides. We note that the disease induced by BLV has characteristics similar to those associated with HTLV-I, namely, a long latent period sometimes preceded by persistent lymphocytosis, an absence of chronic viremia in target organs preceding disease, and an absence of preferred integration sites in tumor cells (*18*). These features could be expected of viruses that contain an LOR product mediating transformation.

Fig. 1 (facing page) Nucleotide sequence of the HTLV-II 3′ terminal region and predicted amino acid sequence of its potential product. Plasmid DNA containing the 3′ portion of MO15A, an HTLV-II proviral clone (*7*), was cleaved with either Cla I or Bgl II, which cut the plasmid uniquely at a single site. After timed digestion with Bal 31 exonuclease, the ends were blunted with T4 DNA polymerase and synthetic linkers were added prior to recloning. Linker sites separated by increments of 100 to 200 nucleotides were end-labeled and the fragments sequenced by the method of Maxam and Gilbert (*19*). The sequence of the 3′ portion following the termination codon for the envelope gene is presented for HTLV-II and HTLV-I. The HTLV-II sequence is numbered according to the nucleotides following the envelope to stop codon. Asterisks represent differences between the DNA sequences. The positions of a conserved splice acceptor consensus sequence and the 5′ end of the LTR are noted. Note that the sequence is not well conserved 5′ to the putative splice acceptor site but is very well conserved 3′ to this site. The latter sequence corresponds to a long open reading frame (LOR) region. The predicted amino acid sequences of the potential products of the HTLV-I and HTLV-II 3′ open reading frames are optimally aligned. Boxed regions indicate amino acid identity or conservative amino acid substitutions between the sequences.

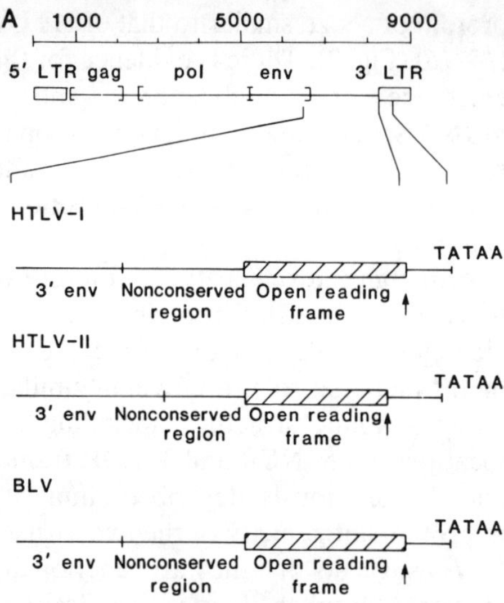

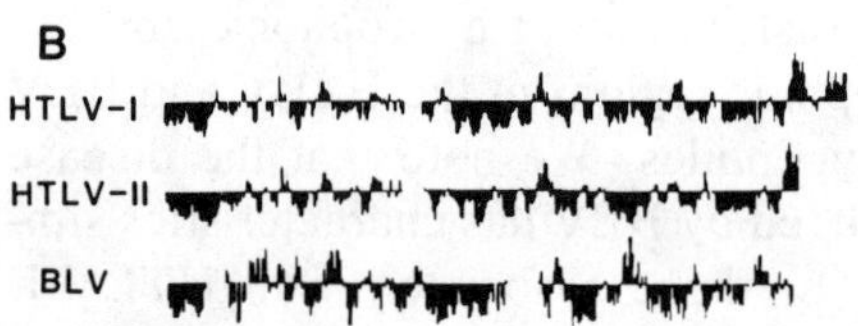

Fig. 2. The open reading frames of the HTLV and BLV genomes. (A) The position of 3' open reading frames in the genomes of HTLV-I and -II and of BLV. The 3' end of the envelope gene is shown, as well as the 5' terminus of the LTR ($\uparrow$) and the promoter (TATAA) sequence. The positions of the nonconserved regions and the open reading frames (hatched boxes) are displayed. (B) The relative hydrophilicity of the 3' open reading frame products of HTLV-I, HTLV-II, and BLV calculated according to the method of Hopp and Woods (20). Hydrophilic regions are shown above the axis, hydrophobic regions below. Dotted lines represent gaps introduced to maintain maximal alignment of protein sequence.

The biology, structure, and pathology of HTLV and BLV differ from other transforming retroviruses such that we propose that they be considered a new subgroup of retroviruses distinct from both the nonacute transforming viruses that contain only the *gag*, *pol*, and *env* genes and the acute transforming viruses that encode oncogenes.

References and Notes

1. B. J. Poiesz *et al.*, *Proc. Natl. Acad. Sci. U.S.A.* **77**, 7415 (1980); V. S. Kalyanaraman, M. Sargadharan, P. Bunn, J. Minna, R. C. Gallo, *Nature (London)* **294**, 271 (1981); M. Robert-Guroff *et al.*, *J. Exp. Med.* **154**, 1957 (1981); M. Yoshida, I. Miyoshi, Y. Hinuma, *Proc. Natl. Acad. Sci. U.S.A.* **79**, 2031 (1982).
2. V. S. Kalyanaraman *et al.*, *Science* **218**, 571 (1982).
3. M. Popovic, M. G. Sarngadharan, E. Read, R. C. Gallo, *Science* **224**, 497 (1984); R. C. Gallo *et al.*, *ibid.*, p. 500; J. Schüpbach *et al.*, *ibid.*, p. 503; M. Sarngadharan, M. Popovic, L. Bruch, J. Schüpbach, R. C. Gallo, *ibid.*, p. 506.
4. M. Seiki, S. Hattori, Y. Hirayama, M. Yoshida, *Proc. Natl. Acad. Sci. U.S.A.* **80**, 3618 (1983).
5. G. M. Shaw *et al.*, *ibid.*, in press.
6. G. Franchini, F. Wong-Staal, R. C. Gallo, in preparation.
7. E. P. Gelman, G. Franchini, V. Manzari, F. Wong-Staal, R. C. Gallo, *Proc. Natl. Acad. Sci. U.S.A.* **81**, 993 (1984).
8. J. Sodroski *et al.*, *Science* **225**, 421 (1984); T. H. Lee *et al.*, in preparation.
9. L. Ratner and F. Wong-Staal, in preparation.
10. J. Brady, J. B. Bolen, M. Radonovich, N. Salzman, G. Khoury, *Proc. Natl. Acad. Sci. U.S.A.* **81**, 2040 (1984).
11. N. Jones and T. Shenk, *ibid.* **76**, 3665 (1979); J. R. Nevins, *Cell* **26**, 213 (1981); A. Berk, F. Lee, T. Harrison, J. Williams, P. A. Sharp, *ibid.* **17**, 935 (1979); R. B. Gaynor, D. Hillman, A. Berk, *Proc. Natl. Acad. Sci. U.S.A.* **81** 1193 (1984).
12. I. Miyoshi *et al.*, *Nature (London)* **294**, 770 (1981); M. Popovic, G. Lange-Wantzin, P. S. Sarin, D. Mann, R. C. Gallo, *Proc. Natl. Acad. Sci. U.S.A.* **80**, 5402 (1983); N. Yamamoto, M. Okada, Y. Koyanagi, M. Kannagi, Y. Hinuma, *Science* **217**, 737 (1982).
13. B. Hahn *et al*, *Nature (London)* **305**, 340 (1983).
14. R. C. Gallo and F. Wong-Staal, *Blood* **60**, 545 (1982).
15. A. Burny, personal communication.
16. N. R. Rice *et al.*, *Virology*, in press.
17. J. Ghysdael, R. Kettmann, A. Burny, *J. Virol.* **29**, 1087 (1979).
18. J. F. Ferrer, D. A. Abt, D. M. Bhatt, R. R. Marshak, *Cancer Res.* **34**, 893 (1974); P. S. Paul *et al.*, *Am. J. Vet. Res.* **38**, 873 (1977); R. Kettmann *et al.*, *J. Virol.* **47**, 146 (1983); D. Gregoire *et al.*, *ibid.* **50**, 275 (1984); J. Deschamp, R. Kettman, A. Burny, *J. Virol.* **40**, 605 (1981); R. C. Gallo *et al.*, *Proc. Natl. Acad. Sci. U.S.A.* **79**, 5680 (1982).
19. A. Maxam and W. Gilbert, *Proc. Natl. Acad. Sci. U.S.A.* **74**, 564 (1977).
20. T. P. Hopp and K. R. Woods, *ibid.* **78**, 3824 (1981).
21. We thank A. Burny for providing the sequence of the 3' region of the BLV, N. R. Rice *et al.* for a preprint of their manuscript, and R. C. Gallo, M. Essex, and J. Coffin for helpful discussions. Supported by an American Cancer Society Directors Grant. J.G.S. was supported by NIH postdoctoral fellowship CA07094.

31 May 1984; accepted 21 June 1984

Report

27 July 1984

44. Sequence of the Envelope Glycoprotein Gene of Type II Human T Lymphotropic Virus

Joseph Sodroski, Roberto Patarca, Dennis Perkins, Debra Briggs, Tun-Hou Lee, Myron Essex, John Coligan, Flossie Wong-Staal, Robert C. Gallo, and William A. Haseltine

Human T-cell leukemia viruses have been implicated as the etiological agents of several human diseases. The most prevalent type, HTLV-I, is associated with a high incidence of an aggressive form of adult T-cell leukemia (ATLL) and several unusual forms of mycosis fungoides and Sezary syndrome (*1*). A second member of the family, HTLV-II, has been isolated from a patient with benign hairy cell leukemia of T-cell origin (*2*). Recently, a new group of viruses, HTLV-III, was isolated from patients with acquired immune deficiency syndrome (AIDS) (*3*).

The envelope glycoprotein is the major antigen recognized by the serum of persons infected with HTLV (*4*). In this respect HTLV resembles several other retroviruses for which the envelope glycoprotein is typically the most antigenic viral polypeptide (*5*). Moreover, most neutralizing antibodies are directed toward the envelope glycoproteins of retroviruses (*5, 6*).

The envelope glycoproteins of HTLV-I, HTLV-II, and HTLV-III have common antigenic determinants. Serum samples from patients infected with HTLV-II recognize the envelope glycoproteins of HTLV-I (*8*). Samples from AIDS patients, some of whom are known to be infected with HTLV-III, also frequently immunoprecipitate the envelope glycoproteins of HTLV-I and -II (*4, 7, 8*). These antigenic cross-reactions motivated us to a study of the HTLV-II envelope glycoprotein gene. Here we present the complete nucleotide sequence of this gene (Fig. 1).

The *env* gene sequence contains an open reading frame 484 amino acids long. The predicted amino acid sequence of the *env* glycoprotein precursor protein is shown in Fig. 2. The most direct evidence that the predicted sequence is the *env* gene is derived from the partial amino acid sequence of the amino terminal regions of the 67,000, 52,000, and 21,000 dalton glycoproteins (gp67, gp52, and gp21) seen in immunoprecipitates of HTLV-II–infected cells (*8*). These proteins represent the fully glycosylated envelope precursor, the processed exterior glycoprotein, and the transmembrane glycoprotein, respectively (*4, 8, 9*). The location of the cysteine and serine residues of the gp67 and gp52, and of the valine residues of gp21 relative to the amino termini, has been determined (*8*). There is an exact correspondence of the residues with the amino acids if one assumes that the amino terminus of the mature exterior glycoprotein is located at amino acid 21 in the precursor protein, and that the amino terminus of the trans-

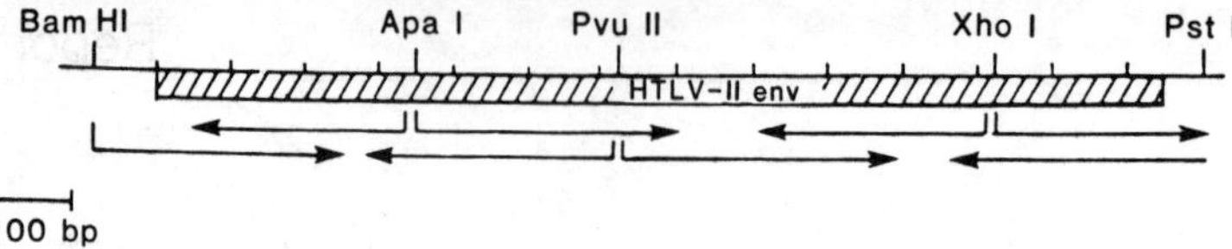

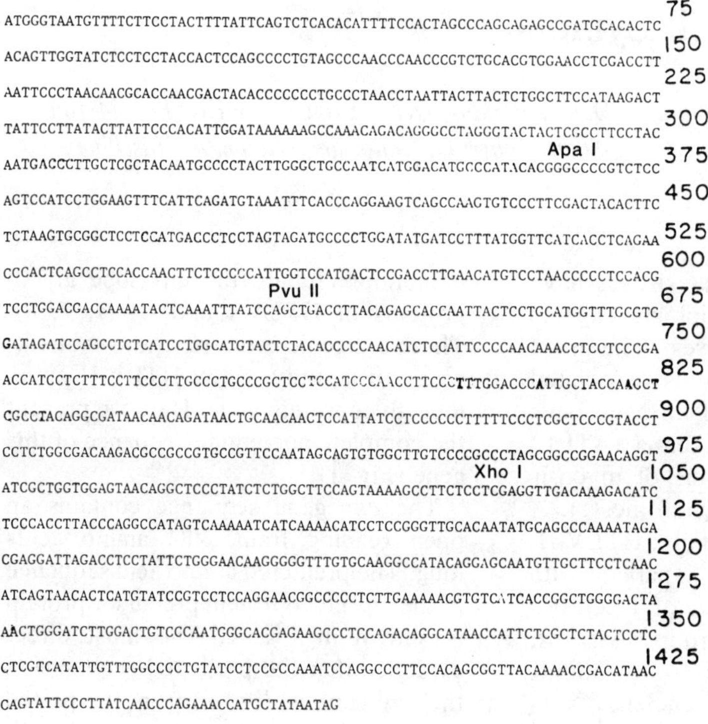

Fig. 1. Nucleotide sequence of the HTLV-II *env* gene. The strategy for sequencing the MO15A (*10*) *env* gene is shown in the top figure. Sites depicted were 5′ and 3′ end-labeled and sequenced according to the procedure of Maxam and Gilbert (*11*). The lower figure depicts the nucleotide sequence of the entire envelope gene with restriction endonuclease sites denoted above the sequence line.

membrane protein is located at amino acid 309. The molecular weight of the unglycosylated precursor protein, 53,000, is close to that predicted by this sequence (53,856) (*9*).

The exterior glycoprotein. A number of structural features of the *env* gene products can be deduced from the predicted primary amino acid sequence. Useful for such analysis is computation of the hydrophobic and hydrophilic properties of subdomains of the protein. Such a display is presented in Fig. 3. Potential glycosylation sites and location of cysteine residues are also indicated.

The first 20 amino acids of the postulated *env* precursor of HTLV II are hydrophobic. This region probably constitutes the leader sequence. The partial amino acid sequence of gp67 and gp52 indicates that the first 20 amino acids are cleaved to generate the mature protein.

Amino acids 21 to 309 probably constitute the exterior glycoprotein. This is sufficient to encode a protein of molecular weight 33,000, the size of the unglycosylated version of gp52 (*9*). This region contains four potential glycosylation sites. Overall the protein is hydrophobic. The hydrophilic regions of this protein

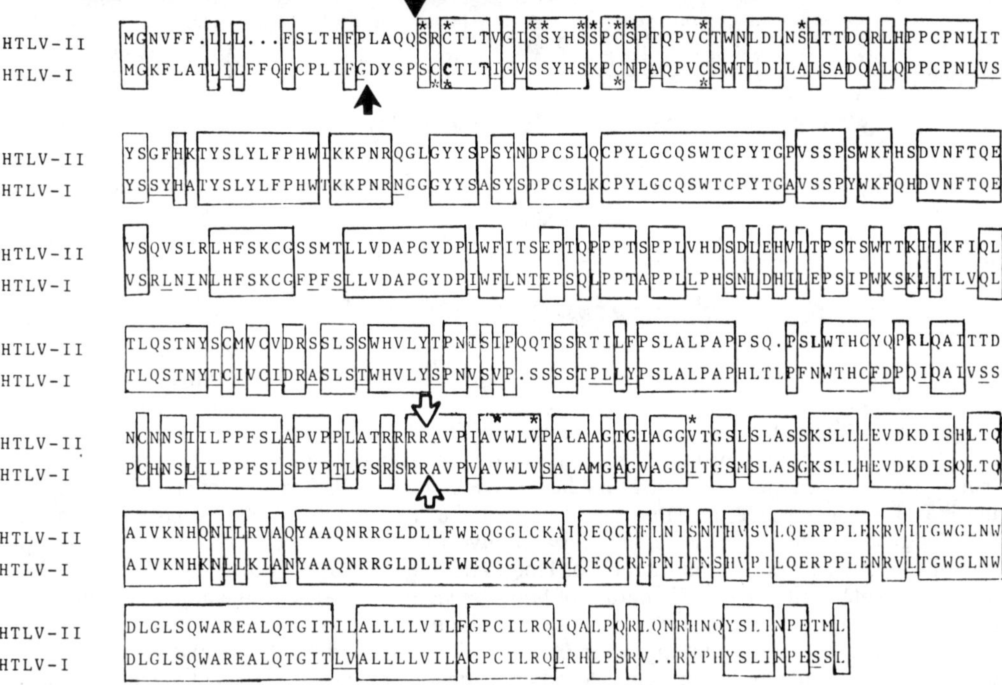

Fig. 2. Amino acid sequence of the HTLV-II and HTLV-I envelope proteins as deduced from the nucleic acid sequence. The HTLV-I sequence is derived from Seiki *et al.* (*12*). Identical amino acids between the two envelope proteins are boxed. Conservative amino acid changes are underlined. Dark arrows indicate the site where the leader sequence is cleaved from the mature envelope glycoprotein. The position of this site has been verified by protein sequencing of envelope proteins labeled with cysteine and serine (for HTLV-II) and with cysteine (for HTLV-I) (*4, 8*). The positions of these labeled residues are indicated by asterisks. The open arrows indicate the point of cleavage of the exterior glycoprotein from the transmembrane protein. The position of this site has also been confirmed by protein sequencing the transmembrane protein after radioactive labeling with valine (shown by asterisks) (*8*). Dots indicate gaps in the sequence placed to maximally align the type I and type II envelope sequences.

are small, one located near the amino terminus of the protein (residues 85 to 93) and one located at the extreme carboxyl terminus of the protein. Two other short hydrophilic regions are located in the center of the protein. The solubility of the exterior glycoprotein in aqueous medium must depend in large measure on glycosylation.

The transmembrane protein. The transmembrane protein begins at residue 309 and is 178 amino acids long, suffi-cient to encode a polypeptide of molecular weight 19,500. The sequence contains one potential glycosylation site.

The transmembrane protein contains two long hydrophobic regions, one located near the amino terminus, 26 amino acids long, and a second located at the carboxyl terminus, 27 amino acids long. There are three cysteine residues located near the potential glycosylation site. The extreme carboxyl terminal domain of the protein is hydrophilic.

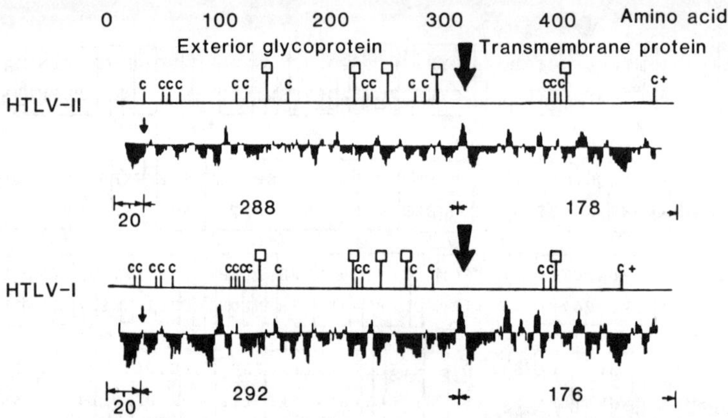

Fig. 3. Schematic representation of the HTLV-II and HTLV-I envelope proteins based on the predicted amino acid sequence. Numbers on top represent amino acid residues from the amino terminus of the complete envelope precursor. The positions of the cysteine residues (c) and potential glycosylation sites (□) are shown. Large arrows above the line drawings depict the site of cleavage of the exterior glycoprotein from the transmembrane protein. The + notes the position of a positively charged amino acid that is positioned on the inner side of the host cell membrane. The small arrowheads underneath the line drawings depict the site of cleavage of the hydrophobic leader sequence from the exterior glycoprotein. The hydrophilic (up) and hydrophobic (down) character of the envelope proteins as determined by the method of Hopp and Woods (*13*) is shown underneath the line drawings. Note the hydrophobic nature of both the leader sequence at the amino terminus and the transmembrane region near the carboxyl terminus of the protein. Also note the alternating hydrophobic and hydrophilic character of the region surrounding the cleavage site between exterior and transmembrane proteins. Numbers beneath each figure represent the lengths of the leader sequence, the mature exterior glycoprotein, and the transmembrane protein, respectively.

Comparison of the sequence of HTLV-I and -II. The structure of the envelope glycoproteins of HTLV-I and -II deduced from the predicted amino acid sequence is very similar (Figs. 2 and 3). The envelope precursor proteins are 488 and 486 amino acids long, respectively. The hydrophobic leader sequences are both 20 amino acids long; the exterior glycoproteins are 292 and 288 amino acids long; and the transmembrane proteins are 176 and 178 amino acids long. The proteins share the same amino acids at 336 of the 488 positions, and 68 of the 152 differences represent conservative changes in protein sequence. The greatest divergence in protein sequence occurs at the extreme amino terminal and carboxyl terminal regions in the *env* gene precursor, both regions that may be absent from the mature protein. The trans-

membrane protein is more highly conserved—85 percent similarity—than is the exterior glycoprotein—65 percent similarity. The overall similarity in protein sequences is also reflected at the DNA level, with 50 percent of the nucleotides being identical, although the regions encoding the extreme amino and carboxyl termini show little or no similarity in DNA sequence.

The distribution of hydrophobic and hydrophilic regions is strikingly similar for HTLV-I and HTLV-II *env* gene products (Fig. 3). Sites of three of the four potential glycosylations of the exterior glycoprotein are shared. The location of the fourth potential glycosylation site near the carboxyl terminus differs in HTLV-I and -II. The location of the single glycosylation site in the transmembrane protein is the same for

HTLV-I and -II. The location of the cysteine residues is also conserved throughout the length of the envelope precursors of HTLV-I and -II.

The location of several cysteine residues is well conserved among this family of proteins. Especially well conserved are cysteine residues spaced eight amino acids apart in the central domain of the transmembrane protein of all the retroviruses, and cysteine residues spaced four amino acids apart that are located near one of the three conserved potential glycosylation sites (the conserved glycosylation site located nearest the carboxyl terminus of the exterior glycoprotein). Because these cysteine residues are invariant among the glycoproteins, we suspect that they play a key role in the structural properties of the *env* genes, and are probably the sites at which disulfide bonds between the transmembrane protein and the exterior glycoprotein are formed.

The conserved spacing of cysteine residues suggests that the shape and rigidity of the exterior glycoprotein is determined by specific disulfide bonds. The similarity in placement of the potential glycosylation sites also suggests that these proteins assume a similar tertiary configuration. The likelihood of overall structural similarity, as well as the identity of much of the primary amino acid sequence, provides a natural explanation for the antigenic cross-reactivity between the envelope glycoproteins of HTLV-I and -II. On the basis of these considerations, the two proteins ought to have common sequence-specific and configuration-specific epitopes. Antigenic differences between the HTLV-I and HTLV-II envelope proteins detected by neutralization of vesicular stomatitis virus pseudotypes (*14*) are probably due to differences in primary amino acid sequence in a limited region of the exterior glycoprotein. The cross-reactivity of the serum of AIDS patients, who are presumably infected with HTLV-III, with the envelope glycoproteins of HTLV-I and -II (*4, 7, 8*) may be explained by similar structural conservation of the envelope glycoprotein of all known members of this retrovirus family.

References and Notes

1. B. J. Poiesz *et al.*, *Proc. Natl. Acad. Sci. U.S.A.* **77**, 7415 (1980); V. S. Kalyanaraman, M. Sarngadharan, P. Bunn, J. Minna, R. C. Gallo, *Nature (London)* **294**, 271 (1981); M. Robert-Guroff, F. Ruscetti, L. Posner, B. Poisz, R. C. Gallo, *J. Exp. Med.* **154**, 1957 (1981); M. Yoshida, I. Miyoshi, Y. Hinuma, *Proc. Natl. Acad. Sci. U.S.A.* **79**, 2031 (1982).
2. V. S. Kalyanaraman *et al.*, *Science* **218**, 571 (1982).
3. M. Popovic, M. G. Sarngadharan, E. Read, R. C. Gallo, *ibid.* **224**, 497 (1984); R. C. Gallo *et al.*, *ibid.*, p. 500 (1984); J. Schüpbach *et al.*, *ibid.*, p. 503; M. Sarngadharan, M. Popovic, L. Bruch, J. Schüpbach, R. C. Gallo, *ibid.*, p. 506.
4. T. H. Lee *et al.*, *Proc. Natl. Acad. Sci. U.S.A.*, in press; J. Schüpbach, M. G. Sarngadharan, R. C. Gallo, *Science* **224**, 607 (1984).
5. T. Taniyama and H. T. Holden, *J. Exp. Med.* **150**, 1367 (1979); D. C. Flyer, S. J. Burakoff, D. V. Faller, *Nature (London)* **305**, 815 (1983).
6. J. Zavada, *J. Gen. Virol.* **15**, 183 (1972); D. N. Love and R. A. Weiss, *Virology* **57**, 271 (1974); D. Boettiger, D. N. Love, R. A. Weiss, *J. Virol.* **15**, 108 (1975); R. A. Weiss and P. Bennett, *Virology* **100**, 252 (1980); A. S. Huang, P. Besmer, L. Chu, D. Baltimore, *J. Virol.* **12**, 659 (1973); T. G. Krontiris, R. Soeiro, B. N. Fields, *Proc. Natl. Acad. Sci. U.S.A.* **70**, 2549 (1973); J. C. Chan, J. L. East, J. M. Bowen, R. Massey, G. Schochetman, *Virology* **120**, 54 (1982); T. J. Schnitzer, R. A. Weiss, J. Zavada, *J. Virol.* **23**, 4449 (1977); L. Thiry *et al.*, *J. Gen. Virol.* **41**, 587 (1978).
7. M. Essex *et al.*, *Science* **221**, 1061 (1983).
8. T. H. Lee *et al.*, *Proc. Natl. Acad. Sci. U.S.A.*, in press.
9. T. H. Lee, unpublished data.
10. E. P. Gelman, G. Franchini, V. Manzari, F. Wong-Staal, R. C. Gallo, *Proc. Natl. Acad. Sci. U.S.A.* **81**, 993 (1984).
11. A. Maxam and W. Gilbert, *ibid.* **74**, 564 (1977).
12. M. Seiki, S. Hattori, Y. Hirayama, M. Yoshida, *ibid.* **80**, 3618 (1983).
13. T. P. Hopp and K. R. Woods, *ibid.* **78**, 3824 (1981).
14. P. Clapham, K. Nagy, R. A. Weiss, *ibid.* **81**, 2886 (1984).
15. Supported by an American Cancer Society Research Development Program grant RD-186 and NIH grant CA-18216. J.G.S. was supported by an NIH postdoctoral fellowship.

31 May 1984; accepted 21 June 1984

45.   Interleukin 2 Regulates Expression of Its Receptor and Synthesis of Gamma Interferon by Human T Lymphocytes

Gabrielle H. Reem and Ning-Hsing Yeh

Earlier studies conducted in our laboratory have provided evidence that expression of interleukin 2 (IL-2) receptors could be induced on thymocytes by agents that induce the synthesis of gamma interferon (IFN-γ) (*1*). We have also shown that cyclosporin A, an immunosuppressant agent, inhibits synthesis of IFN-γ by thymocytes and T lymphocytes and synthesis of IL-2 by thymocytes (*2*). Other investigators reported that cyclosporin A inhibits the synthesis of IL-2 by T cells (*3*). IL-2 has been reported to augment IFN-γ synthesis by human thymocytes and mononuclear cells and to induce synthesis by unstimulated T cells (*1, 4*). In view of the importance of the function of IL-2 and IFN-γ in mounting an immune response, we investigated the role of IL-2 on the expression of IL-2 receptors and synthesis of IFN-γ. The effect of dexamethasone (Dex) on IFN-γ synthesis has not, to our knowledge, been reported. Anti-Tac, a monoclonal antibody that binds at or near the binding site of IL-2, has been found to block the binding of IL-2 and to down-regulate the expression of IL-2 receptors (*5*). Its effect on IFN-γ synthesis is not known. Anti-Tac does not inhibit IL-2 synthesis (*6*). The tumor promoter phorbol myristate acetate (PMA) exerts a synergistic effect with lectins on prolif-

eration of thymocytes and T cells and on synthesis of IL-2 and IFN-γ. Synthesis of both IL-2 and IFN-γ precedes the mitogenic effect of the inducing agents (*1, 2*).

To study the relation between IL-2, the expression of IL-2 receptors, and synthesis of IFN-γ, we isolated mononuclear cells from peripheral blood by density centrifugation on a Ficoll-Hypaque gradient and removed macrophages by incubation on a plastic surface for 60 minutes. The cells were then passed through a nylon wool column and nonadherent cells (T cells) were washed and incubated (6×10^6 cells per milliliter) in complete RPMI 1640 medium (bovine calf serum, 10 percent; glutamine, 2mM; penicillin, 100 U/ml; streptomycin, 100 μg/ml; Amphotericin B, 0.25 μg/ml) or in complete medium containing PMA (1 ng/ml) for 3 hours at 37°C in a humidified atmosphere containing 5 percent CO_2. Cells were plated into flat-bottomed microtiter plates (96 wells, 200 μl) at a density of 6×10^6 cells per milliliter and cultured with agents that induce IL-2 synthesis [concanavalin A (Con A)] or with agents that either inhibit IL-2 synthesis (Dex) or inhibit IL-2 from binding to its receptors (anti-Tac). Cells were harvested and tested for viability and proliferative activity (data not shown).

The expression of IL-2 receptors was determined by staining with immunoperoxidase as described (*1*). The concentration of IFN-γ was determined by a radioimmunoassay with two monoclonal antibodies to IFN-γ (*7*). An IFN-γ standard was included in each assay.

We found evidence that IL-2 modulates the expression of IL-2 receptors and IFN-γ production. IL-2 enhanced the percentage of receptor-bearing cells of activated T cells and increased IFN-γ synthesis. Conversely, T cells deprived of IL-2 by the combined effects of anti-Tac and Dex expressed IL-2 receptors only on a small percentage of cells, and their production of IFN-γ was inhibited.

T cells cultured with either Con A or PMA were induced to express IL-2 receptors (Table 1). The addition of exogenous IL-2 resulted in a threefold increase in the number of receptor-bearing cells. This increase was already detectable after 24 hours, before an increase in the proliferative rate could be detected (data not shown). The number of receptor-bearing cells could be increased further by incubating T cells with PMA and then adding Con A to cultures. PMA in combination with Con A produced a synergistic effect on the expression of receptors. IL-2 added to cultures of cells treated with PMA and Con A further increased the percentage of receptor-bearing cells, and most of the cells in culture were induced to express receptors for IL-2. The addition of IFN-γ to cultures of activated T cells had no significant effect on the expression of IL-2 receptors, indicating that the promotion of the expression of IL-2 receptors was not mediated by IFN-γ (data not shown).

Table 1. Relation between IL-2, the expression of Tac$^+$ cells, and IFN-γ synthesis. Interleukin 2 (100 U/ml), Con A (10 μg/ml), Dex (10^{-6}M), and anti-Tac ascites (diluted to a final concentration of 10^{-4}) were added as indicated. (The IL-2 concentration used results in maximum stimulation of T cell proliferation under these conditions.) Cultures were incubated for 3 days. Tac$^+$ cells were determined with the monoclonal antibody anti-Tac and peroxidase-labeled goat antibody to mouse immunoglobulin G (BioRad Laboratories, Richmond, California). The IFN-γ titers were measured by a solid-phase radioimmunossay. An IFN-γ standard was included in each assay.

Additions	Tac$^+$ cells (%)		IFN-γ (U/ml)	
	Without IL-2	With IL-2	Without IL-2	With IL-2
Complete RPMI 1640 medium				
None	1	6	9	55
Con A	10	30	479	640
Con A + Dex	2	19	62	518
Con A + anti-Tac	8	28	128	324
Con A + Dex + anti-Tac	1	15	18	262
*Complete medium + PMA**				
None	2	9	108	1018
Con A	46	82	4070	5076
Con A + Dex	44	86	1364	1777
Con A + anti-Tac	48	43	3022	3888
Con A + Dex + anti-Tac	16	31	951	1036

*PMA (phorbol myristate acetate) at 1 ng/ml.

Dex and anti-Tac reduced the number of receptor-bearing cells in cultures supplemented with Con A alone. T cells treated with PMA and then cultured with Con A were more resistant to the inhibitory effect of Dex on the expression of IL-2 receptors. This inhibitory effect on cells activated with lectin could be reversed by exogenous IL-2. IL-2 also increased the number of receptor-bearing cells in cultures supplemented with Dex and induced with PMA and Con A. The combined effect of Dex (inhibition of IL-2 synthesis) and anti-Tac (blockage of IL-2 receptors) was synergistic. The expression of receptors induced with Con A alone or in combination with PMA was almost completely abrogated by anti-Tac in combination with Dex. Exogenous IL-2 had only a moderate effect in preventing this inhibition.

Synthesis of IFN-γ was modulated by IL-2 in a manner resembling the effect of IL-2 on its receptors. IL-2 served as an amplifying signal by augmenting IFN-γ synthesis. T cells cultured in complete medium produced low amounts of IFN-γ in culture, and exogenous IL-2 moderately increased their production of IFN-γ. This low degree of synthesis was increased by PMA and Con A. Maximum synthesis of IFN-γ was observed in cultures induced with Con A and PMA to which IL-2 was added. Maximum inhibition was achieved by the combined effects of Dex and anti-Tac. Dex inhibited synthesis of IFN-γ by T cells induced with Con A alone or in combination with PMA. This inhibition was readily overcome by IL-2 in cultures supplemented with Con A and was partially reversed in cultures containing PMA and Con A. Anti-Tac inhibited IFN-γ synthesis more effectively in T cells activated with Con A than in T cells cultured with PMA and

Con A. Once the expression of IL-2 receptors was blocked by anti-Tac, IL-2 was not effective in reversing the inhibitory effect.

In conclusion, IL-2 has an important role in augmenting the expression of IL-2 receptors and in the synthesis of IFN-γ activated by T cells. In cultures of T cells whose supply of IL-2 has been cut off by Dex and anti-Tac, the number of cells displaying receptors and the density of receptors are decreased, and synthesis of IFN-γ ceases. This regulatory effect of IL-2 precedes T cell proliferation. The observation that Dex, an effective immunosuppressant drug, interferes with IFN-γ synthesis may be of clinical significance. Patients treated with glucocorticoids such as Dex risk infection partly because Dex inhibits the bacteriocidal effect of macrophages. Since IFN-γ is an activator of macrophages, these patients could be protected from infections by administration of IFN-γ.

Note added in proof: A similar observation that IL-2 was required for the optimal expression of IL-2 receptors on activated T cells has been made (8).

References and Notes

1. G. H. Reem, L. A. Cook, D. M. Henriksen, J. Vilček, *Infect. Immun.* **37**, 216 (1982); N.-H. Yeh, M. Dipre, G. H. Reem, *Thymus*, in press.
2. G. H. Reem, L. A. Cook, J. Vilček, *Science* **221**, 63 (1983); G. H. Reem, L. A. Cook, M. A. Palladino, *Transplant. Proc.* **15**, 2387 (1983); *J. Biol. Resp. Modif.*, in press.
3. D. Bunjes, C. Hardt, M. Rollinghoff, H. Wagner, *Eur. J. Immunol.* **11**, 657 (1981); E.-L. Larsson, *J. Immunol.* **124**, 2828 (1980).
4. T. Kasahara, J. J. Hooks, S. F. Dougherty, J. J. Oppenheim, *J. Immunol.* **130**, 1784 (1983); K. T. Pearlstein, M. A. Palladino, K. Welte, J. Vilček, *Cell. Immunol.* **80**, 1 (1983); G. H. Reem, L. A. Cook, J. Vilček, *Fed. Proc. Fed. Am. Soc. Exp. Biol.* **42**, 447 (1983); W. L. Farrar, H. M. Johnson, J. J. Farrar, *J. Immunol.* **126**, 1120 (1981).
5. W. J. Leonard *et al.*, *Nature (London)* **300**, 267 (1982); R. J. Robb and W. C. Greene, *J. Exp. Med.* **158**, 1332 (1983); M. Tsudo, T. Uchiyama, K. Takatsuki, H. Uchino, J. Yodoi, *J. Immunol.* **129**, 592 (1982); T. Uchiyama, S. Broder, T. A.

Waldmann, *ibid.* **126**, 1393 (1981); T. Uchiyama, D. L. Nelson, T. A. Fleisher, T. A. Waldmann, *ibid.*, p. 1398.
6. J. M. Depper, W. J. Leonard, R. J. Robb, T. A. Waldmann, W. C. Greene, *J. Immunol.* **131**, 690 (1983).
7. J. Le, B. S. Barrowclough, J. Vilček, *J. Immunol. Meth.* **69**, 61 (1984).
8. F. W. Ruscetti, personal communication.
9. We thank K. Welte and K. A. Smith for purified IL-2, T. Uchiyama for anti-Tac, and T.-W. Chang for help with the determination of IFN-γ. This work was supported by NIH grant RO 1 CA 33653-01A1.

28 March 1984; accepted 15 May 1984

Report

17 August 1984

46. Lymphoma in Macaques: Association with Virus of Human T Lymphotrophic Family

T. Homma, P.J. Kanki, N.W. King, Jr., R.D. Hunt, M.J. O'Connell, N.L. Letvin, M.D. Daniel, R.C. Desrosiers, C.S. Yang, and M. Essex

Human T-cell leukemia virus (HTLV) is a type C retrovirus that was first identified by Gallo and his colleagues in a patient with cutaneous T-cell lymphoma (*1*). Numerous isolates of HTLV were subsequently made from cases of adult T-cell types of leukemia-lymphoma (ATLL) from various parts of the world (*2*). Subsequent serological surveys for antibodies to HTLV have shown a strong association between HTLV and ATLL. Natural antibodies to HTLV have been demonstrated in more than 90 percent of the patients with ATLL as well as in 4 to 37 percent of the healthy adults in areas where ATLL is endemic (*3–7*). In areas where ATLL is not endemic, less than 1 percent of the healthy adults have antibodies (*4–8*).

Evidence that an agent similar to HTLV might be present in nonhuman primates was first reported in Japanese macaques (*Macaca fuscata*) by Miyoshi

and his colleagues (*9*). This observation was further extended to indicate that many Asian and African species of Old World primates have antibodies to HTLV (*10–12*). Most extensively studied were species of the genus *Macaca*. Rates of seropositivity ranging from 9 to 44 percent have been reported in healthy macaques (*10–12*). The geographic distribution of seropositive macaques in Japan does not seem to be correlated with seropositivity in human populations (*11, 12*), suggesting an independent origin for the virus in humans and macaques. To our knowledge, there has been no evidence thus far linking lymphoma or other disease with the HTLV-related agent in nonhuman primates.

A seroepidemiological survey of macaques from Taiwan and the New England Regional Primate Research Center (NERPRC), Southborough, Massachusetts, was conducted. Included were sera from three species of healthy macaques and macaques diagnosed with malignant lymphoma (ML) or lymphoproliferative disease (LPD) at the NERPRC. Serum samples examined for antibodies were obtained from 95 healthy macaques and 13 macaques with ML or LPD. Of these, 20 were from healthy adult *M. cyclopis* captured and housed in Taipei, Taiwan. All other samples were from captive macaques at the NERPRC. Included among these were: 14 healthy *M. cyclopis* and 4 with LPD; 31 healthy *M. mulatta*, 5 with ML and 1 with LPD; and 30 healthy *M. fascicularis* and 3 with ML. Both LPD and ML have been described in conjunction with macaque immunodeficiency syndrome at the NERPRC. Lymphoproliferative disease is a lesion characterized by the presence of nodular aggregates of well-differentiated lymphocytes in the liver, kidney, or bone marrow (*13*); ML is the most common spontaneous neoplasm of macaques at the NERPRC observed over the past 12 years (*14*). All the ML cases were of the non-Hodgkin's type with variability in organ distribution, cellular morphology, and grade of malignancy. The diseased monkeys in this study were the same animals whose pathology was described earlier (*13*).

Sera were examined for antibodies to membrane antigens of HTLV-infected cells (HTLV-MA) as described (*8*). This procedure detects antibodies to two glycoproteins expressed on HTLV-infected cells that are encoded by the *env* gene of HTLV (*7*). Sera were tested on two reference HTLV-I–infected cell lines, Hut 102 and MT-2. Those that scored positive were tested on uninfected T (8402) and B (NC 37) lymphoid cell line to exclude false positives as described earlier (*7, 8*). Antibodies to HTLV-MA

were identified in four of 34 healthy *M. cyclopis* (Table 1). Two of the seropositive macaques were from Taiwan, and the other two were from the healthy population at the NERPRC. In contrast, three of four *M. cyclopis* with LPD were positive for antibodies to HTLV-MA. Of 31 healthy *M. mulatta* from the NERPRC only one was seropositive. Five of six *M. mulatta* with ML or LPD had HTLV-MA antibodies. In *M. fascicularis*, two of 30 healthy individuals had HTLV-MA antibodies while all three with ML were positive. Overall, 11 of 13 (84.6 percent) macaques with ML or LPD had antibodies to HTLV-MA whereas seven of 95 (7.4 percent) of the healthy controls were seropositive. The results obtained on Hut 102 and MT-2 were similar. None of the positive sera reacted with the uninfected cells. Macaques with ML or LPD had antibodies to HTLV-MA significantly more often than healthy macaques ($P < 6.27 \times 10^{-9}$; Fisher's exact test).

Representative serum samples were subjected to radioimmunoprecipitation and sodium dodecyl sulfate–polyacrylamide gel electrophoresis (SDS-PAGE) to analyze the reactivity of the antibodies for known HTLV proteins. Sera were reacted with whole cell lysate of Hut 102 cells since the major *gag* and *env* proteins have been defined in this line (Fig. 1A). A human reference serum positive for antibodies to HTLV-MA and HTLV proteins precipitated proteins with sizes of 24,000 daltons (p24), 45,000 daltons (gp45), and 61,000 daltons (gp61), as described (*7, 8*) (see Fig. 1A). Sera from healthy *M. cyclopis*, one from Taiwan and one from the NERPRC, recognized the same proteins. A serum sample from a *M. fascicularis* with ML showed the same reactivity (Fig. 1A). The same sera

Table 1. Presence of antibodies to HTLV-MA in macaques from Taiwan and the NERPRC. Antibodies to HTLV-MA were detected as described (8). Reference HTLV-infected cell lines, Hut 102 (1) and MT-2 (20) were harvested at the peak phase of logarithmic growth. One million cells were washed twice with phosphate-buffered saline (PBS) and reacted with 40 μl of a 1:4 dilution of serum at 37°C for 30 minutes. Preparations were then washed twice with PBS and exposed to 20 μl of a 1:20 dilution of fluorescein-conjugated immunoglobulin G fraction of goat antiserum to monkey immunoglobulin G (Cappel, Cochranville, Pennsylvania). The samples were incubated at 37°C for 30 minutes, washed twice with PBS, and examined for fluorescence. Samples were considered positive when more than 40 percent of the target cells showed fluorescence. Positive and negative human reference sera were included in each test. Sera that initially scored positive were tested on two uninfected human lymphoid cell lines, 8402, a T-cell line (21), and NC 37, a B-cell line which lacks surface immunoglobulin in (22), to confirm specificity.

Species	Clinical status	Origin	Number tested	Number positive	Percent positive
M. cyclopis	Healthy	Taiwan	20	2	10.0
	Healthy	NERPRC	14	2	14.3
	LPD	NERPRC	4	3	75.0
M. mulatta	Healthy	NERPRC	31	1	3.2
	LPD	NERPRC	1	1	100.0
	ML	NERPRC	5	4	80.0
M. fascicularis	Healthy	NERPRC	30	2	6.7
	ML	NERPRC	3	3	100.0
Total*	Healthy		95	7	7.4
	ML/LPD		13	11	84.6

*Difference between healthy and ML or LPD significant at $P < 6 \times 10^{-9}$ with Fisher's exact test.

were also reacted with glycoproteins prepared from Hut 102 cells by using lentil-lectin affinity chromatography (Fig. 1B). Two proteins presumed to be gp45 and gp61, which migrated at the positions expected for the *env* gene en-coded proteins, were precipitated with sera positive for HTLV-MA antibodies but not with negative sera (Fig. 1B).

Our results extend previous observations that infections with an HTLV-related agent occur in macaques. Of 20 *M. cyclopis* captured and housed in their natural habitat, Taiwan, 10 percent had antibodies to HTLV-MA. The rate of seropositivity among healthy *M. cyclopis* raised in captivity at the NERPRC was similar. Of greater interest, however, is the correlation between exposure

to HTLV and the presence of ML or LPD in macaques. Spontaneous ML has been observed in macaques during the last 12 years at the NERPRC, and successful transmission of ML was reported (14). An LPD has been described in animals with the macaque immunodeficiency syndrome described at the NERPRC. Macaques that developed either of these spontaneous lymphoproliferative abnormalities had higher rates of exposure to HTLV than healthy controls. Earlier reports have described infections with a type D retrovirus in macaques that develop immunodeficiency syndrome (15). However, antibodies directed to the HTLV gp61 and gp45 should not cross-react with the type D retroviruses.

The association between HTLV and

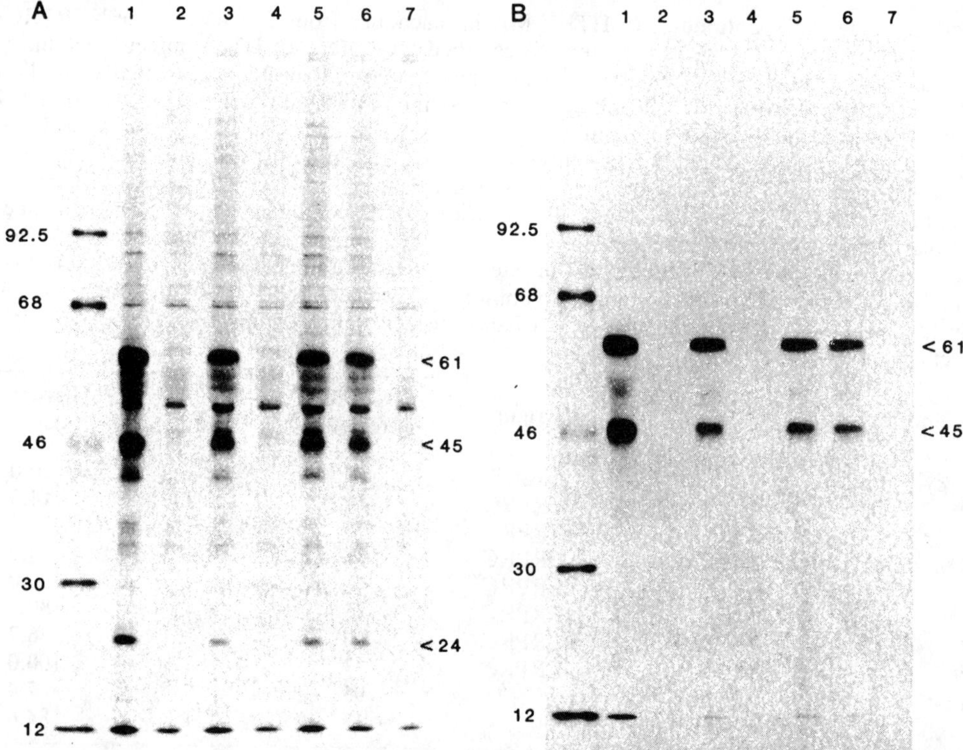

Fig. 1. (A) Reactivity of serum samples from macaques positive for antibodies to HTLV-MA was determined by radioimmunoprecipitation in conjunction with SDS-PAGE as described (7, 8). Hut 102 cells were harvested at their peak of log-phase growth and were exposed to [^{35}S]cysteine [100 μCi/ml; specific activity 1000 to 1050 Ci/mmol; New England Nuclear (NEN)] for 8 to 10 hours. A soluble cell lysate was prepared by disrupting cells with RIPA buffer (0.15M NaCl, 0.05M tris-HCl, pH 7.2, 1 percent Triton X-100, 1 percent sodium deoxycholate, and 0.1 percent SDS) and clearing by centrifugation for 1 hour at 100,000g. The cell lysate was reacted with 10 μl of the following test sera bound to Protein A–Sepharose CL-4B (Protein A beads, Pharmacia, Sweden): (Lane 1) A human reference serum positive for antibodies to HTLV-MA; (lane 2) a human serum negative for antibodies to HTLV-MA; (lane 3) serum from a healthy adult *M. cyclopis* from Taiwan that is positive for antibodies to HTLV-MA; (lane 4) serum from a representative healthy adult *M. cyclopis* from Taiwan that is negative for antibodies to HTLV-MA; (lane 5) serum from a representative *M. fascicularis* with malignant lymphoma; (lane 6) serum from healthy adult *M. cyclopis* from the NERPRC that is positive for antibodies to HTLV-MA; (lane 7) serum from a representative healthy adult *M. cyclopis* from the NERPRC that is negative for antibodies to HTLV-MA. The precipitates were eluted in a sample buffer containing 0.1M Cleland's reagent, 2 percent SDS, 0.08M tris-HCl, pH 6.8, 10 percent glycerol, and 0.2 percent bromophenol blue by boiling at 100°C for 2 minutes. Samples were analyzed in a 12.5 percent acrylamide resolving gel with 3.5 percent stacking gel according to the discontinuous buffer system of Laemmli (23). (B) Reactivity of serum samples with the glycoprotein preparation of Hut 102; the procedure was described in detail (7). The glycoproteins were prepared from a soluble cell lysate of Hut 102 made with RIPA buffer excluding sodium deoxycholate and by passing through a Lentil Lectin–Sepharose CL-4B (Pharmacia) column at the ratio of 20 × 10⁶ cells to 1 to 2 ml of undiluted Lentil Lectin–Sepharose CL-4B. The glycoproteins were eluted from the column with a buffer consisting of 0.15M NaCl, 0.05M tris-HCl, pH 7.2, 1 percent Triton X-100, and 0.2M methyl-α-D-mannoside. The eluted bound fraction was reacted with 10 μl of test serum bound to Protein A beads. Samples of the same serum were used in the same lanes 1 to 7 as described in (A). The precipitates were eluted from Protein A beads and subjected to SDS-PAGE as described above.

ATLL in people represents a strong case for an etiological relation between a given virus and a human cancer (*5, 16*). The reported cases of lymphoid malignancies in macaques are not numerous (*17, 18*). However, there have been reports of multiple cases that occurred over brief intervals of time, suggesting that a transmissible agent could be involved (*14, 18, 19*).

The LPD observed in macaques have not been characterized according to the subpopulations of lymphocytes involved. Nevertheless, the seroepidemiological pattern we observed parallels that seen in people where the presence of antibodies to HTLV is associated with a greatly increased risk for the development of a particular form of lymphoma. Our current results indicate that an agent similar to HTLV is present in colonies of macaques where outbreaks of ML have been reported, and that more consideration should be given to the possible involvement of these agents in the causation of lymphoproliferative abnormalities in macaques.

References and Notes

1. B. J. Poiesz, F. W. Ruscetti, A. F. Gazdar, P. A. Bunn, J. D. Minna, R. C. Gallo, *Proc. Natl. Acad. Sci. U.S.A.* **77**, 7415 (1980); B. J. Poiesz, F. W. Ruscetti, M. S. Reitz, V. S. Kalyanaraman, R. C. Gallo, *Nature (London)* **294**, 268 (1981).
2. I. Miyoshi *et al.*, *Nature (London)* **294**, 770 (1981); R. C. Gallo *et al.*, *Proc. Natl. Acad. Sci. U.S.A.* **79**, 5680 (1982); V. S. Kalyanaraman *et al.*, *Science* **218**, 571 (1982); M. Yoshida, I. Miyoshi, Y. Hinuma, *Proc. Natl. Acad. Sci. U.S.A.* **79**, 2031 (1982); B. F. Haynes *et al.*, *ibid.* **80**, 2054 (1983); M. Popovic *et al.*, *Science* **219**, 856 (1983).
3. Y. Hinuma *et al.*, *Proc. Natl. Acad. Sci. U.S.A.* **78**, 6476 (1981); M. Robert-Guroff *et al.*, *Science* **215**, 975 (1982); W. A. Blattner *et al.*, *Int. J. Cancer* **30**, 257 (1982); J. Schüpbach *et al.*, *Cancer Res.* **43**, 886 (1983).
4. Y. Hinuma *et al.*, *Int. J. Cancer* **29**, 631 (1982).
5. R. C. Gallo *et al.*, *Cancer Res.* **43**, 3892 (1983).
6. M. Essex, M. F. McLane, N. Tachibana, D. P. Francis, T. H. Lee, in *Human T-Cell Leukemia Viruses*, R. C. Gallo, M. Essex, L. Gross, Eds. (Cold Spring Harbor Laboratory, Cold Spring Harbor, N.Y., 1984), pp. 355–362.
7. T. H. Lee *et al.*, *Proc. Natl. Acad. Sci. U.S.A.* **81**, 3856 (1984).
8. M. Essex *et al.*, *Science* **220**, 859 (1983); *ibid.* **221**, 1061 (1983).
9. I. Miyoshi *et al.*, *Lancet* **1982-II**, 658 (1982).
10. M. Hayami *et al.*, *ibid.* **1983-II**, 620 (1983); G. Hunsmann, J. Schneider, J. Schmitt, N. Yamamoto, *Int. J. Cancer* **32**, 329 (1983); T. Ishida, K. Yamamoto, R. Kaneko, E. Tokita, Y. Hinuma, *Micobiol. Immunol.* **27**, 297 (1983); N. Yamamoto, Y. Hinuma, H. ZurHausen, J. S. G. Hunsmann, *Lancet* **1983-I**, 240 (1983).
11. I. Miyoshi *et al.*, *Int. J. Cancer* **32**, 333 (1983).
12. M. Hayami *et al.*, *ibid.* **33**, 179 (1984).
13. N. W. King, R. D. Hunt, N. L. Letvin, *Am. J. Pathol.* **113**, 382 (1983); N. L. Letvin, *et al.*, *Proc. Natl. Acad. Sci. U.S.A.* **80**, 2718 (1983); L. V. Chalifoux, N. W. King, N. L. Letvin, *Lab. Invest.*, in press.
14. R. D. Hunt *et al.*, *Proc. Natl. Acad. Sci. U.S.A.* **80**, 5085 (1983).
15. M. D. Daniel *et al.*, *Science* **223**, 602 (1984); P. A. Marx *et al.*, *ibid.*, p. 1083.
16. R. C. Gallo *et al.*, *Proc. Natl. Acad. Sci. U.S.A.* **79**, 5680 (1982); M. Yoshida, I. Miyoshi, Y. Hinuma, *ibid.* **72**, 2031 (1982); W. A. Blattner *et al.*, *J. Infect. Dis.* **147**, 406 (1983); M. S. Reitz *et al.*, *ibid.* p. 399; M. Robert-Guroff and R. C. Gallo, *Blut* **47**, 1 (1983).
17. R. W. O'Gara and R. H. Adamson, in *Pathology of Simian Primates*, R. N. T. W. Fiennes, Ed. (Karger, Basel, Switzerland, 1972), pp. 190–238.
18. J. R. S. Manning and R. A. Griesemer, *Lab. Animal Sci.* **24**, 204 (1974).
19. R. E. Stowell, E. K. Smith, C. Espana, V. G. Nelson, *Lab. Invest.* **25**, 476 (1971).
20. M. Yoshida, I. Miyoshi, Y. Hinuma, *Proc. Natl. Acad. Sci. U.S.A.* **72**, 203 (1982).
21. C. C. Huang, Y. Hou, L. K. Woods, G. E. Moore, J. Minowada, *J. Natl. Cancer Inst.* **53**, 655 (1974).
22. F. E. Durr, J. H. Monroe, R. Schmitter, K. A. Traul, Y. Hirshaut, *Int. J. Cancer* **6**, 436 (1970).
23. J. K. Laemmli, *Nature (London)* **227**, 680 (1970).
24. Supported in part by NIH grants CA 18216 and RR00168. P.J.K. was supported by NIH Institutional Research Service Award 5TRRR07000. We thank T. H. Lee and M. F. McLane for advice and discussion.

7 June 1984; accepted 27 June 1984

Report

24 August 1984

47. Isolation of Lymphocytopathic Retroviruses from San Francisco Patients with AIDS

Jay A. Levy, Anthony D. Hoffman, Susan M. Kramer, Jill A. Landis, Joni M. Shimabukuro, and Lyndon S. Oshiro

Acquired immune deficiency syndrome (AIDS) has affected more than 4000 individuals in the world; in San Francisco, over 600 cases have been reported (*1*). In addition, there are many patients with unexplained chronic lymphadenopathy which may be caused by the agent responsible for AIDS (*1*). Last year, two different retroviruses were isolated from AIDS patients. One of these, human T cell leukemia virus (HTLV-I) (*2*), which is associated with T cell leukemias in man (*3*), has a type C morphology as determined by electron microscopy; this virus can immortalize T cells to produce continuous cell lines and is primarily cell-associated (*3*). The other, lymphadenopathy-associated retrovirus (LAV), was isolated from the lymph node of a patient with lymphadenopathy (*4*) and has subsequently been recovered from patients with AIDS (*5*). LAV has a type D morphology, causes cytopathic changes in T cells, and is infectious in culture fluids. A third retrovirus, HTLV-III, was recently reported in AIDS patients and related syndromes (*6*). This virus has some cross-reactivity with HTLV-I and HTLV-II but, like LAV, has a type D morphology and causes cytopathic changes in lymphocytes.

In attempts to isolate the infectious agent responsible for AIDS in homosex-ual patients from San Francisco, we have identified lymphocytopathic retroviruses that are similar to LAV. In addition, serologic studies show a high prevalence of antibodies to these AIDS-associated retroviruses (ARV) in individuals from San Francisco.

Using interleukin-2 and phytohemagglutinin stimulation (*3*), we established more than 100 cultures of peripheral mononuclear cells (PMC), which after 1 week in culture, were primarily of the T cell lineage (*7*). When supernatants from cultures prepared from 41 homosexual AIDS patients were examined, 22 were positive for Mg^{2+}-dependent reverse transcriptase activity (Table 1). The viruses were found primarily in PMC of patients in the early stages of disease. The reverse transcriptase activity was detected in the PMC usually within the first 2 weeks of culture, with the peak of activity observed by 12 to 16 days (Fig. 1A). When bone marrow aspirates were cultured, three of nine cultures from AIDS patients showed evidence of retroviruses (data not shown). With some cell cultures, the use of antiserum to interferon helped to demonstrate the presence of virus (*4*). When reverse transcriptase activity diminished in the cultures after 2 to 3 weeks, the addition of fresh lymphocytes from normal donors sometimes re-established this activity (see legend to Fig. 1A). Supernatant fluids from positive cultures (some stored at −70°C for more than 3 months) also induced reverse transcriptase activity in uninfected fresh lymphocyte cultures. Mg^{2+}-dependent reverse transcriptase activity was also observed repeatedly in PMC cultures from patients with lymphadenopathy syndrome, steady male sexual partners of AIDS patients, clinically healthy homosexual men, and one healthy young heterosexual man (Table 1).

The viruses detected in seven of the PMC cultures were grown in high titer

Table 1. Peripheral mononuclear cell (PMC) cultures were established from 10 to 30 ml of heparinized blood from individuals seen at the Kaposi's sarcoma clinic, University of California, San Francisco, or the AIDS clinic, San Francisco General Hospital. Patients were selected at random intervals from the sequence of individuals appearing at the clinics for evaluation. All patients and most of the clinically healthy individuals had lived in San Francisco for at least 2 years. The PMC were separated on Ficoll-Hypaque gradients (9). Washed cells were plated at approximately 2×10^6 per milliliter in RPMI 1640 containing 10 percent fetal bovine serum and antibiotics (penicillin, 100 unit/ml; streptomycin 100 μg/ml). To this medium was added interleukin-2 (Meloy) (0.5 μg/ml) and Polybrene (1 μg/ml). At initiation of the cultures, phytohemagglutinin (Wellcome), approximately 2.5 μg/ml, was added. Some cultures also received $10^{-5}M$ β-mercaptoethanol and sheep antisera to interferon-α (4) provided by the National Institutes of Health (lot 61220); K. Cantell, Helsinki; or F. Barré-Sinoussi, Paris. These antisera were used at a dilution that neutralized 700 to 1000 units of interferon-α per milliliter of culture. The culture supernatants were routinely assayed for Mg^{2+}-dependent reverse transcriptase activity (see legend to Fig. 1) every 3 to 6 days. The cells were studied for the presence of HTLV-I and LAV antigens by standard indirect immunofluorescence assays. For these studies, cells were put on glass slides, air dried, and fixed in cold acetone for 15 minutes. A monoclonal antibody to HTLV p19 provided by Robert-Guroff and Gallo, National Institutes of Health, and a monoclonal antibody to adult T cell leukemia virus (ATLV) p19/p28 provided by Y. Hinuma, Kyoto, Japan (10), were used. For detection of LAV, human serum (from patient B.R.U.) provided by Barré-Sinoussi, Paris, was used (4). Peripheral mononuclear cells producing ARV were also tested for reactivity with sera from AIDS patients from San Francisco. For the sera we examined, the results were the same as those obtained with the B.R.U. serum. The fluorescein-conjugated antibodies for these immunofluorescence assays were either goat antiserum to mouse immunoglobulin G or goat antiserum to human immunoglobulin G. Some cultures were examined for virus by electron microscopy (see legend to Fig. 2). Any cultures that gave positive results repeatedly by any of these tests were considered positive for virus.

Subjects	No. tested	Positive results	
		No.	Percent
Patients with diagnosis of			
AIDS with Kaposi's sarcoma	41	22	53.6
AIDS with opportunistic infection	4	0	0
Lymphadenopathy syndrome	10	5	50.0
Other individuals			
Male sexual partners of AIDS patients*	14	3	21.4
Clinically healthy homosexual men†	9	2	22.2
Clinically healthy heterosexual individuals†	23	1	4.0

*Clinically healthy individuals who had steady sexual contact with a patient for at least 6 months before the patient became ill.   †Some of these individuals volunteered for the study.

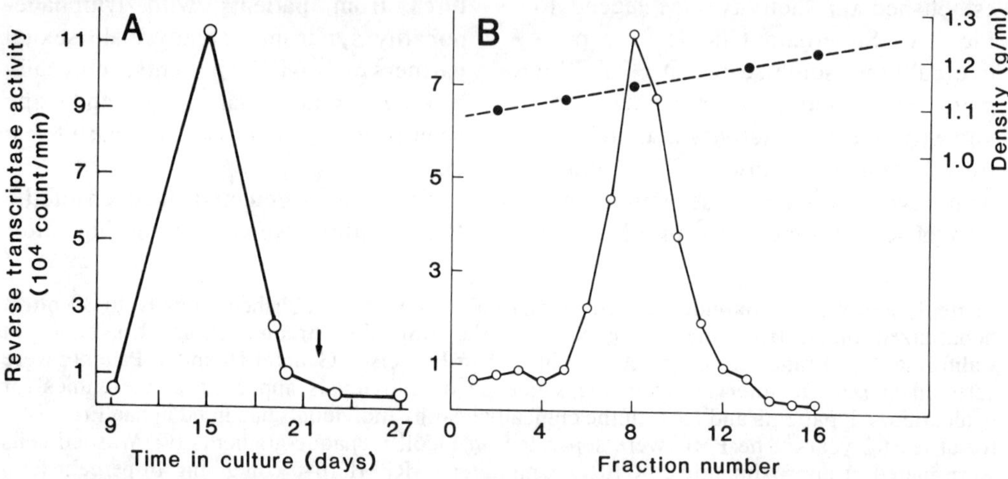

Fig. 1. (A) Kinetics of reverse transcriptase activity detected in peripheral mononuclear cell (PMC) cultures as illustrated by a representative culture. Culture medium (1 to 5 ml) from PMC was centrifuged (Beckman SW41 rotor; 40,000 rev/min, 4°C, 45 minutes). The pellets were assayed in 50 μl of a mixture containing 40 mM tris-HCl (pH 7.8), 60 mM KCl, 2.2 mM dithiothreitol, 10 mM MgCl$_2$, 0.1 percent Triton X-100, 30 μCi of [^{3}H]thymidine triphosphate (specific activity, 78 Ci/mmole), and poly(rA) · oligo(dT) (50 μg/ml) (P-L Biochemicals). Samples were incubated at 0°C for 15 minutes; the reaction was then run for 1 hour at 37°C and stopped with 4 ml of a mixture of 5 percent trichloroacetic acid, 0.005M sodium pyrophosphate, and 0.5N HCl. Precipitates were collected on filters (Whatman GF/A), washed, dried, and counted in a liquid scintillation counter (LKB). A high level of reverse transcriptase activity was seen in the culture on day 15. On day 22 (arrow), when the reverse transcriptase activity was low, the supernatant fluid was removed and inoculated onto fresh human PMC stimulated 3 days before with phytohemagglutinin. Supernatants from this culture, within 6 days, contained reverse transcriptase activity at levels of 650,000 cpm/ml and yielded the virus isolate ARV-2. (B) Density of retrovirus particles. Supernatant from a culture of ARV-infected PMC was concentrated by centrifugation (Beckman SW55 rotor; 45,000 rev/min, 4°C, 30 minutes). The pellet was suspended in 100 μl of a mixture containing 10 mM tris-HCl (pH 8.0), 100 mM NaCl, and 1 mM EDTA (pH 8.0) and layered on a 20 to 60 percent (by weight) sucrose gradient in the same mixture, and centrifuged (Beckman SW55 rotor; 35,000 rev/min, 4°C, 16 hours). Fractions (200 μl) were collected from the top and assayed for reverse transcriptase activity. Density of sucrose was determined by refractive index measurements.

and had similar characteristics. One virus (ARV-2) was recovered within 2 weeks directly from the PMC of a patient approximately 1 month before the onset of AIDS (Fig. 1A). AIDS-associated retroviruses were isolated from subsequent cultures taken 2 and 6 months later, after the onset of AIDS. Multiple time-spaced samplings from five of six other patients with AIDS have also yielded retroviruses (data not shown).

The reverse transcriptase activity of these viruses was associated with particles banding in a sucrose gradient at 1 : 14 to 1 : 16 g/ml (Fig. 1B). With poly(rA) · oligo(dT) or poly(rC) · oligo (dG) as template primers, the viral enzyme had up to an eightfold cation preference for Mg^{2+} over Mn^{2+}. With Mg^{2+}, reverse transcriptase levels higher than 3.5×10^6 cpm per milliliter of culture supernatant could be reached.

The isolated viruses induced multinucleated cells in lymphocyte cultures and did not immortalize the cells. Particles with characteristic type D retrovirus morphology were detected by electron microscopy (Fig. 2). Budding forms showed early features of both type C and type D particles, but only mature type D particles were observed in the cultures.

When antibodies to HTLV-I and LAV were used to detect viral antigens in the cultures infected with these seven isolates (see legend to Table 2), only the antibody to LAV (serum from patient B.R.U.) reacted with cells; up to 20 percent of the cells in these cultures had LAV-related antigens. Sera from AIDS patients in San Francisco reacted with the infected cells in a similar manner (see below).

In attempts to establish ARV in continuous culture, we infected human T cell lines in the presence of antiserum to interferon and Polybrene. The MOLT-4 and CCRF-CEM lines could not be successfully infected, but in the HUT-78 line (8) virus was replicated in substantial titer. This cell line has been useful for the continuous propagation of ARV and the detection of antibodies against virus-infected cells.

A HUT-78 line infected for several weeks with ARV-2 was used to look for antibodies to ARV in sera from patients with AIDS or lymphadenopathy syndrome and in sera from other individuals. The sera were also examined for antibodies to HTLV-I and LAV (Table 2). The results indicated a high prevalence of antibodies to ARV in sera from patients with AIDS and lymphadenopathy syndrome and in sera from steady sexual partners of AIDS patients and healthy homosexual men. When the antibody-negative sera from patients with AIDS and lymphadenopathy syndrome were tested at a lower dilution, all sera from AIDS patients and all but two sera from lymphadenopathy patients reacted with the ARV-infected cells (footnote to Table 2). No antibodies were detected in the sera of healthy heterosexual individ

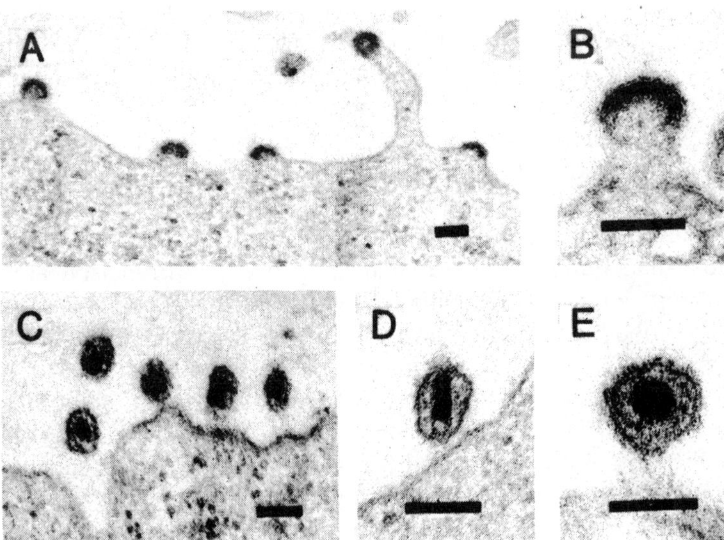

Fig. 2. Transmission electron microscopy of thin sections of peripheral mononuclear cells producing ARV. Cells were fixed in glutaraldehyde, washed, postfixed in osmium tetroxide, and embedded in Araldite. Thin sections were stained in uranyl acetate and lead citrate. (A and B) Budding forms typical of type C and D particles; (C to E) complete extracellular forms of type D morphology. Scale bar, 100 nm.

258

Table 2. The presence of antibodies to HTLV-I in sera from patients and controls was assessed with slides containing acetone-fixed smears of the M-2 cell line (provided by Y. Hinuma) in which 100 percent of the cells demonstrate HTLV or ATLV antigens (*3*). The controls for this experiment included the M-1 line (from Y. Hinuma), which has less than 1 percent positive cells, and the HUT-78 cell line (provided by A. Gazdar, Bethesda) (*8*), which lacks expression of HTLV (*11*). The cells were fixed in acetone and then assayed by standard indirect immunofluorescence procedures; heated (56°C, 30 minutes) sera from AIDS patients and other patients and controls were used at an initial dilution of 1:10. Antibodies to LAV were detected with fixed cells obtained from Barré-Sinoussi. About 10 percent of these lymphocytes were infected with LAV. Antibodies to ARV were detected with an HUT-78 line in which 40 percent of the cells were infected with ARV-2. Most sera were tested as coded samples. The data are the number of individuals showing positive results as a fraction of the number of individuals tested, with the corresponding percentages given in parentheses.

Subjects	HTLV-I	LAV	ARV
Patients with diagnosis of			
AIDS with Kaposi's sarcoma	7/55 (13)	20/38 (53)	59/67* (88)
AIDS with opportunistic infection	1/5 (20)	2/2 (100)	19/19 (100)
Lymphadenopathy syndrome	1/13 (8)	1/4 (25)	22/27* (81)
Other individuals			
Male sexual partners of AIDS patients	1/19 (5)	7/18 (39)	13/14 (93)
Clinically healthy homosexual men	1/13 (8)	1/4 (25)	27/47* (57)
Clinically healthy heterosexual individuals	0/12 (0)	0/9 (0)	0/56* (0)

*When antibody negative–sera were tested at a 1:5 dilution against the ARV-infected cells, all eight AIDS patients (giving 67 of 67, or 100 percent positive), three of five lymphadenopathy syndrome patients (giving 25 of 27, or 92 percent positive), and 3 of 20 healthy homosexual controls (giving 30 of 47, or 64 percent positive) showed reactivity. None of the sera from healthy heterosexual individuals was positive at this dilution.

uals from San Francisco. All available sera of individuals from whom ARV was isolated had antibodies to the virus. Some patients' sera titered at 1:640. The high frequency of these antibodies in healthy homosexuals may reflect a bias resulting from the use of some volunteers for these studies. Nevertheless, these results indicate the close association of ARV with AIDS and lymphadenopathy syndrome, the widespread presence of ARV in the homosexual community, and the detection of greater numbers of individuals with antibodies to ARV than with infectious virus. The data support the contention that lymphadenopathy syndrome is related to AIDS. The prevalence of antibodies to LAV in the patients is in agreement with data from others (*4*). The lower frequency of antibodies to LAV than of antibodies to ARV could be related to the difficulty in reading the results of the immunofluorescence tests, with only 10 percent of the cells infected. All sera that reacted with LAV also contained antibodies to ARV. The low incidence of antibodies to HTLV-I in our patients was consistent with previous reports (*5, 6*).

These studies indicate that patients with AIDS and lymphadenopathy syndrome as well as the steady sexual partners of these patients and healthy homosexual men in the San Francisco area have retroviruses in their PMC and bone marrow (Table 1). The retroviruses studied in detail have the characteristics of LAV. Serologic examination showed a high prevalence of antibodies to ARV and LAV in randomly selected patients and healthy homosexual men in the San Francisco area. We have also detected antibodies to ARV in sera from AIDS patients living elsewhere in the world.

These results are the first independent confirmation of LAV-like viruses in patients outside Europe. Our data cannot reflect a contamination of our cultures with LAV since the original French isolate was never received in our laboratory. The relation of ARV to the recently described HTLV-III is still unknown. However, the similarity of the San Francisco isolates to LAV, the same reverse transcriptase cation preference, the same morphology under electron microscopy, and cytopathic effects similar to those of HTLV-III, suggest that all three virus types belong to the same retrovirus subfamily. Although no conclusion can yet be made concerning their etiologic role in AIDS, their biologic properties and prevalence in AIDS patients certainly suggest that these retroviruses could cause this disease.

References and Notes

1. H. W. Jaffe *et al.*, *Ann. Int. Med.* **99**, 145 (1983); H. W. Jaffe, D. J. Bregman, R. M. Selih, *J. Infect. Dis.* **148**, 339 (1983); D. I. Abrams, B. J. Lewis, J. H. Beckstead, C. A. Casavant, W. L. Drew, *Ann. Int. Med.* **100**, 801 (1984).
2. J. W. Pape *et al.*, *N. Engl. J. Med.* **309**, 945 (1983); N. Clumeck *et al.*, *ibid.* **310**, 492 (1984); E. P. Gelmann *et al.*, *Science* **220**, 862 (1983); R. C. Gallo *et al.*, *ibid.*, p. 865.
3. B. J. Poiesz *et al.*, *Proc. Natl. Acad. Sci. U.S.A.* **77**, 7415 (1980); Y. Hinuma *et al.*, *ibid.* **78**, 6476 (1981); W. L. Drew *et al.*, *J. Infect. Dis.* **143**, 188 (1981).
4. F. Barré-Sinoussi *et al.*, *Science* **220**, 868 (1983).
5. L. Montagnier *et al.*, *Cold Spring Harbor Symp. Quant. Biol.*, in press; E. Vilmer *et al.*, *Lancet* **1984-I**, 753 (1984).
6. M. Popovic, M. G. Sarngadharan, E. Read, R. C. Gallo, *Science* **224**, 497 (1984); R. C. Gallo *et al.*, *ibid.*, p. 500.
7. J. A. Levy, in preparation.
8. A. F. Gazdar *et al.*, *Blood* **55**, 409 (1980).
9. A. Boyum, *Scand. J. Clin. Lab. Invest.* **21**, 51 (1968).
10. M. Robert-Guroff *et al.*, *J. Exp. Med.* **154**, 1957 (1981); Y. Tanaka *et al.*, *Gann* **74**, 327 (1983).
11. V. S. Kalyanaraman *et al.*, *J. Virol.* **38**, 906 (1981).
12. Supported by NIH grant CA-34980 and by a grant from the California State University-wide AIDS Task Force. We thank M. Conant, P. Volberding, D. Abrams, D. Miner, H. Banghart, B. Miller, J. Campbell, J. Greenspan, D. Stites, and J. Delameter, San Francisco, for providing the clinical specimens and sera used for these studies. We thank L. Tobler for some of the tissue culture studies, B. Banapour for help with the reverse transcriptase assays, L. Kaminsky for assistance in the serologic studies, and C. Beglinger for preparation of the manuscript.

31 May 1984; accepted 20 June 1984

Report

31 August 1984

48. Homology of Genome of AIDS-Associated Virus with Genomes of Human T-Cell Leukemia Viruses

Suresh K. Arya, Robert C. Gallo, Beatrice H. Hahn, George M. Shaw, Mikulas Popovic, S. Zaki Salahuddin, Flossie Wong-Staal

Human T-cell leukemia virus (HTLV) was first identified as an infectious agent etiologically associated with adult T-cell leukemia (ATL) (*1*). A related but distinct retrovirus was isolated from a T-cell variant of hairy cell leukemia (*2*). These viruses, known, respectively, as HTLV-I and HTLV-II, show a tropism for human T cells, particularly OKT4$^+$ cells, and have the capacity to immortalize and transform normal T cells in culture (*3*), alter certain T-cell immune functions in vitro (*4*), induce the formation of giant multinucleated T cells (*5*), and, in some cases, selectively kill certain T cells (*6*). These properties and data from epidemiologic studies of the acquired immune deficiency syndrome (AIDS), which is uniformly associated with OKT4$^+$ helper cell depletion (*7*), led us and others to speculate (*8*) that a member of the HTLV family might be the etiological agent of this disease. In support of this hypothesis was the finding that up to 80 percent of AIDS patients, but less than 1 percent of non-AIDS patients from similar risk groups, have serum antibodies that react with the envelope protein of HTLV (*9*). However, actual isolations of the known subgroups of HTLV (that is, HTLV-I and HTLV-II) from AIDS patients were infrequent (*10*).

Recently, we reported repeated isolations of a T lymphotropic retrovirus with cytopathic but not immortalizing activity from patients with AIDS (*11*). This virus can be grown in a previously immortalized T-cell line (HT) that is relatively resistant to the cytopathic effects of the virus and can grow in the absence of T-cell growth factor (interleukin-2) (*12*). Using the infected cells as well as purified virus particles in immunological assays, we found that the serum of 80 to 100 percent of AIDS patients and 70 to 80 percent of patients with lymphadenopathy syndrome reacted positively (*13*). On the basis of its T-cell tropism, the size and Mg^{2+} preference of its reverse transcriptase, the size of its major core protein (24,000 daltons) (*14*), some antigenic cross-reactivity of its proteins with HTLV-I and HTLV-II (*14*), and its capacity to induce formation of giant multinucleated cells (*12*), we considered this virus to be a member of the HTLV family and designated it HTLV-III. Here

we show that certain sequences of the genome of HTLV-III and both HTLV-I and HTLV-II are homologous, with the most conserved sequences being located within the *gag-pol* region and less but detectable homology occurring in the *env* and pX region.

Virus particles were purified from supernatant fluids of HT cells, clone 9 (H9) infected with HTLV-III (HTLV-III$_B$) by centrifugation through a sucrose density gradient at equilibrium (*12*). HTLV-III$_B$ was originally obtained from pooled supernatants of short-term lymphocyte cultures of AIDS patients. Virus particles were also purified from normal peripheral blood lymphocytes newly infected by virus of a primary leukocyte culture of another AIDS patient (HTLV-III$_Z$) (*11*). The particles were lysed with sodium dodecyl sulfate (SDS), digested with proteinase K, and directly chromatographed on an oligo(dT) cellulose column. The resulting polyadenylate [poly(A)]-containing RNA was used as template to synthesize ^{32}P-labeled complementary DNA (cDNA) in the presence of oligo(dT) primers. The size of the resultant cDNA ranged from 0.1 to 10 kb (not shown). When these labeled cDNA's were hybridized to poly(A)-containing RNA purified from infected and uninfected H9 cells as well as other uninfected human cell lines, only the infected H9 cells contained homologous RNA sequences as evidenced by discrete RNA bands after Northern hybridization. Figure 1 shows that cDNA preparations from HTLV-III$_B$ and HTLV-III$_Z$ gave identical patterns, detecting RNA species of about 9.0, 4.2, and 2.0 kb. These bands are similar in size to those corresponding to genomic size messenger RNA (mRNA) and spliced mRNA's of *env* and pX sequences previously observed in cells infected with HTLV-I

(*15*), consistent with the anticipated relatedness of these viruses. Furthermore, viral mRNA bands of HTLV-II–infected cells were detected with an HTLV-III cDNA probe (Fig. 1b, lane 6) and again the sizes of the mRNA were like those with HTLV-I.

To determine directly the homology between HTLV-III and HTLV-I and HTLV-II, we hybridized HTLV-III cDNA to cloned genomes of HTLV-I and HTLV-II digested with specific restriction endonucleases. Complete genomes of a prototype HTLV-I (*16*), an HTLV-I variant called HTLV-Ib (*16*), and HTLV-II were digested with two restriction enzymes as indicated in the legend to Fig. 2 and blot-hybridized to ^{32}P-labeled HTLV-III$_B$ cDNA. A region spanning the *gag* and *pol* genes showed the greatest homology. For the prototype HTLV-I, this corresponds to the 1.7-kb Pst I–Pst I fragment and 5.3-kb Sst I–Sal I fragment. HTLV-Ib, which lacks a Pst I site indicated in parentheses in Fig. 2, revealed the expected 3.0-kb Pst I–Pst I fragment instead. Similarly, strong hybridization to the *gag-pol* sequences of HTLV-II also occurred. This is reflected in the 4.2-kb Bam HI–Xho I fragment and the 4.0-kb Bam HI–Eco RI fragment (Fig. 2, lanes 5 and 6).

Fragments corresponding to the *env* and pX sequences of HTLV-I and HTLV-II also hybridized weakly with HTLV-III$_B$ cDNA (see the 2.4-kb Pst I–Pst I and the 2.1-kb Sst I–Pst I fragment in Fig. 2, lane 1) as did the 1.4-kb Pst I fragment of HTLV-Ib containing only pX sequences (Fig. 2, lane 4). The ease of detection of these sequences varied with different preparations of cDNA, probably because of variable representations of the 3′ end of the virus genome. We used cDNA from both HTLV-III$_B$ and HTLV-III$_Z$. Figure 3 shows the results for HTLV-III$_Z$ cDNA. Subclones of HTLV-I containing different regions of the genome were hybridized to

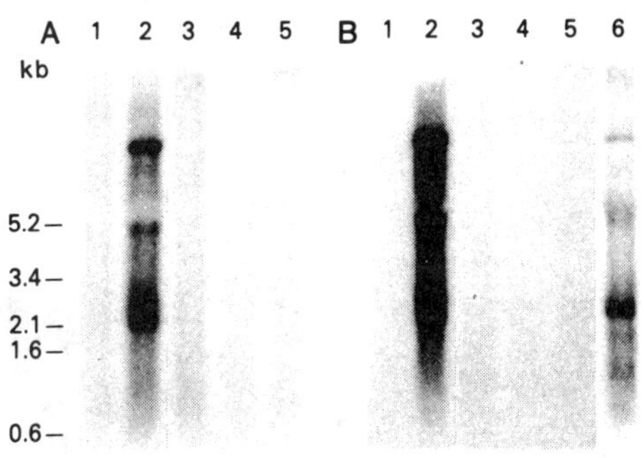

Fig. 1. HTLV-III–specific sequences in cellular RNA from HTLV-infected cells. Poly(A)-selected cellular RNA was size-separated by formaldehyde-agarose gel electrophoresis, transferred to Zeta probe membrane (Bio-Rad Labs) by electroelution and hybridized to (A) HTLV-III$_B$ cDNA and (B) HTLV-III$_Z$ cDNA. (A and B) Lane 1, uninfected H9 cells (5 μg); lane 2, HTLV-III$_B$–infected H9 cells (10 μg); lane 3, leukemic Jurkat cells (10 μg); lane 4, HTLV-I–infected C5/MJ cells (5 μg); and lane 5, HTLV-II–infected MO cells (5 μg). (B) Lane 6, a longer exposure of lane 5 in (B). Poly(A)-selected RNA was prepared by guanidine-HCl extraction and cesium chloride centrifugation followed by oligo(dT) cellulose chromatography as described (*24*). The cDNA was transcribed from poly(A)-selected virus-associated RNA with the use of oligo(dT) as a primer and avian myeloblastosis virus RNA-directed DNA polymerase as described (*25*). The hybridization was performed at 37°C for 16 hours in a mixture containing 40 percent formamide, 5× standard sodium chloride and sodium citrate (SSC; 0.15*M* NaCl and 0.015*M* sodium citrate, *p*H 7), 0.05*M* sodium phosphate buffer (*p*H 7), 5× PM (0.02 percent each of bovine serum albumin, polyvinylpyrrolidone, and Ficoll 400), yeast RNA (200 μg/ml), denatured salmon sperm DNA (20 μg/ml), 0.1 percent SDS, and 10 percent dextran sulfate. The membrane was subsequently repeatedly washed with 2× SSC and 0.1 percent SDS at 62°C, air-dried, and exposed to a Kodak XAR film with the use of intensifying screens.

HTLV-III$_Z$ cDNA (Fig. 3A). With the exception of fragment c, which corresponds to an internal portion of the *pol* gene, all fragments were detected by hybridization, including fragment a (LTR-*gag*) after long exposure of the

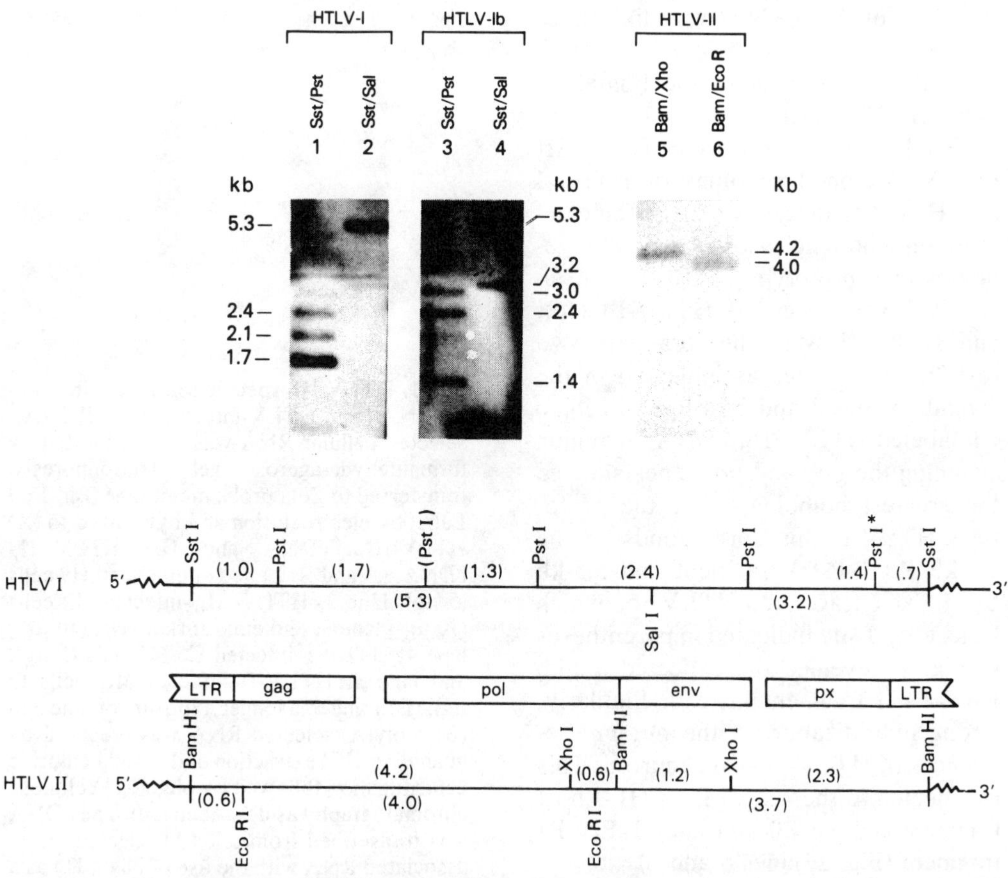

Fig. 2. Relatedness of the genome of HTLV-III$_B$ with the genomes of HTLV-I and HTLV-II. Sites of digestion by the relevant restriction enzymes and the expected sizes of the fragments are shown below the gels. Cloned HTLV-I (λST), HTLV-Ib (λMC), and HTLV-II (pMO) DNA's were digested with the indicated restriction enzymes and fragments were separated by agarose gel electrophoresis, transferred to a nitrocellulose membrane (23), and hybridized with HTLV-III$_B$cDNA. Lanes 1 and 2, HTLV-I (λST) DNA digested with Sst I plus Pst I and Sst I plus Sal I, respectively; lanes 3 and 4, HTLV-Ib (λMC) DNA digested with Sst I plus Pst I and Sst I plus Sal I, respectively; lanes 5 and 6, HTLV-II (pMO) DNA digested with Bam HI plus Xho I and Bam HI plus Eco RI, respectively. HTLV-I (λST) and HTLV-I (λMC) clones were obtained from the genomic libraries of DNA's from ATL patients S.T. and M.C., respectively. Both cellular DNA's were cloned at the Sst I site of phage λgtWES · λB DNA (16). HTLV-I (λST) is a prototype HTLV-I and HTLV-Ib (λMC) is a variant of HTLV-I that contains some divergent restriction enzyme sites, including the lack of the second Pst I site from the 5' end of the viral genome (16). HTLV-II (pMO) was obtained by subcloning λMO15A (26) at the Bam HI site of plasmid pBR322 DNA. The cDNA was synthesized as described in Fig. 1 and hybridization was performed at 37°C for 16 hours in a mixture containing 30 percent formamide, 5× SSC, 5× PM, denatured DNA (100 μg/ml), 0.1 percent SDS, and 10 percent dextran sulfate. The membrane was subsequently washed and exposed as described in Fig. 1.

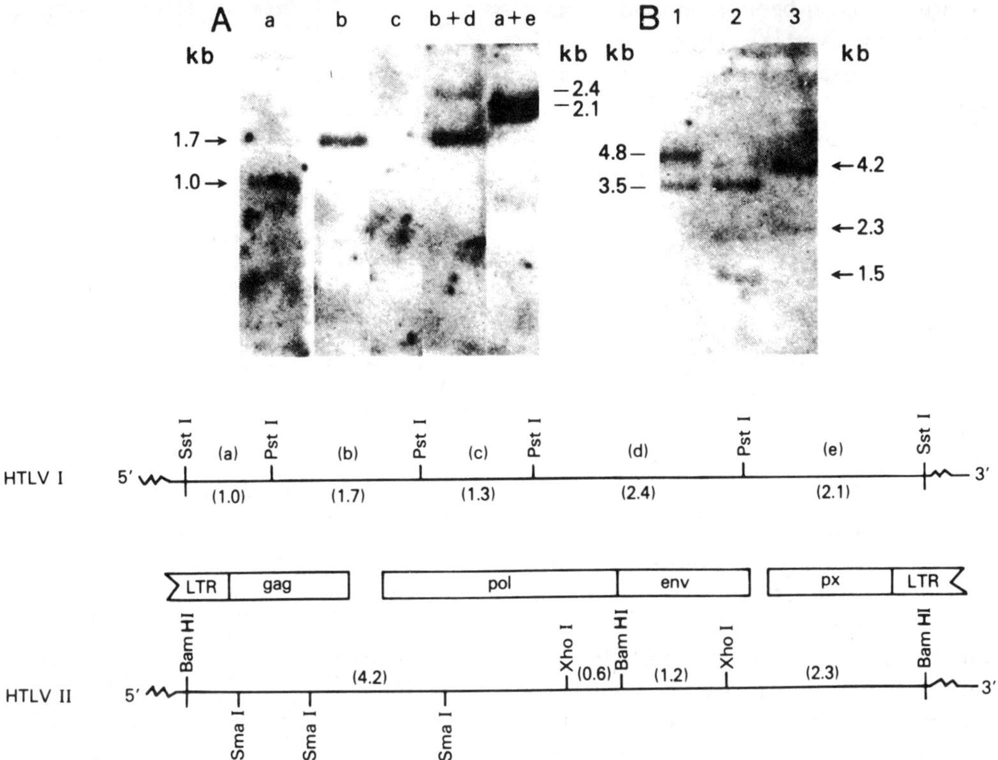

Fig. 3. Relatedness of the genome of HTLV-III$_Z$ with the genomes of HTLV-I and HTLV-II. DNA from subclones of HTLV-I$_{ST}$ and HTLV-II$_{MO}$ was digested with the indicated restriction enzymes. Fragments were separated by agarose gel electrophoresis, transferred to a nitrocellulose membrane (24), and hybridized with HTLV-III$_Z$ cDNA. (A) HTLV-I subclones were constructed by "shotgun" cloning of fragments generated by codigestion with Pst I and Sst I into pBR322 containing fragments designated a to e on the illustrated restriction map of HTLV-I. The viral inserts were released by digestion with the appropriate enzymes. (B) HTLV-II (pMO) DNA: Lane 1, digested with Bam HI; lane 2, digested with Bam HI plus Sma I; lane 3, digested with Bam HI plus Xho I. The cDNA was synthesized as in Fig. 1 and hybridization was performed as in Fig. 2, except that the hybridization mixture contained 40 percent formamide.

autoradiogram. Similarly, the 3' half of HTLV-II contained in the 3.5-kb Bam HI–Bam HI fragment and the 2.3-kb Bam HI–Xho I fragment could be detected with this particular HTLV-III cDNA probe (Fig. 3B).

Retroviruses called LAV (or sometimes IDAV$_1$ and IDAV$_2$) have been isolated from patients with lymphadenopathy syndrome and AIDS (17). Although LAV has been reported to lack relatedness to HTLV-I and -II (17), further characterization of its proteins and

nucleic acids may reveal that LAV is related to these viruses and is identical to or related to HTLV-III.

The present data showing that certain nucleotide sequences of HTLV-III are homologous to sequences of HTLV-I and HTLV-II support our proposal that this virus should be classified within the HTLV family. However, HTLV-III is much less related to HTLV-II and HTLV-I than HTLV-II and HTLV-I are to each other. It is of interest that still other HTLV-related T lymphotropic ret-

264

roviruses have been identified in Old World monkeys (*18*). These primate viruses are closely related to HTLV-I and only minimally to HTLV-II (*19*). Although the most conserved sequences of HTLV-III are in the region spanning the junction of the predicted *gag* and *pol* genes, other weakly homologous sequences are also detected in the *env* and pX genes. Homology in the *gag* and *env* coding sequences has already been suggested by immunological cross-reactivity between these antigens derived from the three subgroups (*14*). Homology in the pX region is an additional demonstration that HTLV-III belongs to the HTLV family, which is unique among retroviruses in its possession of the pX genes (*20, 21*). It is interesting that pX is the most conserved region between HTLV-I and HTLV-II (*21*) and that both of these viruses can transform T cells in vitro. In contrast, the pX region is much less conserved in HTLV-III, a cytopathic virus that lacks transforming activity (*11, 12*).

Comparisons of the LTR regions between HTLV-I and HTLV-II have revealed a conserved 21-bp repeat sequence in two otherwise very divergent LTR's (*22*). The location of this sequence upstream of promoter sequences suggests that it is similar to other viral enhancer sequences. In view of the tropism of HTLV-III for OKT4$^+$ lymphocytes, it will be interesting to see if this virus also has such an enhancer sequence in its LTR. Our present study does not allow us to compare specifically the LTR of HTLV-III to those of HTLV-I and -II. However, the weak signal obtained with 5' and 3' ultimate fragments containing the LTR suggest that these elements have minimal or no homology.

References and Notes

1. R. C. Gallo and F. Wong-Staal, *Blood* **60**, 545 (1982); R. C. Gallo, in *Cancer Surveys*, L. M. Franks, L. M. Wyke, R. A. Weiss, Eds. (Oxford Univ. Press, Oxford, 1984), vol. 3, pp. 113–159.
2. V. S. Kalyanaraman *et al.*, *Science* **218**, 571 (1982).
3. I. Miyoshi *et al.*, *Nature (London)* **294**, 770 (1981); M. Popovic, G. Lange-Wantzin, P. S. Sarin, D. Mann, R. C. Gallo, *Proc. Natl. Acad. Sci. U.S.A.* **80**, 5402 (1983); P. D. Markham *et al.*, *Int. J. Cancer* **31**, 413 (1983); I. S. Y. Chen *et al.*, *Nature (London)* **305**, 502 (1983); M. Popovic *et al.*, in *Human T-Cell Leukemia Viruses*, R. C. Gallo, M. Essex, L. Gross, Eds. (Cold Spring Harbor Laboratory, Cold Spring Harbor, N.Y., in press).
4. M. Popovic *et al.*, in preparation.
5. M. Popovic, F. Wong-Staal, P. S. Sarin, R. C. Gallo, *Adv. Viral Oncol.* **4**, 45 (1984); K. Nagy, P. Clapham, R. Cheingson-Popov, R. A. Weiss, *Int. J. Cancer* **32**, 321 (1983).
6. H. Mitsuya *et al.*, *Science* **223**, 1293 (1984).
7. Centers for Disease Control Task Force on Kaposi's Sarcoma and Opportunistic Infections, *N. Engl. J. Med.* **306**, 248 (1982); J. P. Hanragan, G. P. Wormser, C. P. Macquire, L. J. DeLorenzo, G. Davis, *ibid.* **307**, 498 (1982); J. W. Curran *et al.*, *ibid.* **310**, 69 (1984).
8. R. C. Gallo, P. S. Sarin, W. A. Blattner, F. Wong-Staal, M. Popovic, in *Seminars in Oncology: AIDS*, J. E. Groopman, Ed. (Grune & Stratton, San Diego, 1984), pp. 12–17; M. Essex *et al.*, in *Human T-Cell Leukemia Viruses*, R. C. Gallo, M. Essex, L. Gross, Eds. (Cold Spring Harbor Laboratory, Cold Spring Harbor, N.Y., in press).
9. M. Essex *et al.*, *Science* **220**, 859 (1983); *ibid.* **221**, 1061 (1983); T. H. Lee *et al.*, *Proc. Natl. Acad. Sci. U.S.A.*, in press.
10. R. C. Gallo *et al.*, *Science* **220**, 865 (1983); B. H. Hahn *et al.*, in *Acquired Immune Deficiency Syndrome, UCLA Symposia on Molecular and Cellular Biology*, M. S. Gottlieb and J. E. Groopman, Eds. (Liss, New York, in press).
11. R. C. Gallo *et al.*, *Science* **224**, 500 (1984).
12. M. Popovic, M. G. Sarngadharan, E. Read, R. C. Gallo, *ibid.*, p. 497.
13. M. G. Sarngadharan, M. Popovic, L. Bruch, J. Schupbach, R. C. Gallo, *ibid.*, p. 506; M. G. Sarngadharan *et al.*, in preparation.
14. J. Schüpbach *et al.*, *Science* **224**, 503 (1984).
15. G. Franchini, F. Wong-Staal, R. C. Gallo, *Proc. Natl. Acad. Sci. U.S.A.*, in press.
16. B. Hahn *et al.*, *Int. J. Cancer*, in press.
17. F. Barre-Sinoussi *et al.*, *Science* **220**, 868 (1983); E. Vilmer *et al.*, *Lancet* **1984-I**, 753 (1984); L. Montagnier, personal communication.
18. I. Miyoshi *et al.*, *Gann* **74**, 323 (1983); C. W. Saxinger *et al.*, in *Human T-Cell Leukemia Viruses*, R. C. Gallo, M. Essex, L. Gross, Eds. (Cold Spring Harbor Laboratory, Cold Spring Harbor, N.Y., in press).
19. H.-G. Guo, F. Wong-Staal, R. C. Gallo, *Science* **223**, 1195 (1984).
20. M. Seiki, S. Hattori, Y. Hirayama, M. Yoshida, *Proc. Natl. Acad. Sci. U.S.A.* **80**, 3618 (1983).
21. G. M. Shaw *et al.*, *ibid.* **81**, 4544 (1984).
22. J. Sodroski *et al.*, *ibid.*, in press.

23. E. M. Southern, *J. Mol. Biol.* **98**, 503 (1973).
24. R. A. Cox, *Methods Enzymol.* **12**, 120 (1967); S. L. Adams *et al.*, *Proc. Natl. Acad. Sci. U.S.A.* **74**, 3399 (1980).
25. T. Maniatis, E. F. Fritsch, J. Sambrook, *Molecular Cloning. A Laboratory Manual* (Cold Spring Harbor Laboratory, Cold Spring Harbor, N.Y., 1983), pp. 23–233.
26. E. P. Gelmann *et al.*, *Proc. Natl. Acad. Sci. U.S.A.* **81**, 993 (1984).
27. We gratefully acknowledge the help and advice of Dr. P. Markham and the expert editorial assistance of A. Mozzuca.

1 May 1984; accepted 30 May 1984

Letter to the Editor

7 September 1984

49. Haitians and AIDS

Jean W. Pape, Bernard Liautaud, Franck Thomas, Jean-Robert Mathurin, Marie-Myrtha A. St. Amand, Madeleine Boncy, Vergniaud Pean, Molière Pamphile, A. Claude LaRoche, and Warren D. Johnson, Jr.

Gallo *et al.* (*1*) report that HTLV-III is the most likely candidate virus for the acquired immune deficiency syndrome (AIDS). The test for HTLV-III antibodies will help define more accurately the populations at risk of developing AIDS. In the Research News article about the work by Gallo *et al.* (*Science*, 4 May 1984), Jean L. Marx projects that "there may be an enormous demand for the test." She notes that among the 20 million homosexual males in the United States an unknown number are promiscuous and therefore at high risk of developing AIDS. However, she also includes half a million Haitians, virtually all Haitians living in the United States, in the group of people who will need to be tested for HTLV-III. We are not aware of data in the literature that show an association of HTLV-III and healthy Haitians, or even Haitian patients with AIDS. In our most recent experience in Haiti, we have found accepted risk factors in 67 percent of our patients with AIDS (*2*), indicating that not all Haitians are at risk for AIDS, as Marx implies, but rather a selected subgroup.

References

1. R. C. Gallo *et al.*, *Science* **224**, 500 (1984); M. Popovic *et al.*, *ibid.*, p. 497; J. Schüpbach *et al.*, *ibid.*, p. 503; M. G. Sarngadharan *et al.*, *ibid.*, p. 506.
2. J. W. Pape *et al.*, *Clin. Res.* **32**, 379A (1984).

50. Crash Development of AIDS Test Nears Goal

Barbara J. Culliton

The recent discovery of a virus that is almost surely the cause of AIDS (acquired immune deficiency syndrome) has turned the need for a highly visible AIDS crusade on the part of the federal government into a real political imperative. Ever since the devastating immune system disease was first identified in homosexual men 3 years ago, the Reagan Administration has been criticized by "gay" activists for its alleged failure to mount a well financed war on AIDS. So this spring, when Administration officials learned that Robert C. Gallo, a government scientist with the National Cancer Institute, had isolated and grown the AIDS virus, they were quick to seize the moment to do something visible and to do it fast.

The 23rd of April was a landmark day. That morning, government attorneys filed patent applications covering the Gallo work. Hours later, news that the AIDS virus had been discovered made headlines around the world following a press conference in Washington, D.C., at which Gallo reported that acquired immune deficiency syndrome is caused by a human retrovirus called HTLV-III, which is a variant of a class of human tumor viruses that were previously discovered in his laboratory.* Four papers on HTLV-III by Gallo and his many colleagues appeared in the 4 May 1984 issue of *Science*.

Margaret M. Heckler, the former Republican congresswoman who is now Secretary of the Department of Health and Human Services (HHS), and whose office orchestrated the press conference, stood by Gallo's side. Lauding him for his achievement, she went on to promise that within 6 months there would be a test to screen the U.S. blood supply for evidence of the AIDS virus. Although AIDS occurs primarily in promiscuous homosexual men and intravenous drug users, it also afflicts hemophiliacs who become infected by contaminated blood products. And, to date, at least 50 cases of AIDS have been diagnosed in persons who most likely became infected when they received transfusions of AIDS-posi-

*At present, research on the viral etiology of AIDS focuses on the putative role of two viruses: HTLV-III (human T-cell lymphotropic virus) found by National Cancer Institute scientists and a closely related agent, LAV (lymphadenopathy virus), which was reported a year ago by researchers from the Pasteur Institute in Paris. (A set of papers on AIDS virus by American and French scientists was published in the 20 May 1983 issue of *Science*. Papers on HTLV-III appeared in the 4 May 1984 issue.) Whether HTLV-III and LAV are in fact the same virus, as many virologists expect, ought to be known for certain within a matter of weeks. Whether they match up nucleotide for nucleotide under molecular analysis or not, there is little doubt that from a clinical point of view, these nearly identical viruses cause the disease. The outcome of disputes over priority for finding the AIDS virus has implications not only in terms of scientific credit but also with regard to patent rights and commercial activity. However, the HTLV-III/LAV question does not appear to be central in the short run to the results of the crash program to develop a simple assay for detecting evidence of AIDS virus in the blood supply.

tive blood. Thus, a blood test for AIDS would be useful for diagnosing early disease among high-risk populations and for screening the nation's blood supply. Secretary Heckler promised not only that the test would be available within 6 months but also that it would provide "100 percent certainty."

The Secretary promised. This is an election year and AIDS is a significant public health problem that could figure in the campaign. Out of a combination of scientific accomplishment and political necessity, HHS has launched its own campaign to make the Secretary's promise come true. Five U.S. drug and biotechnology companies have been awarded licenses by the government which give them access to HTLV-III for commercial development. Competition among them to come out with a test kit is fierce and there is every reason to bet success is not far off.

The five competitors, selected from a field of some 20 corporate applicants, are Abbott Laboratories, North Chicago; Electro-Nucleonics, Columbia, Maryland; E. I. du Pont de Nemours, Wilmington, Delaware, in collaboration with Biotech Research Laboratories. Rockville, Maryland; Litton Bionetics, Kensington, Maryland; and Travenol Genentech Diagnostics, Cambridge. In June, each of the five received 25 liters of HTLV-III infected cells, which are being produced in large quantities at the cancer institute's facility in Frederick, Maryland. It is expected that most of them will be ready to file "investigational new drug applications" any day now with the Food and Drug Administration (FDA) which must approve clinical trials of the test kits and which has ultimate say over their approval for commercial marketing. (For a discussion of how the five

companies were chosen, see following article.)

While federal health officials are monitoring the progress toward development of a mass screen for the blood supply, they are also anxiously trying to put in place a relatively large-scale study that will also contribute answers to crucial questions about the transmissibility of the disease. Is AIDS spreading beyond what is currently identified as the high-risk population to the population at large? If so, how? Although there is evidence that the disease is transmitted by the transfusion of AIDS-positive blood, frankly little is known about how great a risk that is. Will most people who receive contaminated blood come down with AIDS or only a few?

To answer questions about the natural history and epidemiology of the disease, the National Heart, Lung and Blood Institute began designing a study several months ago (before Gallo reported on HTLV-III) to enable investigators to track the distribution of blood from four of the country's largest voluntary blood banks, namely those in New York, Miami, Los Angeles, and San Francisco, cities where the incidence of AIDS is highest. The idea behind the study is to collect blood samples now for subsequent testing so that it will be possible in a 6- to 7-year follow-up to see what happens to patients who receive a unit or more of transfused AIDS-positive blood. Will they get AIDS? Or a milder "pre-AIDS" infection? Or might they be unaffected?

Researchers concerned with the natural history and epidemiology of AIDS recognize an urgent need to get at these questions—a need that, for ethical reasons, has been made all the more urgent now that a means of screening blood before it is transfused is so close on the horizon. Using the argot of the space program, HHS officials talk about a brief "window of opportunity" for this study which will close once mass screening removes from the blood supply those units that test positive for AIDS.

"Between now and the time a test is commercially available, we have a unique scientific opportunity to learn about the transmission of this disease," says heart institute director Claude Lenfant. "But it is important to emphasize that this study can only take place because the blood we want to collect and screen will be used in the usual course of blood banking now whether we do our study or not. An informed consent form must clearly explain that we are not deliberately transmitting AIDS."

The design of the first phase of the study is this. Some 200,000 normal, healthy blood donors, who do not fall into any of the high-risk groups for AIDS, will be asked now to consent to having a sample of their blood stored at the blood bank for testing a few months from now. Meanwhile, their blood will be available for transfusion just as is usually the case. Then, when test kits are in hand, the samples will be screened. Researchers expect that somewhere between one-half and one percent of the blood from these normal donors will test AIDS-positive. Both the donors and the patients who received their blood will then become part of a long-term research project.

From a medical point of view, this study makes an enormous amount of sense. If AIDS is spreading slowly among the general population through the blood supply, it is vital to know that. But from an ethical and public relations point of view, this study, which has been under intense—virtually daily—discussion by federal health officials for the past 8 weeks, is creating terrible dilemmas.

For weeks, government scientists and blood bank officials have been arguing over the informed consent form that the blood donors will be asked to sign. A major sticking point was the question of notification of donors. According to one source at the National Institutes of Health (NIH) representatives of three of the blood banks argued vigorously against notifying the donor that his or her blood tested positive for AIDS. The argument was twofold. Weighing the duty to do no harm against the good to be done, some believe notification can only be harmful at present because the meaning of an AIDS-positive test is unclear. Full-blown AIDS is a baffling and nearly 100 percent fatal disease for which there is at present no known cure. It also carries a heavy social stigma. Because the first mass screening tests will be able only to detect antibody to AIDS in the blood, they will provide little clear information about whether the person is at risk of getting a full-blown infection or whether he has simply been exposed to HTLV-III and mounted a successful immune response. Heterosexual blood donors who test AIDS-positive could be falsely labeled homosexuals if the information leaked out. Healthy, nonpromiscuous homosexuals also worry about the stigma that an AIDS-positive test would attach to them. All around, there is concern about what the information would mean to prospective employers or health insurance companies. The issue of confidentiality has been central but is not easily resolved, especially in states where AIDS is a reportable disease. Thus, for many reasons, the likelihood that giving the donor complex, unclear, but frightening information will cause at least psychological stress is very high. The consent form itself will include a statement that says, "the significance of a positive finding and the reliability of the test are not known at this time."

A second argument raised against informing the donor rested on concern that members of high-risk populations who are not readily identifiable as such will lie about their status and donate blood just to find out whether they have AIDS antibodies. By telling the donor, one in effect turns the test into a diagnostic service. Were this to happen, not only would the validity of the data be altered but the risk of actually attracting high-risk donors and contaminating the blood supply increases.

Arguments in favor of informing the donor, espoused by the majority of HHS and NIH scientists involved in the debate, were equally strong and, apparently, have prevailed. As things stand now, for several reasons the decision has been made to tell the donors who agree to participate in the study that they will be notified if the test shows them to be AIDS-positive. First, a positive test will have to be confirmed and the individuals will be closely followed medically for several years for symptoms of AIDS or pre-AIDS. Second, they must be told not to donate blood any more. And third, even though the significance of a positive test is presently unclear, it was agreed that persons have a legal right to know and, in this case, medical professionals have an ethical duty to tell them.

Now that federal officials and blood bank representatives have agreed to the wording of the informed consent, the study has to clear one final hurdle before any blood can actually be collected and stored. Ethical approval of human ex-perimentation rests legally with Institutional Review Boards composed of professionals and laymen who scrutinize research proposals at their respective institutions. If they give their okay, the first stages of this study may begin within a few weeks—a couple of months later than investigators hoped but nonetheless in time to collect samples before the window of opportunity slams shut. Says Amoz Chernoff of the heart institute, "I'm optimistic that the study will go forward."

If it does, unresolved issues will be put on hold for the time being. One crucial matter which has found no consensus yet is the question of what to tell the unwitting recipient of an AIDS-positive transfusion. The arguments about creating anxiety with sketchy information versus a person's right to know and to be medically followed pertain here as they did in the case of the donor. But the recipient, unlike the donor, cannot be asked for prior informed consent because there is no way of knowing in advance that he or she would get AIDS-positive blood. According to Robert Gordon of NIH, the decision about notifying the recipient is being held in abeyance in the hope that by the time the issue has to be faced, enough knowledge will have accrued in this rapidly moving field to permit researchers to convey more useful, clear information than they could now. For instance, within several months it might be possible to screen widely for the presence of viral antigen, rather than just antibody, in the recipient, which would give a better indication of his exposure and risk.

The ethical dilemmas surrounding the consent form in the heart institute's proposed long-term study will be echoed to a degree when the five competing U.S.

companies begin clinical trials of the test kits they are now rushing to develop. Estimates are that as many as 20,000 blood samples will be screened as part of the investigational new drug clearance that precedes FDA approval for marketing. Likewise, once a test is available commercially so that the entire blood supply can be tested, questions of what to tell an AIDS-positive donor will be troublesome until the time comes that individuals either can be reassured that the presence of AIDS antibody is not an inevitable harbinger of serious infection or that successful therapy is at hand. However, health officials point out, despite the thorny issues that rapid test development is raising, the goal of trying to safeguard the blood supply is paramount.

News and Comment

14 September 1984

51.   Five Firms with the Right Stuff

Barbara J. Culliton

On 23 April 1984, the Department of Health and Human Services (HHS) filed patent applications covering the discovery by National Cancer Institute scientists of a virus called HTLV-III that causes AIDS (acquired immune deficiency syndrome). Isolation and characterization of HTLV-III was made by Robert C. Gallo and his colleagues at the cancer institute. Driven by determination to turn that achievement in basic science into a medically useful tool that would be evidence of the Reagan Administration's commitment to fighting AIDS, HHS quickly made plans to grant private companies licenses to use HTLV-III and the cells in which it grows for commercial development of a test to detect evidence of the virus in human blood.

It is standard practice for the federal government to award licenses to private companies, but the extraordinary speed and special attention that was devoted to the licenses for HTLV-III–related techniques bespeak the Administration's desire to refute allegations that it is moving too slowly in its effort to combat this devastating, infectious immune system disorder that primarily afflicts promiscuous homosexuals, intravenous drug users, and hemophiliacs and others who may contract AIDS from transfused blood.

Exactly 2 weeks after government patent applications were filed, a request for proposals appeared in the *Federal Register* and *Business Commerce Daily*. Companies interested in developing a test to screen the nation's entire blood supply were given 10 days to get their applications in. According to Lowell Harmison, science adviser to HHS assistant secretary for health Edward Brandt, some 20 companies were standing in line for a license before the application deadline closed on 17 May.

Meanwhile, scientists at the NCI's facility in Frederick, Maryland, were gearing up for large-scale production of HTLV-III–infected cells to distribute to the companies that would soon be awarded licenses. Frederick scientists with long experience in growing viruses proved remarkably successful at moving into large-scale production but, nonetheless, it was clear that supplies of HTLV-III would be relatively limited. For this reason, and in order to guarantee success by distributing HTLV-III with companies most likely to come through, tough criteria were established for getting a license and, thereby, access to the government's store of AIDS virus. An officer of one competing biotechnology firm said, "They were looking for the companies with the right stuff."

Ten criteria were established, among them these: i) Experience in handling human retroviruses, a family of RNA tumor viruses of which HTLV-III is a subgroup. The government wanted companies that already know how to purify, characterize, and grow these viruses. ii) Because biosafety was a major concern, the companies were required to have existing P–3 containment facilities. iii) The first diagnostic test will most likely be based on a radioimmunoassay system known as EL-ISA (enzyme-linked immunosorbent assay). A technique for detection of antibodies in AIDS and pre-AIDS patients using the HTLV-III core protein, p24, in an ELISA test is covered by one of the federal patent applications. Experience in using ELISA and related tests was another important criteria.

Another criteria of paramount importance, Harmison noted, was proved ability to produce and market a product for mass distribution. There are some 1700 blood banks in the United States and estimates of the numbers of units of blood that might be tested per year range as high as 20 million. Clearly, the potential for profit is enormous, but in order to compete successfully in the race to meet HHS's goal of a mass screening test to be ready within months, the ability to operate on a national scale is also obvious. Any company that failed to meet even one of the ten criteria

was scrubbed from the list of potential licensees, which meant that several of the smaller biotechnology companies with skill in science but not in marketing lost out.

"Seven or eight of the applicants met the criteria," Harmison reports and HHS officials then site-visited the companies to verify such things as the existence of a P-3 facility and a staff of experienced retrovirologists. "If all of the applicants had met the criteria, all would have been awarded a license," Harmison said. But as it turned out, only five had enough of the right stuff: Abbott Laboratories, which already commands a major share of the market for testing blood for hepatitis B; Electro-Nucleonics; DuPont, in collaboration with Biotech Research Laboratories, which was working in collaboration with NCI's Gallo before HTLV-III was nailed down; Litton Bionetics, another biotechnology company with which Gallo has close scientific ties; and Travenol Genetech Diagnostics.

Accuracy, reliability, and cost will play important roles in determining which of the five companies ultimately wins the greatest share of the commercial market once one or more tests are given final approval by the Food and Drug Administration. From a technical point of view, each is taking a slightly different and closely guarded tack, while government officials meet with them regularly to monitor progress as investigational new drug applications to FDA are prepared. Harmison is betting that some of the companies will be ready for clinical trials of test kits by October. Indeed, on a strictly experimental basis, some already are testing blood at the rate of 1000 or more samples a day with assays that can be completed in a matter of hours. Once the test kits are on the market, blood banks will choose which of the approved tests they want to use as the companies vie for their business and for profit.

Another scientifically important challenge in AIDS that also has commercial implications is the development of a vaccine. A number of the companies that failed to win licenses in June now want access to the government's supply of HTLV-III for use in vaccine studies. Although work can proceed without a government license, access to its store of cells confers an advantage. At present, HHS officials are designing criteria for a new round of license awards. Harmison notes that the government is not trying to be unduly

restrictive (a contested view) but, rather, is interested in making sure that a limited resource is distributed to people who have the capacity to make good scientific use of it. Unless something quite unexpected happens, it is a good bet that in the short term the market for a blood test will be captured by one or more of the five present licensees. But the contest for vaccine development is wide open. That's another story.

Report

28 September 1984

52. Human T-Cell Leukemia Virus (HTLV-I) Antibodies in Africa

W. Saxinger, W.A. Blattner, P.H. Levine, J. Clark, R. Biggar, M. Hoh, J. Moghissi, P. Jacobs, L. Wilson, R. Jacobson, R. Crookes, M. Strong, A.A. Ansari, A.G. Dean, F.K. Nkrumah, N. Mourali, and R.C. Gallo

The human T-cell leukemia-lymphoma viruses (HTLV) are a family of related retroviruses originally isolated in the United States from patients with T-cell lymphoma and cutaneous manifestations (*1*). A particular subgroup of the family, HTLV type I, is linked to the cause of these malignancies, which share clinical and epidemiologic features with the disease called adult T-cell leukemia-lymphoma (ATL) that occurs in certain regions of Japan (*2, 3*) and in persons of African ancestry in the Caribbean Basin (*4*) and in the southeastern United States (*5*). An atypical chronic lymphocytic leukemia in Nigeria is also suggestive of an association with HTLV (*6*), as is the high incidence of antibodies cross-reactive

with HTLV-I in Old World primates captured in Kenya and Ethiopia and housed in West Germany (*7*) and the United States and Russia (*8*). Although the mechanism of transmission of HTLV is currently unknown, horizontal transmission is clearly implicated by molecular and epidemiologic analyses (*9, 10*). HTLV seropositivity in regions endemic for ATL is elevated overall in the general population and further elevated among close family members of cases and in recipients of blood transfusions (*11, 12*).

The present study, which is mainly descriptive, was undertaken to investigate the occurrence of antibodies to HTLV-I in various groups of people in widely distributed areas of the African continent. We studied serum samples that had been collected for surveys of diseases with no known association with HTLV-I and samples from hospital-based clinic patients. We used a highly sensitive enzyme-linked immunosorbent assay (ELISA) to detect antibodies to HTLV-I (*13*) (see Table 1). Because of the diversity of the test groups, our data cannot be used to make strict epidemiological comparisons, but can be used as a means to compare the distribution of virus antibody positivity with previously reported studies of exposure to the virus (*2, 12, 14*) in similar or analogous groups.

The testing procedure was performed in two steps (legend to Table 1). In step 1, all samples were screened to determine quantitative levels of antibody binding to HTLV-I. In step 2, "candidate" positive sera were selected and tested for specificity in one or more confirmatory steps. The screen-test results are expressed as a ratio (*R*) to a standard reference normal serum to control daily variations in test results (*13*). The threshold level, $R \geq 2$, was not expected to exclude negative sera. The use of this cutoff for confirmation was based on prior experience with normal U.S. blood donors where samples with a screening ratio of <2 are negative in the confirmation assay. This reference normal serum level and the threshold for detection of sera confirmed as being positive for antibody to HTLV-I were derived from an analysis of 1210 U.S. blood donors (*15*).

Specificity was considered confirmed when sera passed either one of the confirmatory tests described in Table 1. The accuracy and precision of the antibody-blocking procedure was verified by measuring the fractional reduction of antibody binding for mixtures containing a predetermined ratio of HTLV-positive

antibodies to the reference normal serum. The results plotted in Fig. 1 show excellent agreement with the predicted results at low levels of positive antibody and deviation within acceptable limits due to incomplete blockade at the higher levels of human antibody. Of those sera failing confirmation by antibody blocking, only three were confirmed by absorption with virus-positive cells.

The values for the numbers of sera from the groups exceeding the screen-test threshold and for the numbers of confirmed positive sera in each of these groups are presented in Table 1. The median values for screen ratio (*R*) within the groups were in most cases close to the median value of 1.17 found for U.S. donors (*15*). However, median values of *R* for samples from Tunisia and Ghana were two to three times higher. This reflected the absence of a simple correlation between the prevalence of confirmed positive sera and the proportion of sera exceeding the screen threshold level ($R \geq 2$); for example, the proportion of confirmed positive donors in the Ugandan group (21 percent, which was highest of all groups) was two times higher, while the proportion of samples exceeding $R \geq 2$ was only one-half that of the Ghanaian groups.

We investigated some of the reasons for this apparent high rate of false positivity. Among the Ghanaian samples, 28 out of 67 with high ratios ($R \geq 6$) were nonconfirmed. The mean and median immunoglobulin G (IgG) levels of these 28 samples were, respectively, 130 and 106 mg/ml compared to 9 mg/ml for the standard control serum (measured by ELISA with immunopurified goat antiserum to human IgG). Reconstitution experiments showed that these concentrations of IgG could account for elevation in *R* values in all but three cases (*16*).

Table 1. Distribution of HTLV-I antibody among African donors. An indirect ELISA microtest to detect serum antibodies was used (13). Briefly, HTLV-I was purified by rate-zonal ultracentrifugation, disrupted, and coated into the wells of microtiter plates. Portions (5 μl) of test sera, control positive sera, and control negative human sera were incubated overnight at 4°C in wells containing 100 μl of 20 percent heat-inactivated normal goat serum and were quantitated by measurement of absorbance at 490 nm after reaction with peroxidase-labeled goat antiserum to human IgG. Sera with absorbance values two times greater than the normal control level were verified primarily by confirmatory neutralization, which involved the same procedure as the screening test but included an additional 2-hour incubation period before the test sample was incubated with the antigen-coated wells. During this extra 2 hours of incubation, the wells were exposed to unlabeled sheep antibody to HTLV-I which reacted with and saturated HTLV antigen sites on the well, thus preventing the test serum from attaching to the well in the subsequent step. As a control in the test, adjacent wells were exposed to normal sheep serum during the additional incubation period. Sheep antiserum was used at a dilution of 1:2 and had a titer of 100,000 or more. Sheep antiserum showing reactivity with proteins from phytohemagglutinin (PHA)–stimulated human lymphocyte preparations coated on microtiter plate wells were absorbed with PHA lymphocyte preparations until the reactivity was removed. The sheep antiserum used in these experiments required absorption with one volume of cell equivalents per three volumes of serum to reach the end point. A suppression of the absorbance by >50 percent in the sample exposed to the unlabeled sheep antiserum to HTLV-I, relative to a standard normal human serum, was considered a positive confirmatory result for the presence of antibody to HTLV-I. Sera failing the confirmatory test were absorbed with detergent-released cytosols prepared from PHA-stimulated normal human lymphocytes and with HTLV-I–producing cells and retested for binding to HTLV-I (13). Samples were scored positive if the difference between absorption with virus-positive and -negative cell preparations was >50 percent. Titers of positive sera were determined by serial dilution, regression analysis of the titration curves, and solving for the dilution giving results equivalent to a 1:20 dilution of the reference negative control serum tested in wells of the same plate. R is the ratio of the sample to the negative control; all groups followed log-normal distributions of R.

Geographic and racial background of donors	Group characteristics	Number tested	R median	Number with $R \geqslant >2$	Number positive
Egypt, white*	Infectious disease clinic (no malignancies)	101	0.90	12	2
Tunisia, white†	Malignant lymphoma	22	1.31	7	2
	Mammary carcinoma	256	2.10	136	6
Ghana, black‡	Burkitt's patients	510	3.32	336	52
	Normal comparison population	236	3.30	200	19
Uganda, black‖	Burkitt's patients and normal comparison population	86	1.71	31	18
Nigeria, black§	T-cell lymphoma	9	1.60	2	2

Table 1. (continued)

South Africa					
Cape Town, black and white¶	All donors	283	0.90	38	15
	Lymphoid malignancy	22	0.86	2	1
	Myeloid malignancy	104	0.84	16	9
	Solid tumors	59	1.02	11	3
	Nonmalignant disease and healthy blood donors	98	0.80	9	2
Johannesburg, black#	Healthy blood donors	104	0.9	5	0

*Sera from Egypt were collected from infectious disease patients, Navy Medical Research Unit No. 3, Cairo, Egypt.   †Sera from Tunisia were provided through the Collaborative Breast Cancer Project between the Institut Salah Azaiz and the National Cancer Institute in Bethesda (27). These sera were collected as part of an epidemiologic survey of inflammatory breast carcinoma and incidental cases of non-Hodgkin's lymphoma of Mediterranean origin. The latter were diagnosed as B cell ($n = 16$), T cell ($n = 2$), and uncertain ($n = 4$).   ‡These Burkitt's lymphoma patients were being followed by the Burkitt's Tumor Project, Korle Bu Hospital, University of Ghana, and were chosen on the basis of clinical status (divided between untreated patients and patients in remission) and availability of sufficient sera to perform confirmation studies. Comparison groups were family and community study subjects matched to a subset of Burkitt's cases (17).   ‖Sera from Uganda were from Burkitt's lymphoma patients reported to the Burkitt's lymphoma project in Arua, Uganda, and seen at Kuluva Hospital (18). Comparison subjects were matched by age and sex.   §Sera from Nigeria were collected prospectively for this study over a period of 2 months at the University College Hospital, Ibadan, Nigeria (19) from available patients with lymphoid malignancy.   ¶Sera were from unselected patients with leukemias and solid tumors at the University of Cape Town Medical School, Department of Hematology, Clinical Science and Immunology. Racial backgrounds of the patients were: white, 76; black, 9; mixed, 41; and unknown, 157; of the patients with positive sera, white, 9; black, 0; mixed, 2; and unknown, 4. The lymphoid malignancies were diagnosed as acute leukemia ($n = 18$) and chronic leukemia and lymphoma ($n = 4$).   #These sera were collected at the South African Blood Transfusion Service serving the Baragwanath Hospital, which is the major general hospital serving the black community of Johannesburg.

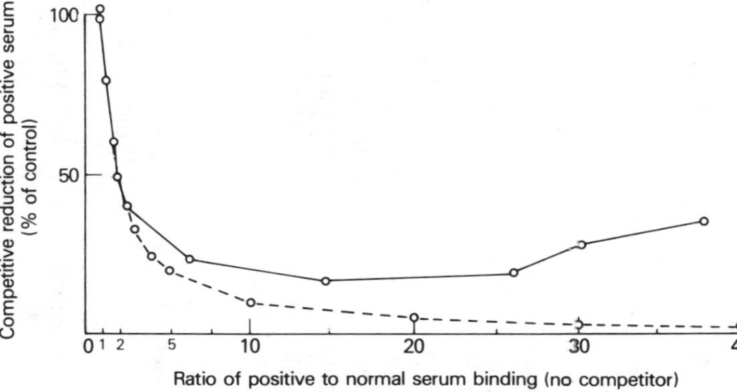

Fig. 1. Correlation between specific antibody binding and its susceptibility to competition by HTLV-specific antiserum. A dilution series containing varying ratios of serum positive for HTLV-I antibodies to serum negative for antibodies was constructed by diluting a positive serum (serum F4608, titer = 3000) with our standard negative serum (serum F4660). Each dilution and the negative control serum were tested for HTLV-binding in wells pretreated with unlabeled sheep antiserum to HTLV-I and normal sheep serum as described in Table 1. The ELISA absorbances at 490 nm were measured and expressed as the ratio to negative human serum treated with normal sheep serum (abscissa); and the relative reduction of each diluted positive human serum after incubation with sheep antiserum to HTLV-I (ordinate). Solid line: a theoretical curve was constructed on the basis of the expected relationship between the fractional content of specific antibodies (abscissa); broken line: the maximum achievable reduction (ordinate).

While it is possible that cross-reacting antibodies with different HTLV subtype specificities may be a source of apparent nonspecificity in some cases, we view this as unlikely since a cross-reactive antibody should be susceptible to competition by the HTLV-I–specific antiserum used in the confirmation test. A possible improvement might be to use a purified viral protein as test antigen. While the confirmatory tests are able to circumvent nonspecificity in the sense of excluding sporadic false positive reactions, for example, reactivity with contaminants of cellular debris or a nonrelevant elevation of serum IgG level, true positive sera would tend to be underestimated in the presence of generalized nonspecific elevation of the test background because of the stringency of the confirmatory test. Thus far, the ELISA with a purified, unfractionated virus preparation has resulted in greater sensitivity and specificity than purified p24 core antigen. These assays may be improved as more purified HTLV proteins become available for testing and more generally applicable confirmatory procedures are developed.

As summarized in Table 1, 131 (6.9 percent) of 1890 sera tested were positive for HTLV-I antibodies. Since this study was not designed to systematically explore disease relationships, positive results may only be interpreted as establishing exposure to HTLV-I in the groups tested. Furthermore, rates of positivity in some of the groups may vary from rates in the general population.

Two serum collections from Ghana collected over the years 1968 to 1981 by the Burkitt Tumor Project, Accra (17) were tested for HTLV-I antibodies. One represented a group of 510 Burkitt's lymphoma patients and the other a group of 236 normal persons from the same families and communities as the patients (17). The numbers positive for HTLV-I antibody in these two groups (not corrected for age) were 10 and 8 percent, respectively (Table 1). Controlling for age, there were no statistically significant differences in HTLV-I antibody rate between these groups. Both groups contained high titers of antibodies to HTLV-I (Table 2). Since there is no known association between HTLV-I and Burkitt's lymphoma and since there was only a slight difference between the values for these groups, this prevalence probably reflects the general population prevalence for that age group. These positivity rates are high given the young age of the persons studied (mean, 13 years) compared to endemic populations in Japan where the antibody positive rate for the equivalent age group is approximately 5 percent (14).

The highest rate of antibody positivity, 21 percent, was found in a serum collection from Uganda (Table 1). The sera had been collected from patients with Burkitt's lymphoma and from normal comparison groups in the West Nile region of Uganda over the years 1970 to 1972 as described previously (18). Since we were unable to discern any difference in the positivity rates between these groups they are listed together in Tables 1 and 2.

In a survey of patients with T-cell leukemia-lymphoma diagnosed in Nigeria (19), two cases fitting the typical characteristics of HTLV-associated disease were identified. The first case, a 19-year-old male student from Lagos, had an aggressive T-cell lymphoma with a high count of white blood cells that included cells of pleomorphic morphology, cutaneous involvement, and hypercalce-

Table 2. Comparison of titers of antibodies to HTLV-I in African groups. Procedures and subject groups are described in Table 1.

Origin and condition of serum donors	Titers (reciprocal serum dilution)				
	20	100	1000	>9999	Range (low-high)
Egypt	1	1			95–960
Tunisia	6	2			30–122
Ghana					
Burkitt's patients	24	23	5		30–4,915
Normal comparison population	5	13		1	46–100,000
Nigeria			2		1,700–4,000
Uganda	3	14		1	40–22,500
Cape Town					
Lymphoid malignancy		1			120
Myeloid malignancy	3	5		1	50–10,000
Nonhematopoietic malignancy		3			400–540
Nonmalignant disease and healthy blood donors	1	1			32–200

mia. The second, a 57-year-old woman, had a clinically aggressive leukemia-lymphoma with generalized adenopathy and visceral involvement. She died shortly after diagnosis. Sera from both patients contained a high titer of antibodies to HTLV-I (see Table 2). One additional patient with ATL with high HTLV antibody titer, a native of Zaire, has been observed in Paris (20).

In Cape Town, 5 to 10 percent of patients with various malignant diseases had HTLV antibody (Table 1). There were no reported cases of ATL, and the greatest number of HTLV-I antibody-positive cases occurred among the myeloid malignancies (10 percent), although one patient with T-cell leukemia was positive. In areas of southwestern Japan that are endemic for ATL, the frequency of HTLV among patients with myeloid leukemias was 16 percent (2). Our present results with regard to the distribution of HTLV-I antibody within disease categories agree very well with the pattern

found in the Kanto district, a nonendemic area of Japan (12). In that district, two important factors contributed to the high rate of HTLV-I antibody positivity in patients with diseases not linked with this virus. One was that the patient population largely originated from an endemic area and the other was the frequent use of blood transfusions in the management of myeloid leukemias (12).

With one exception, serum samples positive for HTLV antibodies were found in groups from all of the African subcontinental regions tested: Tunisia; Ghana; Nigeria; Uganda; Cape Town, South Africa; and Egypt. The absence of HTLV-I antibody in sera from the Johannesburg group may be related only to sample size and probably indicates a lower prevalence than in the other African groups. Race did not appear to be a disposing factor since positive serum samples from Cape Town were mainly of white origin. Although antibody-positive samples were detected in the Tunisian

278

(taken as a whole) and Egyptian groups, the combined factors of frequency and titer found (Tables 1 and 2) were not significantly higher than the baseline for normal donors in the United States (*15, 21*). Both of the positive samples from Tunisian patients with lymphomas had very low titers, that is, 30 and 37, and the lymphomas were of B-cell origin. For reference purposes, among normal blood donors determined by comparable techniques, the HTLV-I antibody positivity rates between nonendemic and endemic regions of Japan range from 2 to 12 percent (*2*) and in the United States, 0.9 to 2.8 percent (*15, 21*).

The typical HTLV-I–associated disease as it occurs endemically in Japan, the Caribbean Basin, and sporadically elsewhere (*22*) is characterized by the occurrence of malignant cells of varying size and pleomorphic morphology with deformed nuclei and mature T-cell surface marker phenotype. It is often characterized by its onset at a relatively young age; by its aggressive clinical course with poor prognosis; and by the enlargement of lymph nodes, spleen, or liver; elevation of white blood cell count; hypercalcemia; and occasional skin involvement. Our data reveal increased levels of HTLV-I–specific antibodies in diverse African groups [compare with (*23*)] and suggest that the antibody levels in regions of South Africa, Ghana, Nigeria, and Uganda equal or exceed those found in previously described areas where HTLV-I and ATL coexist. It would be interesting to conduct systematic surveys of patients with adult non-Hodgkin's lymphoma in various regions of the African continent, with an emphasis on clinical, pathologic, and immunopathologic features of the disease. A study of sera from African patients with

known or suspected T-cell malignancies, including the acquired immune deficiency syndrome (AIDS) (*24*), would help to clarify the distribution of the HTLV family and the diseases associated with it, especially in view of the high HTLV-I antibody level in the Ugandan group, the occurrence of AIDS in neighboring Zaire (*25*), and the occurrence of Kaposi's sarcoma along the equatorial region of Africa with its highest prevalence in eastern Zaire and western Uganda (*26*).

References and Notes

1. B. J. Poiesz, F. W. Ruscetti, A. F. Gazdar, J. D. Minna, R. C. Gallo, *Proc. Natl. Acad. Sci. U.S.A.* **77**, 5415 (1980); B. J. Poiesz, F. W. Ruscetti, M. S. Reitz, V. S. Kalyanaraman, R. C. Gallo, *Nature (London)* **294**, 268 (1981).
2. R. C. Gallo *et al.*, *Cancer Res.* **43**, 3892 (1983); R. C. Gallo, in *Cancer Surveys*, L. M. Franks *et al.*, Eds. (University Press, Oxford, in press); W. A. Blattner, K. Tokatsuki, R. C. Gallo, *J. Am. Med. Assoc.* **250**, 1074 (1983).
3. K. Takatsuki, J. Uchiyama, K. Sagawa, J. Yodoi, in *Topics in Hematology*, S. Seno, F. Takaku, S. Irino, Eds. (Excerpta Medica, Amsterdam, 1977), p. 73.
4. W. Blattner *et al.*, *Int. J. Cancer* **30**, 257 (1982); D. Catovsky *et al.*, *Lancet* **1982-I**, 639 (1982).
5. D. W. Blayney *et al.*, *J. Am. Med. Assoc.* **250**, 1048 (1983).
6. A. F. Fleming, *Lancet* **1983-I**, 69 (1983).
7. N. Yamamoto, Y. Hinuma, H. zur Hausen, J. Schneider, G. Hunsmann, *ibid.*, p. 240.
8. W. C. Saxinger *et al.*, in preparation.
9. M. Robert-Guroff, F. W. Ruscetti, L. W. Posner, B. J. Poiesz, R. C. Gallo, *J. Exp. Med.* **154**, 1957 (1981).
10. R. C. Gallo *et al.*, *Proc. Natl. Acad. Sci. U.S.A.* **79**, 5680 (1981).
11. M. Robert-Guroff *et al.*, *J. Exp. Med.* **157**, 248 (1983).
12. M. Shimoyama *et al.*, *Jpn. J. Clin. Oncol.* **12**, 109 (1982).
13. W. C. Saxinger and R. C. Gallo, *Lab. Invest.* **49**, 371 (1983).
14. Y. Hinuma *et al.*, *Int. J. Cancer* **29**, 631 (1982).
15. In a study of 1788 normal U.S. blood donors from Burlington, Vt.; Birmingham, Ala.; and Houston, Tex.; the rates of positive HTLV-I antibody-positive sera were 0.9, 2.1, and 2.8 percent, respectively. The range of titers was 20 to 530. The median value of R for all groups was 1.17, and 13 percent of sera with $R \geq 2$ were positive [W. C. Saxinger *et al.*, in preparation].
16. We expect that these and other types of indirect assays currently applied without a specific confirmatory step, including immunofluorescence assays that rely on the use of live or fixed

HTLV-I–infected lymphocytes, would also be sensitive to such drastic elevations in IgG and could lead to overestimation of seropositivity in similar cases.

17. R. J. Biggar, F. K. Nkrumah, W. Henle, P. H. Levine, *J. Natl. Cancer Inst.* **66**, 439 (1981).
18. A. G. Dean *et al.*, *Lancet* **1973-II**, 1225 (1973).
19. C. K. O. Williams *et al.*, *Br. J. Haematol.*, in press.
20. Patient was originally seen at the Assistance Publique-Hopitaux de Paris (J. Leibowitch and M. Robert-Guroff, personal communication).
21. W. C. Saxinger and R. C. Gallo, *Lancet* **1982-I**, 1074 (1982).
22. M. Popovic *et al.*, *Science* **219**, 856 (1983).
23. A. Fleming *et al.*, *Lancet* **1983-I**, 334 (1983); G. Hunsmann *et al.*, *Int. J. Cancer* **32**, 329 (1983).
24. R. C. Gallo *et al.*, *Science* **220**, 865 (1983); F. Barré-Sinoussi *et al.*, *ibid.*, p. 868; M. Essex *et al.*, *ibid.*, p. 859; R. C. Gallo *et al.*, *ibid.* **224**, 500 (1984).
25. N. Clumeck *et al.*, *N. Engl. J. Med.* **310**, 492 (1984).
26. A. G. Oettle, *Acta Univ. Int. Cancer* **18**, 330 (1962).
27. P. H. Levine *et al.*, *Int. J. Cancer* **27**, 611 (1981).
28. Supported in part by the University of Cape Town Leukaemia Centre and Staff Research fund, the National Cancer Association, and the Medical Research Council.

17 April 1984; accepted 9 July 1984

Report

28 September 1984

53. Functional Properties of Antigen-Specific T Cells Infected by Human T-Cell Leukemia-Lymphoma Virus (HTLV-I)

Hiroaki Mitsuya, Hong-Guang Guo, Jeffrey Cossman, Mary Megson, Marvin S. Reitz, Jr., and Samuel Broder

The term human T-cell leukemia-lymphoma virus (HTLV) refers to a unique family of T-cell tropic retroviruses. Viruses belonging to the HTLV family play a vital role in the pathogenesis of certain adult T-cell neoplasms (*1, 2*) and are believed to be the etiologic agents of acquired immune deficiency syndrome (AIDS) (*3, 4*). A well-recognized property of some subtypes of HTLV is the ability to infect and transform T cells from normal umbilical cord blood and bone marrow in vitro (*5, 6*). However, the effects of HTLV on antigen-driven T-cell responses are not well understood.

We established a tetanus-toxoid reactive T-cell line from a normal blood donor by repeated cycles of in vitro stimulation with soluble antigen and irradiated autologous peripheral blood mononuclear cells (PBM) as a source of accessory cells (*7*). The cells were continuously exposed to T-cell growth factor (TCGF or interleukin-2). We then attempted to propagate clones from this immune T-cell line in the presence and absence of HTLV-I. In the absence of virus, the cloning efficiency was approximately one in 64; however, in the presence of the virus, it was one in five, as detected by Poisson analysis of large numbers of replicate microcultures set up with varying numbers of antigen-responsive cells. The most rapidly growing clones were YTA1, which was derived from a well without virus, and YTH3 and YTH5, which were derived from wells containing virus. These clones, which were obtained by limiting dilution under conditions of one cell per well and have been maintained in continuous culture for more than 160 days after cloning, are the subject of the present report.

Clone YTA1 exhibited a substantial proliferative response against soluble antigen but only in the presence of irradiated autologous PBM that served as accessory cells. In contrast, YTH3 and YTH5 replicated spontaneously without TCGF or accessory cells. Moreover, YTH3 and YTH5 substantially increased their rate of proliferation in response to tetanus toxoid in the presence and also the absence of irradiated autologous PBM (Fig. 1). The overall magnitude of response was generally greater in the presence of accessory cells.

The antigen specificity of the proliferation of these clones was studied by using tetanus toxoid, purified protein derivative, streptokinase and streptodornase, and Formalin-inactivated, zonally purified A2/Aichi/68 influenza virus. None of the clones tested responded to antigens other than tetanus toxoid (data not shown). These data taken together suggest that immune T cells cloned in the presence of HTLV-I retained the capacity to recognize and respond to soluble antigen while acquiring the capacity to respond in the absence of accessory cells.

We then infected YTA1 by recloning in the presence of HTLV-I as described earlier. The resultant T cell population, which was propagated under starting conditions of one cell per well by limiting dilution, is referred to as YTA1H. This HTLV-I–infected clone, unlike the original YTA1 clone, replicated spontaneously without TCGF. YTA1H increased its rate of replication upon exposure to soluble antigen in a dose-dependent fashion, and an antigen-driven response was observed in the absence of accessory cells (Table 1).

Clone YTH3 retained the antigen-specific reactivity described above for approximately 120 days in culture following cloning, but the magnitude of the response gradually decreased. Clone YTH5, in contrast, developed within 60 days a high spontaneous rate of replication in the absence of TCGF. The observable antigen-driven proliferative response was lost and could not be restored by recloning (data not shown).

We wished to know whether clones YTH3 and YTH5 were themselves capable of serving as accessory cells in presenting soluble antigen to normal T cells. We observed that irradiated YTH3 and YTH5 cells (8) did not function as accessory cells in the response of the normal immune T-cell clone YTA1 to soluble antigen (Fig. 2). The addition of purified interleukin-1 did not permit these HTLV-I–infected cells to serve an antigen-presenting function (data not shown). These observations provide evidence that there were no functional accessory cell subsets in the YTH3 and YTH5 populations.

We then confirmed that YTH3 and YTH5 were infected with HTLV-I and determined the characteristics of the proviruses integrated in the genome. DNA from YTA1, YTH3, and YTH5 was analyzed by Southern blot hybridization. No proviral sequences could be

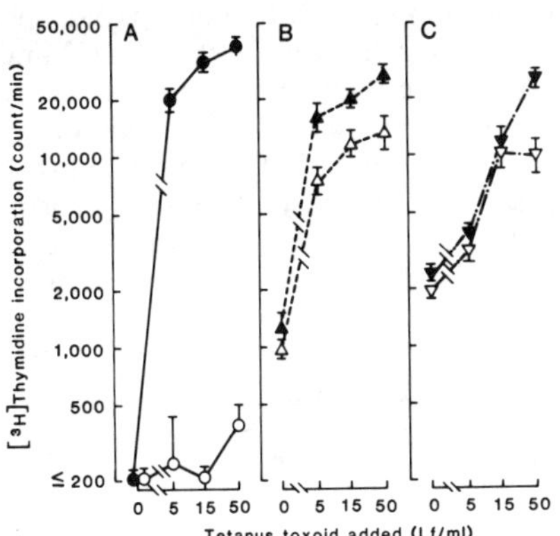

Fig. 1. Stimulation of T-cell clones by soluble tetanus toxoid in the absence of accessory cells. Peripheral blood mononuclear cells (PBM) (10^6) from a normal volunteer (7) were cultured with 25 limit flocculation units (Lf) per milliliter of tetanus toxoid (TT) (Commonwealth of Massachusetts Department of Public Health, Jamaica Plain) in 24-well microculture plates (Costar) at 37°C in 5 percent CO_2-containing humidified air in ml of RPMI 1640 medium supplemented with 10 percent autologous plasma, 4 mM L-glutamine, and per milliliter, 50 units of penicillin and 50 μg of streptomycin (complete medium). After 7 days in culture, the cells were continuously exposed to 15 percent TCGF (by volume) (Cellular Products); on day 14 and beyond, 10 percent heat-inactivated fetal calf serum (FCS) was substituted for the autologous plasma. The cells were stimulated every 7 days with the addition of TT (25 Lf/ml) and irradiated (4000 rad) autologous PBM. On day 31 in culture, the cultured cells were cloned by limiting dilution; 0.1-ml portions containing one cell in 15 percent TCGF-containing complete medium were distributed into round-bottomed 96-well microtiter plates (Limbro) with 10^4 irradiated (4000 rad) autologus PBM and TT (25 Lf/ml) in the presence and the absence of 10^4 irradiated (12,000 rad) HTLV-I–producing MJ tumor cells derived from a patient with HTLV-I–associated lymphoma (5). The plates were incubated at 37°C in 5 percent CO_2-containing humidified air and fed with 0.1 ml of 15 percent TCGF-containing complete medium every 4 to 5 days. Growing colonies were selected on days 10 to 30 and transferred to 24-well Costar plates. Clones exposed to HTLV-I–producing cells could be expanded in 15 percent TCGF-containing complete medium without further addition of TT and PBM, in contrast to cells not exposed to HTLV-I, which required stimulation with TT and irradiated autologous PBM every 10 to 14 days. Cells (10^5) of the unexposed clone YTA1 (○) (A) and HTLV-I–exposed clones YTH3 (△) (B), and YTH5 (▽) (C) were cultured with various concentrations of tetanus toxoid in the presence (closed symbols) and the absence (open symbols) of 5 × 10^4 irradiated autologous PBM in 180 μl of complete medium for 4 days, and then exposed to 0.5 μCi of [³H]thymidine for 5 hours and harvested as described (9). When cultured alone, irradiated autologous PBM did not proliferate. Each symbol represents the mean ± 1 standard deviation of triplicate determinations. The experiments were performed when cells had been in culture for 36 days after cloning.

detected in the DNA from YTA1 (Fig. 3). (These cells were also negative for the HTLV-I *gag* proteins p19 and p24 as assessed by cytoplasmic indirect immunofluorescence.) In contrast, DNA from YTH3 and YTH5 had, respectively, four and two separate clonally integrated proviruses present, since digestion with Eco RI, which does not cut within the HTLV-I provirus, gave four bands with YTH3 and two with YTH5. Digestion with Bam HI resulted in the presence of a band of 1.1 kb detected with the *pol-env-pX* probe. This is common to all HTLV-I–infected cells, and represents an internal fragment of the provirus, indicating that there is not a large internal deletion of the proviruses. These two clones (YTH3 and YTH5) were also tested for viral protein expression. YTH3 contained 2 to 5 percent cells which were highly positive for the HTLV-I *gag* proteins p19 and p24, while 5 to 10 percent of the cells of YTH5 were highly positive

Table 1. Dose-dependent proliferative response of HTLV-I–infected, tetanus toxoid–specific clone YTA1H to soluble antigen in the absence of accessory cells. Cells (10^5 YTA1H and 10^5 YTA1) were cultured with various concentrations of soluble tetanus toxoid in the presence or absence of irradiated (4000 rad) autologous PBM for 3 days, exposed to [^{3}H]thymidine, and harvested as described in Fig. 1. YTA1H had never been exposed to autologous PBM (accessory cells) after cloning; while YTA1 (the uninfected counterpart) had been exposed to irradiated autologous PBM for 7 to 10 days prior to these experiments as part of a cycle of restimulation. The data are expressed as means ± 1 standard deviation of triplicate determinations. N.D., not determined.

Clone	Days after cloning	Irradiated PBM	Tetanus toxoid (Lf/ml)			
			0	4	8	16
YTA1H	20	−	1740 ± 156	N.D.	5240 ± 1261	N.D.
	33	−	4181 ± 75	9830 ± 1368	11286 ± 360	8826 ± 385
YTA1	65	−	149 ± 28	218 ± 109	195 ± 88	318 ± 127
	65	+	156 ± 27	19424 ± 743	11914 ± 566	8091 ± 1599
	82	+	230 ± 18	N.D.	26605 ± 1885	N.D.

for those proteins (data not shown). As has been observed in other settings (9), there appears to be some restriction of viral expression in these cells, since the majority of the cells in these cultures seems to be infected but only a minority is expressing *gag* proteins.

We then analyzed the surface membrane antigens expressed by uninfected and infected antigen-specific T-cell clones by fluorescence-activated cell sorter analysis (10). Clones YTA1, YTH3, and YTH5 reacted with OKT3, OKT4, anti-Tac, and anti-HLA-DR monoclonal antibodies. The cells in each population were negative for OKT8 or OKM1. Thus, both the uninfected and infected antigen-specific T-cell clones have the phenotype of mature, activated helper-inducer cells. It is worth noting that this is the phenotype generally expressed in neoplastic cells obtained from patients with HTLV-I–associated leukemias (2, 11).

It is a general rule that T cells are not stimulated by soluble antigen alone, and that T-cell activation requires a process of associative recognition that depends on accessory cells bearing major histocompatibility complex (MHC) determinants of the appropriate haplotype (12–14). This process is still imperfectly understood despite the dramatic advances in characterizing antigen receptor genes and molecules (15–17).

Rao *et al.* (18) have shown that murine T-cell clones reactive against the *p*-azobenzenearsonate hapten express specific binding sites for radioactively labeled arsanylated ovalbumin. Binding can take place in the absence of accessory cells. Under certain conditions, several structurally related haptens, conjugated to ovalbumin, can competitively inhibit the activation of T cells reactive to the *p*-azobenzenearsonate hapten, although antigen binding per se does not result in T-cell activation. Moreover, Carel *et al.* (19) have obtained a T-cell hybridoma that specifically reacts with soluble cytochrome *c* peptide. This hybridoma binds the peptide antigen in the absence of accessory cells, resulting in production of TCGF (19). These data imply that some antigenic determinants may bind to specific sites on T-cell clones in the absence of accessory cells. However, it is difficult to categorize the functional consequences of binding alone.

To our knowledge, the HTLV-I–infected T cells generated in the current studies provide the first example of a specific human T-cell proliferative response to a soluble antigen without the addition of accessory cells. It is possible that the integration of HTLV-I into the genome of an antigen-specific T cell qualitatively or quantitatively alters the expression of antigen receptors and class II major histocompatibility (MHC) antigens, thereby conferring on the T cell a self-sufficient capacity for associative recognition. However, these HTLV-I–infected T cells have not gained the ability to present antigen to uninfected, antigen-specific T cells in our experimental conditions. Alternatively, HTLV-I infection might obviate an external signal mediated by MHC proteins, allowing the simple engagement of the T-cell antigen-binding receptors by soluble antigen to serve as a sufficient stimulus for a proliferative response. The avail-

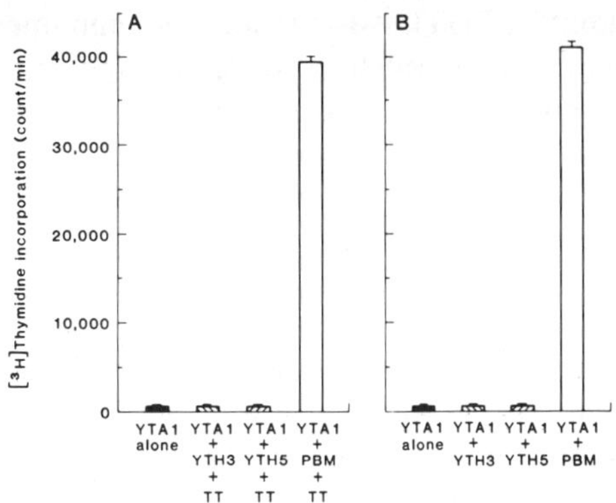

Fig. 2. YTH3 and YTH5 do not present antigen to tetanus toxoid (TT)-specific T cells. (A) 5×10^4 YTH3, YTH5, or autologous fresh PBM [which were irradiated (8) with 4000 rad] were cultured with 10^5 YTA1 cells in the presence of TT (7.5 Lf/ml). (B) Clones YTH3 and YTH5 and fresh autologous PBM were incubated with TT (25 Lf/ml) at 37°C for 3 hours, washed extensively, and irradiated with 4000 rad. These YTH3, YTH5; and PBM (5×10^4) were cultured with 10^5 YTA1 cells without further addition of soluble antigen for 4 days, exposed to [³H]thymidine, and harvested as described in Fig. 1. Irradiated YTH3, YTH5, and PBM, when cultured alone, failed to incorporate [³H]thymidine. Each bar represents the mean ± 1 standard deviation of triplicate determinations.

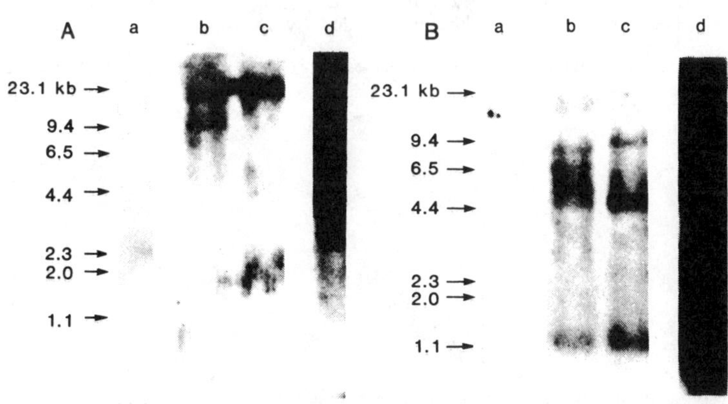

Fig. 3. Proviral sequences of HTLV-I in clones YTH3 and YTH5. The DNA was digested with Bam HI (A) and Eco RI (B), and analyzed by the Southern blotting technique with an HTLV-I probe as described (9, 20). The DNA was from YTA1 (lane a), YTH3 (lane b), YTH5 (lane c), or HTLV-I–producing MJ-tumor cells (lane d). Arrows on the left-hand side show the position of the Hind III fragments of λ phage DNA as a marker. DNA digested with Bam HI and Eco RI was subjected to electrophoresis, transferred to nitrocellulose, and hybridized with a ³²P nick-translated DNA insert from a subclone in pBR322 of the portions of the HTLV-I genome defined by the Cla I and Hind III sites of λCR-1 (21) and containing *pol*, *env*, and *pX* sequences.

ability of HTLV-I–transformed immune lymphocytes might provide an important resource for analyzing antigen recognition by human T cells at a molecular and cellular level. Moreover, it is likely that the capacity of the virus to bring about an altered requirement for accessory cells coupled in some situations with a progressive loss of antigen-specific reactivity in vitro will have relevance in understanding the consequences of HTLV-I infection in vivo.

References and Notes

1. B. J. Poiesz *et al.*, *Proc. Natl. Acad. Sci. U.S.A.* **77**, 7415 (1980); R. C. Gallo *et al.*, *ibid.* **79**, 5680 (1982).
2. S. Broder *et al.*, *Ann. Int. Med.* **100**, 543 (1984).
3. M. Popovic, M. G. Sarngadharan, E. Read, R. C. Gallo, *Science* **224**, 497 (1984); R. C. Gallo *et al.*, *ibid.*, p. 500; J. Schüpbach, M. Popovic, R. V. Gilden, M. A. Gonda, M. G. Sarngadharan, R. C. Gallo, *ibid.*, p. 503; M. G. Sarngadharan, M. Popovic, L. Bruch, J. Schüpbach, R. C. Gallo, *ibid.*, p. 506.
4. Z. Trainin, D. Wernicke, H. Unger-Waron, M. Essex, *Science* **220**, 858 (1983); B. L. Evatt *et al.*, *Lancet* **1984-II**, 698 (1984).
5. M. Popovic *et al.*, *Science* **219**, 856 (1983).
6. P. Markham, S. Z. Salahuddin, B. Macchi, M. Robert-Gurrof, R. C. Gallo, *Int. J. Cancer* **33**, 13 (1984).
7. Peripheral blood mononuclear cells were isolated by Ficoll-Isopaque gradient centrifugation from heparinized blood of a 29-year-old normal male who had been immunized with tetanus toxoid and whose serum was negative for antibodies to HTLV-I. The HLA phenotype of the donor was A24, A32, Bw5, Bw61, Cw1, Cw4, DR2, and DR4 (data kindly provided by D. Mann).
8. For the antigen-presenting assays (see Fig. 2) we used a radiation dose of 4000 rad. Clones YTH3 and YTH5 similarly failed to present tetanus toxoid after irradiation with 500, 1000, 1500, and 2000 rad.
9. H. Mitsuya *et al.*, *Science* **223**, 1293 (1984).
10. The reactivity of cells with OKT3, OKT4, OKT8, OKM1 (Ortho Diagnostics), anti-Tac (a gift of T. A. Waldmann), and anti-HLA–DR (Becton-Dickinson) monoclonal antibodies was determined by fluorescence-activated cell sorter analysis (BD FACS II Systems). YTA1 cells were 98, 98, <1, <1, 61, and 96 percent positive; YTH3 cells were 99, 99, <1, <1, 95, and 99 percent positive; and YTH5 cells were 99, 97, <1, <1, 85, and 87 percent positive for OKT3, OKT4, OKT8, OKM1, anti-Tac, and anti-HLA-DR antibodies, respectively.
11. T. Hattori, T. Uchiyama, T. Toibana, K. Takatsuki, H. Uchino, *Blood* **58**, 645 (1981).
12. B. Benacerraf, *J. Immunol.* **120**, 1809 (1978).
13. R. M. Zinkernagel and P. C. Doherty, *Adv. Immunol.* **27**, 51 (1979).
14. J. A. Berzofsky, in *Biological Regulation and Development*, R. F. Goldberger, Ed. (Plenum, New York, 1980), pp 467–594.
15. Y. Yanagi *et al.*, *Nature (London)* **308**, 145 (1984); S. M. Hedrick, D. I. Cohen, E. A. Nielsen, M. M. Davis, *ibid.*, p. 149.
16. E. L. Reinherz, S. C. Meuer, S. F. Schlossman, *Immunol. Today* **4**, 5 (1983); O. Acuste *et al.*, *Cell* **34**, 717 (1983); S. C. Meuer *et al.*, *Proc. Natl. Acad. Sci. U.S.A.* **81**, 1509 (1984).
17. K. Haskins *et al.*, *J. Exp. Med.* **157**, 1149 (1983).
18. A. Rao, W. W.-P. Ko, S. J. Faas, H. Cantor, *Cell* **36**, 879 (1984); A. Rao, S. J. Faas, H. Cantor, *ibid.*, p. 889.
19. S. Carel, C. Bron, G. Corradin, *Proc. Natl. Acad. Sci. U.S.A.* **80**, 4832 (1983).
20. C. D. Trainor, F. Wong-Staal, M. S. Reitz, Jr. *J. Virol.* **41**, 298 (1982).
21. V. F. Manzari *et al.*, *Proc. Natl. Acad. Sci. U.S.A.* **80**, 1574 (1983).
22. We thank R. Yarchoan for providing the influenza virus and J. Oppenheim for the interleukin-1. We also thank R. C. Gallo for advice and J. A. Berzofsky, W. Strober, and R. Yarchoan for critical reading of the manuscript.

15 May 1984; accepted 10 July 1984

Report

5 October 1984

54. Antigens Encoded by the 3′-Terminal Region of Human T-Cell Leukemia Virus: Evidence for a Functional Gene

T.H. Lee, J.E. Coligan, J.G. Sodroski, W.A. Haseltine, S.Z. Salahuddin, F. Wong-Staal, R.C. Gallo, and M. Essex

The human T-cell leukemia viruses (HTLV) are a family of exogenous human retroviruses with three known types (*1, 2*). HTLV type I (HTLV-I) is etiologically associated with adult T-cell leukemia-lymphoma (ATLL) (*2, 3*). HTLV type II (HTLV-II) was isolated from a patient with a T-cell variant of hairy cell leukemia (*4*). HTLV type III (HTLV-III) refers to prototype virus isolated from patients with acquired immune deficiency syndrome (*5*).

HTLV-I and HTLV-II have several unusual features that distinguish them from the replication-competent retroviruses of mice and chickens. These include lack of chronic viremia in infected individuals, absence of common proviral integration sites in tumors (*6*), *trans*-activation of HTLV long terminal repeat (LTR)–directed transcription in infected cells (*7*), and ability to immortalize T cells in vitro (*8*). In addition to the *gag, pol,* and *env* genes of animal retroviruses, the HTLV genome contains a 1.5-kilobase region, initially described as the "X" region, and located between the *env* gene and the 3′ LTR (*9*). Sequence comparisons of this region between HTLV-I and HTLV-II demonstrate that it can be divided into a 5′ nonconserved

region and a 3′ highly conserved region designated LOR (*10*).

In a previous study, serum samples from adult T-cell leukemia-lymphoma patients and from healthy carriers living in the HTLV-I endemic area of Japan were examined for the presence of antibodies to HTLV-associated membrane antigen (HTLV-MA). We reported that HTLV-specific antigens detected in an HTLV-I–infected tumor cell line, Hut 102, could be grouped into three categories (*11*). These included unglycosylated antigens encoded by the *gag* gene, glycosylated antigens encoded by the *env* gene, and an unglycosylated 42-kilodalton species (p42) whose coding origin was unknown. Antigens sharing biochemical and immunological properties with the *gag* antigens and *env* antigens of Hut 102 cells were also expressed in four other HTLV-I–infected cell lines, although antigens encoded by the *env* gene varied somewhat in size and number in different cells, and the unglycosylated antigens of the p42 class exhibited slight variations in size (*11, 12*). Since p42 did not appear to be recognized products of the *gag* or *env* genes, we investigated the possibility that it might be encoded by the "X" region of HTLV. Using radiolabel sequence analysis (*13*), we found that a portion of the p42 protein appears to be encoded by LOR.

To analyze the generality of p42 expression, we used a competition assay in which 200 times more nonlabeled cell lysate from different cell lines was used to compete with [^{35}S]cysteine-labeled p42 of Hut 102 for specific antibody. As shown in Fig. 1A, antigens that were serologically related to p42 of Hut 102 appeared to be expressed in MT2, MJ, C5/MJ, and C91/PL cell lines (lanes 7 to 10) and in a nonproducer cell line, C81-66-45 (lane 11). The C81-66-45 cell line, also designated C63/CR$_{II}$-4, was defined as nonproducer by its lack of expression of *gag* antigens and the absence of reverse transcriptase activity and viral particles in the spent culture media (*14*). Lymphoid cell lines of different lineage and different stages of differentiation, but not infected with HTLV (lanes 3 to 6), did not complete with p42, thus reaffirming the HTLV-specific nature of this antigen.

Further studies of the p42 protein were done with the C81-66-45 cell line. Immunoprecipitation of [^{35}S]cysteine-labeled proteins with sera from people infected with HTLV-I reveals that a 42-kD antigen is the only major HTLV-specific antigen readily detected in this cell line. This is consistent with the observation that extracts of C81-66-45 cells compete for p42 but not for HTLV *gag*- or *env*-encoded proteins (Fig. 1A). When total cell lysate was applied to a lentil lectin–Sepharose 4B column, the p42 species was detected in the effluent (Fig. 1B) but not in the eluent (data not shown). Sera from individuals who do not have antibodies to HTLV-MA could not precipitate the p42 antigen from C81-66-45 (Fig.

1B) or from other HTLV-producer cell lines (*11, 12*).

To determine the coding sequence of p42, we labeled C81-66-45 cells with selected amino acids. The radiolabeled p42 was isolated by sodium dodecyl sulfate–polyacrylamide gel electrophoresis (SDS-PAGE) and then subjected to automated Edman degradation to determine the NH$_2$-terminal protein sequence. For this purpose, 30×10^6 to 40×10^6 cells were metabolically labeled for 10 to 12 hours with either 5 mCi of [^{35}S]cysteine plus 10 mCi of [^{3}H]serine or 5 mCi of [^{35}S]cysteine plus 10 mCi of [^{3}H]alanine, or 5 mCi of [^{35}S]cysteine plus 10 mCi of [^{3}H]proline, in 25 ml of RPMI 1640 medium with 15 percent fetal bovine serum and depleted with the appropriate amino acids. Radiolabeled cell lysates prepared as described earlier (*11*) were precipitated with a reference human serum known to have antibody to p42. The detailed procedures for immunoprecipitation, electroelution, dialysis, and automated protein sequence analysis were described earlier (*11, 13*). In three trials, no radiolabeled amino acids were detected in the first 35 degradation cycles, indicating that either the NH$_2$-terminus of p42 was inaccessible to Edman degradation or there were no cysteine, serine, proline, and alanine residues present in the first 35 NH$_2$-terminal residues of p42.

To obtain protein sequence information for p42, we subsequently prepared cyanogen bromide (CNBr) fragments from radiolabeled p42 for protein sequence analysis. For this purpose, p42 was isolated from C81-66-45 cells which were metabolically labeled with [^{35}S]cysteine, [^{3}H]leucine, [^{3}H]isoleucine, and [^{3}H]lysine (using the amounts and procedures listed above for the other amino

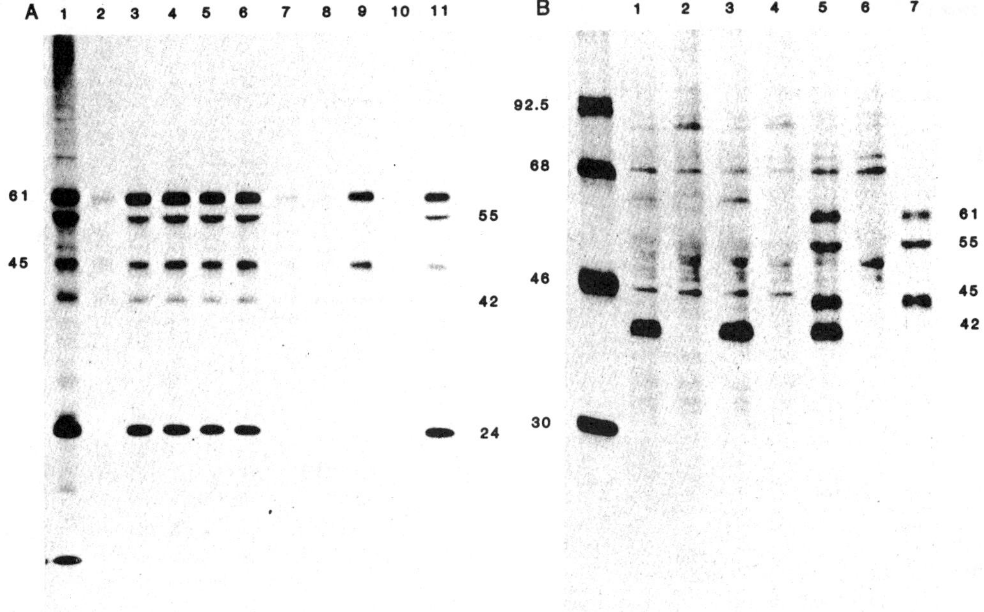

Fig. 1. (A) Expression of antigens related to p42 of Hut 102 in other HTLV-I–infected cells. Detailed procedures for radioimmunoprecipitation assay, SDS-PAGE analysis, and competition assay were described (*11*, *12*). Briefly, 5 μl of reference serum known to have antibody to p42 from a Japanese healthy carrier was preabsorbed to protein A–Sepharose 4B. Approximately 100×10^6 cells equivalent of nonradiolabeled cell lysates from the following cell lines, Hut 102 (lane 2), T8402 (lane 3), NC37 (lane 4), Jurkat (lane 5), Hut 78 (lane 6), MT2 (lane 7), MJ (lane 8), C5/MJ (lane 9), C91/pL (lane 10), C81-66-45 (lane 11), and phosphate-buffered saline (lane 1) were incubated with the positive reference serum absorbed to protein A–Sepharose 4B for 1 hour at 4°C before 0.5×10^6 cells equivalent of [^{35}S]cysteine-labeled cell lysate from Hut 102 was added. After 1 to 4 hours of incubation with intermittent gentle swirling, antigen-antibody complexes were washed and then eluted from immunoprecipitates by boiling for 2 minutes; they were analyzed in a 11.5 percent SDS–polyacrylamide gel. (B) Detection of p42 in C81-66-45 cells. Radioimmunoprecipitation, competition assay, and SDS-PAGE were done exactly as described above. [^{35}S]Cysteine-labeled soluble cell lysate used in lanes 1 and 2 was from C81-66-45 cells. [^{35}S]Cysteine-labeled soluble cell lysate from C81-66-45 cells was also incubated with lentil lectin–Sepharose 4B (Pharmacia) at the ratio of 10×10^6 cells to 0.2 ml of lectin for 1 to 2 hours. The unbound fraction was used as the source of antigen for lanes 3 and 4. [^{35}S]Cysteine-labeled Hut 102 cells prepared as described (*11*, *12*) was the source of antigen for lanes 5, 6, and 7, except that in lane 7 nonradiolabeled cell lysate from 30×10^9 C81-66-45 cells was incubated with the serum for 1 hour before a portion of radiolabeled Hut 102 cell lysate (0.5×10^6 cells equivalent) was added. A positive reference serum from a healthy Japanese carrier (*11*, *12*) was used in lanes 1, 3, 5, and 7. A negative reference serum (*11*, *12*) from a healthy Japanese subject was used in lanes 2, 4, and 6.

acids). Radiolabeled p42 in 0.5 ml of 70 percent formic acid was cleaved with 0.01 mg of CNBr for 24 hours at room temperature. Cyanogen bromide–cleaved fragments of p42 were separated by Sephacryl S-200 chromatography (Fig. 2A). Five pooled fractions, A to E, of estimated size 15, 12, 10, 3, and 1 kD, respectively, were obtained from this separation. The results of automated Edman degradation for pools C to E are presented in Table 1. As shown in Table 2, at least five CNBr fragments, designated CNBr-1 to CNBr-5, can be expected for the CNBr cleavage products encoded by the LOR region of HTLV-I (*10*). Comparison of radioactive protein sequence data with the deduced amino acid sequence for the LOR region reveals that pool E contains the CNBr-2 fragment, pool D contains CNBr-3 fragment, and pool C contains both CNBr-4

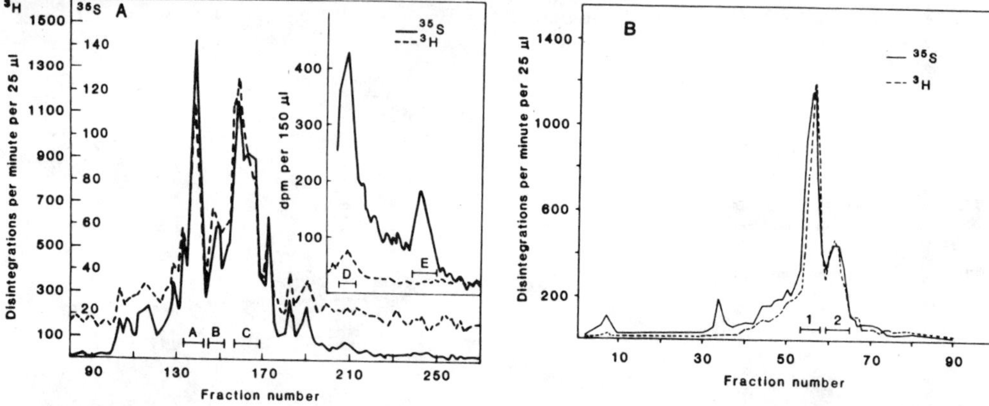

Fig. 2. (A) Sephacryl S-200 chromatography of CNBr fragments of [^{35}S]cysteine-, [^{3}H]leucine-, [^{3}H]isoleucine-, and [^{3}H]lysine-labeled p42. The column (2 by 195 cm) was equilibrated in 6M guanidine HCl plus 0.5 percent acetic acid. Fraction size was 2.0 ml, and the flow rate was 0.2 ml/min. Fractions were pooled as indicated. (B) Purification of CNBr fragments of [^{35}S]cysteine- and [^{3}H]serine-labeled p42 by RPLC. The CNBr fragments of p42 were dissolved in 0.3 ml of 6M guanidine HCl and chromatographed on a Beckman RPSC C-3 column with a Spectra-Physics model 8000B HPLC. Solvent A was 0.01M trifluoroacetic acid (TFA) in H$_2$O, and solvent B was 0.01M TFA in acetonitrile. The solvent program was 0 to 70 percent solvent B in 60 minutes, hold for 10 minutes, 70 to 100 percent solvent B in 10 minutes, and hold for 10 minutes. Flow rate was 0.5 ml/min; 0.5 ml fractions were collected; 10 to 30 µl of each fraction was counted in a liquid scintillation counter (Beckman LS-9000). Fractions were pooled as indicated (fractions A through E in (A) and fractions 1 and 2 in (B)].

and CNBr-5 fragments. Repetitive yield analysis indicated that the amounts of the two CNBr fragments in pool C occurred at a ratio of 4 to 1. Sequence analysis of the NH$_2$-terminal positions of pool A yielded no radioactive peaks in the first 18 degradation cycles. Sequence analysis of pool B suggested that it contained a mixture of CNBr fragments. Although not enough radioactivity was present for high-performance liquid chromatographic (HPLC) analyses of the phenylthiohydantoin (PTH) amino acid derivatives, radioactive peaks occurred at positions where amino acids were identified in pools C to E, suggesting that pool B contained partial cleavage products.

The CNBr cleavage products of radio-labeled p42 were also separated by reverse phase liquid chromatography (RPLC). The profile of RPLC separation of [^{35}S]cysteine- and [^{3}H]serine-labeled CNBr fragments of p42 is shown in Fig. 2B. Two major pooled fractions, designated pool 1 and pool 2, were obtained. Automated protein sequence analysis of pool 1 indicated that pool 1 contained the CNBr-5 fragment (Table 1). Repetitive yield analysis of radiosequence indicated that pool 2 contained a mixture of CNBr-2, CNBr-4, and CNBr-5 fragments.

A summary of radiolabel sequence analysis of p42 is presented in Table 3. The probabilities of observing such a match for pool E, pool D, pool C, and pool 1 by chance alone are no more than $(1/17)^1 \times (16/20)^{11-1}$, that is 6.3 $\times$ 10^{-3};

$(1/17)^6 \times (16/20)^{34-6}$, or 8.0×10^{-11}; $(1/17)^{10} \times (16/20)^{20-10}$, or 5.3×10^{-14}; and $(1/19)^8 \times (18/20)^{38-8}$, or 2.5×10^{-12}, respectively. Since it is highly improbable that the observed matches, which are located in a contiguous stretch of 245 amino acid residues in the LOR region, could occur by chance alone, we conclude that p42 is at least partially encoded by the LOR region of HTLV.

Table 1. Amino terminal radiosequence of CNBr fragments of p42. The probabilities of having the observed sequence to occur by chance alone are: 5.3×10^{-4} (pool C), 8.0×10^{-11} (pool D), 6.3×10^{-3} (pool E), and 2.5×10^{-12} (pool 1). All assignments were made by HPLC analysis of PTH amino acid derivatives (13). The one-letter designations for the amino acids are I, isoleucine; C, cysteine; K, lysine; L, leucine; and S, serine.

Chromato-graphy	Pooled fractions	Position of radiolabeled amino acid																	
		1	2	3	4	5	6	7	8	9	10	11	12	13	14	15	16	17	18	19
S-200	Pool C (major)*	I				C		K						L		L				
S-200	Pool C (minor)		L			L				I				(L)†	(L)†				I	
S-200	Pool D				L					L			L						L	
S-200	Pool E		K																	
RPLC	Pool 1		S			C								S				S	S	S

*The major sequence was present at four times the level of the minor sequence.   †Although leucine residues were anticipated in these positions (see Table 2), definitive assignments could not be made because of the presence of the leucine residue at positions 13 and 15 in the major sequence.

Chromato-graphy	Pooled fractions	Position of radiolabeled amino acid																	
		20	21	22	23	24	25	26	27	28	29	30	31	32	33	34	35	36	37	38
S-200	Pool C (major)*																			
S-200	Pool C (minor)	C																		
S-200	Pool D				L		L													
S-200	Pool E																			
RPLC	Pool 1														S				S	

*The major sequence was present at four times the level of the minor sequence.   †Although leucine residues were anticipated in these positions (see Table 2), definitive assignments could not be made because of the presence of the leucine residue at positions 13 and 15 in the major sequence.

Table 2. Amino terminal protein sequence for the predicted CNBr-cleavage products encoded by the LOR region of HTLV. The one-letter symbols for the amino acids are: A, alanine; R, arginine; N, asparagine; D, aspartic acid; C, cysteine; Q, glutamine; E, glutamic acid; G, glycine; H, histidine; I, isoleucine; L, leucine; K, lysine; M, methionine; F, phenylalanine; P, proline; S, serine; T, threonine; W, tryptophan; Y, tyrosine; and V, valine.

CNBr-1 NH₂	——— P† C L L S A H F P G‡ F G Q S L L F G Y P V Y V F G N C V
CNBr-2	R K Y S P F R N G Y M
CNBr-3	E P T L G Q H L P T L S F P D P G L R P Q N L Y T L W G G S V V C M
CNBr-4	Y L Y Q L S P P I T W P L L P H V I F C H P G Q L G A F L T N V P Y
CNBr-5	I S G P C P K D G Q P S L V L Q S S S F I F H K F Q T K A
	Y H P S F L L S H G

*Residues determined by radiolabel sequence analysis.   †Corresponding to the nucleotide sequence 7286 to 7288 in (9).   ‡A consensus splice acceptor site lies in the nucleotide sequence bearing this residue.

Table 3. Summary of radiolabel sequence analysis of CNBr fragments of p42.

Item	Gel filtration (S-200)				Total	RPLC
	Pool E (CNBr-2)	Pool D (CNBr-3)	Pool C* (CNBr-4)	Pool C† (CNBr-5)		Pool 1 (CNBr-5)
Residues analyzed	11	34	20	20	85	38
Residues expected‡	1	6	7	5	19	8
Observed						
Matched	1	6	5§	5	17	8
Unmatched	0	0	0	0	0	0

*Minor sequence. †Major sequence. ‡Expected from nucleotide sequence in (*10*). §See second footnote to Table 1.

Since the protein sequence of the amino terminus of p42 was not available, we cannot rigorously discuss the origin of the amino terminus of the LOR-encoded protein. However, it is likely that the amino terminus of an LOR protein is encoded by another region of the HTLV genome, possibly the *gag* region. There is at least one potential splice donor site present in the 5′ end of the p19 *gag* coding region and one potential splice acceptor site present in the 5′ end of the LOR region that could conceivably yield an in-frame spliced transcript encoding a *gag*-LOR fusion product of 42 kD (*10*). Oroszlan and co-workers reported that the amino terminus of the HTLV *gag* gene products was inaccessible to Edman degradation, apparently due to myristylation of the *gag* product, p19, at its second residue (*15*). Thus, the inability to sequence the amino terminus of p42 may be due to the presence of amino terminal *gag* sequences containing similar posttranslational modifications.

The 42-kD product of the HTLV LOR region is a novel retroviral protein, distinct from both the viral *gag* and *env* proteins and from oncogene products exhibiting homology to host cell species. The presence of p42 in a large number of HTLV-I–immortalized cells indicates the generality of its production. The ab-sence of other previously characterized HTLV structural proteins in the nonproducer cell line, C81-66-45, provides circumstantial evidence for the importance of p42 in the maintenance of the immortalization in vitro and *trans*-acting transcriptional activation observed in this cell line (*7*). A 38-kD protein, which shares immunochemical properties with p42 and appears to be the LOR region product of HTLV-II, has also been identified in a HTLV-II–immortalized cell line, C3-44/MO (*16*). Further work aimed at characterizing the function of these proteins is likely to yield insight into the transformation-related properties of the HTLV family of retroviruses.

References and Notes

1. R. C. Gallo *et al.*, *Cancer Res.* **43**, 3892 (1983); R. C. Gallo, in *Human T-Cell Leukemia Viruses*, R. C. Gallo, M. E. Essex, L. Gross, Eds. (Cold Spring Harbor Laboratory, Cold Spring Harbor, N.Y., 1984), p. 1.
2. B. J. Poiesz *et al.*, *Proc. Natl. Acad. Sci. U.S.A.* **77**, 7415 (1980).
3. M. Yoshida, I. Miyoshi, Y. Hinuma, *ibid.* **79**, 2031 (1982).
4. V. S. Kalyanaraman *et al.*, *Science* **218**, 571 (1982); I. S. Y. Chen *et al.*, *Nature (London)* **305**, 502 (1983).
5. M. Popovic *et al.*, *Science* **224**, 497 (1984); R. C. Gallo *et al.*, *ibid.*, p. 500; J. Schüpbach *et al.*, *ibid.*, p. 503; M. G. Sarngadharan *et al.*, *ibid.*, p. 506.
6. M. Seiki *et al.*, *Nature (London)* **309**, 640 (1984).
7. J. G. Sodroski, C. A. Rosen, W. A. Haseltine, *Science* **225**, 381 (1984).
8. M. Popovic *et al.*, *Science* **219**, 856 (1983).
9. M. Seiki *et al.*, *Proc. Natl. Acad. Sci. U.S.A.* **80**, 3618 (1983).

10. W. A. Haseltine, J. Sodroski, R. Patarca, D. Briggs, D. Perkins, F. Wong-Staal, *Science* **225**, 419 (1984).
11. T. H. Lee, J. E. Coligan, T. Homma, M. F. McLane, N. Tachibana, M. Essex, *Proc. Natl. Acad. Sci. U.S.A.* **81**, 3856 (1984).
12. T. H. Lee *et al.*, in *Human T-Cell Leukemia Viruses*, R. C. Gallo, M. E. Essex, L. Gross, Eds. (Cold Spring Harbor Laboratory, Cold Spring Harbor, N.Y., 1984), p. 111.
13. J. E. Coligan *et al.*, *Methods Enzymol.* **91**, 413 (1983).
14. S. Z. Salahuddin *et al.*, *Virology* **129**, 51 (1983).
15. S. Oroszlan *et al.*, in *Human T-Cell Leukemia Viruses*, R. C. Gallo, M. E. Essex, L. Gross, Eds. (Cold Spring Harbor Laboratory, Cold Spring Harbor, N.Y., 1984), p. 101; L. E. Henderson, H. C. Kurtzch, S. Oroszlan, *Proc. Natl. Acad. Sci. U.S.A.* **80**, 339 (1983).
16. T. H. Lee *et al.*, unpublished data.
17. We thank G. Franchini for sharing her unpublished data, P. Markham for helpful discussions, and B. Valas for valuable technical assistance. T. H. Lee was supported by Institutional Research Service award 2-T32-CA0903; J. G. Sodroski was supported by NIH postdoctoral fellowship CA07094. The research was supported in part by grants CA13885, CA18216, and CA37466 from the National Institutes of Health, and in part by an American Cancer Society directors grant.

27 August 1984; accepted 5 September 1984

Report

5 October 1984

55. Identification of the Putative Transforming Protein of the Human T-Cell Leukemia Viruses HTLV-I and HTLV-II

Dennis J. Slamon, Kunitada Shimotohno, Martin J. Cline, David W. Golde, and Irvin S.Y. Chen

Human T-cell leukemia virus type I (HTLV-I) and type II (HTLV-II) are closely associated with specific human leukemias and lymphomas involving T lymphocytes (*1–4*). Both of these retroviruses transform normal T lymphocytes in vitro, lending credence to their etiologic role in these human malignancies (*5–8*). Most of the known oncogenic retroviruses belong to one of two general groups, depending on the mechanisms by which they induce malignancy (*9*). The long latency of the chronic transforming retroviruses, such as the avian leukosis viruses and the murine mammary tumor virus, is thought to be due to transformation by insertional mutagenesis, a mechanism whereby the proviral genome is integrated at sites near a cellular gene with subsequent activation of the cellular gene (*10, 11*). The second group, known as the acutely transforming retroviruses, carry specific transforming sequences (viral oncogenes) derived from a cohort of normal cellular genes (cellular oncogenes or proto-oncogenes) (*9*). HTLV appears to be unique among the transforming retroviruses in that it does not have a viral oncogene with a normal cellular homolog, nor does it integrate at any preferential sites in tumors or in cells transformed in vitro

292

(*12, 13*). These observations argue against a mechanism involving insertional mutagenesis, and the absence of sequences homologous to normal cellular DNA sequences separate HTLV from the acutely transforming retroviruses.

The nucleotide sequences of HTLV-I and HTLV-II contain a highly conserved region between *env* and the 3′ long terminal repeat (LTR) of the viruses. Such sequences have not been observed in animal retroviruses except for a similar sequence in bovine leukemia virus (*14–17*). This region, termed "X" by Seiki *et al.* (*14*) has no definitely assigned function but is believed to participate in HTLV-induced cellular transformation (*14, 16, 17*). Protein products encoded by this region have not been reported previously; however, the existence of such proteins has been predicted on the basis of four open reading frames (called X-I to X-IV) in HTLV-I (*14*) and three open reading frames (called pX-a to pX-c) in HTLV-II (*16, 17*). Comparison of the nucleotide sequences of the X regions from the two viruses reveals significant sequence homology (about 75 percent) between the X-IV region of HTLV-I and the X-c region of HTLV-II (*16, 17*). The molecular size of the predicted protein encoded by the X-IV region of HTLV-I is 24 kilodaltons if initiation of translation occurs at the first methionine codon of the X-IV region (*14*). Analysis of the sequence, however, reveals that the reading frame remains open for some 100 amino acid codons upstream from the methionine. A similar open reading frame is found in HTLV-II (*16, 17*). This extended open reading frame is sufficient to encode a protein of 39.6 kD in HTLV-I and 36.8 kD in HTLV-II. The high degree of conservation between the HTLV-I and HTLV-II genomes in this region suggested that this reading frame might encode a protein of functional importance, perhaps one involved in cellular transformation. We therefore undertook to identify such proteins by developing specific antisera to potential proteins encoded by this area of the viral genome.

Previous studies have shown that some antigenic determinants of a protein can be represented by short peptides and that antibodies directed against such peptides are frequently of use in identifying the native protein (*18–26*). On the basis of nucleic acid sequence data, the predicted amino acid sequence of individual proteins can be deduced, and oligopeptides with the required amino acid sequences can be synthesized. Such peptides have been useful in generating antisera to a wide variety of proteins, including the transforming gene products of a number of oncogenic retroviruses (*25–35*). We therefore prepared three synthetic peptides termed pX-IV-1, pX-IV-5, and pX-IV-6 (Fig. 1) based on the amino acid codon sequence of the X region of the HTLV-I virus. The peptides were selected from regions in the sequence found to be relatively hydrophilic by the method of Hopp and Woods (*36*) and were synthesized by Peninsula Laboratories, Belmont, California. All of the peptides were from areas which are highly conserved in HTLV-II. These peptides were coupled to a carrier protein (keyhole limpet hemocyanin) and were used to generate polyclonal antisera in rabbits as described (*19*). To screen for the putative proteins encoded by the X region, we used lymphoid cells transformed by, or infected with, either HTLV-I or HTLV-II. The criterion used to identify a protein as X-encoded was that the same protein be immunoprecipi-

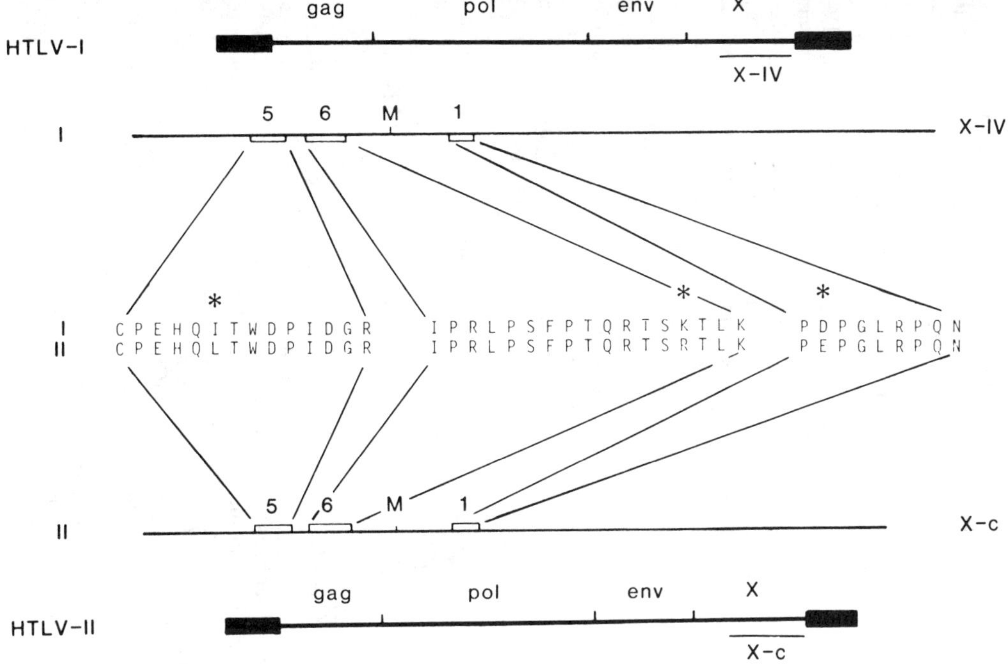

Fig. 1. Schematic representation of the following: the complete HTLV-I and HTLV-II genomes (top and bottom lines, respectively), with the relative positions of the X-IV and X-c regions shown; the X-IV region of the X gene of HTLV-I and the X-c region of the X gene of HTLV-II are immediately below and above their respective genomes, with the relative positions of the synthetic peptides shown. (M marks the position of the first methionine in the X-IV and X-c codon sequence); the amino acid sequence of the synthesized peptides pX-IV-5, pX-IV-6, and pX-IV-1 of HTLV-I and the corresponding amino acid sequence of these peptides in the pX-c region of HTLV-II are shown in the center. Asterisks mark the positions of amino acid differences. The one letter symbols for the amino acids are A, alanine; R, arginine; N, asparagine; D, aspartic acid; C, cysteine; Q, glutamine; E, glutamic acid; G, glycine; H, histidine; I, isoleucine; L, leucine; K, lysine; M, methionine; F, phenylalanine; P, proline; S, serine; T, threonine; W, tryptophan; Y, tyrosine; and V, valine.

tated by antisera to at least two peptides representing separate areas of the amino acid codon sequence, thus greatly decreasing the possibility that the immunoprecipitation was due to chance sequence homology between the synthesized peptide and another cellular protein.

The SLB-I cell line is derived from normal human adult peripheral blood cells transformed in vitro with HTLV-I (37, 38). A protein of 40 kD was consist-

ently immunoprecipitated from these cells with antisera directed to the pX-IV-5 and pX-IV-6 peptides (Fig. 2, lanes b and f). Immunoprecipitation of this protein could be completely competed away with the relevant peptide, indicating a specific antigen-antibody reaction (Fig. 2, lanes c and g). A faint band of similar migration was detected in SLB cells by unimmunized sera (Fig. 2, lanes a and e), but this protein was not competed away by the specific peptide, indicating a lack

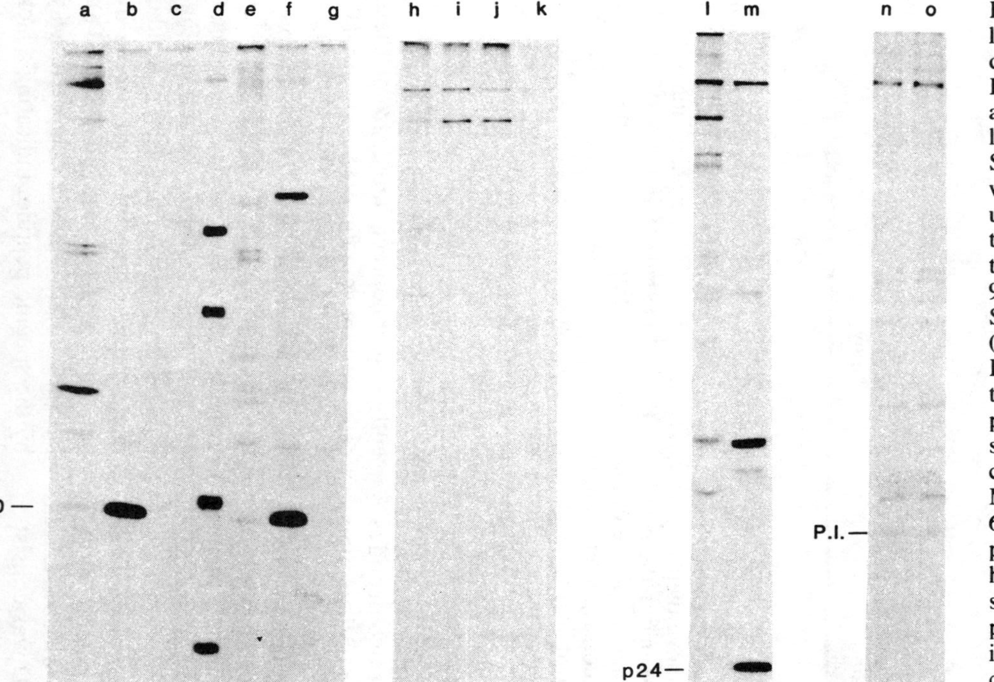

Fig. 2. Immunoprecipitation from various cell lines with antisera directed against peptides derived from the X-IV region of HTLV-I. Indicated lanes are: (lane a) SLB-I cell lysate and unimmunized serum; (lane b) SLB-I cell lysate and antiserum to pX-IV-5; (lane c) SLB-I cell lysate and antiserum to pX-IV-5 which was previously incubated for 30 minutes at 4°C with 10 μl of solution (1 mg/ml) of the pX-IV-5 peptide; (lane d) [14C]-labeled protein standard markers (top to bottom: 200 kD, 92.6 kD, 68 kD, 43 kD, and 25.7 kD); (lane e) SLB-I cell lysate and unimmunized serum; (lane f) SLB-I cell lysate and antiserum to pX-IV-6; (lane g) SLB-I cell lysate and antiserum to pX-IV-6 previously incubated with peptide pX-IV-6 as above; (lane h) MOLT-4 cell lysate and antiserum to pX-IV-5; (lane i) HL-60 cell lysate and antiserum to pX-IV-5; (lane j) MOLT-4 cell lysate and antiserum to pX-IV-6; (lane k) HL-60 cell lysate and antiserum to pX-IV-6; (lane l) SLB-I cell lysate and normal human serum; (lane m) SLB-I cell lysate and serum from a patient with adult T-cell lymphoma (HTLV-I–associated), demonstrating immunoprecipitation of p24^{gag} in the infected cells; (lane n) SLB-I cell lysate and unimmunized serum; and (lane o) SLB-I cell lysate and unimmunized serum previously incubated with both the pX-IV-5 and pX-IV-6 peptides. Total cellular proteins were metabolically labeled with [35S]methionine by culturing cells at a concentration of 1×10^6 cells per milliliter in methionine-free Earle's modified minimal essential medium (Flow Laboratories) supplemented with 2 percent glutamine, 10 percent dialyzed fetal calf serum, and [35S]methionine (100 μCi/ml; >600 Ci/mmol; Amersham) at 37°C for 4 to 5 hours. The cells were then washed twice in cold (4°C) phosphate-buffered saline (pH 7.4) and lysed at a concentration of 4×10^6 cells per milliliter in radioimmunoprecipitation assay (RIPA) buffer [150 mM NaCl, 1 percent sodium deoxycholate, 1 percent Triton X-100, 0.1 percent sodium dodecyl sulfate (SDS), 10 mM tris-HCl (pH 7.6), and 1 mM phenylmethylsulfonyl fluoride (PMSF)]. The cell extracts were clarified by centrifugation at 100,000g for 60 minutes at 4°C. The immunoprecipitation reaction mixture consisted of 10 μl of the indicated sera and clarified cell lysate (8×10^6 count/min) in a final volume of 250 μl of RIPA buffer containing bovine serum albumin (2 mg/ml) and 0.07 percent SDS. The antigen-antibody reaction was carried out overnight at 4°C. Immunoprecipitates were collected by addition of 60 μl of a 10 percent suspension of Pansorbin (Calbiochem) for 30 minutes at 4°C. The samples were then washed four times in RIPA buffer and analyzed on 7.5 percent SDS-polyacrylamide gels as described by Laemmli (47). Gels were then subjected to fluorography (P.I. indicates comigrating protein seen with unimmunized serum in SLB cells).

of relevance to the immunogenicity of the peptides used (Fig. 2, lanes n and o). Furthermore, the 40-kD protein was not found in control hematopoietic cell lines, including MOLT-4, a transformed T-lymphoblast cell line which is not infected with HTLV, and HL-60, a human promyelocytic cell line (Fig. 2, lanes h and k).

The JLB-I cell line is an HTLV-II–transformed T-cell line that was derived from the normal donor whose cells were used to establish the SLB-I cell line (7). In these cells, a protein of 37 kD was found with the same antisera, that is, the antiserum to pX-IV-5 and the antiserum pX-IV-6 (Fig. 3, lanes c and g). Again, immunoprecipitation of this protein could be completely inhibited by the relevant peptide, indicating a specific antigen-antibody reaction (Fig. 3, lanes d and h). The 37-kD protein was not found in control hematopoietic cells that were not infected with HTLV-II (Fig. 2, lanes h to k), nor was it identified by unimmunized sera (Fig. 3, lanes b and f). A second protein of lower molecular weight (approximately 30 kD) was also

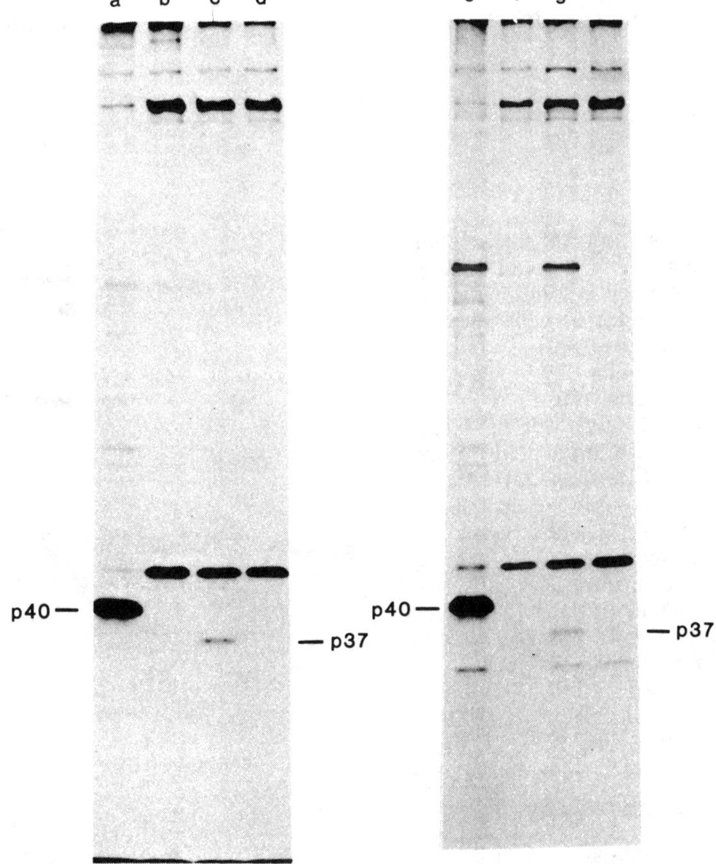

Fig. 3. Immunoprecipitation from cells infected with HTLV-I (SLB-I) and HTLV-II (JLB-I). (Lane a) SLB-I cell lysate and antiserum to pX-IV-5; (lane b) JLB-I cell lysate and unimmunized serum; (lane c) JLB-I cell lysate and antiserum to pX-IV-5; (lanc d) JLB-I cell lysate and antiserum to pX-IV-5 previously incubated with pX-IV-5 peptide as described in Fig. 2; (lane e) SLB-I cell lysate and antiserum to pX-IV-6; (lane f) JLB-I cell lysate and unimmunized serum; (lane g) JLB-I cell lysate and antiserum to pX-IV-6; and (lane h) JLB-I cell lysate and antiserum to pX-IV-6 previously incubated with pX-IV-6 peptide.

identified in the JLB-I cell line with antiserum to pX-IV-6 (Fig. 3, lane g). This protein, however, was not recognized by antiserum to pX-IV-5 (Fig. 3, lane c) and its immunoprecipitation was not competed away by peptide (Fig. 3, lane h).

We demonstrated earlier that HTLV-II productively infects B cells and that the virus produced from these cells maintains the ability to transform T cells (*39*). To demonstrate unambiguously the specific association of the 37-kD protein with HTLV-II infection, we examined uninfected and infected cells of the same B-cell line, 729. The 37-kD protein was seen in infected 729 B-cell lysates and not in uninfected 729 cells (Fig. 4, lanes a, b, e, and f). Again, immunoprecipitation of the 37-kD protein found in the HTLV-II–infected B cells could be inhibited by prior incubation of the antisera with the appropriate synthetic peptide, and unimmunized sera did not recognize the protein (Fig. 4, lanes c, d, g, and h).

Antisera directed against peptide pX-IV-1 (Fig. 1) failed to recognize any unique protein in cells infected with either HTLV-I or HTLV-II (data not shown). The failure of this serum to recognize the 40-kD or 37-kD proteins may be related to the size of the pX-IV-1 peptide. We have found that shorter synthetic peptides (fewer than ten amino acids) are considerably less effective in

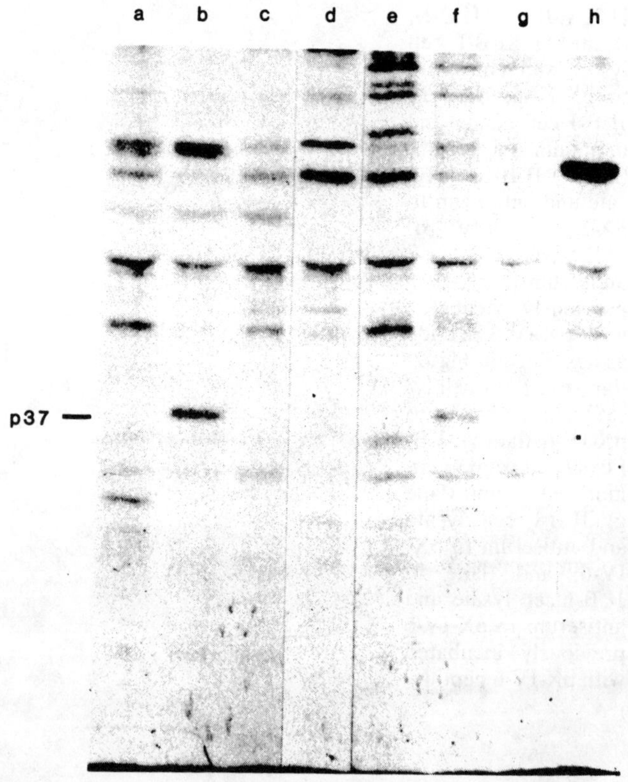

Fig. 4. Immunoprecipitation from uninfected and HTLV-II–infected B cells. (Lane a) 729 (uninfected) cell lysate and antiserum to pX-IV-5; (lane b) 729i (HTLV-II-infected) cell lysate and antiserum to pX-IV-5; (lane c) 729i cell lysate and antiserum to pX-IV-5 first incubated with pX-IV-5 peptide as described in Fig. 2; (lane d) 729i cell lysate and unimmunized serum; (lane e) 729 cell lysate and antiserum to pX-IV-6; (lane f) 729i cell lysate and antiserum to pX-IV-6; (lane g) 729i cell lysate and antiserum to pX-IV-6 previously incubated with pX-IV-6 peptide; and (lane h) 729i cell lysate and unimmunized serum.

generating antisera that recognize the native protein from which they were derived (40).

The conclusion that the 40-kD HTLV-1–related protein and the 37-kD HTLV-II–related proteins are X-encoded is supported by the following.

1) The proteins are identified by antisera to at least two peptides representing different regions of the predicted amino acid sequence of the X region.

2) Transformation with either HTLV-I or HTLV-II resulted in recognition of proteins of different sizes in T cells from the same donor, indicating that the proteins were of viral origin rather than being cellular proteins associated with T-cell transformation. The degree of homology between the portions of the HTLV-I and HTLV-II X regions from which the peptides were prepared is almost complete. There is a single amino acid difference in each peptide in comparison with the HTLV-II codon sequence in these areas (7, 15). In each instance the change is conservative; that is, isoleucine replaces leucine in pX-IV-5, and lysine replaces arginine in pX-IV-6 (Fig. 1). This degree of homology should allow recognition of the HTLV-II X-encoded protein when peptides based on the HTLV-I X sequence are used. Review of the data, however, clearly shows a difference in the amounts of the 40-kD and 37-kD proteins found in the HTLV-I– and HTLV-II–infected cells, repectively (Fig. 3, lanes a, c, e, and g), even though the same amount of [^{35}S]methionine-labeled cell lysate was used in all immunoprecipitation reactions. This finding may reflect a difference in the relative amounts of the proteins in the infected cells. Alternatively, it may be due to a difference in the avidity of the antisera for the proteins.

The amino acid sequences used for the synthesis of the peptides were derived from the codon sequence of the HTLV-I X-IV region rather than the HTLV-II X-c region (Fig. 1). The resulting antisera might therefore be expected to better recognize a protein in which the peptide is conserved with complete fidelity than one in which there are amino acid mismatches.

3) The sizes of the 40-kD and 37-kD immunoprecipitated proteins is close to the sizes predicted from the X regions of HTLV-I (39.6 kD) and HTLV-II (36.8 kD), excluding glycosylation or other posttranslational modifications. Since the antisera recognizing the 40-kD and 37-kD proteins were derived from sequences upstream from the first methionine in the pX-IV open reading frame, we predict that both the 40-kD and 37-kD proteins represent the products of spliced messenger RNA's (mRNA's) consisting predominantly of pX-IV and pX-c sequences, as well as some 5' viral sequences that supply the methionine initiation codon. Indeed, recent results indicate that the X region of both HTLV-I and HTLV-II is transcribed into a 2.0- to 2.2-kb spliced subgenomic mRNA (41). This message would easily accommodate a 37- to 40-kD protein.

4) The fact that the same 37-kD protein is seen in HTLV-II–infected B cells as in HTLV-II–infected T cells, which are transformed, strongly suggests that the 37-kD protein is a virally encoded protein occurring with viral infection and not solely in T-cell transformation. Furthermore, neither the 40-kD nor the 37-kD proteins are found in control hematopoietic cell lines that are transformed but are not infected by HTLV—that is, a human leukemia T-cell line (MOLT-4), a human myeloid leukemia cell line (HL-

298

60), and an Epstein-Barr virus–transformed human B-cell line (729).

It has been suggested that the X region of HTLV is responsible for the transforming potential of the virus (*14, 16, 17, 42*). On the basis of data presented in our study, and in accordance with the accepted convention on naming the putative transforming regions of oncogenic retroviruses (*43*), we propose calling the X-region proteins of HTLV-I and HTLV-II, $p40^{xI}$ and $p37^{xII}$, respectively.

The function of the *xI* and *xII* genes in HTLV-mediated transformation is not clear. Recent evidence suggests that the region may play a role in regulation of viral RNA expression (*44*). It is possible that the $p40^{xI}$ and $p37^{xII}$ proteins may function in a manner analogous to the papova virus T antigens or the adenovirus EIA proteins. These viral proteins serve an important regulatory role in viral replication as well as being necessary for cell transformation (*45, 46*). The mechanisms by which the $p40^{xI}$ and $p37^{xII}$ proteins might facilitate viral transcription and induce cellular transformation, however, remain uncertain.

With the availability of specific antisera for the *xI* and *xII* products, investigations on the subcellular localization and isolation of the proteins are now possible. Such studies should provide important insights into the role of these proteins in HTLV-induced transformation and disease.

References and Notes

1. B. J. Poiesz, F. W. Ruscetti, A. F. Gazdar, P. A. Bunn, J. D. Minna, R. C. Gallo, *Proc. Natl. Acad. Sci. U.S.A.* **77**, 7415 (1980).
2. Y. Hinuma *et al.*, *ibid.* **78**, 6476 (1981).
3. V. S. Kalyanaraman *et al.*, *Science* **218**, 571 (1982).
4. A. Saxon, R. H. Stevens, D. W. Golde, *Ann. Intern. Med.* **88**, 323 (1978).
5. I. Miyoshi, I. Kubonishi, S. Yoshimoto, T. Akagi, Y. Ohtsuki, Y. Shiraishi, K. Nagata, Y. Hinuma, *Nature (London)* **294**, 770 (1981).
6. N. Yamamoto, M. Okada, Y. Koyanagi, M. Kannagi, Y. Hinuma, *Science* **217**, 737 (1982).
7. M. Popovic *et al.*, *ibid.* **219**, 856 (1983).
8. I. S. Y. Chen, S. G. Quan, D. W. Golde, *Proc. Natl. Acad. Sci. U.S.A.* **80**, 7006 (1983).
9. J. M. Bishop, *Annu. Rev. Biochem.* **52**, 301 (1983).
10. W. S. Hayward, B. G. Neel, S. M. Astrin, *Nature (London)* **290**, 475 (1981).
11. R. Nusse, A. van Ooyen, D. Cox, Y. K. T. Fung, H. Varmus, *ibid.* **307**, 131 (1984).
12. B. Hahn, V. Manzari, S. Colombini, G. Franchini, R. C. Gallo, F. Wong-Staal, *ibid.* **303**, 253 (1983); B. Hahn *et al.*, *ibid.* **305**, 340 (1983).
13. M. Seiki, R. Eddy, T. B. Shows, M. Yoshida, *ibid.* **309**, 640 (1984).
14. M. Seiki, S. Hattori, Y. Hirayama, M. Yoshida, *Proc. Natl. Acad. Sci. U.S.A.* **80**, 3618 (1983).
15. A. Burny, personal communication.
16. W. A. Haseltine, J. Sodroski, R. Patarca, D. Briggs, D. Perkins, F. Wong-Staal, *Science* **225**, 419 (1984).
17. K. Shimotohno *et al.*, *Proc. Natl. Acad. Sci. U.S.A.*, in press.
18. R. A. Lerner, *Nature (London)* **299**, 592 (1982).
19. ______, N. Green, H. Alexander, F.-T. Liu, J. G. Sutcliffe, T. M. Shinnick, *Proc. Natl. Acad. Sci. U.S.A.* **78**, 3403 (1981).
20. J. G. Sutcliffe, T. M. Shinnick, N. Green, F.-T. Liu, H. L. Niman, R. A. Lerner, *Nature (London)* **287**, 801 (1980).
21. G. Walter, K.-H. Scheidtmann, A. Carbone, A. P. Laudano, R. F. Doolittle, *Proc. Natl. Acad. Sci. U.S.A.* **77**, 5197 (1980).
22. G. Walter, M. A. Hutchinson, T. Hunter, W. Eckhart, *ibid.* **78**, 4882 (1981).
23. M. H. Baron and D. Baltimore, *Cell* **28**, 395 (1982).
24. E. Pfaff, M. Mussgay, H. O. Böhm, G. E. Schulz, H. Schaller, *EMBO J.* **1**, 869 (1982).
25. J. G. Sutcliffe, R. J. Milner, T. M. Shinnick, F. E. Bloom, *Cell* **33**, 671 (1983).
26. R. Harvey *et al.*, *EMBO J.* **1**, 473 (1982).
27. B. M. Sefton and G. Walter, *J. Virol.* **44**, 467 (1982).
28. T. W. Wong and A. R. Goldberg, *Proc. Natl. Acad. Sci. U.S.A.* **78**, 7412 (1981).
29. J. Papkoff, I. M. Verma, T. Hunter, *Cell* **29**, 417 (1982).
30. T. Tamura, H. Bauer, C. Birr, R. Pipkorn, *ibid.* **34**, 587 (1983).
31. S. Sen, R. A. Houghten, C. J. Sherr, A. Sen, *Proc. Natl. Acad. Sci. U.S.A.* **80**, 1246 (1983).
32. L. E. Gentry, L. R. Rohrschneider, J. E. Casnellie, E. G. Krebs, *J. Biol. Chem.* **258**, 11219 (1983).
33. W. J. Boyle, J. S. Lipsick, E. P. Reddy, M. A. Baluda, *Proc. Natl. Acad. Sci. U.S.A.* **80**, 2834 (1983).
34. T. Curran, A. D. Miller, L. Zokas, I. M. Verma, *Cell* **36**, 259 (1984).
35. S. R. Hann, H. D. Abrams, L. R. Rohrschneider, R. N. Eisenman, *ibid.* **34**, 789 (1983).
36. T. P. Hopp and K. R. Woods, *Proc. Natl. Acad. Sci. U.S.A.* **78**, 3824 (1981).
37. H. P. Koeffler, I. S. Y. Chen, D. W. Golde, *Blood* **64**, 482 (1984).
38. J. C. Gasson, I. S. Y. Chen, C. A. Westbrook, D. W. Golde, in *Normal and Neoplastic Hematopoiesis*, D. W. Golde and P. A. Marks, Eds.

(Liss, New York, 1983), p. 129.
39. I. S. Y. Chen, J. McLaughlin, D. W. Golde, *Nature (London)* **309**, 276 (1984).
40. T. Tanaka, D. J. Slamon, M. J. Cline, in preparation.
41. W. Wachsman *et al.*, *Science*, in press.
42. I. S. Y. Chen *et al.*, in preparation.
43. J. M. Coffin *et al.*, *J. Virol.* **40**, 953 (1981).
44. J. G. Sodroski, C. A. Rosen, W. A. Haseltine, *Science* **225**, 381 (1984).
45. R. B. Gaynor, D. Hillman, A. Berk, *Proc. Natl. Acad. Sci. U.S.A.* **81**, 1193 (1984).
46. J. Brady, J. B. Bolen, M. Radonovich, N. Salzman, G. Khoury, *ibid.*, p. 2040.
47. U. K. Laemmli, *Nature (London)* **227**, 680 (1970).

48. Supported by a grant from Triton Biosciences, by grants CA 32737 and RR 00865 awarded by the National Cancer Institute, and by Cancer Center support grant CA 16042. We gratefully acknowledge the technical assistance of L. Rodriguez, D. Keith, S. Quan, A. Healy, and R. Cortini. We thank L. Kim, B. Colby, and J. Gasson for their advice and encouragement during this study and B. Koers and G. Helfan for their assistance in preparing this manuscript.

30 August 1984; accepted 5 September 1984

Report

12 October 1984

56. Suramin Protection of T Cells in Vitro Against Infectivity and Cytopathic Effect of HTLV-III

Hiroaki Mitsuya, Mikulas Popovic, Robert Yarchoan, Shuzo Matsushita, Robert C. Gallo, and Samuel Broder

Approximately 3 years ago, an apparently new and unexplained disorder called acquired immune deficiency syndrome (AIDS) was recognized (*1–3*). The disorder is a pandemic immunosuppressive disease that predisposes to life-threatening infections with opportunistic organisms and to certain neoplasms (especially Kaposi's sarcomas and occasionally lymphomas), which may be signs of the underlying immune impairment. Characteristically, AIDS is associated with a progressive depletion of T cells, especially the helper-inducer subset bearing the OKT4 surface marker (*2*). No therapy is known to cure AIDS.

The hypothesis that AIDS is caused by a member of the human T-cell leukemia virus (HTLV) family of retroviruses first received direct empirical support in 1983 (*4, 5*). For example, Essex and Lee and their colleagues discovered the presence of antibodies to cell membrane antigen of HTLV-I–infected T cells in serum samples from more than 40 percent of patients with AIDS (in the most sensitive range of their assay) (*6*). This antigen is now known to be expressed on the envelope of HTLV-I (*7*). At the same time, three observations reinforced the possibility that a then-uncharacterized member of the HTLV family might be playing a role in the pathogenesis of AIDS: (i) The report by Barré-Sinoussi *et al.* (*5*) of a new retrovirus, termed lymphadenopathy-associated virus (LAV), isolated from a homosexual man, who was thought to have a possible prodrome of

AIDS. These workers, in the first paper describing their findings, concluded that the new retrovirus belonged in the HTLV family but that it was distinct from the other members then defined. (ii) Detection of AIDS sera containing antibodies to a membrane (HTLV envelope) protein but lacking antibodies to certain internal core structural proteins of HTLV-I and HTLV-II (4). (iii) The infrequent isolation of HTLV-I and HTLV-II from AIDS patients, even in the presence of antibodies to HTLV-I envelope determinants (4).

In the spring of 1984 several converging lines of investigation linked a cytopathic member of the HTLV family of retroviruses to the pathogenesis of AIDS (8, 9). The retrovirus, which is now known to play a role in the etiology of AIDS, is referred to as HTLV-III; this virus preferentially infects and destroys OKT4$^+$ (helper-inducer) T cells (10). Detectable viral replication in vivo characterizes the HTLV-III infection seen in AIDS, at least early in the disease. By contrast, only on rare occasions (11) has it been possible to detect viral replication in vivo in adult T-cell leukemia, which is caused by HTLV-I, the prototypical member of the HTLV family. The discovery of HTLV-III offers researchers new strategies for the experimental therapy of the disease, including the use of drugs that inhibit reverse transcriptase (12).

All retroviruses (including HTLV-III) require the enzyme called reverse transcriptase in their natural cycle of replication (13). The reverse transcriptases of retroviruses infecting humans and animals have similar amino acid sequences (14). In 1979, de Clercq reported that suramin (molecular weight, 1429)—a drug used to treat Rhodesian trypanoso-

miasis and onchocerciasis—was a potent competitive inhibitor of the reverse transcriptase of a number of animal retroviruses (15). Since the first paper by Gallo and his colleagues describing HTLV-I in adult T-cell leukemia was not published until 1980 (16), this finding generated little clinical interest. Moreover, in this human retrovirus–associated disease, a role for an inhibitor of reverse transcriptase is not easy to envision, since the virus induces a monoclonal transformation (17). By the time frank malignancy is evident, there would appear to be no further need for viral replication, and therefore, for reverse transcriptase activity, in the disease process. However, the situation in AIDS appears very different. Retroviral infection of many cells appears to be necessary for the development of this disease. Therefore, inhibitors of reverse transcriptase are worth exploring as new modalities of therapy.

We now report that suramin can block the in vitro infectivity of HTLV-III (in the form of cell-free virions) when assayed in the H9 target population, a line which expresses mature T-cell markers but is permissive for HTLV-III replication and only partially susceptible to its cytopathic effect (8). Also, the drug blocked the cytopathic effect of HTLV-III against a normal OKT4$^+$ (helper-inducer) T-cell clone cultured together with HTLV-III–bearing H9 cells at concentrations of 50 μg/ml (3.5×10^{-5} mol) or greater, levels that are clinically attainable in human beings (18). Our results with suramin might lead to an in vitro model for screening other pharmaceuticals with potential activity against HTLV-III.

In our first experiments (Fig. 1), we used clone H9 cells to investigate the inhibitory effect of suramin on the infec-

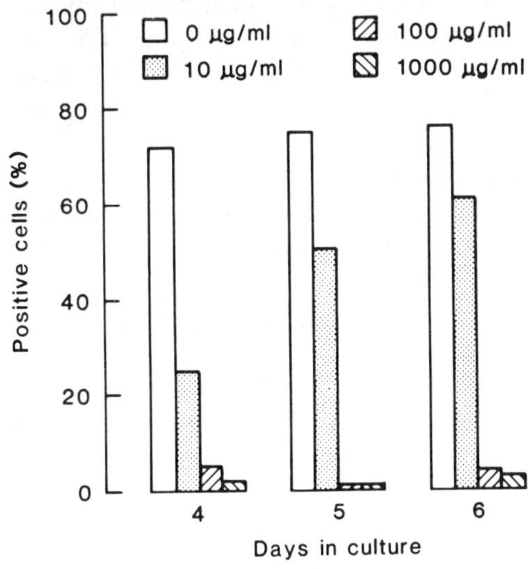

Fig. 1. Inhibition of HTLV-III$_B$ infectivity in H9 cells by suramin. Infection of H9 cells by HTLV-III$_B$ was performed as follows: The target H9 cells were exposed to suramin (10, 100, or 1000 μg/ml) for 2 hours, then to polybrene (2 μg/ml) for 30 minutes before HTLV-III$_B$ infection; control H9 cells were treated similarly but were not exposed to the drug. The H9 cells were then centrifuged (800g) and exposed to HTLV-III$_B$ virus (0.5 ml containing 7.5×10^7 viral particles) for 45 minutes and resuspended in fresh culture medium [RPMI 1640 supplemented with 20 percent heat-inactivated fetal calf serum, 4 mM L-glutamine, penicillin (50 unit/ml), and streptomycin (50 μg/ml)] and cultured in flasks at 37°C in humidified air containing 5 percent CO_2. The cells were continuously exposed to suramin at each concentration. On days 4, 5, and 6 in culture, the percentage of the target H9 cells containing p24 *gag* protein of HTLV-III$_B$ was determined by indirect immunofluorescence microscopy (*8*). Cells were washed with phosphate-buffered saline (PBS) and suspended in the same buffer at a concentration of 10^6 cells per milliliter. Approximately 50 μl of cell suspension was placed on a slide, air-dried, and fixed in acetone for 10 minutes at room temperature. Slides were stored at −20°C until use. Twenty microliters of rabbit antiserum to the p24 *gag* protein of HTLV-III (diluted 1:2000 in PBS) were applied to these preparations and incubated for 50 minutes at 37°C. Then fluorescein-conjugated goat antiserum to rabbit immunoglobulin G (Cappel) was diluted and applied to the fixed cells for 30 minutes at room temperature. Slides were then washed extensively before microscopic examination under ultraviolet illumination (Nikon; HBO 100 W; filter 450 nm NCB10; magnification ×320). Suramin was obtained from Mobay Chemical Corporation FBA Pharmaceuticals, lot No. FL 551J.

tivity of the HTLV-III. H9 cells are permissive for the replication of HTLV-III, as described in detail earlier (*8*). When the target H9 cells were exposed to the HTLV-III$_B$ isolate (in the form of cell-free virions) and cultured for 4 to 6 days in the absence of suramin, 72 to 76 percent of the target H9 cell population became infected and began to produce the virus, as determined by an indirect immunofluorescence assay in which rabbit antibodies were used to detect expression of the HTLV-III$_B$ p24 *gag* protein. A modest, but temporary, protective effect was observed when the H9 cells were cultured in the presence of suramin at a concentration of 10 μg/ml. However, at concentrations of 100 and of 1000 μg/ml, a striking protective effect was observed throughout the 6-day interval of culture. In addition, at these higher doses, the H9 population did not develop multiple-nucleated giant cells with ring formation. The latter is a characteristic feature of HTLV-III infection in these target cells (*8*).

We then asked whether suramin could block the cytopathic effect of HTLV-III$_B$ against a normal helper-inducer T-cell growth factor (TCGF)–dependent T-cell clone, cultured with H9 cells producing HTLV-III$_B$. The normal T-cell clone

(YTA1) used for this purpose has been described (*19*) and displays the following surface membrane phenotype: OKT3$^+$, OKT4$^+$, HLA-DR$^+$, Tac-antigen$^+$, and OKT8$^-$. In addition, YTA1 produces substantial quantities of TCGF and undergoes a proliferative reaction in response to antigen in the presence of appropriate accessory cells. Moreover, YTA1 shows helper activity for immunoglobulin production by normal B cells (*20*).

The results shown in Fig. 2 illustrate the protective effect of suramin on the survival and growth of a cloned normal T-cell population exposed to HTLV-III$_B$ in vitro. The YTA1 target cells were exposed to various doses of suramin for 12 hours and then cultured with irradiated (10,000 rad) HTLV-III$_B$–bearing H9 cells, with the dose of suramin kept constant during the entire time in culture. (Irradiation at this dose eliminates proliferation of H9 cells but not the infectivity of HTLV-III virions.) As a control, uninfected irradiated H9 cells were added to YTA1 cells under the same conditions. All cultures contained 15

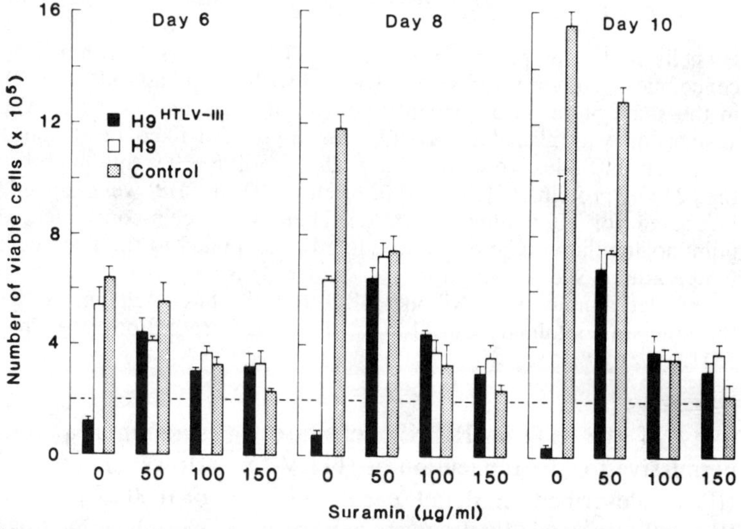

Fig. 2. Inhibition of cytopathic effect exerted by HTLV-III$_B$-bearing H9 cells against a normal helper-inducer T-cell clone (YTA1) by suramin. YTA1 cells (2×10^5) were exposed to suramin at various concentrations (0 to 150 µg/ml) for 12 hours in culture tubes (Falcon 3033) containing 2 ml of 15 percent (by volume) TCGF (Cellular Products) in the culture medium [RPMI 1640 supplemented with 15 percent heat-inactivated fetal calf serum, 4 mM L-glutamine, penicillin (50 unit/ml), and streptomycin (50 µg/ml)]. Culture tubes were kept at 37°C in humidified air containing 5 percent CO_2. Then these YTA1 cells were added with the equal number of irradiated (10,000 rad) HTLV-III$_B$-bearing H9 or uninfected H9 cells. Control cells were cultured without any cells added. Cells were continuously exposed to suramin and TCGF. The assays were all performed in duplicate. On days 6, 8, and 10, the viable cells were counted in a hemocytometer under the microscope by the trypan blue exclusion method. When cultured alone in the presence of TCGF, none of irradiated HTLV-III$_B$–bearing H9 or uninfected H9 cells were alive on day 6 in culture. Normal YTA1 cells could be readily distinguished from neoplastic H9 cells by morphology. The YTA1 target cells had been stimulated by soluble tetanus toxoid antigen plus irradiated (4000 rad) autologous accessory cells 6 days before these experiments as part of a cycle of restimulations. Each bar represents the mean number of viable cells (± 1 standard deviation) of duplicate determinations. The dashed horizontal line shows the starting number of YTA1 cells.

percent (by volume) lectin-free TCGF. We determined the total numbers of viable YTA1 cells as a function of time in culture. In the absence of suramin, the HTLV-III$_B$–producing H9 cells had exerted a substantial cytopathic effect on the YTA1 population by day 6 in culture, and by day 10 the YTA1 population was almost completely killed. The addition of suramin at concentrations of 50 μg/ml or greater enabled the YTA1 target population to survive and grow in the presence of HTLV-III$_B$. (At concentrations of 100 μg/ml or higher, the drug clearly blocked the cytopathic effect of the virus but did exert an inhibitory effect on the normal target T-cell growth.) Thus, suramin can block the replication of HTLV-III$_B$ in permissive H9 cells and can also inhibit the cytopathic effect of HTLV-III$_B$ on an OKT4$^+$ T-cell clone.

Most of what is known about the clinical pharmacology of suramin derives from its use in the therapy of trypanosomiasis and onchocerciasis. After intravenous injection, the drug combines with serum proteins, and much of it circulates in the blood (18). It persists in the bloodstream for very long periods [for example, Hawking (18) has suggested that it may be detected up to 6 months], and its excretion in the urine is very slow. The therapeutic regimens in use result in considerable accumulation in the plasma (frequently in excess of 100 μg/ml) (18, 21). Indeed, concentrations as high as 340 μg/ml may be reached under some conditions (18). These concentrations exceed those found to block the infectivity (Fig. 1) and cytopathic effect (Fig. 2) of HTLV-III in the studies reported here.

The capability of suramin to inhibit the reverse transcriptases of animal retroviruses was reported in 1979 (15), and we recently confirmed that this agent can inhibit the reverse transcriptases of diverse retroviruses including that of HTLV-III (22). However, the drug is not widely viewed as an agent with antiviral therapeutic potential.

We believe the current results provide a rationale for a carefully monitored experimental trial of suramin in patients with AIDS to determine whether the drug can inhibit HTLV-III replication in vivo, and if so, whether clinical improvement takes place. However, we wish to stress several points. First, suramin has a number of recognized toxicities in human beings (18, 21). Renal damage is the most common toxicity, but the drug may be associated with other acute life-threatening reactions, including shock and coma. Second, it is possible that the administration of suramin to patients with AIDS could lead to side effects not currently known, or to unexpectedly severe forms of the known side effects. Third, it is possible that interfering with HTLV-III infection will not substantially benefit patients with late-stage AIDS, since at that point the damage to the immune system might be irreversible. Therefore, there may be a rationale for using this agent for experimental trials early in the disease. Finally, we believe that the administration of this agent should be undertaken only in a research facility capable of monitoring the patient's clinical, immunologic, and virologic status.

References and Notes

1. M. S. Gottlieb et al., Morbid. Mortal. Weekly Rep. 30, 250 (1981); A. Friedman-Kien et al., ibid., p. 305.
2. M. S. Gottlieb et al., N. Engl. J. Med. 305, 1425 (1981).
3. H. Masur et al., ibid., p. 1431; F. P. Siegal et al., ibid., p. 1439; CDC Task Force on Kaposi's Sarcoma and Opportunistic Infections, ibid., 306, 248 (1982).

4. M. Essex *et al.*, *Science* **220**, 859 (1983); E. P. Gelmann *et al.*, *ibid.*, p. 862; R. C. Gallo *et al.*, *ibid.*, p. 865; R. C. Gallo, *Cancer Surveys* **3**, 113 (1984).
5. F. Barré-Sinoussi *et al.*, *Science* **220**, 868 (1983).
6. M. Essex *et al.*, *ibid.* **221**, 1061 (1983); B. L. Evatt *et al.*, *Lancet* **1983-II**, 698 (1983).
7. J. Schüpbach, M. G. Sarngadharan, R. C. Gallo, *Science* **224**, 607 (1984).
8. M. Popovic, M. G. Sarngadharan, E. Read, R. C. Gallo, *ibid.*, p. 497.
9. R. C. Gallo *et al.*, *ibid.*, p. 500; J. Schüpbach, M. Popovic, R. V. Gilden, M. A. Gonda, M. G. Sarngadharan, R. C. Gallo, *ibid.*, p. 503; M. G. Sarngadharan, M. Popovic, L. Bruch, R. C. Gallo, *ibid.*, p. 506.
10. S. Z. Salahuddin and R. C. Gallo, unpublished data.
11. J. Schüpbach, V. S. Kalyanaraman, M. G. Sarngadharan, P. A. Bunn, D. W. Blayney, R. C. Gallo, *Lancet* **1984-I**, 302 (1984).
12. R. C. Ting, S. S. Yang, R. C. Gallo, *Nature (London) New Biol.* **236**, 163 (1972).
13. D. Baltimore, *Nature (London)* **226**, 1209 (1970); H. M. Temin and S. Mizutani, *ibid.*, p. 1211.
14. H. Toh, H. Hayashida, T. Miyata, *ibid.* **305**, 827 (1983); R. Patarca and W. A. Haseltine, *ibid.* **309**, 728 (1984).
15. E. de Clercq, *Cancer Lett.* **8**, 9 (1979).
16. B. J. Poiesz, F. W. Ruscetti, A. F. Gazdar, P.

A. Bunn, J. D. Minna, R. C. Gallo, *Proc. Natl. Acad. Sci. U.S.A.* **77**, 7415 (1980); B. J. Poiesz, F. W. Ruscetti, M. S. Reitz, V. S. Kalyanaraman, R. C. Gallo, *Nature (London)* **294**, 268 (1981).
17. M. Yoshida, I. Miyoshi, Y. Hinuma, *Proc. Natl. Acad. Sci. U.S.A.* **79**, 2031 (1982); F. Wong-Staal *et al.*, *Nature (London)* **302**, 626 (1983).
18. F. Hawking, *Trans. R. Soc. Trop. Med. Hyg.* **34**, 37 (1940); *Adv. Pharmacol. Chemother.* **15**, 289 (1978).
19. H. Mitsuya, H.-G. Guo, J. Cossman, M. Megson, M. S. Reitz, Jr., S. Broder, *Science* **225**, 1484 (1984).
20. S. Matsushita, H. Mitsuya, S. Broder, unpublished data.
21. B. O. L. Duke, *Bull. W.H.O.* **39**, 157 (1968); H. Fuglsang and J. Anderson, in "Research and Control of Onchocerciasis in the Western Hemisphere" (Scientific publication of the Pan American Health Organization, 1974), No. 298, pp. 54–56; M. H. Satti and R. Kirk, *Bull. W.H.O.* **16**, 531 (1957).
22. L. Arthur, R. Gilden, S. Broder, P. Fischinger, unpublished data; P. Sarin and R. C. Gallo, unpublished data.
23. We thank J. F. Berzofsky and J. Hoofnagle for helpful discussions.

29 August 1984; accepted 11 September 1984

Report

12 October 1984

57. Expression of the 3′ Terminal Region of Human T-Cell Leukemia Viruses

William Wachsman, Kunitada Shimotohno, Steven C. Clark, David W. Golde, Irvin S.Y. Chen

The human T-cell leukemia viruses (HTLV) types I and II are lymphotropic retroviruses that have been isolated from patients with specific T-cell malignancies (*1–4*). Infection of normal leukocytes by HTLV-I or HTLV-II in vitro results in the transformation of mature T cells, as shown by their continued proliferation (*5–8*). The mechanism of HTLV-induced leukemogenesis remains obscure. No known viral oncogene has been identified in HTLV. However, analyses of HTLV-I and HTLV-II nucleic acid sequences have identified a region, termed X, whose function is, as yet, unknown (*9–11*). The X region is bounded by *env* and the 3′ terminal repeat (LTR), is approximately 1.6 kilobase pairs long, and contains several open reading frames. The conservation of the X sequence in both HTLV-I and HTLV-II suggests that it encodes a protein that may play a critical role in HTLV replication or HTLV-induced cellular transformation, or both.

The HTLV-II–infected Mo-T cell line was established by primary culture of splenic tissue from a patient with a T-cell variant hairy cell leukemia (*12, 13*). Mo-T cell RNA was assayed for the presence of X-specific sequences by the hybridization–S_1 nuclease technique. Nucleic acid sequence analyses of the HTLV X region revealed three open reading frames in HTLV-II (X-a to X-c) and four open reading frames in HTLV-I (X-I to X-IV) (*9–11*). Three of the open reading frames in HTLV-I are homologous with those in HTLV-II, namely, X-II with X-a, X-III with X-b, and X-IV with X-c. Comparison of nucleic acid sequences in the X region of HTLV-I and HTLV-II reveals only 33 percent homology in the first third of the sequences and an abrupt shift to 75 percent homology in the 3' two-thirds, where the homologous open reading frames are located (*10, 11*). The Hha I–Cla I probe prepared from cloned HTLV-II DNA (see Fig. 1B) is a 431–base-pair fragment that spans the junction between the high- and low-homology X sequences. Figure 1A shows the DNA fragments protected by hybridization to Mo-T cell RNA. A band indicative of a 174-nucleotide protected fragment is observed. This fragment terminates close to the 5' end of the X-c open reading frame near the junction between sequences of low and high homology. The large protected fragment of 431 nucleotides corresponds to hybridization of full-length probe with either genomic HTLV-II RNA or a subgenomic messenger RNA (mRNA) species, such as *env*, that would encompass the entire probe. Control S_1 nuclease studies with RNA from uninfected cell lines did not reveal any protected fragments (data not shown).

JLB-II is an HTLV-II–transformed T-cell line, derived by cocultivation of lethally irradiated Mo-T cells with normal human leukocytes (*8, 14, 15*). In contrast to Mo-T, which harbors multiple proviruses that differ in nucleic acid sequence (*11, 14*), JLB-II contains only the wild-type, replication-competent HTLV-II genome (data not shown). The protected fragments at 174 and 431 nucleotides are again observed in the S_1 nuclease assay with JLB-II RNA. These data suggest that a potential splice acceptor site is located at approximately 174 nucleotides upstream of the Cla I site. The other minor bands in Mo-T cells may be due to variant proviruses or to nonspecific cleavage of the hybrid.

Because of the high homology between the nucleic acid sequences of HTLV-I and HTLV-II in the distal two-thirds of the X region, an X splice acceptor site should also be present in an analogous position of the HTLV-I genome. The Cla I restriction enzyme site is conserved in homologous sequences of HTLV-I and HTLV-II (Fig. 1B). Thus, we prepared a 396-nucleotide probe utilizing the Cla I site in HTLV-I, allowing a direct comparison of the S_1 mapping data.

RNA was extracted from the SLB-I cell line, which was derived by infection of normal human leukocytes with HTLV-I in vitro (*15, 16*). As in the S_1 nuclease assay of HTLV-II RNA, a fragment that is virtually coincident with the 174-nucleotide HTLV-II fragment is protected in the HTLV-I system (Fig. 1A).

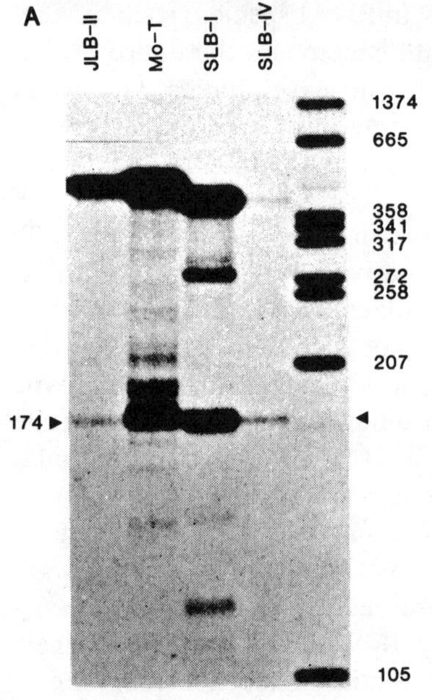

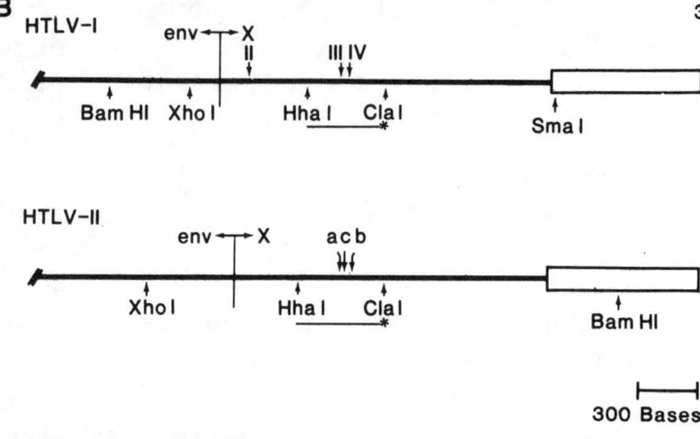

Fig. 1. Detection of X mRNA expression. (A) Hybridization-S_1 nuclease analysis of HTLV-infected cell lines was performed by standard methods (*23, 24*). RNA was extracted from the HTLV-II–infected Mo-T and JLB-II cell lines and the HTLV-I–infected SLB-I and SLB-IV cell lines. Cytoplasmic RNA (30 μg) was hybridized to the 5′ ^{32}P-labeled probe (see B) at 53° to 54°C for 12 to 14 hours. S_1 nuclease (BRL) (150 units) was used for a 1-hour digestion at room temperature. Electrophoresis was performed on an 8 percent acrylamide–8*M* urea sequencing gel. The size of the marker DNA fragments is shown in nucleotides. The 174-base fragment is indicated by the arrow. Control S_1 nuclease studies with RNA from uninfected cells and either HTLV probe reveal no protected DNA fragment (data not shown). (B) Partial restriction enzyme map of the pHT-1 HTLV-I and pH-6 HTLV-II DNA clones. The 3′ long terminal repeat is shown by an open box. The division between X and *env* sequences is indicated. The 5′ ends of the open reading frames are shown for HTLV-I X-II, X-III, and X-IV and for HTLV-II X-a, X-b, and X-c. The Hha I–Cla I hybridization probe utilized for S_1 nuclease analysis is shown as a thin line below the map with an asterisk denoting the site of 5′ ^{32}P-labeling. The sizes of the HTLV-I pHT-1 and HTLV-II pH-6 probes are 396 and 431 nucleotides, respectively.

Analysis of RNA from the HTLV-I–infected SLB-IV cell line resulted in a similar pattern of hybridization.

Taken together, the identity of the S_1 nuclease–resistant fragment seen with HTLV-I and HTLV-II RNA suggests that the X sequences are transcribed into a processed mRNA species. To confirm the presence and determine the size of the subgenomic mRNA predicted from the S_1 nuclease analysis, we performed further studies with size-fractionated polyadenylated [poly(A)$^+$] Mo-T cell RNA (Fig. 2). Northern hybridization data reveal three major species of RNA (Fig. 2A). The 9-kb band in fractions 8 and 9 is the size expected for genomic HTLV-II RNA. The 4.5-kb band in fractions 11 to 13 has been observed with probes specific for the *env* region of HTLV-II (data not shown). The third band, most prominent in fraction 15, is 2.0 to 2.3 kb in size. S_1 nuclease analysis of the fractions used for Northern hybridization demonstrate that the 2.0- to 2.3-kb species corresponds to the fractions containing the protected 174-nucleotide fragment (Fig. 2B).

Analysis of the HTLV-I and HTLV-II nucleic acid sequences in the vicinity of

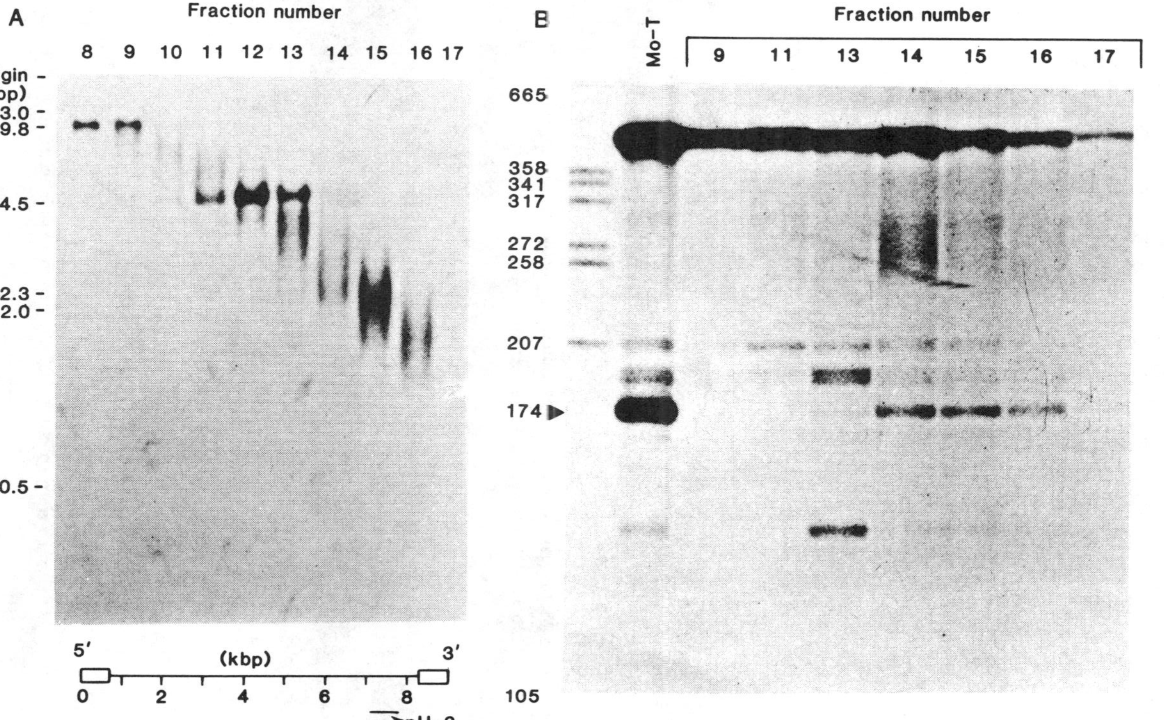

Fig. 2. Determination of X mRNA size. Poly(A)+ cytoplasmic RNA from Mo-T cells (150 μg) was sedimented on a 15 to 30 percent sucrose density gradient in a Beckman SW41 rotor. Twenty-three fractions were collected. (A) Northern hybridization of 10-μl portions of selected gradient RNA fractions was performed on a formaldehyde gel by standard methods (25). The nick-translated hybridization probe was prepared from the HTLV-II pH-3 subclone, which is shown diagramatically below the HTLV-II genome. The molecular size markers are indicated in kilobase pairs. (B) S_1 nuclease analysis of 30-μl portions of selected gradient RNA fractions. The methods are as described in Fig. 1A with the following modifications: 18 μg of L-cell RNA was added to each S_1 assay before the hybridization step and the amount of S_1 nuclease was reduced to 100 units. Control S_1 nuclease assay of uninfected Mo-T RNA is shown in parallel. The molecular size markers are shown in nucleotides. The protected fragment of 174 nucleotides is indicated.

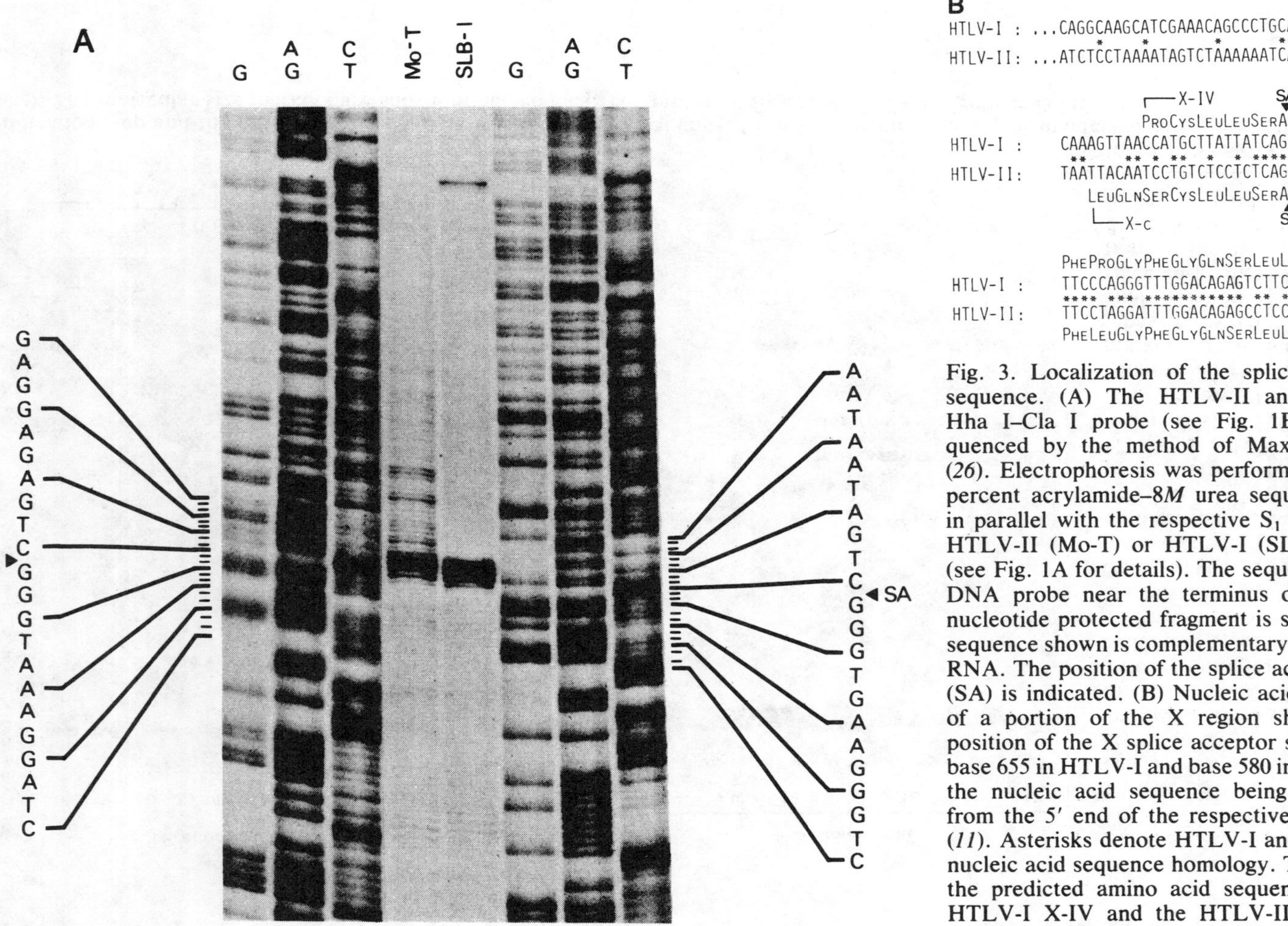

Fig. 3. Localization of the splice acceptor sequence. (A) The HTLV-II and HTLV-I Hha I–Cla I probe (see Fig. 1B) was sequenced by the method of Maxam-Gilbert (26). Electrophoresis was performed on an 8 percent acrylamide–8M urea sequencing gel in parallel with the respective S_1 analysis of HTLV-II (Mo-T) or HTLV-I (SLB-I) RNA (see Fig. 1A for details). The sequence of the DNA probe near the terminus of the 174-nucleotide protected fragment is shown. The sequence shown is complementary to the viral RNA. The position of the splice acceptor site (SA) is indicated. (B) Nucleic acid sequence of a portion of the X region showing the position of the X splice acceptor site (SA) at base 655 in HTLV-I and base 580 in HTLV-II, the nucleic acid sequence being numbered from the 5′ end of the respective X regions (11). Asterisks denote HTLV-I and HTLV-II nucleic acid sequence homology. The start of the predicted amino acid sequence for the HTLV-I X-IV and the HTLV-II X-c open reading frames is shown.

the splice acceptor site identified above reveals two potential consensus splice acceptor sites (*10, 11*). Each probe was sequenced by the method of Maxam-Gilbert and subjected to electrophoresis in parallel with the respective S_1 nuclease–resistant fragments. The data (Fig. 3) reveal the splice acceptor site in HTLV-I to be ACTCAG/CCCA at base pair 655 and in HTLV-II to be CTCAG/CCCA at base pair 580, consistent with consensus sequences for mRNA splice acceptor sites (*17*).

These results are direct evidence for expression of the X region in HTLV. The high homology of HTLV-I and HTLV-II distal to the splice acceptor site (Fig. 3) makes it likely that these sequences encode an X-derived protein. On the basis of the position of the splice site, we predict that these X-encoded products will be from the longest open reading frame, X-IV and X-c in HTLV-I and HTLV-II, respectively. Although other reading frames cannot be excluded, the identification of 40- and 37-kilodalton proteins encoded by X-IV and X-c, respectively, are consistent with this interpretation (*18*).

The location of the first methionine start codons in the X-IV and X-c open reading frames are more than 300 nucleotides downstream from the splice acceptor site (*9–11*), which would be expected to occur nearly midway in the 2- to 2.3-kb X mRNA. Consequently, we believe that the true methionine start codon for both the HTLV-I and HTLV-II X mRNA will be derived from the upstream donor sequencs. Primer extension analyses can be used to determine these leader sequences and identify the methionine start codon for the X message.

HTLV-I and HTLV-II are atypical among replication-competent retroviruses in both their functional and structural features. These viruses have a limited host range (*8, 19, 20*) and exclusively transform T cells. They do not contain known viral oncogenes, nor are they found to be specifically integrated near cellular oncogenes in tumors or transformed cells (*21, 22*). The HTLV-I and HTLV-II genomes are distinguished by the presence of the X sequences. It is likely that the protein encoded by these sequences is related to the unusual biology of HTLV. The expression of these sequences as a unique subgenomic mRNA species supports the classification of these sequences as a new gene distinct from other genes of naturally occurring retroviruses.

References and Notes

1. B. J. Poiesz, F. W. Ruscetti, A. F. Gazdar, P. A. Bunn, J. D. Minna, R. C. Gallo, *Proc. Natl. Acad. Sci. U.S.A.* **77**, 7415 (1980).
2. Y. Hinuma *et al.*, *ibid.* **78**, 6476 (1981).
3. W. A. Blattner *et al.*, *Int. J. Cancer* **30**, 257 (1982).
4. V. S. Kalyanaraman *et al.*, *Science* **218**, 571 (1982).
5. I. Miyoshi *et al.*, *Nature (London)* **294**, 770 (1981).
6. N. Yamamoto, M. Okada, Y. Koyanagi, M. Kannagi, Y. Hinuma, *Science* **217**, 737 (1982).
7. M. Popovic *et al.*, *ibid.* **219**, 856 (1983).
8. I. S. Y. Chen, S. G. Quan, D. W. Golde, *Proc. Natl. Acad. Sci. U.S.A.* **80**, 7006 (1983).
9. M. Seiki, S. Hattori, Y. Hirayma, M. Yoshida, *ibid.*, p. 3618.
10. W. A. Haseltine, J. Sodroski, R. Patarca, D. Briggs, D. Perkins, F. Wong-Staal, *Science* **225**, 419 (1984).
11. K. Shimotohno *et al.*, *Proc. Natl. Acad. Sci. U.S.A.*, in press.
12. A. Saxon, R. H. Stevens, D. W. Golde, *Ann. Intern. Med.* **88**, 323 (1978).
13. A. Saxon, R. H. Stevens, S. G. Quan, D. W. Golde, *J. Immunol.* **120**, 777 (1978).
14. I. S. Y. Chen, J. McLaughlin, J. C. Gasson, S. C. Clark, D. W. Golde, *Nature (London)* **305**, 502 (1983).
15. J. C. Gasson, I. S. Y. Chen, C. A. Westbrook, D. W. Golde, in *Normal and Neoplastic Hematopoiesis*, D. W. Golde and P. A. Marks, Eds. (Liss, New York, 1983), p. 129.
16. H. P. Koeffler, I. S. Y. Chen, D. W. Golde, *Blood* **64**, 482 (1984).
17. S. M. Mount, *Nucleic Acids Res.* **10**, 459 (1982).
18. D. J. Slamon, K. Shimotohno, M. J. Cline, D. W. Golde, I. S. Y. Chen, *Science* **226**, 61 (1984).
19. I. S. Y. Chen, J. McLaughlin, D. W. Golde, *Nature (London)* **309**, 276 (1984).

20. J. G. Sodroski, C. A. Rosen, W. A. Haseltine, *Science* **225**, 381 (1984).
21. M. Seiki, R. Eddy, T. B. Shows, M. Yoshida, *Nature (London)* **309**, 640 (1984).
22. J. Gasson, personal communication.
23. A. J. Berk and P. A. Sharp, *Cell* **12**, 721 (1977).
24. R. Weaver and C. Weissman, *Nucleic Acids Res.* **7**, 1175 (1979).
25. H. Lehrach, D. Diamond, J. M. Wozney, H. Boedtker, *Biochemistry* **16**, 4743 (1977).
26. A. M. Maxam and W. Gilbert, *Proc. Natl. Acad. Sci. U.S.A.* **74**, 560 (1977).
27. We thank J. Gasson, R. Gaynor, and D. Slamon for useful discussions and J. Fujii, J. McLaughlin, C. Nishikubo, and S. Quan for technical assistance. Supported by NCI grants CA 30388, CA 32737, CA 09297, and CA 16042 and by grants PF-2182 and JFRA-99 from the American Cancer Society. W.W. is a Bank of America–Giannini Foundation fellow.

4 September 1984; accepted 11 September 1984

Report

26 October 1984

58.   HTLV-III in Saliva of People with AIDS-Related Complex and Healthy Homosexual Men at Risk for AIDS

Jerome E. Groopman, S. Zaki Salahuddin, M.G. Sarngadharan, Phillip D. Markham, Matthew Gonda, Ann Sliski, and Robert C. Gallo

The acquired immune deficiency syndrome (AIDS) is a transmissible disorder of the cellular immune system resulting in frequently fatal opportunistic infections or neoplasms (*1*). The groups at high risk for AIDS include homosexual or bisexual men and their partners, hemophiliacs, Haitians, Central Africans, and intravenous drug abusers (*2*). In addition, children of high-risk mothers and recipients of random blood products have developed AIDS (*3*). Epidemiological studies indicate that AIDS may be transmitted by an agent in blood and possibly other body fluids. Public health recommendations designed to limit the spread of the AIDS epidemic need to be based on data showing the presence or absence of the agent in each body fluid or excretion (*4*).

A primary pathogenic role for HTLV-III in AIDS and in the AIDS-related complex (ARC) has been demonstrated (*5*). HTLV-III is cytopathic for T4 helper-inducer lymphocytes (this population of cells decreases in function and in absolute number as the disease progresses), and has been isolated from peripheral blood lymphocytes of approximately 50 percent of AIDS patients and 80 percent of ARC patients (*5, 6*). In addition, 90 to 100 percent of AIDS and ARC patients have antibody to the 41,000-dalton HTLV-III antigen (*7*). HTLV-III appears to be serologically closely related to the virus named LAV that was independently isolated from AIDS and pre-AIDS patients in France (*8*). Although LAV was less frequently serologically associated with AIDS in earlier studies (*9*), recent data from Kalyanaraman *et al.* (*10*) indicate that 70 to 95 percent of AIDS and ARC patients are positive for LAV antibodies by an enzyme-linked immunosorbent assay (ELISA). Here we report a study of peripheral blood mononuclear cells and saliva from four patients with AIDS, ten patients with ARC, and six healthy asymptomatic homosexual males at risk for AIDS.

Samples of serum, heparinized peripheral blood, and saliva were obtained from the 20 individuals. The serum samples were tested for antibody to HTLV-III by means of ELISA with whole disrupted virus and by a more sensitive Western electroblot technique (*7, 11*). Mononuclear cells were obtained from heparinized peripheral blood banded in Ficoll-Hypaque, and cell cultures were initiated in complete medium supple-

Table 1. Detection and isolation of HTLV-III from peripheral blood cells or saliva. Heparinized peripheral blood was obtained by venipuncture, and mononuclear cells were isolated by Ficoll-Hypaque density gradient centrifugation and cultured with interleukin-2 as described (*13*). Saliva was obtained at the time of venipuncture, diluted to a final volume of 2 ml in complete growth medium, and incubated for 2 hours at 37°C. It was then filtered through a 0.45-μm filter (Millipore) and added to cultures of interleukin-2–stimulated peripheral blood mononuclear cells. Seropositivity for antibody to HTLV-III was determined by means of ELISA with whole disrupted virus and the Western electroblot technique as previously described (*7, 11*). HTLV-III was identified by assay for reverse transcriptase, electron microscopy, and specific antisera to viral proteins (*14*); PBL, peripheral blood lymphocytes.

Patient or donor	Diagnosis*	Antibody to HTLV-III†		Isolation of HTLV-III	
		ELISA	Western	PBL	Saliva
1	AIDS-KS	+/−	+	−	−
2	AIDS-KS	+/−	+	−	−
3	AIDS-KS	+/−	+	+	−
4	AIDS-OI	+	ND	−	−
5	ARC	+	ND	−	+
6	ARC	+/−	+	−	+
7	ARC	+	ND	−	−
8	ARC	+/−	+	+	+
9	ARC	+/−	+	+	−
10	ARC	+	ND	−	+
11	ARC	+/−	+	−	−
12	ARC	+/−	+	−	−
13	ARC	−	+	+	−
14	ARC	+	ND	+	−
15	HHM	+	ND	+	+
16	HHM	+	ND	−	+
17	HHM	+	ND	+	+
18	HHM	+	ND	−	+
19	HHM	−	−	−	−
20	HHM	−	−	−	−

*KS, Kaposi's sarcoma; OI, opportunistic infection; HHM, healthy homosexual male.　†Symbols: +, present; −, absent; ND, not done; +/−, equivocal result.

312

mented with T-cell growth factor (inter-leukin-2). HTLV-III production was monitored as previously described (5). Saliva samples were diluted to a final volume of 2 ml in complete growth medium, incubated for 2 hours at 37°C, and centrifuged at 1000g for 10 minutes at 4°C. Pelleted materials were fixed for electron microscopy and supernatant fluids were filtered (0.45 μm) and used for transmitting virus to fresh peripheral blood lymphocytes (5). HTLV-III production by infected cells was monitored by means of assays for reverse transcriptase (RT), by electron microscopic observation, and by immunofluores-cence and competition radioimmunoassays with the use of HTLV-III–specific antisera.

As shown in Table 1, all of the AIDS and ARC patients and four of the six healthy homosexuals were positive for antibody to HTLV-III structural proteins. HTLV-III was isolated from the peripheral blood cells of seven of the 18 subjects who were positive for HTLV-III antibody but from neither of the two seronegative healthy homosexuals. Virus was also isolated from the saliva of eight of the 18 individuals who were seropositive for HTLV-III–specific antibodies. As shown in Fig. 1, virus was observed in leukocytes pelleted directly from the saliva of one ARC patient. Cells infected by virus from saliva were tested for the presence of HTLV-III proteins by a homologous competition radioimmunoassay (Fig. 2). The competition patterns thus obtained demonstrated the identity of this virus with HTLV-III.

The inability to recover virus from some seropositive individuals, as noted here and elsewhere (5), may indicate prior exposure to viral antigens without infection or lack of current viremia due to restrictions on HTLV-III replication. Alternatively, HTLV-III may occur in a reservoir other than saliva or peripheral blood lymphocytes in certain persons or at a certain stage of the disease.

Studies of the biological activity of HTLV-III and its role in AIDS and associated clinical disorders have just begun. Transmission of two members of the HTLV family involved in the development of T-cell leukemias and lymphomas, that is, HTLV-I and HTLV-II, usually requires cocultivation procedures, indicating that these viruses are highly cell-associated. HTLV-III, in contrast, is efficiently transmitted by cell-free vi-

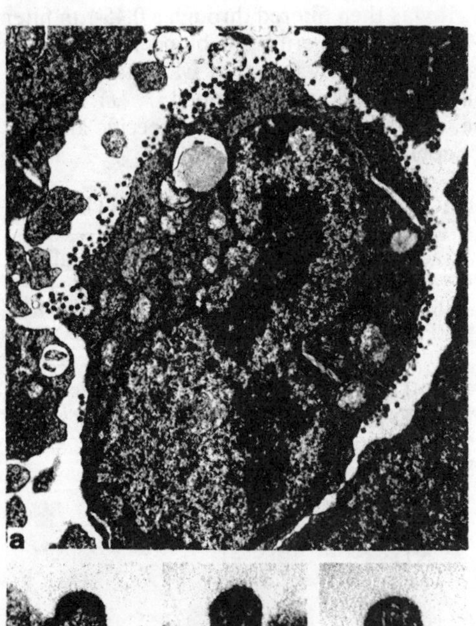

Fig. 1. Transmission electron micrograph of fixed cells obtained from the saliva of patient No. 8. Procedures for preparation of saliva are described in the legends to Table 1. (a) Leukocyte-expressing HTLV-III (×10,000). (b) Budding virus (×150,000). (c) Mature virus particles (×150,000).

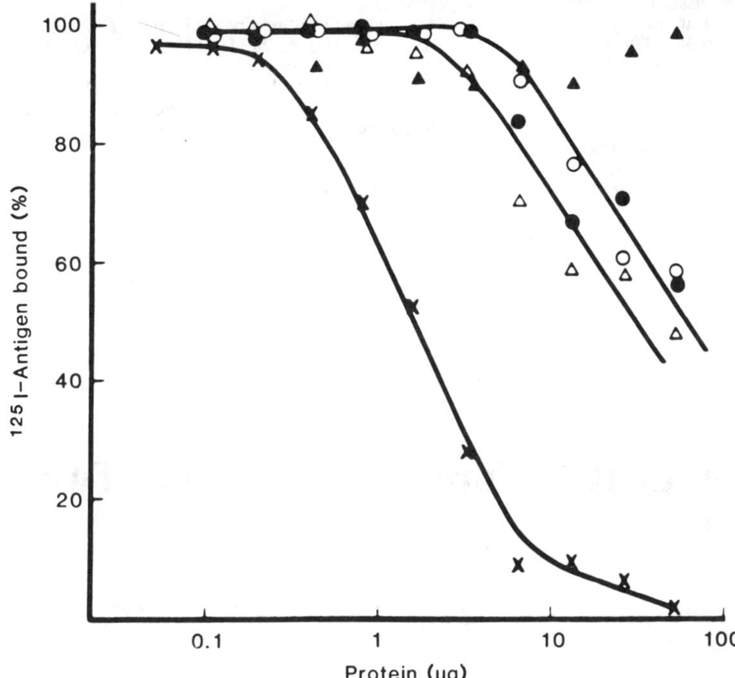

Fig. 2. Homologous competition radioimmunoassay of lysates of cells infected by virus from saliva. The indicated concentrations of disrupted cell proteins were used to compete with the precipitation of ^{125}I-labeled p24 of HTLV-III by antibody to this virus. Cell lysates from: x, H9 cells producing HTLV-III; ▲, H9 control cells; ●, ARC patient No. 8; ○, ARC patient No. 10; and △, HHM healthy homosexual male donor No. 16.

rus making it feasible to study its distribution in body fluids. Studies of feline leukemia viruses, which are associated with both a T-cell leukemia and a profound immunodeficiency, indicate that cell-free fluids, specifically saliva, contain infectious virus (*12*). The mechanism of virus survival in saliva has not been determined either in cats or in the HTLV-III–positive patients. However, cells producing virus (Fig. 1), as well as cell-free virus, were observed in the saliva of the patients described here.

These data should be taken into account in designing recommendations to limit the spread of AIDS. The recovery of HTLV-III from saliva suggests that direct contact with this body fluid should be avoided since saliva may form a protective matrix to support cell-free virus or virus-positive cells and could facilitate horizontal transmission.

References and Notes

1. Centers for Disease Control Task Force of Kaposi's Sarcoma and Opportunistic Infections, *N. Engl. J. Med.* **306**, 248 (1982).
2. M. Gottlieb *et al.*, *ibid.* **305**, 1425 (1981); H. Masur *et al.*, *ibid.*, p. 1431; F. P. Siegal, C. Lopez, G. S. Hammer, *ibid.*, p. 1439; H. B. Hymes *et al.*, *Lancet* **1982-II**, 598 (1982); J. Groopman and P. Volberding *Nature (London)* **307**, 211 (1984); A. S. Fauci *et al.*, *Ann. Intern. Med.* **100**, 92 (1984); M. Gottlieb *et al.*, *ibid.* **99**, 208 (1983); J. Pape *et al.*, *N. Engl. J. Med.* **309**, 945 (1983); J. Vieira *et al.*, *ibid.* **308**, 125 (1983); A. E. Pitchenik *et al.*, *Ann. Intern. Med.* **98**, 277 (1983); N. Blumeck *et al.*, *N. Engl. J. Med.* **310**, 492 (1984).
3. J. W. Curran *et al.*, *N. Engl. J. Med.* **310**, 69 (1984); H. W. Jaffe *et al.*, *Science* **223**, 1309 (1984); J. Oleske *et al.*, *J. Am. Med. Assoc.* **249**, 2345 (1983).
4. H. W. Jaffe *et al.*, *Ann. Intern. Med.* **99**, 145 (1983).
5. M. Popovic, M. G. Sarngadharan, E. Read, R. C. Gallo, *Science* **224**, 497 (1984); R. C. Gallo *et al.*, *ibid.*, p. 500.
6. R. Redfield *et al.*, *N. Engl. J. Med.*, in preparation. ARC has also been termed pre-AIDS, AIDS syndrome, and lymphadenopathy syndrome.
7. J. Schüpbach *et al.*, *Science* **224**, 503 (1984); M. G. Sarngadharan *et al.*, *ibid.*, p. 506.
8. F. Barré-Sinoussi *et al.*, *Science* **220**, 868 (1983).
9. J. C. Montagnier *et al.*, in *Human T-Cell Leuke-*

mia Viruses, R. C. Gallo, M. Essex, L. Gross, Eds. (Cold Spring Harbor Laboratory, Cold Spring Harbor, N.Y., 1984), p 363–379.
10. V. S. Kalyanaraman *et al.*, *Science* **225**, 321 (1984).
11. B. Safai *et al.*, *Lancet* **1984-I**, 1438 (1984).
12. D. P. Francis, M. Essex, W. D. Hardy, *Nature (London)* **269**, 252 (1977); D. P. Francis *et al.*, *J. Clin. Microbiol.* **9**, 154 (1979).
13. P. D. Markham *et al.*, *Int. J. Cancer* **33**, 13 (1984).
14. H. Towbin, T. Staehlin, J. Gordon, *Proc. Natl. Acad. Sci. U.S.A.* **76**, 4350 (1979); M. G. Sarngadharan *et al.*, in preparation.
15. J.E.G. is supported in part by a grant (JFRA 44) from the American Cancer Society. M.G. is supported by PHS contract NOI-CO-23910.

4 September 1984; accepted 21 September 1984

Report

26 October 1984

59. HTLV-III in Cells Cultured from Semen of Two Patients wth AIDS

D. Zagury, J. Bernard, J. Leibowitch, B. Safai, J.E. Groopman, M. Feldman, M.G. Sarngadharan, and R.C. Gallo

Several findings indicate that the primary cause of the acquired immune deficiency syndrome (AIDS) is an infection with the human T-cell leukemia (lymphotropic) virus type III (HTLV-III) (*1–5*). Almost all patients with AIDS and related conditions have detectable specific serum antibodies to a member or members of this retrovirus family (*4–6*), and 48 isolates of HTLV-III were reported in one study (*3*). More than 95 isolates of HTLV-III have since been obtained (*7*). Epidemiological data indicate that transmission of the AIDS agent is through blood or blood products (*8*) or through intimate contact between homosexual males (*9*) or between heterosexual females and their male partners that have been exposed to the agent (*10*). Such data, obtained mostly from surveys of populations at risk within the United States, together with the observed lymphotropism of the causative virus, led us to suspect that lymphocytes infected with HTLV-III might be found in the semen of AIDS patients. In the study reported here we attempted to answer the following question: Can the lymphocytes from the seminal fluid of AIDS patients be grown in vitro and, if so, can HTLV-III be detected in and isolated from these cells?

Semen was obtained from two patients with AIDS and stored frozen in 10 percent dimethyl sulfoxide in liquid nitrogen. Both patients had disseminated Kaposi's sarcoma, low numbers of circulating T4 lymphocytes, and reversed T4/T8 ratios (0.5 and 0.2, respectively). Semen was also obtained from three healthy heterosexual males. The semen was collected under sterile conditions, thawed at 37°C, and subjected to low-speed centrifugation. Cell pellets were resuspended in RPMI 1640 medium containing 10 percent fetal calf serum. After thawing, a mononuclear cell–enriched fraction was isolated over Ficoll-Hypaque (Seromed, München, FRG). The number of cells obtained in this manner varied from 0.8×10^5 to 3×10^5 per milliliter in the semen of normal donors. The mononuclear cell–enriched fractions from AIDS patients 1 and 2 yielded 0.06×10^5 and 0.9×10^5 cells per milliliter, respectively. These fractions contained 70 percent of adherent macrophage-monocytes and 20 to 30 percent lymphocytes and residual spermatozoa (Fig. 1). The lymphocytes from the normal individuals consisted of 17 percent $T4^+$ cells (OKT4), 30 percent $T8^+$ cells (OKT8) and 14 percent mature B cells (OKB7). The lymphocytes in the AIDS patients consisted of 20 to 50 percent $T4^+$ cells and 2 to 18 percent $T8^+$ cells. The nonproliferating, uncultured semen mononuclear cells from the healthy donors and the two AIDS patients did not express HTLV-III antigens by fixed-cell indirect immunofluorescence with the use of either rabbit polyclonal antiserum to HTLV-III (2) or murine monoclonal antibody to the p15 and p24 proteins of HTLV-III (Table 1).

Portions (10^3) of mononuclear cells from the semen of the AIDS patients and the normal donors were seeded in 200 μl round-bottom wells (Nunk) containing culture medium. Cells were activated by phytohemagglutinin (0.1 percent; Gibco) for 24 hours and cultured in the presence of semipurified lectin-free T-cell growth factor interleukin-2 (IL-2) and a feeder layer containing 1.5×10^5 irradiated (4000 rad) lymphoid cells as described (11).

Proliferating cultures, monitored by inverted microscopy, were transferred and seeded at 3×10^5 to 4×10^5 cells per milliliter in round-bottom tubes (Falcon) containing 1.5 ml of culture medium and 10 percent IL-2. These cells prolifer-

ated only in the presence of IL-2; they were subcultured periodically and growth was maintained for at least 6 weeks under these conditions.

These cultured cells were tested for HTLV-III antigens by fixed-cell indirect immunofluorescence with the use of rabbit antiserum to HTLV-III. By day 6 a few HTLV-III–positive cells were detectable in cultures from the two AIDS patients. However, the positive reaction was transient; it was not observed on cells cultured 12 days or longer. No positive cells were observed at any time in cultures derived from the semen of the three normal individuals.

Cells cultured from the semen of the AIDS patients were cocultivated with clone H9, an HTLV-III permissive T-cell line derived from a parental human leukemic T-cell line (2). Cocultivation was initiated after the primary semen mononuclear cells had been cultured for 6 days, at which time HTLV-III–positive cells were present. The medium containing IL-2 was then replaced by normal culture medium containing 0.5 percent sheep antiserum to human α-interferon (α-IFN) (neutralizing titer, 6 IU at 10^{-5} dilution), and 1.5×10^4 H9 cells were added per 200-μl well. The cocultures, H9/AIDS, were transferred after 48 hours to 2-ml round-bottom tubes and seeded at a concentration of 3×10^5 cells per milliliter in culture medium containing antiserum to α-IFN. The cultures were subcultured when the population reached a concentration of 10^6 cells per milliliter.

Ten days after the initiation of cocultivation the cell population was examined by light microscopy and the cells were tested for various immunological markers. The results were compared with those obtained with the reference H9 and H9/HTLV-III cell lines (2, 3). We observed a number of large cells (12 to 20

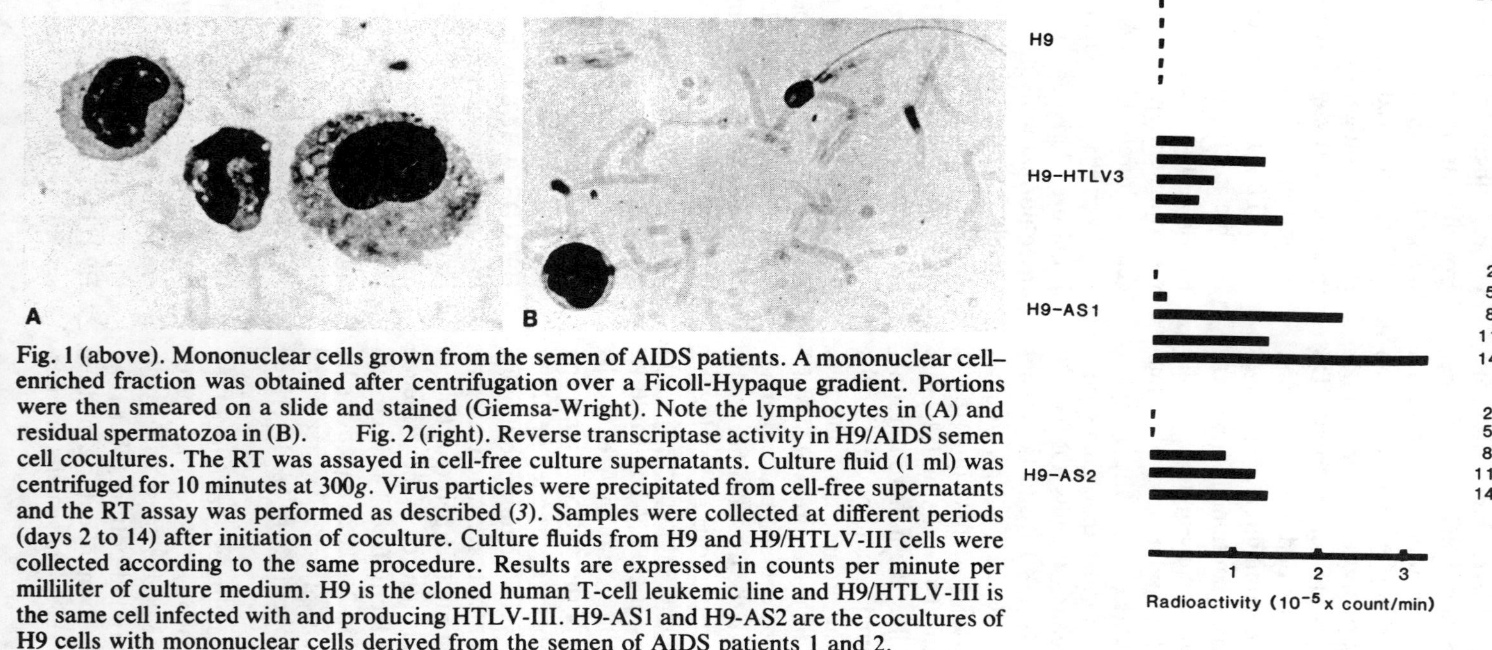

Fig. 1 (above). Mononuclear cells grown from the semen of AIDS patients. A mononuclear cell–enriched fraction was obtained after centrifugation over a Ficoll-Hypaque gradient. Portions were then smeared on a slide and stained (Giemsa-Wright). Note the lymphocytes in (A) and residual spermatozoa in (B).   Fig. 2 (right). Reverse transcriptase activity in H9/AIDS semen cell cocultures. The RT was assayed in cell-free culture supernatants. Culture fluid (1 ml) was centrifuged for 10 minutes at 300g. Virus particles were precipitated from cell-free supernatants and the RT assay was performed as described (3). Samples were collected at different periods (days 2 to 14) after initiation of coculture. Culture fluids from H9 and H9/HTLV-III cells were collected according to the same procedure. Results are expressed in counts per minute per milliliter of culture medium. H9 is the cloned human T-cell leukemic line and H9/HTLV-III is the same cell infected with and producing HTLV-III. H9-AS1 and H9-AS2 are the cocultures of H9 cells with mononuclear cells derived from the semen of AIDS patients 1 and 2.

Table 1. HTLV-III Antigens in H9/AIDS semen cocultures. The presence of HTLV-III antigens was assayed by fixed-cell indirect immunofluorescence as described (*3*). In brief, cells of the H9 clone were cocultured with mononuclear cells derived from semen of AIDS patients (H9/AIDS) previously cultured for 15 days and from the reference (control) H9 and H9/HTLV-III lines. They were then spotted on a slide, dried, and fixed in acetone for 10 minutes at room temperature. Twenty microliters of either rabbit polyclonal antiserum to HTLV-III (diluted 1:2000 in phosphate-buffered saline) or murine monoclonal antibody to p15 (1:100) or to p24 (1:100) was applied and the cells were incubated for 50 minutes at 37°C (*16*). After three washes the fluorescein-conjugated antiserum (1:100) was applied and the cells were incubated for 30 minutes at room temperature. Technical controls consisted of (i) spots treated with rabbit serum or with a murine monoclonal antibody to immunoglobulin in place of the specific antibodies and (ii) spots treated only with the fluorescein conjugate. No fluorescence was detected in these control samples.

| | Cells positive (%)* | | | |
Antibody reagent	H9/ AIDS semen 1	H9/ AIDS semen 2	H9	H9/ HTLV-III
Rabbit polyclonal antiserum to disrupted HTLV-III	20	22	0	42
Monoclonal antibody to HTLV-III p15 (*14*)	20	26	0	75
Monoclonal antibody to HTLV-III p24 (*14*)	30	40	0	90

*Percentage of positive cells. This number represents the mean percentage found on three samples.

μm in diameter) with basophilic cytoplasm surrounding a large Golgi region and containing an indented nucleus; giant multinucleated syncytial cells; and numerous cells in mitosis. This morphological pattern is very similar to that seen with the reference H9/HTLV-III cell line, and all three types of cultured cells (the coculture, the H9/HTLV-III reference line, and the uninfected H9 reference line) showed a similar lymphocytic phenotype. No cells expressed T4 or T8 antigens in the cocultures. Thirty-five to 45 percent of the cells expressed HLA-DR antigen (OKI$_2$). The uninfected H9 cell cultures differed by showing less cellular degeneration and fewer multinucleated cells.

Cocultures were monitored for reverse transcriptase (RT) activity. Such activity was detectable as of day 8 of the coculture (Fig. 2). In contrast, RT activity was not detectable in long-term cultures (12 to 40 days) of semen T cells (not shown). Furthermore, 20 to 40 percent of the cells from 15-day-old cocultures expressed HTLV-III antigens (Table 1 and Fig. 3). Cell samples from the cocultures were also examined by electron microscopy. Retrovirus particles were observed at the surface of some cells (Fig. 4).

This study shows that semen from normal individuals and from patients with AIDS contains a number of mononuclear cells that proliferate at low cell densities in vitro in the presence of IL-2 and a feeder cell layer. We found that some cells from semen derived from the two AIDS patients contained HTLV-III that replicated in the culture system. However, expression was transient. Semen cell cultures older than 12 days contained neither HTLV-III antigens nor RT activity. In previous studies, long-

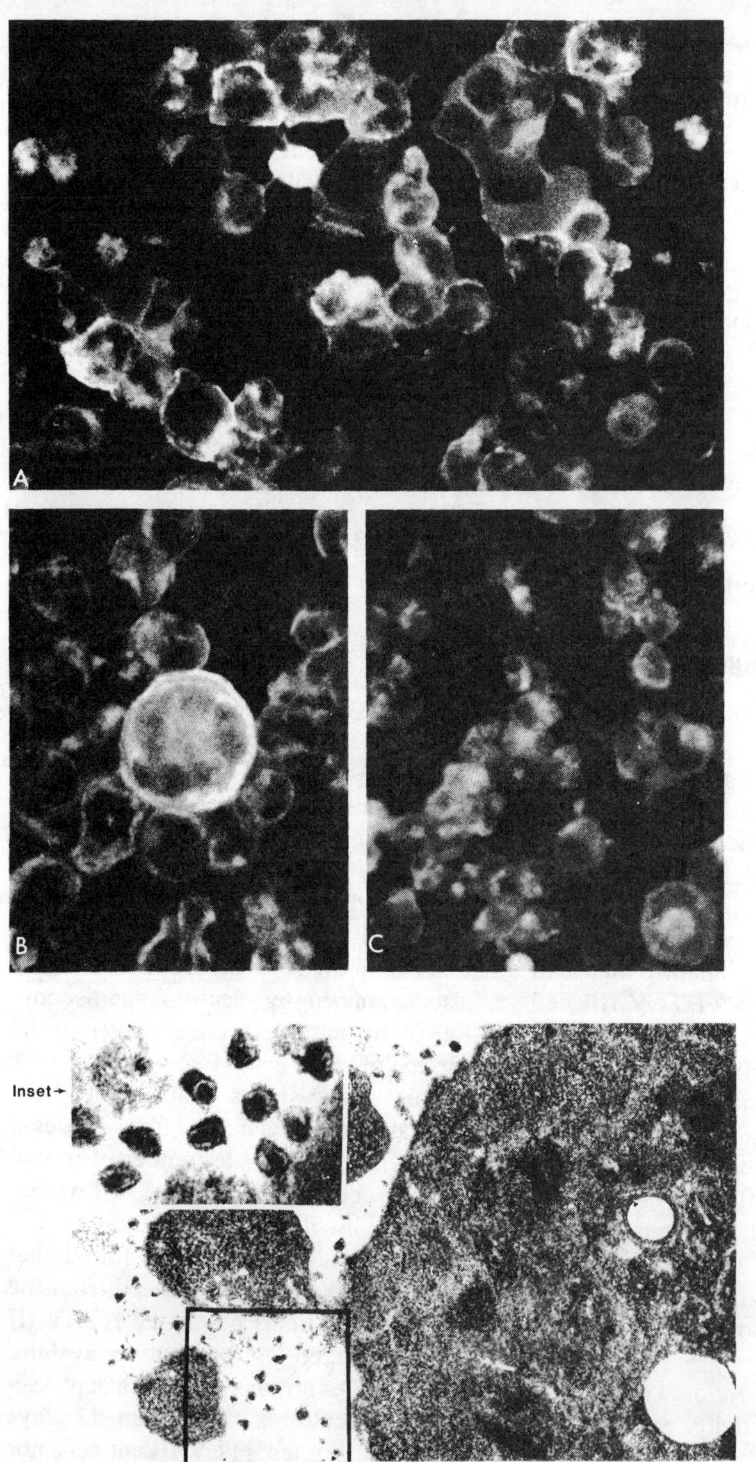

Fig. 3 (top). Detection of HTLV-III antigens by fixed-cell indirect immunofluorescence. Cells were treated as described in Table 1. (A and B) Cells from H9/AIDS semen coculture. (C) Cells from H9. Note the fluorescence localized on the surface of cells in (A) and (B). In (C) the cells are all negative. Fig. 4 (bottom). Retrovirus particles observed by electron microscopy at the surface of a cell from a 15-day-old H9/AIDS semen cell coculture. The cell preparation was fixed in glutaraldehyde-osmium and embedded in Epon. Ultrathin sections were prepared, mounted in grids, and stained with uranyl acetate lead citrate. Magnification: ×10,000; inset in upper left corner, ×76,000.

term cultures derived from blood, bone marrow, or lymph node cells from AIDS patients were also frequently negative for HTLV-III (3). When the semen mononuclear cells from the primary short-term cultures were cocultured with H9, definitive results were obtained because of transmission and amplification of the virus. That the virus isolated belongs to the HTLV-III subgroup is indicated by its morphology (Fig. 4) and, more important, by the positive results with HTLV-III specific antisera (12). Thus, these results are consistent with the epidemiological data implicating semen as a source of the AIDS etiological agent (9, 10) and with results (2–5, 8–10, 12–15) indicating that HTLV-III is the agent.

References and Notes

1. F. Barré-Sinoussi *et al.*, *Science* **220**, 868 (1983).
2. M. Popovic, M. G. Sarngadharan, E. Read, R. C. Gallo, *ibid.* **224**, 497 (1984).
3. R. C. Gallo *et al.*, *ibid.*, p. 500.
4. M. G. Sarngadharan *et al.*, *ibid.*, p. 506.
5. B. Safai *et al.*, *Lancet* **1984-I**, 1438 (1984).
6. V. S. Kalyanaraman *et al.*, *Science* **225**, 321 (1984).
7. S. Z. Salahuddin, P. Markham, M. Popovic, R. Gallo, in preparation.
8. J. W. Curran *et al.*, *N. Engl. J. Med.* **310**, 69 (1984); J. Groopman *et al.*, in preparation.
9. J. Goedert *et al.*, *Lancet*, in press; H. W. Jaffe *et al.*, *Ann. Intern. Med.* **99** 145 (1983).
10. J. Groopman *et al.*, in preparation.
11. D. Zagury *et al.*, *J. Immunol. Methods* **43**, 67 (1981).
12. J. Schüpbach *et al.*, *Science* **224**, 503 (1984).
13. S. Broder and R. C. Gallo, *N. Engl. J. Med.*, in press.
14. D. Mathez *et al.*, *Lancet*, in press.
15. M. G. Sarngadharan, L. Bruch, M. Popovic, R. C. Gallo, in preparation.
16. The rabbit polyclonal antiserum has been described (*15*). The monoclonal antibodies to p15 (BT2) and p24 (BT3) were provided by M. G. Sarngadharan [see (*17*)].
17. F. Veronese *et al.*, in preparation.
18. We acknowledge the contributions of Professor Chany, Dr. Lebon, and Mme. Robert (Hôpital Saint Vincent de Paul, Paris) for their help in performing RT assays and providing goat antiserum to human α-IFN. We also thank Professor Caulet and Dr. Tessier (Riems) for providing normal semen from volunteers. This work was supported in part by grants from ARC-Villejuif; Ligue Nationale Contre le Cancer; DRET and Institut Jean Godinot.

4 September 1984; accepted 21 September 1984

Report

26 October 1984

60. HTLV-III in the Semen and Blood of a Healthy Homosexual Man

David D. Ho, Robert T. Schooley, Teresa R. Rota, Joan C. Kaplan, Theresa Flynn, Syed Z. Salahuddin, Matthew A. Gonda, and Martin S. Hirsch

The acquired immune deficiency syndrome (AIDS) was first recognized in 1981 as a generally fatal disorder of cell-mediated immunity manifested clinically by opportunistic infections or Kaposi's sarcoma (*1–3*). More than 6000 cases of AIDS have been reported to the Centers for Disease Control to date. Epidemiologic data in male homosexuals (*4, 5*) and female sexual partners of men with the syndrome (*6*) suggest that the disease can be transmitted sexually, possibly through contact with semen. Recently, a novel retrovirus, the human T-lymphotropic virus type III (HTLV-III), has been shown to be the likely etiologic agent for AIDS (*7, 8*). The lymphadenopathy-associated virus (LAV), initially isolated in France (*9*), appears to be closely related or identical to HTLV-III (*10*). Both viruses are now frequently isolated from blood of persons with AIDS or the AIDS-related complex (ARC) (*11*). Here we report the isolation of HTLV-III from semen of a healthy homosexual man who is seropositive for HTLV-III.

The subject, a 30-year-old homosexual male, has been evaluated at the Massachusetts General Hospital every 3 months since June 1983 as a participant in a prospective study of homosexual men with or without AIDS. His past medical history includes gonorrhea, hepatitis, and sexual contacts in 1982 with a man who subsequently developed Kaposi's sarcoma. However, he has shown no constitutional or localized signs or symptoms of AIDS. His peripheral blood leukocyte counts, lymphocyte proliferative responses to concanavalin A, and allogeneic cytotoxicity responses have been consistently normal. The subject's T helper/T suppressor (T4/T8) ratios have ranged from 1.0 to 2.4 (normal 1.7 ± 0.5) on five serial determinations. Four semen and four urine cultures for cytomegalovirus (CMV) have been negative. Serologically he is antibody positive for CMV (1:32 by complement fixation) and for Epstein-Barr viral capsid antigen (1:320) and nuclear antigen (1:80), and is negative for HTLV-I membrane antigen by an indirect immunofluorescence technique (*12*).

Tests for antibodies to HTLV-III were performed on five serum samples obtained from our study participant between June 1983 and August 1984. Approximately 1×10^4 H9 cells (*13*) infected with HTLV-III were placed in each 12-mm^2 well on glass slides. After fixation with acetone, 15 μl of a 1:10 dilution of serum were added to each well for 30 minutes. The samples were washed three times in phosphate-buffered saline (PBS), 15 μl of fluorescein-conjugated goat antibody to human immunoglobulin (Electronucleonics) was added for another 30 minutes, and the samples were again washed three times in PBS before being examined under ultraviolet light. Appropriate positive and negative control sera were included in each assay. All five serum samples were positive for antibodies to HTLV-III, with over 80 percent of the cells showing fluorescence.

In August 1984, semen and blood were obtained from the subject for virus isolation. The semen sample (3 ml) was immediately diluted 1:10 in RPMI 1640 medium with 20 percent fetal calf serum (FCS) in order to lessen the semen's toxic effect on cells. Ficoll-Hypaque (density of 1.078 g/ml) separation was then performed on the diluted semen preparation, which yielded 1.3×10^6 viable mononuclear cells. This low cell count prohibited adequate phenotypic analysis. However, the cells were heterogeneous with approximately 30 percent resembling lymphocytes. After treatment with phytohemagglutinin-P (PHA-P, 10 μg/ml; Sigma), the mononuclear cells were cultured in RPMI 1640 medium with 20 percent FCS and 10 percent interleukin-2 (Electronucleonics). No cellular proliferation was seen by day 2 of culture. Therefore, after treatment with Polybrene (Sigma; 2 μg/ml) the mononuclear cells were cocultivated with 3 × 10⁶ H9 cells, a mature T-cell clone derived from an adult with lymphoid leukemia (*13*).

This cocultivation culture was examined every 2 to 3 days for cytopathic effects (CPE). On day 11 of culture, a few of the H9 cells were noted to be enlarged, "ballooned," and multinucleated. The changes were similar to those described by Popovic *et al.* for H9 cells infected with HTLV-III (*13*). Fixed-cell indirect immunofluorescence tests with a known HTLV-III–positive serum from another homosexual man demonstrated HTLV-III antigens in approximately 1 percent of the H9 cells (Fig. 1A). By day 15, the CPE and positive immunofluorescence were observed in 25 percent of the cells in culture. These progressed to 75 percent by day 19 (Table 1). We subsequently obtained murine monoclonal antibodies to the HTLV-III core proteins p15 and p24 (*14*). Tests with these antibodies in similar fixed-cell indirect immunofluorescence preparations were also positive (Table 1). The affected H9 cells were negative for antigens of Epstein-Barr virus (EBV) and cytomegalovirus and for p19 and p24 of HTLV-I by indirect immunofluorescence. Assays for reverse transcriptase (RT) activity were done as described (*13, 15*). Serial culture supernatant fluids were positive for RT activity beginning on day 11 (Table 1). In addition, on day 15, transmission electron microscopy showed many budding and mature viral particles consistent with HTLV-III (Fig. 1B).

Peripheral blood mononuclear cells (PBMC) were obtained by centrifugation

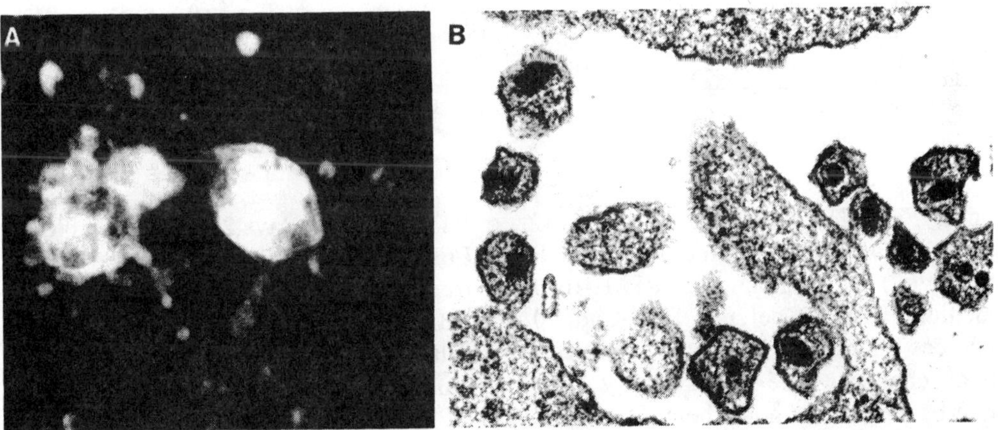

Fig. 1. (A) Multinucleated H9 cells showing positive immunofluorescence for HTLV-III antigens. H9 cells, cocultivated with mononuclear cells from the subject's semen, were placed on glass slides and fixed with acetone. The test serum was antibody positive for HTLV-III by an enzyme-linked immunosorbent assay (ELISA) and Western blot (*8*) but negative for HTLV-I by membrane immunofluorescence (*12*). Fifteen microliters of a 1:64 dilution of this serum were added to each well for 30 minutes. After three successive washes in PBS, 15 μl of a fluorescein conjugated goat antiserum to human immunoglobulin was added for an additional 30 minutes. The slides were then washed, dried, mounted, and examined with ultraviolet light (×500). (B) Transmission electron micrograph showing viral particles (×45,000).

Table 1. Detection of HTLV-III in semen and blood. Indirect immunofluorescence tests were performed with monoclonal antibodies against HTLV-III p15 and p24 antigens. Techniques were described in the legend to Fig. 1, except that the monoclonal antibodies were used at 1:200 dilutions and we used rabbit antiserum to mouse Fab_2-fluorescein isothiocyanate conjugate (1:40; Cappel). Before being assayed for RT, virus particles were precipitated from 5 ml of culture fluid by the addition of 2.5 ml of a solution containing 30 percent (w/v) polyethylene glycol (Fisher Carbowax 8000) in $0.4M$ NaCl. The suspension was placed at 0°C overnight and then centrifuged at 2100 rev/min at 4°C for 45 minutes. The precipitate was resuspended in 300 μl of 50 percent glycerol, 25 mM tris-HCl, pH 7.5, 5 mM dithiothreitol, 150 mM KCl, and 0.025 percent Triton-X 100. Virus particles were disrupted by the addition of 0.9 percent Triton-X 100 and $1.5M$ KCl (100 μl). The RT activity was assayed as described (*13, 15*) with the use of poly(rA)-oligo(dT)$_{12-18}$ (2.5 μg/ml, P-L Biochemicals). Results are expressed as counts per minute of methyl-[^{3}H]deoxythymidine triphosphate (16 to 18 Ci/mmol; New England Nuclear) incorporated per milliliter of culture fluid; NT, not tested.

Test	Days					
	5	11	15	19	25	29
H9-semen mononuclear cell cocultivation						
Cytopathic effects	−	+	+	+	+	+
Immunofluorescence (percent positive)						
Human serum positive for HTLV-III	0	1	25	75	90	90
Monoclonal antibodies to HTLV-III p15 and p24	0	0	N.T.	90	90	90
Reverse transcriptase activity (10^5 cpm/ml)	0	0.2	8	52	32	40
Peripheral blood mononuclear cell culture						
Immunofluorescence (percent positive)						
Monoclonal antibodies to HTLV-III p15 and p24	0	0	N.T.	0	5	5
Reverse transcriptase activity (10^4 cpm/ml)	N.T.	N.T.	0	0	1.0	0.8*

*Result from day 33.

on a Ficoll-Hypaque gradient. PBMC (5×10^6) were then treated with PHA-P (10 μg/ml) and maintained on RPMI-1640 medium with 20 percent FCS and 10 percent interleukin-2. No abnormal cellular changes were observed by light microscopy throughout the culture period. However, after day 25, PBMC expressed HTLV-III antigens as detected by indirect immunofluorescence with a human serum positive for HTLV-III or with monoclonal antibodies to HTLV-III p15 and p24 (Table 1), but they were consistently negative for EBV, CMV, and HTLV-I antigens. The corresponding supernatant fluids showed significant RT activity on days 25 and 29 (Table 1). Furthermore, on day 12, addition of cell-free supernatant fluid (2 ml) from the PBMC culture to Polybrene-treated H9 cells (3×10^6) resulted in characteristic morphologic changes 14 days later. The CPE were similar to those induced by the mononuclear cells from the subject's semen described above. These H9 cells also become positive for HTLV-III antigens, and their supernatant fluids showed RT activity (0.4×10^5 to 4.8×10^5 cpm/ml).

That our isolates are HTLV-III is indicated by their (i) antigen expression, (ii) RT characteristics, (iii) morphology on electron microscopy, and (iv) ability to induce unique CPE in H9 cells (*7, 13*). That the isolates are not HTLV-I or HTLV-II is shown by the positive staining obtained with the HTLV-III–specific monoclonal antibodies (*14*) and the negative results with the HTLV-I–specific monoclonal antibodies.

HTLV-III was recovered from the mononuclear-cell fraction of semen. Attempts to find virus in the spermatozoa fraction of semen from 11 individuals have yielded negative results. Because of the toxic effects of semen on target cells used for these isolations, it is unclear whether there is also cell-free HTLV-III in seminal plasma. The coexistence of other viruses in semen, such as CMV (*16, 17*), may also interfere with the successful cultivation of HTLV-III.

The demonstration of HTLV-III in the semen of an asymptomatic individual who is at risk for AIDS supports epidemiologic data suggesting that AIDS can be sexually transmitted. It is unknown why one HTLV-III carrier remains well while another develops AIDS. Asymptomatic carriers should be closely followed for the possible development of AIDS. Recent surveys suggest that the prevalence of HTLV-III/LAV seropositivity in urban male homosexuals may be as high as 65 percent (*18*). Most of these men are healthy and without obvious immune deficits. The frequency of HTLV-III carriers in this population is unknown. These issues need to be addressed by careful prospective analyses of asymptomatic HTLV-III seropositive individuals.

References and Notes

1. M. S. Gottlieb *et al.*, *Morbid. Mortal. Weekly Rep.* **30**, 250 (1981).
2. ______, *N. Engl. J. Med.* **305**, 1425 (1981).
3. A. E. Friedman-Kien *et al.*, *Ann. Intern. Med.* **96**, 693 (1982).
4. H. W. Jaffe *et al.*, *Ann. Intern. Med.* **99**, 145 (1983).
5. D. M. Auerbach, W. M. Darrow, H. W. Jaffe, J. W. Curran, *Am. J. Med.* **76**, 487 (1984).
6. C. Harris *et al.*, *N. Engl. J. Med.* **308**, 1181 (1983).
7. R. C. Gallo *et al.*, *Science* **224**, 500 (1984).
8. M. G. Sarngadharan, M. Popovic, L. Bruch, J. Schüpbach, R. C. Gallo, *ibid.*, p. 506.
9. F. Barré-Sinoussi *et al.*, *ibid.* **220**, 868 (1983).
10. M. G. Sarngadharan, personal communication; R. Cheingsong-Popov *et al.*, *Lancet* **1984-II**, 477 (1984).
11. V. S. Kalyanaraman *et al.*, *Science* **225**, 321 (1984); S. Z. Salahuddin *et al.*, in preparation.
12. M. Essex *et al.*, *Science* **220**, 859 (1983).
13. M. Popovic, M. G. Sarngadharan, E. Read, R. C. Gallo, *ibid.* **224**, 497 (1984).
14. F. V. DiMarzo *et al.*, in preparation.
15. B. J. Poiesz *et al.*, *Proc. Natl. Acad. Sci. U.S.A.* **77**, 7415 (1980).
16. D. J. Lang, J. F. Kummer, D. P. Hartley, *N. Engl. J. Med.* **291**, 121 (1974).
17. L. Mintz, L. Drew, R. C. Miner, F. H. Braff, *Ann. Intern. Med.* **99**, 326 (1983).
18. D. C. Des Jarlais *et al.*, *Morbid. Mortal. Weekly Rep.* **33**, 377 (1984).
19. We thank M. Popovic and R. Gallo for the H9 cells, A. Bodner for HTLV-III p15 and p24 monoclonal antibodies, and B. Haynes for HTLV-I p19 and p24 monoclonal antibodies. This work is supported in part by NIH grants CA 12464, CA 35020, CA 37461, contract NOI-CO-23910, and the Mashud A. Mezerhane B. Fund. D.D.H. is a fellow of the American Cancer Society, Massachusetts Division.

13 September 1984; accepted 27 September 1984

Report

26 October 1984

61. Prevalence of Antibodies to Lymphadenopathy-Associated Retrovirus in African Patients with AIDS

F. Brun-Vézinet, C. Rouzioux, L. Montagnier, S. Chamaret, J. Gruest, F. Barré-Sinoussi, D. Geroldi, J.-C. Chermann, J. McCormick, S. Mitchell, P. Piot, H. Taelman, Kapita Bila Mirangu, Odio Wobin, Mbendi N. Mazebo P., Kayembe Kalambayi, C. Bridts, J. Desmyter, F.M. Feinsod, and T.C. Quinn

The isolation of a new lymphotropic retrovirus from cultured lymphocytes of a patient with lymphadenopathy syndrome (LAS) was reported in May 1983 (*1*). This virus, named lymphadenopathy-associated virus (LAV), differed from the previous isolates of human T-cell leukemia virus (HTLV-I) by the lack of antigenic relatedness of its major core protein (p25) to HTLV-I p24 and by a peculiar morphology of mature virions, which was similar to those of D type particles and equine infectious anemia virus (*2*). In addition, antibodies produced in horses infected by the latter virus precipitated the p25 of the human virus (*2*).

Similar isolates have been made from AIDS or LAS patients belonging to the groups that are at risk for the disease: four from homosexuals, two from two hemophiliac siblings, two from Haitians, and three from Zairians (*3–6*). Such viruses display selective tropism for the T4$^+$ subset of lymphocytes, both in vitro and in vivo, in which they induce a depression of cell growth and a cytopathic effect (*3, 7*) upon activation. A high prevalence of antibodies to viral structural proteins was found in AIDS and LAS patients hospitalized in France, including patients of African origin (*3, 8*). By contrast, only one of 330 controls (French blood donors, laboratory workers, and prisoners) was serologically positive for these antibodies (*6, 8*). These data suggest that such a group of viruses could play a role in the etiology of AIDS, with the possible help of other antigenic stimuli activating latently infected lymphocytes (*3, 4*).

We now report the results of a study to determine the presence of LAV antibodies in sera of AIDS patients diagnosed in 1983 in Zaire by an international team (*9*). The results show a high prevalence of antibodies in the AIDS group, as compared to control groups, and correlation with a decrease in the ratio of T4 to T8 cells and in the absolute number of T4 cells.

For antibody detection, two assays were used in parallel:

1) A radioimmunoprecipitation assay (RIPA), followed by sodium dodecyl sulfate–polyacrylamide gel electrophoresis

(SDS-PAGE) analysis, which detects immunoglobulin G antibodies to LAV p25 protein after metabolic labeling of the virus with [^{35}S]methionine (*3, 8*).

2) An enzyme-linked immunosorbent assay (ELISA) for LAV antibodies which has been described in detail (*3, 8*). Each serum was analyzed in duplicate at a 1:40 dilution. In order to eliminate nonspecific binding of immunoglobulins, which often occurs in the sera of AIDS patients, we performed a control adsorption on lysates of uninfected lymphocytes at the same protein concentration for each serum. To improve the sensitivity of the test, we introduced the following modifications: The virus was purified three times in sucrose gradients and disrupted with 1 percent Triton and 0.1 percent sodium deoxycholate in RIPA buffer (*1*) lacking SDS. Two hundred nanograms of virus-associated proteins were coated in each well. Only when the optical density difference between control and virus was higher than 0.4 was a response considered positive.

As the source of virus, the original strain of LAV (LAV-1) grown on stimulated T lymphocytes of an adult healthy donor (F.R.) was used at the beginning of these studies. Later, virus was produced in a more convenient way from a lymphoblastoid cell line from the same donor, persistently infected with the virus. Although the original strain of LAV did not grow on normal B cells, we found that LAV, after being passaged several times on cultured lymphocytes, could grow readily on a lymphoblastoid line (FR8) obtained by transformation of FR's B lymphocytes with Epstein-Barr virus (*10*). The virus grown on this line (B-LAV-1) has retained the original tropism of LAV for T4 lymphocytes, although it is also able to grow in some other lymphoblastoid lines, including one derived from umbilical cord (LCo). It could not be distinguished from LAV-1 by ultrastructural morphology and its major proteins. The validity of using B-LAV-1 antigens for detection of antibodies to LAV type viruses was assessed with RIPA and ELISA by comparing results obtained on the same sera with the antigens of LAV grown on T cells, and those with the antigens of B-LAV grown on the lymphoblastoid line FR8. In the ELISA against B-LAV, the control for nonspecific binding was performed with a cytoplasmic lysate of the uninfected FR8 line. No contamination by Epstein-Barr virus antigens (EA and VCA) could be detected by precipitation of gradient-purified B-LAV with the corresponding specific antisera. Without exception, results obtained with both viral strains were the same. The sensitivity of ELISA was within the same range as that of RIPA, whether lysed LAV-1 or B-LAV-1 was used.

The criteria, both clinical and immunological, for AIDS diagnosis in the Zaire patients are described in detail elsewhere (*9*). Briefly, a patient with AIDS was a previously healthy adult under 60 years of age, who had evidence of an opportunistic infection or disseminated Kaposi's sarcoma, no underlying history of immunosuppressive disease or immunosuppressive drug use, and in addition fulfilled at least two of the following three immunologic criteria: skin test anergy to multiple antigens, an absolute number of helper T lymphocytes (OKT4) less than 400 per cubic millimeter and a ratio of helper to suppressor T cells (OKT4/OKT8) less than 0.7. Most of the Zaire patients were diagnosed in the Mama Yemo Hospital and the University Hospital. Sera from 37 of the 38 patients who were diagnosed as having AIDS during a 3-week period were available for testing. In addition, 26 sera from a control group of concurrently hospitalized patients with other diagnoses were also screened for LAV antibodies. Of these control patients, 14 had noninfectious diseases, eight had tuberculosis, three had acute malaria, and one had acute nonbacterial meningoencephalitis. For each case, the absolute number of leukocytes and T lymphocytes and the T4/T8 ratio were determined. The coded sera were tested independently by RIPA (L.M. and S.C.) and ELISA (C.R. and F.B.-V.).

The high percentage of LAV seropositivity (94 percent) was demonstrated in the AIDS patients (Table 1). A few sera were weakly positive by RIPA (as exemplified in Fig. 1) and borderline by ELISA, and they were not considered positive in the latter test. One serum (patient 27) was frankly positive by ELISA, and negative by RIPA. In addition, sera from four patients with AIDS-related complex were also positive. Sera from two women who were sexual partners of men who died of AIDS were also weakly positive. Both women were healthy, but one women had a T4/T8 ratio of 0.11 with 122 T4 cells per cubic millimeter whereas the other woman had a ratio of 1.39.

By contrast, only 23 percent of patients in the control group showed positive results for LAV (Table 1; $P = 0.0001$); of the six patients with LAV antibodies, five had a T4/T8 ratio less than 0.7 (three with lung tuberculosis and two with acute falciparum malaria), whereas only one of the 18 patients with T4/T8 $>$ 1.0 had antibodies to LAV ($P = 0.02$ by Fisher's exact test). The mean T4/T8 ratio of the six controls with LAV antibodies was 0.37 (range, 0.09 to 0.42), compared to 1.79 (range, 0.6 to 5.4) for the 20 controls lacking antibodies ($P < 0.001$, Student's t-test). The LAV-positive control patient with a T4/T8

Table 1. LAV antibodies in Zairian groups.

Subjects	Positive for LAV antibodies	
	RIPA	ELISA
1983 (Mama Yemo and University hospitals, Kinshasa)		
AIDS patients*	35/37	32/36
AIDS-related complex	4/4	4/4
Sexual partners of AIDS patients	2/2	2/2
Controls (Mama Yemo and University hospitals, Kinshasa)	6/26	5/26
T4/T8 $<$ 0.7†	5/8	4/8
T4/T8 $>$ 0.7	1/18	1/18
T4 cells $<$ 400/mm^3‡	4/8	
T4 cells $>$ 400/mm^3	2/18	
1980 Controls (mothers)	N.D.	5/100
1983 Controls (hospitalized patients, Ngaliema Hospital)	N.D.	7/100

*Association between presence of LAV antibodies and AIDS (1983), $P = 0.0001$ (χ^2 test). †Association of LAV antibodies with lower T4/T8 ratio in the control group, $P = 0.02$ (Fisher test). ‡Association of LAV antibodies with absolute T4 number $<$ 400/mm^3 in control group, $P = 0.03$ (Fisher's exact test).

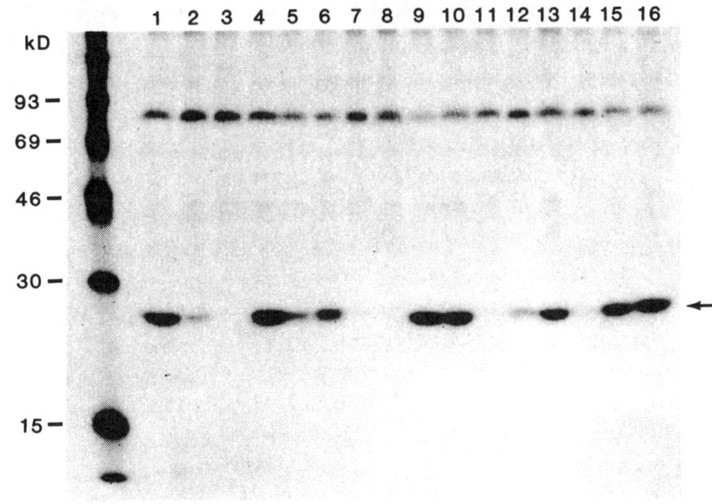

Fig. 1. Radioimmuno-precipitation assay of patient antibody by LAV p25. Virus produced by LCo cells was metabolically labeled with [^{35}S]methionine as described (*1*). The pelleted virus was not further purified and was lysed in RIPA buffer containing 5 percent Zymofren (Specia) and diluted in 50-μl portions of the same buffer. Each portion of viral lysate was incubated with 5 μl of serum to be tested for 1 hour at 37°C and 18 hours at 4°C. Immune complexes were adsorbed on protein A–Sepharose beads, washed, denatured, and subjected to electrophoresis in 12.5 percent polyacrylamide-sodium dodecyl sulfate slab gel as described (*1*). Numbers on the left are molecular size markers in kilodaltons. (Lanes 1, 4, 6, 9, 10, 13, 15, and 16) Highly positive sera; (lanes 2, 5, 12) weakly positive sera; and (lanes 3, 7, 8, 11, and 14) negative sera. In contrast to HTLV-III (*16*), the main protein specifically precipitated is p25. The 43-kD band and the 84-kD band are cellular contaminants that are immunoprecipitated in all the tested sera.

ratio of 1.05 was a 20-year-old woman suffering from arterial hypertension and recent weight loss. Seronegative patients included 14 with noninfectious diseases, five with pulmonary tuberculosis, and one with meningoencephalitis of probable viral origin.

Titers of antibody to LAV in both groups were measured by ELISA. A control positive serum was tested at four dilutions (1/40 to 1/320) on each plate, and the standard curve obtained was used to determine the antibody titer of the patients' sera, according to a computerized program (*8*). Of the 32 AIDS patients, 14 had titers higher than 1/400, seven had titers between 1/100 and 1/400, and 11 had titers between 1/40 and 1/100. The latter were weakly positive by RIPA. In the control group, two had a titer higher than 1/400, including the pa-

tient with arterial hypertension, and three had titers between 1/40 and 1/100.

Sera of African patients hospitalized in Belgium from 1977 until 1983 were also found to have LAV antibodies. These include three Zairians and three Rwandeses with AIDS, and two Zairians and one Rwandese with LAS. Two additional control groups were sampled in 1980 and 1983. Sera from 100 healthy mothers living in Kinshasa, Zaire, were collected in April to July 1980 for hepatitis B studies; five of these were found to have LAV antibodies by ELISA (Table 1). In another group of 100 patients with noninfectious disease treated at the Ngaliema Hospital in Kinshasa in 1983, seven had positive results for LAV (Table 1).

One case deserves particular notice, since it shows that LAV-associated AIDS was already present in Zaire in

1977, and it suggests familial transmission. The patient was a Zairian mother who died in 1978 and whose clinical signs of illness in 1977 were retrospectively considered to fulfill the criteria of AIDS (*11*). Her serum from 1977 contained antibodies to LAV. She had a female infant who, throughout her first year of life, had recurrent extensive candidiasis and depressed mitogen responses. The girl has completely recovered and is now a healthy 7-year-old living in Belgium. Her serum taken at age 6 years was weakly positive by RIPA for LAV antibody.

The prediction that a single infectious agent is at the origin of AIDS implies that all those with proven AIDS show signs of infection. Failures to show infection by the agent should be rare or must be reasonably attributed to lack of sensitivity for demonstrating virus or antibody. In the case of a lymphotropic, lymphocytolytic agent such as LAV, failure to show antibody may also be due to eventual depletion of cells that are a necessary link in immune reaction. Evidence for secondary antibody failure in AIDS was presented earlier (*4*). The prediction does not imply that all those infected by the agent proceed to clinical AIDS but, unless additional factors outweigh the direct role of the agent in the causation of AIDS, it does imply that the agent is relatively infrequent in the healthy population at risk for AIDS, and the frequency of infection in that population parallels, at a lower level, the frequency of AIDS cases.

The incidence of AIDS in Zaire has recently been found to be very high in Kinshasa, ranging from 15 to 20 cases per 100,000 population (*9*). Our data, showing LAV infection in 94 percent of Zairian AIDS cases and in at least 5 percent of control populations, support

the hypothesis that retroviruses of the LAV type are universally involved in this disease. The finding of seropositivity in healthy individuals in 1980 (5 percent in Zairian mothers) suggests that almost as many individuals were carrying LAV in 1980 as in 1983 (7 percent). Indeed this rate in Zaire is much higher than that observed in European countries, which have a lower incidence of AIDS (0.3 percent positive for antibody to LAV in healthy French control populations in 1983). However, LAV-associated AIDS in Africa is not solely restricted to Zaire, but it extends to other countries of equatorial or subequatorial Africa. We and others (*12*) have also found a high degree of LAV seropositivity in AIDS patients in Rwanda and the Central African Republic.

Further evidence of the causal relationship between LAV and AIDS is the high prevalence of LAV antibody in AIDS among Caucasian homosexuals, hemophiliacs, parenteral drug users, and Haitians, and its rarity in control groups (*8, 13*). In addition, viruses with characteristics similar to LAV have also been isolated from lymphocytes from each of the above risk groups, as well as from Zairian AIDS patients diagnosed in France and in Kinshasa (*13–15*).

The observation of LAV seropositivity in heterosexual partners and children of AIDS patients is consistent with earlier observations of heterosexual and familial (vertical) transmissions of AIDS in Zairian patients (*9*). These epidemiologic features are different from those observed in the United States and Europe and will require further studies for confirmation.

Finally, the significance of the higher rate of LAV seropositivity in hospitalized patients without AIDS but with tuberculosis or malaria and the significance of the correlation of seropositivity with lowered T4/T8 ratios and decreased T4 lymphocytes are still unknown. One possibility is that these patients may have had early clinical manifestations of AIDS, but which did not fulfill our strict definition of AIDS. Larger prospective studies, including culture and serology for LAV, will be required to confirm these associations, to examine the high rates of infection in various populations in Africa, to identify groups at special risk, and to determine the modes of LAV and AIDS transmission in Africa, which may be more diverse than those observed in Europe and the United States.

References and Notes

1. F. Barré-Sinoussi *et al. Science* **220**, 868 (1983).
2. L. Montagnier *et al., Ann. Virol. (Inst. Pasteur)* **135E**, 119 (1984).
3. L. Montagnier *et al.,* in *Human T Cell Leukemia Lymphoma Viruses,* R. C. Gallo, M. E. Essex, L. Gross, Eds. (Cold Spring Harbor Laboratory, Cold Spring Harbor, N.Y., 1984), p. 363.
4. E. Vilmer *et al., Lancet* **1984-I**, 753 (1984).
5. J. C. Chermann *et al., UCLA Symposia on Molecular and Cellular Biology* (New Series 16), M. S. Gottlieb and J. E. Groopman, Eds. (Liss, New York, 1984).
6. L. Montagnier, F. Barré-Sinoussi, J. C. Chermann, in *Proceedings of the Meeting of the European Group for Immunodeficiencies* (Elsevier/North-Holland, Amsterdam, 1984), p. 367.
7. D. Klatzmann *et al., Science* **225**, 59 (1984).
8. F. Brun-Vézinet *et al., Lancet* **1984-I**, 1253 (1984).
9. P. Piot *et al., ibid.* **1984-II**, 65 (1984).
10. L. Montagnier *et al., Science* **225**, 63 (1984).
11. J. Vandepitte *et al., Lancet* **1983-I**, 925 (1983).
12. C. George *et al.,* in preparation.
13. G. Rouzioux *et al.,* in preparation.
14. J. L. Vilde *et al.,* in preparation.
15. A. Ellrodt *et al., Lancet* **1984-I**, 1383 (1984).
16. M. G. Sarngadharan *et al., Science* **224**, 506, 1984.
17. We thank M. Tamfum, University of Kinshasa, and F. Beets, Clinic of Ngaliema in Kinshasa, for providing part of the sera; and F. Rey and M. T. Nugeyre for skillful technical assistance. Viral Oncology Unit members also belong to Research Team 147 of C.N.R.S.

14 May 1984; accepted 27 July 1984

Report

26 October 1984

62. Alteration of T-Cell Functions by Infection with HTLV-I or HTLV-II

M. Popovic, N. Flomenberg, D.J. Volkman, D. Mann, A.S. Fauci, B. Dupont, and R.C. Gallo

Since the first isolation of a human retrovirus (*1*), designated human T-cell leukemia-lymphoma virus subgroup I (HTLV-I), a large number of human T-lymphotropic retroviruses (HTLV) have been isolated (*2–6*). This was made possible by the development of sensitive methods for virus detection (*7*) and growth of the T cells with T-cell growth factor (TCGF) (*8*). HTLV-I is closely associated with malignancies of mature T cells occurring in adults of various countries (*2*), particularly with clusters of adult T-cell leukemia (ATL) in Japan (*4*) and a related syndrome in the Caribbean (*5*). The disease has an aggressive clinical course frequently accompanied by opportunistic infections (*9*), including

Table 1. Properties of KLH-specific helper T-cell clone and the cytotoxic T-cell clones before and after infection with HTLV. The development, growth properties in vitro, and functional characterization of KLH-specific and cytotoxic T-cell clones have been described (12, 13). The T-cell clones were infected by cocultivation with three different HTLV isolates: HTLV-I$_{TK}$ isolated from the mother of a Japanese patient with ATL (3); HTLV-I$_{EP}$ from a patient with AIDS (2) and HTLV-II$_{MO}$ from a patient with a T-cell variant of hairy cell leukemia (14). The cocultivation assay and identification of the HTLV-infected T-cell population by histocompatibility (data not shown) and karyotyping have been described (3, 18). Cell-surface markers were identified in three independent experiments and representative data are shown. The percentage and mean fluorescent units (mfu) of positive cells reacting with monoclonal antibodies OKT4 (helper-inducer), OKT8 (suppressor-cytotoxic), antibody to TAC (TCGF receptor), and 4D12 (detecting an epitope common to the HLA-B cross-reactive group antigens) were described (3, 18, 20). Positive cells are those that show greater fluorescence than the P-3 myeloma protein. The values are lower than previously described (18, 20) because of P-3 binding. However, there are no essential changes in reaction with OKT4 and OKT8 monoclonal antibodies before and after HTLV infection. The percentage of HTLV-infected T cells was determined by immunofluorescence assay (IFA) with a mouse monoclonal antibody against HTLV p19 (16). The core protein p24 was detected by homologous radioimmunoprecipitation assay (RIPA) with goat serum directed against HTLV-I p24 (17) and by heterologous RIPA with rabbit serum directed against HTLV-II p24 (14). RIPA was carried out with ^{125}I-labeled HTLV-I p24 and a limiting dilution of the goat (homologous) or the rabbit (heterologous) antibodies to p24. Reverse transcriptase (RT) activity in culture fluids was assayed (15) and the activity expressed as picomoles of ^{3}H-labeled deoxythymidine monophosphate incorporated into trichloracetic acid-precipitable DNA per milliliter of 20-fold-concentrated culture fluids. Virus particles were detected by electron microscopy. N.D., none detected.

T-cell clone	Sex chro-mo-somes	Cell surface markers								HTLV expression				
		OKT4		OKT8		TAC		4D12		IFA for p19 (% posi-tive)	RIPA for HTLV p24 (% competition)		RT (pmol/ml)	Virus parti-cles
		%	mfu	%	mfu	%	mfu	%	mfu		Homol-ogous	Heterol-ogous		
SR-2	XX	69	773	0.6	21	30	245	0	1.0	0	0	N.D.	0	N.D.
SR-2/HTLV-I$_{TK}$	XX	74	881	1.2	26	48	773	45	588	85	100	100	50	+
						Cytotoxic to HLA-DR2								
DM322A-13	XX	51	599	6	56	27	689	7.3	59	0	0	N.D.	0	N.D.
DM32A-13/HTLV-I$_{TK}$	XX	61	781	6	49	72	2158	25	386	18–75	100	100	25	+
DM322A-13/HTLV-I$_{EP}$	XX	44	408	4.3	57	48	883	23	315	75	100	100	12	+
DM322A-13/HTLV-II$_{MO}$	XX	46	621	3.7	50	42	1229	7.4	39	18–72	<50	100	32	+
						Cytotoxic to HLA-DR7								
AE15.3	XY	62	489	4	56	35	306	22	189	0	0	N.D.	0	N.D.
AE15.3/HTLV-I$_{TK}$	XY	37	564	12	174	39	2456	58	2081	45–90	100	100	410	+
AE15.3/HTLV-II$_{MO}$	XY	65	502	6	33	46	448	43	210	15–45	<50	100	22	+

Pneumocystis carinii pneumonia (*9*), which is also a common opportunistic infection in acquired immune deficiency syndrome (AIDS) (*10*). Some earlier results were consistent with the notion that a member of the HTLV family causes AIDS (*11*), and there is now evidence that a new subgroup of HTLV (HTLV-III) is the primary cause (*6*). It is possible that infection of a certain subset of lymphocytes with the leukemogenic HTLV's (HTLV-I and HTLV-II) can occur in vivo, ultimately leading to an immunological deficiency by abrogation of the specific functions of the lymphocytes or by selective cell killing. This, combined with the ability of HTLV-I to immortalize some infected T cells, may explain the apparent efficient leukemogenic activity of these viruses.

The ability of HTLV-I or HTLV-II to alter specific T-cell functions was studied by in vitro infection of T-cell clones of predefined function. One T-cell clone, SR-2, both proliferates and provides "help" to B lymphocytes when exposed to the soluble antigen keyhole limpet hemocyanin (KLH) in association with antigen-presenting cells (APC) expressing a defined histocompatible (HLA) class II antigen (DR4 and LD40). Two other clones, DM322A and AE15.3, exhibit specific cytotoxic responses toward cells expressing the HLA DR2 and DR7 target antigens, respectively. Their development and characterization in vitro have been described (*12, 13*). The properties of these clones, virus expression, karyotype, and cell-surface characteristics before and after infection with HTLV are summarized in Table 1. All three T-cell clones were infected by cocultivation with different HTLV isolates (*3*). The SR-2 clone was infected with an isolate of HTLV-I known as HTLV-I$_{TK}$ (*3*). The cytotoxic DM322A T-cell clone was infected with the HTLV-I$_{TK}$ and HTLV-I$_{EP}$, which is an isolate from a patient (E.P.) with AIDS (*2*); and with HTLV-II$_{MO}$, a virus belonging to a separate subgroup of HTLV and, therefore, called subgroup II (*14*). The cytotoxic clone AE15.3 was infected with HTLV-I$_{TK}$ and HTLV-II$_{MO}$.

Table 1 shows that HTLV was fully expressed in all three T-cell clones, as determined by reverse transcriptase activity in culture fluids (*15*) and by electron microscopic examinations. The identity of HTLV-infected clones and their normal (noninfected) counterparts was determined by HLA typing (data not shown) and chromosomal analysis. The percentage of HTLV-infected cells was determined by an indirect immunofluorescence assay in which monoclonal antibodies to the HTLV structural protein p19 were used (*16*). The major core protein, p24, was detected by homologous and heterologous radioimmunoprecipitation assays performed with goat and rabbit sera directed against p24 of HTLV-I and HTLV-II, respectively (*17*). In addition, the expression of new antigens related to HLA class I antigens was induced by the HTLV-I$_{EP}$ and HTLV-I$_{TK}$ isolates and not by HTLV-II (*18*). These findings taken together demonstrated that the cells were infected by particular isolates of each subgroup.

The blastogenic responses of the uninfected and HTLV-infected KLH-specific T-cell clone SR-2 were studied next. Uninfected SR-2 showed little or no thymidine incorporation (Fig. 1A). Low levels of thymidine incorporation occurred with APC alone, but increased by a factor of more than 14 in the presence of both KLH and compatible APC. Moreover, the T cells did not respond to KLH in association with incompatible APC. In contrast, HTLV-I–infected cells (SR-2/

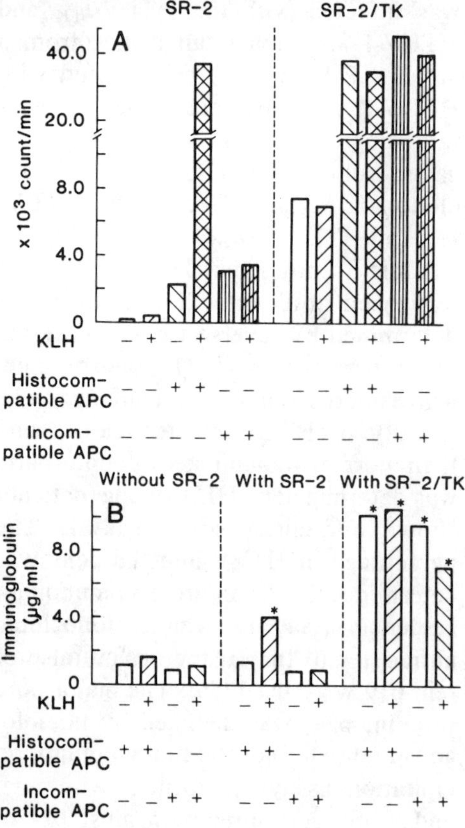

Fig. 1. Function of a KLH-specific human T-cell clone (SR-2) before and after infection with HTLV. (A) Proliferative responses of (i) normal (uninfected) KLH-specific SR-2 and (ii) HTLV-I$_{TK}$–infected SR-2 cells (SR-2/TK) were determined in the presence (+) or absence (−) of KLH and histocompatible or incompatible APC. Briefly, 2.5×10^5 irradiated (3500 rad) mononuclear cells were incubated with 10^4T cells, with or without KLH (100 µg/ml). After 3 days, cultures were treated with 1 µCi of [^{3}H]thymidine for 18 hours. Data represent mean counts per minute of triplicate cultures. Mononuclear cells from compatible or incompatible persons above, with or without KLH, gave ≤700 count/min. (B) Immunoglobulin production of B cells in presence (+) or absence (−) of KLH and histocompatible or incompatible APC was followed (i) without KLH-specific SR-2 cells, (ii) with SR-2 cells, and (iii) with HTLV-I$_{TK}$–infected SR-2/TK cells. In the assay, 2.5×10^5 T cells (SR-2 or SR-2/TK) for 10 days and the supernatant was measured for immunoglobulins G and M. Data represent mean immunoglobulin levels of triplicate cultures. Cultures with added SR-2 or SR-2/TK cells were compared to those without added T cells, and the significance of the values was determined by Student's t-test (*$P < 0.05$). The standard error of the mean was less than 20 percent of the total immunoglobulin level in each case.

TK) proliferated in the absence of both KLH and APC. The addition of KLH alone had a negligible effect, but the presence of APC increase proliferation more than fivefold whether histocompatible (DR4 and LD40) or incompatible APC were used, with or without KLH antigen. Thus, HTLV infection of SR-2 alters these cells so that they proliferate spontaneously and are further stimulated by allogeneic APC in an unregulated fashion regardless of the presence of histocompatibility or antigen. HTLV-I–transformed T cells can respond to a common structure of HLA class II antigens by proliferation (19); this would explain the ability of irradiated APC to augment proliferation of SR-2/TK cells. Further studies are needed to determine whether the nonspecific stimulation of these cells could be mediated through soluble lymphokines.

The ability of SR-2 and SR-2/TK to stimulate polyclonal B-cell activation is illustrated in Fig. 1B. Both compatible and incompatible allogeneic mononuclear cells containing B- and T-lymphocytes and monocytes were obtained from individuals who were not immune to KLH. These cells were cultured alone with uninfected SR-2 helper cells or with infected SR-2/TK cells. Supernatant immunoglobulin production was measured (see legend to Fig. 1B). Immunoglobulin production increased by a factor of almost 3 when SR-2 cells were cultured with compatible APC in the presence of KLH but not when incompatible APC were used or when compatible or incompatible APC were used in the absence of KLH antigen. In contrast, the SR-2 cells infected with HTLV-I$_{TK}$ (SR-2/TK) stimulated B-cell immunoglobulin production to a greater degree, and this did not depend on activation of the infected T cells by KLH or on the presence of histocompatible APC. The nonspecific nature of the B-cell help shown by the HTLV-infected helper T cells indicates that these cells stimulate in an unregulated manner, independent of either the HLA or antigen recognition that were characteristic of the uninfected clone.

Two T-cell clones, DM322A and AE15.3, with specific cytotoxic activity directed toward HLA class II antigens DR2 and DR7, respectively, were infected with HTLV, and their cytotoxic function was compared to that of the uninfected clones. The percentage of HTLV-positive T cells (measured as the percentage of cells positive for the HTLV-specific antigen p19) and cytotoxic activity were determined in parallel experiments at various intervals after infection. As the number of HTLV-positive cells increased, there was a parallel decrease in cytotoxic activity in both HTLV-infected clones (Fig. 2). When the percentage of virus-infected cells was over 70 percent, cytotoxic T-cell activity decreased to 1/10 or less. In some instances there was complete loss of function. The cytotoxic activity in both T-cell clones could not be restored by restimulation with antigen-specific cells. The data indicate that cytotoxic function in both the T-cell clones infect-

ed with different virus isolates is irreversibly lost.

Previous studies of human T cells infected with HTLV-I and HTLV-II showed that some of the infected T cells are transformed and differ from normal uninfected T cells in several well-defined characteristics in vitro (*20*). In addition, as we have shown with two types of functionally defined T-cell populations, the morphologic, growth, and cell-surface alterations of HTLV-infected T cells are accompanied by alterations in function in the case of KLH-specific helper T cells and by significant decrease or complete loss of cytotoxic function in the case of cytotoxic T cells. Although proliferation and B-cell help in uninfected, KLH-specific SR-2 cells are regulated by the presence of both the soluble antigen and the histocompatibility of APC, cells infected with HTLV manifest a loss of this regulation of induction. Thus, functions of SR-2 cells such as proliferation and B-cell help become indiscriminant after HTLV-I infection, resulting in polyclonal induction of immunoglobulin production. If HTLV-III, the apparent cause of AIDS, has effects similar to those of HTLV-I in these systems, the results might be relevant to the observation that AIDS patients exhibit polyclonal activation of B cells (*21*). The capability of HTLV-I and HTLV-II to induce loss of specific responses of the infected T cells is consistent with observations suggesting that HTLV-I–associated T-cell malignancies are linked with immune deficiency manifested in various opportunistic infections, including those produced by agents like *Pneumocystis carinii* (*9*), and, as recently shown, with an increased risk of B-cell lymphoid malignancies (*22*).

Retroviruses associated with neoplas-

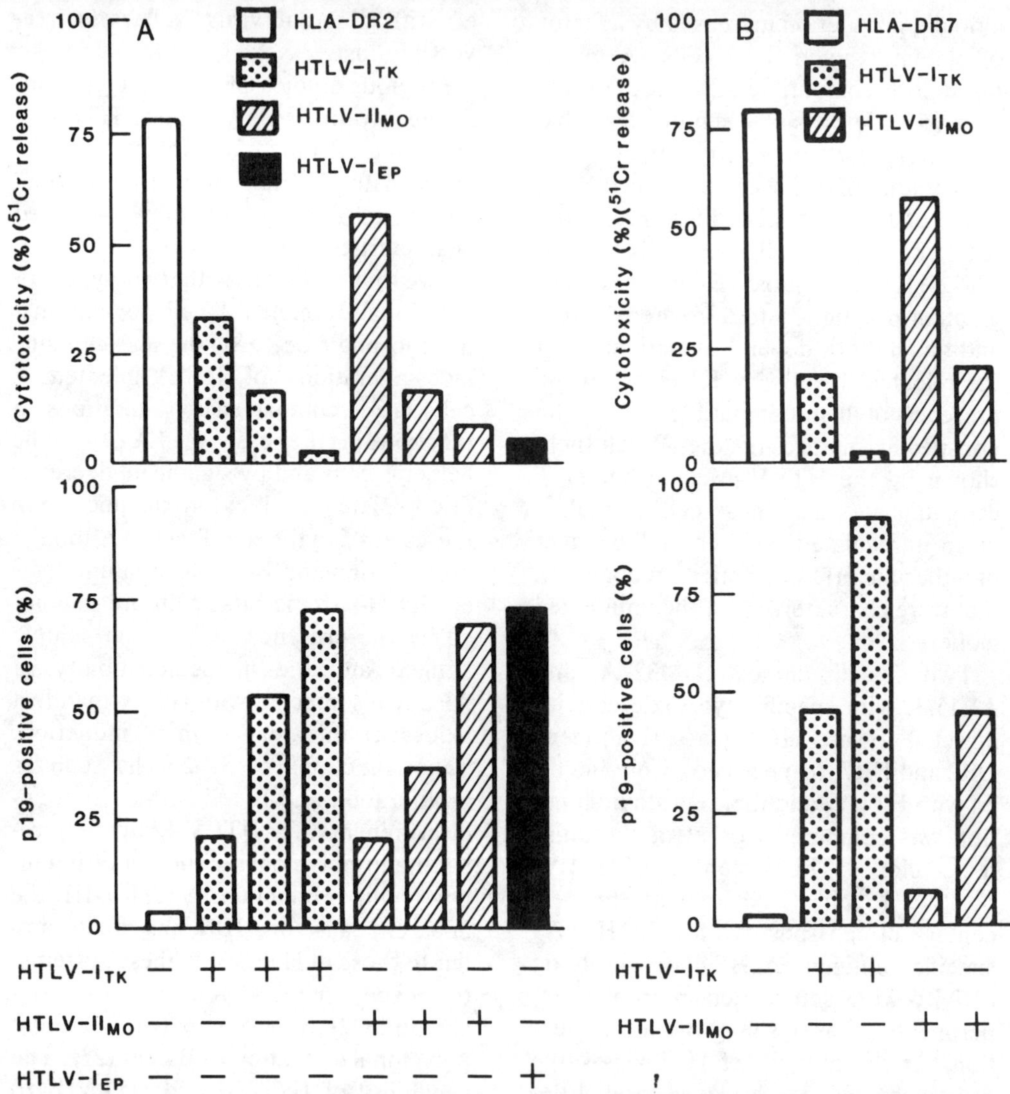

Fig. 2. Cytotoxic activity of DM322A-13 and AE15.3 T-cell clones before and after HTLV infection. Cytotoxicity assays and immunofluorescence assays for HTLV p19 were performed as described (*17, 21*). Cytotoxic T-cell clones infected with particular HTLV isolates were analyzed for cytotoxicity and for HTLV p19 from the same cultures and compared at various intervals after infection to normal (uninfected) counterparts. (A) Clone Dm322A-13 with cytotoxicity directed toward HLA-DR2 was infected with HTLV-I$_{TK}$, HTLV-II$_{MO}$, and HTLV-I$_{EP}$, respectively. (B) Clone AE15.3 with cytotoxicity directed toward HLA-DR7 was infected with HTLV-I$_{TK}$ and HTLV-II$_{MO}$ isolates, respectively. (−) Negative for particular HTLV isolate; (+) positive for particular HTLV isolate. Data represent the mean of triplicate determinations of ^{51}Cr release, and variability for each value does not exceed 20 percent.

tic diseases may also cause other diseases. In cats, for example, an acquired immune deficiency may result from infection with feline leukemia virus (FeLV) (23), and abrogation of lymphocyte functions in vitro by FeLV has also been demonstrated (23). Clinical observations as well as in vitro data suggest that the now widening family of human T4 lymphotropic retroviruses can induce alterations in T cells that could lead to an immune deficiency. In addition, our present results show that HTLV-I and HTLV-II can infect and immortalize T cells having a specific immune function. HTLV-infected T cells cultured in vitro are frequently mono- or oligoclonal, representing a selected cell population (20). Therefore, it is possible that, at the time of infection of the normal clones, some T cells were in "a nonfunctional phase," and these HTLV-transformed T cells became dominant. However, this is unlikely because the alteration of specific function after HTLV infection followed the same pattern in six independent experiments with three different HTLV isolates (Figs. 1 and 2). It is of interest to attempt immortalization of various types of functional human T cells for molecular analysis of various specific T-cell structures. For instance, Mitsuya et al. (24) recently provided evidence for only partial abrogation of a specific cytotoxic T-cell function in a T-cell clone positive for HTLV-I. Thus, the establishment of immortalized T-cell clones with various degrees of altered T-cell function originated from functionally defined T-cell populations could provide a system suitable for the molecular analysis of T cells with specific function.

References and Notes

1. B. J. Poiesz, F. W. Ruscetti, A. F. Gazdar, P. A. Bunn, J. D. Minna, R. C. Gallo, *Proc. Natl. Acad. Sci. U.S.A.* **77**, 7415 (1980); B. J. Poiesz, F. W. Ruscetti, M. S. Reitz, V. S. Kalyanaraman, R. C. Gallo, *Nature (London)* **294**, 268 (1981).
2. R. C. Gallo, in *Cancer Surveys*, L. M. Franks, L. M. Wyke, R. Weiss, Eds. (Oxford Univ. Press, Oxford, 1984), vol. 3, p. 112.
3. M. Popovic *et al.*, *Science* **219**, 856 (1983); P. S. Sarin *et al.*, *Proc. Natl. Acad. Sci. U.S.A.* **80**, 2370 (1983).
4. Y. Hinuma *et al.*, *Proc. Natl. Acad. Sci. U.S.A.* **78**, 6476 (1981); V. S. Kalyanaraman, M. G. Sarngadharan, Y. Nakao, Y. Ito, T. Aoki, R. C. Gallo, *ibid.* **79**, 1654 (1982); M. Yoshida, I. Miyoshi, Y. Hinuma, *ibid.*, p. 2031; M. Robert-Guroff, Y. Nakao, K. Notake, Y. Ito, A. Sliski, R. C. Gallo, *Science* **215**, 975 (1982).
5. D. Catovsky *et al.*, Lancet **1982-I**, 639 (1982); W. A. Blattner *et al.*, *Int. J. Cancer* **30**, 257 (1982); R. C. Gallo *et al.*, *Cancer Res.* **43**, 3892 (1983); M. F. Greaves *et al.*, *Int. J. Cancer* **33**, 795 (1984).
6. F. Barré-Sinoussi *et al.*, *Science* **220**, 868 (1983); M. Popovic, M. G. Sarngadharan, E. Read, R. C. Gallo, *ibid.* **224**, 497 (1984); R. C. Gallo *et al.*, *ibid.*, p. 500; M. G. Sarngadharan, M. Popovic, L. Bruch, J. Schüpbach, R. C. Gallo, *ibid.*, p. 506.
7. R. C. Gallo, F. W. Ruscetti, R. E. Gallagher, in *Hematopoietic Mechanisms*, B. Clarkson, P. A. Marks, J. Till, Eds. (Cold Spring Harbor Laboratory, Cold Spring Harbor, N.Y., 1978), vol. 5, p. 671.
8. D. A. Morgan, F. W. Ruscetti, R. C. Gallo, *Science* **193**, 1007 (1976); J. W. Mier and R. C. Gallo, *Proc. Natl. Acad. Sci. U.S.A.* **77**, 6134 (1980).
9. K. Kinoshita *et al.*, in *Adult T-Cell Leukemia and Related Diseases*, M. Hahaoka, K. Takatsuki, M. Shimoyama, Eds. (Plenum, Tokyo, 1982), p. 167; N. Ueda *et al.*, *Acta Pathol. Jpn.* **29**, 221 (1979).
10. "Pneumocystis pneumonia—Los Angeles," *Morbid. Mortal. Weekly Rep.* **30**, 250 (1981); "Kaposi's sarcoma and pneumocystis pneumonia among homosexual men—New York City and California" *ibid.*, p. 305.
11. M. Essex *et al.*, *Science* **220**, 859 (1983); M. Essex *et al.*, in *Human T-Cell Leukemia/Lymphoma Virus*, R. C Gallo, M. Essex, L. Gross, Eds. (Cold Spring Harbor Laboratory, Cold Spring Harbor, N.Y., 1984), p. 335.
12. B. Sredni, D. Volkman, R. M. Schwartz, A. S. Fauci, *Proc. Natl. Acad. Sci. U.S.A.* **78**, 1858 (1981).
13. N. Flomenberg, E. Duffy, B. Dupont, *Scand. J. Immunol.* **19**, 237 (1984).
14. V. S. Kalyanaraman *et al.*, *Science* **218**, 571 (1982); I. S. Y. Chen *et al.*, *Nature (London)* **305**, 502 (1983); E. P. Gelmann, G. Franchini, V. Manzari, F. Wong-Staal, R. C. Gallo, *Proc. Natl. Acad. Sci. U.S.A.* **81**, 993 (1984).
15. H. M. Rho, B. J. Poiesz, F. W. Ruscetti, R. C. Gallo, *Virology* **112**, 355 (1981).
16. M. Robert-Guroff *et al.*, *J. Exp. Med.* **154**, 1957 (1981).
17. V. S. Kalyanaraman, M. G. Sarngadharan, B. J. Poiesz, F. W. Ruscetti, R. C. Gallo, *J. Virol.* **38**, 906 (1981).
18. D. Mann *et al.*, *J. Immunol.* **131**, 2021 (1983); D. Mann *et al.*, *Nature (London)* **305**, 58 (1983); M. Popovic, V. S. Kalyanaraman, D. Mann, E. Richardson, P. S. Sarin, R. C. Gallo, in *Human*

336

T-Cell Leukemia/Lymphoma Virus, R. C. Gallo, M. Essex, L. Gross, Eds. (Cold Spring Harbor Laboratory, Cold Spring Harbor, N.Y., 1984), p. 217.
19. N. Suciu-Foca, A. Lewison, M. Popovic, R. C. Gallo, D. W. King, *Nature (London)*, in press.
20. M. Popovic, G. Lange-Wantzin, P. S. Sarin, D. Mann, R. C. Gallo, *Proc. Natl. Acad. Sci. U.S.A.* **80**, 5402 (1983); M. Popovic, F. Wong-Staal, P. S. Sarin, R. C. Gallo, in *Advances in Viral Oncology*, G. Klein, Ed. (Raven, New York, 1984), p. 45.
21. H. C. Lane, H. Masur, L. C. Edgar, G. Whalen, A. H. Rook, A. S. Fauci, *N. Engl. J. Med.* **309**, 453 (1983).
22. W. A. Blattner *et al.*, in *Human T-Cell Leukemia/Lymphoma Virus*, R. C. Gallo, M. Essex, L. Gross, Eds. (Cold Spring Harbor Laboratory, Cold Spring Harbor, N.Y., 1984), p. 267.
23. M. Essex, W. D. Hardy, Jr., S. M. Cotter, R. M. Jakowski, A. Sliski, *Infect. Immun.* **11**, 470 (1975); R. G. Olsen *et al.*, in *Viruses in Naturally Occurring Cancers*, M. Essex, G. Todaro, H. zur Hausen, Eds. (Cold Spring Harbor Laboratory, Cold Spring Harbor, N.Y., 1980), p. 665; W. D. Hardy, Jr. *et al.*, *Cancer Res.* **36**, 582 (1976); L. J. Anderson, O. Jarrett, H. M. Lair, *J. Natl. Cancer Inst.* **47**, 807 (1971); S. M. Cotter, W. D. Hardy, Jr., M. Essex, *J. Am. Vet. Med. Assoc.* **166**, 499 (1975).
24. H. Mitsuya, H. G. Guo, M. Megson, C. Trainor, M. S. Reitz, Jr., S. Broder, *Science* **223**, 1293 (1983).
25. We thank V. S. Kalyanaraman for performing the radioimmunoprecipitation assays. B. Kramarsky for electron microscopic examination, F. Bach for lymphocyte tissue typing, and N. Suciu-Foca for valuable comments on the manuscript. We also thank E. Richardson and E. Read for technical help and A. Mazzuca for editorial assistance. Supported in part by an interagency agreement with the Uniformed Services University of Health Sciences (Y01-CP-30500).

21 May 1984; accepted 10 July 1984

Report

2 November 1984

63. Transmission of HTLV-III Infection from Human Plasma to Chimpanzees: An Animal Model for AIDS

Harvey J. Alter, Jorg W. Eichberg, Henry Masur, W. Carl Saxinger, Robert Gallo, Abe M. Macher, H. Clifford Lane, and Anthony S. Fauci

Originally identified in male homosexuals and abusers of intravenous drugs (*1*), the acquired immune deficiency syndrome (AIDS) has more recently been recognized as a potential consequence of blood transfusion (*2*). Our investigation, designed to determine whether there was a transmissible agent in human blood capable of inducing AIDS and to establish an animal model in which the pathogenesis, treatment, and prevention of AIDS could be studied, began before the virologic investigations (*3–5*) that linked human AIDS to a type C retrovirus. Retroviruses designated human T-cell leukemia virus type III (HTLV-III) (*3*) and lymphadenopathy-associated virus (LAV) (*5*) have been reproducibly recovered from patients with AIDS and the AIDS-related syndrome. Whether or not HTLV-III and LAV are identical viruses remains to be determined. Common to both these agents is tropism for the T4 lymphocyte, a cell whose depletion is the focal point of the chain of immunologic and clinical events that comprises AIDS (*1*).

In experiments to maximize the potential for AIDS transmission to chimpanzees, each of three study animals (CH132, CH114, and CH133) was sequentially infused with plasma from three different patients selected to represent the spectrum of AIDS-related disorders (specifically, the lymphadenopathy syndrome, Kaposi's sarcoma, and life-threatening opportunistic infection) as defined by the Centers for Disease Control (*6*). One animal served as a control and received 3 units of normal donor plasma. To enhance further the potential for transmission of an agent with a low titer of antibody and to simulate the human transfusion experience, inocula were given in large volume (50 to 150 ml) to each chimpanzee. Plasmas were ABO-compatible, and no adverse reactions were associated with this interspecies transfusion program. The chimpanzees were housed individually in an isolation hut at the Southwest Foundation for Biomedical Research (SFBR) in San Antonio, Texas. Their clinical status was monitored by biweekly physical examination, and their immunologic status was assessed by biweekly determination of absolute lymphocyte counts, the number of T3, T4, and T8 subsets, B cells, natural killer cell activity, lymphocyte mitogen responsiveness, interleukin-2 activity, and reactions in mixed lymphocyte culture by means of established techniques (*7*).

Antibodies to HTLV-III were determined in a solid-phase ELISA (enzyme-linked immunosorbent assay) with the H9 HTLV-III clone (*3*) as described (*8*). Assays were performed in duplicate, and results were expressed as a ratio of the absorbance of the test sample compared to the average of four negative controls. A ratio greater than 6.0 was considered as indicating the presence of antibody to HTLV-III. Positive samples in the screening assay were subsequently titered, and selected samples were tested for the presence of immunoglobulin M (IgM) antibodies to HTLV-III (*6*). All samples were tested under code.

Before inoculation, all chimpanzees were seronegative for antibodies to HTLV-III and had normal T4 numbers, T4:T8 ratios, and mitogen responses. The first animal (CH132, Fig. 1A) received 150 ml of plasma from each of three donors (P_6, P_7, and P_8), who were seropositive for antibodies to HTLV-III (titers were more than 1:1,000,000 for P_6, 1:770,000 for P_7, and 1:73,000 for P_8). The early appearance of antibodies to HTLV-III was followed by a continuous decline to baseline by week 28 after inoculation (Fig. 1A). This is a pattern of passive transfer of antibody from donor to recipient and does not indicate HTLV-III infection. In view of the susceptibility to HTLV-III infection of other chimpanzees in this study (see below), the absence of infection in CH132 implies that some AIDS patients positive for antibodies to HTLV-III are not infectious or that susceptibility to AIDS is governed by factors other than the presence or absence of humoral antibody to HTLV-III (or both).

The next animal (CH114, Fig. 1B) received 150 ml of plasma from each of three donors (P_1, P_2, and P_3) over a 3-day period. Donor P_1 had lymphadenopathy and immunologic abnormalities consistent with AIDS but was asymptomatic and remains well 1 year after initiation of this study. Donor P_2 had Kaposi's sarcoma, and donor P_3 had life-threatening

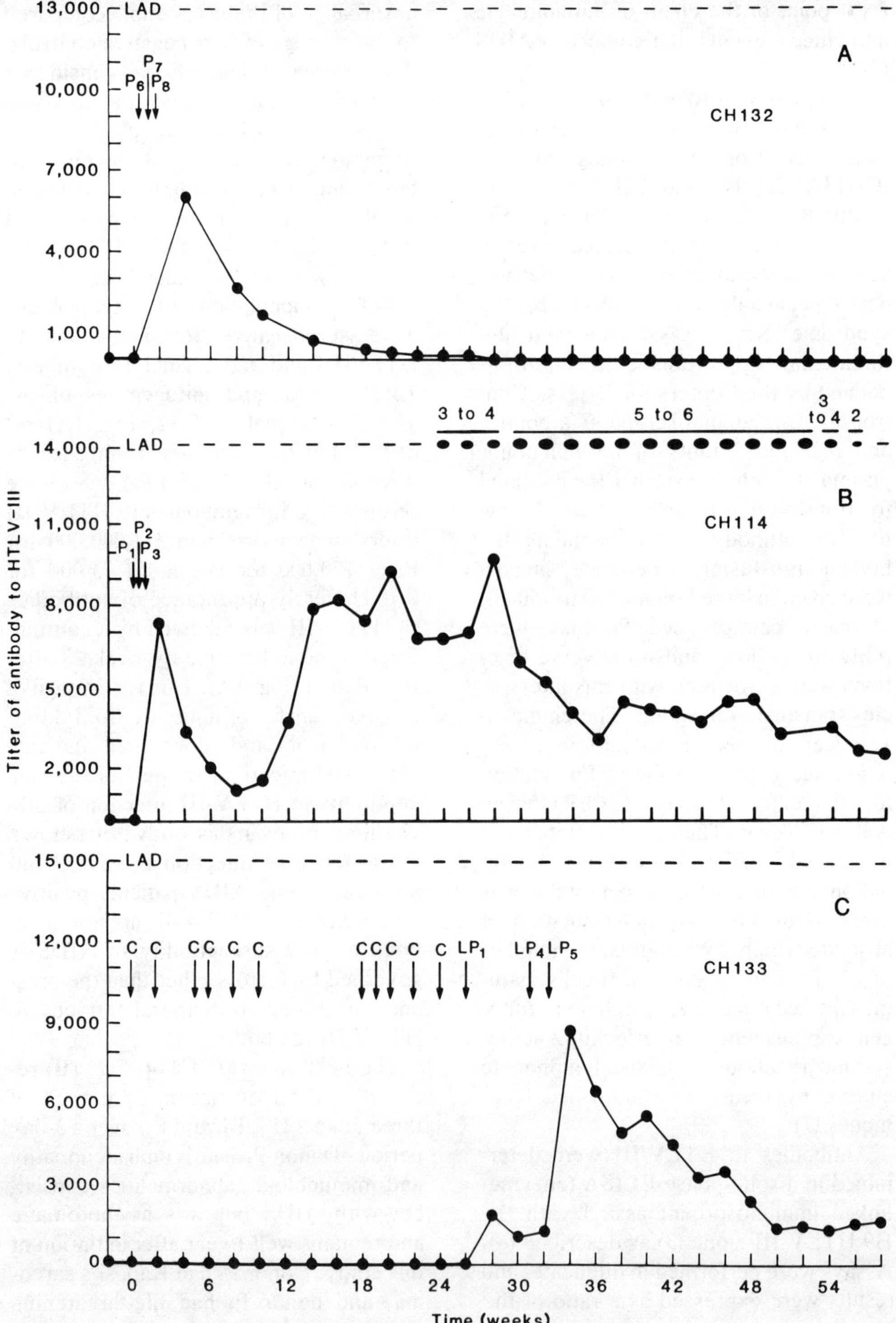
LAD
13,000
10,000
7,000
4,000
1,000
P6 P7 P8
CH132
A
3 to 4
5 to 6
3 to 4
2
LAD
14,000
11,000
8,000
5,000
2,000
P1 P2 P3
CH114
B
Titer of antibody to HTLV-III
LAD
15,000
12,000
9,000
6,000
3,000
0
C C C C C C
C C C C C LP1
LP4 LP5
CH133
C
0 6 12 18 24 30 36 42 48 54
Time (weeks)

opportunistic infections; both died within 6 months of their apheresis procedure. All three donors had antibody to HTLV-III with titers of 1:215,000, 1:48,000, and 1:930,000, respectively.

Antibodies to HTLV-III in CH114 were detectable at a titer of 1:7300 in the first sample obtained 2 weeks after inoculation (Table 1 and Fig. 1B). Antibody titers then diminished in each biweekly sample, reproducing the pattern of passive transfer observed in CH132 (Fig. 1A). During week 10, however, the titer of antibodies to HTLV-III began to rise steeply to 1:7900 and then reached a plateau with fluctuation to a peak at 1:9700. Antibody then diminished but has persisted at titers of 1:4000 to 1:6000 throughout 1 year of follow-up examinations. The specificity of this antibody for HTLV-III was confirmed by Western blot analysis (9) and by blocking the ELISA reactivity with HTLV-III–specific sheep antiserum (10). At week 24, 14 weeks after antibody seroconversion,

CH114 was first noted to develop bilateral inguinal lymphadenopathy (4 by 2 cm) and a lesser degree of cervical adenopathy. Inguinal nodes progressed in size to 6 by 3 cm and persisted at this size for 22 weeks before gradually diminishing; the total duration of adenopathy was 32 weeks. This degree of adenopathy had never been observed in any of the chimpanzees housed at SFBR (11). An inguinal lymph node biopsy specimen obtained at week 33 showed severe lymphoid hyperplasia (Fig. 2). An inguinal node biopsy done before the inoculation had not revealed these hyperplastic changes. Special stains, including Giemsa, periodic acid–Schiff, methenamine silver, and Fite, did not reveal mycobacteria, fungi, *Pneumocystis carinii*, or other microorganisms. Also, CH114 did not show antibody seroconversion for the cytomegalovirus or Epstein-Barr virus.

Coincident with the adenopathy, the percentage of T4 cells, the T4:T8 ratio,

Fig. 1 (facing page). Clinical and serologic events in chimpanzee 132 (A), 114 (B), and 133 (C). Antibody to HTLV-III was measured in an ELISA and is expressed as the reciprocal titer. LAD relates to the degree of lymphadenopathy expressed either as none (−) or as a figure representative of the relative size (in centimeters) of the largest node palpated. Arrows indicate the date of transfusion; P represents plasma (150 ml), LP represents lymphocyte-rich plasma (150 ml), and C represents single donor cryoprecipitate (each arrow represents 3 to 4 units, each unit being the amount of cryoprecipitate derived from 300 ml of plasma). Donor P_1 and LP_1 were the same donor with the lymphadenopathy syndrome. All other donors were different AIDS patients. (A) CH132 (50 kg in weight, 9 years of age) had antibodies to HTLV-III in the first specimen after inoculation, and the antibody level declined progressively to zero, a pattern consistent with the decay of passively transfused antibody. No evidence of HTLV-III infection was noted despite inoculation of the animal with large volumes of plasma from donors positive for antibodies to HTLV-III. (B) In CH114 (51 kg in weight, 8 years of age) a similar pattern of passive antibody transfer was noted but with active production of antibody beginning at weeks 10 to 12. Antibodies to HTLV-III persisted throughout the course of follow-up examinations. Twelve weeks after the appearance of antibody, the chimpanzee developed substantial lymphadenopathy which persisted for 32 weeks. (C) CH133 (43 kg in weight, 7 years of age) showed no serologic response to repeated infusions of cryoprecipitate. The presence of active antibody to HTLV-III is indicated by the plateau of antibody titer beginning at week 50, a pattern inconsistent with the continuous decay of passively acquired antibody. In addition, IgM antibody to HTLV-III was detected at weeks 32 to 40 (see text). CH133 did not develop adenopathy or clinical illness.

and lymphocyte response to mitogens (particularly phytohemagglutinin) all decreased (Table 1). The decrease in the percentage of T4 cells and in the T4:T8 ratio was transient but was observed over a 4-week interval (weeks 30 to 34),

Table 1. Clinical, serologic, and immunologic events in chimpanzee 114. Week 0 is a 3-day period during which CH114 received sequential plasma transfusions (150 ml each) from three human donors (P_1, with lymphadenopathy; P_2, with Kaposi's sarcoma; and P_3, with opportunistic infection). LAD is lymphadenopathy: (−) none, (+) 1 cm, (++) 2 cm, (+++) 3 to 4 cm, and (++++) 5 to 6 cm. T4:T8 is the ratio of the number of T4 helper lymphocytes to T8 suppressor lymphocytes (the normal number of T4 is 43.5 ± 7.5, and the normal ratio is 0.96 ± 0.27). Phytohemagglutinin (PHA) and pokeweed mitogen (PWM) responses are expressed as the stimulatory ratio (13); note that this ratio consistently diminished during the period of peak adenopathy. Titers of antibody to HTLV-III were measured by serial dilutions in the ELISA as described (6). Absorbance and dilution data were fitted with a least-squares procedure, and an end point was determined by the value of a normal control serum diluted 1:20. N.D., not done.

Week	LAD	Reciprocal titer of antibody to HTLV-III	Total lymph (per cubic millimeter)	T4 (%)	T8 (%)	T4:T8	Mitogen response	
							PHA	PWM
−2	−	<40	3696	55.0	55.0	1.00	1.0	0.4
0	−	<40	5016	52.2	44.6	1.17	0.8	1.3
2	−	7300	6579	29.5	43.1	0.68	N.D.	N.D.
4	−	3300	4928	42.8	44.7	0.95	1.5	2.1
6	−	2000	4416	36.0	47.6	0.76	0.2	0.7
8	−	1100	4015	41.7	50.4	0.83	1.5	1.4
10	−	1500	4355	51.0	44.8	1.14	0.7	1.2
12	−	3600	3835	51.0	45.8	1.11	1.0	0.9
14	−	7900	4480	40.8	45.3	0.90	N.D.	N.D.
16	−	8100	4029	49.0	45.3	1.08	2.0	2.9
18	−	7100	6228	44.7	47.2	0.94	0.3	0.2
20	−	9200	5580	38.6	45.2	0.85	0.7	1.2
22	−	6700	4154	38.1	45.3	0.84	1.4	2.1
24	+++	6700	5544	28.2	50.9	0.55	0.4	1.1
26	+++	7000	3102	39.8	44.6	0.89	0.3	0.5
28	+++	9700	6790	39.3	45.1	0.87	0.2	0.3
30	++++	5900	4620	19.3	44.8	0.43	0.5	0.6
32	++++	5120	5440	26.4	52.0	0.51	0.6	0.4
34	++++	4000	6003	28.2	44.0	0.64	0.1	0.2
36	++++	3000	3330	41.5	43.6	0.95	0.4	0.6
38	++++	4400	5280	38.1	42.3	0.90	0.3	0.6
40	++++	4100	3672	34.6	45.9	0.75	0.4	1.3
42	++++	4000	5360	36.6	40.4	0.91	0.5	0.3
44	++++	3600	5076	36.5	48.0	0.76	0.6	0.5
46	++++	4400	4275	26.6	46.4	0.57	0.5	1.2
48	++++	4500	3689	43.1	47.0	0.92	2.5	2.4
50	++++	3100	5593	44.9	36.9	1.22	0.4	1.3
54	+++	3480	4599	32.4	48.9	0.66	0.3	0.2
56	++	2650	5005	30.1	52.9	0.57	1.2	0.8
58	−	2550	4465	34.9	46.8	0.75	1.6	1.1

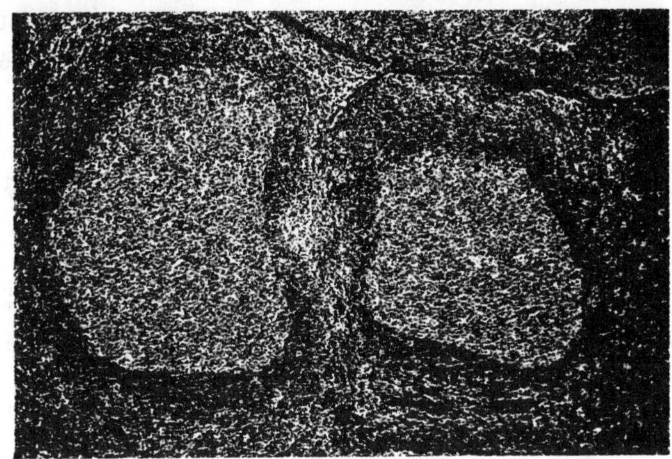

Fig. 2. Photomicrograph of a lymph node biopsy specimen from CH114 showing severe lymphoid hyperplasia with markedly enlarged germinal centers populated by cells with large vesicular nuclei and an indistinct eosinophilic cytoplasm. Mitotic figures are numerous. A biopsy done before inoculation did not show these hyperplastic changes.

which coincided with the early period of peak adenopathy. Thereafter, immunologic factors returned to baseline levels. Despite the development of antibodies to HTLV-III, the adenopathy, and the immune defects, CH114 remained clinically well throughout 1 year of follow-up studies. In essence, this chimpanzee developed a syndrome similar to that of donor P_1 (asymptomatic lymphadenopathy syndrome) except that the immune defects were more transient.

The last animal (CH133, Fig. 1C) was used in a two-phase experiment. First, repeated inoculations of single-donor cryoprecipitate were given to determine whether the immunologic abnormalities frequently observed in hemophiliac patients (12) could be induced in this manner and whether stimulation with foreign protein might enhance susceptibility to subsequent doses of plasma or lymphocytes contaminated with the AIDS agent. The intermittent administration of 39 units of single-donor cryoprecipitate did not result in depression of the T4:T8 ratio or in the development of antibodies to HTLV-III (Fig. 1C). In the second phase of the study, beginning at week 26, CH133 received 150 ml of lymphocyte-rich plasma (LP) from donor LP_1 (the same donor whose plasma was given to CH114). On week 31, CH133 received lymphocyte-rich plasma from donor LP_4, a patient with Kaposi's sarcoma (HTLV-III antibody titer, 1:24,000). On week 32, plasma and lymphocytes from donor LP_5, a patient with an extensive lymphadenopathic form of Kaposi's sarcoma (HTLV-III antibody titer, >1:1,000,000), were administered.

The interpretation of HTLV-III antibody response in CH133 is confounded by the intervals between transfusions and the large volume of passively administered antibody. Nonetheless, it appears that this animal developed an active HTLV-III antibody response on the basis of (i) the plateau of antibody titer beginning at week 50, a pattern inconsistent with the continuous decay curve of passively administered antibody as seen in CH132 (Fig. 1A), and (ii) the initial appearance of IgM antibodies to HTLV-III at week 32, which persisted through week 40 when last tested. An IgM antibody to HTLV-III was not observed in CH132 (which showed only passive transfer of antibody) but was detected early in the course of HTLV-III antibody production in HTLV-III–infected CH114. CH133 manifested no clinical or immunologic evidence of AIDS.

The control animal, CH140, received plasma from three normal donors negative for antibodies to HTLV-III. No clinical or immunologic evidence of AIDS was noted, and no specific HTLV-III antibody response developed. As additional controls, 15 uninoculated chimpanzees housed at SFBR were tested, and all were found to be negative for antibody to HTLV-III.

Our results show that (i) the chimpanzee is susceptible to HTLV-III infection and can thus serve as an infectivity model for the study of AIDS; (ii) in addition to HTLV-III antibody seroconversion, the chimpanzee can develop a clinical syndrome of lymphadenopathy and immunologic impairment providing a disease model that simulates the human AIDS-related lymphadenopathy syndrome; and (iii) HTLV-III infection can be transmitted by lymphocyte-poor plasma, substantiating the potential AIDS risk of noncellular blood components such as pooled clotting-factor concentrates. The susceptibility of the chimpanzee to HTLV-III infection will provide an animal model of AIDS in which to assess antiviral agents and biologic response modifiers and, most importantly, in which to test the safety, immunogenicity, and efficacy of future vaccines.

References and Notes

1. A. S. Fauci *et al.*, *Ann. Int. Med.* **100**, 92 (1984).
2. J. W. Curran *et al.*, *N. Engl. J. Med.* **310**, 69 (1984); H. W. Jaffe *et al.*, *Science* **223**, 1309 (1984).
3. M. Popovic, M. G. Sarngadharan, E. Read, R. C. Gallo, *Science* **224**, 497 (1984); R. C. Gallo *et al.*, *ibid.*, p. 500.
4. M. G. Sarngadharan *et al.*, *ibid.*, p. 506.
5. J. F. Barré-Sinoussi *et al.*, *ibid.* **220**, 868 (1983); L. B. Montagnier *et al.*, in *Human T-Cell Leukemia Viruses*, R. C. Gallo, M. Essex, L. Gross, Eds. (Cold Spring Harbor Laboratory, Cold Spring Harbor, N.Y., in press).
6. Centers for Disease Control Task Force on Kaposi's Sarcoma and Opportunistic Infections, *N. Eng. J. Med.* **306**, 248 (1982).
7. J. W. Eichberg *et al.*, *Dev. Comp. Immunol.* **4**, 135 (1981); R. L. Siegel and R. W. Fox, *Adv. Exp. Med. Biol.* **166**, 295 (1983).
8. W. C. Saxinger and R. C. Gallo, *Lab. Invest.* **49**, 371 (1983).
9. H. Towbin, T. Staehelin, J. Gordon, *Proc. Natl. Acad. Sci. U.S.A.* **76**, 4350 (1979).
10. W. C. Saxinger *et al.*, *Science*, in press.
11. J. W. Eichberg, personal communication.
12. Centers for Disease Control, *Morbidity Mortality Wkly. Rep.* **31**, 365 (1982).
13. The stimulatory ratio was calculated as follows. A stimulatory index, representing the amount of label (in counts per minute) of cells plus mitogen divided by that of cells plus medium, was calculated in each test for each animal. The stimulatory ratio is that of the index for CH114 to the index for CH140 (a control animal), the index of each being determined simultaneously in the identical assay.
14. We thank G. Nemo and L. Barbosa for helpful advice; A. Bodner, F. Laurent, M.-W. Hoh, and D. Lawlor for technical assistance; and the staffs of the Medicine Branch (NCI), Critical Care Medicine Department (NIH), and the National Institute of Allergy and Infectious Diseases for care of the patients. Supported by the Division of Blood Diseases and Resources of the National Heart, Lung, and Blood Institute, NIH.

16 August 1984; accepted 17 September 1984

64. The AIDS Connection

Gina Kolata

Sleeping sickness is caused by African trypanosomes, which are protozoa. AIDS seems to be caused by a type of RNA virus. At first glance, the two diseases seem to have little in common. But several groups of investigators are currently looking to see if the trypanosomes may have similar effects to those of the AIDS viruses on the immune system and, if so, whether that can lead to new insights into either disease.

John Mansfield of the University of Louisville, for example, finds that trypanosomes produce immune system changes in mice that very much resemble the changes seen with AIDS. Whether the same effects occur in humans is unclear, but a team of scientists from the Centers for Disease Control, the National Institutes of Health, and Zaire are currently in Zaire testing and comparing patients with AIDS to patients with any of several parasitic diseases, including sleeping sickness, to see how these parasites affect immune functions. Results should be available in December, according to Thomas Quinn of Johns Hopkins University School of Medicine and the NIH.

The investigators in Zaire are not just looking to see if sleeping sickness and AIDS produce the same immune suppression. They are also investigating a hypothesis that AIDS is prevalent in Zaire because trypanosomiasis and other parasitic infections that occur in Zaire render patients less able to fight off the AIDS virus.

A final AIDS connection is with suramin, a drug that is commonly used to treat sleeping sickness. Recently, Robert Gallo and his associates at the NIH discovered that it is effective against the putative AIDS virus in vitro (*Science*, 12 October 1984). They are now beginning studies to see if it can be administered to AIDS patients. Samuel Broder, a member of the NIH group, attributes the drug's effectiveness against both African trypanosomes and AIDS viruses to serendipity. But it is another intriguing link between the ancient disease of trypanosomiasis and the recently discovered AIDS.

65.   AIDS Amendment Angers Cancer Institute

Barbara J. Culliton

Just before Congress recessed for the presidential election, it passed an amendment to the Health and Human Services' appropriations bill that added $14.6 million to the Administration's budget request for research on AIDS (acquired immune deficiency syndrome). The amendment, which was proposed on the floor of the Senate by Alan Cranston (D–Calif.), provides an extra $11.2 million for the Centers for Disease Control (CDC), $2.6 million for the National Institute of Allergy and Infectious Diseases, $822,000 for the National Institute of Mental Health, and nothing at all for the National Cancer Institute (NCI), where virologists identified the AIDS virus last spring.

Senator Cranston, who sees his amendment as an indication of congressional support for AIDS research, suddenly found himself in the cross fire of an intra-HHS dispute when cancer researchers accused him of favoring other health agencies to the exclusion of the NCI, which has done a great majority of the pioneering work on this deadly and still-spreading disease. Although NCI officials are tight-lipped on the subject, their irritation was expressed for them by members of the cancer community who serve in various advisory capacities. For example, on behalf of the Board of Scientific Counselors of the NCI's cancer etiology division, G. Barry Pierce of the University of Colorado Medical Center wrote Cranston that he was "dismayed" by the Senator's "oversight" in leaving NCI out of the largesse of his amendment.

On the one hand, cancer scientists who are not involved in AIDS research were distressed to find NCI denied additional funds because they believe that the money the institute currently is spending on AIDS is money that otherwise would go for other areas of cancer research. In part, this reflects the idea some people have that AIDS isn't really a *cancer* problem at all and, therefore, that whatever NCI spends on it should come from funds separate from the rest of the budget.

On the other hand, AIDS researchers who have NCI support were stunned to see Congress appropriating extra money for research in other health agencies which, they think, are not as much in the forefront as they. That the competitive spirit between NCI scientists and those in the allergy institute and at CDC is alive and well is evident from off-the-record comments about Congress being inveigled to neglect the NCI.

For his part, Cranston, who appears to have been caught in the middle, denies any such intent. In a response to Pierce he laid responsibility at the feet of HHS officials whose budget recommendations formed the basis of the figures in his amendment. "Our amendment was derived directly from the budget recommendations made by the Assistant Secretary for Health, Edward N. Brandt, Jr., in his May 25, 1984 memorandum to HHS Secretary Heckler," Cranston wrote. In short, said a Cranston aide, the senator was taking his cues from the experts in HHS and, if NCI was not slated for additional funds, it was because of decisions made by HHS officials and by persons in the office of the director of the National Institutes of Health. In fact, that is where the cancer community's ire is directed, not at the senator himself.

Brandt's memo, which was never formally passed on to Congress as an approved Administration request for supplemental funds, asked for a $20 million add-on for AIDS for FY 1984 and an additional $36 million for FY 1985. The Administration chose instead to "reprogram" funds for AIDS from other research in order to avoid an across-the-board increase in the President's budgetary requests. By the time Cranston was drawing up his own amendment, in collaboration with Senators Edward Kennedy, Patrick Moynihan, and Donald Riegle, the amount slated for AIDS research in the cancer institute had grown from the Administration's original request of $18.9 million to $26.8 million. Of that, $2 million was added in the congressional appropriations process but $5.9 million was "reprogrammed" from other NCI activities, just as NCI supporters claim.

At issue is why Cranston, in drafting his amendment, did not put it back. According to the Senator, nothing in the HHS documents he obtained indicated that the reprogramming represented a real problem. "As to the possibility that my amendment should have sought to restore that $5.9 million for other research purposes, I note that the Administration had very recently made the determination, reflected in the NIH allocation sheet, that that amount could be freed up for AIDS research and there was no documentation—such as the Assistant Secretary's May 25 memorandum, which was available to support additional AIDS funding—to support restoring it to the other programs."

From the point of NCI backers on this issue, the cancer institute was left in the lurch by HHS and NIH officials who could have made a case for NCI but failed to. Feelings are particularly strong because it is likely that Cranston would have included money for NCI's AIDS studies if a case had been pressed. However, in light of the fact that the cancer institute's budget is by far the largest of all the NIH institutes, it is hard for NCI to win much sympathy when it pleads for more funds.

Although the Cranston amendment is a fait accompli, the issue of AIDS versus other research programs in the cancer institute budget is sure to come up again. One NIH official, commenting privately on the matter, said, "There is some truth to what the cancer people are saying, but I do think they can absorb this."

66. The Interleukin-2 Receptor Gene is Cloned

Jean L. Marx

Persistence, it seems, pays off. The secrets of the T cell, once a major source of frustration for immunologists, are now being resolved at an accelerating pace. Researchers have taken two major steps toward understanding the activation of T cells, which play a central role in bringing about immune responses. The long elusive T-cell receptor for antigen is finally in hand (see following article). And three groups of investigators have now cloned DNA's that correspond to the gene coding for the receptor for the lymphokine interleukin-2.

Whereas the receptor for antigen is part of the first stage of T-cell activation, in which certain T cells are specifically primed to begin working, the interleukin-2 receptor is part of the common pathway that they must then follow to mount an effective immune attack. Interleukin-2, by binding to the receptors that appear on the antigen-stimulated cells, causes the cells to proliferate, thus greatly enlarging the active population. "Expression of the interleukin-2 receptor is pivotal to whether the T-cell response succeeds or fails," notes Warner Greene of the National Cancer Institute (NCI).

Not only will cloning of the interleukin-2 receptor gene greatly facilitate the study of normal T-cell responses, but it may also aid in the understanding of diseases in which T-cell proliferation is abnormal. In particular, it may help to understand adult T-cell leukemia, which is caused by human T-cell leukemia virus I (HTLV-I). The leukemic cells carry greatly increased numbers of the interleukin-2 receptor, which may contribute to their uncontrolled division. Moreover, another member of the HTLV family, HTLV-III, causes AIDS (acquired immune deficiency syndrome), which is characterized by T-cell death rather than proliferation, and it will be interesting to determine whether this virus has any effect on production of the receptor.

The three groups that cloned DNA's corresponding to the interleukin-2 receptor gene all used similar approaches and obtained comparable results. They first isolated the receptor by precipitating it with a monoclonal antibody. Greene, Warren Leonard, and their NCI colleagues and also Tasuku Honjo and his colleagues at Kyoto University in Japan* used the same monoclonal antibody, which was prepared by Takashi Uchiyama of the Kyoto group when he was working in Thomas Waldmann's NCI laboratory. The third group, from Immunex Corporation in Seattle, which has not yet published their data, isolated the receptor with their own monoclonal antibody.

The investigators then determined the sequence of amino acids on the amino terminus of the receptor protein, con-

---

*W. J. Leonard *et al.*, *Nature (London)* **311**, 626 (1984); T. Nikaido *et al.*, *ibid.*, p. 631.

structed DNA probes corresponding to that sequence, and used the probes to pick out the cDNA's (DNA's copied from the messenger RNA's of cells that make the receptor) with the complementary structure.

The investigators have determined the nucleotide sequence of the cloned cDNA's and from it deduced the amino acid sequence of the receptor protein. The protein consists of 251 amino acids and has a molecular weight of about 28,500, but this is brought up to 55,000 by the addition of sugars and sulfate groups, among other things. Neither the receptor gene nor the protein shares any significant homologies with other known normal genes or oncogenes.

The structural organization of the receptor protein is somewhat unusual. The largest portion, consisting of some 220 amino acids on the amino terminus, is on the outer portion of the cell where it can bind interleukin-2. Then there is a very hydrophobic segment of 19 amino acids that is embedded in the membrane. The surprising feature is the small size of the region that projects into the cell cytoplasm. It consists of only 13 amino acids on the carboxyl end of the protein.

The intracytoplasmic regions of receptors for other growth factors, including epidermal growth factor, are much larger and are kinases, enzymes that attach phosphate groups to cellular proteins, usually to tyrosine residues in the case of growth factor receptors. This activity is probably important for transmitting the growth factor signals to the cell interior. But as Greene points out, "The intracytoplasmic domain of the interleukin-2 receptor is probably too small for an enzymatic function. It is very different from all the other growth factor receptors that are tyrosine kinases." How this

receptor transmits its signals to the cell interior remains a puzzle.

Expression of the gene also displays some interesting features. Although there appears to be only one copy of the gene per haploid cell, both the NCI and Kyoto workers find two major size classes of messenger RNA (mRNA) transcripts. These are 1500 and 3500 base pairs long, and both appear capable of producing a functional receptor protein. The gene contains at least two sites at which transcription may be terminated, and the use of alternative sites apparently gives rise to the two size classes of mRNA. Whether the RNA's have different functions is currently unclear.

In addition, Leonard, Greene, and their colleagues have noted that both major mRNA groups contain a subclass of transcripts that have lost a segment of 216 nucleotides from within the protein coding sequence. Because the missing segment is bordered by sequences that typically mark the boundaries of regions to be cut from mRNA molecules, the investigators propose that it has been spliced out of the messengers. Somewhat surprisingly they find that only the unspliced version can produce a functional receptor. Ordinarily, the spliced messenger produces the active protein.

Studying the control of interleukin-2 receptor synthesis is one of the major goals of the investigators. In contrast to the situation with most receptor systems, the formation both of interleukin-2 and its receptor must be induced. The receptor appears on the surfaces of T cells only after they have been specifically activated by antigen binding. This presumably helps to ensure that only the activated cells proliferate in response to the growth factor. Interleukin-2 itself induces an increase in the receptor number. Eventually, however, the number of receptors declines. The decrease, which may contribute to the normal termination of the immune response, results from a decrease in transcription of the receptor gene, according to Greene and Leonard. The unusual splicing pattern also raises the possibility that receptor number may be partially controlled by regulating splicing of the mRNA's.

Of special interest are the interleukin-2 receptors of cells that have been made leukemic by HTLV-I. These receptors are present in high numbers, some five to ten times more than appear on normal, activated T cells. They may also show qualitative differences. In some leukemic cell lines they are slightly smaller than normal, although this difference is in the carbohydrate and sulfate residues, not in the protein portion of the molecule. However, until receptor genes of normal and HTLV-I–transformed cells are compared, slight differences in amino acid sequence can not be ruled out. All three groups originally cloned the gene from transformed cell lines. Work on the normal gene is under way.

Current work suggests that HTLV-I may transform cells by producing a protein that increases gene transcription. For example, the uncontrolled proliferation of the cells might result if genes that regulate cell division are abnormally switched on. One obvious candidate for this is the interleukin-2 receptor gene. The cloning work means that this hypothesis can now be readily tested.

67. More on the T-Cell Receptor

Jean L. Marx

The remarkable progress in characterizing the T-cell receptor for antigen continues. Two groups, one from Mark Davis's laboratory at Stanford University School of Medicine and the other including Susumu Tonegawa, Herman Eisen, and their colleagues at the Massachusetts Institute of Technology, have just reported the cloning of what they carefully call "a third type of T-cell receptor gene" (*1*). However, there can be very little doubt that the investigators have in fact cloned genes for the α-chain of the T-cell receptor, which, as other investigators have shown, consists of two protein chains. Davis, in collaboration with Stephen Hedrick of the University of California at San Diego, and, independently, Tak Mak, Yusuke Yanagi, and their colleagues at the Ontario Cancer Institute in Toronto, cloned the first β-chain genes about a year ago. With the α-chain gene now in hand, immunologists are getting their first look at both T-cell receptor proteins.

The new clones displace another cloned gene that the MIT workers had proposed earlier this summer as a candidate α-chain gene. This gene has many of the predicted characteristics of a T-cell receptor gene. It is expressed only in T cells, is structurally related to the β-chain and immunoglobulin genes, and, like these genes, rearranges to produce the active form as T cells mature. Further work has made it extremely unlikely that this is an α-chain gene, however. In particular, the protein it encodes lacks sites for attaching the *N*-linked sugar residues that are commonly found on receptor proteins and have now been shown by various investigators to be present on α-chains from several sources. Moreover, John Kappler and Philippa Marrack of the National Jewish Hospital in Denver and their colleagues have determined portions of the amino acid sequence of a human α-chain and find little resemblance to the protein encoded by the earlier MIT clone *(2)*.

The evidence that the new clones represent α-chain genes appears unassailable. They meet all the criteria listed above and their proteins have appropriate glycosylation sites. The structural organization of their products resembles those of the β-chain and antibody proteins. The β-chain, like the heavier of the two chains of which antibodies are composed, consists of four separately encoded regions, which have been designated as the V (for variable), D (diversity), J (joining), and C (constant) regions. The current work shows that the α-chain consists at least of V, J, and C regions. It may also contain a D region, although this is not yet certain. Moreover, the clone prepared by the Stanford group from helper T cells, and the one prepared by the MIT group from cytotoxic T cells, contain the same C-region coding sequence. Their V regions are different, which is to be expected because the cells of origin recognize different antigens.

In addition, an α-chain peptide with 17 amino acids that was sequenced by the Kappler-Marrack group is almost identical to corresponding segments of the proteins encoded by the clones of the Stanford and MIT groups. Finally, Davis and his colleagues note that comparison of their murine α-chain sequence with that of a human α-chain studied in Jack Strominger's laboratory at Harvard University suggests that the two are species variants of the same molecule *(3)*.

The function of the gene represented by the earlier MIT clone remains an intriguing puzzle. The gene has a number of interesting features. According to Tonegawa, it varies slightly in structure from one T-cell line to another, which is one of the predicted characteristics of a gene coding for a receptor, such as the T-cell receptor, that must recognize many different antigens. The T-cell receptor recognizes antigens only in conjunction with appropriate histocompatibility molecules. For many years there has been a debate over whether there are two separate receptors on the T cell, one for antigen and one for the histocompatibility molecule, or a single receptor that recognizes both together. The evidence generally favors the single receptor hypothesis but, Tonegawa suggests, the variability of the mystery gene raises the possibility that it might encode a second receptor. More work will be required to resolve this issue.

Meanwhile, Davis and his Stanford colleague Phillip Patten have evidence suggesting that the β-chain may have sites for recognizing both the antigen and histocompatibility molecule *(4)*. They have compared the amino acid sequences of three recently determined β-chain variable regions with the four that were already known and find that β-chains appear to have seven especially variable subregions, in contrast to the three hypervariable regions found in antibody chains, which are part of the antigen-binding site. The corresponding segments of the β-chain may also bind antigen, the Stanford work suggests, whereas the remaining

350

hypervariable regions may be involved in contacts with the histocompatibility molecule—provided, of course, that one receptor recognizes both.

Additional Reading

1. Y-H. Chien *et al.*, *Nature (London)* **312**, 31 (1984); H. Saito *et al.*, *ibid.*, p. 36.
2. C.H. Hannum *et al.*, *ibid.*, p. 65.
3. N. Jones *et al.*, *Science*, in press.
4. P. Patten *et al.*, *Nature (London)* **312**, 40 (1984).

Report

30 November 1984

68. Diagnostic Potential for Human Malignancies of Bacterially Produced HTLV-I Envelope Protein

Kenneth P. Samuel, James A. Lautenberger, Cheryl L. Jorcyk, Steven Josephs, Flossie Wong-Staal, and Takis S. Papas

Human T-cell leukemia virus subgroup I (HTLV-I) is a retrovirus causatively linked to certain adult lymphoid malignancies, notably adult T-cell leukemia-lymphoma (ATL) (*1*). Many isolates of this virus, identified in the United States, the Caribbean basin (*2*), southwestern Japan (*3*), Israel (*2*), Europe (*4*), and Africa (*5*), have been shown to be nearly identical (*6*). Two other isolates (HTLV-II), including one from a patient with T-cell hairy cell leukemia (*7*), are related to HTLV-I but differ significantly in antigen assays and in their genomes (*8*). A third subgroup of HTLV (HTLV-III) that is associated with the acquired immune deficiency syndrome (AIDS) has been described (*9*).

Antibodies that react with HTLV-I proteins have been found in the sera of ATL patients. These antibodies recognize both the *gag* core antigens and the envelope proteins of the virus (*10*). Viral core proteins were purified (*11*), sequenced (*12*), and used extensively in immunoassays (*13*); however, progress with the more important viral envelope proteins was slow. A limiting factor, therefore, in studies of the immune response to these viruses has been the difficulty in isolating the viral envelope proteins in pure form and in quantity.

As an alternative approach, we expressed the virus envelope protein in a bacterial vector. This procedure has the advantage that only a single viral product as defined by the structure of the input DNA is made by the bacteria. HTLV-I was suitable for such an approach because the integrated proviral DNA has been cloned (*14, 15*) and sequenced (*16*). We chose to express the HTLV-I envelope by placing it into the pJLA16 derivative (*17*) of plasmid pJL6 (*18*). This plasmid contains the 13 amino terminal codons of the bacteriophage λ *c*II gene placed under the transcriptional control of the well-regulated phage λ p_L promoter. This plasmid has been used to express sequences from *myc*, *myb*, and *ras* oncogenes (*18, 19*).

Initial attempts to express the entire HTLV-I envelope were unsuccessful, possibly because this protein can interact with the bacterial cell membrane in such a way as to be toxic to the cell. Therefore, individual fragments coding for specific regions of the envelope were inserted into pJLA6 by use of polynucleotide linkers (Fig. 1). Such plasmids were introduced into *Escherichia coli* MZ1, a strain that contains a partial λ prophage bearing the mutant cI857 temperature-sensitive repressor. At 32°C the repressor is active, and the p_L promoter on the plasmid is repressed. At 42°C the repressor is inactive and the p_L promoter is induced, allowing a high level of expression of genes under its transcriptional control. When lysogens carrying either of the two plasmids containing different portions of the HTLV-I envelope gene were grown at 32°C and induced by shifting the temperature to 42°C, prominent bands were revealed by sodium dodecyl sulfate–polyacrylamide gel electrophoresis (SDS-PAGE) that were not found in uninduced cells or in induced cells containing the pJL6 vector alone (Fig. 2). These proteins were observed in gels of isotopically labeled bacterial extracts and in gels stained for total protein. On the basis of DNA sequence data of the envelope gene fragments, the calculated molecular sizes of the pKS300 and pKS400 proteins are 12.84 and 15.88 kilodaltons (kD), respectively. These sizes include the 1.56-kD coding sequence contributed by the amino terminal codons of the λ cII gene. The molecular weights of both proteins determined by SDS-PAGE are consistent with those calculated for a 321-base-pair (pKS300

insert) and a 397-base-pair (pKS400 insert) coding sequence.

The HTLV-I *env* gene codes for a glycoprotein (gp61) of molecular weight 61,000 (61K) that is cleaved into the 46K exterior glycoprotein (gp46) and the 21K transmembrane protein (gp21E) (*20*). The precise site of proteolytic cleavage has been determined by locating isotopically labeled valine residues with respect to the amino terminal end of gp21 (*21*). The cleavage of the *env* gene precursor is adjacent to the residues Arg-Arg that are also next to the proteolytic cleavage sites in the bovine leukemia virus and mouse mammary tumor virus *env* precursor (*22*). Because the Bam HI site separating the inserted fragments is close to the region coding for the proteolytic cleavage site that separates gp46 from p21E, the protein from pKS300 contains sequences corresponding to the carboxyl terminal portion of gp46, and the protein from pKS400 predominantly consists of sequences from p21E.

Sera from many patients with HTLV-I–associated ATL and certain other lymphoid malignancies contain antibodies to proteins that have been shown to be the product of the viral *env* gene (*10*). In experiments to determine whether such antibodies can recognize a bacterially synthesized envelope product, a lysate of induced MZ1[pKS400] cells containing this protein was fractionated by SDS-PAGE and transferred to nitrocellulose by electrophoretic (Western) blotting. Strips containing the transferred proteins were reacted with diluted human serum, and the antigen-antibody complexes formed were detected by incubation of the strips with ^{125}I-labeled *Staphylococcus aureus* protein A and subsequent autoradiography. Prominent bands corresponding to reaction of antibody to the

15-kD bacterial envelope product developed when the serum used was from patients with HTLV-I–associated ATL or from HTLV-I antigen (positive) individuals (Fig. 3). No such reactions were observed with sera from healthy control individuals. This procedure was used to screen a group of 28 coded sera. Anti-

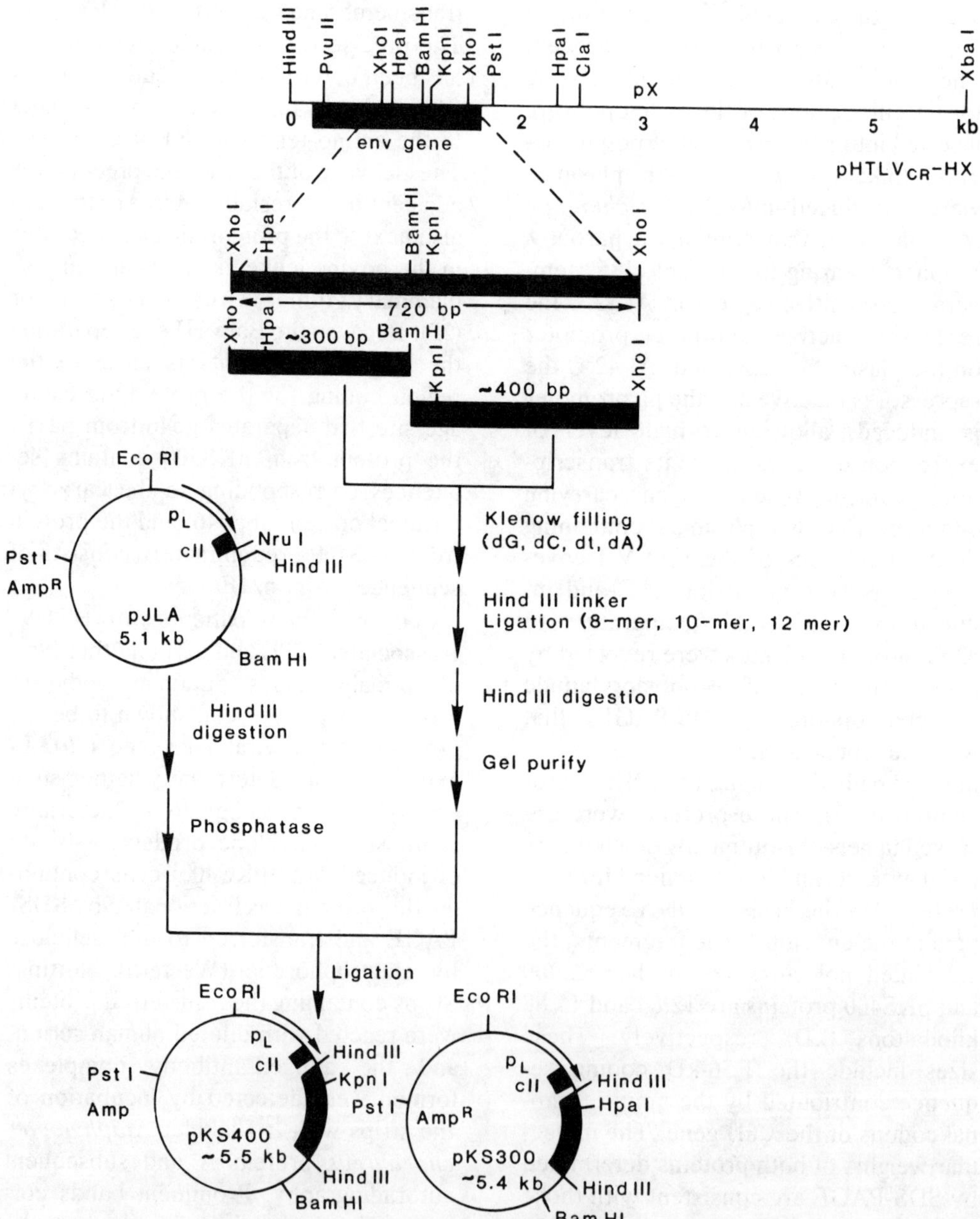

Fig. 1. Construction of plasmids pKS300 and pKS400. Plasmid pHTLV-I HX-CR was obtained by subcloning the 5.7-kb Hind III–Xba I fragment of λ CR1 (*15*) that contains envelope, pX, and long terminal repeat sequences. Recombinant DNA procedures were as described (*24*).

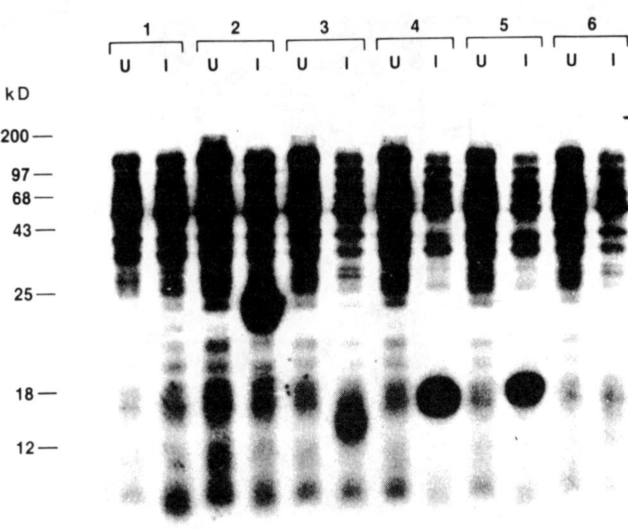

Fig. 2. Expression of the HTLV-I envelope gene in *E. coli* MZ1 cells. Cells were grown at 32°C, induced by shifting the temperature to 41°C, labeled with [^{35}S]cysteine, and lysed (*18*). Proteins were resolved by SDS-PAGE and visualized by autoradiography. Uninduced (U) and induced (I) cell extracts of expression plasmid vectors: (lane 1) pJL6 vector without insert; (lane 2) pJLcII *ras*; (lane 3) pKS300; (lane 4) pKS400.1; (lane 5) pKS400.2; (lane 6) 400-bp fragment in wrong orientation.

bodies that recognized the bacterially synthesized HTLV-I envelope protein sequences were found in all sera that had been shown to have antibodies to HTLV-I by an ELISA (enzyme-linked immunosorbent assay) with disrupted virions as antigen (Table 1). None of the normal control sera were found to have reacting antibodies. Antibodies from a patient (Mo) with a hairy cell leukemia (*23*), whose disease is associated with HTLV-II (*7*), strongly reacted to the protein coded for in pKS400. This indicates that there is a high degree of relatedness between the p21E region of HTLV-I and HTLV-II.

Because the bacterially synthesized HTLV-I *env* protein was recognized by antibodies in sera from an HTLV-II (positive) patient, it was of interest to see if this assay could be used to screen for HTLV-III, an even more distantly related subgroup. Therefore, we examined a number of serum samples from AIDS

Table 1. Antibody recognition of bacterially synthesized HTLV-I envelope in human sera. An ELISA was used to determine the presence (+) or absence (−) of antibody to HTLV-I or HTLV-II in the sera.

Donor status	Antibody	Sera tested (No.)	Sera positive (No.)
Clinically normal heterosexual	+	2	2 of 2
	−	8	0 of 8
Clinically normal homosexual	−	5	0 of 5
AIDS patients	+	2	2 of 2
	−	2	0 of 2
ATL patients	+	5	5 of 5
Mycosis fungoides patient	+	1	1 of 1
Hairy cell leukemia patient Mo	+	1	1 of 1
Lymphadenopathy syndrome patients	−	2	0 of 2

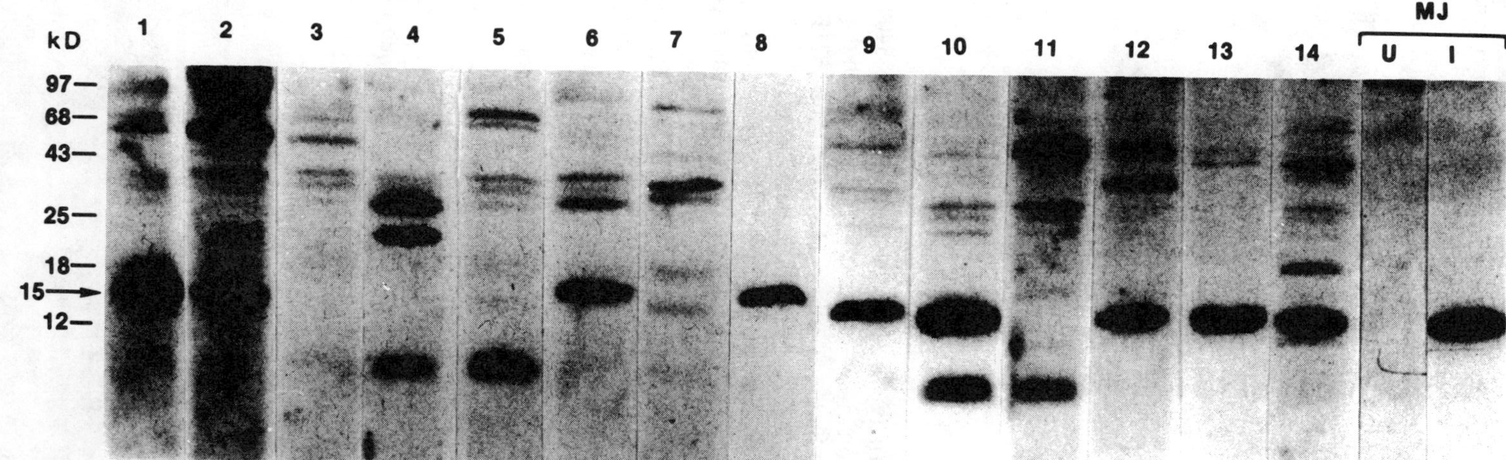

Fig. 3. Recognition of bacterially synthesized HTLV-I envelope protein by antibodies in human serum. MZ1[pKS400] cells were grown at 32°C, induced at 42°C, and lysed in the presence of 1 percent SDS and 0.1 percent β-mercaptoethanol. Protein in the extracts was resolved by SDS-PAGE and transferred to nitrocellulose by the Western blot procedure (25). Serum samples were from the following donors: (lane 1) American ATL patient; (lane 2) T-cell hairy cell leukemia patient Mo; (lanes 3 to 5) healthy normal donors; (lane 6) healthy relative of the ATL patient; (lane 7) healthy normal donor; (lane 8) Japanese ATL patient; (lane 9) AIDS patient found to be HTLV-II(+) by the ELISA (disrupted virus antigen); (lane 10) AIDS patient found to HTLV-I(+) by ELISA (disrupted virus antigen); (lane 11) healthy normal donor; (lane 12) American ATL patient; (lane 13) mycosis fungoides patient; (lane 14) healthy normal donor found to be HTLV-I(+) by ELISA (disrupted virus antigen). Uninduced (U) and induced (I) extracts pKS400 reacted with serum from ATL patient MJ (HTLV-I positive by ELISA). The ELISA assays were performed as described (26) by using HTLV-I disrupted virions.

patients, some of whom were also seropositive for HTLV-I. The sera positive for AIDS that reacted with HTLV-I in the ELISA contained antibodies that recognized the bacterially synthesized HTLV-I *env* protein. None of the sera from AIDS patients that were HTLV-I negative contained antibodies that reacted with this protein. Because antibodies that react with HTLV-III proteins can be found in the serum of more than 90 percent of all AIDS patients (9), this result indicates that there is little or no cross-reaction between the carboxyl terminal portion of the envelope proteins of HTLV-I and HTLV-III. We have not completely analyzed the pKS300 protein product for reactivity in serum of leukemia patients.

These results show the importance of using bacterially synthesized proteins to study the properties of antibodies in human serum. Because the structure of the genes for such proteins can be controlled by recombinant DNA techniques, the antigens produced by these methods have a defined structure. Such antigens could be used in competition experiments to study the structure of natural antigens. The antigens we studied differ from the presumed viral envelope protein in several respects. They consist only of a small fragment of the envelope and are fused to an unrelated phage sequence at their amino terminal end. Furthermore, they may differ in secondary structure since they were synthesized in a bacterial cell and, during the immobilization process of the Western blot procedure, may have undergone denaturation. Our results show that, in spite of these factors, structures are preserved that are recognized by the antibodies to the native viral protein. Because protein can be produced in this manner in less time and for less expense, this approach should be important for large-scale epidemological surveys and for blood-bank assays.

References and Notes

1. B. J. Poiesz *et al.*, *Proc. Natl. Acad. Sci. U.S.A.* **77**, 7415 (1980); B. J. Poiesz, F. W. Ruscetti, M. S. Reitz, V. S. Kalyanaraman, R. C. Gallo, *Nature (London)* **294**, 268 (1981); R. C. Gallo *et al.*, *Proc. Natl. Acad. Sci. U.S.A.* **79**, 5680 (1982).
2. W. A. Blattner *et al.*, *Int. J. Cancer* **30**, 257 (1982); M. Popovic *et al.*, *Science* **219**, 856 (1983); R. C. Gallo *et al.*, *Cancer Res.* **43**, 3892 (1983).
3. M. Robert-Guroff *et al.*, *Science* **215**, 975 (1982); V. S. Kalyanaraman *et al.*, *Proc. Natl. Acad. Sci. U.S.A.* **79**, 1653 (1982).
4. F. A. Vyth-Dreese, P. Rumke, M. Robert-Guroff, G. de Lange, R. C. Gallo, *Int. J. Cancer* **32**, 337 (1983); D. Catovsky *et al.*, *Lancet* **1982-I**, 639 (1982); W. Blattner *et al.*, *Int J. Cancer* **30**, 257 (1982).
5. A. Fleming *et al.*, *Lancet* **1983-II**, 334 (1983); W. Saxinger *et al.*, *Science* **225**, 1473 (1984).
6. F. Wong-Staal *et al.*, *Nature (London)* **302**, 626 (1983); R. C. Gallo, in *Cancer Surveys*, J. Wyke and R. Weiss, Eds. (Oxford University Press, Oxford, 1984), p. 113.
7. V. S. Kalyanaraman *et al.*, *Science* **218**, 571 (1982).
8. G. M. Shaw *et al.*, *Proc. Natl. Acad. Sci. U.S.A.* **81**, 4544 (1984); W. A. Haseltine *et al.*, *Science* **225**, 419 (1984).
9. M. Popovic, M. G. Sarngadharan, E. Read, R. C. Gallo, *Science* **224**, 497 (1984); R. C. Gallo *et al.*, *ibid.*, p. 500; M. G. Sarngadharan *et al.*, *ibid.*, p. 506; B. Safai *et al.*, *Lancet* **1984-II**, 1438 (1984).
10. M. Essex *et al.*, *Science* **221**, 1061 (1983); P. Clapham, K. Napy, R. A. Weiss, *Proc. Natl. Aca. Sci. U.S.A.* **81** 2886 (1984).
11. V. S. Kalyanaraman, M. G. Sarngadharan, B. Poiesz, R. W. Ruscetti, R. C. Gallo, *J. Virol.* **38** 906 (1981).
12. S. Oroszlan *et al.*, *Proc. Natl. Acad. Sci. U.S.A.* **79**, 1291 (1982).
13. V. S. Kalyanaraman, M. G. Sarngadharan, P. A. Bunn, J. D. Minna, R. C. Gallo, *Nature (London)* **294**, 271 (1981).
14. M. Seiki, S. Hattori, M. Yoshida, *Proc. Natl. Acad. Sci. U.S.A.* **79**, 6899 (1982).
15. V. Manzari *et al.*, *ibid.* **80**, 1574 (1983).
16. M. Seiki, S. Hattori, Y. Hirayama, M. Yoshida, *ibid.*, p. 3618.
17. J. A. Lautenberger, A. Seth, C. Jorcyk, T. S. Papas, *Gene Anal. Techniques* **1**, 63 (1984).
18. J. A. Lautenberger, D. Court, T. S. Papas, *Gene* **23**, 75 (1983).
19. J. A. Lautenberger, L. Ulsh, T. Y. Shih, T. S. Papas, *Science* **221**, 858 (1983); J. A. Lautenberger, N. C. Kan, D. Court, T. Pry, S. Showalter, T. S. Papas, in *Gene Amplification and Analysis*, T. S. Papas, M. Rosenberg, J. Chirikjian, Eds. (Elsevier, New York, 1984), vol. 3, pp. 147–174.
20. J. Schupbach, M. G. Sarngadharan, R. C. Gallo,

21. *Science* **224**, 607 (1984).
21. T. H. Lee, unpublished data.
22. A. M. Schultz, T. D. Copeland, S. Oroszlan, *Virology* **135**, 417 (1984).
23. A. Saxon, R. H. Stevens, D. W. Golde, *Ann. Intern. Med.* **88**, 323, 1978.
24. T. Maniatis, E. F. Fritsch, J. Sambrook, *Molecular Cloning: A Laboratory Manual* (Cold Spring Harbor Laboratory, Cold Spring Harbor, N.Y., 1982), pp. 392–397.

25. H. Towbin, T. Staehlin, G. Julian, *Proc. Natl. Acad. Sci. U.S.A.* **76**, 4350 (1979).
26. W. C. Saxinger and R. C. Gallo, *Lab. Invest.* **49**, 371 (1983).
27. We thank M. Robert-Guroff for providing reagents, data, and test serum and R. Gallo for helpful discussions.

24 August 1984; accepted 2 October 1984

Research Article

7 December 1984

69. Molecular Characterization of Human T-Cell Leukemia (Lymphotropic) Virus Type III in the Acquired Immune Deficiency Syndrome

George M. Shaw, Beatrice H. Hahn, Suresh K. Arya, Jerome E. Groopman, Robert C. Gallo, and Flossie Wong-Staal

The human retrovirus that has been isolated repeatedly from patients with the acquired immune deficiency syndrome (AIDS) and from persons at risk for the disease (*1–5*) shares many of the biological and physicochemical properties common to the human T-cell leukemia (lymphotropic) viruses (HTLV). These properties include tropism for T-lymphocytes, induction of multinucleated giant cells, a Mg^{2+} preferring reverse transcriptase of high molecular weight, a relatively small major core protein (molecular weight 24,000; p24), distant antigenic and nucleic acid homology, and a likely African origin (*1–4, 6–10*). Because of these similarities, and because of the uniform nomenclature adopted for the HTLV family of retroviruses (*11*), the

AIDS associated virus was called HTLV-III.

Detailed characterization of HTLV-III and serologic testing of large numbers of patients with AIDS or AIDS-related complex (ARC) became possible when it was found that the virus could be transmitted to a human T-cell line, H9, that is largely resistant to the cytopathic effects of the virus but is a good virus producer (*1*). This cell line has served as the principal source of viral reagents for several seroepidemiological studies of HTLV-III in AIDS (*3–5, 12–16*), and as the source of virus in the present study of the molecular biology of the AIDS agent. In this article, we describe the molecular cloning of two full-length integrated proviral DNA forms of HTLV-III and an analysis of the HTLV-III genome in cell lines and fresh tissues from patients with AIDS or ARC.

Molecular Cloning of the HTLV-III Provirus

Sequences of HTLV-III were first detected in DNA of infected H9 cells (H9/HTLV-III) by Southern blot analysis with the use of a ^{32}P-labeled complementary DNA (cDNA) probe prepared from HTLV-III virions. There was no evidence of such sequences in uninfected H9 cells. The identity of these sequences in H9/HTLV-III was subsequently confirmed by using as a probe the cloned genome of HTLV-III derived from unintegrated linear viral DNA (9). Preliminary analyses of Southern digests of H9/HTLV-III DNA revealed that the virus was present in this cell line both as unintegrated DNA and as proviral DNA integrated into the cellular genome at multiple different sites. Since the HTLV-III provirus was found to lack Xba I restriction sites, a genomic library was constructed by using Xba I–digested H9/HTLV-III DNA, and this was screened with an HTLV-III cDNA probe (8) to obtain molecular clones of full-length integrated provirus with flanking cellular sequences. Fourteen such clones were obtained from an enriched library of 10^6 recombinant phage, and two of these were plaque-purified and characterized.

Figure 1 illustrates the restriction maps of these two clones, designated λHXB-2 and λHXB-3. The overall length of the HTLV-III provirus is approximately 10 kilobases (kb). The identical restriction cleavage site patterns (Bgl II–

Sst I–Hind III) spaced 9 kb apart in the two clones suggested that these regions represent the viral long terminal repeat (LTR) elements. This was confirmed by hybridizing a cloned 0.9-kb cDNA fragment corresponding to the 3′ terminus of HTLV-III to these terminal regions (data not shown). To show that the restriction enzyme cleavage sites depicted in Fig. 1 for clones λHXB-2 and λHXB-3 were actually present in the viral DNA of HTLV-III–infected H9 cells, we digested DNA from the H9/HTLV-III cell line with various restriction enzymes and analyzed it by the Southern blot technique. As shown in Fig. 2 (lanes b), the restriction fragments for Sst I, Eco RI, Hind III, Pst I, Bam HI, and Bgl II predicted from the restriction maps of λHXB-2 and λHXB-3 (Fig. 1) are indeed present in the Southern blots of HTLV-III–infected cellular DNA.

To determine whether the HTLV-III genome contains sequences homologous to normal human DNA, the viral insert of λHXB-2 (5.5 kb and 3.5 kb Sst I–Sst I fragments) was isolated, nick translated, and used to probe HTLV-III–infected and uninfected cellular DNA. Under standard conditions of hybridization [washing conditions: 1 × SSC (standard saline citrate), 65°C; annealing temperature (T_m), −27°C], this probe hybridized to DNA from H9/HTLV-III cells as well as other HTLV-III–infected cells, but not to DNA from uninfected H9 cells, uninfected HT cells (the parent cell line from which H9 was cloned), or normal human tissues (data not shown). This finding is in agreement with the results of other experiments in which the unintegrated (replicative intermediate) form of HTLV-III was used as probe (9) and demonstrates that HTLV-III, like

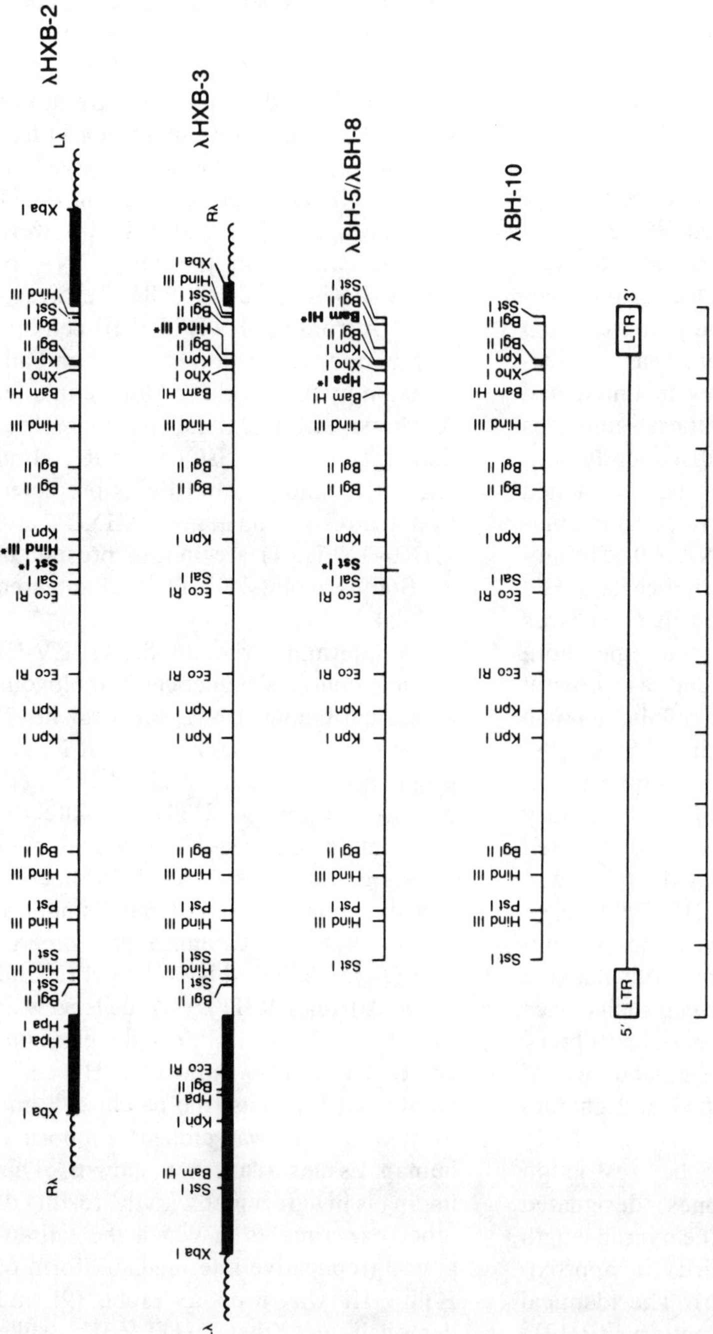

Fig. 1. Restriction endonuclease maps of four closely related clones of HTLV-III. λHXB-2 and λHXB-3 represent full-length integrated proviral forms of HTLV-III obtained from a λ phage library of H9/HTLV-III DNA (36). These clones contain the complete provirus (thin lines) including two LTR regions plus flanking cellular sequences (heavy lines). The LTR regions are known to contain the three restriction enzyme sites Bgl II, Sst I, and Hind III as shown, but their overall lengths are estimated. Clones λBH-10 and λBH-5/λBH-8 were derived from the linear unintegrated replicative intermediate form of HTLV-III in acutely infected H9 cells and have been reported elsewhere (9). Their restriction maps are shown here for comparison with λHXB-2 and λHXB-3 and with Southern blots of genomic DNA from other HTLV-III containing cells. It should be noted that λBH-5/λBH-8 consists of two separately cloned Sst I fragments (λBH-5 and λBH-8) which together constitute one HTLV-III genomic equivalent but which are not necessarily derived from the same viral molecule (9). Also, because λBH-10 and λBH-5 were cloned with the restriction enzyme Sst I (9), they lack 5' LTR sequences as shown. Other differences in the restriction maps between these HTLV-III clones are indicated by bold letters and asterisks, with λBH-10 being used as a reference.

HTLV-I and HTLV-II, is an exogenous retrovirus lacking nucleic acid sequences derived from human DNA.

As noted above, we previously cloned and analyzed the unintegrated linear DNA form of HTLV-III from H9 cells acutely infected with this virus (9). These clones, designated λBH-5, λBH-8, and λBH-10, were characterized in the same way as λHXB-2 and λHXB-3 and are shown for comparison in Fig. 1. The clones of integrated proviral DNA and unintegrated linear DNA are similar to each other yet are distinguishable by differences in several restriction cleavage sites. We know from recent analyses that λBH-10 and λBH-5/λBH-8 are incomplete viral clones that lack a short Sst I–Sst I segment of approximately 190 base pairs in the 5' LTR-leader sequence region as a consequence of the use of Sst I in their cloning. The other differences between these clones must represent differences in the viral DNA restriction patterns since the predicted fragments unique to each clone can be identified in digests of H9/HTLV-III cellular DNA [see Fig. 2 and (9)].

Genomic Diversity of HTLV-III

The finding of different forms of HTLV-III in a cell line originally infected with viral isolates from different patients suggested that the restriction pattern of the HTLV-III genome could vary from isolate to isolate. To test whether such diversity was a common occurrence, we examined the restriction patterns of HTLV-III in a number of different T-cell lines derived from individual patients with AIDS or ARC. In Fig. 2 we compare the restriction pattern of HTLV-III from a Haitian man (R.F.) with AIDS to that of the virus in the H9/

HTLV-III cell line. As shown, the provirus from R.F. contains two Sst I sites, presumably in the LTR regions, which generate a 9-kb fragment indistinguishable in size from that in H9/HTLV-III, λHXB-3, or λBH-10 (Figs. 1 and 2). However, the HTLV-III in R.F. is substantially different from the predominant viral forms in H9/HTLV-III in most other restriction sites, including enzymes known to generate internal viral fragments in H9/HTLV-III DNA (for example, Eco RI, Hind III, and Bgl II). Because of these differences, and because most of the viral DNA in the HTLV-III$_{RF}$ line is polyclonally integrated (and therefore would not produce flanking bands), we conclude that the restriction map of HTLV-III$_{RF}$ must differ substantially from that of the viral forms in H9/HTLV-III cells.

We confirmed these differences by analyzing full-length clones of the HTLV-III$_{RF}$ provirus and showing that they differ from H9/HTLV-III in at least 19 out of 31 restriction sites. Despite these differences in restriction pattern, HTLV-III$_{RF}$ proviral DNA hybridized to λBH-10 probe under conditions of relatively high stringency ($T_m - 27°C$), indicating that the genomes of these viruses overall are similar. This conclusion is further supported by the finding that the major core protein of HTLV-III$_{RF}$ is similar in size (p24) and in antigenic reactivity to other HTLV-III isolates as determined by homologous radioimmunoprecipitation assays (15). Nevertheless, important differences may occur in the genomes of these viruses, for example, in the envelope glycoprotein which is a major determinant of antigenicity for most retroviruses.

In Fig. 3 we compare three more HTLV-III infected cell lines, one derived from a healthy homosexual man

(R.H.) and two others from a child with ARC (M.N.). The isolates from M.N. were transmitted into the uninfected H9 cell line and also into the JM line (*17*), a human T-cell line that is unrelated to H9. Restriction digests with Hind III and Bgl

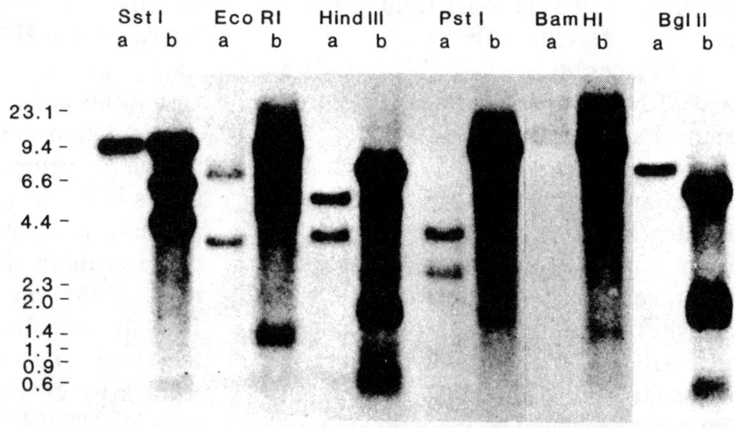

Fig. 2. Southern blot analysis of DNA from an HTLV-III–infected cell line established by coculturing uninfected H4 cells [another cloned cell line from HT cells; see (*1*)] with fresh peripheral blood mononuclear cells of a heterosexual Haitian man (R.F.) with AIDS (lanes a). For comparison, identical digestions of cellular DNA from the H9/HTLV-III line are shown (lanes b). The major internal restriction fragments predicted from clones λHXB-2, λHXB-3, λBH-10, λBH-5 and λBH-8 are apparent in blots of the H9/HTLV-III DNA (for example, see Sst I bands of 9, 5.5, and 3.5 kb, Eco RI band of 1.1 kb, and Hind III bands of 6.4, 4.5, 2, and 1 kb). In contrast, the restriction fragments generated by these same enzymes are quite different for HTLV-III$_{RF}$, indicating that the genome of this isolate is substantially different from the viral genomes in H9/HTLV-III cells. The experimental conditions have been described (*36–38*).

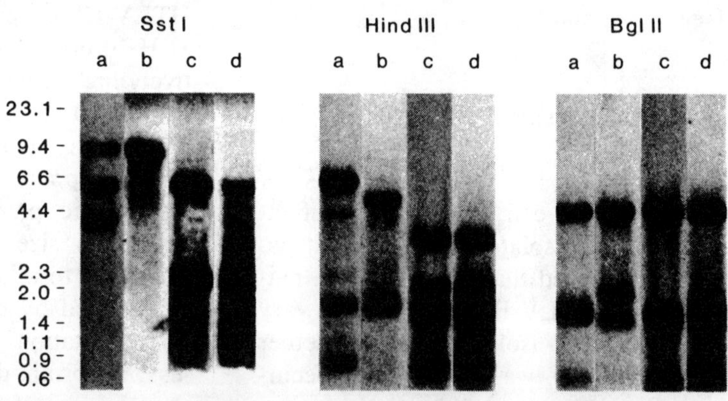

Fig. 3. Southern blot analysis of restriction endonuclease digested DNA from (lanes a) H9/HTLV-III cells and (lanes b, c, and d) from three other HTLV-III–infected cell lines. (Lanes b) DNA from a primary T-cell line established from peripheral blood lymphocytes of a healthy HTLV-III seropositive homosexual man (R.H.). (Lanes c and d) DNA from cell lines MN-1 and MN-2 established by transmission of the viral isolate HTLV-III$_{MN}$ into (lanes c) H9 cells or (lanes d) JM cells. As shown, the restriction patterns of the viral isolates from patients R.H. and M.N. are different from each other and from the H9/HTLV-III viral forms. HTLV-III$_{MN-1}$ and HTLV-III$_{MN-2}$ are identical to each other, indicating that the viral genome was not detectably altered as a consequence of its replication in a particular host cell type. The experimental conditions for this experiment, including the probe (λBH-10i), are the same as described for Fig. 2.

II (as well as Eco RI, which is not shown), indicated that isolate HTLV-III$_{RH}$ is different from H9/HTLV-III. Similarly, HTLV-III$_{MN}$ is different from H9/HTLV-III in its restriction pattern for Sst I and Hind III as well as for Eco RI and Xho I. Moreover, these differences in restriction patterns are not the result of selective pressures associated with H9 cells, since similar patterns were observed for HTLV-III$_{MN}$ grown in H9 or JM cells and digested with a total of seven different restriction enzymes, three of which are shown in Fig. 3.

To determine whether similar variability of the HTLV-III genome occurs in vivo, we examined the restriction enzyme cleavage patterns of HTLV-III DNA in freshly biopsied lymph nodes from one patient with ARC (K.C.) and another with AIDS (F.O.). In the HTLV-III viral DNA from patient K.C. (Fig. 4A), two major Sst I bands were present, as in H9/HTLV-III cells and in λHXB-2. However, the Hind III and Bgl II fragments did not correspond to fragments in any of the other isolates or clones of HTLV-III, and the cut made by Xba I within the provirus was unlike that in any other HTLV-III so far studied. In contrast to the viral DNA in isolate HTLV-III$_{KC}$, the viral DNA in HTLV-III$_{FO}$ (Fig. 4B) corresponds in its major Sst I, Eco RI, Hind III, and Bgl II fragments to those in λBH-10 and λHXB-3. We assume that the small bands are present but too faint to be seen in this blot and that the Eco RI band is a doublet generated by cutting two internal Eco RI sites in predominantly unintegrated linear viral DNA (see Fig. 5). In one other HTLV-III–containing fresh tissue specimen the virus was similar to λHXB-2 in its Sst I and Bgl II patterns but different in its Hind III pattern (data not shown). In all, we examined 12 different HTLV-III isolates from either fresh or cultured cells. Five of them could be distinguished from each other by substantial differences in their restriction cleavage patterns. Seven others, including the four highly related forms cloned from the H9/HTLV-III cell line, were similar to (but not necessarily identical with) one of the first five. From these results it was not possible to differentiate between isolates from patients with AIDS and ARC on the basis of their restriction patterns.

The diversity in the genomic restriction maps of different HTLV-III isolates stands in contrast to the high degree of conservation in the genomes of HTLV-I and HTLV-II. For example, Wong-Staal et al. (18) reported that ten out of ten HTLV-I isolates from different regions of the world had conserved internal Pst I and Bam HI cleavage sites. Similarly, in a survey of 88 patients with adult T-cell leukemia (ATL) in Japan, Yoshida et al. (19) found that the Pst I sites in the HTLV-I proviruses were similar in 79 (90 percent) of them. Preliminary analysis of the exceptional nine cases indicated that these represented defective proviruses and not complete HTLV-I proviruses with divergent restriction patterns. These investigators also compared isolates of HTLV-I from Japan and the United States and found them to be quite similar (19). We have cloned and analyzed HTLV-I proviruses from two patients with ATL and have found them to be very similar to each other and to a Japanese clone of HTLV-I whose sequence has been reported (20–22). We have also compared the full-length clones of HTLV-II from two different individuals and have found them to be identical in 25 out of 25 restriction sites (21). Thus, we conclude that the genomes of different isolates of HTLV-III

Fig. 4. Detection by Southern blot hybridization of HTLV-III sequences in DNA from freshly biopsied lymph nodes of (A) a patient with ARC (K.C.) and (B) another with AIDS (F.O.). (A) Five micrograms of DNA from cell line H9/HTLV-III (H9+), 25 μg of DNA from the uninfected cell line H9 (H9−), and 50 μg of DNA from the lymph node cells of

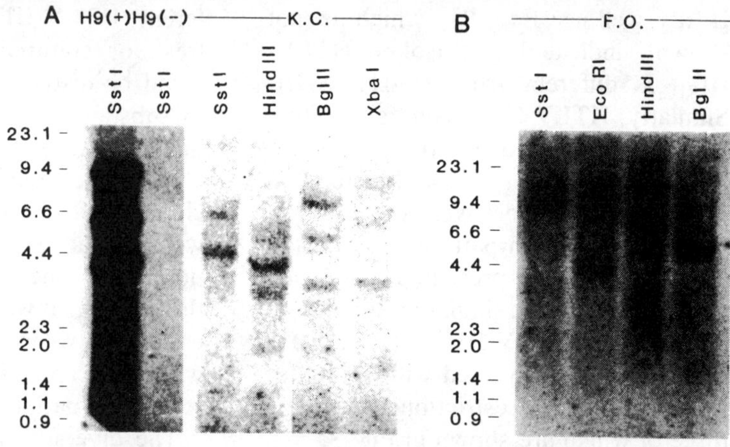

patient K.C. were digested with the indicated restriction enzymes. HTLV-III sequences were detected in the DNA of H9/HTLV-III cells (H9+) and lymph node cells of K.C. but not in the DNA from uninfected H9 cells (H9−). (B) HTLV-III sequences were also detected in the DNA (25 μg per lane) from lymph node cells of patient F.O. [see (35) for methods]. The long exposure time (7 days) and the presence of some degraded DNA account for the heavy background smear in the first lane (H9+).

vary considerably more than do those of either HTLV-I or HTLV-II.

Unintegrated Viral DNA and Cytopathic Effects

In the life cycle of a retrovirus, the single-stranded RNA genome must be copied by reverse transcriptase into an unintegrated linear DNA form prior to its integration into the host cell's chromosomal DNA (23). The linear unintegrated DNA duplex contains a copy of the viral genome in a nonpermuted order and can generally be detected only as a short-lived replication intermediate in the cytoplasm of infected cells shortly after viral infection. Persistence of the unintegrated form of viral DNA has been observed uncommonly in certain animal retroviral systems (24, 25) and has been correlated with the cytopathic effects of these retroviruses (24). In cells freshly

infected with HTLV-III, in chronically infected cells, and even in biopsied lymph node tissue from a patient with AIDS, we have found that a substantial amount of HTLV-III DNA persists in the unintegrated form, mostly as linear double-stranded DNA but also in much lesser amounts as closed and nicked circular DNA (Fig. 5). Although we have not quantified the actual numbers of unintegrated as opposed to integrated viral DNA forms per cell, we have found, in most cell lines examined, that the intensity of hybridization of the 10-kb band representing unintegrated linear DNA is much greater than that of the high molecular weight smear representing polyclonally integrated proviral DNA and is similar in intensity to internal viral bands generated by enzymes such as Sst I, Bgl II, and Hind III. We have found this relative abundance of unintegrated viral DNA in seven out of eight cell lines and in one out of three fresh tissue specimens, all of which contained detectable amounts of HTLV-III. The importance of this unintegrated DNA in the cytopathic effects of HTLV-III in vitro and in vivo requires further study.

Detection of HTLV-III DNA in

Fresh Tissue

Antibodies to HTLV-III can be detected in most patients with AIDS or ARC (*12*), and HTLV-III can be isolated from a large proportion of these patients (*1, 2, 13*). In the present study, we examined by Southern hybridization a variety of fresh tissue specimens from 65 patients with ARC or AIDS for the presence of HTLV-III DNA. Representative blots of lymph node DNA from a patient with ARC and another with AIDS are shown in Fig. 4. Sequences of HTLV-III were detectable in both tissue specimens but in small amounts. For example, in Fig. 4A, the signal intensity for 5 μg of H9/HTLV-III DNA is much greater than that for 50 μg of lymph node DNA. It should be noted, however, that H9/HTLV-III cells contain many HTLV-III DNA molecules per cell (*26*).

In all, HTLV-III sequences were detected in only 9 out of 65 patients evaluated (Table 1). Roughly the same proportion of ARC patients (3 out of 26) as AIDS patients (6 out of 39) was positive for HTLV-III, and viral sequences were detected most commonly in lymph node (7 of 34) and spleen (2 of 11). None of five Kaposi's sarcoma tissue specimens examined was positive for HTLV-III DNA sequences. These specimens had been obtained from the skin of three patients and from lymph node of two others and had been estimated by histopathologic examination to consist of between 30 and 90 percent Kaposi's sarcoma cells. Since we have found that our Southern hybridizations can detect less

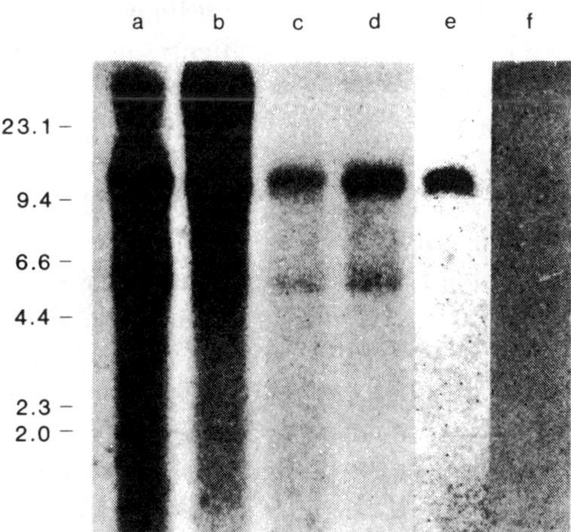

Fig. 5. Demonstration by Southern analysis of unintegrated HTLV-III DNA in cell lines and fresh tissue derived from patients with AIDS or ARC. High molecular weight DNA was extracted as described (*35, 37*). Samples (10 to 20 μg) were then subjected to electrophoresis in standard horizontal 0.8-cm-thick, 0.7 percent agarose gels without prior restriction enzyme digestion and blotted and hybridized to λBH-10i probe as described (*39*). The bands migrating at approximately 10 kb represent the unintegrated linear form of the virus and the smaller bands at approximately 5 kb, the unintegrated closed circular form. Identical bands were obtained when these DNA's were digested with Xba I (which does not cut the HTLV-III genomes in these samples) and when undigested low molelcular weight (Hirt) DNA was examined. (Lane a) Normal peripheral blood mononuclear cells 4 days after infection with concentrated H9/HTLV-III virions (*9*); (lane b) H9/HTLV-III cells 6 months after infection with HTLV-III (*1*); (lane c) JM cells 3 months after infection with HTLV-III (*17*); (lane d) primary RH lymphocytes after 3 months of culture; (lane e) lymphocytes from freshly biopsied lymph node of patient F.O.; and (lane f) normal uninfected human lymphocytes.

Table 1. Survey by Southern hybridization of fresh tissue specimens from patients with AIDS or ARC for HTLV-III DNA sequences. Tissue samples were obtained from 65 patients, and DNA was extracted as described (35). A sample of each DNA (25 to 50 μg) was digested with Sst I (alone) and with Bgl II (alone), both of which generate internal viral DNA fragments in all HTLV-III isolates that we have studied. All other experimental conditions and methods were as described for Fig. 4. A positive and negative control (H9/HTLV-III and normal lymphocyte DNA, respectively) was included on each filter. The DNA on the filters was also hybridized to nick-translated λ phage and pBR322 (lacking HTLV-III sequences) to rule out the possibility that the bands observed could be due to contamination of the fresh tissue DNA's with either of these vectors.

Clinical diagnosis	Number of patients		Number of tissue samples		Tissue tested*
	Tested	Positive	Tested	Positive	
ARC	26	3	7	0	PBC
			18	3	LNC
			1	0	BMC
AIDS	39	6	15	1	PBC
			16	4	LNC
			8	0	BMC
			11	2	SPL
			5	0	KS

*Abbreviations: PBC, peripheral blood mononuclear cells; BMC, bone marrow mononuclear cells; LNC, lymph node cells; SPL, spleen; KS, Kaposi's sarcoma.

than one viral DNA copy per ten cells, we interpreted these data to indicate that the three Kaposi's sarcoma lesions did not contain HTLV-III sequences. To ensure that the Kaposi's sarcoma DNA was of good quality and was adequately digested, we rehybridized the DNA on the nitrocellulose filters to an HLA class I gene probe which readily detected the expected HLA gene fragments (data not shown). Of the nine patients positive for HTLV-III sequences in this fresh tissue survey, more than one tissue type was examined in three. In the first patient, HTLV-III DNA sequences were detected in a cervical lymph node on one occasion (see Fig. 4B) but not in an axillary lymph node or in peripheral blood lymphocytes from the same patient 2 months later. In another patient, HTLV-III DNA sequences were detect-

ed in both lymph node and spleen, and in the third patient, viral sequences were detected in spleen but not lymph node.

In most of the patients in which HTLV-III DNA sequences were detected in fresh tissue, the signal intensities were weak. From dilution experiments with known amounts of HTLV-III–containing DNA, we have estimated that, in the nine positive patients reported here, HTLV-III DNA was present at a level of less than one copy per 10 cells (data not shown). Theoretically, this low signal intensity could also be explained by the presence of a virus distantly homologous to HTLV-III in these cells. This is unlikely, however, because cell lines derived from these tissues are productively infected with HTLV-III (as determined by both nucleic acid and immunologic characterization) and because the restriction fragments in the Southern blots of DNA derived from fresh and cultured cells correspond to many of those present in the cloned genomes of HTLV-III. Furthermore, the genomes of HTLV-III and of the virus referred to as LAV [lymphadenopathy-associated virus (27)] are highly related, so any presumed differences between them could not account for the weak signals detected in AIDS and ARC tissues. We have also hybridized full-length HTLV-I and HTLV-II probes to these infected DNA's and they do not detect viral sequences, thus indicating that the weak signals detected by the HTLV-III probe are not due to hybridization to HTLV-I or HTLV-II sequences.

Discussion

We have described here the molecular cloning and analysis of the full-length HTLV-III proviral genome from the cell line H9/HTLV-III. Since this cell line is the principal source of viral reagents for the seroepidemiological studies of HTLV-III in AIDS (12), and since these H9/HTLV-III–derived viral clones detect viral sequences in fresh and cultured tissues from patients with this disease, we conclude that λHXB-2 and λHXB-3 are representative of the virus that causes AIDS. This conclusion is further substantiated by the fact that these cloned HTLV-III probes detect viral sequences in cells infected with LAV under stringent hybridization conditions (28).

From an analysis of the HTLV-III proviral clones, it is apparent that the viral genome is approximately 10 kb in length (slightly larger than HTLV-I and HTLV-II) and possesses redundant se-

quences, presumably the LTR elements, at each end. Comparison of these full-length proviral clones of HTLV-III with two clones of linear unintegrated viral DNA derived from the same HTLV-III–infected H9 cells (9) indicates that they are colinear and very similar in restriction pattern. These clones of HTLV-III lack any sequences homologous to DNA from uninfected human cells as determined by blot hybridization at moderately high stringency ($T_m - 27°C$).

We have used both biochemical (9) and electron microscopic (26) heteroduplex techniques to determine homology between HTLV-III and HTLV-I and HTLV-II and have found significant homology in the *gag-pol* region. This finding is in agreement with our earlier observations for which we used HTLV-III cDNA (8) and with the immunologic studies of Sarngadharan *et al.* (7). It is interesting that very minimal, if any, homology has been detected between the HTLV-III genome and the pX region of HTLV-I and HTLV-II, since it is the pX region which is most highly conserved between HTLV-I and HTLV-II and is thought to be involved in their transforming properties (20, 29). This difference in relative homologies may be related to the different biological properties of these viruses, HTLV-I and HTLV-II being primarily transforming and HTLV-III cytopathic.

The finding of substantial diversity in the restriction cleavage patterns of different HTLV-III isolates is probably related to the highly replicative nature of this virus (1) and the well-recognized infidelity of retroviral replication (30, 31). This characteristic distinguishes HTLV-III from HTLV-I, the latter being predominantly a transforming virus that exists for long periods in a proviral form that is generally not expressed (*32*). The true extent of the genomic differences in HTLV-III is not known, but for many of the isolates tested the majority of restriction enzyme cleavage sites were different from those found in the HTLV-III clones and in the H9/HTLV-III DNA. In fact, we recently cloned the complete HTLV-III provirus from cell line H9/HTLV-III$_{RF}$ (see Fig. 2) and found that this provirus differs from the proviruses in H9/HTLV-III cells in at least 19 out of 31 mapped restriction sites. Since even a single base pair substitution in a critical region of a retroviral genome can have drastic effects on its biologic function (*31*), further studies involving the expression of HTLV-III genes (such as attempts to express envelope sequences for vaccine production) will need to take into account the genomic diversity of different HTLV-III isolates. However, it may be possible to take advantage of this diversity by evaluating different isolates of HTLV-III for regions of conserved nucleotide sequences. Similar studies have been done with HTLV-I and HTLV-II and have led to new insights regarding the biologic properties of these viruses (*20, 29*). It may also be possible to exploit this diversity in following the transmission of specific HTLV-III viruses both in vivo and in vitro.

Unlike most other retroviruses, HTLV-III appears to persist in both integrated and unintegrated forms in chronically infected cells. We found proviral DNA integrated at multiple sites in eight chronically infected cell lines, indicating that the cell population was polyclonal with respect to the site of HTLV-III integration. These findings distinguish HTLV-III from HTLV-I and HTLV-II, both of which have predominant transforming effects and lead to the proliferation, in vitro and in vivo, of monoclonal-ly expanded populations of cells (*6*). Since HTLV-III has not been shown to possess transforming properties but is cytopathic, it is not surprising that even chronically infected cells contain polyclonally integrated provirus. It is not known whether this polyclonality is due to the continuous reinfection of neighboring cells or to the stable growth of a population of immortalized cells having HTLV-III integrated at random sites. Seven of the eight cell lines, as well as one of the three fresh tissue samples, also contained unintegrated linear viral DNA. The relative proportion of unintegrated HTLV-III DNA and its location (that is, in the cytoplasm, nucleus, or both) have not been determined, and it is not known whether this form of the virus is responsible for its cytopathic effects. Such a mechanism has been proposed to explain the cytopathic effects of certain other retroviruses (*24*).

We have previously been able to isolate HTLV-III from peripheral blood or lymph node tissue from most patients with AIDS or ARC (*12*), in concordance with the 85 to 100 percent seropositivity for HTLV-III in these groups. However, as shown herein, HTLV-III DNA is usually not detected by standard Southern hybridization of these same tissues and, when it is, the bands are often faint. This must mean that only a minor population of cells is infected with HTLV-III at any one time. Thus, the lymph node enlargement commonly found in ARC or AIDS patients cannot be due directly to the proliferation of HTLV-III–infected cells (as occurs with HTLV-I in adult T-cell leukemia). Whether the lymphocytic proliferation in lymph nodes occurs in response to infection with HTLV-III or another agent, or both, is not known. Similarly, the absence of detectable HTLV-III sequences in Kaposi's sarcoma tissue of AIDS patients suggests that this tumor is not directly induced by infection of each tumor cell with HTLV-III. Furthermore, the observation that HTLV-III sequences are found rarely, if at all, in peripheral blood mononuclear cells, bone marrow, and spleen provides the first direct evidence that these tissues are not heavily or widely infected with HTLV-III in either AIDS or ARC. However, on the basis of our ability to culture virus successfully from these various tissues (*13*), it is apparent that each does harbor the virus in a small population of cells. It is likely that the use of more sensitive techniques will increase the frequency of detection of HTLV-III sequences in fresh tissues from patients.

The availability of molecular clones of HTLV-III will now permit the direct comparison of this virus to other retroviruses detected in patients with AIDS or ARC. These viruses, named variously as LAV, IDAV$_1$, IDAV$_2$, and ARV (*27, 33*), are morphologically indistinguishable from HTLV-III and, for those isolates tested, immunologically indistinguishable as well (*34*). On the basis of these results and of our detecting viral sequences in LAV-infected cells using HTLV-III probes (*28*), we believe that HTLV-III, LAV, IDAV$_1$, IDAV$_2$, and the most recently described AIDS-associated viral isolate, ARV, are all essentially the same virus. However, given the diversity in the genomic restriction pattern of HTLV-III reported herein, we would expect similar differences to be present in these other viral isolates.

References and Notes

1. M. Popovic, M. G. Sarngadharan, E. Read, R. C. Gallo, *Science* **224**, 497 (1984).
2. R. C. Gallo *et al.*, *ibid.*, p. 500.
3. J. Schüpbach *et al.*, *ibid.*, p. 503.
4. M. G. Sarngadharan, M. Popovic, L. Bruch, J. Schüpbach, R. C. Gallo, *ibid.*, p. 506.
5. B. Safai *et al.*, *Lancet* **1984-I**, 1438 (1984).
6. R. C. Gallo, *Cancer Surv.* **3**, 114 (1984).
7. M. G. Sarngadharan, L. Bruch, M. Popovic, R. C. Gallo, in preparation.
8. S. K. Arya *et al.*, *Science* **225**, 927 (1984).
9. For a report of the cloning and analysis of the unintegrated linear (replicative intermediate) DNA form of HTLV-III, see B. H. Hahn *et al.*, *Nature (London)*, in press.
10. W. C. Saxinger *et al.*, in preparation.
11. T. Watanabe, M. Seiki, M. Yoshida, *Science* **222**, 1178 (1983); R. C. Gallo, M. Essex, L. Gross, Eds., *Human T-Cell Leukemia/Lymphoma Virus* (Cold Spring Harbor Laboratory, Cold Spring Harbor, N.Y., 1984).
12. From 88 to 100 percent of AIDS patients, approximately 85 to 90 percent of ARC patients, and in one series, 21 percent of healthy homosexual men possess serum antibodies to HTLV-III, whereas less than 1 percent of normal heterosexuals have these antibodies (*3–5, 13–15*). Furthermore, antibodies to HTLV-III have been detected in most hemophiliacs and children with AIDS and in ten out of ten pairs of transfusion-associated donor-recipient AIDS cases (*4, 13, 15, 16*).
13. S. Z. Salahuddin *et al.*, in preparation.
14. J. Schüpbach *et al.*, in preparation.
15. M. G. Sarngadharan, unpublished data.
16. J. Groopman *et al.*, *N. Engl. J. Med.*, in press.
17. S. Z. Salahuddin and P. D. Markham, unpublished data.
18. F. Wong-Staal *et al.*, *Nature (London)* **302**, 626 (1983).
19. M. Yoshida, M. Seiki, K. Yamaguchi, K. Takatsuki, *Proc. Natl. Acad. Sci. U.S.A.* **81**, 2534 (1984); T. Watanabe, M. Seiki, M. Yoshida, *Virology* **133**, 238 (1984).
20. G. M. Shaw *et al.*, *Proc. Natl. Acad. Sci. U.S.A.* **81**, 4544 (1984).
21. G. M. Shaw *et al.*, in *Acquired Immune Deficiency Syndrome: UCLA Symposium on Molecular and Cellular Biology*, M. J. Gottlieb and J. E. Groopman, Eds. (Liss, New York, 1984), p. 59.
22. M. Seiki, S. Hattori, Y. Hirayama, M. Yoshida, *Proc. Natl. Acad. Sci. U.S.A.* **80**, 3618 (1983).
23. J. M. Bishop, *Annu. Rev. Biochem.* **47**, 35 (1978); J. M. Bishop, *ibid.* **52**, 301 (1983).
24. E. Keshet and H. M. Temin, *J. Virol.* **31**, 376 (1979); S. K. Weller, A. E. Joy, H. M. Temin, *ibid.* **33**, 494 (1980).
25. S. Molineaux and J. E. Clements, *Gene* **23**, 137 (1983).
26. F. Wong-Staal, unpublished data.
27. F. Barré-Sinoussi *et al.*, *Science* **220**, 868 (1983); L. Montagnier *et al.*, in *Human T-Cell Leukemia/Lymphoma Virus*, R. C. Gallo, M. Essex, L. Gross, Eds. (Cold Spring Harbor Laboratory, Cold Spring Harbor, N.Y., 1984), p. 363; E. Vilmer *et al.*, *Lancet* **1984-I**, 753 (1984).
28. F. Wong-Staal *et al.*, in preparation.
29. J. G. Sodroski, C. A. Rosen, W. A. Haseltine, *Science* **225**, 381 (1984); W. A. Haseltine *et al.*, *ibid.*, p. 419; J. Sodroski *et al.*, *ibid.*, p. 421.
30. S. Goff, P. Trakman, D. Baltimore, *J. Virol.* **38**, 239 (1981).
31. J. J. O'Rear and H. M. Temin, *Proc. Natl. Acad. Sci. U.S.A.* **79**, 1230 (1982).
32. G. Franchini *et al.*, *ibid.* **81**, 6207 (1984).
33. P. M. Feorino *et al.*, *Science* **225**, 69 (1984); V. S. Kalyanaraman *et al.*, *ibid.*, p. 321; J. A.

Levy, A. D. Hoffman, S. M. Kramer, J. A. Landis, J. M. Shimabukuro, L. S. Oshiro, *ibid.*, p. 840.

34. M. G. Sarngadharan *et al.*, in preparation.

35. Freshly biopsied lymph nodes were minced with a scalpel in 2 ml of isotonic phosphate buffered saline (*p*H 7.4). This cell suspension was made up to 20 ml in tris (20 m*M*, *p*H 7.4), EDTA (5 m*M*), sodium dodecyl sulfate (5 mg/ml), and proteinase K (100 μg/ml) and incubated at 50°C for 3 hours. The DNA was then extracted three times with phenol and chloroform (1:1 by volume) saturated with 50 m*M* tris (*p*H 9.0) and once with chloroform alone, adjusted to 0.3*M* Na$^+$ with sodium acetate (*p*H 6.0), and precipitated with two volumes of absolute ethanol. High molecular weight DNA was dissolved in TE buffer (20 m*M* tris, *p*H 7.4; and 1 m*M* EDTA). The indicated amount of DNA was digested with 150 units of each restriction enzyme for 8 hours at 37°C and then subjected to electrophoresis in 0.7 percent agarose. The probe (λBH-10i) and other experimental conditions were the same as described for Fig. 2 except that 10 × 10^6 dpm of probe per milliliter of hybridization solution was used and the blots were exposed to x-ray film for 7 days.

36. A λ phage library was constructed according to standard methods (*37*) using the cloning vector J1λ (*38*) and Xba I digested H9/HTLV-III DNA which had been enriched by sucrose gradient centrifugation for 10- to 15-kb fragments. Phage plaques (10^6) were screened with cDNA prepared from doubly banded HTLV-III virions (*8*), and 14 positive signals were obtained. Two of these were plaque purified and their restriction maps determined according to standard methods (*37*).

37. T. Maniatis *et al.*, Eds., *Molecular Cloning—A Laboratory Manual* (Cold Spring Harbor Laboratory, Cold Spring Harbor, N.Y., 1982).

38. J. Mullins *et al.*, *Nature (London)* **308**, 856 (1984).

39. High molecular weight DNA was prepared from RF and H9/HTLV-III cells by standard methods (*37*). We used 15 μg of DNA for each restriction enzyme digestion, performed according to manufacturers' recommendations; the DNA was subjected to electrophoresis through 0.8-cm-thick 0.7 percent agarose slab gels. Gels were blotted in 10× SSC onto 0.1-μm nitrocellulose filters (Schleicher and Schuell) (*37*). Hybridizations were performed at 37°C for 18 hours in 2.4× SSC, 40 percent formamide, 10 percent dextran sulfate, 1 mg/ml each of bovine serum albumin, polyvinylpyrollidone, and Ficoll, and 20 μg/ml transfer RNA. Filters were washed for 2 hours at 65°C in 1× SSC. The probe used was the Sst I/Sst I insert from λBH-10, 3 × 10^6 dpm/ml (specific activity approximately 2 × 10^8 dpm/μg). Blots were exposed to Kodak XAR-5 film for 2 days.

40. We thank M. Popovic, P. D. Markham, and Z. Salahuddin for providing the HTLV-III–infected cell cultures. We thank S. Broder, J. Oleske, J. Hoxie, and D. Miller, as well as the staff of the NIH Medicine Branch, for supplying us with clinical specimens, E. Read for technical assistance, and A. Mazzuca for typing the manuscript. G.M.S. was funded through the Intergovernmental Personnel Act of the National Institutes of Health in conjunction with the Ohio State University College of Medicine. B.H.H. was supported by the German Science Foundation and the Fogarty Center for International Studies.

4 September 1984; accepted 16 October 1984

IV

January – September 1985

70. More Progress on the HTLV Family

Jean L. Marx

Human T-cell leukemia viruses (HTLV's) have been linked to two serious and as yet incurable diseases—adult T-cell leukemia and acquired immune deficiency syndrome (AIDS)—and are therefore the targets of an intense research effort. On 6 and 7 December of last year, investigators discussed the status of this research at an "HTLV symposium" that was sponsored by the National Cancer Institute (NCI) and held at the National Institutes of Health in Bethesda, Maryland. There clearly has been rapid progress in understanding the molecular biology of these viruses. The structures of the viral genomes are being elucidated and researchers are beginning to understand how the viruses may alter infected cells to produce the uncontrolled proliferation seen in the leukemia or the immune cell destruction characteristic of AIDS. The new work also suggests that it may be necessary to define a new virus category to accommodate the HTLV's and their relatives.

A major question in AIDS research over the past several months concerns whether lymphadenopathy-associated virus (LAV), which was isolated and causally linked to the disease by Luc Montagnier of the Pasteur Institute and his colleagues, is the same as HTLV-III, which was isolated and causally linked to AIDS by Robert Gallo's group at the NCI. There now appears to be little room for doubt on this issue. The results obtained by the two groups are so similar that it is difficult to imagine how they could be dealing with different viruses.

The structures of the LAV and HTLV-III particles look identical. They both have the same cylindrical cores, for example. Both viruses are transmitted only by close contact. Both show the same strong preference for infecting T4 cells, a subclass of T lymphocytes that includes the helper cells needed for many immune responses. Both kill the T4 cells, which is the apparent cause of the profound immune suppression of AIDS patients. In collaborative studies, the NCI and Pasteur workers have found that the core proteins of HTLV-III and LAV are antigenically indistinguishable and the genomes are highly related as shown by molecular hybridization studies.

The NCI workers now have isolated HTLV-III from more than 100 patients with AIDS or AIDS-related complex, a condition that includes lymphadenopathy as a prominent symptom and may be a mild or early form of AIDS. The Pasteur group has isolated LAV from more than 30 such patients. Researchers on both sides of the Atlantic have generally found that 90 percent or more of patients with AIDS or lymphadenopathy carry antibodies to HTLV-III or LAV, an indication that they were infected with the virus. Less than 1 percent of healthy, nonhomosexual controls have the antibodies.

The final proof that HTLV-III and LAV are the same depends on the results of a comparison of the nucleotide sequences of the viral genomes. This will soon be possible. At least three groups have determined the genome sequence of one or the other or both viruses, although the investigators in question are reluctant to discuss the data before they are published.

Despite the likelihood that HTLV-III and LAV are essentially the same virus, the genomes of the French and U.S. isolates may not prove to be absolutely identical. Work by Gallo, with Flossie Wong-Staal and George Shaw, also of NCI, and their colleagues, has already shown that the genomes of different HTLV-III isolates can show sequence variations, a finding of some concern to those who are trying to develop a vaccine to protect against the virus. If the genome variations are reflected in antigenic differences, a single vaccine may not protect against all virus variants.

Need for a vaccine to protect against AIDS is great. So far, more than 7200 cases from the United States have been reported to the Centers for Disease Control in Atlanta, and the reported number of cases lags behind the actual number by 15 percent, according to James Curran, who heads the CDC's task force on AIDS. The CDC predicts that another 8500 individuals will be stricken in 1985, Curran told the meeting participants.

One of the many puzzling aspects of AIDS has been the high frequency of degenerative brain changes, which cause dementia and other neurological problems and do not appear to be the result of the patients' opportunistic infections. New data* presented at the symposium

*See also M. A. Gonda *et al.* and G. M. Shaw *et al.* in *Science*, 11 January 1985.

suggest that HTLV-III itself may be the cause of the brain degeneration, which afflicts about as many as 75 percent of the patients in the later stages of the disease.

According to Matthew Gonda of the NCI–Frederick Cancer Research Facility, who obtained the results with the Gallo group, the HTLV-III particle is very similar structurally to that of visna virus, which causes a slowly progressing, degenerative brain disease in sheep and goats. "In all stages of development it is difficult to distinguish HTLV-III from visna virus," Gonda says. Moreover, the genomes of the two viruses are partially homologous.

Not only does HTLV-III resemble visna virus structurally but it also infects the brains of AIDS patients, according to data presented at the symposium by Wong-Staal. The viral DNA could be detected in brain cells from 5 of 15 individuals who had died of AIDS and had showed neurological symptoms.

Whereas HTLV-III causes the death of the T4 cells it infects, HTLV-I and -II cause them to undergo malignant transformation and uncontrolled growth. About 6 months ago, researchers began getting their first clues to how HTLV-I and -II might produce these effects. William Haseltine at Harvard's Dana-Farber Cancer Institute and his colleagues obtained evidence indicating that the two viruses each produce a protein with the ability to *trans*-activate, that is, to increase the expression of genes attached to appropriate viral control sequences, whether or not those genes are integrated in the cellular genome. A protein with the ability to stimulate viral gene expression in this way might do the same for cellular genes, including genes participating in the control of cell division.

The investigators suggested that the proteins were likely to be encoded near the 3′ ends of the viral genomes in a region that had been designated "pX" because its coding function was unknown. The 3′ half of that region, which they now call the "long open reading frame" (LOR), is highly conserved between the two viruses and capable of coding for a protein. Shortly thereafter, Haseltine and his collaborators, and, independently, Irvin Chen and his colleagues at the University of California School of Medicine in Los Angeles, demonstrated that the LOR regions of the two viruses are active, directing the synthesis of proteins having a molecular weight of approximately 40,000.

Now Haseltine and his colleagues, in collaboration with Wong-Staal and Gallo, have evidence that HTLV-III also produces a factor with *trans*-activating abilities in infected cells.† The virus is about ten times more active in this regard than HTLV-I and -II. The "exuberant" *trans*-activation by HTLV-III may help to explain why this virus kills infected cells, Haseltine suggests, whereas infection by HTLV-I and -II causes transformation. HTLV-I and -II may have been infecting humans long enough to become attenuated, with the result that they reproduce poorly in cells and are less likely to kill them. Instead the viral genome integrates into the cellular genome and eventually causes transformation of some cells. Meanwhile, HTLV-III, especially if it has arisen more recently, may be less attenuated and still have cell-killing as its dominant effect.

It remains to be seen which cellular

---

†J. Sodroski *et al.* in *Science*, 11 January 1985.

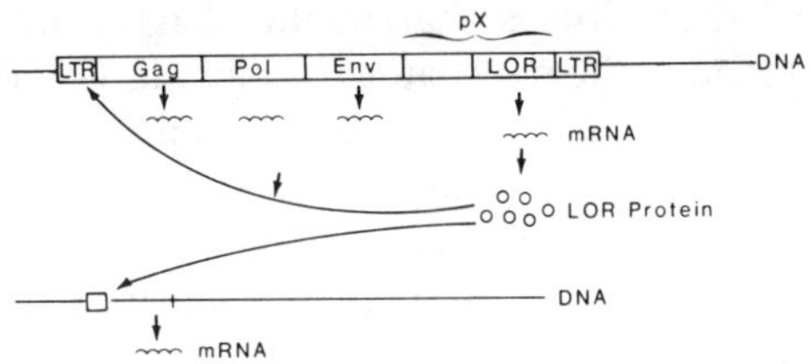

Trans-activation model

genes, if any, are regulated by the *trans*-activating factors of the various HTLV's, and whether these differ from virus to virus. The factors might be specific for different cellular genes, the identities of which would be of great interest to anyone studying the control of cell division. "These viruses may have put their fingers on the pulse of the replicative cycle of the T4 cell," as Haseltine puts it.

The HTLV's are retroviruses, meaning that they have RNA as their genetic material and that the life cycles include a step in which the RNA genomes are copied into DNA. Until recently, they have generally, although somewhat uneasily, been considered to be members of the type C oncornavirus (cancer-causing RNA virus) subgroup of the retroviruses. However, the structures of the HTLV particles are somewhat different from those of other type C retroviruses and they appear to transform by a different mechanism, namely by *trans*-activation. Of course, HTLV-III apparently does not transform at all. For these reasons, many of the researchers in the field are now proposing that the HTLV's ought to be included in a newly defined category of retroviruses. The name HTLV is also being changed to human T-cell *lymphotropic* virus in recognition of the fact that HTLV-III is not a leukemia virus, although it, like HTLV-I and -II, prefers to infect T cells.

374

Other viruses that might also be included in the new category include visna virus, which had previously been placed in the lentivirus (slow virus) subgroup of retroviruses. In addition to its other similarities to HTLV-III, recent work from Janice Clements' laboratory at Johns Hopkins University School of Medicine indicates that visna virus produces a *trans*-activating factor.

Another candidate for inclusion is bovine leukemia virus, which resembles the HTLV's in a number of ways, according to Arséne Burny of the University of Brussels. "It induces in cows a disease that is very like adult T-cell leukemia in humans," he explains, "although in cows it is a B-cell leukemia." The overall arrangement of the RNA genome of bovine leukemia virus is very similar to that of HTLV-I and -II. It also contains a LOR region near the 3' end, for example. Although the exact nucleotide sequence of the bovine leukemia virus genome shows considerable variation from those of the two HTLV's, Burny and others find that the protein products of the bovine virus genes can be antigenically similar to HTLV gene products, including those of HTLV-III. "There is significant divergence at the nucleic acid level, but at the protein level there are regions that are well conserved," he concludes. Finally, Burny with the Haseltine group has evidence for *trans*-activation by bovine leukemia virus, although it is less effective in this regard than HTLV-I and -II.

David Derse and James Casey of the NCI–Frederick Cancer Center and Salvatore Caradonna of Louisiana State Medical Center in New Orleans have made observations concerning bovine leukemia virus that are similar to those of Burny and Haseltine. They, too, find that expression of genes linked to the viral control sequence only occurs in infected cells. However, they propose a different interpretation of the result, namely, that such gene expression requires specific cellular, rather than viral, *trans*-activating factors. They base this interpretation partly on the biological behavior of the virus in tumor cells from infected animals. These cells do not make viral products even though the viral genome is present and integrated in the cellular genome.

This seems hard to reconcile, Casey points out, with the hypothesis that the virus itself makes a factor that stimulates transcription of viral genes, which might be expected to produce explosive viral reproduction. In addition, there must be a way to account for the initial production of a viral *trans*-activating factor. Casey suggests that just certain types of infected cells, perhaps only rarely and at a particular stage of development, can produce the correct activating factor. Subsequently, a product of a viral gene, most likely to be a pX (LOR) region gene, might initiate cancerous transformation but would not be required for maintenance of the transformed state. In previous work, Chen had also proposed that cell-specific factors might contribute to activation of HTLV-II transcription.

Haseltine takes issue with these proposals. He concedes that the question of why there is no viral gene expression in tumor cells is a good one—and an active subject of investigation in his laboratory and elsewhere. But he maintains that for bovine, leukemia virus and all three HTLV's, "the *trans*-activation effect is manifest whether or not the cell is a target cell."

These matters may take some time to resolve. In any event, even if cellular factors participate in the original activation of viral genes, a virus might still produce its own *trans*-activating factor. Infection by certain DNA-containing tumor viruses, including adenovirus and SV40, features both types of events. As Burny points out, "The [HTLV and BLV] family is structurally similar to the RNA viruses, but functionally they are much more reminiscent of the DNA viruses."

Report

11 January 1985

71. *Trans*-Acting Transcriptional Regulation of Human T-Cell Leukemia Virus Type III Long Terminal Repeat

Joseph Sodroski, Craig Rosen, Flossie Wong-Staal, S. Zaki Salahuddin, Mikulas Popovic, Suresh Arya, Robert C. Gallo, and William A. Haseltine

The human T-cell leukemia viruses (HTLV) are retroviruses associated with disorders of the OKT4$^+$ (helper) subset of T lymphocytes. HTLV type I (HTLV-I) is the probable etiologic agent of adult T-cell leukemia (*1*). HTLV type II (HTLV-II) is a rare isolate originally derived from a patient with a T-cell variant of hairy cell leukemia (*2*). HTLV-III is the probable etiologic agent of the acquired immune deficiency syndrome (AIDS), a disease characterized by depletion of the OKT4$^+$ cell population (*3*). In cells infected with HTLV-I or HTLV-II, the rate of transcription of heterologous genes directed by the viral long terminal repeat (LTR) sequences is greatly augmented (*4*). This phenomenon, called *trans*-acting transcriptional regulation, is also shared by bovine leukemia virus (BLV), a virus that appears to be structurally and functionally related to HTLV-I and -II (*5*). The genomes of HTLV-I, HTLV-II, and BLV have a long open reading frame (LOR) located between the *env* gene and the 3' LTR that is not related by primary sequence to vertebrate genomic DNA (*6*). Proteins encoded by the LOR region of HTLV-I and II were recently identified (*7*). We have proposed that the protein product of the LOR region mediates *trans*-acting transcriptional regulation as well as some of the biological effects of virus infection (*4*). HTLV-III is distantly related to HTLV-I and -II by primary nucleotide sequence (*3, 8*) and by antigenic cross reactivity between the 24,000 dalton (p24) proteins and envelope proteins (*9*). In addition, there is a sequence distantly related to the LOR genes of HTLV-I and II near the 3' terminus of the HTLV-III genome (*8*). These observations prompted us to examine the ability of the HTLV-III LTR to function in uninfected cell lines and cell lines infect-

Table 1. Relative CAT activity in transfected cells. The percentage conversion of chloramphenicol to its acetylated forms in cells transfected with HTLV-CAT recombinants was normalized against the percentage conversion in similar cells transfected with pSV2CAT. The values represent the percentage acetylation per unit time relative to that directed by pSV_2CAT. The pU3R-I, pU3-II, and pBLV-CAT plasmids contain the U3 sequences of the LTR's of HTLV-I, HTLV-II and BLV, respectively, located 5' to the CAT gene as described (*4, 5*). The experiments were repeated a minimum of two times each with less than 20 percent variation in the values reported. ND, not determined.

Cell line	Description	pU3R-III	pU3R-I	pU3-II	pBLV-CAT	pSV_2CAT
	Cells not infected with HTLV-III					
HOS	Human osteosarcoma cells	2.0	0.9			1.0
HOS/PL	HTLV-I–infected HOS cell line	1.6	75			1.0
FLK	Fetal lamb kidney cells	1.9	1.6			1.0
FLK-BLV	BLV-infected FLK cells	2.5	0.9			1.0
CCC S+L–	Feline epithelial cells	1.2	0.7			1.0
Raji	Human B-lymphocyte line	2.5	2.0			1.0
MT2	HTLV-I–infected human T lymphocyte line	1.4	130			1.0
C81-66-45	HTLV-I–immortalized nonproducer T-lymphocyte line	2.8	76			1.0
C3-44	HTLV-II producer T-lymphocyte line	1.7	105			1.0
	Uninfected and HTLV-III–infected cell lines					
H9	Human T lymphocytes	3.6	2.5	<0.1	<0.1	1.0
H9/HTLV-III	Human T lymphocytes infected with HTLV-III	1160	3.2	<0.1	<0.1	1.0
L8460D Jurkat	Human T lymphocytes	1.8	ND	ND	ND	1.0
L8460D Jurkat HTLV-III	Human T lymphocytes infected with HTLV-III	500	ND	ND	ND	1.0

ed with members of the HTLV-BLV family.

The transcriptional control elements of retroviruses lie within the U3 region of the LTR (*10*). To examine the ability of the HTLV-III LTR to act as a promoter, we inserted the entire U3 and about 75 nucleotides of the R region from an HTLV-III complementary DNA (cDNA) clone (*11*) 5′ to a chloramphenicol acetyltransferase (CAT) gene (Fig. 1) (*12*). This plasmid (pU3R-III) was introduced into eukaryotic cells via transfection and the level of CAT activity, which is correlated with steady-state CAT messenger RNA levels (*4, 12, 13*), was measured 48 hours after transfection. The CAT activity was normalized to that observed following transfection of pSV$_2$CAT, a plasmid that contains the SV40 early region promoter 5′ to the CAT gene (*12*), to control for differences in the ability of different cell types to take up and express foreign DNA.

The results show that the HTLV-III LTR functions as an efficient promoter in a variety of animal and human lymphoid and nonlymphoid cell lines (Table 1). Apparently, the HTLV-III LTR, like the HTLV-I LTR (*4*), is not dependent on virus-associated *trans*-acting factors for efficient promoter activity, and is not functionally restricted to lymphoid cells. There was no significant stimulation of CAT activity directed by pU3R-III in cells infected with HTLV-I, HTLV-II, or BLV. We conclude that the *trans*-acting transcriptional factors associated with HTLV-I, HTLV-II, or BLV (*4, 5*) do not stimulate gene expression directed by the HTLV-III LTR.

We then examined whether the HTLV-III LTR might be transcriptionally activated by factors present in HTLV-III-infected cells. The pU3R-III plasmid was transfected into uninfected human T-cell lines and matched cell lines infected in vitro with HTLV-III (*3*) (Table 1 and Fig. 2). The HTLV-III LTR was about three to four times as efficient as the SV40 early promoter at directing CAT activity in the uninfected H9 lym-

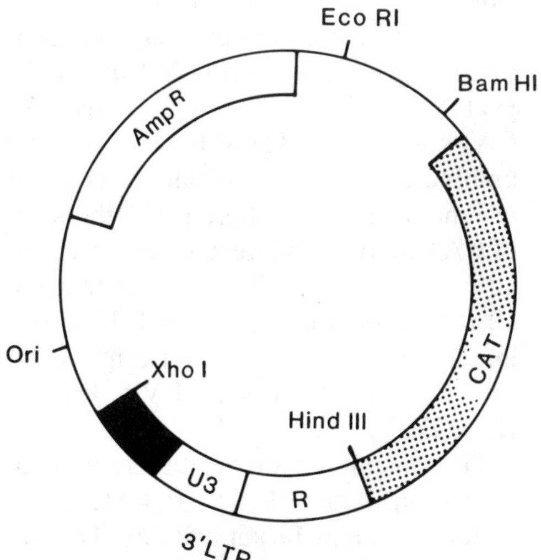

Fig. 1. Construction of pU3R-III plasmid. The diagram depicts the pU3R-III plasmid (Amp^R, ampicillin resistance gene; ori, bacterial origin of replication). The pU3R-III plasmid was constructed by isolating from the HTLV-III LTR cDNA clone C15 an Xho I–Hind III fragment containing the entire U3 and approximately 75 nucleotides of the R region (*11*). This fragment was inserted into the Xho-I–Hind III vector fragment of pSVIXCAT as previously described (*4*). Approximately 180 nucleotides of viral sequence 5′ to the LTR are included in the inserted fragment (solid black box). All recombinant DNA techniques were performed according to the enzyme manufacturer's specifications. Plasmids were purified by centrifugation in CsCl$_2$ gradients prior to transfection.

378

Fig. 2. Transient expression of the CAT gene in uninfected and HTLV-III–infected cells. Uninfected and HTLV-III–infected H9 cells (*3*) were transfected by a modification of the DEAE-dextran technique (*16*). Approximately 5×10^6 cells were washed once in serum-free medium and resuspended in 3 ml of serum-free medium containing 250 μg of DEAE-dextran per milliliter and 50 m*M* tris-chloride, *p*H 7.3 to which 5 to 10 μg of plasmid DNA had been added. After incubation at 37°C for 1 hour, cells were centrifuged, rinsed in serum-free medium, and resuspended in medium supplemented with fetal bovine serum. Cells were harvested 48 hours after transfection and cellular extracts were prepared by freeze-thawing three times. After removal of cell debris by centrifugation, ex-

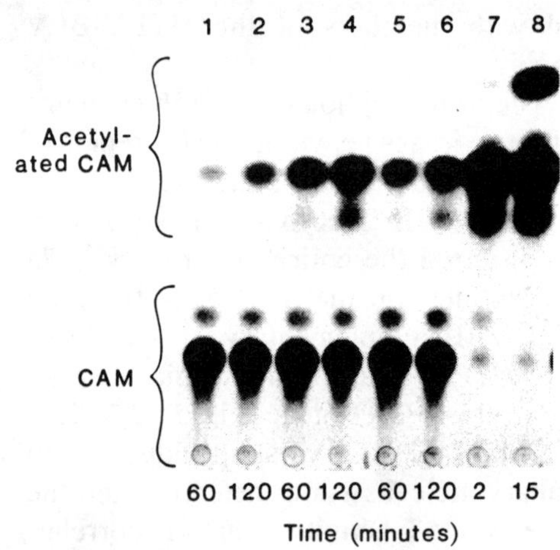

tracts (100- to 200-μg protein content) were analyzed for CAT activity as described (*12*), with 3 m*M* acetyl coenzyme A being used in the reaction mix. Percentage conversion of chloramphenicol to the acetylated forms was determined by ascending thin-layer chromotography and liquid scintillation counting of spots cut from the plate. The figure depicts a typical CAT assay. Lanes 1 to 4, uninfected H9 cells; lanes 5 to 8, H9 cells infected with HTLV-III. The plasmids used for transfection and the duration of the CAT enzymatic assay were as follows: pSV₂CAT, 60 minutes (lane 1) and 120 minutes (lane 2); pU3R-III, 60 minutes (lane 3) and 120 minutes (lane 4); pSV₂CAT, 60 minutes (lane 5) and 120 minutes (lane 6); and pU3R-III (lanes 7 and 8). Note that the time course of the CAT enzymatic assay for lanes 7 and 8 was only 2 minutes and 15 minutes, respectively.

phocytes. In contrast, there was a dramatic increase in the CAT activity directly by the HTLV-III LTR in the infected H9 cells. The level of CAT activity of pU3R-III in HTLV-III–infected H9 cells was more than 1100 times that of pSV₂CAT. This relative increase in the ability of the pU3R-III plasmid to direct CAT gene expression was also seen in another lymphocyte line, Jurkat L8460D, infected in vitro with HTLV-III (*14*) (Table 1). As the majority of transiently expressing DNA is extrachromosomal, factors present in HTLV-III–infected H9 cells that modulate gene expression by the HTLV-III LTR must act in *trans*. We conclude that factors associated with HTLV-III viral infection *trans*-activate transcription directed by the HTLV-III LTR.

To examine whether the *trans*-acting factors present in HTLV-III–infected cells could stimulate CAT gene expression directed by other HTLV-BLV LTR's, we introduced plasmids that contain the U3 region of HTLV-I (pU3R-I), HTLV-II (pU3-II), and BLV (pBLV-CAT) (*4, 5*) into HTLV-III–infected and uninfected H9 cells. In all cases there was no significant difference in the level of CAT activity in infected and uninfected cells (Table 1). We conclude that the viral *trans*-acting factors in HTLV-III–infected H9 cells do not transcriptionally activate the LTR's of HTLV-I, HTLV-II, or BLV.

The magnitude of the transcriptional activation of the HTLV-III LTR in the infected H9 and Jurkat cell lines is noteworthy. Relative to the activity of the

SV40 promoter, the level of CAT activity directed by the HTLV-III LTR in the infected cells was about five to ten times the maximum level of CAT activity directed by the HTLV-I or HTLV-II LTR's and about 50 to 100 times that observed for the BLV LTR in the appropriate infected cell type (*4*, *5*). Efficient *trans*-activation of the viral LTR may be related to the high levels of virus production observed in some HTLV-III–infected cell lines (*3*). High levels of virus production may be responsible, at least in part, for the ability of HTLV-III to establish a chronic viremia, which is unusual for the other HTLV's or BLV (*1*, *15*).

Transcriptional *trans*-activation of the LTR in infected cells places HTLV-III in the retroviral family that includes HTLV-I, HTLV-II, and BLV, in accord with demonstrated similarities among the genomes and proteins of these viruses (*3*, *8*, *9*). The ability of these viruses to alter the transcriptional environment of the host cell suggests that they might exert their phenotypic effects via transcriptional regulation of specific host cellular genes. The specific activation of LTR sequences of the infecting virus suggests that sequences recognized by HTLV-III–associated *trans*-acting factors differ from those recognized by factors present in HTLV-I– or HTLV-II– infected cells. The cellular genes regulated by such factors might also differ, leading to cell death consequent to infection by HTLV-III and to cell proliferation following infection by HTLV-I or HTLV-II.

References and Notes

1. B. J. Poiesz *et al.*, *Proc. Natl. Acad. Sci. U.S.A.* **77**, 7415 (1980); V. S. Kalyanaraman, M. Sarngadharan, P. Bunn, J. Minna, R. C. Gallo, *Nature (London)* **294**, 271 (1981); M. Robert-Guroff, F. Ruscetti, L. Posner, B. Poiesz, R. C. Gallo, *J. Exp. Med.* **154**, 1957 (1981); M. Yoshida, I. Miyoshi, Y. Hinuma, *Proc. Natl. Acad. Sci. U.S.A.* **79**, 2031 (1982); M. Popovic *et al.*, *Nature (London)* **300**, 63 (1982).
2. V. S. Kalyanaraman *et al.*, *Science* **218**, 571 (1982); I. S. Y. Chen, J. McLaughlin, J. C. Glasson, S. C. Clark, D. S. Golde, *Nature (London)* **305**, 502 (1983); E. P. Gelmann, G. Franchini, V. Manzari, F. Wong-Staal, R. C. Gallo, *Proc. Natl. Acad. Sci. U.S.A.* **81**, 993 (1984).
3. M. Popovic, M. G. Sarngadharan, E. Read, R. C. Gallo, *Science* **224**, 497 (1984); R. C. Gallo *et al.*, *ibid.*, p. 500; J. Schüpbach *et al.*, *ibid.*, p. 503; M. Sarngadharan, M. Popovic, L. Bruch, J. Schüpbach, R. C. Gallo, *ibid.*, p. 506.
4. J. G. Sodroski, C. A. Rosen, W. A. Haseltine, *ibid.* **225**, 381 (1984).
5. S. Oroszlan *et al.*, *Proc. Natl. Acad. Sci. U.S.A.* **79**, 1291 (1982); C. A. Rosen, J. G. Sodroski, R. Kettman, A. Burny, W. A. Haseltine, *Science*, in press.
6. M. Seiki, S. Hattori, Y. Hirayama, M. Yoshida, *Proc. Natl. Acad. Sci. U.S.A.* **80**, 3618 (1983); W. A. Haseltine *et al.*, *Science* **225**, 419 (1984); N. R. Rice *et al.*, *Virology*, in press.
7. T. H. Lee *et al.*, *Science* **226**, 57 (1984); D. J. Slamon *et al.*, *ibid.*, p. 61.
8. S. K. Arya *et al.*, *ibid.* **225**, 927 (1984).
9. M. Essex *et al.*, *ibid.* **221**, 1061 (1983).
10. H. M. Temin, *Cell* **27**, 1 (1981); *ibid.* **28**, 3 (1982).
11. S. K. Arya and F. Wong-Staal, unpublished data. Clone C15 was derived from a cDNA library prepared from poly(A)selected HTLV-III RNA that was reverse transcribed with the use of an oligo-dT primer. The cDNA's were cloned into the Pst I site of pBR322 by dG-dC tailing and screened with ^{32}P-labeled cDNA from homologous cells. Clone C15 consists of approximately one kilobase of viral insert containing the entire U3 and R regions of the HTLV-III LTR and about 500 nucleotides of viral sequence 5' to U3.
12. C. M. Gorman, L. F. Moffat, B. H. Howard, *Mol. Cell. Biol.* **2**, 1044 (1982); C. M. Gorman, G. T. Merlino, M. C. Willingham, I. Pastan, B. Howard, *Proc. Natl. Acad. Sci. U.S.A.* **79**, 6777 (1982).
13. M. D. Walker, T. Edlund, A. M. Boulet, W. J. Rutter, *Nature (London)* **306**, 557 (1983).
14. Single-cell clones of the human Jurkat T-cell line JM were established by limiting dilution. These JM clones were infected with a single HTLV-III isolate (HTLV-IIIMN) obtained from the peripheral blood of a juvenile with pre-AIDS [R. C. Gallo *et al.*, *Science* **224**, 500 (1984)]. The cloned cells were treated with DEAE-Dextran (25 µg/ml) for 30 minutes at 37°C, then rinsed and incubated with cell-free supernatant from the virus-producing peripheral blood cells. After infection, these cells were maintained in RPMI 1640 medium supplemented with 10 percent fetal bovine serum and 2 m*M* glutamine.
15. V. S. Kalyanaraman *et al.*, *Science* **225**, 321 (1984); D. D. Ho *et al.*, *ibid.* **226**, 451 (1984).
16. C. Queen and D. Baltimore, *Cell* **33**, 729 (1983).
17. We thank R. Weiss for gifts of cell lines, M. F. McLane and M. Essex for use of their facilities, D. Celander and W. C. Goh for helpful discussions, N. Shiomi for expert technical assistance, and D. Artz for help in manuscript preparation. This work was supported by an American Can-

cer Society director's grant and by grant CA36974 from the National Institutes of Health. J.S. and C.R. were supported by grants CA07094 and CA07580, respectively.

12 October 1984; accepted 1 November 1984

Report

11 January 1985

72. Sequence Homology and Morphologic Similarity of HTLV-III and Visna Virus, a Pathogenic Lentivirus

Matthew A. Gonda, Flossie Wong-Staal, Robert C. Gallo, Janice E. Clements, Opendra Narayan, and Raymond V. Gilden

The family Retroviridae consists of animal viruses that contain an RNA-dependent DNA polymerase (or reverse transcriptase). These viruses replicate by way of DNA intermediates and often integrate into the host genome and can, in some instances, be transmitted through the germ line. Their gross morphogenesis is similar in that an encapsidated viral RNA genome is released from infected cells by budding from the plasma membrane; however, they also show fine morphological as well as biochemical differences that enable one to differentiate between individual members of this family.

At present, the family Retroviridae is composed of three subfamilies: Oncovirinae, Spumivirinae, and Lentivirinae (*1*). Of these, only the Oncovirinae and Lentivirinae produce pathologic disorders germane to this study. The oncoviruses, which can be further subdivided into intercisternal type A, and types B, C, and D, and which include certain tumor-causing viruses, are the only retroviruses that can be transmitted both as exoge-

nous infectious viruses and as endogenous genetic elements. Lentiviruses, in contrast, are exogenous viruses which, to date, are only known to infect ungulate (hoofed) mammals, in particular, domestic sheep (*2*), goats (*3*), cattle (*4*), and horses (*5*). The lentiviruses cause persistent but debilitating infections, replicate at a slow but progressive rate, and have been demonstrated to have pathogenic potential in vitro, causing syncytia, cell lysis, and death of susceptible cells during virus replication (*4–6*).

Several isolates of human retroviruses, known collectively as human T-cell leukemia (lymphotropic) viruses (HTLV), have been obtained from patients with certain T-cell malignancies (*7*). Initially, two major types (HTLV-I and HTLV-II) were identified. HTLV-I is strongly associated with adult T-cell leukemia (*7, 8*) while HTLV-II was first detected and isolated from cultured cells from a patient with hairy cell leukemia (*9*). Another type, HTLV-III, is believed to be the etiologic agent of the acquired immune deficiency syndrome (AIDS) (*10, 11*).

Particles of HTLV-I and -II observed by thin-section electron microscopy have been likened to oncoviruses of type C morphology (8). HTLV-III, however, is morphologically distinct from HTLV-I and -II and type C viruses (10–15). Whereas HTLV-III, during maturation of its extracellular particles, shows the formation of bar-shaped nucleoids, HTLV-I, -II, and type C viruses show round, central, variably electron-dense cores. Differences between HTLV types I and II and type C viruses are found in the thickness and spacing of the electron-dense core material in both budding and mature particles and the diameter of mature particles. Morphologically, HTLV-III resembles visna and equine infectious anemia viruses, both members of the lentivirus family, more closely than HTLV-I or -II or type C viruses (15–18). Other workers (14) have pointed out a resemblence between mature virions of lymphadenopathy associated virus (LAV), which may be similar or identical to HTLV-III, and both equine infectious anemia virus (EIAV) and type D retroviruses; however, we emphasize that there is a clear distinction in morphogenesis between HTLV-III and type D viruses. It has also been reported that the core protein of LAV was precipitated by sera from horses infected with EIAV (14, 19). This observation, along with the demonstrated cytopathic effect of HTLV-III in vitro (10), further suggested the possibility of a taxonomic link to pathogenic lentiviruses.

Analysis of the structural and evolutionary relation between HTLV-III and other retroviruses has been facilitated by the ability to isolate and amplify their genomes by molecular cloning techniques (20–22). In the present study, we used thin-section electron microscopy, molecular hybridization, and heteroduplex nucleotide sequence analysis to detect structural similarities and identify regions of homology between HTLV-III and visna virus.

HTLV-III was grown in an established human T-cell line (H9) (10–12), and, after being washed and pelleted by centrifugation, the infected cells were fixed in glutaraldehyde and embedded in epoxy resins for electron microscopy. Visna virus, strain 1514, was propagated in sheep choroid plexus cells. The infected cells were harvested 5 days after cytopathic effects were observed and similarly processed for electron microscopy. Examination of thin sections revealed striking similarities between HTLV-III and visna virus at all stages of maturation (Fig. 1, A–J). Buds (120 to 140 nm in diameter) with crescent or semicircular cores appeared at the cell membranes in both cultures. The double-membrane envelope and electron-dense laminar core were separated by a lighter electron-dense intermediate layer (Fig. 1, A, B, C, and G). The electron-lucent region between the core and the double-membrane envelope that is typical of type C viruses was not evident in these viruses (18). Free, extracellular immature particles were observed in both cultures (Fig. 1, C and H). These had a similar distribution of virus-specific layers as budding virus and frequently had an electron-lucent center, which was also seen in some budding forms. In the mature extracellular particles (90 to 130 nm in diameter), the cores condensed, often forming a bar-shaped nucleoid (Fig. 1, D and I) which, in cross sections, appeared smaller, circular, and most often eccentrically located (Fig. 1, E and J).

Molecular clones of HTLV-I, -II, -III, and visna virus (20–22) were used in heteroduplex mapping studies to determine the relative conservation and loca-

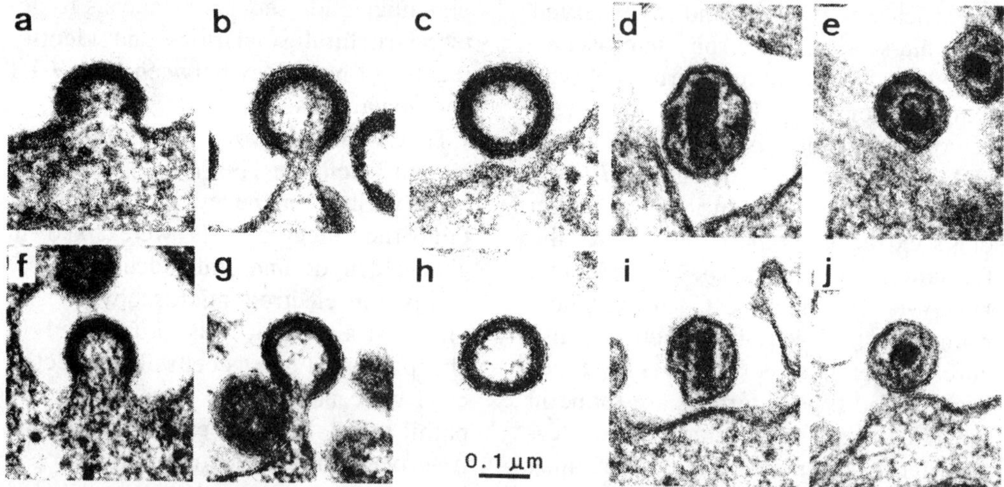

Fig. 1. Electron microscopy (×100,000) of thin sections of cells infected with HTLV-III and visna virus (strain 1514). Cell pellets were fixed in 1.25 percent buffered glutaraldehyde and then in 1 percent osmium tetroxide, dehydrated in graded alcohols, and embedded in epoxy resins. Thin sections were cut and stained with uranyl acetate and lead citrate. (A to E) HTLV-III–infected H9 human lymphocytes. (F to J) Visna virus–infected sheep choroid plexus cells. (A, B, F, and G) Bud formation of virus particles at the plasma membrane. (C and H) Free immature, extracellular virus particles. (D and I) Free mature, extracellular virus particles with bar-shaped nucleoid. (E and J) Free mature extracellular virus particles with condensed circular, eccentric cores.

tion of any sequence homology. We used the technique of thermal melt analysis, whereby the relative stringency of spreads is varied by increasing or decreasing the concentrations of formamide and salt in the spreading solution [see (23) and legend to Fig. 2]. The analysis was performed at T_m −52°C and T_m −45°C (with 20 and 30 percent formamide, respectively, in hyperphases containing 0.2M TES, pH 8.5). The relative conservation of sequences was expressed as a percentage, with the amount of duplexed DNA in the heteroduplex being used as the numerator and 9.0 kilobases (kb) as the denominator [9.0 kb being the size of a cloned HTLV-III genome containing one long terminal repeat (LTR) sequence as determined separately in gel electrophoresis experiments].

All heteroduplex analyses were performed with inserts in bacteriophage λ DNA cloned in the opposite orientation of the plus strand of the λ DNA arms. This configuration allowed the highly homologous λ DNA arms to drive the reaction and bring in close proximity the cloned inserts for base pairing. In heteroduplexes of HTLV-I and HTLV-III (Fig. 2A) or HTLV-I and visna virus (Fig. 2B), in spreads from 20 percent formamide, less than 6 percent of the HTLV-I genome was homologous to sequences in HTLV-III, and only 3 percent of the HTLV-I genome formed a duplex with visna virus. Most of the homologous sequences were within the 5′ one-third of the inserts (*gag* or *gag/pol* gene region), and were limited to two or three small regions of approximately 0.1 to 0.3 kb each. When the stringency was in-

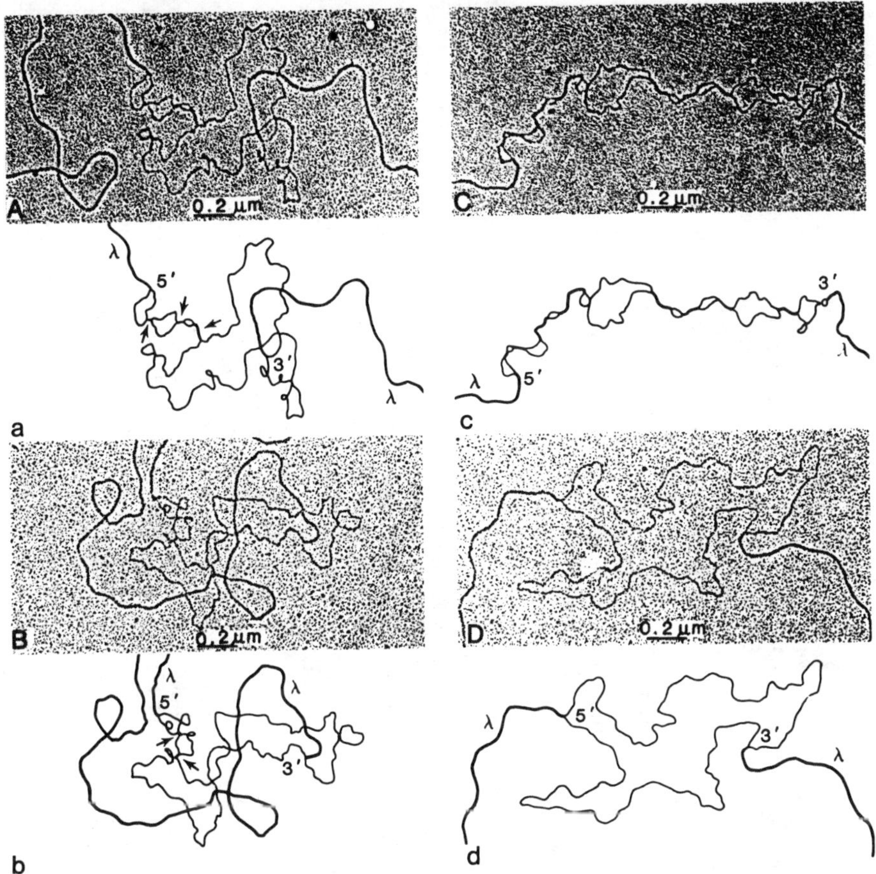

Fig. 2. Heteroduplex analysis of HTLV-I, -II, and -III and visna virus. Heteroduplexes were prepared between HTLV-III and visna virus and each of these to HTLV-I and -II. Heteroduplexes were prepared according to the method of Davis *et al.* (*33*). When thermal melt analyses were performed, only the formamide concentrations in the hyperphase were adjusted. Spreads typically contained DNA (0.01 to 0.02 μg), cytochrome C (30 μg/ml), 0.2*M* TES, and 0.02*M* EDTA, *p*H 8.5. The concentration of formamide was varied from 20 to 30 percent. Hypophases contained one-tenth the electrolyte and 0.001 percent *n*-octyl β-*d*-glucopyranoside. The stringency of hybridization was calculated from the known guanine plus cytosine (G + C) content of HTLV-I (53.9 percent) derived from Seiki *et al.* (*25*) and the following relation (*34*): $T_m = 81.5 + 16.6 (\log M) + 0.41 (\text{percent G + C}) - 0.72 (\text{percent formamide})$ in which M is the monovalent salt molarity and (percent G + C) is the percentage G + C residues in the DNA. The effective temperatures (which are expressed at $T_m - \Delta T$, in which ΔT is the difference between T_m and the temperature at which the heteroduplex was mounted for microscopy) for 20 and 30 percent formamide hyperphases were $T_m - 52°C$ and $T_m - 45°C$, respectively. All heteroduplex analysis were performed with inserts in bacteriophage λ. (A to D) Actual heteroduplexes. (a to d) Interpretive drawings. (A) Heteroduplex of HTLV-I and HTLV-III. (B) Heteroduplex of HTLV-I and visna virus. (C) Heteroduplex of HTLV-III and visna virus. (D) Heteroduplex of negative control HTLV-III and visna virus in which the HTLV-III insert was in the opposite orientation of the HTLV-III insert in phage λ used in (C). The 5′ and 3′ ends of the inserts and the λ arms are indicated. Regions of homology in (A) and (B) are noted by solid arrows. All micrographs are at the same magnification.

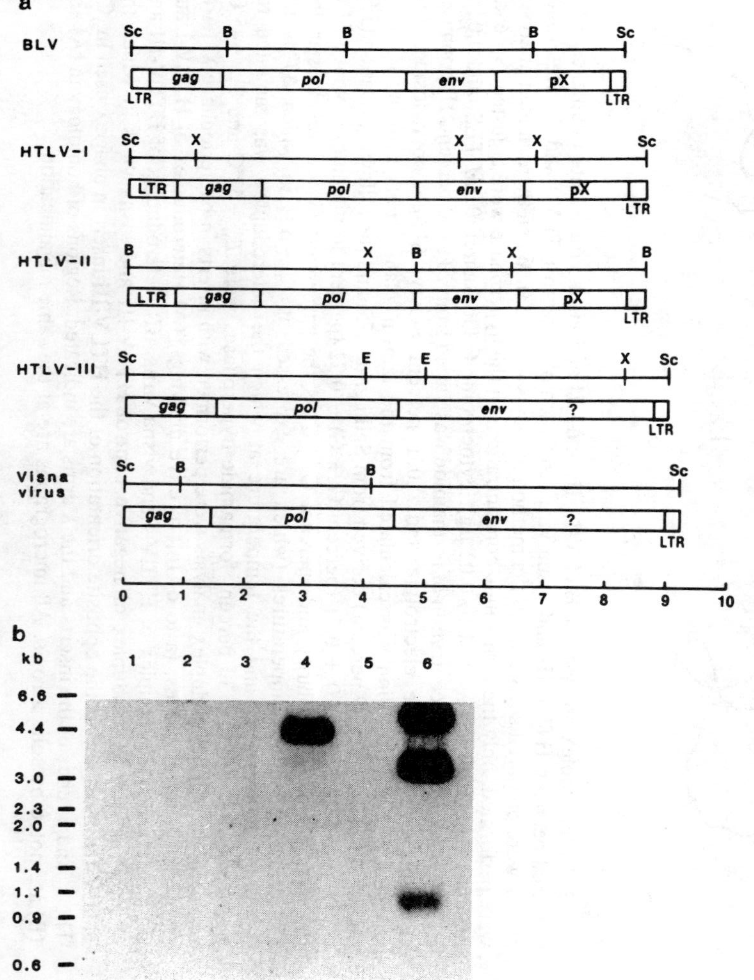

Fig. 3. Related nucleotide sequences detected by ^{32}P-labeled nick-translated probes (*35*) in HTLV-I, -II, -III, visna virus, and BLV. Viral DNA inserts were purified free of their cloning vectors (pBR322 or λWES) by restriction enzyme digestion and gel electrophoresis in low-melt agarose. The purified inserts were again digested with appropriate enzymes to molecularly dissect the genomes, separated on an agarose gel (0.9 percent), and transferred to Gene Screen Plus (New England Nuclear) by the method of Southern (*36*). The blots were hybridized under nonstringent conditions (T_m −39°C) as determined according to the equation in Fig. 2 in a solution containing 1M NaCl, salmon sperm DNA (100 μg/ml), 0.5 percent sodium dodecyl sulfate (SDS), and 20 percent deionized formamide with a ^{32}P-labeled nick-translated probe (either HTLV-III or visna virus; 1 × 10^7 cpm/ml) at 37°C for 36 hours. The filters were then washed initially in 3× SSC (1× SSC = 0.15M NaCl and 0.015M sodium citrate) and 0.5 percent SDS at 50°C (T_m − 49°C). One microgram of DNA was loaded into each lane except the homologous DNA lane (visna virus), which contained 0.05 μg. (a) Limited restriction enzyme maps show subgenomic fragments and the relative genomic complexity of each virus clone where known. Restriction enzyme digestions were Sac I (Sc), Eco RI (E), Xho (X), and Bam HI (B). The size of cloned inserts are drawn to scale. Restriction enzyme sites are accurate to ±0.1 kb. The sequence data for *env* regions of HTLV-III and visna virus are not complete and, therefore, their entire coding capacities are not known. By using one or more of the above enzymes, fragments were obtained of 3.2, 2.0, 1.7, and 1.2 kb for BLV; 4.4, 1.7, 1.3, and 1.1 kb for HTLV-I; 4.0, 2.2, 1.6, and 0.8 kb for HTLV-II; 4.0, 3.3, 1.0, and 0.7 kb for HTLV-III; and 5.1, 3.2, and 0.9 kb for visna virus. (b) The viruses tested were BLV (lane 1), HTLV-I (lane 2), HTLV-II (lane 3), HTLV-III (lane 4), no DNA (lane 5), and visna virus (lane 6). The ^{32}P-labeled nick-translated probe in (b) was visna virus. Hybridized filters were exposed to x-ray film for 16 hours at −70°C before development. Molecular size standards are depicted in kilobases.

creased to 30 percent formamide, less than 3 percent of the HTLV-I genome was homologous to HTLV-III and none of the genome was homologous to visna virus (data not shown). Heteroduplexes between HTLV-II and HTLV-III revealed no regions of identity in spreads from either 20 to 30 percent formamide (data not shown). In contrast, heteroduplexes formed between λ clones of HTLV-III and visna virus (Fig. 2C) revealed a striking amount of homology. In spreads from 20 percent formamide, approximately 35 percent of the HTLV-III genome was duplexed with visna virus, with the homology dispersed over the entire genome. In spreads from 30 percent formamide, 15 percent of the HTLV-III genome was duplexed with visna virus, with the conserved sequences occurring largely, but not exclusively, in the *gag/pol* region (data not shown). To verify that the conditions (20 percent formamide, 0.2*M* TES, *p*H 8.5) for heteroduplexing were not so mild as to allow nonspecific hybridization over short stretches of DNA, we hybridized to the λ visna clone a clone of HTLV-III that was in the reverse orientation of the clone used in Fig. 2C. No regions of hybridization were observed in any of these heteroduplexes (Fig. 2D).

To confirm and extend these findings, we performed reciprocal hybridizations using HTLV-III or visna virus as the probes under relaxed conditions (T_m −39°C; see legend to Fig. 3). The cloned viral DNA's studied included HTLV-I, -II, and -III, visna virus, and bovine leukemia virus (BLV), an exogenous virus of cattle associated with leukemia and lymphosarcoma. In its genomic complexity and organization, BLV is similar to both HTLV-I and HTLV-II and it shows a clear but distant relation to these viruses (*24*). Viral DNA inserts were separated from their cloning vectors by restriction enzyme digestion and gel electrophoresis. Purified inserts were again digested with restriction enzymes to molecularly dissect the genomes, and were subjected to gel electrophoresis and Southern blotting. A limited restriction enzyme map is shown in Fig. 3A, which depicts the subgenomic fragments of each viral clone and the relative genomic complexity where known. The location and extent of homology between HTLV-III or visna virus and each of these genomes was quantitated visually by autoradiography after hybridization of a ^{32}P-labeled nick-translated probe.

When visna virus was used as the probe, it hybridized most strongly to itself and to a 4.0-kb fragment in HTLV-III that included most of the *gag* and *pol* genes (Fig. 3B). In the reciprocal blot in which HTLV-III was used as the probe, it hybridized most strongly to itself and a 3.2-kb fragment in visna virus (data not shown). This fragment included most of the visna *gag* and *pol* genes. Under mild washing conditions (T_m −49°C), low, but specific, hybridization of both the visna and HTLV-III probes was detected with HTLV-I and -II and with BLV, but only when the exposure times were two to three times longer than those used in Fig. 3B (data not shown). As the washing stringencies were increased (T_m −39°C to −29°C), the heterologous hybridization intensities were reduced while the homologous reactions remained undiminished.

The genomes of HTLV-I and -II and BLV are structurally similar in that they have *gag*, *pol*, and *env* genes and a unique segment, termed pX, located between the *env* gene and the 3′ LTR (*21, 24, 25*). The 3′ 1-kb coding sequences of the pX regions (also referred to as long open reading frames, or LOR) of HTLV-I and -II are highly related (*21*) and believed to code for a protein that stimulates viral replication; these sequences may also activate transcription of cellular genes relevant to the transformation activity of these viruses (*26*). HTLV-III also codes for a protein analogous in function to that coded for by the LOR of HTLV-I and -II (*27*). Less is known about the genomic complexity and coding capacity of lentiviruses. Results from our previous study (*28*), as well as the present data, indicate a low, but significant, hybridization between HTLV-III and HTLV-I and -II. In other studies (*22*), minimal reactions were seen with type C virus reagents. The strong reactions seen here between visna and HTLV-III (tenfold greater than between HTLV-III and HTLV-I and -II) and the homology among all members of the HTLV family suggest a link between these viruses and lentiviruses.

On the basis of their morphology, the viruses now classified as Lentivirinae are indistinguishable from HTLV-III. There are also other features that the lentiviruses have in common with HTLV-III, such as their cytopathic (cell-killing) effects in vitro and their ability to produce persistent debilitating diseases in vivo. In contrast, HTLV-I and -II cause T-cell malignancies, immortalizing the infected cell.

If HTLV-III is related to the Lentivirinae, as these data suggest, studies of the mechanism by which HTLV-III was initially transmitted to humans and when and where this transmission occurred may prove interesting. Humans have long been closely associated with domestic ungluates, and the transmission of certain lentiviruses to human cells in vitro was recently demonstrated experimentally (*29*).

Lentiviruses persist in their ungulate hosts by various mechanisms. Although they induce the formation of binding antibodies to all of their respective polypeptides, they vary greatly with respect to the induction of neutralizing antibodies to envelope proteins. For example, visna and EIAV readily induce neutralizing antibodies; however, by a process called "antigenic drift," these viruses mutate rapidly in the *env* gene, thus allowing variants to escape the immune system and induce a new cycle of disease (*30*). Caprine arthritis encephalitis virus, in contrast, does not induce the formation of neutralizing antibodies during natural or experimental infections (*31*). Isolates of HTLV-III also show heterogeneitey in the *env* gene region, as indicated by restriction enzyme and heteroduplex analyses (*22*). This further similarity between HTLV-III and lentiviruses indicates that development of a vaccine to prevent AIDS may prove to be a considerable challenge. A recent study indicating the presence of HTLV-III in brain tissue of AIDS patients (*32*) further links this virus with lentiviruses (*3*).

References and Notes

1. F. Fenner, *Intervirology* **6**, 1 (1975–76); *Acta Virol. (Praha)* **20**, 170 (1976); R. E. Matthews, *Intervirology* **12**, 234 (1979).
2. B. Sigurdsson, *Brit. Vet. J.* **110**, 225 (1954); ______, P. A. Paulsson, H. Grimsson, *J. Neuropathol. Exp. Neurol.* **16**, 389 (1957); B. Sigurdsson and P. A. Paulsson, *J. Exp. Neurol.* **39**, 519 (1958).
3. T. B. Crawford, D. S. Adams, W. P. Cheevers, L. C. Cork, *Science* **207**, 997 (1980); D. S. Adams, T. B. Crawford, P. Kelvjer-Anderson, *Am. J. Pathol.* **99**, 257 (1980); L. C. Cork, W. J. Hadlow, J. R. Gorham, R. C. Piper, T. B. Crawford, *J. Infect. Dis.* **129**, 134 (1974); L. C. Cork and O. Narayan, *Lab. Invest.* **42**, 596 (1980).
4. M. J. Van Der Maaten, A. D. Boothe, C. L. Seger, *J. Natl. Cancer Inst.* **49**, 1649 (1972); A.

D. Boothe and M. J. Van Der Maaten, *J. Virol.* **13**, 197 (1974).

5. T. B. Crawford, W. P. Cheevers, P. Klevjer-Anderson, T. C. McGuire, in *Persistent Viruses, ICN/UCLA Symposium on Molecular and Cellular Biology*, J. Stevens, G. Todaro, C. F. Fox, Eds. (Academic Press, New York, 1978), vol. 11, pp. 727–749; Y. Kono, K. Kobayashi, Y. Fukunaga, *Arch. Virol.* **34**, 202 (1971); *ibid.* **41**, 1 (1973).

6. A. T. Haase, *Curr. Top. Microbiol. Immunol.* **72**, 101 (1975); D. Narayan, D. E. Griffin, A. M. Silverstein, *J. Infect. Dis.* **135**, 800 (1977); R. C. Kennedy, E. M. Eklung, C. Lopez, W. J. Hadlow, *Virology* **35**, 483 (1968); H. Thormar and P. A. Paulsson, *Perspect. Virol.* **5**, 291 (1967); O. Narayan *et al.*, *J. Gen. Virol.* **59**, 345 (1982).

7. For a brief review, see M. G. Sarngadharan *et al.*, in *Human Carcinogenesis*, C. C. Harris and H. H. Autrup, Eds. (Academic Press, New York, 1983), p. 679; R. C. Gallo, in *Cancer Surveys*, L. M. Frank, J. Wyke, R. A. Weiss, Eds. (Oxford Univ. Press, Oxford, 1984), vol. 3, pp. 113–159; F. Wong-Staal, *Blood*, in press.

8. V. S. Kalyanaraman *et al.*, *Proc. Natl. Acad. Sci. U.S.A.* **79**, 1653 (1982); M. Robert-Guroff *et al.*, *Science* **215**, 925 (1982); Y. Hinuma *et al.*, *Int. J. Cancer* **29**, 631 (1982); W. A. Blattner *et al.*, *ibid.* **30**, 257 (1982); J. Schüpbach, V. S. Kalyanaraman, M. G. Sarngadharan, Y. Nakao, R. C. Gallo, *Int. J. Cancer* **32**, 583 (1983); J. Schüpbach *et al.*, *Cancer Res.* **43**, 886 (1983); B. J. Poiesz *et al.*, *Proc. Natl. Acad. Sci. U.S.A.* **77**, 7415 (1980); B. J. Poiesz, F. W. Ruscetti, M. S. Reitz, V. S. Kalyanaraman, R. C. Gallo, *Nature (London)* **294**, 268 (1981).

9. V. S. Kalyanaraman *et al.*, *Science* **218**, 571 (1982); A. Saxons, R. H. Stevens, D. W. Golde, *Ann. Intern. Med.* **88**, 323 (1978).

10. M. Popovic, M. G. Sarngadharan, E. Read, R. C. Gallo, *Science* **224**, 497 (1984); *ibid.*, p. 500; J. E. Groopman *et al.*, *ibid.* **226**, 447 (1984); D. Zagury *et al.*, *ibid.*, p. 449; D. D. Ho *et al.*, *ibid.*, p. 451.

11. R. C. Gallo *et al.*, *ibid.* **224**, 500 (1984).

12. J. Schüpbach *et al.*, *ibid.*, p. 503.

13. M. G. Sarngadharan, M. Popovic, L. Bruch, J. Schüpbach, R. C. Gallo, *ibid.*, p. 504 (1984).

14. F. Brun-Vézinet *et al.*, *ibid.* **226**, 453 (1984).

15. M. A. Gonda, S. Z. Salahuddin, M. Popovic, R. C. Gallo, R. V. Gilden, in preparation.

16. H. Thormar, *Virology* **14**, 463 (1961); J. E. Coward, D. H. Harter, C. Morgan, *ibid.* **40**, 1030 (1970); K. K. Takemoto, C. F. Mattern, L. B. Stone, J. E. Coe, G. Lavelle, *J. Virol.* **7**, 301 (1971).

17. M. A. Gonda, H. P. Charman, J. L. Walker, L. Coggins, *Am. J. Vet. Res.* **39**, 731 (1978).

18. G. Schidlovsky, in *Cancer Research: Cell Biology, Molecular Biology, and Tumor Virology*, R. C. Gallo, Ed. (CRC Press, Cleveland, 1977), pp. 189–245.

19. L. Montagnie *et al.*, *Science* **225**, 63 (1984); L. Montagnier *et al.*, in *Human T-Cell Leukemia Lymphoma Virus*, R. C. Gallo, M. E. Essex, L. Gross, Eds. (Cold Spring Harbor Laboratory, Cold Spring Harbor, N.Y., 1984).

20. S. Molineaux and J. E. Clements, *Gene* **23**, 137 (1983).

21. G. W. Shaw *et al.*, *Proc. Natl. Acad. Sci. U.S.A.* **81**, 4544 (1984); G. W. Shaw *et al.*, *Acquired Immune Deficiency Syndrome*, M. S. Gottlieb and J. E. Groopman Eds. (Liss, New York, in press), vol. 16; E. P. Gelman, G. Franchini, V. Manzari, F. Wong-Staal, R. C. Gallo, *Proc. Natl. Acad. Sci. U.S.A.* **81**, 993 (1984); M. Clarke, E. P. Gelman, M. S. Reitz, *Nature (London)* **292**, 31 (1983).

22. B. H. Hahn *et al.*, *Nature (London)* **312**, 166 (1984); B. H. Hahn *et al.*, in preparation.

23. R. W. Davis and R. W. Hyman, *J. Mol. Biol.* **62**, 287 (1971).

24. N. R. Rice *et al.*, *Virology* **138**, 82 (1984); N. R. Rice, R. M. Stephens, A. Burny, R. V. Gilden, *Virology*, in press; S. Oroszlan *et al.*, *Proc. Natl. Acad. Sci. U.S.A.* **79**, 1291 (1982); T. D. Copeland, M. H. Morgan, S. Oroszlan, *FEBS Lett.* **156**, 37 (1983); T. D. Copeland, S. Oroszlan, V. S. Kalyanaraman, M. S. Sarngadharan, R. C. Gallo, *ibid.* **162**, 390 (1983); A. M. Schultz, T. D. Copeland, S. Oroszlan, *Virology* **135**, 417 (1984).

25. M. Seiki, S. Hattori, Y. Hirayama, M. Toshida, *Proc. Natl. Acad. Sci. U.S.A.* **80**, 3618 (1983).

26. D. J. Slamon, K. Shimotohno, M. J. Cline, D. W. Golde, I. S. Y. Chen, *Science* **226**, 61 (1984); T. H. Lee *et al.*, *ibid.*, p. 57 (1984); J. G. Sodroski, C. A. Rosen, W. A. Haseltine, *ibid.* **225**, 381 (1984); I. Chen, J. McLaughlin, D. W. Golde, *Nature (London)* **309**, 276 (1984).

27. J. Sodroski *et al.*, *Science* **227**, 171 (1985).

28. S. K. Arya *et al.*, *ibid.* **225**, 927 (1984).

29. J. A. Georgiades, A. Billiau, B. Vanderschueren, *J. Gen. Virol.* **38**, 375 (1978).

30. O. Narayan, D. E. Griffin, J. Chase, *Science* **197**, 376 (1977); O. Narayan, D. E. Griffin, J. E. Clements, *J. Gen. Virol.* **41**, 343 (1978); S. Payne, B. Parekh, R. C. Montelaro, C. J. Issel, *ibid.* **65**, 1395 (1984); J. E. Clements, N. D'Antonio, O. Narayan, *J. Mol. Biol.* **158**, 415 (1982).

31. P. Klevjer-Anderson and T. C. McGuire, *Infect. Immun.* **38**, 455 (1982); O. Narayan *et al.*, *J. Virol.* **49**, 349 (1984).

32. G. W. Shaw *et al.*, *Science* **227**, 77 (1985).

33. R. W. Davis, M. Simon, N. Davidson, *Methods Enzymol.* **21**, 413 (1971).

34. B. L. McConaughy, C. D. Laird, B. J. McCarthy, *Biochemistry* **8**, 3289 (1969).

35. P. W. J. Rigby, M. Diekmann, C. Rhodes, P. Berg, *J. Mol. Biol.* **113**, 237 (1977).

36. E. M. Southern, *ibid.* **98**, 503 (1975).

37. We thank K. Nagashima, J. Shumaker, and J. E. Elser for technical contributions and M. Fanning for assistance in preparing the manuscript. Supported by NCI under contract No. N01-CO-23910 with Program Resources, Inc. (M.A.G. and R.V.G.).

13 November 1984; accepted 6 December 1984

Report

11 January 1985

73. HTLV-III Infection in Brains of Children and Adults with AIDS Encephalopathy

George M. Shaw, Mary E. Harper, Beatrice H. Hahn, Leon G. Epstein, D. Carleton Gajdusek, Richard W. Price, Bradford A. Navia, Carol K. Petito, Carl J. O'Hara, Jerome E. Groopman, Eun-Sook Cho, James M. Oleske, Flossie Wong-Staal, and Robert C. Gallo

The acquired immune deficiency syndrome, or AIDS, is frequently complicated by central nervous system (CNS) dysfunction (*1–5*). In some patients, this is due to well-defined focal lesions in the brain such as those resulting from toxoplasmosis or lymphoma. However, far more common than these focal disturbances is the development of a more generalized encephalopathy that includes dementia as a dominant feature (*1, 2*). Indeed, many adult AIDS patients eventually develop this encephalopathy which characteristically begins with impaired concentration and mild memory loss and progresses to severe global cognitive impairment. Motor signs, including generalized hyperreflexia and increased tone may accompany the dementia, and some patients develop a spastic-ataxic gait or frank paraparesis. These neurological symptoms and signs usually progress over a course of several weeks to months (*1, 2*). In children with AIDS, a similar constellation of neurologic abnormalities occurs (*3*). Although the prevalence of dementia or other unexplained generalized CNS abnormalities in AIDS is uncertain, it is believed to occur to some degree in a substantial number, if not the majority, of patients (*1–5*).

The histopathological substrate of AIDS encephalopathy has not been defined. Gross cerebral atrophy and scattered microglial nodules consisting of aggregates of microglia and astrocytes are the most common findings in these patients but are not present in every case (*1, 2*). Disseminated infection of brain by cytomegalovirus has been found in a minority of affected individuals (*1, 2*).

It is now generally accepted that a newly discovered human retrovirus, human T-cell leukemia (lymphotropic) virus type III (HTLV-III), is the causative agent of AIDS (*6–8*). HTLV-III possesses a variety of biological and physicochemical properties in common with HTLV types I and II, among which are distant nucleic acid similarities and a striking tropism for T lymphocytes (*6, 9, 10*). However, recent studies (*11*) indicate that the genome of HTLV-III is more closely related to visna virus, a lentivirus that causes a chronic degenerative neurologic disease in sheep (*12*), than it is to HTLV-I or HTLV-II (*9*). Because of the frequency of unexplained dementia or encephalopathy observed in patients with AIDS and because brain cells and T lymphocytes are known to share common cell surface antigens (*13–16*), we examined the brains of 15 AIDS patients for evidence of HTLV-III infection. This report shows that in five of these patients HTLV-III sequences were detectable in the brain.

Table 1 summarizes the clinical and pathological characteristics of the 15 AIDS patients. These patients were studied because they had evidence of dementia or encephalopathy before death. Their neuropathological findings were variable in nature and degree and included histologically normal brains, mild to severe microglial nodules, vacuolar myelopathy, and cytomegalovirus or *Toxoplasma gondii* infections. As shown here and elsewhere (*1, 2*), histologic abnormalities were not consistently correlated with the presence or degree of dementia in these patients.

We examined, by Southern blot hybridization, DNA samples obtained from the cerebral cortex (containing both grey and white matter) of each of the 15 patients. HTLV-III DNA sequences were detected in five of them (patients 1, 2, 3, 4, and 5), as shown in Table 1 and Fig. 1. HTLV-III was not detected in the brains of the other ten AIDS patients or in four other control patients who were either healthy or suffered from Alzheimer's disease (Fig. 1) (*17*). In each of the five positive brain samples, the restriction-enzyme Sst I generated one of two different hybridization patterns. For example, brain DNA from patients 1, 2, 3, and 5 contained HTLV-III sequences that gave two bands of 5.5 kb and 3.5 kb when digested with Sst I, whereas the viral sequences in patient 4 generated a single 9-kb band when digested with the same enzyme. These differences in restriction patterns result from restriction site polymorphisms and correspond to two highly related but distinct forms of HTLV-III which are similar to ones we previously identified, cloned, and char-

acterized (*9, 18*). Both of these forms of the virus were also evident in DNA from the T-cell line H9/HTLV-III (*9, 18*), which was included in this experiment as a positive control (Fig. 1, lane j). The DNA samples were also digested with Bgl II and Hind III. These restriction enzymes generated many of the same bands found in other HTLV-III isolates (*18, 19*) as well as other bands that were different (for example, see the Hind III digestion of H9/HTLV-III DNA compared to brain DNA in Fig. 2). These findings showing different but highly related forms of HTLV-III in brain are in keeping with our previous demonstration that diversity in the viral genome is a characteristic feature of HTLV-III (*18–20*).

To estimate the relative abundance of HTLV-III DNA sequences present in brain compared to other body tissues, we examined DNA from spleen, lymph node, liver, lung, and brain of one patient (Fig. 2). As shown, very small amounts of viral DNA were detectable in DNA from lymph node and spleen, and the sizes of the bands, as expected, corresponded exactly to those generated by the same restriction enzyme digestion of brain DNA from this patient (see Fig. 1, lane a). When the same amount of DNA from brain and the other tissues from this patient were compared directly, it was apparent that brain was by far the most heavily infected with HTLV-III (Fig. 2).

We did not have the opportunity to examine other tissues besides brain from the remaining four positive cases in this study. However, from Fig. 2 and from an earlier survey of different lymphoid tissues from AIDS patients (*18*) we conclude that the abundance of HTLV-III in these brains samples was generally equivalent to, and sometimes greater

Table 1. Fifteen patients who had AIDS and encephalopathy were evaluated for the presence of HTLV-III in brain tissue. Clinical findings were documented before death by the patients' physicians; histopathologic findings were confirmed by a neuropathologist; and Southern analyses and in situ hybridizations were performed as described (30–32). All brain specimens were coded and analyzed independently by Southern analysis and in situ hybridization in a blinded manner; N.D., not done. Abbreviations: KS, Kaposi's sarcoma; PCP, *Pneumocystis carinii* pneumonia; dCMV, disseminated cytomegalovirus infection; MAI, *Mycobacterium avium intracellulare*; cTOX, cerebral toxoplasmosis; NHL, non-Hodgkins lymphoma; ARC, AIDS-related complex; BTR, blood transfusion recipient, CMV, cytomegalovirus.

Pa-tient	Age	Sex	Risk factors	Systemic diagnoses	Neurologic findings	Neuropathology	Detection of HTLV-III	
							South-ern anal-ysis	In situ
1	33 years	M	Homosexual	MAI, dCMV, PCP	Dementia (severe)	Microglial nodules (severe), CMV, gemistocytic astrocytosis (grey matter)	+	+
2	34 years	M	Homosexual	Oral *Candida*	Dementia (severe), paraparesis	Microglial nodules (severe), gemistocytic astrocytosis, perivascular lymphocytes and macrophages	+	+
3	4 months	M	Mother was intravenous drug abuser, BTR	PCP, oral *Candida*	Loss of developmental milestones, secondary microcephaly	Microglial nodules (mild), gross cerebral atrophy	+	+
4	6 years	M	Mother with ARC	dCMV, oral *Candida*	Loss of developmental milestones, hypertonia, ataxia, seizures	Gross cerebral atrophy, neuronal loss, microglial nodules	+	+
5	34 years	M	Homosexual	KS, PCP, MAI, dCMV	Dementia (moderate)	Microglial nodules (mild), gemistocytic astrocytosis (white matter), white matter vacuolation	+	–
6	44 years	M	Homosexual	KS, PCP, MAI, dCMV	Dementia (mild)	Microglial nodules (mild), vacuolar myelopathy	–	–
7	34 years	M	Homosexual	KS	Dementia (mild)	Healed toxoplasmosis	–	–
8	41 years	M	Homosexual	PCP, dCMV	Dementia (mild)	Microglial nodules (moderate)	–	–
9	37 years	M	Homosexual	MAI, dCMV, PCP	Dementia (severe), paraparesis	Normal brain, vacuolar myelopathy	–	–
10	8 months	F	Haitian parents	PCP, CMV, pneumonia	Loss of developmental milestones, seizures, hypertonia	Normal brain (terminal hypoxic change)	–	–
11	37 years	F	Intravenous drug abuser	PCP	Dementia, seizures	Cerebral atrophy	–	–
12	10 months	M	Mother was intravenous drug abuser, BTR	Oral *Candida*	Loss of developmental milestones, secondary microcephaly	Gross cerebral atrophy, perivascular lymphocytes	–	–
13	46 years	M	Homosexual	KS, PCP, dCMV	Dementia	Microglial nodules, CMV	–	N.D.
14	43 years	M	Homosexual	KS, NHL	Dementia	Demyelination inflammation (non-specific leukoencephalopathy)	–	N.D.
15	49 years	F	Sexual partner with ARC	KS, PCP, cTOX	Ataxia, seizures, dementia	Toxoplasmosis with necrosis and inflammation	–	N.D.

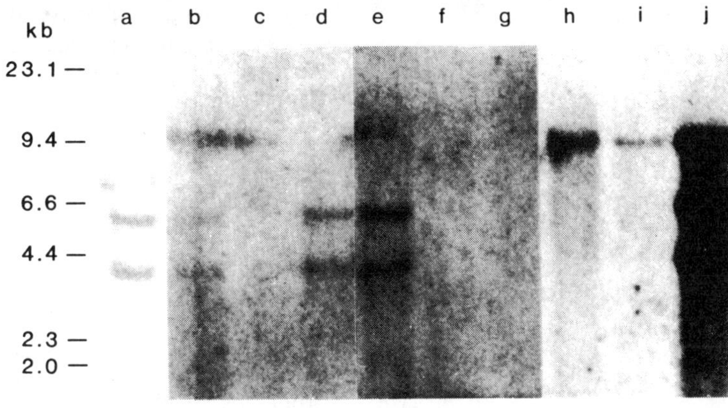

Fig. 1. Southern blot analysis of brain DNA from patients with AIDS. High molecular weight DNA was extracted, digested with Sst I, and blot-hybridized to an HTLV-III–specific probe as described (*30*). Lane a, patient 3; lane b, patient 1; lane c, patient 10; lane d, patient 5; lane e, patient 2; lane f, patient 8; lane g, patient 9; lanes h and i, the parietal and occipital cortex, respectively, of patient 4; lane j, HTLV-III–infected T-cell line (H9/HTLV-III) (*9, 18*). Not shown are the blot hybridizations of brain DNA from patients 6 and 11 to 15, and from four non-AIDS control individuals, all of which were negative. As shown, HTLV-III sequences were detected in brain DNA from patients 1 to 5. Two Sst I patterns were evident (5.5 kb and 3.5 kb in lanes a, b, d, and e and 9 kb in lanes h and i) which, as discussed in the text, correspond to two distinguishable but highly related forms of HTLV-III (*9, 18*). Both of these forms of the virus are evident in the DNA from H9/HTLV-III cells shown in lane j.

than, that found in other tissues including peripheral blood, lymph node, spleen, and bone marrow of other AIDS and ARC patients.

To define further the nature of HTLV-III infection in brain, we used in situ hybridization to examine brain cells directly for viral-specific RNA. Frozen sections of brain from 12 of the 15 patients already evaluated by Southern analysis (Table 1 and Fig. 1) were examined in a coded fashion without knowledge of the results of the blot-hybridization. There was nearly complete agreement between the results obtained by the two techniques (Table 1). Four of five specimens positive for HTLV-III by Southern analysis were also positive by in situ hybridization, indicating that the HTLV-III genome was being expressed in these tissues. Similarly, all seven specimens negative for viral sequences by Southern analysis were also scored negative by in situ analysis. The discrepancy between the results of the Southern and in situ hybridizations in patient 5 could have resulted from degradation of RNA (which is more labile than DNA), a lack of expression of the viral genome in that sample, or the presence of virus in one region of the cerebral cortex but not others.

Figure 3, A and B, shows numerous silver grains representing HTLV-III viral RNA in the brain cells of two of the AIDS patients. Such grains were not present in brain from a control, non-AIDS patient (Fig. 3D). As an additional control, a probe lacking HTLV-III sequences was hybridized to sections of brain from each of the 12 AIDS patients; no positively hybridizing cells were found (Fig. 3C). The specimens shown in Fig. 3, A and C, were taken from a region of the cerebral cortex of patient 3 immediately adjacent to that which was used to make high molecular weight DNA for Southern analysis (Fig. 1, lane

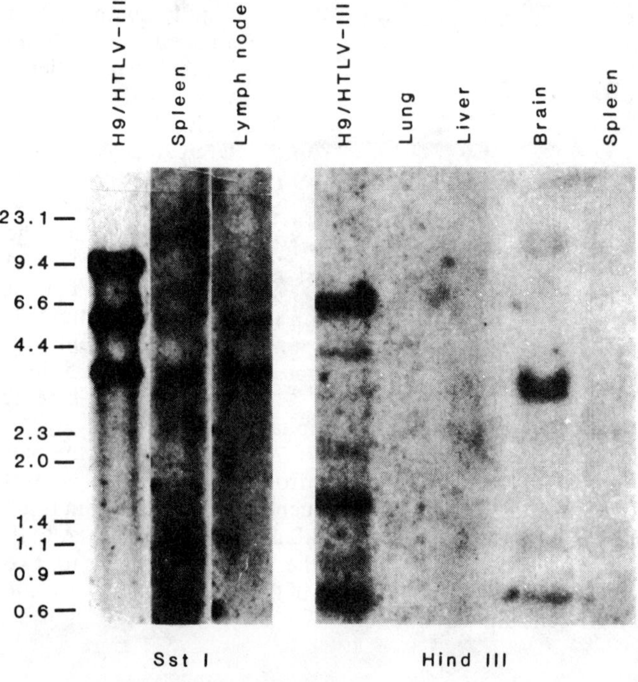

Fig. 2. Detection of HTLV-III DNA in brain and other tissues from patient 3 (see Table 1 and lane a in Fig. 1). DNA was extracted from brain, spleen, lymph node, liver, and lung, digested with the indicated restriction endonucleases, and blot-hybridized as described (*30*). DNA (30 μg) from each tissue was used so that the relative abundance of HTLV-III DNA in each could be ascertained. DNA (3 μg) from the H9/HTLV-III cell line was included as a positive control [note that H9/HTLV-III cells each contain many HTLV-III molecules (*9, 18*)]. The Sst I blot (left) was exposed to x-ray film for 7 days whereas the Hind III blot (right) was exposed for only 1 day. This blot hybridization demonstrates that the abundance of HTLV-III was much greater in brain than in any of the other tissues from this patient. It is also evident that the restriction pattern for Hind III is different in the HTLV-III isolate from this patient compared with those forms present in H9/HTLV-III cells (see text for discussion).

a). We estimate from both techniques that from 1 to 10 percent of cells in this specimen were infected with HTLV-III.

The specific type of brain cell infected with HTLV-III could not be determined from these studies, but it is clear that the positive hybridization was not due to the infiltration of brain by HTLV-III infected lymphocytes. We base this conclusion on (i) the histologic characteristics of the brain samples used for the Southern and in situ hybridizations (lymphocytes were scant or absent in all but one brain specimen), (ii) the cellular morphology of the virally infected cells identified by in situ hybridization (nuclear and cytoplasmic dimensions were not those of lymphocytes), and (iii) the fact that only very few lymphocytes in lymph node, spleen, and peripheral blood (less than one in ten) are infected with HTLV-III at any one time [see Fig. 2 and (*18, 21*)]. Further studies with the use of in situ hybridization and immunocytochemical techniques are needed to determine the cell type or types infected with HTLV-III, be they of neuronal, glial, or macrophage lineage.

The true incidence of HTLV-III brain infection in AIDS patients with encephalopathy is not yet known. Nor is it known whether HTLV-III brain infection may occur in patients with AIDS or AIDS-related complex (ARC) without encephalopathy. The brain specimens used in this study were taken from different cortical regions (for example, frontal, parietal, or occipital lobes) and, except for one patient (number 4), we were able to examine only a single region of each brain for HTLV-III sequences. Thus, although HTLV-III was detected in frontal (patient 2), parietal (patients 4 and 5), and occipital (patients 1 and 4) lobes, it is possible that viral infection could have been anatomically restricted at certain points in the disease course in some of the patients studied and thus were not detected by our limited sampling. Moreover, a number of brain specimens had been less than optimally preserved, so it is possible that low-level infection with HTLV-III could have gone undetected.

Thus the cellular and anatomic distribution of the virus, its histopathological correlate, and its relation to the patients' clinical signs and symptoms, if any, remain to be determined.

Our finding of HTLV-III in brains of 5 out of 15 AIDS patients (33 percent) is comparable to results in lymphoid tissues examined by the same Southern blot technique (18). Moreover, the abundance of HTLV-III DNA in brain appears to be equal to, and sometimes greater than, that in lymphoid tissues

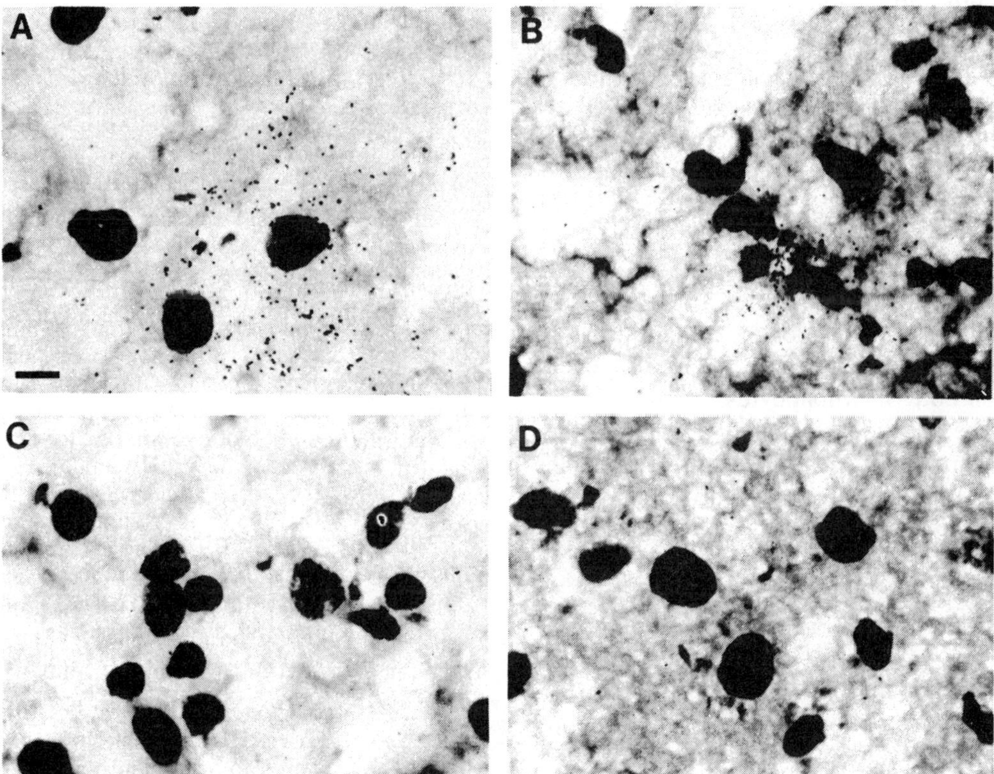

Fig. 3. Detection of HTLV-III viral RNA in the brains of AIDS patients by in situ hybridization. Brain section from (A) patient 3, hybridized with HTLV-III–specific probe, (B) patient 4, hybridized with HTLV-III–specific probe, (C) patient 3, hybridized with control phage λ-specific probe lacking HTLV-III sequences, and (D) non-AIDS (control) patient hybridized with HTLV-III–specific probe. In situ hybridization was carried out as described (31). Exposure, 2 days. Scale bar, 10 μm.

394

(Fig. 2) (*18*). We have also observed that the relative abundance of HTLV-III RNA per cell as determined by in situ hybridization is generally greater in brain than in lymph node, peripheral blood, or bone marrow (*21*).

The finding of HTLV-III DNA and RNA in brain indicates that not only is the virus present in this tissue compartment but that it is being expressed there.

Furthermore, we have shown, by using restriction enzymes that cleave the viral genome only once or not at all, that in brain, as in other tissues (*18*), HTLV-III DNA occurs in substantial amounts in both chromosomally integrated and unintegrated forms (*17*). Since unintegrated DNA represents a replicative intermediate stage in the life cycle of retroviruses, this finding suggests that HTLV-III is actively replicating in the brains of these AIDS patients.

The finding of HTLV-III in brain and its apparent enrichment there is of considerable interest aside from its possible clinical implications. Certain surface antigens, such as Thy-1 (*13–16*), occur on both T lymphocytes and brain cells. The question of whether there are other shared antigens between lymphocytes and brain cells, both neuronal and glial, is controversial (*15, 16, 22–24*). It is possible that the dual tissue tropism of HTLV-III is the result of similarities in surface membrane determinants of T lymphocytes and certain brain cells, and the characterization of such common viral receptors on these cells could define further their antigenic relatedness.

This apparent tropism for brain by a retrovirus is not without precedence. Certain strains of murine leukemia virus induce both lymphoma and neurologic disease in wild mice (*25*). These animals experience a slowly progressive paralytic disease characterized pathologically by spongiform degeneration of the gray matter, particularly in the anterior horns of the spinal cord. As in AIDS encephalopathy, there is a characteristic absence of inflammatory reaction in the involved neural tissue.

Another retrovirus, visna, causes a chronic degenerative CNS disease in sheep (*12*). Like HTLV-III, visna virus infects both brain and lymphocytes (*12*), has pronounced cytopathic activity (*26*), has morphologic and genetic similarities with HTLV-III (*11*), and persists in cells in substantial amounts as unintegrated viral DNA (*27*). This last property is very unusual for retroviruses and is a particular feature of HTLV-III and other cytopathic retroviruses (*18, 28*). Unlike the noninflammatory lesions described in AIDS encephalopathy, the CNS disease resulting from visna virus is associated with an intense mononuclear cell inflammatory response (*29*). This difference between the histopathologic characteristics of visna infection and that of AIDS encephalopathy, however, must be considered in light of the profound cellular immunodeficiency that occurs in patients with AIDS but not in animals infected with visna virus.

Our results indicate that HTLV-III, in addition to its role in causing the immune deficiency of AIDS (*6–8*), may also have a role in the pathogenesis of AIDS encephalopathy. It will be important to determine which CNS cell types are infected with HTLV-III and how the virus affects these cells in vitro and in vivo. Finally, in attempting to develop therapeutic agents for the treatment of AIDS, investigators will now have to allow for the presence of HTLV-III within the sanctuary of the CNS.

References and Notes

1. W. D. Snider *et al.*, *Ann. Neurol.* **14**, 403 (1983); B. D. Jordan, B. A. Navia, C. Petito, E-S. Cho, and R. W. Price, *Front. Radiat. Ther. Oncol.*, in press.
2. B. A. Navia *et al.*, in preparation.
3. L. G. Epstein *et al.*, *Ann. Neurol.*, in press.
4. K. Welch *et al.*, *J. Am. Med. Assoc.* **252**, 1152 (1984).
5. P. Gapen, *ibid.* **248**, 2941 (1982).
6. M. Popovic *et al.*, *Science* **224**, 497 (1984).
7. R. Gallo *et al.*, *ibid.* **224**, 500 (1984); J. Schüpbach *et al.*, *ibid.* **224**, 503 (1984); M. G. Sarngadharan *et al.*, *ibid.* **224**, 506 (1984); B. Safai *et al.*, *Lancet* **1984-I**, 1438 (1984); J. Groopman *et al.*, *N. Engl. J. Med.* **311**, 1419 (1984).
8. S. Z. Salahuddin *et al.*, in preparation.
9. B. H. Hahn *et al.*, *Nature (London)* **312**, 166 (1984).
10. R. C. Gallo, *Cancer Surv.* **3**, 114 (1984); R. C. Gallo *et al.*, *Proc. Natl. Acad. Sci. U.S.A.* **79**, 4680 (1982).
11. M. A. Gonda *et al.*, *Science* **227**, 173 (1985).
12. J. E. Clements *et al.*, *Proc. Natl. Acad. Sci. U.S.A.* **77**, 4454 (1980); J. E. Clements, O. Narayan, L. C. Cork, *J. Gen. Virol.* **50**, 423 (1980); O. Narayan *et al.*, *ibid.*, p. 69.
13. A. E. Reif and J. M. V. Allen, *J. Exp. Med.* **120**, 413 (1964); M. C. Raff, *Nature (London)* **224**, 378 (1969); H. G. Thiele, R. Stark, D. Keese, *Eur. J. Immunol.* **2**, 424 (1972); W. Stohl and N. K. Gonatas, *ibid.* **119**, 422 (1977); J. McKenzie and J. W. Fabre, *Brain Res.* **230**, 307 (1981).
14. R. C. Seeger *et al.*, *J. Immunol.* **128**, 983 (1982).
15. S. Szuchet, J. Antel, B. G. W. Arnason, *Nature (London)* **295**, 66 (1982).
16. J. A. Garson *et al.*, *ibid.* **298**, 375 (1982).
17. G. Shaw *et al.*, unpublished data.
18. G. M. Shaw *et al.*, *Science* **226**, 1165 (1984).
19. F. Wong-Staal *et al.*, in preparation.
20. The ability to detect proviral DNA integrated into the host cells' genome at multiple sites depends on the generation of internal viral restriction fragments of the same size that appear as discreet bands on Southern blots. Enzymes that cut the provirus only once, or not at all, will not generate such discreet bands. Given the recognized diversity, or polymorphism, in the restriction patterns of different HTLV-III isolates (*18*), the number of cleavage sites for any particular restriction enzyme could not be known a priori. Thus, to diminish the likelihood of false-negative hybridization results, we digested each of the 15 DNA samples described in this report with two different restriction enzymes (Sst I alone and Bgl II alone) that had been found to generate internal fragments in every HTLV-III isolate previously tested (*18, 19*). As an additional control, the quality of the DNA extracted from each brain sample and the completeness of each restriction enzyme digestion were both assured by rehybridizing the filters to HLA class II probes and demonstrating the expected bands. Conversely, to ensure that the observed bands in the DNA from positive brains were not due to contaminating phage or pBR322, filters were also hybridized to each of these vector DNA's and shown to be negative. Moreover, we could be sure that the positive brain specimens were not contaminated accidentally with cloned HTLV-III DNA, since the viral sequences in the different specimens of brain differed from each other and from other isolates and clones of HTLV-III (*18*) by at least some restriction sites.
21. M. E. Harper, unpublished observations.
22. M. Hirayama *et al.*, *Nature (London)* **301**, 152 (1983).
23. U. Traugott, E. L. Reinherz, C. S. Raine, *J. Neuroimmunol.* **3**, 365 (1982); S. L. Hauser *et al.*, *ibid.* **5**, 197 (1983).
24. C. S. Raine, personal communication.
25. M. B. Gardner *et al.*, *J. Natl. Cancer Inst.* **51**, 1243 (1973); M. B. Gardner, *Curr. Top. Microbiol. Immunol.* **79**, 216 (1978).
26. B. Sigurdsson, H. Thormar, P. A. Palsson, *Arch. Ges. Virusforsch.* **10**, 368 (1960).
27. J. E. Clements and O. Narayan, *Virology* **113**, 412 (1981); S. Molineaux and J. E. Clements, *Gene* **23**, 137 (1983).
28. E. Keshet and H. M. Temin, *J. Virol.* **31**, 376 (1979); S. K. Weller, A. E. Joy, H. M. Temin, *ibid.* **33**, 494 (1980).
29. G. Petursson *et al.*, *Lab. Invest.* **35**, 402 (1976).
30. Specimens of brain were obtained from 15 AIDS patients (see Table 1) either at necropsy or open biopsy and were frozen at $-70°C$ for subsequent analysis. All specimens were from cerebral cortex containing grey and white matter, but in only some instances was the exact region of the cerebrum known. Frozen brain tissue (approximately 1 g) was pulverized under liquid nitrogen, made up to 20 ml in tris (20 mM, pH 7.4), EDTA (5 mM) sodium dodecyl sulfate (5 mg/ml), and proteinase K (100 μg/ml), and incubated at 50°C for 3 hours. The DNA was then adjusted to 0.3M Na$^+$ with sodium acetate (pH 6.0), extracted three times with a solution of phenol and chloroform (1:1 by volume) saturated with 50 mM tris (pH 9.0), extracted once with chloroform alone, and then precipitated with two volumes of absolute ethanol. High molecular weight DNA was dissolved in TE buffer (20 mM tris, pH 7.4; and 1 mM EDTA). The DNA (20 μg) was digested with 150 units of Sst I for 8 hours at 37°C and then subjected to electrophoresis through 0.7 percent agarose slab gels. Gels were blotted in 10$\times$ SSC onto 0.1 μm nitrocellulose filters (Schleicher and Schuell). Hybridizations were performed at 37°C for 18 hours in 2.4$\times$ SSC, 40 percent formamide, 10 percent dextran sulfate, 1 mg/ml each of bovine serum albumin, polyvinylpyrrollidone, and Ficoll, and 20 μg of transfer RNA per milliliter. Filters were washed for 3 hours at 65°C in 1 $\times$ SSC. The probe used was the 8.9-kb-long Sst I–Sst I insert from λBH-10 (*9*), 10 $\times$ 10^6 dpm/ml (approximately 2 $\times$ 10^8 dpm/μg). Blots were exposed to Kodak XAR-5 film for 3 days.
31. In situ hybridization was carried out as described by Harper *et al.* (*32*). Briefly, frozen sections were prepared from OCT-embedded brain tissue, mounted on microscope slides, fixed in 4 percent paraformaldehyde, and stored in 70 percent ethanol at 4°C until hybridized. Slide preparations were then acetylated, treated with 0.1M tris-HCl (pH 7.0) and 0.1M glycine, and hybridized with 10^6 count/min of ^{35}S-labeled RNA transcribed from pBH10-R3 [8.9-kb-long Sst I–Sst I viral insert from HTLV-III clone λBH-10 (*9*) subcloned into pSP64]. Hybridiza-

tion was performed in 50 percent formamide, 2× SSC, and 10 mM DTT for 3 hours at 50°C. Slides were rinsed in 50 percent formamide, 2× SSC at 52°C, treated with ribonucleases A and T$_1$ for 30 minutes, and dehydrated in ethanol. Preparations were autoradiographed with Eastman NTB2 emulsion, exposed at 4°C for 2 days, developed in Dektol developer, and stained with Wright stain. For these in situ hybridization studies, sections were not subjected to DNA strand separation (denaturation), thereby ensuring that hybridization of the HTLV-III probe was to viral RNA and not DNA.
32. M. E. Harper *et al.*, in preparation.
33. We thank L. Rankin and A. B. Minnefor for

providing clinical data and postmortem material, L. Marselle for technical assistance, and R. Singer for discussions. G.M.S. was funded through the Intergovernmental Personnel Act of the National Institutes of Health in conjunction with the Ohio State University College of Medicine, and B.H.H. was supported by the German Science Foundation and the Fogarty Center for International Studies. R.W.P. was supported, in part, by New York AIDS institute grant number A0159. L.G.E. is an assistant professor of Neuroscience and Pediatrics at the University of Medicine and Dentistry of New Jersey and is currently a visiting scientist at the NIH.

13 November 1984; accepted 6 December 1984

Report

18 January 1985

74. Bovine Leukemia Virus Long Terminal Repeat: A Cell Type–Specific Promoter

David Derse, Salvatore J. Caradonna, and James W. Casey

Bovine leukemia virus (BLV) is a B-cell lymphotropic retrovirus associated with a disease complex termed "enzootic bovine leukosis" (*1*). Unlike most other avian and mammalian retroviruses, BLV transcripts have not been detected in tumors or lymphocytes of infected animals (*2*). In addition, BLV displays a highly restricted infectivity in vitro (*3, 4*). Nucleotide sequence data have revealed that BLV, like the human T-cell leukemia viruses types I and II (*5*) (HTLV-I and HTLV-II) possesses an unusual long terminal repeat (LTR) structure (*6, 7*). The LTR's bordering retroviral proviruses contain sequences required for viral integration, replication, and expression (*8*), and determine to a large extent the pathological consequences of infection. Because the LTR encompasses a promoter unit analogous to that controlling cellular gene expression, we suspected that the restricted expression and infectivity of BLV were functional manifestations of an atypical LTR. To examine this possibility, we tested the ability of the BLV LTR to promote the expression of a heterologous gene placed under its control in various cellular environments.

The BLV-infected fetal lamb kidney (FLK-BLV) cell line is one of only a few lines characterized that produce significant amounts of BLV (*3*). The four BLV proviruses harbored by FLK-BLV cells were cloned into bacteriophage lambda L47 (*9*). Restriction fragments containing each of the four proviral 5′ LTR's, as well as a single 3′ LTR, were inserted into the plasmid pSV0cat (*10*) as outlined in Fig. 1. The transcriptional utilization of the BLV LTR's were assessed by comparing the levels of CAT activity transiently expressed in cells transfected with pBL-cat and pRSVcat plasmids. The latter plasmid contains a CAT gene controlled by the Rous sarcoma virus LTR (*10*). Results from typical transfection experiments are shown in Table 1 and Fig. 2. In monkey kidney (CV-1), bovine kidney (MDBK), mouse fibroblast (LTK⁻), or human rhabdomyosar-

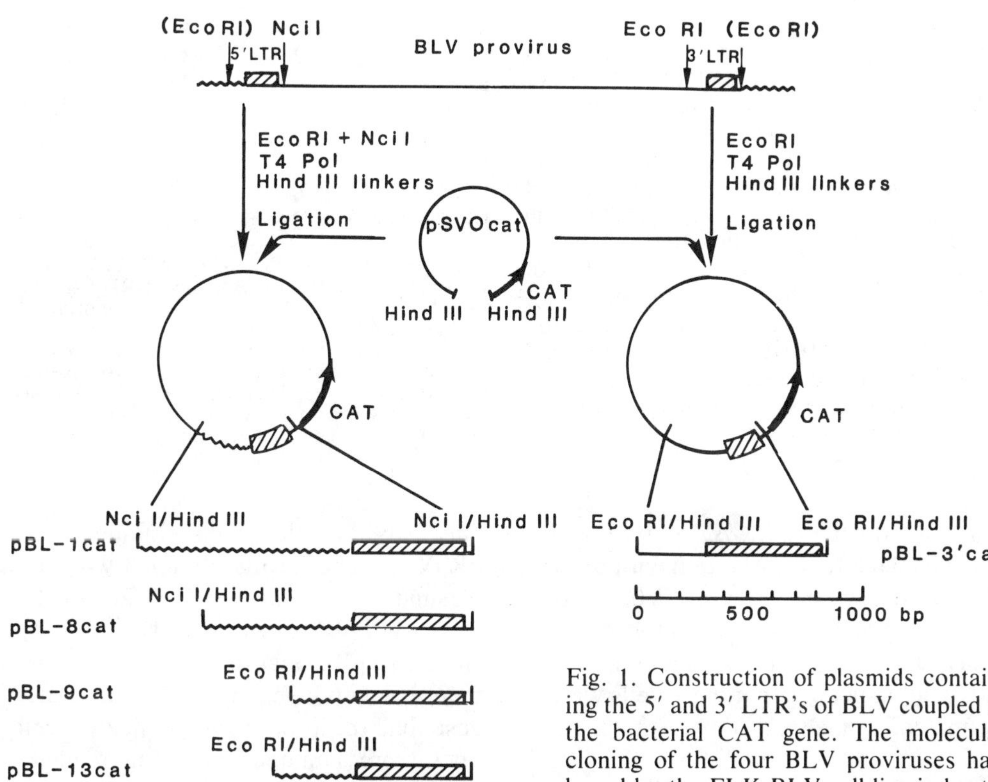

Fig. 1. Construction of plasmids containing the 5′ and 3′ LTR's of BLV coupled to the bacterial CAT gene. The molecular cloning of the four BLV proviruses harbored by the FLK-BLV cell line in bacteriophage λ L47 (*9*). Phage λ clones containing each of the four BLV proviruses with flanking cellular DNA were obtained and are identified B1, B8, B9, and B13. At the top of the figure is shown provirus B13 (solid lines) bounded by its LTR's (hatched boxes) and flanked by cellular DNA (wavy lines). The Eco RI sites in parentheses refer to sites unique to the flanking cellular DNA of proviral clone B13. The Nci I site is located 16 bp downstream of the 5′ LTR. Restriction enzyme fragments containing 5′ or 3′ LTR's derived from each proviral clone were purified by polyacrylamide gel electrophoresis then modified by filling in the ends and adding synthetic Hind III linkers. The fragments were then ligated to Hind III–digested and bacterial alkaline phosphatase–treated pSVOcat (*10*). The resulting plasmids thus contain CAT coding sequences whose expression in eukaryotic cells is controlled by transcriptional regulatory signals present in the BLV LTR. For the plasmids shown here, the viral RNA start site is located approximately 370 bp upstream of the first AUG codon in the CAT sequence.

Table 1. Comparison of CAT expression in mammalian cells transfected with pBL-9cat, pRSVcat, and pSVOcat. All cells were at low passage number and were maintained in Temin's modified minimum essential medium supplemented with 10 percent fetal calf serum. Plasmid DNA was transfected onto cells as a calcium phosphate coprecipitate exactly as described previously (10, 11). DNA (10 μg) was applied to 6×10^5 cells grown in 10-cm culture dishes. Forty-eight hours after transfection the cells were collected and extracts were prepared and assayed for CAT activity (10). The CAT reaction mixtures contained in a volume of 180 μl: 100 μl of 0.25M tris-HCl, pH 7.5; 5 μl of ^{14}C-labeled chloramphenicol (1 mCi/ml, 49 mCi/mmol); 20 μl of 10 mM acetyl coenzyme A; and cell extract. The volumes of cell extract and the incubation times were varied for each cell line to ensure that measurements of CAT activity were in the linear range of the reaction. CAT activities were determined in at least two transfection experiments and, in most instances, with different preparations of a plasmid. The data are expressed as the percentage of the total radioactivity comigrating with monoacetate products with 20 μl of the 100-μl cell extracts. Incubation times were: LTK$^-$, 1 hour; CV-1, BLV-bat$_2$, and RD-4, 2 hours; MDBK, 5 hours; FLK and Tb1Lu, 6 hours. For FLK-BLV cell extracts the incubation time was 10 minutes, with 2 μl of cell extract.

Cell type	Conversion (%)		
	pBL-9cat*	pRSVcat	pSVOcat
CV-1	0.2	11.0	0.9
MDBK	0.2	4.2	0.2
RD-4	0.2	18.8	0.2
LTK$^-$	0.4	7.6	0.8
FLK	0.2	10.4	0.4
Tb1Lu	0.2	7.5	0.2
FLK-BLV	25.0	2.2	0.2
BLV-bat$_2$	32.2	0.9	0.2

*The other BLV LTR–containing CAT plasmids shown in Fig. 1 were also examined in RD-4, LTK$^-$, and FLK-BLV cells. These plasmids gave negligible levels of CAT activity in RD-4 and LTK$^-$ cells. When tested on FLK-BLV cells in the same experiment shown for pBL-9cat above, the plasmids pBL-1cat, pBL-8cat, pBL-13cat, and pBL-3′ cat yielded levels of CAT activity which gave, respectively, 28.0, 21.5, 23.2, and 20.4 percent conversion.

coma (RD4) cell lines, CAT activity was not detected after transfection with pBL-9cat or the promoterless pSV0cat. In these same cell lines, CAT activity was easily detected after transfection with pRSVcat, indicating that these cells were competent to take up DNA. Similar results were obtained in transfections of primary fetal lamb kidney (FLK) cells and a bat lung cell line, Tb1Lu (Table 1). In contrast, the BLV LTR directed high levels of CAT activity in the productively infected cell lines FLK-BLV and BLV-bat$_2$ (Table 1 and Fig. 2). These cells were previously established after infection of FLK and Tb1Lu cells with BLV (3, 4). The plasmid pBL-9cat yielded levels of enzyme activity that were tenfold higher in FLK-BLV cells and approximately 30-fold higher in BLV-bat$_2$ cells than the levels obtained with pRSVcat. The results obtained with the plasmids pBL-1cat, pBL-8cat, pBL-13cat, and pBL-3′ cat (Fig. 1) were very similar to pBL-9cat in the above experiments (data not shown). These data suggest that the productively infected cell lines express unique factors that regulate promoter activity by interacting with specific sequences in the BLV LTR.

Using the permissive FLK-BLV cell line as the host for transfections, we next sought to identify regions in the BLV LTR required for optimal expression of the heterologous gene. FLK-BLV cells accumulated nearly identical levels of CAT activity after transfections with pBL-1cat, pBL-8cat, pBL-9cat, pBL-13cat, or pBL-3′cat (data not shown), indicating that all of the transcriptional control sequences are contained entirely within the LTR; 5'-host or virus sequences flanking the LTR's in these constructs did not affect promoter activity. As shown in Fig. 3, sequences from the 5' and 3' ends of the LTR were deleted at the indicated restriction enzyme sites and the remainder of the LTR was then inserted into pSVOcat. Removal of 25 bp from the 5' end and 30 bp from the 3' end of the LTR did not adversely affect promoter function manifested as CAT activity (pBL-H2cat, Fig. 3). In pBL-P2cat, 61 bp has been deleted from the 5' end of the LTR, resulting in a 68 percent reduction of CAT activity compared to levels produced by pBL-9cat. The removal of an additional 26 bp from the 5' end (that is, deletion of nucleotides 1 through 88 in the LTR) caused a 91 percent decrease in the expression of CAT activity (pBL-P1cat, Fig. 3). It thus appears that sequences contained approximately between nucleotides numbered 30 to 100 in the BLV LTR (Fig. 3), 100 bp to 170 bp upstream of the RNA start site, are essential for optimal transcriptional activity. The position of this region, relative to the site of RNA initiation, is similar to where enhancer sequences have been identified in several other LTR's (*12, 13*).

Although this region contains several short (8 to 10 bp) direct and inverted repeats (*6, 7*), there is no extensive homology with other enhancer sequences. Weiher has proposed the existence of a core enhancer sequence, 5'-GTGG$^{AAA}_{TTT}$-3', which is found near a number of promoter units but whose functional significance is still unknown (*14*). Several related sequences are present in the region 100 to 170 bp upstream of the BLV RNA start site. As shown by the nucleotide numbering of the LTR in Fig. 3,

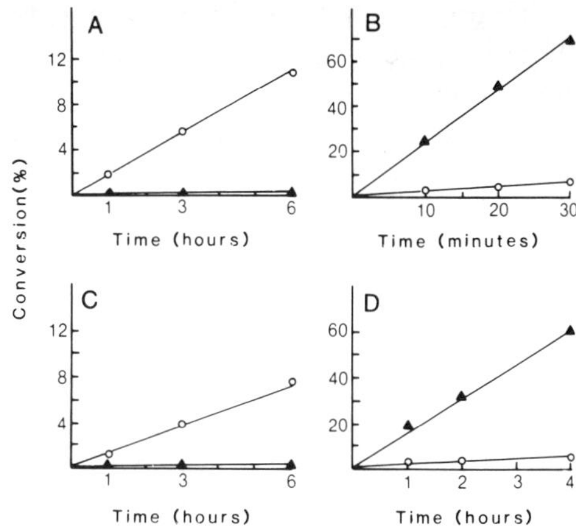

Fig. 2. Differential expression of CAT activity directed by BLV and RSV LTR's in uninfected and BLV-producer cells. Transfections and CAT assays were performed as described in Table 1. The percentage of ^{14}C-labeled chloramphenicol converted to monoacetate products is plotted as a function of incubation time with extracts of (A) FLK cells, (B) FLK-BLV cells, (C) bat lung TB1Lu cells, and (D) BLV-bat$_2$ cells transfected with pBL-9cat (△), pRSVcat (○), and pSVOcat (baseline).

these sequences are: 5'-CTGGTGA-3' (nucleotides 74 to 80), 5'-GTGGCTA-3' (nucleotides 93 to 99), and, in inverted form, 5'-AAACCAG-3' (nucleotides 44 to 50). Delineation of functionally significant sequences within this area of U3 must await more extensive analysis.

As stated above, removal of 30 bp from the 3' end of the LTR did not reduce CAT expression (pBL-H2 cat, Fig. 3). However, deletion of 176 bp of DNA from the 3' end of the LTR produced a 78 percent decrease in the expression of CAT activity (pBL-S2cat) and removal of 276 bp of 3' terminal LTR sequences, spanning the region between 50 bp downstream of the RNA start site and the 3'-end of the LTR, caused an 87 percent reduction in the transient accumulation of CAT activity (pBL-S1cat). The influence of LTR sequences located downstream of the RNA start site on heterologous gene expression has not previously been observed with other retroviral LTR's. Finally, the plasmid pBL-Hcat (Fig. 3), possessing 100 nucleotides on the 5′ side and 185 nucleotides on the 3′ side of the RNA start site, yielded a level of CAT activity that was only 3 percent of that obtained with pBL-9cat, suggesting that sequences located 5′ and

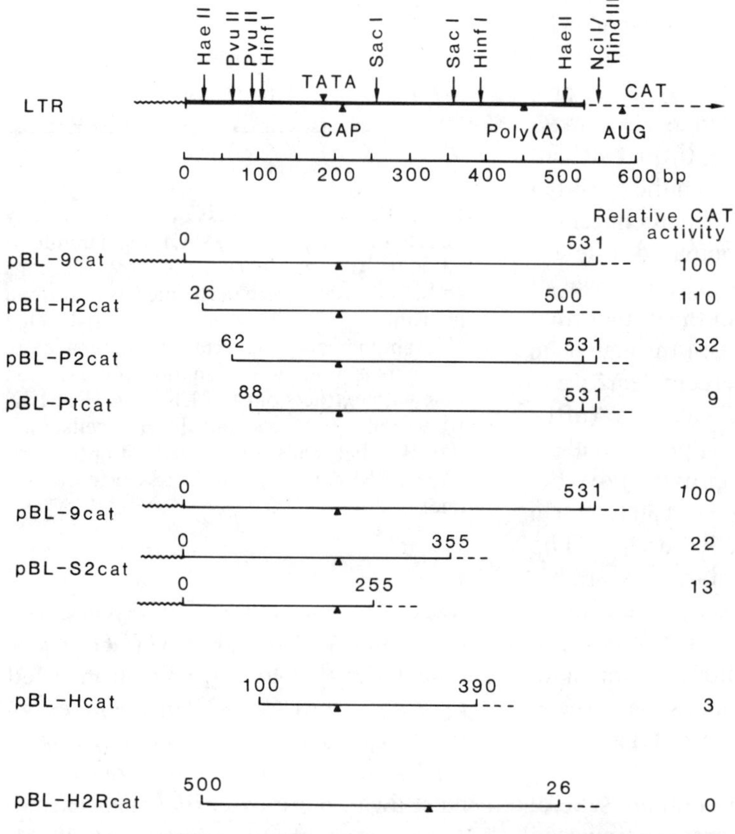

Fig. 3. Deletion mapping of LTR sequences that regulate the expression of CAT activity in FLK-BLV cells. The top line shows restriction enzyme sites in the 531-bp BLV LTR (heavy line) used to generate the deletions of the LTR sequences shown below. For reference, the viral poly(A) addition site (at nucleotide number 445) and the RNA start site (position number 205 ± 5) are shown (6, 7); the latter is indicated by an arrowhead in all of the deleted LTR's. The construction of pBL-9cat is described in the legend to Fig. 1. The remainder of the plasmids shown here were constructed by inserting restriction fragments into the Hind III site of pSVOcat as already outlined. The plasmids pBL-H2cat and pBL-H2Rcat were derived by cloning the 473-bp Hae II LTR fragment into pSVOcat in sense (pBL-H2cat) and antisense (pBL-H2Rcat) polarities with respect to the CAT gene. pBL-P2cat and pBL-P1cat were prepared by partial digestion of pBL-3′cat with Pvu II, followed by addition of Hind III linkers. After Hind III digestion, the 480-bp and 453-bp LTR fragments were purified by polyacrylamide gel electrophoresis and inserted into pSVOcat. pBL-S2cat and pBL-S1cat were generated from pBL-9cat by partial digestion with Sac I, end repair with T4 DNA polymerase, and addition of Hind III linkers. The 635-bp and 535-bp LTR fragments, obtained by gel electrophoresis of Hind III digests, were again inserted into pSVOcat. pBL-Hcat contains a 290-bp Hinf I LTR fragment cloned into the Hind III site of pSVOcat after Hind III linker addition. The transfections and assays were performed as described in Table 1. For the CAT assays we used 2 μl of cell extract incubated for 10, 20, and 30 minutes. Activities are expressed as percentages relative to the levels measured in extracts of cells transfected with pBL-9cat.

3′ to the RNA start site independently influence heterologous gene expression. It is unlikely that the 3′ deletion effect is solely the result of shortening the distance between the RNA start site and CAT coding sequences (in pBL9-cat this distance is 370 bp and in pBL-S2cat the distance is approximately 80 bp). The transcriptionally active LTR's contained within pRSVcat (*11*) and pMS-LTR2 (*12*) (carrying the Mo-MSV LTR coupled to the CAT gene) lack U5 and R sequences, and the viral RNA start sites are located 60 to 70 bp from the first AUG codon in the CAT gene. Our results indicate that the BLV LTR may contain two independent promoter control sequences (one in U3 and one in R), perhaps explaining why BLV has such an unusually long R region (*6, 7*). An alternative explanation that should not be overlooked is that deletion of U5 and parts of R may adversely affect post-transcriptional stages of gene expression.

While we anticipated that the BLV LTR would direct CAT expression in the cells known to produce BLV, it was surprising to observe a total lack of activity in all other cell lines tested. This cell type–specificity is reminiscent of the promoters controlling expression of insulin, chymotrypsin (*15*), and immunoglobulin (*16*) genes and is analogous to the cell-specific or response-specific expression previously observed with other retroviruses. Transcription of mouse mammary tumor virus is induced in response to glucocorticoids and mediated through an interaction of the activated hormone receptor with sequences in the LTR (*17*). Moloney murine leukemia virus is expressed in fibroblasts but not in F9 embryonal carcinoma (EC) cells (*18*). The transcriptional block in the latter cell line can be overcome by substituting

a variant enhancer element for its normal counterpart in the viral LTR, suggesting that the permissive and nonpermissive cells express different sets of regulatory proteins that interact with specific enhancer sequences (*18*). That BLV expression is also regulated by cellular *trans*acting factors in vivo is suggested by the biological behavior of the virus. For example, viral RNA cannot be detected in lymphocytes taken directly from infected animals (*19*). However, virus is transiently produced shortly after these cells are transferred to short-term culture (*20*), implying that BLV expression is regulated by cellular factors responsive to environmental stimuli.

Recently, the LTR's derived from HTLV-I and HTLV-II were examined with respect to promoter function (*21, 22*). In a manner similar to the BLV LTR, the HTLV-I and HTLV-II LTR's functioned at high levels only in cell lines known to express HTLV information. According to an alternative interpretation of this phenomenon, virus expression is activated by a viral gene product (*22*). In this model, a low-frequency transcriptional event would initiate a positive feedback scheme resulting in the production of virus at a high and uncontrolled level. For BLV, at least, this model seems inconsistent with the biologic properties of the virus in nature. We are inclined to believe that the events and factors that initiate the primary transcription of BLV are identical to those which allow its sustained expression in the producer cell lines. This raises the question of how the productively infected cell lines in our experiments acquired the ability to utilize the BLV promoter when the parental FLK and bat lung cells could not. This question is related to the problem of establishing cell lines productively infected with BLV, an apparently rare occurrence (3, 4). One explanation consistent with both of these observations is that the original cell populations contain rare variants that express the factor or factors that allow BLV promoter function and, thus, productive infection. Regardless of the type or origin of these regulatory factors, they probably interact with specific sequence elements in the LTR's.

We have observed that the BLV LTR functions as a highly restricted promoter unit and possesses sequences 5′ and 3′ to the RNA start site that influence gene expression. The expression of BLV in vivo is probably restricted to a specific cell type in the B-cell lineage or to a specific state of response of that cell to environmental stimuli. Characterization of the unique transcriptional regulatory factors present in the productively infected cell lines, which confer activity on the BLV promoter unit, should clarify the mechanisms of restricted viral expression seen in nature. Retroviral LTR's contain promoters that must be analogous to those of cellular genes, and cellular gene expression is highly regulated by a variety of mechanisms. Thus it is not surprising to observe tissue-specific or response-specific (hormonally regulated) retrovirus expression. BLV and HTLV are unusual biologically and structurally compared with all other RNA tumor viruses and it seems probable that they belong to a unique class of retroviruses whose other members have not yet been identified because of their highly restricted infectivity and expression.

References and Notes

1. A. Burny *et al.*, in *Viral Oncology*, G. Klein, Ed. (Raven, New York, 1980), pp. 231–289.
2. R. Kettmann *et al.*, *Proc. Natl. Acad. Sci. U.S.A.* **79**, 2465 (1982).
3. M. J. Van der Maaten and J. M. Miller, *Biblio. Haematol.* **43**, 360 (1976).
4. D. C. Graves and J. F. Ferrer, *Cancer Res.* **36**, 4152 (1976).
5. M. Seiki, S. Hattori, M. Yoshida, *Proc. Natl. Acad. Sci. U.S.A.* **79**, 6899 (1982); K. Shimotohno, D. W. Golde, M. Miwa, T. Sugimura, I. S. Y. Chen, *ibid.* **81**, 1079 (1984).
6. D. Couez *et al.*, *J. Virol.* **49**, 615 (1984); A. Tsimanis *et al.*, *Nucleic Acids Res.* **17**, 6079 (1983).
7. D. Derse, A. J. Diniak, J. Casey, P. L. Deininger, *Virology*, in press.
8. H. E. Varmus, *Science* **216**, 812 (1982).
9. J. W. Casey *et al.*, unpublished data.
10. C. M. Gorman, L. F. Moffat, B. H. Howard, *Mol. Cell. Biol.* **2**, 1044 (1982).
11. C. M. Gorman, G. T. Merlino, M. C. Willingham, A. Pastan, B. H. Howard, *Proc. Natl. Acad. Sci. U.S.A.* **79**, 6777 (1982).
12. L. A. Laimins, P. Gruss, R. Pozzatti, G. Khoury, *J. Virol.* **49**, 183 (1984).
13. A. Srinivasan, E. P. Reddy, C. Y. Dunn, S. A. Aaronson, *Science* **223**, 286 (1984).
14. H. Weiher, M. Konig, P. Gruss, *ibid.* **219**, 626 (1983).
15. M. D. Walker, T. Edlund, A. M. Boulet, W. J. Rutter, *Nature (London)* **306**, 557 (1983).
16. J. Stafford and C. Queen, *ibid.*, p. 77; S. D. Gillies, S. L. Morrison, V. T. Oi, S. Tonegawa, *Cell* **33**, 717 (1983); J. Banerji, L. Olson, W. Schaffner, *ibid.*, p. 729.
17. V. L. Chandler, B. A. Maler, K. R. Yamamoto, *Cell* **33**, 489 (1983).
18. E. Linney, B. Davis, J. Overhauser, E. Chao, H. Fan, *Nature (London)* **308**, 470 (1984).
19. R. Kettmann *et al.*, *Leuk. Res.* **4**, 509 (1980).
20. V. Baliga and J. F. Ferrer, *Proc. Soc. Exp. Biol. Med.* **156**, 388 (1977).
21. I. S. Y. Chen, J. McLaughlin, D. W. Golde, *Nature (London)* **309**, 276 (1984).
22. J. G. Sodrowski, C. A. Rosen, W. A. Haseltine, *Science* **225**, 381 (1984).
23. We thank B. Howard for the plasmids pSVOcat and pRSVcat and N. Rice for critical review of the manuscript. D.D. is supported by NIH postdoctoral fellowship CA07392.

5 October 1984; accepted 27 November 1984

Report

18 January 1985

75. *Trans* Activation of the Bovine Leukemia Virus Long Terminal Repeat in BLV-Infected Cells

Craig A. Rosen, Joseph G. Sodroski, Richard Kettman, Arsene Burny, and William A. Haseltine

The genome of bovine leukemia virus (BLV) contains the long terminal repeat (LTR), *gag*, *pol*, and *env* sequences characteristic of all retroviruses (*1*). In addition, like the human T-cell leukemia virus (HTLV), the BLV genome has a long open reading frame (LOR) region of approximately 1600 nucleotides 3' to the envelope gene (*2*). We have previously proposed that the HTLV LOR region protein mediates transcriptional *trans* activation of the HTLV LTR (*3*). Therefore, it was of interest to determine whether factors present in BLV-infected cells mediate *trans* activation of the BLV LTR.

The transcription initiation signals for retroviruses lie within the long terminal repeat (LTR) sequences that flank the integrated provirus (*4*). To test the transcriptional capabilities of the BLV LTR sequences, we constructed plasmids in which the BLV LTR was placed 5' to the bacterial chloramphenicol acetyltransferase (CAT) gene (Fig. 1) (*5*). To assay for transcriptional activity, we introduced the recombinant plasmids into eukaryotic cells via transfection (*6*). Levels of CAT enzymatic activity are closely correlated with levels of CAT messenger RNA, thereby providing a measure of the ability of the sequences 5' to the

CAT gene to promote transcription (*5, 7*).

The ability of the BLV LTR sequences to function as transcriptional elements in uninfected murine fibroblasts and human epithelial lines was tested. Parallel experiments were done with several other plasmids in which the CAT gene was under control of other promoter sequences. Upon transfection these additional plasmids all yielded appreciable levels of CAT activity (Table 1), indicating that the transfection procedures used resulted in efficient uptake and expression of DNA. No CAT activity was detected in extracts prepared from those cells that were transfected with the plasmid containing the BLV LTR sequences. Similar results were obtained after transfection of human T and B lymphocytes (Table 1). These results show that the BLV transcriptional elements do not function as a transcriptional promoter in these cells.

The ability of the BLV LTR sequence to function as a transcriptional element in BLV-infected and uninfected fetal lamb kidney (FLK) cells was examined. The CAT activity directed by the BLV LTR sequences was not detected in the uninfected cells, suggesting that the BLV LTR was inactive in these cells. In

Table 1. Relative CAT activity in transfected cells. Non-lymphoid and lymphoid cell lines were transfected by modifications of the $CaPO_4$ and DEAE dextran coprecipitation techniques, respectively (6). Preparation of cellular extracts and CAT assays were as described in the legend to Fig. 2. Plasmid pU3R-III contains the LTR of HTLV-III (3). To control for differences in the ability of different cell types to take up and express foreign DNA, we normalized the percentage conversion of chloramphenicol to its acetylated forms against the percentage conversion in similar cells transfected with pSV2cat taken as 1.0. Thus, the values represent the percentage acetylation per hour relative to that directed by pSV2cat. Plasmid pSV2cat and the other plasmids used are described in the legend to Fig. 2; ND, not done.

Cell line	Description	pSV2cat	pBLVcat	pU3R-I	pU3R-II	pU3R-III	pRSVcat	Reference
NIH 3T3	Murine fibroblast cell line	1.0	<0.05	0.9	ND	ND	ND	
Hela	Human cervical carcinoma line	1.0	<0.05	2.2	ND	ND	1.6	
HUT 78	HTLV-negative human T lymphocyte	1.0	<0.05	4.5	ND	ND	2.1	18
Raji	Human B lymphocyte immortalized by EBV	1.0	<0.05	6.2	ND	2.5	ND	19
FLK, uninfected	Fetal lamb kidney cell	1.0	<0.05	0.9	<0.05	1.9	1.9	
FLK BLV-producer	BLV-producing fetal lamb kidney cells	1.0	7.6	1.6	<0.05	2.5	1.3	20
CCL 88	Bat lung cells	1.0	<0.05	1.1	<0.05	ND	3.6	8
CCL 88 BLV-producer	BLV-producing bat lung cells	1.0	3.8	1.6	<0.05	ND	2.2	8
C 8166/45	HTLV-I immortalized nonproducer	1.0	<0.05	75	ND	2.8	ND	21
C3-44	HTLV-II producer T-cell line	1.0	<0.05	140	95	1.7	ND	18
MT2	HTLV-I immortalized producer T-cell line	1.0	<0.05	180	ND	1.4	2.5	21
H9	HTLV-negative human T lymphocyte	1.0	<0.05	2.5	<0.05	3.6	ND	22
H9/HTLV-III	H9 T-lymphocytes infected with HTLV-III	1.0	<0.05	3.2	<0.05	1,160	ND	22

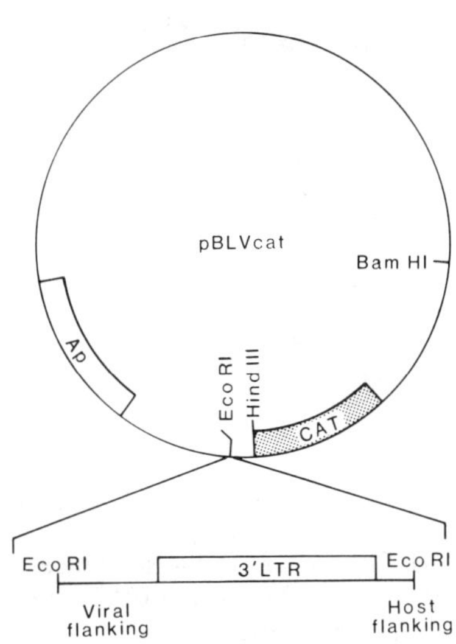

Fig. 1. Construction of pBLVcat. The BLV LTR sequences used in this study were those of the LTR subclone T15-4, obtained from an Eco RI tumor DNA fragment of a bovine lymphosarcoma (*14*). Subclone T15-4 was digested with Eco RI and the 890-base-pair fragment containing the BLV LTR was isolated from a low-melting agarose gel and ligated into the Eco RI site of plasmid pBR322. DNA was transfected into the *Escherichia coli* strain HB101 and ampicillin-resistant colonies were screened for the presence and orientation of the BLV insert. A positive clone was cleaved with Hind III–Bam HI and the vector fragment was isolated. The Hind III–Bam HI fragment of plasmid pSV2cat containing the CAT coding sequence and SV40 polyadenylation signals was ligated to this BLV fragment. The construction of the final plasmid, pBLVcat, was confirmed by extensive restriction enzyme analysis. Plasmid DNA was purified by banding in CsCI. All recombinant DNA techniques were according to established procedure (*17*). Enzyme digestions were done according to the manufacturers' specifications.

contrast, a high level of CAT activity was detected upon transfection of the BLV-infected producer cells (Table 1 and Fig. 2). The infected cell line used for this experiment produced BLV virions as demonstrated by high reverse transcriptase levels (data not shown). Similar results were obtained with additional uninfected and BLV-infected matched cell lines. The cell lines used were uninfected bat lung cells (CCL88) and a clonal isolate of the CCL88 line that produced BLV (*8*), and FLK cells that were infected with BLV 6 to 8 days prior to transfection (Table 1 and Fig. 2).

From these experiments we conclude that *trans* acting factors, either encoded by the virus or virally induced, activate BLV LTR-controlled gene expression. This effect probably occurs at the level of transcription (*3, 7*).

Gene expression directed by the LTR sequences of HTLV types I, II, and III is augmented by *trans* acting factors present in HTLV-infected cells (*3*). We tested if these factors could activate the BLV transcriptional control sequences. We have previously shown that *trans* acting factors present in HTLV-II–infected cells activate HTLV-1 LTR–directed CAT gene expression.

As indicated in Table 1, the *trans* acting factors present in the HTLV-I, HTLV-II, and HTLV-III infected cell lines were unable to activate BLV LTR–directed CAT gene expression. Similarly, factors present in the BLV-infected cells were unable to increase CAT gene expression directed by the different HTLV-LTR sequences. This suggests that the *trans* acting factors for HTLV-I, -II, and -III are not functionally interchangeable with those factors that activate the BLV LTR sequences; this is not surprising given the lack of primary sequence homology between the HTLV and BLV LTR sequence (*9, 10*).

The major determinant for efficient function of the BLV transcriptional elements may be the presence of BVL-

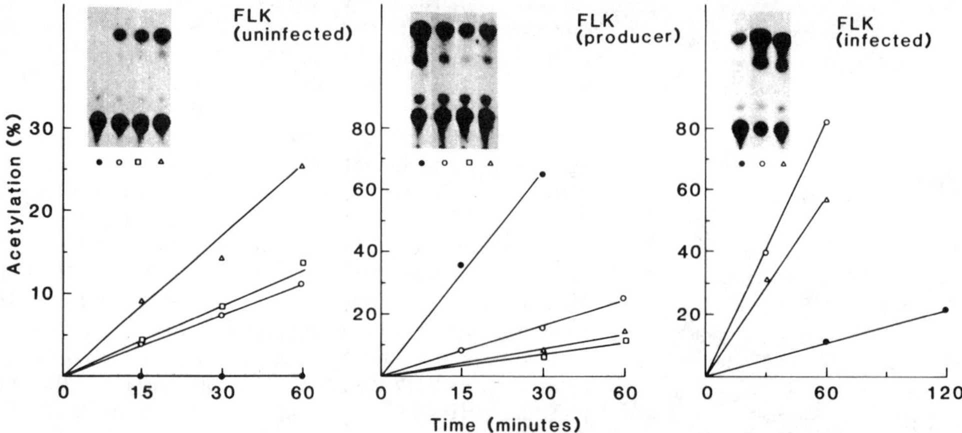

Fig. 2. Transient expression of the CAT gene directed by BLV LTR transcriptional sequences. In addition to the pBLVcat (●) plasmid several other plasmids that contained the CAT gene under control of other promoters were transfected for control purposes. These plasmids include pSV2cat (□), which contains the SV40 early region promoter sequences (5), pRSVCAT (△), which contains the Rous sarcoma virus LTR (5), and pU3R-I (○) and pU3R-II that contain the HTLV-I and HTLV-II LTR sequences, respectively (3). The recombinant plasmids were introduced into the fibroblast and epithelial cells by a modification of the $CaPO_4$ coprecipitation technique (6). Approximately 1×10^6 cells were seeded onto 100-mm dishes 24 hours prior to transfection. One milliliter of the $CaPO_4$ precipitate containing 5 μg of plasmid DNA and 30 μg of carrier salmon sperm DNA was added to the medium. After a 24-hour incubation period at 37°C the medium was removed, cells were washed once with phosphate-buffered saline (PBS), fed again with fresh medium containing 10 percent fetal bovine serum. Lymphocyte cell lines were transfected by the DEAE dextran method as described previously (6). Forty-eight hours after transfection, the cells were centrifuged (lymphocytes) or scraped from dishes, washed once with PBS, resuspended in 150 μl of 250 mM tris, pH 8.0, and subjected to three freeze (−70°C)-thaw (37°C) cycles. Debris was removed by a brief centrifugation and protein determinations were made on the cell extract. Acetyl coenzyme A (final concentration 4 mM) and ¹⁴C-labeled chloramphenicol (0.30 μCi) were added to the cell extracts, and a time-course assay was performed. The percentage conversion of chloramphenicol to its acetylated forms was determined by ascending thin-layer chromotography and liquid scintillation counting of the spots cut from the thin-layer chromatography plate. The graph depicts typical time-course assays obtained from the indicated cell types. The insets show actual autoradiograms of CAT conversions obtained from one time point within the linear range of a time-course assay. All experiments were repeated a minimum of three times and relative CAT activity differed by no more than 20 percent.

associated *trans* acting factors, because CAT gene expression directed by the plasmid that contains the BLV LTR was only observed in BLV-infected cells. In this respect BLV resembles HTLV-II rather than HTLV-I because the activity of the HTLV-II LTR appears to be restricted, for the most part, to HTLV-II–infected cells (3).

The phenomenon of *trans* activation and the presence of a LOR region distinguish both BLV and HTLV from other nonacute retroviruses. Circumstantial evidence suggests that *trans* activation of the HTLV LTR is mediated by the protein product of the HTLV LOR region (3, 11). Because the genome of BLV contains a LOR region 3′ to its envelope gene (2), we propose that the BLV LOR protein product mediates transcriptional activation of the BLV LTR. A 2-kilobase message capable of encoding such a protein has been detected in BLV-infected cells (12).

One question arising from these studies is how viral transcription proceeds after infection if the BLV LTR is nonfunctional in uninfected cells. A possible explanation might be that either small amounts of LOR protein or message are packaged in the virions and serve to initiate transcription upon virus entry into the cell. Alternatively, transcription may be occurring in the uninfected cells, but at a level too low to be detected in our assay. In any event, virus-induced *trans* acting transcriptional activation of the LTR should result in an autostimulatory effect, thus increasing the rate of BLV transcription and replication.

Bovine lymphosarcoma, the disease induced by BLV, is characterized by a long latency often preceded by persistent lymphoblastosis, absence of chronic viremia, and, most important, no site-specific viral integration (13, 14). These characteristics are different from the disease patterns associated with the murine and avian retroviruses yet are similar to the disease induced by HTLV-I (14, 15).

We have proposed that cellular immortalization by HTLV-I is mediated either directly or indirectly by the HTLV LOR product, possibly via *trans* activation of cellular genes involved in lymphocyte growth control. Because the disease characteristics, together with the phenomenon of *trans* activation, distinguish BLV and HTLV from other nonacute retroviruses, we suggest that the product of the BLV LOR region also plays an important role in the transformation process.

Similarities in the virion capsid protein of HTLV-I and -II and of BLV have been detected previously (1). Likewise, certain features of the LTR sequences of BLV resemble more closely those of HTLV-I and -II than they do the LTR regions of other retroviruses (16). Such features include an unusually long R region, the potential to perform a thermodynamically stable loop structure between sequences in the U3 and R regions (this loop includes the site of RNA initiation), and the absence of appropriately located polyadenylation signals (10). These common structural features, together with the functional (that is, *trans*-activation) and pathological similarities of HTLV-I and BLV-induced disease, indicate that these viruses are members of a new family of retroviruses distinct from both the nonacute and the acute (oncogene-containing) transforming retroviruses.

References and Notes

1. S. Oroszlan, T. D. Copeland, L. E. Henderson, J. R. Stephenson, R. V. Gilden, *Proc. Natl. Acad. Sci. U.S.A.* **76**, 2996 (1979).
2. W. A. Haseltine *et al.*, *Science* **225**, 419 (1984); N. R. Rice *et al.*, *Virology*, in press.
3. J. G. Sodroski, C. A. Rosen, W. A. Haseltine, *Science* **225**, 281 (1984); J. G. Sodroski *et al.*, *ibid.* **227**, 171 (1985).
4. H. M. Temin, *Cell* **28**, 3 (1982).
5. C. M. Gorman, G. T. Merlino, M. C. Willingham, I. Pastan, B. Howard, *Proc. Natl. Acad. Sci. U.S.A.* **78**, 6777 (1982).
6. F. L. Graham and A. J. Van der Eb, *J. Virol.* **52**, 456 (1973); C. Queen and D. Baltimore, *Cell* **33**, 741 (1983).
7. S. L. McKnight, E. R. Gavis, R. Kingsbury, *Cell* **25**, 385 (1981); M. D. Walker, T. Edlund, A. M. Boulet, W. J. Rutter, *Nature (London)* **306**, 557 (1983).
8. D. C. Graves and J. F. Ferrer, *Cancer Res.* **36**, 4152 (1976).
9. D. Couez *et al.*, *J. Virol.* **49**, 615 (1984); S. Josephs *et al.*, *Virology*, in press; A. Tsimanis *et al.*, *Nucleic Acid. Res.* **17**, 6079 (1983).
10. J. Sodroski *et al.*, *Proc. Natl. Acad. Sci. U.S.A.* **81**, 4617 (1984).
11. T. H. Lee *et al.*, *Science* **226**, 57 (1984).
12. J. Ghysdael, R. Kettman, A. Burny, *J. Virol.* **29**, 1087 (1979); R. Z. Mamoun, personal communication.
13. A. Burny *et al.*, in *Viral Oncology*, G. Klein, Ed. (Raven, New York, 1974); J. F. Ferrer, C. Auila, N. D. Stock, *Cancer Res.* **32**, 1864 (1977).
14. R. Kettman *et al.*, *Proc. Natl. Acad. Sci.*

U.S.A. **79**, 2465 (1982).
15. V. S. Kalyanaramen *et al.*, *ibid.*, p. 1653; B. J. Poiesz *et al.*, *ibid.* **77**, 7415 (1980); T. Uchiyama, J. Yodoï, K. Sagawa, K. Takasuki, H. Uchino, *Blood* **50**, 481 (1977).
16. N. Sagata, T. Yasunaga, Y. Ogawa, J. Tsuzuku-Kawamura, Y. Ikawa, *Proc. Natl. Acad. Sci. U.S.A.* **81**, 4741 (1984).
17. T. Maniatis, E. F. Fritsch, J. V. Sambrook, in *Molecular Cloning: A Laboratory Manual* (Cold Spring Harbor Laboratory, Cold Spring Harbor, N.Y., 1982).
18. V. Manzari *et al.*, *Proc. Natl. Acad. Sci. U.S.A.* **80**, 11 (1983).
19. R. Glaser and M. Nonoyama, *J. Virol.* **14**, 174 (1974).
20. M. J. Van der Maaten and J. M. Miller, *Bibl. Haematol. (Basel)* **43**, 360 (1976).
21. S. Z. Salahuddin *et al.*, *Virology* **129**, 51 (1983).
22. M. Popovic, G. Sarngadharan, E. Rend, R. C. Gallo, *Science* **224**, 497 (1984); R. C. Gallo *et al.*, *ibid.*, p. 500.
23. We thank N. Shiomi for technical assistance and D. Artz for help in preparation of the manuscript. Supported by American Cancer Society Directors Grant RD-186, and NIH grant CA36974. C.A.R. and J.G.S. were supported by grants CA97580 and CA07094, respectively. R.K. is Cherchour Guslific du Fords National Belge de la Recherche Scientifique.

14 September 1984; accepted 28 November 1984

76.   AIDS Virus Genomes

Jean L. Marx

The molecular characterization of the virus that causes AIDS (acquired immune deficiency syndrome) continues to move at a rapid clip. Four groups have now determined the complete nucleotide sequences of the genetic material of viruses that have been linked to the disease.

Paul Luciw of Chiron Research Laboratories in Emeryville, California, Jay Levy of the University of California, School of Medicine, in San Francisco, and their colleagues report the sequence for the virus they have christened "AIDS-associated retrovirus" (ARV) in the 1 February 1985 issue of *Science*. A second group, including Lee Ratner, Flossie Wong-Staal, and Robert Gallo of the National Cancer Institute, Mark Pearson of E.I. du Pont de Nemours and Company in Wilmington, and William Haseltine of Harvard's Dana-Farber Cancer Institute, report sequences for two isolates of the virus desig-nated "human T-cell lymphotropic virus-III" (HTLV-III) in the 24 January 1985 issue of *Nature*. A group from Genentech, Inc., in San Francisco, is also publishing AIDS virus sequences in the 7 February 1985 issue of *Nature*. And the fourth group, from Luc Montagnier's laboratory at the Pasteur Institute in Paris, published the sequence for the virus they have called "lymphadenopathy-associated virus" (LAV) in the January 1985 issue of *Cell*. Despite the different names given these viruses, there is now general agreement that they are variants of the same virus.

One question that the sequence data can help answer concerns how closely the AIDS virus resembles other retroviruses, especially HTLV-I and -II. All four groups find that there are substantial differences between the genome of HTLV-III and the HTLV-I and -II genomes, although some short segments show resemblances. "ARV is no more closely related to HTLV-I and -II than to other retroviruses," Luciw concludes. Simon Wain-Hobson of the Pasteur Institute presented similar findings for LAV at the recent "HTLV Symposium," which was sponsored by the NCI and held in Bethesda, Maryland, on 6 and 7 December 1984. However, Gallo notes that there are other points of similarity between HTLV-III and the other two HTLV's that would favor including them in the same viral category.

Another important question, one that bears upon the possible mode of action of the AIDS virus as well as its relation to HTLV-I and -II, concerns whether its genome contains a "long-open reading frame" (LOR region) near its right-hand end similar to those in the HTLV-I and -II genomes. The products of the HTLV-I and -II LOR regions increase viral and possibly cellular gene expression, according to Haseltine, and this activity may be what causes the malignant transformation of infected cells. Haseltine, Wong-Staal, and their colleagues also have evidence that HTLV-III produces an analogous factor.

The organization of the ARV genome does not show a LOR region comparable to that of HTLV-I and -II, Luciw says, although it does have a protein-coding sequence about half the size of LOR in an analogous location. He notes that the organization of the ARV genome is very similar to what Wain-Hobson proposes for LAV. The Gallo group has a different interpretation of the coding sequence arrangement in the right-hand region of the HTLV-III genome. Although they do not see a separate LOR region there, their results indicate that the long *env* gene has a dual function. Depending on how the messenger RNA product of the gene is spliced, it can produce either the protein that forms the viral envelope or a protein of size comparable to the HTLV-I and -II LOR products.

Finally, restriction mapping of the genomes of various AIDS virus isolates has already shown that these may vary in structure, a result that is being confirmed by the sequence analyses. For example, the sequence of the long terminal repeat of HTLV-III, which was determined by the Gallo–Wong-Staal group and also appears in the 1 February 1985 issue of *Science*, differs in about 5 percent of its nucleotides from the long terminal repeat of ARV. Sequence analysis may help to identify viral gene segments that are highly conserved, and thus important for viral activities. Moreover, the corresponding peptides might eventually prove useful for producing reagents to detect infection by the virus or a vaccine to protect against AIDS.

Research Article

1 February 1985

77. Nucleotide Sequence and Expression of an AIDS-Associated Retrovirus (ARV-2)

Ray Sanchez-Pescador, Michael D. Power, Philip J. Barr, Kathelyn S. Steimer, Michelle M. Stempien, Sheryl L. Brown-Shimer, Wendy W. Gee, Andre Renard, Anne Randolph, Jay A. Levy, Dino Dina, and Paul A. Luciw

A wide variety of diseases in many animal species are a consequence of infection by retroviruses (*1*). A distinct group of human retroviruses has been isolated from patients with the acquired immune deficiency syndrome (AIDS) and individuals with related conditions, such as persistent lymphadenopathy. Several independent isolates, called lymphadenopathy-associated virus or LAV (*2*), human T-cell lymphotropic virus type III or HTLV-III (*3*), and AIDS-associated retrovirus or ARV (*4*) by the laboratories of origin, are similar with respect to morphology, cytopathology, requirements for optimum reverse transcriptase activity, at least some antigenic properties, and some restriction endonuclease cleavage sites in viral DNA. Epidemiological studies show that infection by one of these viruses may be a necessary condition for the development of AIDS, although predisposing factors may contribute to the onset of the disease (*3–10*).

Molecular clones of HTLV-III, LAV, and ARV-2 have been described (*11, 12*). These clones provide material for analyses of viral structure, viral replication, and mechanisms of pathogenesis as well as for measurements of similarities and differences among the retroviruses asso-

ciated with AIDS and with other retroviruses. In this report, the genetic structure of an ARV isolate is established from the sequences of molecular clones of ARV-2 DNA (*12*) and from the partial sequence of virion proteins.

The DNA sequence of ARV-2. Proviral DNA and circular unintegrated viral DNA species from ARV-2 infected cells have been cloned in bacteriophage λ (*12*), and the structures of five recombinant phage containing ARV-2 DNA were characterized (Fig. 1). The nucleotide sequence of various regions of each of these molecular clones was determined and used to establish the complete sequence of ARV-2 DNA. The sequence variations in ARV-2 DNA in these phage are presented in Table 1.

Long terminal repeat regions (LTR's). The LTR's of retroviruses participate in the integration of the virus with the host cell and in the regulation of transcription of viral ‘genes (*13–15*). To define the precise boundaries of the LTR sequences, we compared the junctions with host-cell DNA in the sequences of λ-9B, λ-7A, λ-8A, and λ-7D (Fig. 1). The LTR of ARV-2 is 636 bp and is bounded by an inverted repeat of 3 bp (CTG) (Fig. 2). The sizes of the inverted repeat at the ends of the LTR's of the other human

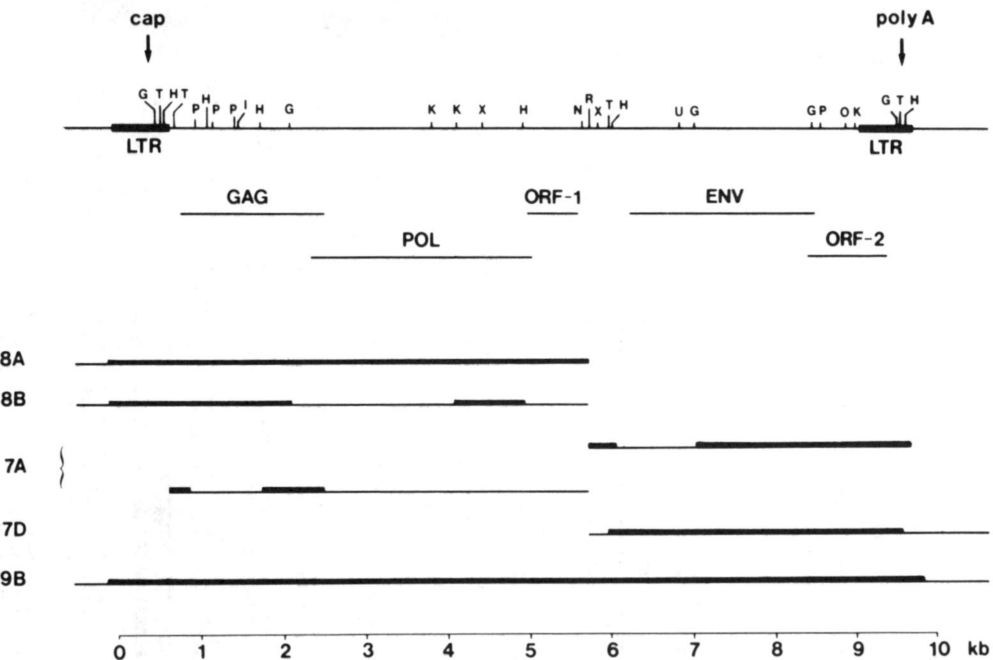

Fig. 1. Restriction endonuclease map of ARV-2. Five recombinant λ clones were isolated (*12*) and used to determine the nucleotide sequence of ARV. Clones 8A, 8B, 7D, and 9B represent integrated DNA. Clone 7A is from unintegrated DNA (*12*). The heavy lines indicate regions that were sequenced in each clone. The regions that encompass the *gag, pol*, and *env* ORF's as well as two additional open reading frames are indicated. G = Bgl II, H = Hind III, I = Sph I, K = Kpn I, N = Nco I, O = Xho I, P = Pst I, R = Eco RI, T = Sst I, U = Pvu II, X = Xba I.

retroviruses, HTLV-I and HTLV-II, are 2 bp (*16, 17*). Integration of proviruses did not occur in a specific site in the host cell genome since adjacent cell DNA sequences in λ-9B, λ-8A, and λ-7D were unique (data not shown). Preceding the rightward (3′) LTR is a polypurine tract of 16 bp beginning at position 8632 (Fig. 2). Polypurine tracts are similarly positioned in other retroviruses and play an important role in the initiation of plus-strand DNA synthesis (*15*). Immediately downstream from the leftward (5′) LTR is a sequence of 18 bp that is complementary to 18 bases of a transfer RNA–lysine (tRNA^{lys}) species (Fig. 2). Initiation of minus-strand DNA synthesis in retrovir-

uses requires a host cell tRNA molecule as a primer (*15*). MMTV (mouse mammary tumor virus) also requires a tRNA^{lys} molecule (*18*), whereas other known mammalian retroviruses includ-

Table 1. Polymorphism of the λ recombinants shown in Fig. 1.

Position*	7A	7D	8A	8B	9B
−123	G		A		G
−115	G		A		G
3789			A	G	
4223			T	C	
5761	G	A			G

*Numbering system as described in Fig. 2.

Fig. 2


```
                                                                                                                              L
       U3→                                                                                                                    T
-453   CTGGAAGGGCTAATTTGGTCCCAAAGAAGACAAGAGATCCTTGATCTGTGGATCTACCACACACAAGGCTACTTCCCTGATTGGCAGAATTACACACCAGGGCCAGGGATCAGATATCCA  R
-333   CTGACCTTTGGATGGTGCTTCAAGCTAGTACCAGTTGAGCCAGAGAAGGTAGAAGAGGCCAATGAAGGAGAGAACAACAGCTTGTTACACCCTATGAGCCTGCATGGGATGGAGGACGCG
-214   GAGAAAGAAGTGTTAGTGTGGAGGTTTGACAGCAAACTAGCATTTCATCACATGGCCCGAGAGCTGCATCCGGAGTACTACAAAGACTGCTGACATCGAGCTTTCTACAAGGGACTTTCCG
                                                                                           ←U3 R→
 -93   CTGGGGACTTTCCAGGGAGGCGTGGCCTGGGCGGGACTGGGGAGTGGCGTCCCTCAGATGCTGCATATAAGCAGCTGCTTTTTGCCTGTACTG GGTCTCTCTGGTTAGACCAGATCTGAG
                                                                                         ←R U5→
  28   CCTGGGAGCTCTCTGGCTAACTAGGGAACCCACTGCTTAAGCCTCAATAAAGCTTGCCTTGAGTGCTTCA AGTAGTGTGTGCCCGTCTGTTGTGTGACTCTGGTAACTAGAGATCCCTCA
                    ←U5
 148   GACCCTTTTAGTCAGTGTGGAAAAATCTCTAGCAG TGGCGCCCGAACAGGGACGCGAAAGCGAAAGTAGAACCAGAGGAGCTCTCTCGACGCAGGACTCGGCTTGCTGAAGCGCGCACAG

                           LysGluArgGluMetGlyAlaArgAlaSerValLeuSerGlyGlyGluLeuAspLysTrpGlu 21
 268   CAAGAGGCGAGGGGCGGCGACTGGTGAGTACGCCAATTTTTGACTAGCGGAGGCTAGAAGGAGAGAGAGATGGGTGCGAGAGCGTCGGTATTAAGCGGGGGAGAATTAGATAAATGGGAA

       LysIleArgLeuArgProGlyGlyLysLysLysTyrLysLeuLysHisIleValTrpAlaSerArgGluLeuGluArgPheAlaValAsnProGlyLeuLeuGluThrSerGluGlyCys 61
 388   AAAATTCGGTTAAGGCCAGGGGGAAAGAAAAAATATAAGTTAAAACATATAGTATGGGCAAGCAGGGAGCTAGAACGATTCGCAGTCAATCCTGGCCTGTTAGAAACATCAGAAGGCTGC

       ArgGlnIleLeuGlyGlnLeuGlnProSerLeuGlnThrGlySerGluGluLeuArgSerLeuTyrAsnThrValAlaThrLeuTyrCysValHisGlnArgIleAspValLysAspThr 101
 508   AGACAAATATTGGGACAGCTACAGCCATCCCTTCAGACAGGATCAGAAGAACTTAGATCATTATATAATACAGTAGCAACCCTCTATTGTGTACATCAAAGGATAGATGTAAAAGACACC

       LysGluAlaLeuGluLysIleGluGluGluGlnAsnLysSerLysLysLysAlaGlnGlnAlaAlaAlaAlaAlaGlyThrGlyAsnSerSerGlnValSerGlnAsnTyrProIleVal 141
 628   AAGGAAGCTTTAGAGAAGATAGAGGAAGAGCAAAACAAAAGTAAGAAAAAGGCACAGCAAGCAGCAGCTGCAGCTGGCACAGGAAACAGCAGCCAGGTCAGCCAAAATTACCCTATAGTG

       GlnAsnLeuGlnGlyGlnMetValHisGlnAlaIleSerProArgThrLeuAsnAlaTrpValLysValValGluGluLysAlaPheSerProGluValIleProMetPheSerAlaLeu 181
 748   CAGAACCTACAGGGGCAAATGGTACATCAGGCCATATCACCTAGAACTTTAAATGCATGGGTAAAAGTAGTAGAAGAAAAGGCTTTCAGCCCAGAAGTAATACCCATGTTTTCAGCATTA

       SerGluGlyAlaThrProGlnAspLeuAsnThrMetLeuAsnThrValGlyGlyHisGlnAlaAlaMetGlnMetLeuLysGluThrIleAsnGluGluAlaAlaGluTrpAspArgVal 221
 868   TCAGAAGGAGCCACCCCACAAGATTTAAACACCATGCTAAACACAGTGGGGGGACATCAAGCAGCCATGCAAATGTTAAAAGAGACTATCAATGAGGAAGCTGCAGAATGGGATAGAGTG

       HisProValHisAlaGlyProIleAlaProGlyGlnMetArgGluProArgGlySerAspIleAlaGlyThrThrSerThrLeuGlnGlnIleGlyTrpMetThrAsnAsnProPro 261
 988   CATCCAGTGCATGCAGGGCCTATTGCACCAGGCCAAATGAGAGAACCAAGGGGAAGTGACATAGCAGGAACTACTAGTACCCTTCAGGAACAAATAGGATGGATGACAAATAATCCACCT

       IleProValGlyGluIleTyrLysArgTrpIleIleLeuGlyLeuAsnLysIleValArgMetTyrSerProThrSerIleLeuAspIleArgGlnGlyProLysGluProPheArgAsp 301
1108   ATCCCAGTAGGAGAAATCTATAAAAGATGGATAATCCTGGGATTAAATAAAATAGTAAGAATGTATAGCCCTACCAGCATTCTGGACATAAGACAAGGACCAAAGGAACCCTTTAGAGAT

       TyrValAspArgPheTyrLysThrLeuArgAlaGluGlnAlaSerGlnAspValLysAsnTrpMetThrGluThrLeuLeuValGlnAsnAlaAsnProAspCysLysThrIleLeuLys 341
1228   TATGTAGACCGGTTCTATAAAACTCTAAGAGCCGAACAAGCTTCACAGGATGTAAAAAATTGGATGACAGAAACCTTGTTGGTCCAAAATGCAAACCCAGATTGTAAGACTATTTTAAAA

       AlaLeuGlyProAlaAlaThrLeuGluGluMetMetThrAlaCysGlnGlyValGlyGlyProGlyHisLysAlaArgValLeuAlaGluAlaMetSerGlnValThrAsnProAlaAsn 381
1348   GCATTGGGACCAGCAGCTACACTAGAAGAAATGATGACAGCATGTCAGGGAGTGGGGGGACCCGGCCATAAAGCAAGAGTTTTGGCTGAAGCCATGAGCCAAGTAACAAATCCAGCTAAC

       IleMetMetGlnArgGlyAsnPheArgAsnGlnArgLysThrValLysCysPheAsnCysGlyLysGluGlyHisIleAlaLysAsnCysArgAlaProArgLysLysGlyCysTrpArg 421
1468   ATAATGATGCAGAGAGGCAATTTTAGGAACCAAAGAAAGACTGTTAAGTGTTTCAATTGTGGCAAAGAAGGGCACATAGCCAAAAATTGCAGGGCCCCTAGGAAAAAGGGCTGTTGGAGA

       CysGlyArgGluGlyHisGlnMetLysAspCysThrGluArgGlnAlaAsnPheLeuGlyLysIleTrpProSerTyrLysGlyArgProGlyAsnPheLeuGlnSerArgProGluPro 461
       PhePheArgGluAspLeuAlaPheLeuGlnGlyLysAlaArgGluPheSerSerGluGlnThrArgAla 23
1588   TGTGGAAGGGAAGGACACCAAATGAAAGATTGCACTGAGAGACAGGCTAATTTTTTAGGGAAGATCTGGCCTTCCTACAAGGGAAGGCCAGGGAATTTTCTTCAGAGCAGACCAGAGCCA

       ThrAlaProProGluGluSerPheArgPheGlyGluGluLysThrThrProSerGlnLysGlnGluProIleAspLysGluLeuTyrProLeuThrSerLeuArgSerLeuPheGlyAsn 501
       AsnSerProThrArgArgGluLeuGlnValTrpGlyGlyGluAsnAsnSerLeuSerGluAlaGlyAlaAspArgGlnGlyThrValSerPheAsnPheProGlnIleThrLeuTrpGln 63
1708   ACAGCCCCACCAGAAGAGAGCTTCAGGTTTGGGGAGGAGAAAACAACTCCCTCTCAGAAGCAGGAGCCGATAGACAAGGAACTGTATCCTTTAACTTCCCTCAGATCACTCTTTGGCAAC
```

G
A
G

```
       AspProSerSerGlnOC
       ArgProLeuValThrIleArgIleGlyGlyGlnLeuLysGluAlaLeuLeuAspThrGlyAlaAspAspThrValLeuGluGluMetAsnLeuProGlyLysTrpLysProLysMetIle 103
1828   GACCCCTCGTCACAATAAGGATAGGGGGGCAACTAAAGGAAGCTCTATTAGATACAGGAGCAGATGATACAGTATTAGAAGAAATGAATTTGCCAGGAAAATGGAAACCAAAAATGATAG

       GlyGlyIleGlyGlyPheIleLysValArgGlnTyrAspGlnIleProValGluIleCysGlyHisLysAlaIleGlyThrValLeuValGlyProThrProValAsnIleIleGlyArg 143
1948   GGGGAATTGGAGGTTTTATCAAAGTAAGACAGTACGATCAGATACCTGTAGAAATCTGTGGACATAAAGCTATAGGTACAGTATTAGTAGGACCTACACCTGTCAACATAATTGGAAGAA

       AsnLeuLeuThrGlnIleGlyCysThrLeuAsnPheProIleSerProIleGluThrValProValLysLeuLysProGlyMetAspGlyProLysValLysGlnTrpProLeuThrGlu 183
2068   ATCTGTTGACTCAGATTGGTTGTACTTTAAATTTCCCCATTAGTCCTATTGAAACTGTACCAGTAAAATTAAAGCCAGGAATGGATGGCCCAAAAGTTAAGCAATGGCCATTGACAGAAG

       GluLysIleLysAlaLeuValGluIleCysThrGluMetGluLysGluGlyLysIleSerLysIleGlyProGluAsnProTyrAsnThrProValPheAlaIleLysLysLysAspSer 223
2188   AAAAAATAAAAGCATTAGTAGAGATATGTACAGAAATGGAAAAGGAAGGGAAAATTTCAAAAATTGGGCCTGAAAATCCATACAATACTCCAGTATTTGCTATAAAGAAAAAAGACAGTA

       ThrLysTrpArgLysLeuValAspPheArgGluLeuAsnLysArgThrGlnAspPheTrpGluValGlnLeuGlyIleProHisProAlaGlyLeuLysLysLysLysSerValThrVal 263
2308   CTAAATGGAGAAAACTAGTAGATTTCAGAGAACTTAATAAAAGAACTCAAGACTTCTGGGAAGTTCAGTTAGGAATACCACACCCCGCAGGGTTAAAAAAGAAAAAATCAGTAACAGTAT

       LeuAspValGlyAspAlaTyrPheSerValProLeuAspLysAspPheArgLysTyrThrAlaPheThrIleProSerIleAsnAsnGluThrProGlyIleArgTyrGlnTyrAsnVal 303
2428   TGGATGTGGGTGATGCATACTTTTCAGTTCCCTTAGATAAAGACTTTAGAAAGTATACTGCATTTACCATACCTAGTATAAACAATGAGACACCAGGGATTAGATATCAGTACAATGTGC

       LeuProGlnGlyTrpLysGlySerProAlaIlePheGlnSerSerMetThrLysIleLeuGluProPheArgLysGlnAsnProAspIleValIleTyrGlnTyrMetAspAspLeuTyr 343
2548   TGCCACAGGGATGGAAAGGATCACCAGCAATATTCCAAAGTAGCATGACAAAAATCTTAGAGCCTTTTAGAAAACAGAATCCAGACATAGTTATCTATCAATACATGGATGATTTGTATG

       ValGlySerAspLeuGluIleGlyGlnHisArgThrLysIleGluGluLeuArgGlnHisLeuLeuArgTrpGlyPheThrThrProAspLysLysHisGlnLysGluProProPheLeu 383
2668   TAGGATCTGACTTAGAAATAGGGCAGCATAGAACAAAAATAGAGGAACTGAGACAGCATCTGTTGAGGTGGGGATTTACCACACCAGACAAAAAACATCAGAAAGAACCTCCATTCCTTT

       TrpMetGlyTyrGluLeuHisProAspLysTrpThrValGlnProIleMetLeuProGluLysAspSerTrpThrValAsnAspIleGlnLysLeuValGlyLysLeuAsnTrpAlaSer 423
2788   GGATGGGTTATGAACTCCATCCTGATAAATGGACAGTACAGCCTATAATGCTGCCAGAAAAAGACAGCTGGACTGTCAATGACATACAGAAGTTAGTGGGAAAATTGAATTGGGCAAGTC

       GlnIleTyrAlaGlyIleLysValLysGlnLeuCysLysLeuLeuArgGlyThrLysAlaLeuThrGluValIleProLeuThrGluGluAlaGluLeuGluLeuAlaGluAsnArgGlu 463
2908   AGATTTATGCAGGGATTAAAGTAAAGCAGTTATGTAAACTCCTTAGAGGAACCAAAGCACTAACAGAAGTAATACCACTAACAGAAGAAGCAGAGCTAGAACTGGCAGAAAACAGGGAGA

       IleLeuLysGluProValHisGluValTyrTyrAspProSerLysAspLeuValAlaGluIleGlnLysGlnGlyGlnGlyGlnTrpThrTyrGlnIleTyrGlnGluProPheLysAsn 503
3028   TTCTAAAAGAACCAGTACATGAAGTATATTATGACCCATCAAAAGACTTAGTAGCAGAAATACAGAAGCAGGGGCAAGGCCAATGGACATATCAAATTTATCAAGAGCCATTTAAAAATC

       LeuLysThrGlyLysTyrAlaArgMetArgGlyAlaHisThrAsnAspValLysGlnLeuThrGluAlaValGlnLysValSerThrGluSerIleValIleTrpGlyLysIleProLys 543
3148   TGAAAACAGGAAAGTATGCAAGGATGAGGGGTGCCCACACTAATGATGTAAAACAGTTAACAGAGGCAGTGCAAAAAGTATCCACAGAAAGCATAGTAATATGGGGAAAGATTCCTAAAT

       PheLysLeuProIleGlnLysGluThrTrpGluAlaTrpTrpMetGluTyrTrpGlnAlaThrTrpIleProGluTrpGluPheValAsnThrProProLeuValLysLeuTrpTyrGln 583
3268   TTAAACTACCCATACAAAAGGAAACATGGGAAGCATGGTGGATGGAGTATTGGCAAGCTACCTGGATTCCTGAGTGGGAGTTTGTCAATACCCCTCCCTTAGTGAAATTATGGTACCAGT

       LeuGluLysGluProIleValGlyAlaGluThrPheTyrValAspGlyAlaAlaAsnArgGluThrLysLeuGlyLysAlaGlyTyrValThrAspArgGlyArgGlnLysValValSer 623
3388   TAGAGAAAGAACCCATAGTAGGAGCAGAAACTTTCTATGTAGATGGGGCAGCTAATAGGGAGACTAAATTAGGAAAAGCAGGATATGTTACTGACAGAGGAAGACAAAAAGTTGTCTCCA

       IleAlaAspThrThrAsnGlnLysThrGluLeuGlnAlaIleHisLeuAlaLeuGlnAspSerGlyLeuGluValAsnIleValThrAspSerGlnTyrAlaLeuGlyIleIleGlnAla 663
3508   TAGCTGACACAACAAATCAGAAGACTGAATTACAAGCAATTCATCTAGCTTTGCAGGATTCGGGATTAGAAGTAAACATAGTAACAGACTCACAATATGCATTAGGAATCATTCAAGCAC

       GlnProAspLysSerGluSerGluLeuValSerGlnIleIleGluGlnLeuIleLysLysGluLysValTyrLeuAlaTrpValProAlaHisLysGlyIleGlyGlyAsnGluGlnVal 703
3628   AACCAGATAAGAGTGAATCAGAGTTAGTCAGTCAAATAATAGAGCAGTTAATAAAAAAGGAAAAGGTCTACCTGGCATGGGTACCAGCACACAAAGGAATTGGAGGAAATGAACAAGTAG

       AspLysLeuValSerAlaGlyIleArgLysValLeuPheLeuAsnGlyIleAspLysAlaGlnGluGluHisGluLysTyrHisSerAsnTrpArgAlaMetAlaSerAspPheAsnLeu 743
3748   ATAAATTAGTCAGTGCTGGAATCAGGAAAGTACTATTTTTGAATGGAATAGATAAGGCCCAAGAAGAACATGAGAAATATCACAGTAATTGGAGAGCAATGGCTAGTGATTTTAACCTGC

       ProProValValAlaLysGluIleValAlaSerCysAspLysCysGlnLeuLysGlyGluAlaMetHisGlyGlnValAspCysSerProGlyIleTrpGlnLeuAspCysThrHisLeu 783
3868   CACCTGTAGTAGCAAAAGAAATAGTAGCCAGCTGTGATAAATGTCAGCTAAAAGGAGAAGCCATGCATGGACAAGTAGACTGTAGTCCAGGAATATGGCAACTAGATTGTACACATCTAG

       GluGlyLysIleIleLeuValAlaValHisValAlaSerGlyTyrIleGluAlaGluValIleProAlaGluThrGlyGlnGluThrAlaTyrPheLeuLeuLysLeuAlaGlyArgTrp 823
3988   AAGGAAAAATTATCCTGGTAGCAGTTCATGTAGCCAGTGGATATATAGAAGCAGAAGTTATTCCAGCAGAGACAGGGCAGGAAACAGCATATTTTCTCTTAAAATTAGCAGGAAGATGGC
```

P O L

(continued)

Fig. 2 (continued).


```
             ProValLysThrIleHisThrAspAsnGlySerAsnPheThrSerThrThrValLysAlaAlaCysTrpTrpAlaGlyIleLysGlnGluPheGlyIleProTyrAsnProGlnSerGln 863
4108   CAGTAAAAACAATACATACAGACAATGGCAGCAATTTCACCAGTACTACGGTTAAGGCCGCCTGTTGGTGGGCAGGGATCAAGCAGGAATTTGGCATTCCCTACAATCCCCAAAGTCAAG

             GlyValValGluSerMetAsnAsnGluLeuLysLysIleIleGlyGlnValArgAspGlnAlaGluHisLeuLysThrAlaValGlnMetAlaValPheIleHisAsnPheLysArgLys 903
4228   GAGTAGTAGAATCTATGAATAATGAATTAAAGAAAATTATAGGACAGGTAAGAGATCAGGCTGAACACCTTAAGACAGCAGTACAAATGGCAGTATTCATCCACAATTTTAAAAGAAAAG

             GlyGlyIleGlyGlyTyrSerAlaGlyGluArgIleValAspIleIleAlaThrAspIleGlnThrLysGluLeuGlnLysGlnIleThrLysIleGlnAsnPheArgValTyrTyrArg 943
4348   GGGGGATTGGGGGATACAGTGCAGGGGAAAGAATAGTAGACATAATAGCAACAGACATACAAACTAAAGAACTACAAAAGCAAATTACAAAAATTCAAAATTTTCGGGTTTATTACAGGG

             AspAsnLysAspProLeuTrpLysGlyProAlaLysLeuLeuTrpLysGlyGluGlyAlaValValIleGlnAspAsnSerAspIleLysValValProArgArgLysAlaLysIleIle 983
4468   ACAACAAAGATCCCCTTTGGAAAGGACCAGCAAAGCTTCTCTGGAAAGGTGAAGGGGCAGTAGTAATACAAGATAATAGTGACATAAAAGTAGTGCCAAGAAGAAAAGCAAAAATCATTA

             ArgAspTyrGlyLysGlnMetAlaGlyAspAspCysValAlaSerArgGlnAspGluAspAM
4588   GGGATTATGGAAAACAGATGGCAGGTGATGATTGTGTGGCAAGTAGACAGGATGAGGATTAGAACATGGAAAAGTTTAGTAAAACACCATATGTATATTTCAAAGAAAGCTAAAGGATGG

4708   TTTTATAGACATCACTATGAAAGTACTCATCCAAGAGTAAGTTCAGAAGTACACATCCCCCTAGGGGATGCTAAATTGGTAATAACAACATATTGGGGTCTGCATACAGGAGAAAGAGAA

4828   TGGCATTTGGGCCAGGGAGTCGCCATAGAATGGAGGAAAAAGAAATATAGCACACAAGTAGACCCTGGCCTAGCAGACCAACTAATTCATCTGCATTATTTTGATTGTTTTTCAGAATCT

4948   GCTATAAAAAATGCCATATTAGGATATAGAGTTAGTCCTAGGTGTGAATATCAAGCAGGACATAACAAGGTAGGATCTCTACAATACTTGGCACTAGCAGCATTAATAACACCAAAAAAG

5068   ACAAAGCCACCTTTGCCTAGTGTTAAGAAACTGACAGAGGATAGATGGAACAAGCCCCAGAAGACCAAGGGCCACAGAGGGAGCCATACAATGAATGGACACTAGAGCTTTTAGAGGAGC

5188   TTAAGAGAGAAGCTGTTAGACATTTTCCTAGGCCATGGCTCCATAGCTTAGGACAATATATCTATGAAACTTATGGGGATACTTGGGCAGGAGTGGAAGCCATAATAAGAATTCTGCAAC

5308   AACTGCTGTTTATTCATTTCAGAATTGGGTGTCAACATAGCAGAATAGGCATTATTCAACAGAGGAGAGCAAGAAGAAATGGAGCCAGTAGATCCTAATCTAGAGCCCTGGAAGCATCCA

5428   GGAAGTCAGCCTAGGACTGCTTGTAACAATTGCTATTGTAAAAAGTGTTGCTTTCATTGCTACGCGTGTTTCACAAGAAAAGGCTTAGGCATCTCCTATGGCAGGAAGAAGCGGAGACAG

5548   CGACGAAGAGCTCCTCAGGACAGTCAGACTCATCAAGCTTCTCTATCAAAGCAGTAAGTAGTAAATGTAATGCAATCTTTACAAATATTAGCAATAGTATCATTAGTAGTAGTAGCAATA

                                                                       GluLysLysGlnLysThrValAlaMetLysVal 11
5668   ATAGCAATAGTTGTGTGGACCATAGTACTCATAGAATATAGGAAAATATTAAGACAAAGAAAATAGACAGATTAATTGATAGAATAAGAGAAAAAGCAGAAGACAGTGGCAATGAAAGTG

             LysGlyThrArgArgAsnTyrGlnHisLeuTrpArgTrpGlyThrLeuLeuLeuGlyMetLeuMetIleCysSerAlaThrGluLysLeuTrpValThrValTyrTyrGlyValProVal 51
5788   AAGGGGACCAGGAGGAATTATCAGCACTTGTGGAGATGGGGCACCTTGCTCCTTGGGATGTTGATGATCTGTAGTGCTACAGAAAAATTGTGGGTCACAGTTTATTATGGAGTACCTGTG

             TrpLysGluAlaThrThrThrLeuPheCysAlaSerAspAlaArgAlaTyrAspThrGluValHisAsnValTrpAlaThrHisAlaCysValProThrAspProAsnProGlnGluVal 91
5908   TGGAAAGAAGCAACTACCACTCTATTTTGTGCATCAGATGCTAGAGCATATGATACAGAGGTACATAATGTTTGGGCCACACATGCCTGTGTACCCACAGACCCCAACCCACAAGAAGTA

             ValLeuGlyAsnValThrGluAsnPheAsnMetTrpLysAsnAsnMetValGluGlnMetGlnGluAspIleIleSerLeuTrpAspGlnSerLeuLysProCysValLysLeuThrPro 131
6028   GTATTGGGAAATGTGACAGAAAATTTTAACATGTGGAAAAATAACATGGTAGAACAGATGCAGGAGGATATAATCAGTTTATGGGATCAAAGCCTAAAGCCATGTGTAAAATTAACCCCA

             LeuCysValThrLeuAsnCysThrAspLeuGlyLysAlaThrAsnThrAsnSerSerAsnTrpLysGluGluIleLysGlyGluIleLysAsnCysSerPheAsnIleThrThrSerIle 171
6148   CTCTGTGTTACTTTAAATTGCACTGATTTGGGGAAGGCTACTAATACCAATAGTAGTAATTGGAAAGAAGAAATAAAAGGAGAAATAAAAAACTGCTCTTTCAATATCACCACAAGCATA

             ArgAspLysIleGlnLysGluAsnAlaLeuPheArgAsnLeuAspValValProIleAspAsnAlaSerThrThrThrAsnTyrThrAsnTyrArgLeuIleHisCysAsnArgSerVal 211
6268   AGAGATAAGATTCAGAAAGAAAATGCACTTTTTTCGTAACCTTGATGTAGTACCAATAGATAATGCTAGTACTACTACCAACTATACCAACTATAGGTTGATACATTGTAACAGATCAGTC

             IleThrGlnAlaCysProLysValSerPheGluProIleProIleHisTyrCysThrProAlaGlyPheAlaIleLeuLysCysAsnAsnLysThrPheAsnGlyLysGlyProCysThr 251
6388   ATTACACAGGCCTGTCCAAAGGTATCATTTGAGCCAATTCCCATACATTATTGTACCCCGGCTGGTTTTGCGATTCTAAAGTGTAATAATAAAACGTTCAATGGAAAAGGACCATGTACA

             AsnValSerThrValGlnCysThrHisGlyIleArgProIleValSerThrGlnLeuLeuLeuAsnGlySerLeuAlaGluGluGluValValIleArgSerAspAsnPheThrAsnAsn 291
6508   AATGTCAGCACAGTACAATGTACACATGGAATTAGGCCAATAGTGTCAACTCAACTGCTGTTAAATGGCAGTCTAGCAGAAGAAGAGGTAGTAATTAGATCTGACAATTTCACGAACAAT

             AlaLysThrIleIleValGlnLeuAsnGluSerValAlaIleAsnCysThrArgProAsnAsnAsnThrArgLysSerIleTyrIleGlyProGlyArgAlaPheHisThrThrGlyArg 331
6628   GCTAAAACCATAATAGTACAGCTGAATGAATCTGTAGCAATTAACTGTACAAGACCCAACAACAATACAAGAAAAAGTATCTATATAGGACCAGGGAGAGCATTTCATACAACAGGAAGA
```

```
          IleIleGlyAspIleArgLysAlaHisCysAsnIleSerArgAlaGlnTrpAsnAsnThrLeuGluGlnIleValLysLysLeuArgGluGlnPheGlyAsnAsnLysThrIleValPhe 371
6748      ATAATAGGAGATATAAGAAAAGCACATTGTAACATTAGTAGAGCACAATGGAATAACACTTTAGAACAGATAGTTAAAAAAATTAAGAGAACAGTTTGGGAATAATAAAACAATAGTCTTT

          AsnGlnSerSerGlyGlyAspProGluIleValMetHisSerPheAsnCysArgGlyGluPhePheTyrCysAsnThrThrGlnLeuPheAsnAsnThrTrpArgLeuAsnHisThrGlu 411
6868      AATCAATCCTCAGGAGGGGACCCAGAAATTGTAATGCACAGTTTTAATTGTAGAGGGGAATTTTTCTACTGTAATACAACACAACTGTTTAATAATACATGGAGGTTAAATCACACTGAA

          GlyThrLysGlyAsnAspThrIleIleLeuProCysArgIleLysGlnIleIleAsnMetTrpGlnGluValGlyLysAlaMetTyrAlaProProIleGlyGlyGlnIleSerCysSer 451
6988      GGAACTAAAGGAAATGACACAATCATACTCCCATGTAGAATAAAACAAATTATAAACATGTGGCAGGAAGTAGGAAAAGCAATGTATGCCCCTCCCATTGGAGGACAAATTAGTTGTTCA

          SerAsnIleThrGlyLeuLeuLeuThrArgAspGlyGlyThrAsnValThrAsnAspThrGluValPheArgProGlyGlyGlyAspMetArgAspAsnTrpArgSerGluLeuTyrLys 491
7108      TCAAATATTACAGGGCTGCTATTAACAAGAGATGGTGGTACAAATGTAACTAATGACACCGAGGTCTTCAGACCTGGAGGAGGAGATATGAGGGACAATTGGAGAAGTGAATTATATAAA

          TyrLysValIleLysIleGluProLeuGlyIleAlaProThrLysAlaLysArgArgValValGlnArgGluLysArgAlaValGlyIleValGlyAlaMetPheLeuGlyPheLeuGly 531
7228      TATAAAGTAATAAAAATTGAACCATTAGGAATAGCACCCACCAAGGCAAAGAGAAGAGTGGTGCAGAGAGAAAAAAGAGCAGTGGGAATAGTAGGAGCTATGTTCCTTGGGTTCTTGGGA

          AlaAlaGlySerThrMetGlyAlaValSerLeuThrLeuThrValGlnAlaArgGlnLeuLeuSerGlyIleValGlnGlnGlnAsnAsnLeuLeuArgAlaIleGluAlaGlnGlnHis 571
7348      GCAGCAGGAAGCACTATGGGCGCAGTGTCATTGACGCTGACGGTACAGGCCAGACAATTATTGTCTGGTATAGTGCAACAGCAGAACAATTTGCTGAGGGCTATTGAGGCGCAACAACAT

          LeuLeuGlnLeuThrValTrpGlyIleLysGlnLeuGlnAlaArgValLeuAlaValGluArgTyrLeuArgAspGlnGlnLeuLeuGlyIleTrpGlyCysSerGlyLysLeuIleCys 611
7468      CTGTTGCAACTCACAGTCTGGGGCATCAAGCAGCTCCAGGCAAGAGTCCTGGCTGTGGAAAGATACCTAAGGGATCAACAGCTCCTAGGGATTTGGGGTTGCTCTGGAAAACTCATTTGC

          ThrThrAlaValProTrpAsnAlaSerTrpSerAsnLysSerLeuGluAspIleTrpAspAsnMetThrTrpMetGlnTrpGluArgGluIleAspAsnTyrThrAsnThrIleTyrThr 651
7588      ACCACTGCTGTGCCTTGGAATGCTAGTTGGAGTAATAAATCTCTGGAAGACATTTGGGATAACATGACCTGGATGCAGTGGGAAAGAGAAATTGACAATTACACAAACACAATATACACC

          LeuLeuGluGluSerGlnAsnGlnGlnGluLysAsnGluGlnGluLeuLeuGluLeuAspLysTrpAlaSerLeuTrpAsnTrpPheSerIleThrAsnTrpLeuTrpTyrIleLysIle 691
7708      TTACTTGAAGAATCGCAGAACCAACAAGAAAAGAATGAACAAGAATTATTAGATAAGTGGGCAAGTTTGTGGAATTGGTTTAGCATAACAAACTGGCTGTGGTATATAAAGATA

          PheIleMetIleValGlyGlyLeuValGlyLeuArgIleValPheAlaValLeuSerIleValAsnArgValArgGlnGlyTyrSerProLeuSerPheGlnThrArgLeuProValPro 731
7828      TTCATAATGATAGTAGGAGGCTTGGTAGGTTTAAGAATAGTTTTTGCTGTGCTTTCTATAGTGAATAGAGTTAGGCAGGGATACTCACCATTGTCATTTCAGACCCGCCTCCCAGTCCCG

          ArgGlyProAspArgProAspGlyIleGluGluGluGlyGlyGluArgAspArgAspArgSerValArgLeuValAspGlyPheLeuAlaLeuIleTrpGluAspLeuArgSerLeuCys 771
7948      AGGGGACCCGACAGGCCCGACGGAATCGAAGAAGAAGGTGGAGAGAGAGACAGAGACAGATCCGTTCGATTAGTGGATGGATTCTTAGCACTTATCTGGGAAGATCTGCGGAGCCTGTGC

          LeuPheSerTyrArgArgLeuArgAspLeuLeuLeuIleAlaAlaArgThrValGluIleLeuGlyHisArgGlyTrpGluAlaLeuLysTyrTrpTrpSerLeuLeuGlnTyrTrpIle 811
8068      CTCTTCAGCTACCGCCGCTTGAGAGACTTACTCTTGATTGCAGCGAGGACTGTGGAAATTCTGGGGCACAGGGGGTGGGAAGCCCTCAAATATTGGTGGAGTCTCCTGCAGTATTGGATT

          GlnGluLeuLysAsnSerAlaValSerTrpLeuAsnAlaThrAlaIleAlaValThrGluGlyThrAspArgValIleGluValAlaGlnArgAlaTyrArgAlaIleLeuHisIleHis 851
8188      CAGGAACTAAAGAATAGTGCTGTTAGCTGGCTCAACGCCACAGCTATAGCAGTAACTGAGGGGACAGATAGGGTTATAGAAGTAGCACAAAGAGCTTATAGAGCTATTCTCCACATACAT

          ArgArgIleArgGlnGlyLeuGluArgLeuLeuLeuOC
8308      AGAAGAATTAGACAGGGCTTGGAAAGGCTTTTGCTATAAGATGGGTGGCAAGTGGTCAAAACGTAGTATGGGTGGATGGTCTGCTATAAGGGAAAGAATGAGACGAGCTGAGCCACGAGC

8428      TGAGCCAGCAGCAGATGGGGTGGGAGCAGTATCTCGAGACCTGGAAAAACATGGAGCAATCACAAGTAGCAATACAGCAGCTACTAATGCTGATTGTGCCTGGCTAGAAGCACAAGAGGA
                                                                                                          U3->
8548      GGAAGAGGTGGGTTTTCCAGTCAGACCTCAGGTACCTTTAAGACCAATGACTTACAAGGCAGCTTTAGATATTAGCCACTTTTTAAAAGAAAAGGGGGGA  CTGGAAGGGCTAATTTGGT

8667      CCCAAAGAAGACAAGAGATCCTTGATCTGTGGATCTACCACACACAAGGCTACTTCCCTGATTGGCAGAATTACACACCAGGGCCAGGGATCAGATATCCACTGACCTTTGGATGGTGCT

8787      TCAAGCTAGTACCAGTTGAGCCAGAGAAGGTAGAAGAGGCCAATGAAGGAGAGAACAACAGCTTGTTACACCCTATGAGCCTGCATGGGATGGAGGACGCGGAGAAAGAAGTGTTAGTGT
                                                                            <-U3 R->
8907      GGAGGTTTGACAGCAAACTAGCATTTCATCACATGGCCCGAGAGCTGCATCCGGAGTACTACAAAGACTGCTGACATCGAGCTTTCTACAAGGGACTTTCCGCTGGGGACTTTCCAGGGA

9027      GGCGTGGCCTGGGCGGGACTGGGGAGTGGCGTCCCTCAGATGCTGCATATAAGCAGCTGCTTTTTGCCTGTACTG GGTCTCTCTGGTTAGACCAGATCTGAGCCTGGGAGCTCTCTGGC
                         <-R U5->
9146      TAACTAGGGAACCCACTGCTTAAGCCTCAATAAAGCTTGCCTTGAGTGCTTCA AGTAGTGTGTGCCCGTCTGTTGTGTGACTCTGGTAACTAGAGATCCCTCAGACCCTTTTAGTCAGT
              ->U5
9265      GTGGAAAAATCTCTAGCAG
```

E N V

L T R

Fig. 2 (pages 412 to 415). Nucleotide sequence of ARV-2 DNA. The predicted amino acid sequences for the products of the *gag, pol*, and *env* genes are indicated. The U3, R, and U5 regions of the LTR's are also designated. The cap site, as determined from the experiment shown in Fig. 3, is position +1. A 3-bp inverted repeat at the ends of the LTR, the TATA box at position −29, the sequence complementary to the 3'-end of the tRNA^{lys} at position 183, and the polyadenylation signal at position 9174 are underlined. The overlines indicate the amino acid sequences determined from virion proteins (Fig. 4). The nucleotides at the beginning of each line are numbered, and the amino acids at the end of each line are indicated. **Methods:** Restriction enzyme DNA fragments of recombinant phage DNA (Fig. 1) were isolated after electrophoresis in polyacrylamide or agarose gels, cloned into M13 vectors, and used as templates for DNA sequencing by the dideoxy chain termination method (50). Oligonucleotide primers for sequencing were chemically synthesized by solid-phase phosphoramidite chemistry on an Applied Biosystems 380A machine. The limits of the LTR's were established by comparing the sequence of both ends of proviral DNA as well as the sequence of a permuted clone (7A in Fig. 1). For protein sequencing, 0.38 mg of purified virus was subjected to electrophoresis on a 12 percent polyacrylamide Laemmli gel and the bands corresponding to p16*gag* and p25*gag* were cut out and electroeluted by the method of Hunkapiller *et al.* (51). NH$_2$-terminal microsequencing of these proteins was carried out as described by Hunkapiller *et al.* (52). COOH-terminal analysis was by the carboxypeptidase digestion procedures of Hayashi (53). The compiled ARV-2 DNA sequence, including both copies of the LTR, is 9737 bp in length. The analysis of the genetic organization of ARV-2 draws on comparisons with other retroviruses. For these comparisons we used computer programs such as MALIGN to identify homologous regions among DNA sequences and protein sequences. Structural relations were also investigated; predicted proteins from ARV-2 open reading frames were analyzed for hydropathy patterns by the method of Hopp and Woods (54) and for specific structural features by a modification of the method of Chou and Fasman (55). These two parameters were combined to determine regions of a protein that may be on the surface, particularly loops composed of hydrophilic residues.

ing HTLV-I and HTLV-II have a tRNA-proline primer (*16, 17, 19*).

Contained within the LTR's of retroviruses are signals that control initiation and processing of viral transcripts (*13–15*). The cap site and a portion of the leader sequence are specified by the LTR. A primer-extension experiment in which we used purified virion RNA identified the 5'-end of ARV-2 RNA (Fig. 3). Thus, the ARV-2 LTR (R-U5 region) contributes 182 bp to the leader (Fig. 2). Many genes of eukaryotic cells and viruses contain a TATA box about 25 bp upstream from the start of the transcript (*20*); the TATA box is important for positioning the start site of transcription (*20, 21*). In the ARV-2 LTR sequence, a TATA box is located at −29 to −25. A 13-bp palindrome, at −25 to −13, overlaps the 3'-end of the ARV-2 TATA box;

the significance of this structural feature is not known. Another common element of eukaryotic transcriptional units, a CAAT box, usually positioned 60 to 70 bp upstream from the cap site (*22*) is not present in the ARV-2 LTR.

A consensus sequence that signals addition of polyadenylated tails, AATAAA (*23*), is located in the rightward ARV-2 LTR at position 9174 to 9179 (Fig. 2). Further downstream, between 9203 to 9224, is a region that is devoid of A residues (Fig. 2). The site of addition of polyadenylated [poly(A)] tails in the LTR's of many retroviruses is followed by a region of 20 to 30 bp that is also deficient in adenylic acid residues (*19*). For several eukaryotic genes and retroviruses, including MuLV (murine leukemia virus), MMTV, RSV (Rous sarcoma virus), and RAV-0 (Rous-associated virus), the dinucleotide CA is located at the poly(A) addition site (*19*). These comparisons were used to propose a tentative poly(A) addition site at posi- tions 9198 in the rightward ARV-2 LTR (Fig. 2).

The enhancer element, generally lo- cated upstream from the TATA box, has

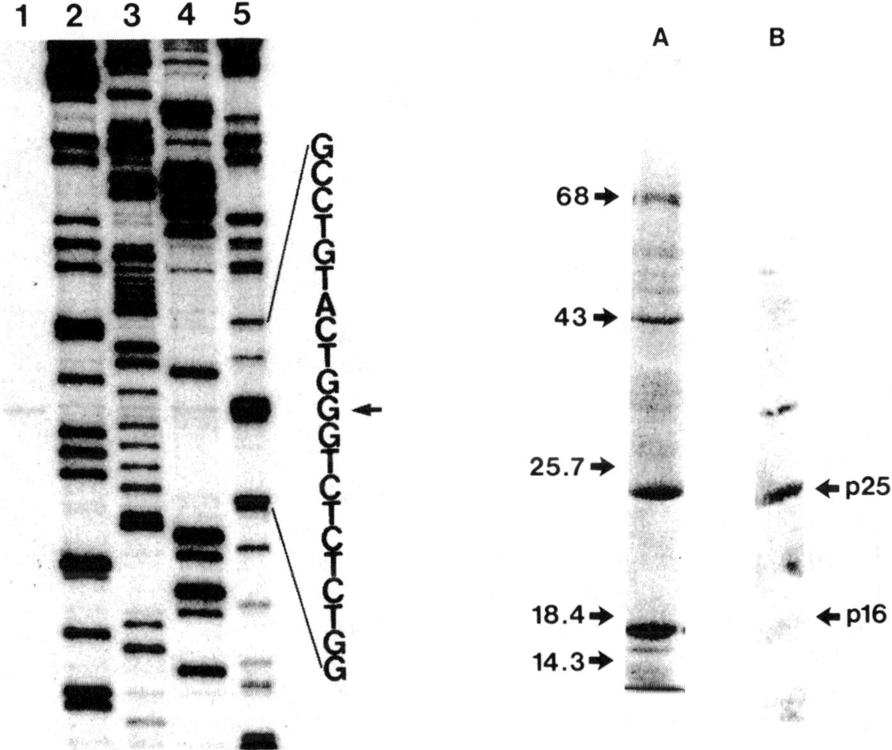

Fig. 3 (left). Identification of the 5'-end of ARV-2 RNA. Viral RNA was isolated from virions (*12*) and used as a template for Klenow fragment of DNA polymerase I with the synthetic oligonucleotide 5'GGGCACACACTACTTGAAGC as a primer. An M13 clone containing the leftward LTR of ARV-2 was also primed with the same oligonucleotide in the presence of dideoxynucleotides (*50*). Both reactions were resolved on a sequencing gel. Lane 1 corresponds to the primer extension reaction with ARV-2 RNA template. Lanes 2, 3, 4, and 5 correspond to C, T, A, and G, respectively, of the sequencing reactions of the M13 recombinant clone.

Fig. 4 (right). Polypeptides of purified virus. Gradient purified ARV-2 (5 μg per lane) was subjected to electrophoresis on a 12 percent polyacrylamide gel according to the method of Laemmli (*56*). Lane A, staining with Coomassie brilliant blue. Lane B (immunoblot), polypep- tides transferred to nitrocellulose (*57*) and treated first with a 1:500 dilution of serum from an AIDS patient (EW5111 reference serum from P. Feorino, Centers for Disease Control, Atlanta, Georgia) and then with a 1:200 dilution of horseradish peroxidase–conjugated goat antiserum to human immunoglobulin G (Cappel Laboratories, No. 3201-0081). The color substrate was HRP Color Development Reagent (containing 4-chloro-1-napthol; Bio-Rad). The molecular weights of protein markers subjected to electrophoresis in parallel lanes are shown in kilodaltons on the left. P25 and p16 indicate the bands that correspond to p25*gag* and p16*gag* that were used as substrates for amino acid sequencing.

been shown to be an important feature of transcriptional regulation for some eukaryotic genes and viruses (*24–28*). Large repeats, characteristic of some retroviral enhancers, are not present in the ARV-2 LTR. A close fit for the proposed consensus sequence for enhancer elements, (G) TGG$^{AAA}_{TTT}$ (G) (*29*), is not found in the ARV-2 LTR.

The gag *gene.* The *gag* region of retroviruses encodes the internal structural proteins of the virion (*30*). A precursor polypeptide is synthesized and subsequently cleaved to yield mature *gag* proteins (*30*). The DNA sequence of ARV-2 predicts a *gag* precursor of 502 codons initiating at the ATG at position 337, the first ATG in the proposed full-length ARV-2 RNA (Fig. 2). To verify the use of this reading frame and to identify virion proteins as products of *gag*, we determined partial amino acid sequences of two virion proteins, p25 and p16, detected with serum from an AIDS patient (Fig. 4) but not with normal human control serum (data not shown). Virion proteins were isolated from a polyacrylamide gel and the first 30 amino acids at the NH$_2$-terminus of p16 and the first 20 of p25 were determined by gas-phase microsequencing. Alignment with the DNA sequence (Fig. 2) suggests that the first *gag* polypeptide is 134 amino acids in length and may correspond to a p12*gag* virion protein species seen on polyacrylamide gels (unpublished results). The NH$_2$-terminus of p25 is generated by a cleavage between Tyr-138 and Pro-139 (Fig. 2). Proline is present at the NH$_2$-terminus of at least three other major retroviral *gag* proteins (p25*gag* of HTLV-I, p27*gag* of RSV, and p30*gag* of MuLV) (*16, 19*). A protease with this cleavage specificity has not yet been identified in ARV-2, but this activity can be encoded by a retrovirus (*30*). The

carboxyl terminus of p25*gag* was determined by digestion with carboxypeptidase and yielded the sequence Arg-Val-Leu (amino acids 367, 368, and 369, respectively). The NH$_2$-terminus of p16 is generated by cleavage between Met-383 and Met-384 (Fig. 2). Processing at this site may involve chymotrypsin or a chymotrypsin-like enzyme, which is believed to process part of the *gag* precursor polypeptide in other retroviruses (*30*). The COOH-terminus of p16 probably occurs at Gln-506 since a translational stop codon follows (Fig. 2), although further proteolytic processing could also be involved.

A small amount of amino acid sequence homology is noted when p25*gag* of ARV-2 is compared to p24*gag* of HTLV-I (*16*) (data not shown). This homology involves the position of two cysteine (C) residues relative to the COOH-terminal of both proteins (Fig. 2). Also, four of five amino acids at the COOH-terminus of p25*gag* of ARV-2 match those at the COOH-terminus of p24*gag* of HTLV-I (Fig. 2) (*16*). A preponderance of hydrophilic residues characterizes these proteins.

Sequence comparisons of p16*gag* of ARV-2 with p16*gag* of HTLV-I (*16*), p12*gag* of RSV (*19*), and p15*gag* of MuLV (*19*) reveal the best homology (Fig. 5). The relative positions of the five Cys residues in each of these three proteins are closely conserved and all three contain a high proportion of hydrophilic residues.

The pol *gene.* The *pol* region encodes the virion RNA-dependent DNA polymerase (reverse transcriptase). Several additional enzymatic functions related to replication are controlled by this region, including ribonuclease H, a DNA endonuclease, and, in some retroviruses, a protease (*15, 30*). An open reading frame

```
                *    *                       *
                393           400                     410
ARV        K C F N C G K E G H I A K N C R A P R
HTLV-I     P C F R C G K A G H W S K D C T Q P R
RSV        L C Y T C G S P G H Y Q A Q C P K K R
MuLV       Q C A Y C K E K G H W A K D C P K K P


                          *    *
                                      420
ARV        K K G - - - - - C W R C G R E G H Q
HTLV-I     P P P G P - - - C P L C Q D P T H W
RSV        K S G N S R E R C Q L C N G M G H N
MuLV       R G P R G P R P Q T S L L T L D D -


                     *
                     429
ARV        M K D C T
HTLV-I     K R D C P
RSV        A K Q C R
MuLV       - - - - -
```

Fig. 5 (left). Homology of amino acids in regions of the *gag* gene of ARV-2, HTLV-I, RSV, and MuLV. Identical amino acid residues are underlined. Positions of cysteines are noted with asterisks. ARV-2: p16*gag*, amino acid 14 to 51 (Fig. 2). HTLV-I: p12*gag*, amino acid 12 to 50 (*10*). RSV: p12*gag*, amino acid 20 to 61 (*16*), MuLV: p10*gag*, amino acid 25 to 60 (*16*). Numbers indicate amino acid positions (Fig. 2).

```
          262           270                 280
ARV     T V L D V G D A Y F S V P L D K D F R K
HTLV    Q T T D L R D A F F Q I P L P K Q F Q P
RSV     M V L D L K D C F F S I P L A E Q D R E
MuLV    T V L D L K D A F F C L R L H P T S Q P


                      290                 300
ARV     Y T A F T I P S I N N E T P G I R Y Q Y
HTLV    Y F A F T V P Q Q C N Y G P G T R Y A W
RSV     A F A F T L P S V N N Q A P A R R F N W
MuLV    L F A F E W - R D P E M G I S G Q L T W


                      310                 320
ARV     N V L P Q G W K G S P A I F Q S S M T K
HTLV    K V L P Q G F K N S P T L F E M Q L A H
RSV     K V L P Q G M T C S P T I C Q L V V G Q
MuLV    T R L P Q G F K N S P T L F D E A L H R


                      330                 340
ARV     T L E P F R K Q N P D I V I Y Q Y M D D
HTLV    I L E P I R Q A F P Q C T I L Q Y M D D
RSV     V L E P L R L K H P S L C M L H Y M D D
MuLV    D L A D F R I Q H P D L I L L Q Y V D D


                      350
ARV     L Y V G S D L E I G Q
HTLV    I L L A S P S H E D L
RSV     L L L A A S S H D G L
MuLV    L L L A A T S E L D C
```

Fig. 6 (right). Homology of amino acids in the NH$_2$-terminal portion of the *pol* genes of ARV-2, HTLV-I, RSV, and MuLV. Identical amino acid residues are underlined. ARV-2: amino acid 262 to 352 (Fig. 2). HTLV-I: amino acid 110 to 196 (*10*). RSV: amino acid 113 to 177 (*16*). MuLV: amino acid 265 to 351 (*16*). Numbers indicate amino acid positions (Fig. 2).

of 1003 codons appears to be the ARV-2 *pol* domain (Fig. 2). Some homology at the protein level is observed in the NH$_2$-terminal portions of the predicted *pol* genes of ARV-2, HTLV-I (*16, 31*), RSV (*19*), and MuLV (*16*) (Fig. 6). This region is also homologous to portions of the putative viral polymerases of hepatitis B viruses and cauliflower mosaic virus (*31*). Analysis of the remainder of the *pol* genes of ARV-2, HTLV-I, RSV, and MuLV demonstrates appreciable homology in protein structure and sequence near the COOH-termini (*16, 19, 32, 33*) (Fig. 7). A 32-kD polypeptide is produced by proteolytic processing near the COOH-terminus of the RSV *pol* polypeptide precursor (*33*). Alignments of shared amino acids in this region of the ARV-2 *pol* gene (in particular, Cys residues) with the defined NH$_2$-terminus of p32 of RSV (*33*) permits tentative identification of a processing site for the counterpart protein (Fig. 7).

The env *gene.* The *env* region encodes the major glycoprotein found in the membrane envelope of the virus and in the cytoplasmic membrane of infected cells (*30*). Retroviral *env* proteins arise generally from a precursor polypeptide

```
           719                 730
ARV     G I D K A Q E E H E K Y H S N W R A M A
HTLV-I  Q L S P A - E L H S F T H C G Q T A L T
RSV     P L R E A K D L H T A L H I G P R A L S
MuLV    Q L T H L S F S K M K A L L E R S H S P

                                       *   *
           740                 750
ARV     S D F N L P P V V A K E I V A S C D K C
HTLV-I  L Q G A T T T E - A S N I L R S C H A C
RSV     K A C N I S M Q Q A R E V V Q T C P H C
MuLV    Y Y M L N R D R T L K N I T E T C K A C

           760                 770
ARV     Q L K G E A M H G Q V D C - - - - - - -
HTLV-I  R G G N P Q H Q M P R G H I R - R G L L
RSV     N S A P A L E A G V N P - - - - R G L G
MuLV    A Q V N A S K S A V K Q G T R V R G H R

                       780
ARV     S P G I W Q L D C T H L E G K I I L - -
HTLV-I  P N K I W Q G D I T H F K Y K N T L T R
RSV     P L Q I W Q T D F T - L E P R M A P R S
MuLV    P G T H W E I D F T E I K P G L Y G Y K

           790                 800
ARV     - - - V A V H V A S G Y I E A E - V I P
HTLV-I  - L H V W V D T F S G A I S A T Q K R K
RSV     W L A V T V D T A S S A I V V T Q H G R
MuLV    Y L L V F I D T F S G W I E A F P T K K

           810                 820
ARV     A E T G Q E T A Y F L L K L A G R - W P
HTLV-I  E T S S E A I S S L L Q A I A H L - G K
RSV     V T S V A V Q H H W A T A I A V L - G R
MuLV    E T A K V V T K K L L E E I F P R F G M

           830                 840
ARV     V K T I H T D N G S Q F T S T T V K A A
HTLV-I  P S Y I N T D N G P A Y I S Q D F L N M
RSV     P K A I K T D N G S C F T S K S T R E W
MuLV    P Q V L G T D N G P A F V S K V S Q T V

           850                 860
ARV     C W W A G I K Q E F G I P Y N - P Q S Q
HTLV-I  C T S L A I R H T T H V P Y N - P T S S
RSV     L A R W G I A H T T G I P G N - S Q G Q
MuLV    A D L L G I - D W K L H C A Y R P Q S S

           870                 878
ARV     G V V E S M N N E L K K I I
HTLV-I  G L V E R S N G I L L K T L
RSV     A M V E R A N R L L K D R I
MuLV    G Q V E R M N R T I K E T L
```

Fig. 7. Homology of amino acids in the COOH-terminal portion of the *pol* genes of ARV-2, HTLV-I, RSV, and MuLV. Identical amino acid residues are underlined. Positions of cysteines are noted with asterisks. ARV-2: 719 to 878 (Fig. 2). HTLV-I: amino acid 599 to 766 (*10*). RSV: amino acid 568 to 743 (*16*). MuLV: amino acid 846 to 1019 (*16*). Numbers indicate amino acid positions (Fig. 2).

that is processed at two or more sites: the first processing event removes a signal peptide of about 30 amino acids and the second yields a COOH-terminal polypeptide containing a hydrophobic stretch (about 22 amino acids) that spans the membrane and is followed by a hydrophilic cytoplasmic anchor (*30*). Results of transient expression experiments in mammalian cells (see Fig. 8) indicate that serologically reactive ARV-2 *env* protein is initiated downstream from the Sst I site at position 5555 to 5560 (Fig. 2). We propose that the ATG at position 5779 (*34*) initiates the *env* precursor, but direct determination of the NH$_2$-termini of the *env* precursor polypeptide and of processed forms will ultimately be required to establish the biogenesis of *env* proteins. Two other potential initiation codons are near the 5'-end of the same long open reading frame (863 codons) proposed to encode the ARV-2 *env* protein (positions 5845 and 5851, Fig. 2).

Secondary structure analysis shows that the COOH-terminal region is organized into predominantly α-helices and β-sheets; the NH$_2$-terminal half appears to have many hydrophilic loop regions (see legend to Fig. 2); similar structural properties characterize the domains of *env* gene products of other retroviruses

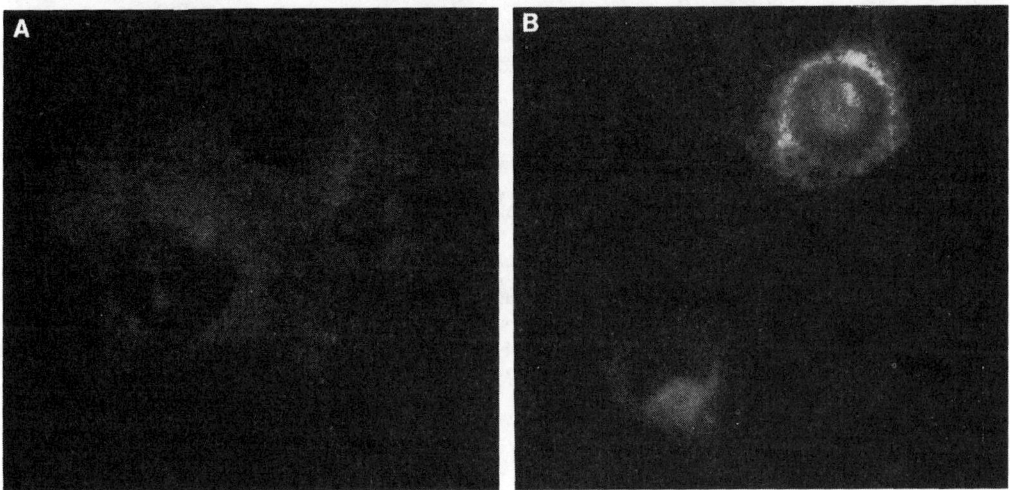

Fig. 8. Expression of cloned ARV genes in mammalian cells. ARV-2 DNA fragments containing the *gag* and *env* genes were prepared as follows: λ-7A DNA (Fig. 1) was digested with Sst I and Kpn I and the 3.1-kb *gag* DNA fragment was purified by electrophoresis in low-melting agarose gels (*7*); λ-7D DNA (Fig. 1) was digested with Sst I and Kpn I and the 3.2-kb *env* DNA fragment was similarly purified. Each of these fragments was cloned into a modified form of a plasmid containing the SV40 origin of DNA synthesis and the promoter and poly(A) addition regions of the SV40 early gene (*58, 59*). Both ARV *gag* and *env* DNA fragments contain ATG start codons. pSV7c/gag utilized a TAA stop codon in SV40 DNA. pSV7c/env has the TAA stop codon at the end of the open reading frame for *env* (Fig. 2). COS-7 monkey cells, expressing the SV40 early gene, were grown on glass microscope slides, transfected with plasmid DNA by the calcium phosphate coprecipitation method (*60*), incubated for 60 hours, and fixed in cold acetone. The fixed cell monolayers were treated for 1 hour at 37°C with a 1:200 dilution (in PBS with 5 percent fetal calf serum) of an AIDS reference serum (Fig. 4) or with a similar dilution of normal human control serum. Cells were washed in PBS and treated for 1 hour at 37°C with fluorescein-labeled goat antiserum to human immunoglobulin G (Cappel Laboratories). In all cases, sera were preadsorbed on normal COS-7 cells that had been fixed with 0.2 percent paraformaldehyde. Shown here are fluorescence photomicrographs (×630) of cells transfected with (A) pSV 7C/gag and (B) pSV7C/env. About 5 percent of cells in a monolayer expressed viral antigens.

(data not shown). A tentative assignment of a processing site for ARV-2 *env* includes the sequences Lys-Arg-Arg or Lys-Arg (Fig. 9). Which of these sites is used remains to be determined. Processing in this region will generate final products of 59 and 42 kD without accounting for carbohydrates residues. The NH$_2$-terminal and COOH-terminal portions contain, respectively, 26 and 5 potential NH$_2$-linked glycosylation sites (Asp-X-Thr, Asp-X-Ser) (Figs. 2 and 9). Cysteine residues are asymmetrically distributed as in other retroviral *env* gene products (*19*). The NH$_2$-terminal domain has 18 Cys residues and the COOH-terminal portion has 3 Cys residues. Two large hydrophobic regions are evident in the COOH-terminal domain (Fig. 9). The rightward hydrophobic stretch is long enough (23 amino acids) to span membranes.

Expression of cloned ARV genes. In an attempt to obtain ARV antigens without the production of infectious virus, an SV40 vector system was used to express

422

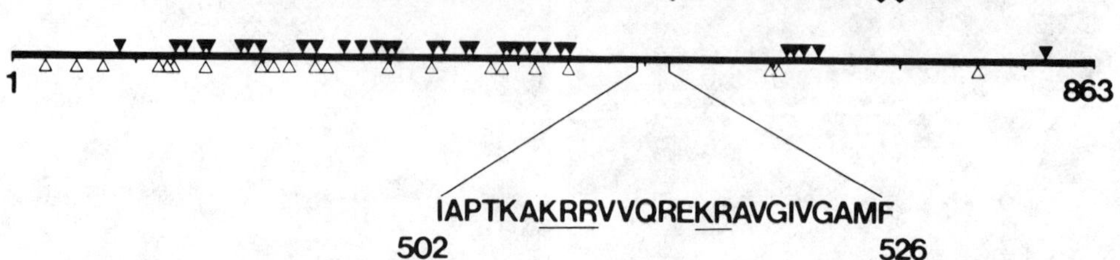

Fig. 9. Schematic diagram of ARV-2 *env* open reading frame. Numbers refer to amino acids in the open reading frame proposed for *env* (nucleotides 5755 to 8346, Fig. 2). Symbols: △, cysteine residues; ▼, potential *N*-glycosylation sites; ◆, hydrophobic regions. The two putative processing sites for generating NH_2- and COOH-terminal domains are underlined.

the candidate *gag* and *env* genes in transfected mammalian cells. The criterion for expression was serological reactivity of fixed cells with serum from AIDS patients in immunofluorescence tests. Recombinant SV40 plasmids containing these genes were transfected into 5×10^4 COS-7 monkey cells growing on microscope slides (Fig. 8); after 60 hours, cell monolayers were fixed and treated with AIDS patients' sera or normal human control sera and then with fluorescein-labeled goat antiserum to human immunoglobulin G (Fig. 8). Approximately 5 percent of cells transfected with pSV7c/gag showed a speckled pattern of immunofluorescence throughout the cytoplasm with AIDS patient serum EW5111 (Fig. 8A). Antiserum MC from a patient in the early stage of AIDS appeared not to react with cells transfected with pSV7c/gag (data not shown). By immunoblot analysis with proteins from purified ARV-2, antiserum MC was shown to have very low levels of antibody to p25*gag*, whereas antiserum EW5111 readily reacted to p25*gag*. Serum from normal individuals gave no appreciable fluorescence (data not shown) in cells transfected with pSV7c/ gag cells transfected with the vector plasmid pSV7c, containing no ARV-2 DNA, did not fluoresce with any serum

samples from AIDS patients. About 5 percent of cells (from 5×10^4 cells per microscope slide) transfected with pSV7c/env and treated with either EW5111 or MC antiserum showed bright immunofluorescence largely confined to the cytoplasm in a netlike pattern (Fig. 8B). These patterns may be a consequence of the fixation procedure or may indicate that viral *env* protein is localized in structures such as endoplasmic reticulum inside the cell. No fluorescence was observed in cells transfected with pSV7c/env and treated with normal human control sera (data not shown).

Discussion. The complete DNA sequence of ARV-2 reveals a fundamental genetic structure similar to that of other retroviruses. Several features of ARV-2 indicate that it is no more closely related to the other human retroviruses HTLV-I and HTLV-II than it is to avian or murine retroviruses.

ARV-2 has an inverted 3 bp repeat (CTG . . . CAG) at the ends of the LTR. All other retrovirus LTR's have TG . . . CA at their ends as part of a 2- to 16-bp inverted repeat (*14*). The MuLV LTR has two direct repeats 72 bp long located in an internal position within the LTR (*19*). HTLV-II has several direct repeats, one of which is 21 bp long and is very similar to a 21-bp repeat in HTLV-I

(*16, 17*). RSV, however, is like ARV-2 and has no large direct repeats in its LTR (*19*). In the ARV-2 LTR, the proposed poly(A) addition site is 20 bp downstream from the consensus poly(A) addition signal, AATAAA (Fig. 2); thus, the R region is 97 bp long [measured from the cap site to the poly(A) site]. The poly(A) addition sites of MuLV and RSV are about 20 bp downstream from AATAAA found in each LTR; these viruses have R regions 68 bp and 21 bp, respectively (*19*). In contrast, in HTLV-I and HTLV-II, the AATAAA sequence is located upstream from the TATA box; R is 229 bp in HTLV-I and 287 bp in HTLV-II (*16, 17*). ARV-2 and MMTV have a $tRNA^{lys}$ for priming minus-strand DNA synthesis (Fig. 2) (*18*); avian retroviruses use $tRNA^{trp}$ and other mammalian retroviruses use $tRNA^{pro}$ (*19*).

The *gag* regions of MuLV and RSV encode precursor polypeptides that are cleaved into at least four and five proteins, respectively (*30*). Both ARV-2 and HTLV-I encode a *gag* precursor that appears to give rise to three proteins (Fig. 2) (*16*). A small amount of homology of amino acid sequences was noted in the COOH-terminal portion of *gag* in these viruses; ARV-2, HTLV-I, and RSV were found to be similarly related

in this assessment (Fig. 5 and Table 2).

Different retroviruses use different mechanisms to synthesize and translate the *pol* gene messenger RNA (*16*). Elucidation of *pol* biogenesis in ARV-2 will require detailed analyses of splicing patterns of viral mRNA in infected cells together with studies of the polypeptide intermediates. ARV may be different from all other retroviruses since the COOH-terminal end of the proposed *pol* gene does not overlap the NH_2-terminal end of the proposed *env* gene.

The predicted ARV-2 *env* polypeptide, like that of other retroviruses, has a hydrophilic NH_2-terminal domain and a COOH-terminal portion characterized by a long stretch of hydrophobic amino acids (23 amino acids long) (Fig. 9). The NH_2-terminal domain of ARV-2 *env* contains 26 potential glycosylation sites, an unusually high number when compared to other retroviruses: HTLV-I has 5 (*17*), HTLV-II has 6 (*35*), RSV has 17 (*24*), and MuLV has 7 (*24*). The extent and function of glycosylation in retroviral *env* proteins remain to be investigated.

In ARV-2 there are two additional open reading frames designated ORF-1 and ORF-2 (Fig. 10). Near the 5'-end of each open reading frame is an ATG that is flanked by purine residues at -3 and

Table 2. Summary of homologies of ARV-2 with other retroviruses. Homologies are given as percentages from the MALIGN program.

Virus	ARV-2 *gag* (amino acid 393 to 429, Fig. 5)		ARV-2 *pol* (amino acid 262 to 352, Fig. 6)		ARV-2 *pol* (amino acid 719 to 878, Fig. 7)	
	Amino acid	Nucleotide	Amino acid	Nucleotide	Amino acid	Nucleotide
HTLV-1	50	7	45	11	32	19
RSV	39	7	42	15	30	12
MuLV	36	10	34	15	17	23

A

```
                 1                                          10                                          20
                 cys gln glu glu lys gln lys ser leu gly ile met glu asn arg trp gln val met ile val trp gln val asp arg met
4551  ATAAAAGTAG  TGC CAA GAA GAA AAG CAA AAA TCA TTA GGG ATT ATG GAA AAC AGA TGG CAG GTG ATG ATT GTG TGG CAA GTA GAC AGG ATG

                 30                                         40                                          50
                 arg ile arg thr trp lys ser leu val lys his his met tyr ile ser lys lys ala lys gly trp phe tyr arg his his tyr glu ser
4642  AGG ATT AGA ACA TGG AAA AGT TTA GTA AAA CAC CAT ATG TAT ATT TCA AAG AAA GCT AAA GGA TGG TTT TAT AGA CAT CAC TAT GAA AGT

                 60                                         70                                          80
                 thr his pro arg val ser ser glu val his ile pro leu gly asp ala lys leu val ile thr thr tyr trp gly leu his thr gly glu
4732  ACT CAT CCA AGA GTA AGT TCA GAA GTA CAC ATC CCC CTA GGG GAT GCT AAA TTG GTA ATA ACA ACA TAT TGG GGT CTG CAT ACA GGA GAA

                 90                                         100                                         110
                 arg glu trp his leu gly gln gly val ala ile glu trp arg lys lys lys tyr ser thr gln val asp pro gly leu ala asp gln leu
4822  AGA GAA TGG CAT TTG GGC CAG GGA GTC GCC ATA GAA TGG AGG AAA AAG AAA TAT AGC ACA CAA GTA GAC CCT GGC CTA GCA GAC CAA CTA

                 120                                        130                                         140
                 ile his leu his tyr phe asp cys phe ser glu ser ala ile lys asn ala ile leu gly tyr arg val ser pro arg cys glu tyr gln
4912  ATT CAT CTG CAT TAT TTT GAT TGT TTT TCA GAA TCT GCT ATA AAA AAT GCC ATA TTA GGA TAT AGA GTT AGT CCT AGG TGT GAA TAT CAA

                 150                                        160                                         170
                 ala gly his asn lys val gly ser leu gln tyr leu ala leu ala ala leu ile thr pro lys lys thr lys pro pro leu pro ser val
5002  GCA GGA CAT AAC AAG GTA GGA TCT CTA CAA TAC TTG GCA CTA GCA GCA TTA ATA ACA CCA AAA AAG ACA AAG CCA CCT TTG CCT AGT GTT

                 180                                        190                                 200     203
                 lys lys leu thr glu asp arg trp asn lys pro gln lys thr lys gly his arg gly ser his thr met asn gly his AM
5092  AAG AAA CTG ACA GAG GAT AGA TGG AAC AAG CCC CAG AAG ACC AAG GGC CAC AGA GGG AGC CAT ACA ATG AAT GGA CAC TAG AGCTTTTAGA

      Translated Mol. Weight = 23707.95
```

Fig. 10. Amino acid and DNA sequence of (A) open reading frame 1 (ORF-1).

B

```
                 1                           10                        20
           his lys glu leu ile glu leu phe ser thr tyr ile glu glu leu asp arg ala trp lys gly phe cys tyr lys met gly
8263 ATAGAAGTAG CAC AAA GAG CTT ATA GAG CTA TTC TCC ACA TAC ATA GAA GAA TTA GAC AGG GCT TGG AAA GGC TTT TGC TAT AAG ATG GGT

                30                          40                        50
           gly lys trp ser lys arg ser met gly gly trp ser ala ile arg glu arg met arg arg ala glu pro arg ala glu pro ala ala asp
8354 GGC AAG TGG TCA AAA CGT AGT ATG GGT GGA TGG TCT GCT ATA AGG GAA AGA ATG AGA CGA GCT GAG CCA CGA GCT GAG CCA GCA GCA GAT

                60                          70                        80
           gly val gly ala val ser arg asp leu glu lys his gly ala ile thr ser ser asn thr ala ala thr asn ala asp cys ala trp leu
8444 GGG GTG GGA GCA GTA TCT CGA GAC CTG GAA AAA CAT GGA GCA ATC ACA AGT AGC AAT ACA GCA GCT ACT AAT GCT GAT TGT GCC TGG CTA

                90                          100                       110
           glu ala gln glu glu glu glu val gly phe pro val arg pro gln val pro leu arg pro met thr tyr lys ala ala leu asp ile ser
8534 GAA GCA CAA GAG GAG GAA GAG GTG GGT TTT CCA GTC AGA CCT CAG GTA CCT TTA AGA CCA ATG ACT TAC AAG GCA GCT TTA GAT ATT AGC

                120                         130                       140
           his phe leu lys glu lys gly gly leu glu gly leu ile trp ser gln arg arg gln glu ile leu asp leu trp ile tyr his thr gln
8624 CAC TTT TTA AAA GAA AAG GGG GGA CTG GAA GGG CTA ATT TGG TCC CAA AGA AGA CAA GAG ATC CTT GAT CTG TGG ATC TAC CAC ACA CAA

                150                         160                       170
           gly tyr phe pro asp trp gln asn tyr thr pro gly pro gly ile arg tyr pro leu thr phe gly trp cys phe lys leu val pro val
8714 GGC TAC TTC CCT GAT TGG CAG AAT TAC ACA CCA GGG CCA GGG ATC AGA TAT CCA CTG ACC TTT GGA TGG TGC TTC AAG CTA GTA CCA GTT

                180                         190                       200
           glu pro glu lys val glu glu ala asn glu gly glu asn asn ser leu leu his pro met ser leu his gly met glu asp ala glu lys
8804 GAG CCA GAG AAG GTA GAA GAG GCC AAT GAA GGA GAG AAC AAC AGC TTG TTA CAC CCT ATG AGC CTG CAT GGG ATG GAG GAC GCG GAG AAA

                210                         220                       230        235
           glu val leu val trp arg phe asp ser lys leu ala phe his his met ala arg glu leu his pro glu tyr tyr lys asp cys OP
8894 GAA GTG TTA GTG TGG AGG TTT GAC AGC AAA CTA GCA TTT CAT CAC ATG GCC CGA GAG CTG CAT CCG GAG TAC TAC AAA GAC TGC TGA CATCGA

GCTT


Translated Mol. Weight = 27147.86
```

Fig. 10. (continued) (B) open reading frame 2 (ORF-2). The molecular weights are given in daltons. Nucleotides are numbered according to Fig. 2.

+4; thus, these ATG codons are potential start codons (*31*). HTLV-I (*16*), HTLV-II (*17*), and BLV (*36*) contain open reading frames that initiate beyond *env* and extend into the rightward LTR; this location is analogous to that of ORF-2 in ARV-2. Comparisons of ORF-2 in ARV-2 with counterpart regions in these other retroviruses revealed no apparent homology at the DNA and protein levels (data not shown). For HTLV-I and HTLV-II, these regions are expressed as proteins that are implicated in viral pathogenesis (*37, 38*). Assessments of patterns of transcription and polypeptide synthesis will be essential to determine whether or not these ARV-2 open reading frames are expressed.

Certain taxonomic issues need to be addressed with respect to the relationships among the human retroviruses at the nucleotide sequence level. A probe representative of ARV-2 anneals under high stringency conditions to restriction enzyme DNA fragments from cells infected with LAV or with HTLV-III (*39*). Thus, these three retroviruses are closely related. In addition, we have shown that the probe to ARV-2 anneals under high stringency conditions to proviral DNA of two independent isolates, ARV-3 and ARV-4 (*12*). At the protein level, very low homology is evident when ARV-2 genes are compared with those of HTLV-I (Figs. 5 to 7 and Table 2); homology at the nucleotide level is even lower because of degeneracy of codons (Table 2). In our assessments, ARV-2 appears to be no more closely related to these other human retroviruses than it is to RSV (Table 2). Subhuman primate endogenous viral sequences (*40, 41*) are also distantly related to ARV *pol* (data not shown). Hybridization and annealing studies under very low stringency conditions demonstrated detectable homology of HTLV-III with HTLV-I and HTLV-II (*11, 42*). Our homology assessments at the nucleotide level (Table 2) indicate that stable hybrids or duplexes cannot be formed between ARV-2 DNA and HTLV-I DNA under these conditions. These issues could be fully resolved by comparing the DNA sequences of the genomes of retroviruses associated with AIDS (LAV, HTLV-III, and ARV).

The pathology that attends ARV infection is a unique aspect of this retrovirus. Selective tropism for human T-helper cells, syncytia formation, and cell killing are characteristics of ARV infection in tissue culture cells (*2–4, 43*). Attachment of virus to cell receptors and fusion of membranes are two properties controlled by the *env* gene that probably play a fundamental role in viral pathogenesis. The predicted sequence of ARV-2 *env* will be used to design mutagenesis experiments aimed at determining the function of *env* in attachment and fusion. LTR's of some avian and mammalian retroviruses have been shown to control tissue tropism, leukemogenicity, and specific disease patterns (*44–48*). Whether or not the ARV LTR plays a role in any of the pathologic manifestations associated with ARV infection remains to be established.

Sequence variations in ARV may be an important feature of viral pathogenesis that would enable the virus to evade host immune responses. Many viruses show sequence variation during passage. Infection of an animal with equine infectious anemia virus (EIAV) leads to differences in the *env* protein of progeny virus, probably as a consequence of immunological selective pressures in the host (*49*). Our studies of ARV have demonstrated sequence differences (i) in separate molecular clones of one ARV-2 isolate (Table 1) and (ii) in independent ARV isolates (*12*). Biological activity of cloned ARV-2 DNA has not yet been assessed by transfection of permissive cells. The generation of sequence variation in the ARV-2 genome can be studied by analyzing viruses recovered from different molecularly cloned ARV-2 DNA's. These approaches could provide insight into methods by which the viral infection could be prevented, modified, or eliminated.

Note added: The percentage of homologies in Table 2 in this chapter do not correspond to those printed in the original publication due to typing errors in the original figures 5, 6, and 7. The table and three figures have been corrected in this volume.

References and Notes

1. N. Teich, J. Wyke, T. Mark, A. Bernstein, W Hardy, in *Molecular Biology of Tumor Viruses. RNA Tumor Viruses*, R. Weiss, N. Teich, H. Varmus, J. Coffin, Eds. (Cold Spring Harbor Laboratories, Cold Spring Harbor, N.Y., 1982), p. 785.
2. F. Barré-Sinoussi *et al.*, *Science* **220**, 868 (1983).
3. M. Popovic, M. G. Sarngadharan, E. Read, R. C. Gallo, *ibid.* **224**, 497 (1984); R. C. Gallo *et al.*, *ibid.*, p. 500.
4. J. A. Levy *et al.*, *ibid.* **225**, 840 (1984).
5. J. A. Levy and J. Ziegler, *Lancet* **1983-II**, 78 (1983).
6. J. Schüpbach *et al.*, *Science* **224**, 503 (1984).
7. M. G. Sarngadharan, M. Popovic, L. Bruch, J. Schüpbach, R. C. Gallo, *ibid.*, p. 506.
8. J. Laurence *et al.*, *N. Engl. J. Med.* **311**, 1269 (1984).
9. J. J. Goedert *et al.*, *Lancet* **1984-I**, 711 (1984).
10. F. Brun-Vezinet *et al.*, *ibid.* **1983-I**, 1253 (1983).
11. B. H. Hahn *et al.*, *Nature (London)* **312**, 167 (1984); M. Alizon *et al.*, *ibid.*, p. 757.
12. P. A. Luciw, S. J. Potter, K. Steimer, D. Dina, J. A. Levy, *ibid.*, p. 760.
13. H. M. Temin, *Cell* **27**, 1 (1981).
14. ______, *ibid.* **28**, 3 (1982).
15. H. E. Varmus and R. Swanstrom, in *Molecular Biology of Tumor Viruses: RNA Tumor Viruses*, R. Weiss, N. Teich, H. Varmus, J. Coffin, Eds. (Cold Spring Harbor Laboratory, Cold Spring Harbor, N.Y., 1982), p. 369.
16. M. Seiki, S. Hattori, Y. Hirayama, M. Yoshida, *Proc. Natl. Acad. Sci. U.S.A.* **80**, 3618 (1983).
17. J. Sodroski *et al.*, *ibid.* **81**, 4617 (1984).
18. G. G. Peters and C. Glover, *J. Virol.* **35**, 31 (1980).
19. Appendix to *Molecular Biology of Tumor Viruses: RNA Tumor Viruses*, R. Weiss, N. Teich, H. Varmus, J. Coffin, Eds. (Cold Spring Harbor Laboratory, Cold Spring Harbor, N.Y., 1982), p. 1321.
20. E. B. Ziff and R. M. Evans, *Cell* **15**, 1463 (1978).
21. T. Yamamoto, D. deCrombrugghe, I. Pastan, *ibid.* **22**, 787 (1980).
22. A. Efstratiadis *et al.*, *ibid.* **21**, 653 (1980).
23. N. J. Proudfoot and G. G. Brownlee, *Nature (London)* **252**, 359 (1974).
24. C. Benoist and P. Chambon, *ibid.* **290**, 304 (1981).
25. P. Gruss, R. Dhar, G. Khoury, *Proc. Natl. Acad. Sci. U.S.A.* **78**, 943 (1981).
26. M. Kriegler and M. Botchan, *Mol. Cell. Biol.* **3**, 325 (1983).
27. L. A. Laimins, G. Khoury, C. Gorman, B. Howard, P. Gruss, *Proc. Natl. Acad. Sci. U.S.A.* **79**, 6453 (1982).
28. P. A. Luciw, J. M. Bishop, H. E. Varmus, M. R. Capecchi, *Cell* **33**, 705 (1983).
29. H. Weiher, M. König, P. Gruss, *Science* **219**, 626 (1983).
30. C. Dickson, R. Eisenman, H. Fan, E. Hunter, N. Teich, in *Molecular Biology of Tumor Viruses: RNA Tumor Viruses*. R. Weiss *et al.*, Eds. (Cold Spring Harbor Laboratory, Cold Spring Harbor, N.Y., 1982), p. 513.
31. H. Toh, H. Hayashida, T. Miyata, *Nature (London)* **305**, 827 (1983).
32. I-M. Chiu, R. Callahan, S. R. Tronick, J. Schlom, S. A. Aaronson, *Science* **223**, 364 (1984).
33. D. P. Grandgenett, R. J. Knaus, P. J. Hippenmeyer, *Virology* **130**, 257 (1983).
34. M. Kozak, *Nucleic Acids Res.* **12**, 857 (1983).
35. J. Sodroski, R. Patarca, D. Perkins, D. Briggs, T.-H. Lee, M. Essex, J. Coligan, F. Wong-Staal, R. C. Gallo, W. A. Haseltine, *Science* **225**, 421 (1984).
36. N. R. Rice *et al.*, *Virology* **138**, 82 (1984).
37. D. J. Slamon, K. Shimotohno, M. J. Cline, D. W. Golde, I.S.Y. Chen, *Science* **226**, 61 (1984).
38. T. H. Lee *et al.*, *ibid.*, p. 57.
39. M. Bryant and M. Gardner, personal communication.
40. T. I. Bonner, C. O'Connell, M. Cohen, *Proc. Natl. Acad. Sci. U.S.A.* **79**, 4709 (1982).
41. T. A. Tamura, *J. Virol.* **47**, 140 (1983).
42. S. K. Arya *et al.*, *Science* **225**, 927 (1984).
43. D. Klatzmann *et al.*, *ibid.*, p. 59.
44. P. A. Chatis, C. A. Holland, J. W. Hartley, W. P. Rowe, N. Hopkins, *Proc. Natl. Acad. Sci. U.S.A.* **80**, 4408 (1983).
45. L. DesGroseillers, E. Rassart, P. Jolicoeur, *ibid.*, p. 4203; J. Lenz and W. A. Haseltine, *J. Virol.* **47**, 317 (1983).
46. P. N. Tsichlis *et al.*, *Mol. Cell. Biol.* **2**, 1331 (1982).
47. W. A. Haseltine *et al.*, *Science* **225**, 419 (1984).
48. S. Y. Chen, J. McLaughlin, D. W. Golde, *Nature (London)* **309**, 276 (1984).
49. R. Montelaro, B. Parekh, C. Issel, A. Orrego, *J. Biol. Chem.* **259**, 10539 (1984).
50. J. Messing and J. Viera, *Gene* **19**, 269 (1982).
51. M. Hunkapiller, E. Lujar, F. Ostrander, L. Hood, *Methods Enzymol.* **91**, 227 (1983).
52. M. Hunkapiller, R. Hewick, W. Dreyer, L. Hood, *ibid.*, p. 399.
53. R. Hayashi, *ibid.* **47**, 84 (1977).
54. P. Hopp and K. R. Woods, *Proc. Natl. Acad.*

Sci. U.S.A. **78**, 3824 (1981).
55. P. Y. Chou, and G. D. Fasman, *Annu. Rev. Biochem.* **47**, 251 (1978).
56. U. Laemmli, *Nature (London)* **227**, 680 (1970).
57. H. Towbin, T. Staehelin, J. Gordon, *Proc. Natl. Acad. Sci. U.S.A.* **76**, 4350 (1979).
58. M. Lusky and M. Botchan, *Nature (London)* **293**, 79 (1981).
59. O. Laub *et al., J. Virol.* **48**, 271 (1983).
60. F. L. Graham and A. J. van de Eb, *Virology* **52**, 456 (1973).
61. We thank R. Blacher and F. Masiarz for viral protein purification and amino acids analysis, R. Najarian for help in the DNA sequencing, M.

Powers for immunoblots, D. Parkes for restriction enzyme analysis, C. T. Lee-Ng for synthetic DNA purification, M. A. Wormstead for assistance in tissue culture, and P. Montes and D. Topping for preparation of the manuscript. We also thank L. Overby and our colleagues at Chiron for comments and support. H. E. Varmus (University of California, San Francisco) is acknowledged for helpful discussions. A. Renard is a visiting scholar from Laboratoire de Genie Gentique, Universite de Liège, 4000 Liège, Belgium.

5 December 1984; accepted 31 December 1984

Report

1 February 1985

78. Characterization of Long Terminal Repeat Sequences of HTLV-III

Bruno Starcich, Lee Ratner, Steven F. Josephs, Takashi Okamoto, Robert C. Gallo, and Flossie Wong-Staal

The human retrovirus termed HTLV-III has been etiologically linked to the acquired immune deficiency syndrome (AIDS) (*1–3*), a disease characterized by opportunistic infections and malignancies such as Kaposi's sarcoma. This syndrome is also characterized by a preferential loss of OKT4$^+$ lymphocytes (*4*), the principal cell target for HTLV-III replication (*2*). In a recent study (*3*), serum samples from 95 percent of patients with AIDS or AIDS-associated disorders reacted with HTLV-III viral proteins, whereas samples from 30 percent of normal homosexuals and less than 1 percent of normal heterosexuals showed such a reaction (*3*). Like the human T-cell leukemia (lymphotropic) virus types I and II, HTLV-III is lymphotropic; shows a particular capacity to

infect T4 lymphocytes; contains a relatively large DNA polymerase (about 90,000 daltons), which is Mg^{2+} dependent; contains a major core protein of 24,000 daltons; induces formation of giant multinucleated cells; and, like HTLV-I and HTLV-II, contains a novel gene at the 3' end of the viral genome referred to as the long open reading frame (LOR) (*5*). Among animal retroviruses, bovine leukemia virus (BLV) also shares many of these characteristics as well as actual protein sequence homologies with HTLV-I (*6*). HTLV-III also shows substantial genomic homology with visna virus (*7*), a retrovirus that causes a chronic neurological disease of sheep.

The availability of recombinant DNA clones of HTLV-III prepared in our laboratory (*8, 9*) has enabled us to study the molecular details of this virus genome. The LTR region of HTLV-III was first analyzed since this region in other retroviruses is known to include regulatory sequences for viral transcription, host cell tropism, and determination of pathogenetic capabilities (*10*). Furthermore, comparison of the HTLV-III LTR with the LTR's of HTLV-I, HTLV-II, BLV, and other retroviruses, especially members of the subfamily Lentiviridae, may provide evidence of the evolutionary origin of this virus.

Figure 1a shows the structural features of the HTLV-III LTR derived from a genomic clone designated HXB2 (*9*). The complete nucleotide sequence of this LTR is shown in Fig. 1b. The complete provirus is flanked by a 7-bp direct repeat TAGTAGT. The LTR begins with the dinucleotide TG at position 1 and terminates with the inverted sequence CA at position 634. The same unusually short inverted repeats are also found in HTLV-I (*11*) and HTLV-II (*12*) LTR's and not in any of 12 other retroviruses examined including avian and mammalian type C retroviruses, the type B mouse mammary tumor virus and type D retroviruses (Table 1). The overall length of the HTLV-III LTR is 634 bp.

The U3 region is 453 bp in length, terminating at the RNA transcription initiation site as determined by S_1 nuclease mapping of the viral RNA (Fig. 2) and by estimation of the size of the (−) strand strong-stop complementary DNA (cDNA) (*13*). Upstream from this site is the proposed promoter signal, TATAA, which at −27 bp is at a position typical for promoters of eukaryotic genes (*14*). No open reading frame is found within U3. Furthermore, we were not able to

Table 1. Comparison of the LTR of HTLV-III to those of other retroviruses. Abbreviations: LTR, long terminal repeat; IR, inverted repeat; HTLV, human T-cell leukemia/lymphoma virus; BLV, bovine leukemia virus; AMV, avian myelocytomatosis virus; ASV, avian sarcoma virus; RSV, Rous sarcoma virus; MoMuLV, Moloney murine leukemia virus; MSV, murine sarcoma virus; FeLV-B, feline leukemia virus B; FeSV, feline sarcoma virus; SNV, spleen necrosis virus; MMTV, mouse mammary tumor virus; SSV, simian sarcoma virus.

Virus	Length in nucleotides					tRNA primer	References
	LTR	IR	U3	R	U5		
HTLV-III	634	2	453	98	83	Lys	
HTLV-I	754	2	353	221	180	Pro	(*11*)
HTLV-II	763	2	314	247	203	Pro	(*12*)
BLV	535	6	215	233	86	Pro	(*15*)
AMV	312	9	217	8	87	Trp	(*24*)
ASV	330	15	229	21	80	Trp	(*25*)
RSV	334	15	233	22	79	Trp	(*26*)
AKR	626	13	479	70	76	Pro	(*27*)
MoMuLV	594	13	449	68	77	Pro	(*28*)
MSV	588	11	444	68	76	Pro	(*29*)
FeLV-B	539	11	394	68	77	Pro	(*30*)
FeSV	482	12	340	68	74	Pro	(*31*)
SNV	570	3	396	79	95	Pro	(*32*)
MMTV	1328	6	1194	11	118	Lys	(*33*)
SSV	504	7	360	70	76	Pro	(*34*)

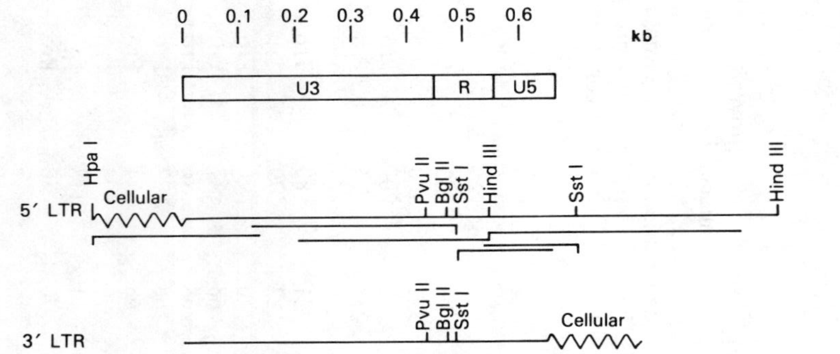

Fig. 1 (left). A schematic drawing of HTLV-III LTR, restriction map of the 5′ and 3′ LTR regions of the HXB2 (9) clone and sequencing strategy. To determine the cell-LTR boundaries we compared the sequencing data from an unintegrated DNA clone BH8 (8), corresponding to the 3′ 3.5-kb portion of the viral genome, with the sequence of HXB2. After restriction enzyme digestions, the labeling of 5′ ends was accomplished with γ-^{32}P-labeled adenosine triphosphate and the T4 polynucleotide kinase; 3′ ends were labeled with α-^{32}P dideoxy-ATP and terminal deoxynucleotidal transferase. The sequence was determined by the method of Maxam and Gilbert (22). The U3-R boundary was localized by S1 nuclease mapping (23) (see Fig. 2) and strong-stop cDNA synthesis. The R-U5 boundary was determined from the sequence of a cDNA clone obtained by using oligo(dT) as primer and viral RNA as template (not shown).

Fig. 2 (right). Complete HTLV-III LTR sequence of the genomic clone obtained from the HTLV-III–producing T-cell line H9 (2).

```
                                                           TAGTAGT
U3
TGGAAGGGCTAATTCACTCCCAACGAAGACAAGATATCCTTGATCTGTGGATCTACCACA   60
--

CACAAGGCTACTTCCCTGATTAGCAGAACTACACACCAGGGCCAGGGGTCAGATATCCAC  120

TGACCTTTGGATGGTGCTACAAGCTAGTACCAGTTGAGCCAGATAAGGTAGAAGAGGCCA  180

ATAAAGGAGAGAACACCAGCTTGTTACACCCTGTGAGCCTGCATGGGATGGATGACCCGG  240

AGAGAGAAGTGTTAGAGTGGAGGTTTGACAGCCGCCTAGCATTTCATCACGTGGCCCGAG  300

AGCTGCATCCGGAGTACTTCAAGAACTGCTGATATCGAGCTTGCTACAAGGGACTTTCCG  360

CTGGGGACTTTCCAGGGAGGCGTGGCCTGGGCGGGACTGGGGAGTGGCGAGCCCTCAGAT  420
    TATA  Pvu II              U3 v R              Bgl II
CCTGCATATAAGCAGCTGCTTTTTGCCTGTACTGGGTCTCTCTGGTTAGACCAGATCTGA  480
    ------------
                                              Hind   III
    SstI                                      Poly(A) s
GCCTGGGAGCTCTCTGGCTAGCTAGGGAACCCACTGCTTAAGCCTCAATAAAGCTTGCCT  540
                                                    ----------
    R  v U5
TGAGTGCTTCAAGTAGTGTGTGCCCGTCTGTTGTGTGACTCTGGTAACTAGAGATCCCTC  600
                            U5 v   tRNA Lys
AGACCCTTTTAGTCAGTGTGGAAAATCTCTAGCAGTGGCGCCCGAACAGGGAC         660
                          -- -------------------
                          TAGTAGT
```

find repetitive sequences in U3 such as were found in HTLV-I (*11*), HTLV-II (*12*), and BLV (*15*). Sequences related to the enhancer core sequence GTGG(A/T)(A/T)(A/T)G (*16*) include TGGTTAG at position 463 and TGGATGG at position 128.

As in the HTLV-I and HTLV-II LTR's, and again unlike that of other known retroviruses, no CAT box was found in the usual location at −70 to −80 bp from the site of RNA initiation. However, a sequence similar to that signal, CCAAT, is located upstream at position 178.

The polyadenylation signal AATAAA is positioned at −24 bp from the polyadenylation site at nucleotide 551. The placement of this signal is typical for those of eukaryotic genes (*14*) but distinct from those of HTLV-I, HTLV-II, and BLV which are positioned much further upstream (*11, 12, 15*). The R–U5 boundary was determined from the sequence of a cDNA clone obtained by using oligo(dT) as primer and viral RNA as template (not shown). The polyadenylation site is also flanked by sequences related to the transcriptional termination consensus signals TTTGCN(G/C)TTGCA and TTGT (*17*); the latter is found 20 bp downstream from this site at position 571. The R region is therefore 98 bp long.

The U5 region is 83 bp long and ends with a CA dinucleotide. This is followed by the primer site which is 18 bp complementary to the 3′ terminus of transfer

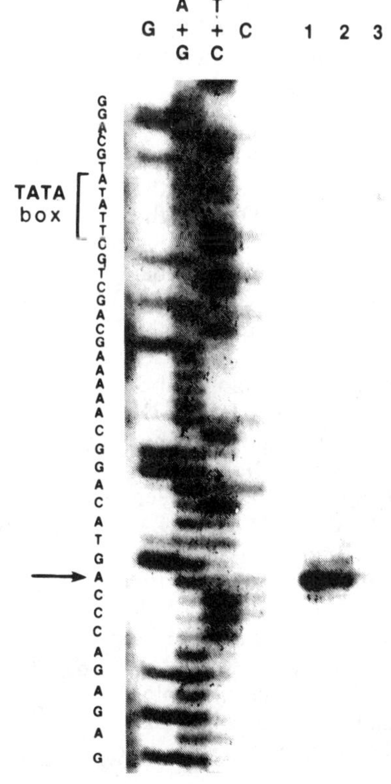

Fig. 3. S1 nuclease mapping of HTLV-III and the RNA initiation site. Procedure: 0.25 µg of HTLV-III virion RNA (lane 1), 5 µg of poly A(+) cellular RNA from HTLV-III infected H9 cells (lane 2), or uninfected H9 cells (lane 3) were hybridized to a Hind III–Hpa I fragment of clone HXB2 at 49°C for 3 hours in 40 m*M* Pipes, *p*H 6.4, 400 m*M* NaCl, 1 m*M* EDTA, and 80 percent formamide. The probe was labeled at the Hind III site with [γ-^{32}P]ATP and T4 polynucleotide kinase (*22*). Samples were then incubated with S1 nuclease (200 U/ml), 280 m*M* NaCl, 30 m*M* sodium acetate, *p*H 4.4, 4.5 m*M* zinc acetate, and denatured calf thymus DNA (20 µg/ml) at 45°C for 30 minutes (*23*). Samples were subjected to electrophoresis on an acrylamide gel. Samples of the same ^{32}P-labeled Hind III–Hpa I DNA fragment were subjected to electrophoresis in parallel after they had undergone sequence reactions (*22*). The (−) strand nucleotide sequence is shown to the left of the figure. Since the chemical cleavage reactions destroy the nucleotide at which the base-specific strand scission occurs (*22*), the actual sequence length of the major S$_1$ nuclease-protected fragment is 1 bp shorter than the corresponding position on the sequence ladder (arrow).

432

RNA–lysine (tRNA[lys]). This is distinct from HTLV-I, HTLV-II, BLV, and all other mammalian type C retroviruses, which utilize tRNA-proline. Mouse mammary tumor virus (MMTV) is the only other retrovirus known to contain a tRNA-lysine primer binding site (Table 1). The structural features of the HTLV-III LTR are compared to those of other retrovirus LTR's in Table 1. The lengths of U5, R, and U3 of HTLV-III are similar to those of other retroviruses thus far described.

As with the HTLV-I LTR (18), the HTLV-III LTR also contains sequences that have some homology to those of human T-cell growth factor (TCGF, or IL-2) (19). One of these sequences, which is located 275 nucleotides upstream from the HTLV-III transcriptional initiation site (CAP site, U3-R boundary), is 70 percent homologous to a sequence at an analogous position 293 nucleotides upstream from the CAP site of the TCGF gene (Fig. 4a). Other homologous (80 percent) sequences are located 20 and 24 bp downstream from the core enhancer consensus signals in the first intron of the TCGF gene and in HTLV-III U3, respectively (Fig. 4b).

A sequence similarity of 83 percent was also found between HTLV-III U3 and intron I of human γ-interferon (γ-IF) (20) (Fig. 4c). The corresponding sequence of the γ-IF gene is also located immediately downstream from an enhancer-like sequence GTGGTTA.

Since the TCGF and γ-IF genes are expressed exclusively in T cells, and since the regions of homology are located downstream from their potential enhancer signals, the corresponding sequences in the HTLV-III LTR could play some role in host cell tropism or transcriptional regulation of this virus.

Some general features of the HTLV-III LTR are similar to those of HTLV-I, HTLV-II, and BLV. A 62 percent ho-

Fig. 4. (a) Sequence homology between the HTLV-III LTR and the TCGF gene. (b) Sequence homology between the HTLV-III LTR U3 region and the TCGF gene. (c) Sequence homology between the HTLV-III LTR U3 region and human γ-IF. (d) Sequence homology between HTLV-III U3 and BLV U3 regions. (e) Sequence homologies among the U3 regions of HTLV-I, HTLV-II, and HTLV-III. Gaps were introduced during complex analyses, to maximize the homologies (35).

```
a)  HTLV-III LTR  180    AAT AAAGGAGAGAACACCAGCTTGTTACA    208
          TCGF     139    AAAGAAAGGAG GAAAAACTGTTTCATACA    167


b)     HTLV-III LTR  152    AGTTGAGCCAGAGAAGATAGAA GAA    176
             TCGF   1656    AGTTGTGCCAGTTAAGAGAGAATGAA   1681


c)       HTLV-III LTR  324    AACTG CTGA TATCGAGCTTGCT    345
               IF      627    AAATGACTGAATATCGA CTTGCT    649


d)      BLV U3   152    TGCTGA CCTCA  CCTGCTGATAAATTAA    178
     HTLV-III U3  405    TGGCGAGCCCTCAGATCCTGC  ATA   TAA  431


e) HTLV-I   U3   307    AATAAACTAGCAGGAGTCTATAAAAGCGTGG    337
   HTLV-II  U3   268    AATAAAAGATGCCGAGTCTATAAAGGCGCAA    298
   HTLV-III U3   172    GATAAGGTAGAAGAGGCCAATAAAGGAGAGA    192
```

mology was found between HTLV-III U3 and BLV U3 sequences (*15*) that include the functional promoters of both viruses (Fig. 4d).

Homologies of 61 and 55 percent were also found between HTLV-III and HTLV-I and HTLV-II U3 sequences, respectively (*11, 12*). These sequences include the functional promoter signals of HTLV-I and HTLV-II and a promoter-like signal of HTLV-III U3 (AATAAA) (Fig. 4e) (position 527 in Fig. 2). One can speculate that this promoter-like sequence was actually utilized in an ancestral virus. If so, the R region of this virus would be extended and thus be more similar in length to those of HTLV-I, HTLV-II, and BLV. Furthermore, in this extended R region a stable loop structure would be positioned similarly to those shown for HTLV-I, HTLV-II, and BLV (*11, 12, 15*). These structural analogies suggest that HTLV-III has evolved from the same ancestor as other members of the HTLV/BLV family. The functional role of the transcriptional regulatory sequences in U3 as well as the involvement of the LTR in the cytopathic effect of HTLV-III remain to be demonstrated.

The recent finding of similarities between HTLV-III and visna virus in morphology, cytopathic potential, ability to infect brain tissue, and nucleotide sequence strongly suggests that these viruses are related (*7, 21*). It would be of interest to determine whether the LTR of visna is similar in structure to the LTR of HTLV-III.

References and Notes

1. R. C. Gallo *et al.*, *Science* **224**, 500 (1984); J. Schüpbach *et al.*, *ibid.*, p. 503.
2. M. Popovic, M. G. Sarngadharan, E. Read, R. C. Gallo, *ibid.*, p. 497.
3. M. G. Sarngadharan, M. Popovic, L. Bruch, J. Schüpbach, R. C. Gallo, *ibid.*, p. 506.
4. M. S. Gottlieb *et al.*, *N. Engl. J. Med.* **305**, 1425 (1981).
5. L. Ratner *et al.*, *Nature (London)*, in press.
6. S. Oroszlan *et al.*, in *Human T-Cell Leukemia/ Lymphoma Virus*, R. C. Gallo, M. Essex, L. Gross, Eds. (Cold Spring Harbor Laboratory, Cold Spring Harbor, N.Y., 1984), p. 101.
7. M. A. Gonda *et al.*, *Science* **227**, 173 (1985).
8. B. H. Hahn *et al.*, *Nature (London)* **312**, 166 (1984).
9. G. M. Shaw *et al.*, *Science* **226**, 1165 (1984).
10. J. Lenz and W. A. Haseltine, *J. Virol.* **47**, 317 (1983); L. Des Groseillers, E. Rassart, P. Jolicoeur, *Proc. Natl. Acad. Sci. U.S.A.* **80**, 4203 (1983).
11. M. Seiki, S. Hattori, Y. Hirayama, M. Yoshida, *Proc. Natl. Acad. Sci. U.S.A.* **80**, 3618 (1983).
12. J. Sodroski *et al.*, *ibid.* **81**, 4617 (1984).
13. L. Ratner *et al.*, unpublished observations.
14. H. W. Temin, *Cell* **27**, 1 (1981).
15. N. Sagata, T. Yasunaga, Y. Owaga, J. Tsuzuku-Kawamure, Y. Ikawa, *Proc. Natl. Acad. Sci. U.S.A.* **81**, 4741 (1984).
16. H. Weiher, M. König, P. Gruss, *Science* **219**, 626 (1983).
17. T. I. Bonner, C. O'Connell, M. Cohen, *Proc. Natl. Acad. Sci. U.S.A.* **79**, 4709 (1982).
18. N. J. Holbrook, M. Lieber, G. R. Crabtree, *Nucl. Acids Res.* **12**, 5005 (1984).
19. T. Fujita, C. Takaoka, H. Matsui, T. Taniguchi, *Proc. Natl. Acad. Sci. U.S.A.* **80**, 7437 (1983).
20. P. W. Gray and D. V. Goeddel, *Nature (London)* **298**, 859 (1982).
21. G. M. Shaw *et al.*, *Science* **227**, 177 (1985).
22. A. M. Maxam and W. Gilbert, *Methods Enzymol.* **65**, 499 (1980).
23. A. J. Berk and P. A. Sharp, *Cell* **12**, 721 (1977).
24. E. P. Reddy *et al.*, *Proc. Natl. Acad. Sci. U.S.A.* **80**, 2500 (1983).
25. R. Swanstrom, W. J. DeLorbe, J. M. Bishop, H. E. Varmus, *ibid.* **78**, 124 (1981).
26. D. E. Schwartz, R. Tizard, W. Gilbert, *Cell* **32**, 853 (1983).
27. R. Villemur, E. Rassart, L. Des Groseillers, P. Jolicoeur, *J. Virol.* **45**, 539 (1983).
28. T. M. Shinnick, R. A. Lerner, J. G. Sutcliffe, *Nature (London)* **293**, 543 (1981).
29. R. Dhar *et al.*, *Proc. Natl. Acad. Sci. U.S.A.* **77**, 3937 (1980).
30. J. H. Elder and J. I. Mullins, *J. Virol.* **46**, 871 (1983).
31. A. H. Hampe, M. Gobet, J. Even, C. J. Sherr, F. Galibert, *ibid.* **45**, 466 (1983).
32. K. Shimotohno, S. Mizutani, H. M. Temin, *Nature (London)* **285**, 550 (1980).
33. N. Kennedy, G. Knedlitschek, B. Groner, N. E. Hynes, P. Herrlich, R. Michalides, A. J. J. van Ooyen, *ibid.* **295**, 622 (1982).
34. S. Devare, E. P. Reddy, J. D. Law, S. A. Aaronson, *J. Virol.* **42**, 1108 (1982).
35. C. L. Queen and L. J. Korn, *Methods Enzymol.* **65**, 595 (1980).
36. We thank G. Shaw, B. Hahn, S. K. Arya, and G. Chan in our laboratory for the HTLV-III clones, W. A. Haseltine for helpful discussions, J. Maizel for secondary structure analysis, and A. Mazzuca and L. Bruening for editorial assistance. B.S. is a fellow of the Italian Association for Cancer Research.

30 November 1984; accepted 31 December 1984

79.   Evidence for Exposure to HTLV-III in Uganda Before 1973

W. Carl Saxinger, Paul H. Levine, A.G. Dean, Guy de Thé, Gunhild Lange-Wantzin, Jasmine Moghissi, Francine Laurent, Mei Hoh, M.G. Sarngadharan, and Robert C. Gallo

The acquired immune deficiency syndrome (AIDS) is known to occur among homosexual or bisexual men, intravenous drug abusers and their infants, female sexual partners of men with the syndrome, Haitians, and patients with hemophilia (*1, 2*). Recently, a retrovirus of the human T-cell leukemia (lymphotropic) virus "family" called HTLV-III was isolated with high frequency in serum samples from patients with AIDS and pre-AIDS (*3*), and antibodies to the virus were found in 88 to 100 percent of AIDS patients and individuals at high risk for AIDS (*4*). Many data indicate that this virus is the cause of AIDS (*5*). Similar or identical retroviruses have also been identified (*6*) and subsequently isolated (*7*). Some of these are now being directly compared to several isolates of HTLV-III.

AIDS, first recognized as a separate disease entity in 1981 (*1*), is diagnosed as a severe, unexplained immune deficiency that usually involves a reduction in the number of helper T lymphocytes and is accompanied by multiple opportunistic infections or malignancies. Where and how the disease arose are open questions, but several observations are consistent with an African origin.

Although the occurrence of AIDS in black central Africans was only recently reported (*8*), Kaposi's sarcoma is highly prevalent there (*9*), and cases in children and young adults with a presentation and course similar to those associated with Kaposi's sarcoma in homosexual men with AIDS were documented in 1971 (*10*). Earlier studies in our laboratory and others indicated that HTLV type 1 (HTLV-I) occurs with high frequency in regions of central Africa (*11–14*), and closely related retroviruses are present in many Old World monkeys (*13, 15*). These and other results led us to suggest an African origin of the HTLV family (*16*). Furthermore, we recently found a high prevalence of serum antibodies recognizing HTLV-I in Ugandan children with Burkitt's lymphoma and in normal family and community members sampled in 1972 and 1973 (*11*). We have now extended our observations to the prevalence of antibodies related to HTLV-III in the West Nile district population of Uganda and have found evidence suggesting the existence of a virus related to HTLV-III present at a time predating or coinciding with the earliest report of cases resembling AIDS.

The Ugandan serum tested was primarily from clinically healthy donors randomly selected as controls for Burkitt's lymphoma patients on the basis of age, sex, and community. All samples were collected between August 1972 and July 1973 (*17*). The mean age of the patient population was 6.4 years (*17*). Samples from this collection were tested for antibodies recognizing HTLV-III in two stages. First, all the samples were tested by indirect enzyme-linked immunosorbent assay (ELISA) for quantitative levels of immunoglobulin G binding to disrupted HTLV-III virions coated onto the wells of microtiter plates (*18*). HTLV-III virions were produced in high quantity by specific clones from a permissive human neoplastic T-cell line (*19*). Test results were normalized to values for a standardized normal human control serum, and all samples with normalized values exceeding a cutoff of the mean + 2 standard deviations (determined from 82 normal donors) (*20*) were confirmed by the demonstration of antibody binding to virus-specific proteins separated by sodium dodecyl sulfate–polyacrylamide gel electrophoresis (SDS-PAGE) and electrophoretically transferred to nitrocellulose strips (*21*).

Of the 75 samples, 50 of 55 that exceeded the cutoff of 2 standard deviations recognized specific viral bands with an overall positive rate of 66 percent. The most prominent reactions were with antigens having molecular weights of 76K, 55K, 41K, and 24K. Less frequently recognized antigens had molecular weights of 64K, 59K, 32K, and 18K. These values coincide with the previously described molecular weights of HTLV-III antigens recognized by serum from AIDS patients or individuals at risk for AIDS (*4, 22*). Representative samples from two consecutive experiments are shown in Fig. 1, aligned in order of ascending screening ratios from left to right. Under the same experimental conditions all 4 of 82 normal donors exceeding the ELISA cutoff were negative in the blotting procedure.

Titers of positive samples were determined and compared with titers determined previously (*11*) for HTLV-I–positive serum from this group (Table 1). The extent of cross-reactivity between HTLV-I antibody–positive serum samples from individuals in regions in which adult T-cell leukemia is endemic and HTLV-III antibody–positive serum from AIDS patients and high-risk groups is shown in Table 2. The data show little or no cross-reactivity between natural antibodies to HTLV-I and HTLV-III under the conditions of our test. Ten of 50 samples (20 percent) showing a positive antibody response to HTLV-III antigens were also positive for HTLV-I, while 10 of 12 samples (83 percent) positive for HTLV-I were positive for HTLV-III. These percentages are in good agreement with the overall rates of 16 percent for HTLV-I and 66 percent for HTLV-III. The agreement might have been closer, but 11 samples of the original group of 86 had been depleted. Of the 11 samples that were removed 5 were positive for HTLV-I antibody. The mean titer of samples positive in both the HTLV-I and HTLV-III tests was two to three times higher than that of samples that were not. Only one sample (out of 10) had a higher titer with respect to HTLV-I (840 versus 80).

The data show that antibodies recognizing a virus related to or identical to HTLV-III were present in most of the Ugandan subjects tested. Since the subjects were chosen to be representative of Burkitt's lymphoma patients by age, sex, and community and since the mean age was low, it is likely that residents of the West Nile region of Uganda have been and continue to be exposed to the virus at a very early age. The immunologic specificity of the tests argues against cross-reactivity resulting from antibodies against HTLV-I (or vice versa) in these cases (Table 2) (*11*); and, since antibodies against HTLV type 2 (HTLV-

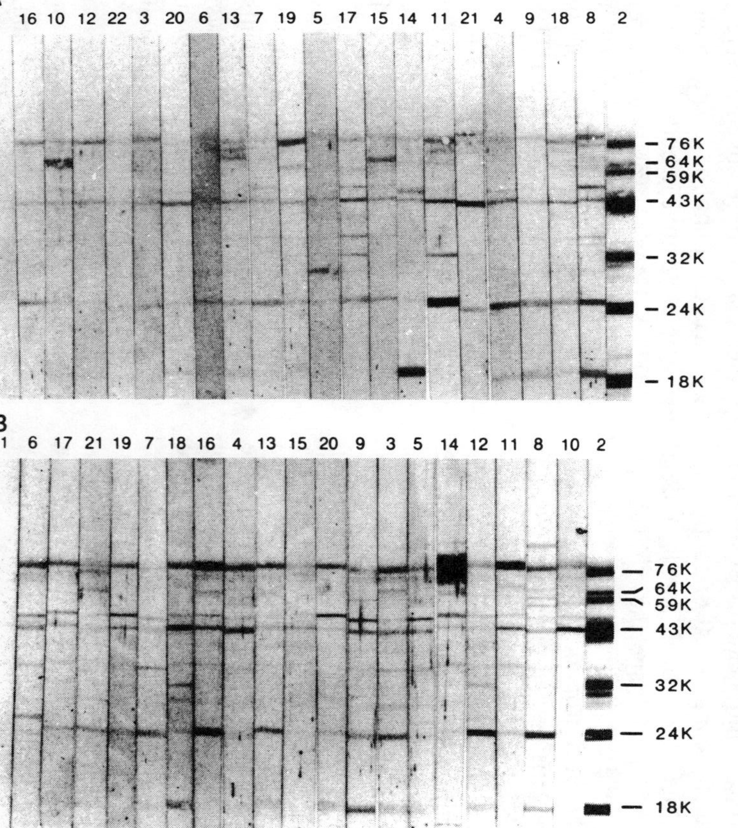

Fig. 1. Identification of HTLV-III antigens recognized by Ugandan serum collected in 1972 and 1973. Absorbance values of samples tested for HTLV-III antibody were expressed in ratio to a standard normal control serum and samples with ratio values greater than the mean + 2 standard deviations = 2.0 for normal donors were subjected to a confirmatory test requiring positive reactivity with the major HTLV-III viral bands separated by SDS-PAGE (200 μg of virus per 12 percent acrylamide slab) and transferred to nitrocellulose sheets by electroblotting (*21*) overnight at 15°C and 30 volts. The sheets were cut into strips and incubated with human test serum diluted 1:400 in 5 percent nonfat dried milk [Blotto (*26*)] containing 0.02 percent merthiolate for 16 hours at 4°C. The strips were washed with wash buffer (*18*), phosphate-buffered saline (PBS) containing 0.5 percent deoxycholate, 0.5 percent Triton X-100, and 1 mM phenylmethylsulfonyl fluoride (PMSF). Next, the strips were incubated at room temperature for 1 hour with goat antiserum to human immunoglobulin G Fc fragment (Cappel) diluted 1:400 in buffer 1 (*18*), 20 mM tris-HCl (*p*H 7.5) containing 1 mM EDTA, 0.2M NaCl, 0.3 percent Triton X-100, bovine serum albumin (2 mg/ml), and 4 percent normal goat serum. The strips were washed as described above and incubated for 1 hour at room temperature with human immunoglobulin G conjugated with horseradish peroxidase (2 μg/ml) (*27*) in PBS containing 0.5 percent Tween 20 and 5 percent normal goat serum. After washing the peroxidase color reaction was developed by incubation in 25 mM tris (*p*H 7.5) containing 0.02 percent hydrogen peroxide and 0.025 percent *o*-dianisidine. (A) and (B) show 39 different sera tested in consecutive experiments. Strips are arranged in order of ascending screening ratios from left to right; lane numbers refer to the original position of the strip within the nitrocellulose blot. Lanes 1 in (A) and (B) contain normal control human serum; lanes 2 in (A) and (B) contain positive control human serum from an AIDS patient. Normal (control) human serum at a tenfold higher concentration (1/40) also showed no visible staining.

Table 1. Antibodies to HTLV-III and HTLV-I in serum collected in 1972 and 1973 from 75 Ugandan children. All samples that were positive by the Western blotting procedure were included in titration analyses. Titration data were obtained from serial dilutions of a test sample in the standard ELISA protocol. The data were analyzed by using the equation in reciprocal form for molecular binding (28). The slope for the regression line where x is serum dilution and y inverse optical density (values of inverse optical density greater than 25 were excluded) was determined and the general equation for a straight line was used to solve for x = titer. The titration end point was the value of y for a 1/20 dilution of standard normal serum. NA, not applicable.

Serum positive for	HTLV III antibodies			HTLV I antibodies		
	Number of samples	Mean titer	Geometric mean titer (coefficient of variation;* range)	Number of samples	Mean titer	Geometric mean titer (coefficient of variation;* range)
HTLV-III	40	421	263 (46; 43 to 1750)	NA	NA	NA
HTLV-III and HTLV-I	10	1328	447 (73; 84 to 7400)	10	264	195 (34; 80 to 840)
HTLV-I	NA	NA	NA	2	83	71 (95; 40 to 125)
Total	50	601	295 (52)	12	236	166 (37)

*×100, analysis performed on log units (titers).

II) (23) would be expected to react more efficiently with HTLV-I than HTLV-III (4, 22), it is unlikely that HTLV-II is responsible for the high prevalence of HTLV-III antibodies seen. As expected, titers of HTLV-III antibody–positive serum against HTLV-II antigens were not significant. Therefore we favor the interpretation that this population subgroup has been exposed to both HTLV-III and, to a lesser extent, HTLV-I (24). Subjects with antibodies reactive with both HTLV-I and HTLV-III had higher titers than those with a single specificity. We believe that certain host or environmental factors may facilitate or enhance exposure, susceptibility, or immune responsiveness to both or even other viruses. Alternatively, it is conceivable that the observed antibody reactivities against HTLV-I and HTLV-III result from unusual cross-reactivity of antibodies against an undescribed variant of HTLV, that is, a type 4. Finally, infection by one of the viruses could increase susceptibility to the other, but studies of areas where HTLV-I is endemic, such as southern Japan and Jamaica, do not support this idea.

If, as we suspect, the antibody reactivities found represent widespread exposure or infection by HTLV-III, then it must be asked why the incidence of AIDS in the Ugandan population (and neighboring Zaire) has gone unnoticed for so long. It is possible that AIDS existed in African populations without being recognized as a separate disease entity. The virus may have originated in Africa in the past and exposure to the virus may be much more common than AIDS itself in some populations. As with

Table 2. Specificity of ELISA tests for HTLV-III and HTLV-I antibodies. Titers were determined as described in Table 1; representative sera are listed individually; ATL, adult T-cell leukemia.

Serum	Titer of antibodies	
	Against HTLV-I	Against HTLV-III
Caribbean black ATL patients		
S0082	76,000	<20
S0180	44,000	120
S0209	100,000	<20
S0310	310,000	40
S0646	81,000	40
S0668	520	<20
S0669	19,000	<20
S1050	19,000	<20
S1089	49,000	40
*AIDS or at-risk patients**		
J8757	<20	29,000
J8759	24	3,400
J8760	<20	100,000
J8783	23	110,000
J8786	<20	29,000
J8800	<20	105,000

*Danish white homosexual males with AIDS (J8757) or "asymptomatic" when presenting with venereal disease (29, 30).

many other infectious diseases, host responsiveness may vary between severe and subclinical. If recent reports of AIDS in central Africa suggesting that the disease is newly evolved and spreading are correct (8), then it is essential to determine which of the various host- and virus-related factors are responsible. For example, it is important to know whether the current spread of AIDS is due to a spread of HTLV-III from nonsusceptible to susceptible populations or to a molecular change in the virus. In this regard, our samples were taken from a sparsely populated subsistence-farming environment (17) where AIDS is not known to occur, while the recent spread in African AIDS appears to be in more densely populated urban environments and heterosexual populations (25). Clearly, epidemiologic and virologic studies are needed to examine changes in the occurrence of AIDS and AIDS-related diseases in healthy individuals (particularly children) in central Africa.

References and Notes

1. M. S. Gottlieb *et al.*, *N. Engl. J. Med.* **305**, 1425 (1981); H. Masur *et al.*, *ibid.*, p. 1431.
2. F. P. Siegal *et al.*, *ibid.*, p. 1439; M. Poon, A. Landay, E. F. Prasthofer, S. Stagno, *Ann. Int. Med.* **98**, 287 (1983); B. Moll *et al.*, *Clin. Immunol. Immunopathol.* **25**, 417 (1982); J. W. Curran *et al.*, *N. Engl. J. Med.* **310**, 69 (1984); A. S. Fauci, *J. Am. Med. Assoc.* **249**, 2375 (1983).
3. R. C. Gallo *et al.*, *Science* **224**, 500 (1984).
4. M. G. Sarngadharan, M. Popovic, L. Bruch, J. Schüpbach, R. C. Gallo, *ibid.*, p. 506.
5. S. Broder and R. C. Gallo, *N. Engl. J. Med.*, in press.
6. F. Barré-Sinoussi *et al.*, *Science* **220**, 868 (1983); L. Montagnier *et al.*, in *Human T-Cell Leukemia/Lymphoma Virus*, R. C. Gallo, M. Essex, L. Gross, Eds. (Cold Spring Harbor Laboratory, Cold Spring Harbor, N.Y., 1984), p. 363.
7. E. Vilmer *et al.*, *Lancet* **1984-I**, 753 (1984); L. Montagnier *et al.*, *Science* **225**, 63 (1984); J. A. Levy *et al.*, *ibid.*, p. 840.
8. N. Clumeck *et al.*, *N. Engl. J. Med.* **310**, 492 (1984).
9. A. G. Oettle, *Acta Unio Int. Contra Cancrum* **18**, 350 (1962).
10. J. F. Taylor, *Lancet* **1973-I**, 883 (1973); ______, A. C. Templeton, C. L. Vogel, J. L. Ziegler, S. K. Kyalwazy, *Int. J. Cancer* **8**, 122 (1971).
11. W. Saxinger *et al.*, *Science* **225**, 1473 (1984).
12. C. K. O. Williams *et al.*, *Br. Med. J.* **288**, 1495 (1984).
13. W. C. Saxinger *et al.*, in *Human T-Cell Leukemia/Lymphoma Virus*, R. C. Gallo, M. Essex, L. Gross, Eds. (Cold Spring Harbor Laboratory, Cold Spring Harbor, N.Y., 1984), p. 323.
14. G. Hunsmann *et al.*, *Int. J. Cancer* **32**, 329 (1983).
15. I. Miyoshi *et al.*, *Lancet* **1982-II**, 658 (1982); N. Yamamoto, Y. Hinuma, H. zur Hausen, J. Schneider, G. Hunsmann, *ibid.* **1983-I**, 240 (1983); I. Miyoshi *et al.*, *Int. J. Cancer* **32**, 333 (1983); T. Ishida *et al.*, *Microbiol. Immunol.* **27**, 297 (1983).
16. R. C. Gallo, A. Sliski, F. Wong-Staal, *Lancet* **1983-II**, 962 (1983).
17. A. G. Dean *et al.*, *ibid.* **1973-II**, 1225 (1973).
18. C. Saxinger and R. C. Gallo, *Lab. Invest.* **49**, 371 (1983).
19. M. Popovic, M. G. Sarngadharan, E. Read, R. C. Gallo, *Science* **224**, 497 (1984).
20. Serum samples were from a larger group of 356 Danish normal volunteer blood donors collected by Henning Sörensen at the Righaspitalet, University Hospital of Copenhagen Blood Bank, serving the Copenhagen area. A detailed description by age and sex is given by W. C. Saxinger, G. Lange-Wantzin, K. Thomsen, M.

Hoh, and R. C. Gallo (in preparation).
21. H. Towbin, T. Staehelin, J. Gordon, *Proc. Natl. Acad. Sci. U.S.A.* **76**, 4350 (1979).
22. J. Schüpbach *et al.*, *Science* **224**, 503 (1984).
23. V. S. Kalyanaraman *et al.*, *Proc. Natl. Acad. Sci. U.S.A.* **79**, 1653 (1982).
24. Although HTLV-III–positive serum samples that cross-react with HTLV-I under the experimental conditions described here are occasionally seen, they have been sufficiently rare to suggest that they could have arisen from coinfection rather than cross-reactivity in the usual sense. The apparent difference between this and a previous report indicating serological cross-reactivity between HTLV-III and HTLV-I [M. Essex *et al.*, *Science* **220**, 859 (1983)] might arise from differences found in target antigens present in live cells versus antigens dissociated from purified virus particles and deposited on a solid surface. In any case, the data presented in the tables are representative of our experience and are clearly different from the relative titers and prevalence of HTLV-I and HTLV-III antibody reactivity in the Ugandan serum.
25. P. Van de Perre *et al.*, *Lancet* **1984-II**, 62 (1984); P. Piot *et al.*, *ibid.*, p. 65.
26. D. A. Johnson, J. W. Gautsch, J. R. Sportsman, J. H. Elder, *Gene Anal. Techn.* **1**, 3 (1984).
27. P. K. Nakane and A. Kawaoi, *J. Histochem. Cytochem.* **22**, 1084 (1974).
28. J. T. Edsall and J. Wyman, Eds., *Biophysical Chemistry* (Academic Press, New York, 1958), p. 616.
29. W. A. Blattner *et al.*, *Lancet* **1983-II**, 61 (1983).
30. G. Lange-Wantzin, W. C. Saxinger, R. C. Gallo, in preparation.

4 September 1984; accepted 7 December 1984

80.   OTA Critical of AIDS Initiative

Constance Holden

The Public Health Service's multi-front battle against acquired immune deficiency syndrome (AIDS) has been hampered by insufficient funds and inadequate planning, according to a report from the Office of Technology Assessment (OTA).

The report, produced at the behest of two congressional committees, says that despite much money—$97.4 million in fiscal 1985—"it has not always been clear...that the amount of support for AIDS activities has been equivalent to the needs identified by PHS agencies." It contends that "except when prodded by Congress, the Department [of Health and Human Services] has maintained that PHS agencies should be able to conduct AIDS research without extra funds"—with the result that, despite extra appropriations, agencies have had to divert money from other activities.

The OTA maintains that planning has been thwarted by personnel cuts and financial uncertainties. It chastises the Administration for not seeking appropriations from the $30 million fund established by the Public Health Emergency Act of 1983.

The report is also critical of the fact that despite the designation of AIDS as the "number one health priority" of the Department of Health and Human Services (HHS), there has been no mechanism to speed up approval and funding of grant applications which take more than a year to process.

Although in the past 4 years PHS-funded researchers have defined the syndrome, found an AIDS virus, devised a test for antibodies to the virus, and are working feverishly to develop a vaccine, the report faults HHS for concentrating almost exclusively on biology. "Psychological and social factors, . . . the service needs of AIDS patients, and public education and prevention have not been considered funding priorities." Education efforts have been directed at professionals, "leaving education of high-risk groups largely up to the leadership of the groups themselves." The education part of the AIDS budget went up to 4 percent in fiscal 1985.

According to the report, former Assistant Secretary for Health Edward Brandt defended the PHS's "massive effort" against AIDS, and said that impediments to planning have been posed more by "the rapidly changing problem" than by inadequate resources. Brandt also expressed the view that "a concerted effort in public education or . . . psychosocial factors cannot take place" until the biomedical puzzle is solved.

Ethical, social, legal, and medical problems relating to AIDS are likely to become increasingly complex as the disease spreads beyond high-risk groups. Over 7000 cases have been reported so far, and the government predicts 40,000 more in the next 2 years.

Report

8 March 1985

81. Subcellular Localization of the Product of the Long Open Reading Frame of Human T-Cell Leukemia Virus Type I

Wei Chun Goh, Joseph Sodroski, Craig Rosen, Max Essex, and William A. Haseltine

Human T-cell leukemia virus type I (HTLV-I) is a retrovirus that is thought to be the etiologic agent of adult T-cell leukemia-lymphoma (ATLL) (*1, 2*). Infection with HTLV-I results in a low incidence of ATLL after a long latent period. The mechanism of disease induction by HTLV-I differs from that of the chronic leukemia viruses (*3*), however, in that no specific chromosomal sites of proviral integration have been detected in HTLV-I–induced tumors (*4*). Moreover, HTLV-I transforms primary cells in culture (*5*), heretofore a property associated only with the acute retroviruses that contain oncogenes derived from the host cell. HTLV-I does not appear to contain an oncogene, because its genome lacks sequences that are similar to conserved cellular genes (*6*). The genomes of HTLV-I and of the related virus HTLV-II contain long open reading frames (LOR) located between the envelope gene and the 3' long terminal repeat (LTR). The LOR region encodes proteins of 42 kilodaltons (kD) (HTLV-I) and 38 kD (HTLV-II) (*6, 7, 8*). This raises the possibility that the product of the LOR region mediates both the transforming activity of these viruses and *trans*-acting transcriptional activation of the viral LTR evident in HTLV-I–infected cells (*9*). To obtain insight into the possible mechanism whereby the LOR product might exert these effects, we characterized the intracellular location of the 42-kD LOR product of HTLV-I.

The lymphocyte cell lines used for this work were HUT 102, a virus-producing line established from a patient with adult T-cell leukemia (*1, 10*), and C81-66-45, a T-cell line derived by fusion of primary umbilical cord blood cells with HUT 102 (*11*). The virus-encoded proteins present in HUT 102 cells include the *gag* gene products (phosphoprotein 19, p24, p15, and p55), and *env* gene products (glycoproteins gp61, gp45, and gp21) (*12, 13*) as well as a 42-kD protein recently demonstrated to be encoded by the LOR region of this genome (Fig. 1) (*7*). Previous studies have shown that the 42-kD protein is neither a phospho- nor a glycoprotein and cannot be iodinated by treatment of the intact cells with lactoperoxidase (*7, 13*). The 42-kD LOR protein is recognized by serum from some ATLL patients and by serum from some infected but asymptomatic HTLV-I carriers (*7, 13*). The C81-66-45 cell line does not produce virus, and the only viral protein detected by serum from ATLL patients in this cell line is the 42-kD LOR product (*7*).

To identify the subcellular location of the HTLV-I LOR region product, we labeled cells of both lines with [^{35}S]cysteine and then separated them into nuclear and membrane-cytoplasmic fractions by treatment with a nonionic detergent in the presence of an iso-osmotic solution under conditions that stabilize the nuclear membrane (*14*). The nuclei were then separated from the other cellular components by differential centrifugation. The membrane-cytoplasmic fraction was further cleared of insoluble material by a high-speed centrifugation.

The nuclear fraction appeared to be free of intact cells under microscopic inspection. Assays for the lysosomal enzyme β-*N*-acetylglucosaminidase (*15*), which provides an independent biochemical marker for cytoplasmic contamination of the nuclear fraction, indicated that only about 7 percent of the total cellular activity of the enzyme was in the nuclear fraction. Moreover, the nuclei remained intact, as most of the DNA is retained in the nuclear fraction as dem-

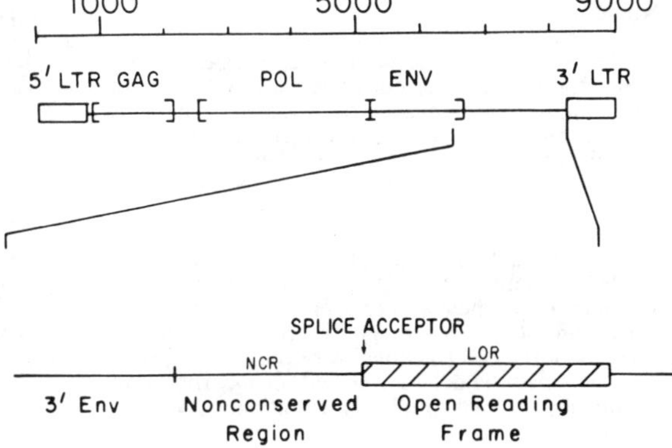

Fig. 1. Open reading frame (LOR) in the 3′ region of the HTLV genome. The positions of the nonconserved region between HTLV-I and HTLV-II and the single open reading frame encoding the p42 LOR product are shown. The splice acceptor site used in production of the LOR message is indicated (*8*).

onstrated by the fractionation of cells labeled with [³H]thymidine (Table 1).

The location of the 42-kD protein in the cell fractions was determined by immunoprecipitation of the labeled proteins with serum from an ATLL patient. This serum had previously been shown to react strongly with the 42-kD protein as well as with HTLV-I *gag* and *env* gene products (7, 13). All three fractions, nuclear, membrane-cytoplasmic (S-100), and the resuspended pellet of the S-100 fraction (P-100) were tested.

The reactivity of the ATLL patient serum for the unfractionated HUT 102 and C81-66-45 cells is compared to that of normal human serum in Fig. 2. The 42-kD LOR protein was evident in both immunoprecipitates. When the different fractions were tested separately, a significant amount of the 42-kD LOR protein was found in the nuclear fraction of both HUT 102 and C81-66-45 cells. By con-

trast, the p24 and p55 *gag* products as well as the gp61 and gp45 *env* gene products were totally absent from the nuclear preparations (Fig. 2), providing further evidence of the lack of cytoplasmic or outer membrane contamination in the nuclear fraction. These viral proteins are known to be present in the cell membrane (gp61 and gp45) and the cytosol (p55, p24) (12, 13). Negligible amounts of viral proteins were detected in the P-100 fractions. Densitometric tracing of the autoradiograms of the immunoprecipitated protein in the subcellular fractions showed that between 50 and 60 percent of the 42-kD LOR protein was present in the nuclear fraction of both the HUT 102 and C81-66-45 cell lines. The actual fraction of the 42-kD protein present in the nucleus is likely to be higher because some of it may have been lost from the nuclei during the isolation procedure.

From these data we conclude that a significant fraction of the 42 kD protein is located within the nucleus of HTLV–I-transformed lymphocytes. The results also suggest that a fraction of the 42-kD protein is located outside the nucleus. Such nuclear localization of a retrovirus-coded protein, other than those proteins encoded by cell-derived oncogenes including the *myc, fos* and *myb* (16), has not, to our knowledge, been reported previously. The product of the HTLV-I LOR region has been implicated in the transcriptional regulation of the LTR, as well as in mediation of cell transformation by this virus, for example, in the immortalization of primary lymphocytes in vitro (6, 9, 17). It has been suggested that the HTLV LOR region product might exert these effects by way of sequence-specific transcriptional regulation of both viral LTR and host cellular

Table 1. Assays for β-*N*-acetylglucosaminidase in subcellular fractions and incorporation of [³H]thymidine.

Fraction	Activity of β-*N*-acetyl-glucos-aminidase* (%)	[³H] Thymidine incorporation† (%)
S-100	93	4
Nuclear	7	96

*Cells were fractionated with buffer A as described in Fig. 2, sonicated and centrifuged at 10,000 rev/min for 10 minutes to remove debris. Lysates from the S-100 and nuclear fractions were incubated in 0.1*M* sodium citrate buffer (*p*H 4.5), 0.16 percent Triton X-100, and 1 m*M* *p*-nitrophenol-β-*N*-acetylglucosaminide for 60 minutes at 37°C. Reactions were stopped by the addition of sodium carbonate buffer and the optical densities at 420 nm were determined. †Cells were labeled with [³H]thymidine at 1 μCi/ml for 16 hours, washed with phosphate-buffered saline thrice, and fractionated as described in Fig. 2. Portions of the cell fractions were precipitated with cold trichloracetic acid and tested for incorporation of radioactivity by scintillation counting.

Fig. 2. Subcelluar localization of the p42 LOR product. HUT 102 and C81-66-45 cells were labeled with [^{35}S]cysteine for 12 hours in RPMI 1640 medium containing 20 percent fetal calf serum. Cells were washed twice with cold phosphate-buffered saline and resuspended (5×10^7 cells per milliliter) in buffer A [10 mM tris-Cl, pH 8.5, 0.25M sucrose, 3.7 mM CaCl$_2$, 12 mM MgCl$_2$, 1 mM phenyl-methylsulfonyl fluoride (PMSF), and 1 percent NP40].

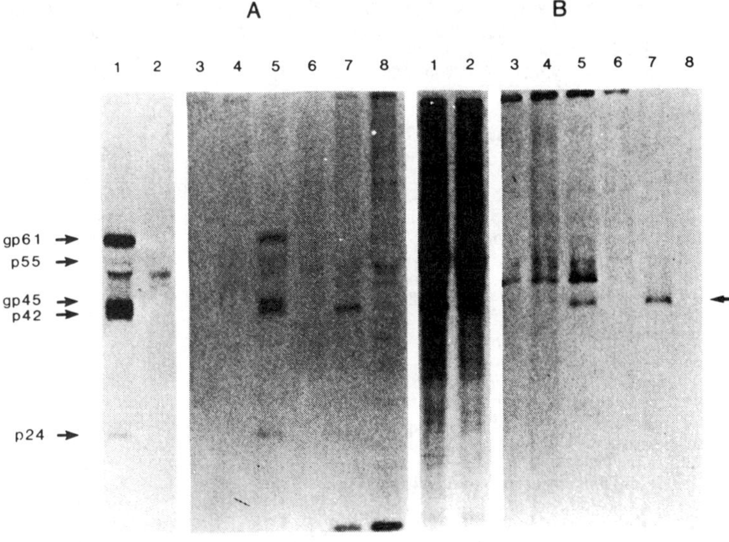

The cells were incubated for 20 minutes on ice and pipetted up and down gently. A portion was removed for microscopic analysis. Nuclei were centrifuged at 600g for 5 minutes at 4°C and washed once with buffer A. The supernatant, termed the S-100 fraction, was further centrifuged at 100,000g. Pelleted debris was called the P-100 fraction. The nuclear and P-100 fractions were resuspended in RIPA lysis buffer (0.15M NaCl, 0.05M tris-HCl, pH 7.2, 1 percent Triton X-100, 1 percent sodium deoxycholate, and 0.1 percent sodium dodecyl sulfate) while the S-100 fraction was adjusted to 1 percent Triton X-100. (A and B) Immunoprecipitations of HUT 102 and C81-66-45 cells, respectively. The amount of the cell fraction used for the immunoprecipitation corresponds to the amount derived from equivalent cell numbers in each experiment. Lanes 1 and 2, total unfractionated cell lysates; lanes 3 and 4, the P-100 fractions, lanes 5 and 6, the S-100 fractions; lanes 7 and 8, the nuclear fractions. Serum samples from ATLL patients (lanes 1, 3, 5, and 7) and normal subjects (lanes 2, 4, 6, and 8) that were described previously (7, 13) were used.

genes (9). The nuclear location of the 42-kD HTLV-I LOR product is consistent with these roles. We note that the transforming proteins of some DNA tumor viruses, which also exert transcriptional regulatory effects, are also located within the nucleus (18).

References and Notes

1. B. J. Poiesz *et al.*, *Proc. Natl. Acad. Sci. U.S.A.* **77**, 7415 (1980).
2. R. C. Gallo, in *Human T-cell Leukemia Viruses*, R. C. Gallo, M. E. Essex, L. Gross, Eds. (Cold Spring Harbor Laboratory, Cold Spring Harbor, N.Y., 1984); B. J. Poiesz, F. W. Ruscetti, M. S. Reitz, V. S. Kalyanaraman, R. C. Gallo, *Nature (London)* **294**, 268 (1981); Y. Hinuma *et al.*, *Proc. Natl. Acad. Sci. U.S.A.* **78**, 6476 (1981); M. Yoshida, I. Miyoshi, Y. Hinuma, *ibid.* **79**, 2031 (1982); M. Popovic *et al.*, *Nature (London)* **300**, 63 (1982); W. A. Blattner *et al.*, *Int. J. Cancer* **30**, 257 (1982); M. S. Robert-Guroff *et al.*, *J. Exp. Med.* **157**, 248 (1983); P. S. Sarin *et al.*, *Proc. Natl. Acad. Sci. U.S.A.* **80**, 2370 (1983); M. Essex *et al.*, *Science* **221**, 1061 (1983); M. Essex, *J. Nat. Cancer Inst.* **69**, 981 (1982); B. F. Haynes *et al.*, *Proc. Natl. Acad. Sci. U.S.A.* **80**, 2054 (1983); D. Slater, S. Bleeken, N. Rooney, A. Hamed, *Br. J. Dermatol.* **109**, 120 (1983).
3. W. S. Hayward, B. G. Neel, S. M. Astrin, *Nature (London)* **290**, 475 (1981); G. S. Payne, J. M. Bishop, H. E. Varmus, *ibid.* **295**, 209 (1982); Y. T. Fung, W. G. Lewis, L. B. Crittenden, H. J. Kung, *Cell* **33**, 357 (1983); P. N. Tsichlis, P. G. Strauss, L. F. Hu, *Nature (London)* **302**, 445 (1983); R. N. A. van Ooyen, D. Cox, Y. K. T. Fung, H. Varmus, *ibid.* **307**, 131 (1984); L. M. Corcoran, J. M. Adams, A. R. Dunn, S. Cory,

Cell **37**, 113 (1984); D. Steffen, *Proc. Natl. Acad. Sci. U.S.A.* **81**, 2097 (1984); H. T. Cuypers *et al.*, *Cell* **37**, 141 (1984).
4. B. Hahn *et al.*, *Nature (London)* **305**, 340 (1983); M. Seiki, R. Eddy, T. B. Shows, M. Yoshida, *ibid.* **309**, 640 (1984).
5. I. Miyoshi *et al.*, *ibid.* **294**, 770 (1981); N. Yamamoto, M. Okada, Y. Koyanagi, M. Kannagi, Y. Hinuma, *Science* **217**, 737 (1982); M. Popovic *et al.*, *ibid.* **219**, 856 (1983); M. Popovic, G. Lange-Wartzin, P. S. Sarin, D. Mann, R. C. Gallo, *Proc. Natl. Acad. Sci. U.S.A.* **80**, 5402 (1983).
6. M. Seiki, S. Hattori, Y. Hirayama, M. Yoshida, *Proc. Natl. Acad. Sci. U.S.A.* **80**, 3618 (1983); W. A. Haseltine *et al.*, *Science* **225**, 419 (1984).
7. T. H. Lee *et al.*, *Science* **226**, 57 (1984); D. J. Slamon, K. Shimotohno, M. J. Cline, D. W. Golde, I. S. Y. Chen, *ibid.*, p. 61.
8. W. Wachsman, K. Shimotohno, S. C. Clark, D. W. Golde, I. S. Y. Chen, *ibid.*, p. 177.
9. J. Sodroski, C. Rosen, W. A. Haseltine, *ibid.* **225**, 381 (1984).
10. A. F. Gazdar *et al.*, *Blood* **55**, 409 (1980).
11. S. Z. Salahuddin *et al.*, *Virology* **129**, 51 (1983).
12. V. S. Kalyanaraman, M. G. Sarngadharan, B. J. Poiesz, F. W. Ruscetti, R. C. Gallo, *J. Virol.* **38**, 906 (1981); M. Robert-Guroff, F. W. Ruscetti, L. E. Posner, B. J. Poiesz, R. C. Gallo, *J. Exp. Med.* **154**, 1957 (1981); M. Robert-Guroff *et al.*, *Virology* **122**, 297 (1982); S. Oroszlan *et al.*, *Proc. Natl. Acad. Sci. U.S.A.* **79**, 1291 (1982); V. S. Kalyanaraman, M. Jarvis-Morar, M. G. Sarngadharan, R. C. Gallo, *Virology* **132**, 61 (1984); T. H. Lee *et al.*, in *Human T-cell Leukemia Viruses*, R. C. Gallo, M. E. Essex, L. Gross, Eds. (Cold Spring Harbor Laboratory, Cold Spring Harbor, N.Y., 1984), p. 111.
13. T. H. Lee *et al.*, *Proc. Natl. Acad. Sci. U.S.A.* **81**, 3856 (1984); T. H. Lee and M. Essex, unpublished observations; T. H. Lee *et al.*, *Proc. Natl. Acad. Sci. U.S.A.*, in press.
14. V. G. Allfrey, *Methods Enzymol.* **31**, 246 (1974); G. M. Lawson *et al.*, in *Laboratory Methods Manual for Hormone Action and Molecular Endocrinology*, W. T. Schroder and B. W. O'Malley, Eds. (Houston Biological Associates, ed. 5, 1981).
15. A. J. Barrett and M. F. Health, *Lysosomal Enzymes in Lysosomes: A Laboratory Handbook*, J. T. Dingle Ed. (Elsevier/North-Holland, ed. 2, 1977), pp. 19–145.
16. P. Donner, I. Greiser-Wilke, K. Moelling, *Nature (London)* **296**, 262 (1982); H. D. Abrams, L. R. Rohrschneider, R. N. Eisenman, *Cell* **29**, 427 (1982); H. Persson and P. Leder, *Science* **225**, 718 (1984); T. Curran, A. D. Miller, L. Zokas, I. M. Verma, *Cell* **36**, 259 (1984); W. J. Boyle, M. A. Lampert, J. S. Lipsick, M. A. Baluda, *Proc. Natl. Acad. Sci. U.S.A.* **81**, 4265 (1984); K. H. Klempnauer, G. Symonds, G. I. Evan, J. M. Bishop, *Cell* **37**, 537 (1984); P. Donner, T. Bunte, I. Greiser-Wilke, K. Moelling, *Proc. Natl. Acad. Sci. U.S.A.* **80**, 2861 (1983).
17. M. Seiki, S. Hattori, Y. Hirayama, M. Yoshida, *Nature (London)* **309**, 640 (1984).
18. J. H. Pope and W. P. Rowe, *J. Exp. Med.* **120**, 121 (1964); D. Kalderon, W. D. Richardson, A. F. Markham, A. E. Smith *Nature (London)* **311**, 33 (1984); L. T. Feldman, J. R. Nevins, *Mol. Cellular Biol.* **3**, 829 (1983); M. Green, K. H. Brackerman, M. A. Cartas, T. Matsuo, *Virology* **42**, 30 (1982); L. A. Lucher *et al.*, *ibid.* **52**, 136 (1984).
19. We thank F. Barin for advice, S. Cook, D. Helland, T. Jorgensen, R. Van Buskirk, R. Crowther, W. Franklin, D. Celander, and R. Ruprecht for discussions; Z. Salahuddin, M. F. McLane, F. Wong-Staal, and R. C. Gallo for providing cell lines and materials; and D. Artz for help in preparing the manuscript. W.C.G. is supported by NIH grant CA09361 and J.S. and C.R. were supported by NIH fellowships CA07094 and CA07580, respectively. This work was supported by a Directors Grant from the American Cancer Society and by NIH grant CA36974.

7 November 1984; accepted 18 December 1984

Report

15 March 1985

82. Suppression of Gamma Interferon Production by Inactivated Feline Leukemia Virus

R.W. Engelman, R.W. Fulton, R.A. Good, and N.K. Day

Feline leukemia virus (FeLV), a contagious retrovirus transmitted primarily through salivary secretions, causes neoplastic or nonneoplastic diseases in the infected cat, including a state of immunodeficiency characterized by diminution of cellular and humoral immunity. Retrovirus-induced immunosuppression, the most frequent sequela of persistent FeLV viremia, predisposes the animal to secondary illness of infectious or autoimmune origin and accounts for most FeLV-related deaths (*1*). Viremic cats have suppressed blastogenic responses to T-cell mitogens, reduced mobility of lymphocyte membrane concanavalin A (Con A) receptors, suppressed antibody responses to synthetic polypeptides, prolonged allograft rejection times, and various degrees of hypocomplementemia, thymic atrophy, and depletion of the paracortical zones of lymph nodes (*2*). In addition, peripheral blood and splenic lymphocytes from FeLV-infected cats, when stimulated with T-cell mitogens, cannot be induced to produce interferon, or when induced produce only low titers thereof (*3*). Although little is known about how FeLV initiates immunosuppression, the virus may mediate immunomodulating events independent of cellular infection, since FeLV inactivated by ultraviolet light and certain FeLV structural proteins have been

shown to impair lymphocyte proliferative responses and membrane receptor capping to Con A in vitro (*4*). This inability of lymphocytes to respond to mitogenic stimuli during incubation with inactivated virus may be due to decreased elaboration of T-cell growth factor (possibly interleukin-2) activity (*5*). We report here that the synthesis in vitro of a gamma-like interferon by normal feline lymphocytes that have been stimulated with *Staphylococcus* enterotoxin A (SEA) is reduced when ultraviolet-inactivated FeLV is also present in culture during the period of stimulation.

Seven healthy, FeLV-free domestic cats maintained in our laboratory served as donors of peripheral blood lymphocytes. The cells were isolated from defibrinated whole blood by Ficoll-Hypaque density centrifugation. Cell viabilities were determined by vital dye exclusion. Lymphocytes (5×10^6 per milliliter) in RMPI 1640 medium supplemented with 10 percent fetal calf serum, antibiotics, antimycotics (Gibco), and $5 \times 10^{-5}M$ 2-mercaptoethanol (Eastman Kodak) were placed in flat-bottom microplate wells (16 mm in diameter). The cells were cultured in the absence of mitogen, in the presence of SEA (1.0 μg/ml; Microbial Biochemistry Branch, Division of Microbiology, Food and Drug Administration, Cincinnati), or with SEA (1.0 μg/ml) plus

Table 1. Titer of interferon-generated (units per milliliter) and viability of peripheral blood lymphocytes after 72 hours of culture. N.D., not done.

Cat	Number of experiments	No mitogen	SEA (1.0 µ/ml)							
				UV-inactivated FeLV (µg/ml)						
				625	400	300	200	100	50	10
301	2	<10	214	N.D.	19	52	61	134	150	196
249	3	<10	168	N.D.	39	67	124	150	141	378
1225	2	<10	47	<10	<10	<10	17	N.D.	N.D.	25
1264	2	<10	200	N.D.	39	43	99	112	83	N.D.
302	2	<10	289	N.D.	35	125	44	119	150	130
248	4	367	768	N.D.	409	89	734	980	875	815
000	2	<10	287	<10	N.D.	N.D.	160	367	N.D.	N.D.
				Viability after culture						
Samples tested		15	28	N.D.	14	11	13	11	6	8
Viability (percent*)		90 ± 10	93 ± 4	N.D.	86 ± 11	90 ± 6	89 ± 6	92 ± 7	95 ± 2	96 ± 2

*Mean ± standard error.

ultraviolet-inactivated KT-FeLV. The KT-FeLV was purified and ultraviolet-inactivated (4). Final culture volume in all cases was 1.0 ml. Microplates were placed in culture boxes, incubated at 37°C in a humidified atmosphere containing 10 percent CO_2, and rocked for 72 hours at eight cycles per minute. Cultures were then harvested, cells were pelleted by slow centrifugation, and supernatants were collected and stored at 4°C. The antiviral activity of supernatant fluids from these cultures were titrated for ability to inhibit the cytopathic effects of approximately 40 plaque-forming units of vesicular stomatitis virus (VSV) on a monolayer of feline lung (FL) cells (American Type Culture Collection, Rockville, Maryland) by means of a plaque reduction method (6). All titrations were carried out in duplicate. Interferon (units per milliliter) was measured as the reciprocal of the dilution that reduced the number of plaque-forming units by 50 percent. A reference sample of feline interferon (162 U/ml) was used to monitor the assays.

To determine whether the inactivated FeLV suppressed mitogen-induced proliferation of lymphocytes, four separate lymphocyte blastogenesis assays were performed by a method previously reported (4), except that Con A (2.5 to 10.0 μg per well) or SEA (0.05 to 0.5 μg per well) served as mitogens and 18.75 μg of inactivated FeLV was used in the test wells. Under these conditions the amount of inactivated virus per lymphocyte was 18×10^{-5} μg per cell and the residual proliferative response, as determined by measuring the incorporation of tritiated thymidine, ranged from 22.4 to 78.5 percent, which is comparable to reported values.

Two, three, or four separate culture series were established with lymphocytes from each of the seven cats. Table 1 shows induced antiviral activity of the supernatant as an average of two to four determinations. A value of <10 U/ml denotes an undetectable interferon level. Supernatant from wells containing only lymphocytes and complete medium had no antiviral activity (except for two of the four cultures of cells from cat 248). Cultures containing SEA-stimulated lymphocytes produced interferon at between 47 and 768 U/ml. When 625 μg of inactivated FeLV was incubated with SEA in lymphocyte cultures, the supernatant showed no antiviral effect. With the addition of 400 μg of virus to SEA-stimulated lymphocyte cultures, the induced antiviral activity of the supernatant was markedly reduced compared to the positive control. Under these conditions there was 8×10^{-5} μg of virus per lymphocyte and the residual antiviral activity ranged from 8.8 to 53.2 percent. With further dilution of the virus the induced antiviral activity of the supernatant increased. In some cases, when small amounts of inactivated FeLV were incorporated in cultures the resultant antiviral effect exceeded that in the positive control (cats 249 and 248).

To characterize the antiviral activity of the supernatant, we conducted separate tests in which they were dialyzed at pH 2, heat-treated at 56°C for 30 minutes, or subjected to ultracentrifugation (110,000g for 90 minutes). No antiviral activity remained in samples dialyzed at pH 2 or subjected to heat, while ultracentrifugation did not reduce the antiviral effect (Table 2). Supernatants that effected plaque reduction when VSV was used as the challenge virus also

Table 2. Characterization of the antiviral activity of culture supernatants as a gamma-like interferon (units per milliliter).

Treatment	Cat					
	248	249	1264	1276	301	302
pH						
*p*H 7.2	767	339	246			
*p*H 2	<10	<10	<10			
Heat						
Control			246	44		
56°C (30 minutes)			<10	<10		
Activity against other viruses						
VSV					150	
FCV					267	
FHV-1					<10	
Heterologous cells						
FL					150	200
MDBK					<10	<10

demonstrated this protective antiviral effect when feline calicivirus (FCV, clone F-9) was substituted as the challenge virus, showing that the antiviral substance effectively inhibited the replication of other viruses. Feline herpesvirus type 1 (FHV-1, clone C27) was insensitive to any antiviral activity in any of the tested supernatants. Variation in the sensitivity of different viruses to interferon has been described (7). Samples with antiviral activity in FL cell monolayers showed no activity in a heterologous system of interferon assay with Madin-Darby bovine kidney (MDBK) cell monolayers (American Type Culture Collection) and VSV as a challenge virus. These findings indicate that the antiviral effect of treating FL cell monolayers with supernatants from cultures containing SEA-stimulated lymphocytes was attributable to an interferon. This interferon was a gamma-like (immune) interferon on the basis of its susceptibility to *p*H 2.

The reduction in interferon production in lymphocyte cultures where cells were incubated with virus and SEA was not solely attributable to a reduction in the number of viable lymphocytes. By resuspending individual cell pellets in 1.0 ml of complete medium after harvesting the supernatants, we determined mean viability after 72 hours of incubation in 106 cultures from three experiments involving four cats (Table 1). Lymphocyte viabilities after culture differed only slightly, regardless of the culture conditions.

To show that the addition of virus did not neutralize the mitogenic properties of SEA, we incubated inactivated FeLV (1250 µg) and SEA (50 µg) together at 37°C for 18 hours in 4.0 ml of complete medium. The virus was then removed by ultracentrifugation (100,000*g* for 90 minutes). The remaining SEA-containing supernatant, used in place of stock SEA for the stimulation of lymphocytes, induced comparable interferon titers when compared to stock SEA (Table 3). To determine whether interferon was produced but subsequently neutralized by the presence of inactivated virus, 400 μg of FeLV was added to SEA-stimulated lymphocyte cultures for the final 2 hours of incubation. Subsequent testing of these supernatants did not show any reduction in antiviral activity (Table 3), suggesting that the FeLV-induced impairment of antiviral activity was a result of reduced interferon synthesis and not reduced effectiveness caused by the presence of FeLV.

The reduction in interferon synthesis mediated by FeLV in vitro may reflect clinically relevant impairment of lymphocyte function in cats persistently infected with FeLV. Gamma interferon appears to occupy a pivotal regulatory position in cellular immune responses, enhances antimicrobial activity of human macrophages, and augments cytotoxic and natural killer cell activities and the expression of interleukin-2 receptors on T cells (8). Deficient synthesis of this lymphokine may play a role in the pathogenesis of immunodeficiency in FeLV-infected cats. This finding is especially provocative in light of the proposed retroviral [human T-cell leukemia (lymphotropic) virus type 3] etiology of the acquired immune deficiency syndrome (AIDS) in humans (9). A recent study of 16 patients with AIDS who had opportunistic infections showed that mononuclear cells from 11 produced subnormal amounts of gamma interferon in response to a mitogen (10). Although this subnormal synthesis of interferon may reflect a quantitative deficiency in the T cells responsible for interferon synthesis, impaired interferon synthesis in the 11 patients and substantial synthesis in the other five cannot be attributed with assurance to alterations in lymphocyte

Table 3. Failure of FeLV to alter the mitogenic properties of SEA or the antiviral activity of SEA-stimulated lymphocyte supernatants. Values are interferon titers (units per milliliter).

Treatment	Cat		
	1276	249	301
Treatment of SEA			
Stock SEA	550	150	
SEA after incubation with FeLV	727	139	
Treatment of culture supernatant			
None			123, 150, 138
FeLV (400 μg)			80, 150, 143

numbers. In addition to or independent of a reduction in the number of interferon-synthesizing cells, the presence of immunosuppressive quantities of retrovirus at the cellular level may markedly impair synthesis of interferon and perhaps other lymphokines in vivo. The immunologic amplification attributable to these mediators would then be significantly reduced, resulting in a diminution of functional immunity and increased susceptibility to serious secondary illness.

References and Notes

1. W. D. Hardy, in *Feline Leukemia Virus*, W. D. Hardy, M. Essex, A. J. McClelland, Eds. (Elsevier/North-Holland, New York, 1980), pp. 3–31; *Springer Semin. Immunopathol.* **5**, 75 (1982).
2. G. L. Cockerell, E. A. Hoover, S. Krakowka, R. G. Olsen, D. S. Yohn, *J. Natl. Cancer Inst.* **57**, 1095 (1976); J. E. Dunlap, W. S. Nichols, L. C. Hebebrand, L. E. Mathes, R. G. Olsen, *Cancer Res.* **39**, 956 (1979); Z. Trainin, D. Wernicke, H. Ungar-Waron, M. Essex, *Science* **220**, 858 (1983); R. G. Olsen, L. E. Mathes, S. W. Nichols, in *Feline Leukemia*, R. G. Olsen, Ed. (CRC Press, Boca Raton, Fla., 1981), pp. 149–165; L. Kobilinsky, W. D. Hardy, N. K. Day, *J. Immunol.* **122**, 2139 (1979).
3. W. T. Liu, R. A. Good, L. Q. Trang, R. W. Engelman, N. K. Day, *Proc. Natl. Acad. Sci. U.S.A.* **81**, 6471 (1984).
4. L. C. Hebebrand, L. E. Mathes, R. G. Olsen, *Cancer Res.* **37**, 4532 (1977); L. E. Mathes *et al.*, *ibid.* **39**, 950 (1979).

5. M. A. Wainberg, S. Vydelingum, R. G. Margolese, *J. Immunol.* **130**, 2372 (1983).
6. W. E. Stewart, in *The Interferon System* (Springer-Verlag, New York, 1981), pp. 13–26.
7. S. Pestka and S. Baron, *Methods Enzymol.* **78**, 3 (1981); R. W. Fulton, D. Y. Cho, M. Downing, N. J. Pearson, R. H. Cane, *Vet. Rec.* **107**, 479 (1980).
8. C. F. Nathan, H. W. Murray, M. E. Wiebe, B. Y. Rubin, *J. Exp. Med.* **158**, 670 (1983); H. M. Johnson and W. L. Farrar, *Cell Immunol.* **75**, 154 (1983); I. Kawase *et al.*, *J. Immunol.* **131**, 288 (1983).
9. M. Popovic, M. G. Sarngadharan, E. Read, R. C. Gallo, *Science* **224**, 497 (1984); R. C. Gallo *et al.*, *ibid.*, p. 500; J. Schupbach *et al.*, *ibid.*, p. 503; H. W. Jaffe *et al.*, *ibid.* **223**, 1309 (1984); J. L. Marx, *ibid.* **224**, 475 (1984).
10. H. W. Murray, B. Y. Rubin, H. Masur, R. B. Roberts, *N. Engl. J. Med.* **310**, 883 (1984).
11. We thank R. G. Olsen and L. E. Mathes for kindly providing the KT-FeLV preparation, L. Q. Trang and L. Burge for technical assistance, and K. Deatherage for preparing the manuscript. Aided by grants awarded by the American Cancer Society (IM-298) and the National Institutes of Health (CA-34103 and CA-31547). This report represents a portion of R.W.E.'s Ph.D. thesis.

26 September 1984; accepted 3 December 1984

83. A Virus by Any Other Name . . .

Jean L. Marx

If any doubt remained, it has now been resolved. Comparison of the genetic material of the viruses that have been isolated and linked to AIDS (acquired immune deficiency syndrome) shows that they are, as expected, variants of the same virus. They are not identical, however, and the differences could affect efforts to develop a vaccine to protect against the disease and also the reliability of the newly developed AIDS tests.

Another issue that has been emphasized by the availability of the sequence data concerns the naming of the AIDS virus. This may be of less practical interest than vaccine development but is nonetheless proving to be a bone of contention.

Currently there are no less than three names for the virus. Luc Montagnier and his colleagues at the Pasteur Institute in Paris call it lymphadenopathy-associated virus (LAV) because they originally isolated it from an individual with lymphadenopathy, a condition characterized by swollen lymph nodes and fever that may be a mild or early form of AIDS. Robert Gallo and his colleagues at the National Cancer Institute (NCI) designated the virus they isolated as human T-cell lymphotropic virus-III (HTLV-III) because they found it to resemble HTLV-I and -II, which cause leukemias or lymphomas in humans. And finally, Jay Levy and his colleagues at the University of California in San Francisco simply called their isolate AIDS-associated retrovirus (ARV). (Retroviruses have RNA as their genetic material and their life cycle includes a step in which the RNA is copied into DNA.)

Although the Pasteur group now prefers the LAV designation, in their original report of the isolation of the virus, which appeared in the 20 May 1983 issue of *Science*, they referred to it as a new member of the HTLV family. They had detected in the patient from whom the virus was isolated antibodies that appeared to react with HTLV-I proteins, a result indicating that HTLV-I and the new viral isolate might be related.

This result turned out to be an artifact, Montagnier says. On further study, he and his colleagues could find no similarity between proteins from HTLV-I and the new virus and concluded that the two viruses were not related after all. The Pasteur group began using the LAV designation in September 1983 when they presented their data at a Cold Spring Harbor meeting on the "Human T-Cell Leukemia/Lymphoma Virus." By then they had obtained three additional isolates, this time from patients with full-blown AIDS, and gave them the designation "immune deficiency–associated virus" (IDAV). According to Montagnier, the designations LAV and IDAV were chosen because the link to AIDS had not yet been firmly established.

For a time at least, Gallo and his colleagues appeared to be following a false trail. In the same *Science* issue in which the Pasteur group described their first LAV isolate, the NCI workers reported a possible connection between AIDS and HTLV-I itself. Gallo had suspected that there might be such a link because HTLV-I and the then still mysterious AIDS agent seemed to be transmitted in a similar manner and they both preferentially infected the same kind of T cell.

By the time these reports were published, however, the NCI workers were being tantalized by indications that T cells from many AIDS patients carried another virus, one which was proving hard to grow in cultured cells, a problem

that was also hindering the Pasteur workers in their studies of LAV/IDAV.

The Gallo group solved the problem first, publishing in the 4 May 1984 issue of *Science* a series of four papers dealing with the propagation and characterization of the virus, which they designated HTLV-III, and presenting strong evidence for a link between it and AIDS. Levy subsequently published his report of the isolation of ARV in the 24 August 1984 *Science*. By the end of 1984 the work from both sides of the Atlantic had coalesced to the point where there seemed to be little doubt that the investigators were all studying the same virus, a conclusion now confirmed by the sequence comparisons.

They show that LAV and HTLV-III differ in only 1.5 percent of their nucleotides (*1, 2*). The proteins they encode would be identical in about 98 percent of their amino acids. The ARV genome shows more variation, diverging in about 6 percent of its nucleotides from the LAV and HTLV-III genomes and encoding proteins that would be about 90 percent identical to those of the other two viruses. Nevertheless, all the viruses are similar enough to be considered variants of the same virus.

The nucleotide differences are not evenly distributed across the viral genomes. They appear to be concentrated in the *env* gene, which codes for the major protein on the exterior of the viral particle. According to Levy, the *env* genes of ARV and HTLV-III differ by more than 20 percent. In addition, the Gallo group has sequenced another HTLV-III isolate and finds that it differs from the first by about as much as ARV does. The greatest divergence is again in the major exterior protein, according to Flossie Wong-Staal of NCI.

This concentration of differences in the *env* gene may complicate the development of an AIDS vaccine. The envelope protein is the likely target of the protective antibodies that would be generated by a vaccine. If the protein varies too much from one virus to the next, a single vaccine might not be able to confer immunity to all strains.

Moreover, the variability that is now being picked up may indicate that the *env* gene of the AIDS virus is particularly susceptible to mutation, much as are the genes for certain of the influenza virus proteins. In that event, a vaccine might be effective to begin with, but then cease to protect as the virus changed. One question the investigators now want to answer is whether there are conserved sequences in the envelope protein that do not show the variations. If there are and if they prove to be antigenic, then it might be possible to design a vaccine that will raise antibodies specifically directed against those portions of the protein.

Variation in the *env* gene might also affect the reliability of diagnostic tests for the presence of the AIDS agent. These currently use viral proteins to identify antibodies to the virus in blood samples from infected individuals. The antibodies might escape detection if they were elicited by a viral strain that differed significantly in its proteins from the one used to make the test reagents.

The tests recently approved for use by the Food and Drug Administration miss roughly 5 percent of the individuals who have been infected by the AIDS virus. Preliminary results suggest, Wong-Staal says, that these false negatives are not caused by viral differences but by a lack of immune response in the individual.

Needless to say, more work, including more sequence comparisons, will be required to determine the impact of the *env* gene variations on vaccine development and test reliability. The Gallo group is willing to give HTLV-III isolates or clones to researchers who wish to pursue these problems.

The continuing debate over the name of the AIDS virus centers around whether HTLV-III is still an appropriate designation. Gallo and his associates think that it is. Montagnier, Levy, and many others think that it is not. They note, for example, that the biological effects of HTLV-I and -II, which cause T-cell proliferation, are the opposite of the effects of the AIDS virus, which causes T-cell death. As Montagnier puts its, "HTLV-III and LAV are very different from HTLV-I and -II. HTLV-III is not a leukemia virus. I think there is a need for another name."

Nevertheless, Gallo maintains that the HTLV-III designation is appropriate for the AIDS virus, partly because it shares with HTLV-I and -II a strong preference for infecting T cells of the helper class. He points out that he has already changed the original meaning of HTLV from "human T-cell *leukemia* virus" to "human T-cell *lymphotropic* virus" in recognition of the cell-killing propensities of the AIDS agent.

Perhaps the best argument in favor of those who desire another name comes from the analysis of the gene sequences of the AIDS virus isolates, which have now been reported by four groups, including one from Chiron Research Laboratories in Emeryville, California, and another from Genentech, Inc., in San Francisco, in addition to the Gallo and Montagnier groups (*3–6*). All four groups, including that of Wong-Staal, Gallo, and their colleagues, find that the nucleotide sequences of the AIDS virus genomes show little resemblance to those of the HTLV-I and -II genomes, except for some short segments primarily in the *pol* gene, which codes for the viral enzyme that copies RNA into DNA. "The AIDS virus is no more closely related to HTLV-I and -II than to Rous sarcoma virus," says Chiron's Paul Luciw.

The organization of the protein-coding segments of the AIDS virus also differs from those of HTLV-I and -II. The AIDS virus has a short coding region (box A in the diagram) of as yet undefined function between the *pol* and *env* genes, which is not found in the HTLV's. Moreover, the HTLV's have a long region, designated pX, between the *env* genes and the right-hand long terminal repeats (LTR's). William Haseltine of Harvard's Dana-Farber Cancer Institute and the Gallo group have evidence that the right-hand half of pX, which they have called the LOR (for long open reading frame region), codes for a protein that activates gene expression and may be involved in the malignant transformation caused by HTLV-I and -II.

The AIDS virus genome does not have a comparable pX region, at least according to the Pasteur, Chiron, and Genentech workers, but has a shorter segment with protein-coding capabilities (box B) that extends into the LTR. This segment can encode a protein containing about 200 amino acids, which would make it considerably shorter than the LOR protein, which has a molecular weight of about 40,000.

Haseltine, Wong-Staal, and Gallo also have evidence that HTLV-III makes a

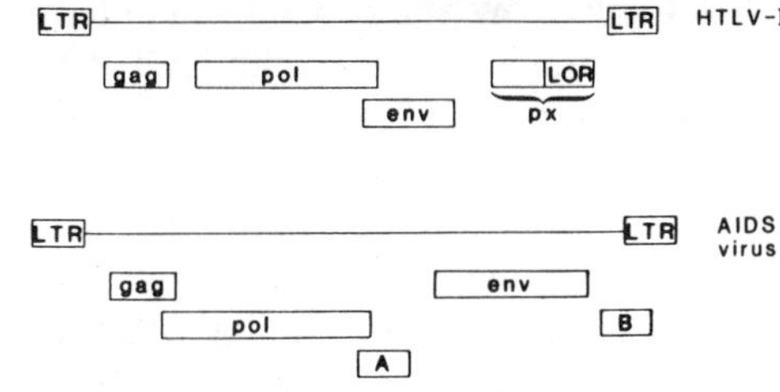

Genomic organization of HTLV-I and the AIDS virus.

protein analogous to the gene-activating LOR products of HTLV-I and -II. In fact, the possibility that all three viruses work by a similar mechanism, even though their final effects are different, is another reason why Gallo thinks that the HTLV-III designation should be maintained.

In any event, the Gallo and Haseltine groups have a different view of the gene organization at the right-hand end of the AIDS virus genome. They propose that the *env* and LOR segments are essentially fused in a single open reading frame that encodes both the envelope protein and the LOR product equivalent. Which of the two possible products will be produced depends on how the messenger RNA that is transcribed from the region is spliced, they suggest. However, according to Daniel Capon, the Genentech group's analysis of the splicing patterns of HTLV-III messenger RNA's does not support such an interpretation, but indicates instead that the open reading frame to the right of the *env* gene encodes a complete protein without *env* sequences. They nonetheless speculate that this protein might have a gene-activating function similar to that of the LOR products of HTLV-I and -II.

454

As things now stand, Gallo maintains his determination to keep the HTLV-III designation for the AIDS virus. "We never claimed that they [the viral gene sequences] had to be highly homologous." He suggests the possibility of combining names, using HTLV-III/LAV for isolates from Montagnier's laboratory or HTLV-III/ARV for Levy's isolates. This suggestion is unlikely to win many supporters.

Meanwhile, Montagnier proposes that the initials LAV be retained while changing the full name to lymphadenopathy/ AIDS virus, now that the connection to the immune deficiency syndrome has been established. "I think that we should keep the name originally given by us because we were the first to isolate it," he asserts. Gallo, incidentally, won the day in an earlier dispute over naming the leukemia viruses because the first HTLV was isolated in his laboratory. Finally, perhaps predictably, Levy is content with the name ARV.

If no one yields, the issue may have to be resolved by an international committee. Harold Varmus of the University of California School of Medicine in San Francisco is currently assembling such a committee in his role as chairman of the Retrovirus Study Group of the International Committee on the Taxonomy of Viruses. It would include some seven of the regular members of the study group, plus a half-dozen additional participants. Gallo, Montagnier, and Levy are among the proposed members. Varmus plans to solicit naming suggestions and then poll the membership for their preferences. A fourth name, unassociated with any particular group, may be the result.

There are apparently no hard and fast rules for determining viral relatedness. A variety of characteristics, including the size and shape of the viral particles, whether they have RNA or DNA as their genetic material, host range, and biological action, have been used. The ability to determine complete gene sequences, a skill which has been acquired relatively recently, adds a new consideration. According to Varmus, the same genetic principles that have been applied to defining species generally may be applicable to viruses. "Members of a virus 'species' would share genetic characteristics and allow genetic intermingling between members of the same 'species' while resisting the influx of information from other 'species,' " he explains.

Varmus expects that it will be sometime in June before the committee can come to a decision about the name of the AIDS virus. Whether it will be accepted remains to be seen. "These deliberations can be irrelevant to the way people behave," he points out. "Nothing we do is binding. If someone wants to ignore it, he can."

References

1. L. Ratner, R. C. Gallo, F. Wong-Staal, *Nature (London)* **313**, 636 (1985).
2. M. Alizon and L. Montagnier, *ibid.*, p. 743.
3. R. Sanchez-Pescador *et al.*, *Science* **227**, 484 (1985).
4. L. Ratner *et al.*, *Nature (London)* **313**, 277 (1985).
5. M. A. Muesing *et al.*, *ibid.*, p. 450.
6. S. Wain-Hobson *et al.*, *Cell* **40**, 9 (1985).

Report

22 March 1985

84. Bovine Leukemia Virus–Related Antigens in Lymphocyte Cultures Infected with AIDS-Associated Viruses

L. Thiry, S. Sprecher-Goldberger, P. Jacquemin, J. Cogniaux, A. Burny, C. Bruck, D. Portetelle, S. Cran, and N. Clumeck

Lymphadenopathy syndrome–associated retroviruses (LAV) have been isolated from patients with the acquired immune deficiency syndrome (AIDS) in France (*1*) and human T-cell leukemia viruses type III (HTLV-III) have been cultivated from AIDS patients in the United States (*2*). There appear to be no differences between the two groups of isolates and their major core proteins (p25) are identical by competitive radioimmunoassay (*3*). That AIDS in Central Africa is probably caused by similar viruses is indicated by studies in which an LAV-related virus was isolated from a Zairian married couple, one with AIDS and one with pre-AIDS (*4*), and antibodies to disrupted virions of LAV were found in most Zairian patients with AIDS (*5*).

We were thus surprised to find that lymphocytes cultivated from tissues of African patients with AIDS treated in Belgium (*6*) reacted with rabbit antiserum to purified antigens of bovine leukemia virus (BLV) when tested by a solid-phase radioimmunoassay. This prompted the study of possible cross-reactions between a BLV-infected ovine cell line and normal lymphocytes inoculated in this laboratory with an LAV strain (*7*).

Cells infected with HTLV-III were not available at the time of this study. Lymphocytes from ten healthy adults were purified in Ficoll-Hypaque and grown for 3 days with purified phytohemagglutinin (PHA; 1 μg/ml). Washed lymphocyte suspensions containing 2×10^6 cells per milliliter and Polybrene (2 μg/ml) were inoculated with LAV in amounts equivalent to a reverse transcriptase activity of 10,000 cpm per milliliter of cell suspension. After a 3- to 4-hour adsorption period, the suspensions were diluted 1:2 and transferred into RPMI 1640 medium with 10 percent fetal calf serum, 10 percent human T-cell growth factor (TCGF or interleukin-2), Polybrene (2 μg/ml), and sheep antibody to α-interferon diluted 1:1000. Unadsorbed virus was removed after 1 day of culture and cells were grown in the same medium. Cell extracts were prepared after 5, 7, and 10 days of LAV infection. Results obtained on day 7 are shown in Table 1. The LAV-infected lymphocytes bound immunoglobulins of a rabbit antiserum that contains antibodies to LAV (*8*); rabbit antisera to purified BLV p24 and gp51 reacted with the LAV-infected cells at least to the same extent as the antiserum to LAV. The monospecificity of these polyclonal antisera to purified BLV p24 and gp51 has been demonstrated previously (9). Of ten virus-free lymphocyte cultures run in parallel, none adsorbed the antisera to BLV, but lymphocytes of patient 7 strongly reacted with the antiserum to LAV. It is possible that the antigen inoculated into the rabbit also contained a histocompatibility polypeptide from the lymphocytes in which LAV was grown.

We also analyzed cross-reactions between cells infected with BLV, LAV, and HTLV-I (Table 2). With radioimmunoassays using ^{125}I-labeled goat antiserum to rabbit immunoglobulins, we demonstrated the binding of rabbit antibodies to BLV p24 with fetal lamb kidney (FLK) cells (a BLV-producing line) and, to a lesser extent, with LAV-infected primary lymphocyte cultures. There was also a low but significant reaction with MT$_2$ cells producing HTLV-I. Antibodies to BLV gp51 bound to LAV-infected lymphocytes and to FLK cells, but not to MT$_2$ cells, while antiserum to LAV

Table 1. Reaction of LAV-infected lymphocytes with antiserum to BLV p24, BLV gp51, and LAV gp13. Lymphocytes grown for 7 days with LAV were adjusted to a concentration of 10^6 cells per milliliter with protease inhibitors (2 mM tosyl lysine chloromethylketone and phenylmethylsulfonyl fluoride); they were frozen at $-80°C$ for at least 2 hours and then thawed and sonicated. Cell extracts were distributed in the wells of Microtest III flexible assay plates (Falcon 3911, 50 μl per well) and left to dry overnight. We then added 50 μl of a 5 percent bovine serum albumin solution. After 1 hour of incubation at 37°C, we added 50 μl of rabbit antiserum diluted 1:1000 in 40 percent fetal calf serum. After 2 hours at 37°C, wells were washed three times with phosphate buffered saline (PBS) and then filled with 50 μl of PBS containing 25,000 cpm of goat antiserum to rabbit immunoglobulin (059-03, ATAB). After 1 hour at room temperature, wells were washed three times, dried for 20 minutes at 70°C, cut, and distributed into tubes for counting in a gamma counter. Antisera and labeled immunoglobulins were diluted and incubated in 40 percent fetal calf serum before use. Results show mean of quadruplicate tests. Standard deviations were ±10 percent, as well as the index of ^{125}I bound calculated as the ratio of counts per minute in test wells to the counts in control wells with no antisera added.

| | Binding of ^{125}I-labeled goat antiserum to rabbit immunoglobulin | | | |
| | With LAV | | Without virus | |
Serum	Radio-activity (cpm)*	Index	Radio-activity (cpm)*	Index
LAV grown in lymphocytes from patient 3				
Antiserum to BLV p24	724	4.2	145	1.2
Antiserum to BLV gp51	481	2.8	138	1.1
Antiserum to LAV	671	4.0	98	0.8
Nonimmune serum	170		123	
LAV grown in lymphocytes from patient 7				
Antiserum to BLV p24	510	6.0	89	0.9
Antiserum to BLV gp51	595	7.0	104	1.0
Antiserum to LAV	935	11	784	8.0
Nonimmune serum	85		98	

*Standard deviations are ±10 percent.

gp13 bound even more to FLK cells than to those infected with LAV.

There are two possible explanations for these results. First, reaction of the antiserum to LAV with FLK cells was not completely specific, since control, virus-free ovine cells (OVK) also reacted with this serum, although significantly

Table 2. Binding of antibodies to various virus-infected and virus-free cells. The LAV-infected lymphocytes were as described in Table 1. The FLK and OVK cell lines are, respectively, BLV producers and virus-free cells. MT_2 is a lymphoid T-cell line producing a Japanese isolate of HTLV-I (ATLV), while the T cells of the HSB_2 line do not produce virus. Of the antibodies, goat antiserum to HTLV-I p24 as well as mouse monoclonal antibody 493 and 12/1-2 were obtained from R. C. Gallo and F. de Noronha; antibody 5G9 was from B. F. Haynes. Bovine and sheep sera of animals with BLV tumors contained antibodies to BLV. Binding of the various antibodies was revealed as in Table 1 or with labeled Protein A (Pharmacia, Uppsala), affinity-isolated goat antiserum to mouse immunoglobulins (TAGO Inc., Burlingame) or rabbit antiserum to goat immunoglobulins (Janssens Pharmaceutica, Belgium). Iodination of these products was performed each month in this laboratory. Results show indices of ^{125}I bound, as defined in Table 1. Some tests were not feasible (NF) because of nonspecific adsorption of Protein A to lymphocytes.

Antibody		Index of binding to different cells					
		Human lymphocytes		FLK/ BLV	OVK	MT_2	HSB_2
Source	Specificity	Infected with LAV	Control				
Goat antiserum to rabbit immunoglobulin							
Rabbit	BLV p24	3.9	1	11	1	2.2	1
	BLV gp51	4.7	1	3	1	1	
	LAV gp13	2.9	1	7.5	2	1	1
Protein A							
Rabbit	BLV p24	NF	NF	30	1	1.8	1
	BLV gp51	NF	NF	3	1	1	1
	LAV	NF	NF	6.5	2.4	2	2
Goat	HTLV-I p24	NF	NF	3	1	28	1
Mouse mo-	493 HTLV-1 p24	NF	NF	2.5	1	3.5	1
noclonal	6G9 HTLV-I p24	NF	NF	1	1	5.9	1
Bovine	With BLV tumor	NF	NF	1.8	1	1	1
	Virus free	NF	NF	1	1	1	1
Goat antiserum to mouse immunoglobulin							
Mouse mo-	493 HTLV-I p24	1	1	1.8	1	2.2	1
noclonal	6G9 HTLV-I p24	1	1	1	1	3	1
	12/1-2 HTLV-I p19	1	1	1.8	1	3	1
Rabbit antiserum to goat immunoglobulin							
Goat	HTLV-I p24	1	1	2.2	1	12	1
Sheep	With BLV tumor	1	1	2	1	1	1
	Virus free	1	1	1	1	1	1

less than did the FLK cells. Second, FLK cells produced more virus particles than LAV-infected lymphocytes, as judged by the amount of released particle-bound reverse transcriptase activity (not shown). When Protein A was used as a labeled reagent, the reaction of the antiserum to LAV was also partly nonspecific, and the nonspecificity was much higher if the antiserum was not diluted in 40 percent fetal calf serum, indicating that this rabbit had been partly immunized against calf serum proteins. By contrast, rabbit antisera to BLV p24 and gp51 did not react with virus-free cells, and the Protein A assay with antiserum to BLV p24 confirmed a small degree of cross-reactivity between FLK and MT$_2$ cells. Conversely, goat antiserum to HTLV-I also bound to some antigens of FLK cells. Of two mouse monoclonal antibodies to HTLV-I p24, one, antibody 493, revealed an epitope common to BLV- and HTLV-I–infected cells.

Serum from an animal with a BLV tumor and containing BLV antibodies reacted specifically with FLK cells, although weakly because of the low affinity of Protein A for bovine immunoglobulins. Protein A could not be used in radioimmunoassays with human lymphocyte primary cultures since this reagent binds directly to Fc fragments of lymphocyte subpopulations. It was possible to study reactions of LAV-infected lymphocytes with mouse and ovine antibodies by using labeled antisera to mouse and goat immunoglobulins. Epitopes for HTLV-1 p24, recognized by the monoclonal antibodies 493 and 6G9, were not detected in LAV-infected lymphocytes, nor were the HTLV-I p19 epitopes recognized by monoclonal antibody 12/1-2. Actually, LAV-infected lymphocytes did not reveal any antigenic

component of HTLV-I p24 when assayed with goat antiserum to HTLV-I p24. Neither did they react with BLV antibodies in the serum from the animal with a BLV tumor.

These results are consistent with data showing that amino acid sequences of HTLV-I p24 are homologous to BLV p24 (*10*). However, immunological cross-reactions between the two viruses have been demonstrated previously, although LAV has been shown to be related to equine infectious anemia virus (EIAV); in particular, LAV p24 was immunoprecipitated by horse sera containing antibodies to EIAV, but not by antibodies to core proteins of various other retroviruses, including BLV (*11*).

Our data do not apply to purified virions. They leave open the possibility that common antigenicity between BLV and HTLV group may be more readily detected in virus-infected cells, possibly because exposition of the shared components depends on the steric configuration of precursor polyproteins.

We found that rabbit antisera to BLV were useful for the early detection of retrovirus markers in lymphocyte cultures from AIDS patients. The four patients studied here belonged to a group of black patients from Central Africa treated in Brussels and documented according to the criteria described (*6*). A specimen from lymph node biopsy and a blood sample were obtained on the same day from patient A, and the lymphocytes were cultivated for 3 days with PHA (1 µg/ml), washed, and grown in RPMI 1640 medium with TCGF and Polybrene. Supernatants were collected periodically for assay of particle-bound reverse transcriptase activity. Cell extracts were prepared and assayed for reactivity with antiserum to BLV p24 (Table 1). Transient expression of an antigen related to

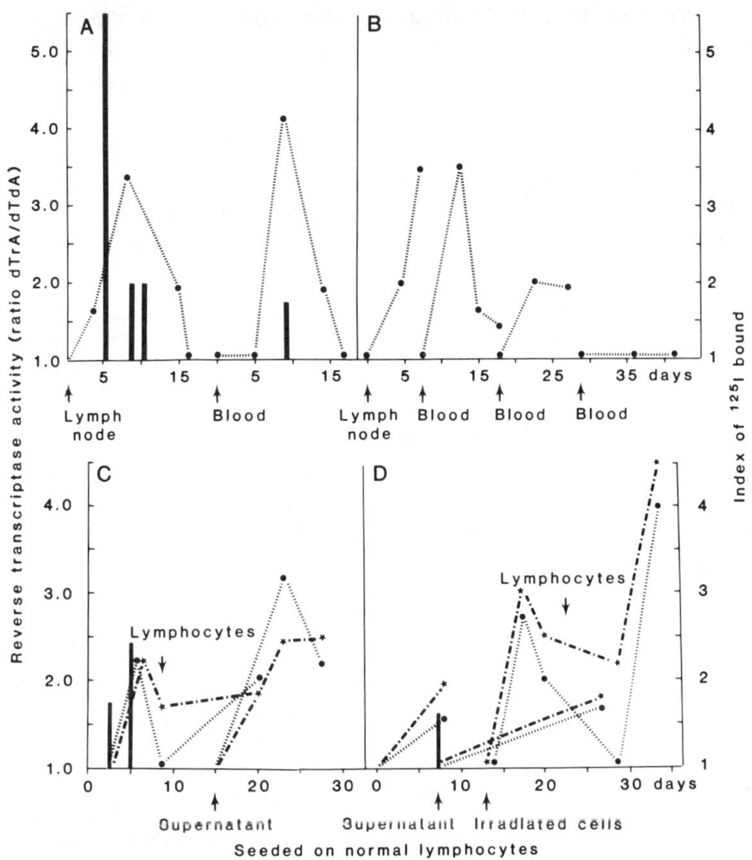

Fig. 1. (A and B) Binding of rabbit antiserum to BLV p24 (●) to lymphocyte cultures from AIDS patients A and B and detection of particle-bound reverse transcriptase in the supernatant (black bars). Antibody binding was assayed as in Table 1 and indices of ^{125}I bound were calculated from the radioactivity (counts per minute) of labeled goat antiserum to rabbit immunoglobulin bound to cell extracts treated with antiserum to BLV p24 divided by the radioactivity bound to cell extracts treated with normal rabbit serum or without rabbit serum. Reverse transcriptase activity was determined on concentrates (100 times) of tissue culture fluids suspended in assay buffer containing Triton X-100 (2 percent) and Tween 80 (0.1 percent). Assays were performed in $0.05M$ tris-HCl buffer, pH 7.9, containing 10 μM ^{3}H-labeled dTTP (50 Ci/mmol), 130 μM deoxyadenosine triphosphate, 50 μg each of $dT_{12-18}rA$ and $dT_{12-18}dA$ per milliliter, 5 mM $MgCl_2$. $0.1M$ NaCl, and bovine serum albumin (5 mg/ml). The assays were carried out at 30°C for 30 minutes. The results were expressed as the ratio of the enzymatic activity obtained on both synthetic template-primers $(dT_{12-18}rA)/(dT_{12-18}dA)$. Standard deviations are ±10 percent. (C and D) Binding of rabbit antisera to BLV p24 (●) and BLV gp51 (★) to lymphocyte cultures of ganglia biopsy from AIDS patient C and blood sample from patient D. Supernatants of the cultures were filtered at the times indicated by arrows and inoculated with Polybrene (2 μg/μl) into normal lymphocyte cultures that had been grown for 3 days with PHA (1 μg/μl). The cells were washed and resuspended in RPMI 1640 medium with 10 percent fetal calf serum, TCGF, and Polybrene before being inoculated with the filtered supernatants. Lymphocytes of the 13-day-old culture of patient D were irradiated with 2000 Rad from a cobalt source, and equivalents of 5 × 10^6 cells were cocultivated with 5 × 10^6 normal target lymphocytes, previously exposed to PHA. Standard deviations are ±10 percent.

460

BLV p24 occurred in both lymph node and blood cultures, with peak expression corresponding to peak reverse transcriptase production (Fig. 1). Disappearance of both retrovirus markers coincided with degeneration of the lymphocyte cultures. Early expression of BLV p24–related antigens within 5 days of culture was also observed with lymph node cells of patient B, as well as with two blood samples from this patient obtained 7 and 17 days later. A third blood sample, taken 1 month after the lymph node biopsy, yielded negative results. For the next two patients, C and D, cell extracts from the lymphocyte cultures were assayed in parallel with antibodies to BLV gp51 and to BLV p24 (Fig. 1, C and D). Lymph node cell culture of patient C simultaneously produced reverse transcriptase and expressed BLV-like gp51 and p24. Fresh lymphocytes from a healthy adult were added after 8 days of culture, at a moment when retrovirus markers were already decreasing. Their synthesis resumed after addition of the fresh target cells. Induction of BLV-related gp51 and p24 could be transferred to other lymphocyte cultures, when filtered supernatant of the 15-day-old original culture was added with Polybrene (2 μg/ml) to a lymphocyte culture from an adult donor. Similar results were obtained with lymphocyte cultures of a blood specimen from patient D. In addition, cells of the 14-day-old original culture were irradiated and cocultivated with normal adult lymphocytes. The production of BLV-related antigens could be sustained provided that fresh target lymphocytes were added to the culture.

Lymphocyte cultures from 25 healthy Belgian donors grown with PHA and TCGF did not bind rabbit antisera to BLV p24 or gp51 but four of these cultures bound the antiserum to LAV gp13. The use of this antiserum to detect viral antigens in crude whole cell extracts is valid only if virus-free control cultures are studied simultaneously.

It is striking that BLV markers were detected in the 20 Zairian patients tested thus far. The markers appeared within 5 to 8 days in the lymph node cultures and in five of six blood samples tested and reported here. Whether the change from positive to negative results in the blood tests for patient B has some prognostic meaning will be interesting to follow. These tests may prove useful in indicating the presence of LAV or HTLV-III in AIDS patients and their healthy contacts.

References and Notes

1. F. Barré-Sinoussi *et al.*, *Science* **220**, 868 (1983); J. C. Chermann *et al.*, *Antibiot. Chemother.* **32**, 48 (1984); E. Vilmer *et al.*, *Lancet* **1984-I**, 753 (1984).
2. M. Popovic, M. G. Sarngadharan, E. Read, R. C. Gallo, *Science* **224**, 497 (1984); R. C. Gallo *et al.*, *ibid.*, p. 500.
3. P. M. Feorino *et al.*, *ibid.* **225**, 69 (1984).
4. A. Elbrodt *et al.*, *Lancet* **1984-I**, 1383 (1984).
5. F. Brun-Vézinet *et al.*, *Science* **226**, 453 (1984).
6. N. Clumeck *et al.*, *Lancet* **1983-I**, 642 (1983); N. Clumeck *et al.*, *N. Engl. J. Med.* **310**, 492 (1984).
7. The LAV strain was received from F. Barré-Sinoussi.
8. J. C. Chermann, personal communication.
9. F. Bex *et al.*, *Cancer Res.* **39**, 1118 (1979); J. Ghysdael *et al.*, *J. Virol.* **29**, 1087 (1979); D. Portetelle *et al.*, *Virology* **105**, 223 (1980).
10. S. Oroszlan *et al.*, *Proc. Natl. Acad. Sci. U.S.A.* **79**, 1291 (1982).
11. L. Montagnier *et al.*, *Ann. Virol. (Inst. Pasteur)* **135E**, 119 (1984).
12. We thank M. Jacques, L. Tack, and J. Stienon for technical assistance and J. Herinckx for preparation of the manuscript. We thank R. C. Gallo for sending MT₂ and HSB₂ cells as well as antibodies to HTLV-I and J. C. Chermann for providing LAV and antiserum to LAV gp13 and for helpful advice on the cultivation of infected lymphocytes. Specimens of patient A were provided by C. Jonas and lymphocytes of healthy donors by P. J. Van Vooren. This work was supported by grants from Caisse Générale d'Epargne et de Retraite and from Fonds de la Recherche Scientifique Médicale.

19 September 1984; accepted 12 December 1984

Report

5 April 1985

85. Expression in *Escherichia coli* of Open Reading Frame Gene Segments of HTLV-III

N.T. Chang, P.K. Chanda, A.D. Barone, S. McKinney, D.P. Rhodes, S.H. Tam, C.W. Shearman, J. Huang, T.W. Chang, R.C. Gallo, and F. Wong-Staal

The human T-cell lymphotropic virus type III (HTLV-III) has been routinely isolated from patients with the acquired immune deficiency syndrome (AIDS) (*1, 2*). More than 100 isolates have been obtained (*3–5*) and, although genetic variants with different restriction enzyme maps have been observed, serum samples from more than 90 percent of patients with AIDS and pre-AIDS contain antibodies reactive with the prototype HTLV-III isolate, H9/HTLV-III-B2, as demonstrated by Western blot analyses and solid phase immunoassays (*6, 7*). These and other results (*8–10*) suggest that the antibodies to HTLV-III are highly cross-reactive with the different genetic variants and that it may be possible to develop diagnostic assays and, perhaps, a preventive vaccine.

The helper T-cell tropism (*11*), the size of some of the viral proteins (*7, 12*), and serological (*6, 13, 14*) and DNA hybridization studies (*15*) indicate that HTLV-III is related to the leukemia-causing HTLV-I and HTLV-II (*16*). This information and sequence data (*17*) suggest that the HTLV-III RNA genome is similar to those of other retroviruses and contains at least (i) a *gag* gene that encodes the internal structural (nucleocapsid or core) proteins, (ii) a *pol* gene that encodes the reverse transcriptase,

and (iii) an *env* gene that encodes the envelope glycoproteins of the virion. In addition, viruses in the HTLV family contain a pX region, which in HTLV-III consists of a coding sequence with one large open reading frame, designated *lor*, located between the *env* gene and the 3′ end of the genome (*18–20*). This *lor* is continuous in the same frame with the *env* and, therefore, is referred to as *env-lor*. It has been suggested that the *lor* is responsible for the unique pathogenic properties of the viruses, namely, the transforming property of HTLV-I and HTLV-II and the cytolytic property of HTLV-III on helper T cells (*18*).

In a study designed to identify peptides encoded by regions of the HTLV-III genome, open reading frame DNA segments were cloned in an expression vector to generate a library of *Escherichia coli* clones, each expressing a different peptide encoded by a DNA segment of one of the four HTLV-III genes mentioned above. We then determined which of these peptides are reactive with antibodies to HTLV-III in sera from AIDS patients.

Fragments of HTLV-III DNA derived from λBH-10, a previously constructed recombinant bacteriophage λ (*21*) containing a 9-kb segment of HTLV-III DNA (Fig. 1A), were inserted into the

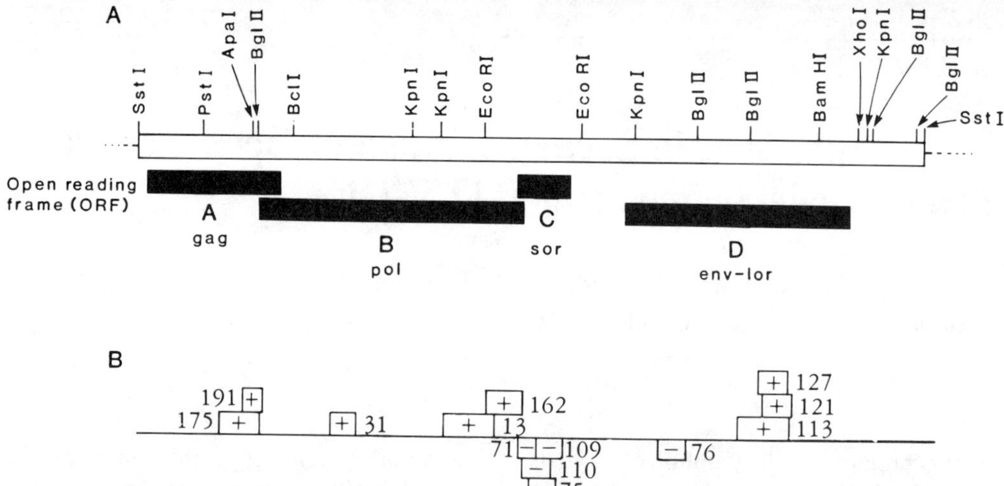

Fig. 1. (A) Restriction map of HTLV-III DNA in λBH-10. (B) Location in HTLV-III genome of DNA inserts in ORF clones. The exact position of each end of the clones is indicated in Table 1. The plus and minus signs indicate that the fusion proteins are or are not, respectively, immunoreactive with sera from AIDS patients, as demonstrated by Western blot analyses.

Table 1. Locations in the HTLV-III genome of ORF clones.

ORF clone number	Coordinates in HTLV-III genome*	
	Left end	Right end
13	3758	4362
31	2486	2808
71	4623	4852
75	4749	5035
76	6260	6603
109	4854	5164
110	4641	4873
113	7077	7716
121	7478	7722
127	7376	7700
162	4229	4617
175	1202	1669
191	1463	1690

*Plasmid DNA from lac^+ clones was digested with Bam HI and the HTLV-III specific insert (plus 10 bp of flanking vector DNA) was purified by agarose gel electrophoresis and cloned into M13mp19 RFI DNA which had also been digested with Bam HI. The nucleotide sequence at each end of the insert DNA was then determined by means of the "dideoxy" sequencing method, and these sequences were located relative to the known nucleotide sequence of the HTLV-III genome (17).

open reading frame (ORF) vector pMR100 (Fig. 2) (22). This vector contains a bacterial *lac* promoter DNA segment linked to a second DNA fragment containing a hybrid coding sequence in which the NH_2 terminus (5′ segment) of the λCI gene of λ is fused to an NH_2-terminally deleted *lac*IZ gene (3′ segment). A short linker DNA fragment containing a Sma I cloning site has been inserted between these two fragments in such a manner that a frameshift mutation has been introduced upstream of the *lac*IZ-coding DNA. As a result, pMR100 shows negligible β-galactosidase activity when introduced into cells of the lac^- host *E. coli* LG90. The insertion of foreign DNA containing an ORF, in this case the HTLV-III DNA, into the Sma I cloning site can reverse the frameshift mutation if the inserted coding sequence is in the correct reading frame with respect to both the λCI leader sequence and the *lac*IZ gene. Such a three-element

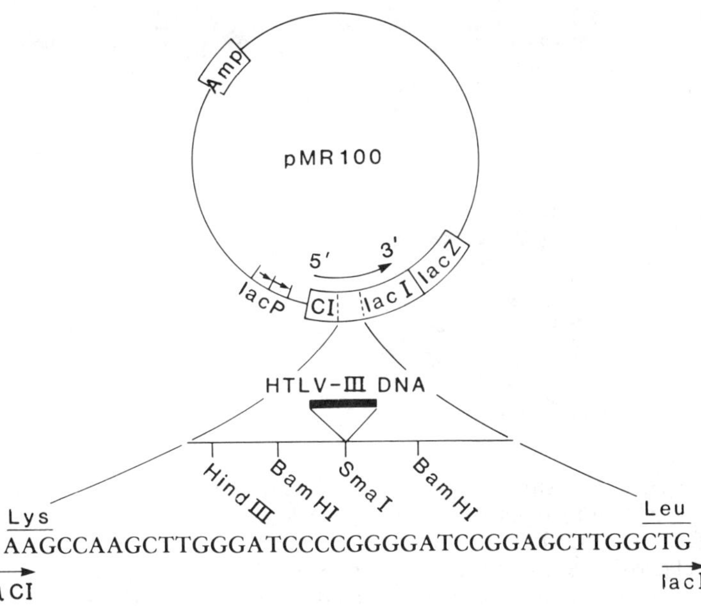

Fig. 2. Construction of the ORF expression vector containing HTLV-III DNA. Ten micrograms of HTLV-III DNA excised from λBH-10 (Fig. 1A) with Sst I were sonicated and end-repaired with T4 DNA polymerase (27). DNA fragments of 200 to 600 bp were isolated by gel electrophoresis. The fragments were then ligated to Sma I–cleaved pMR100 with T4 DNA ligase as described (22) and used to transform *E. coli* strain LG90 which was then plated on MacConkey agar containing ampicillin (50 μg/ml). *Lac*+ (red) colonies were isolated for further study.

fused gene will be expressed as a tripartite fusion protein, having a portion of the λCI protein at the amino terminus, the HTLV-III protein segment in the middle, and the *lac*IZ polypeptide at the COOH terminus. This results in high levels of expression of β-galactosidase activity upon introduction into LG90.

Transformants were screened on MacConkey plates to detect individual clones that express β-galactosidase enzymatic activity in situ (23). Of the 6000 ampicillin-resistant transformants screened, about 300 were found to express β-galactosidase activity. Colony hybridization with the use of ^{32}P-labeled nick-translated HTLV-III DNA as a probe revealed that all these *lac*+ clones contain HTLV-III DNA. The proteins produced by the *lac*+ clones were analyzed by sodium dodecyl sulfate–polyacrylamide gel electrophoresis (SDS-PAGE) along with those of the control *lac*+ clone pMR200,

which produces a λCI-β-galactosidase fusion protein. The *lac*IZ gene in pMR200 is identical to that in pMR100 except that it has a single base pair deletion which brings it in phase with the λCI gene to produce an active β-galactosidase. By virtue of their very large size, β-galactosidase and its fusion proteins are separated from the bulk of proteins in cell lysates on SDS-polyacrylamide gels and can be easily identified by Coomassie brilliant blue staining (Fig. 3A). Approximately half of the *lac*+ clones containing HTLV-III DNA produce polypeptides that are larger (15,000 to 27,000 daltons) than the λCI-*lac*IZ fusion protein of pMR200 (Fig. 3A, lanes 3, 6, and 7).

These findings are consistent with data showing that the DNA inserts are up to 700 bp long. Of the remaining clones, most showed a stained band with electrophoretic mobility similar to that of the

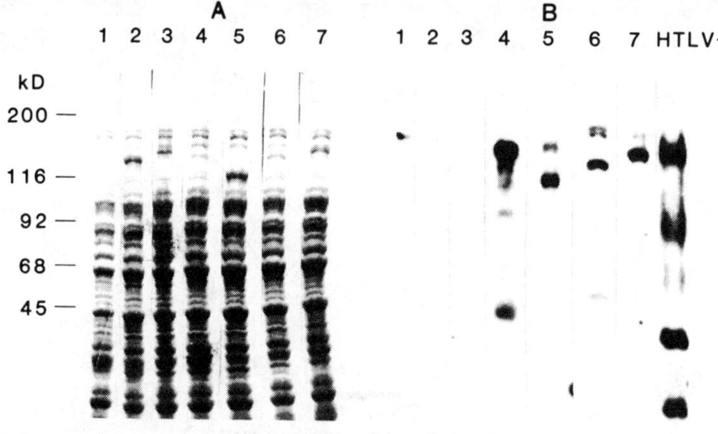

Fig. 3. (A) Gel analysis of λCI–HTLV-III–β-galactosidase fusion proteins. Cells from 1.5-ml cultures [grown in L-broth containing ampicillin (50 μg/ml)] were centrifuged, the pellets were resuspended in 100 μl of 1.2-fold concentrated sample buffer (26), and heated at 100°C for 3 minutes. After the samples were sonicated for 5 minutes to reduce the viscosity, 10 to 20 μl were analyzed on 7.5 percent SDS–polyacrylamide gels (26) and stained with Coomassie brilliant blue R-250. Lanes: 1, pMR100; 2, pMR200; 3, ORF 109; 4, ORF 4; 5, ORF 191; 6, ORF 121; 7, ORF 127. (B) Immunoreactivity of λCI–HTLV-III–β-galactosidase fusion proteins with sera from AIDS patients. Cells containing the recombinant plasmids were lysed and fractionated by electrophoresis on a 7.5 percent SDS–polyacrylamide gel. The proteins were electrophoretically transferred onto nitrocellulose paper. The nitrocellulose sheet was incubated for 2 hours at 37°C with 5 percent nonfat dry milk, 0.1 percent Antifoam A, 0.1 percent sodium azide in 0.9 percent NaCl (milk buffer) and then for 1 to 2 hours at room temperature with 5 percent normal goat serum in milk buffer. A pool of several well-characterized sera from AIDS patients was added and the nitrocellulose sheet incubated overnight at 4°C. The filter was washed twice with a solution containing 0.5 percent deoxycholic acid, 0.1M NaCl, 0.5 percent Triton X-100, 10 mM sodium phosphate, and 0.1 mM phenylmethylsulfonyl fluoride (pH 7.5) (wash buffer) for 30 minutes. After the filter was treated once with milk buffer containing goat serum, ^{125}I-labeled goat antiserum to human immunoglobulin G (1 × 10⁶ cpm/ml) was added and incubation was continued for another 30 minutes at room temperature. The filter was washed three times with wash buffer, 20 minutes each, dried, and autoradiographed. Bands indicate the positions of the immunoreactive proteins.

λCI-β-galactosidase fusion protein of pMR200 and a few showed a greater mobility (Fig. 3A, lane 5). This may be due to a small HTLV-III insert, proteolytic degradation or anomalous electrophoretic mobility of the fusion protein, rearrangement of the recombinant plasmid, or internal initiation of translation within the HTLV insert. Similar anomalies have been observed previously with this expression system (22). In addition, a few clones show a fusion protein with an apparent molecular weight greater than expected (Fig. 3A, lane 4). This may be due to the presence of either a single larger insert or, as we have demonstrated by sequence analysis of several clones, multiple smaller inserts. The β-galactosidase fusion proteins account for about 1 to 2 percent of total cellular protein.

The peptides produced by the *lac*⁺ clones were examined by Western blot analysis (24) for immunoreactivity with sera from AIDS patients (Fig. 3B). The recombinant peptides also reacted with antiserum to β-galactosidase, consistent with the proposition that they had the general structure λCI-HTLV-III peptide-*lac*IZ. From the pattern of immunoreactivity of the negative controls pMR100 and pMR200 (Fig. 3B, lanes 1 and 2), which do not contain HTLV-III DNA inserts, it is evident that these sera from AIDS patients contain antibodies reactive with several bacterial proteins of the host *E. coli*. This is not surprising, since human serum commonly contains antibodies to *E. coli*. When sera from AIDS patients was absorbed with Sepharose 4B conjugated with *E. coli* extract, the background immunoreactivity was reduced but not completely eliminated.

Of the 300 *lac*$^+$ clones analyzed, 20 reacted specifically with sera from AIDS patients. The unreactive clones (Fig. 3B, lane 3) probably contain peptides that fold in such a way that they are not reactive with antibodies or correspond to regions of HTLV-III protein molecules that are not immunogenic in AIDS patients. Alternatively, lack of reactivity may be due to the destruction of epitopes by the immunoblotting procedure.

The HTLV-III DNA inserts from the 20 immunoreactive clones were analyzed by DNA sequencing to determine precise sizes and locations on the HTLV-III genome. The HTLV-III genome consists of four ORF segments designated ORF-A, ORF-B, ORF-C, and ORF-D (Fig. 1A) (*17*). ORF-A and ORF-B, which correspond to the coding regions of the *gag* and *pol* genes, are 1.5 kb and 3.0 kb long, respectively. ORF-C is about 0.6 kb long, slightly overlaps with the ORF-B region, and is capable of encoding a polypeptide of 21 kilodaltons (kD). The location of ORF-C and its overlap with the *pol* gene are reminiscent of the structure of the *env* genes in HTLV-I and -II. However, ORF-C, designated the short ORF, *sor*, is too short to code for the entire envelope protein. ORF-D is 2.5 kb long and could encode both a large precursor of the major envelope glycopro-

tein and another protein derived from the 3′ terminus which may be analogous to the *lor* (pX) products of HTLV-I and -II. This gene region of HTLV-III, designated *env-lor* (*17*), is at least twice as long as the *lor* of HTLV-I and -II and it is unclear whether single or multiple proteins are encoded herein.

As shown in Fig. 1B, the *lac*$^+$ ORF clones expressing fusion proteins immunoreactive with sera from AIDS patients were located in ORF-A (clones 175 and 191), ORF-B (clones 13, 31, and 162), or ORF-D (clones 113, 121, and 127) and not in ORF-C. The 12 immunoreactive clones not included in Fig. 1B were found to be either duplicates of those that are shown or mosaics containing more than a single fragment of HTLV-III. Since none of the immunoreactive clones mapped to ORF-C, the library of *lac*$^+$ ORF clones was screened by in situ colony hybridization with the use of a ^{32}P-labeled nick-translated probe made from the 1.1-kb Eco RI–Eco RI fragment which spans the entire ORF-C region. Several clones (71, 75, 109, and 110) were isolated and none were immunoreactive. When these clones were sequenced, together they were found to cover 180 of the 203 codons in ORF-C. The function of the *sor* (ORF-C) region remains unclear. Either the *sor* is not expressed at the protein level or the encoded peptide may not be immunogenic in patients with AIDS or pre-AIDS.

Analysis of the ORF structures in HTLV-III leads to the question of which such structure corresponds to the *env* gene. It is possible that the *env-lor* region in HTLV-III contains all or a part of the *env* gene in addition to the presumed *lor* gene. Recent evidence suggests that the *lor* in HTLV-I encodes a 42-kD protein involved in the process of viral activation and transformation (*18–20, 25*).

466

When the lysate of one of the ORF clones (121 in Fig. 1B) was tested against serum samples, from 20 AIDS patients and 12 healthy normal subjects in a strip radioimmunoassay based on the Western blot technique, immunoreactivity against the λCI-HTLV-III-β-galactosidase fusion polypeptide was detected in the serum of 19 of the AIDS patients but none of the normal controls. This indicates that the protein encoded by the portion of the *env-lor* region contained in ORF clone 121 is produced in HTLV-III–infected cells and induces antibody production in most if not all AIDS patients.

These and further studies of the expression of the *env-lor* region in other vector systems and of antibodies to different regions of the fusion polypeptides may lead to the development of useful reagents for studying HTLV-III proteins and for preparing means to diagnose and treat AIDS.

References and Notes

1. M. Popovic, M. G. Sarngadharan, E. Read, R. C. Gallo, *Science* **224**, 497 (1984).
2. R. C. Gallo *et al.*, *ibid.*, p. 500.
3. P. D. Markham, G. M. Shaw, R. C. Gallo, in *AIDS*, V. T. DeVita, S. Hellman, S. A. Rosenberg, Eds. (Lippincott, Philadelphia, in press).
4. J. E. Groopman *et al.*, *Science* **226**, 447 (1984).
5. D. Zagury *et al.*, *ibid.*, p. 449; D. D. Ho *et al.*, *ibid.*, p. 451.
6. J. Schüpbach *et al.*, *ibid.* **224**, 503 (1984).
7. M. G. Sarngadharan, M. Popovic, L. Bruch, J. Schüpbach, R. C. Gallo, *ibid.*, p. 506.
8. B. Safai *et al.*, *Lancet* **1984-I**, 1458 (1984).
9. H. J. Alter *et al.*, *Science* **226**, 549 (1984).
10. P. M. Feorino *et al.*, *ibid.* **225**, 69 (1984).
11. D. Klatzmann *et al.*, *ibid.*, p. 59.
12. J. Schüpbach, M. G. Sarngadharan, R. C. Gallo, *ibid.* **224**, 607 (1984).
13. M. Essex *et al.*, *ibid.* **220**, 859 (1983).
14. T. H. Lee *et al.*, *Proc. Natl. Acad. Sci. U.S.A.*, in press.
15. S. K. Arya *et al.*, *Science* **225**, 927 (1984).
16. R. C. Gallo, *Cancer Surv.* **3**, 113 (1984).
17. L. Ratner *et al.*, *Nature (London)* **313**, 277 (1985).
18. J. G. Sodroski, C. A. Rosen, W. A. Haseltine, *Science* **225**, 381 (1984).
19. T. H. Lee *et al.*, *ibid.* **226**, 57 (1984).
20. D. J. Slamon, K. Shemotohno, M. J. Cline, D. W. Golde, I. S. Y. Chen, *ibid.*, p. 61.
21. B. H. Hahn *et al.*, *Nature (London)* **312**, 166 (1984).
22. M. R. Gray *et al.*, *Proc. Natl. Acad. Sci. U.S.A.* **79**, 6598 (1982).
23. J. H. Miller, *Experiments in Molecular Genetics* (Cold Spring Harbor Laboratory, Cold Spring Harbor, N.Y., 1982).
24. H. Towbin, T. Staehelin, J. Gordon, *Proc. Natl. Acad. Sci. U.S.A.* **76**, 4350 (1979).
25. W. A. Haseltine *et al.*, *Science* **225**, 419 (1984).
26. U. Laemmli, *Nature (London)* **227**, 680 (1970).
27. P. L. Deininger, *Anal. Biochem.* **129**, 216 (1983).
28. We thank M. Rosbash for the pMR100 and pMR200 vector plasmids, R. Ting for the purified HTLV-III, and V. R. Zurawski, Jr., for valuable discussions.

21 December 1984; accepted 20 February 1985

86. Characterization of Envelope and Core Structural Gene Products of HTLV-III with Sera from AIDS Patients

W. Gerard Robey, Bijan Safai, Stephen Oroszlan, Larry O. Arthur, Matthew A. Gonda, Robert C. Gallo, and Peter J. Fischinger

Human T-cell leukemia (lymphotropic) virus type III (HTLV-III) is a human retrovirus closely related in a number of its properties to HTLV-I and HTLV-II (*1–8*). In addition, studies have suggested that this cytopathic virus is more closely related to visna virus, a pathogenic retrovirus in the subfamily Lentivirinae, than to any other retrovirus (*9*). HTLV-III is not endogenous to the human genome, and data have revealed that individual viral genomes show degrees of nucleic acid heterogeneity (*7, 8*). Virus isolation studies from patients with acquired immune deficiency syndrome (AIDS) and AIDS-related complex (ARC) and from individuals in several of the groups at high risk for the disease showed a high probability of virus presence, although HTLV-III appeared to be present in a minority of cells within an organ (*2, 8*). Antibody detection by an enzyme-linked immunosorbent assay or electrotransfer tests in individuals with AIDS or ARC and those in the high-risk groups have unambiguously defined the association of HTLV-III to AIDS (*4, 5, 10*).

Although the presence of antibody to HTLV-III in humans defines previous exposure to the virus, the presence of antibody to viral proteins does not impart immunity because advanced AIDS patients have readily detectable antibodies (*3–6, 11*). HTLV-III can be isolated from most antibody-positive subjects (*2*) and occasionally from normal-appearing, high-risk individuals who do not have detectable antibody (*12*). It therefore seems that a protected individual, that is, one with no residual virus and a strong neutralizing or other protective antibody response, has not been identified. In lieu of a simple quantal neutralization test for HTLV-III, we felt it would be advantageous to identify the HTLV-III viral envelope glycoprotein (gp) and antibodies to the glycoprotein in various virus-exposed groups because, for many viruses, the major envelope glycoprotein contains epitopes that elicit protective antibodies (*13*). The identification of the viral glycoprotein is a precondition for understanding the nature of the protective state and consequently the individual who could successfully cope with or overcome infection with HTLV-III.

A tentative description of one or more high molecular weight proteins precipitated by AIDS sera as the possible glycoprotein of HTLV-III has been made (*10*). We have identified the major viral glycoprotein and the major structural group-specific antigen together with their precursor polypeptides by a combination of immunoaffinity chromatography, radioimmunoprecipitation, and two-dimensional peptide mapping techniques. The identification of the envelope and the structural gene products was accomplished by immunoaffinity chromatography of cell culture fluids containing HTLV-III (Fig. 1). Lane 1 shows the immunoreactive polypeptides isolated from virus-containing cell culture fluids from H9 cells infected with HTLV-III (*1*). The immunoaffinity resin used in this experiment was prepared from the immunoglobulin G (IgG) fraction of a serum from an AIDS patient

(serum 149) that had a high reactivity to HTLV-III polypeptide p24. Several polypeptides were identified as related to HTLV-III. Cells infected with HTLV-III were also labeled with [^{14}C]glucosamine, and cell extracts were subjected to immunoprecipitation with serum 149 (Fig. 1, lane 2). The results showed that two of the previously isolated species of polypeptides, gp120 and gp46, were glycoproteins. An additional glycoprotein, gp160, was identified in cell extracts. Isotopically labeled glucosamine was not detected in the region of p75-85.

In a related experiment, detergent extracts of HTLV-III–infected cells were chromatographed over immunoaffinity resins prepared from the IgG fractions of

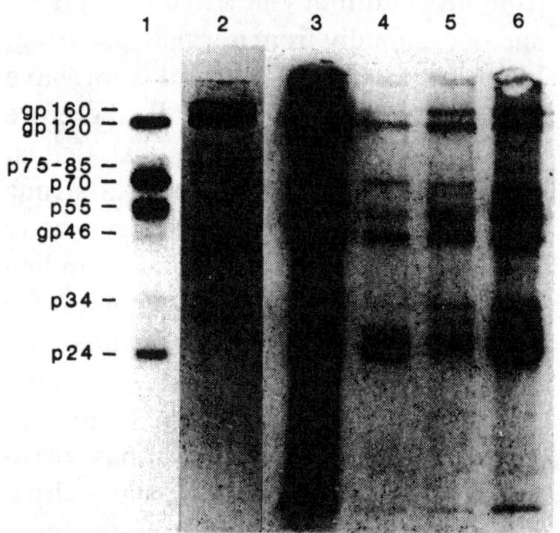

Fig. 1. Detection of HTLV-III–related antigens in extracellular extracts (lane 1) and detergent extracts (lanes 2 and 6) of HTLV-III–infected cells. Clarified cell culture fluids (lane 1) were chromatographed over AIDS IgG–Sepharose, eluted, labeled with ^{125}I by the chloramine-T method, concentrated by immunoprecipitation, and analyzed by sodium dodecyl sulfate–polyacrylamide gel electrophoresis (*18, 21*). HTLV-III–infected H9 cells were labeled with [^{14}C]glucosamine (5 μCi/ml) for 16 hours; lysed with phosphate-buffered saline containing 1 percent Triton X-100, 0.5 percent sodium deoxycholate, and 0.1 percent sodium dodecyl sulfate; and immunoprecipitated with serum 149 after prior treatment with normal human serum (lane 2). HTLV-III–infected H9 cells were extracted with immunoaffinity buffer [1 percent Triton X-100, 1*M* KCl, and 0.01*M* tris (*p*H 8.5)] and chromatographed over AIDS IgG–Sepharose (lane 3), chimpanzee IgG–Sepharose (lane 4), AIDS IgG–Sepharose A3 (lane 5), and A4 (lane 6). The eluted material was labeled with ^{125}I as above and concentrated by immunoprecipitation with the respective homologous serum. The molecular sizes were estimated relative to the migration of the molecular weight standards myosin (200K), β-galactosidase (116K), phosphorylase B (93K), bovine albumin (68K), ovalbumin (46K), carbonic anhydrase (30K), soybean trypsin inhibitor (21K), and lysozyme (14.4K). The molecular weights assigned to gp160 and gp120 are subject to some degree of error because of the nonlinear relation of the migration of molecular weight standards in the upper range of the gel. Also, the polypeptide conventionally designated as p24 is probably somewhat heavier.

serum 149 (Fig. 1, lane 3), serum from a chimpanzee infected with HTLV-III (*14*) (lane 4), and two sera from selected AIDS patients with Kaposi's sarcoma (lanes 5 and 6). Cytoplasmic extracts of virus-infected cells are useful for detecting virion polypeptide precursors. A prominent gp160 was detected in addition to virion gp120. At best, trace quantities of p75-85 were observed, suggesting a virion or extracellular location for this molecule. Additionally, p70, p55, p46, p34, and p24 were detected. In general, sera that were reactive with p24 (149 and chimpanzee) reacted with p70, p55, p34, and p24. The chimpanzee serum was marginally reactive with p24 and p55. In contrast, the two sera not appreciably reactive with p24 (A3 and A4) showed little or no precipitation of p70, p55, p34, or p24. However, gp160 and gp120 were readily detected. The A3 serum may precipitate a trace polypeptide in the region of p70. Additionally, the A3, A4, and chimpanzee sera did precipitate several molecules in the size range of p27 to p32 that were not detected by serum 149.

Two-dimensional oligopeptide mapping was performed to determine whether these molecules reflected a possible precursor-product relation. The trypsin and chymotrypsin peptide maps (Fig. 2A) show that gp160 contains the major gp120 peptides plus substantial additional peptide information. This suggests that gp120 is derived from gp160 after a proteolytic modification. Polypeptide p75-85 showed the same amount of major peptide complexity as detected in gp120. A tentative explanation would be that the lower-weight polypeptide represents the intact peptide chain of gp120 that was deglycosylated in the virion or extracellular spaces. The complexity of

the chymotrypsin map suggests that the gp160 preparation may not be homogeneous. A similar observation was made in a study of visna virus polypeptide processing (*15*). Two major peptides in gp120 and p75-85 (upper right quadrant) are present in the gp160 map as minor peptides. This is probably due to decreased iodination of those peptides as longer exposures of the maps to film revealed their presence. In any case, the two high molecular weight glycoproteins described here and by others (*10*) are related. The gp120's detected in infected cells by the three immunoaffinity resins prepared from human sera (Fig. 1) have been mapped and shown to be identical to the gp120 isolated from virions. Additionally, the group of polypeptides between p27 and p32 detected by the chimpanzee and Kaposi's sarcoma sera are related by peptide maps and appear within the p75-85, gp120, and gp160 molecules. This suggests that the low molecular weight species are likely to be degradation products of gp120 or gp160 or both and are not variants of the p24 *gag* gene product. The maps p27 and p32 appear to be more highly related to the maps of gp120 than to the maps of gp160.

The observation that sera strongly positive for p24 antibodies (serum 149) reacted with p70, p55, and p34 suggests a precursor-product relation between these molecules. The trypsin and chymotrypsin maps (Fig. 2B) support this relation. The proteins were isolated from virions and mapped as described above. The maps, especially chymotrypsin, showed a high degree of homology between p70 and p55. Further, p70 contains several peptides not found in p55, suggesting that p55 is part of p70. The p24 trypsin map is simple, but the three peptides can be located in the structure of both p55 and p70. Likewise, the chymotrypsin map of p24 can be located in p55 and p70, although two peptides (those with the greatest electrophoretic mobility) have somewhat diminished mobilities in the form of the cleaved molecule. The largest polypeptide *gag*

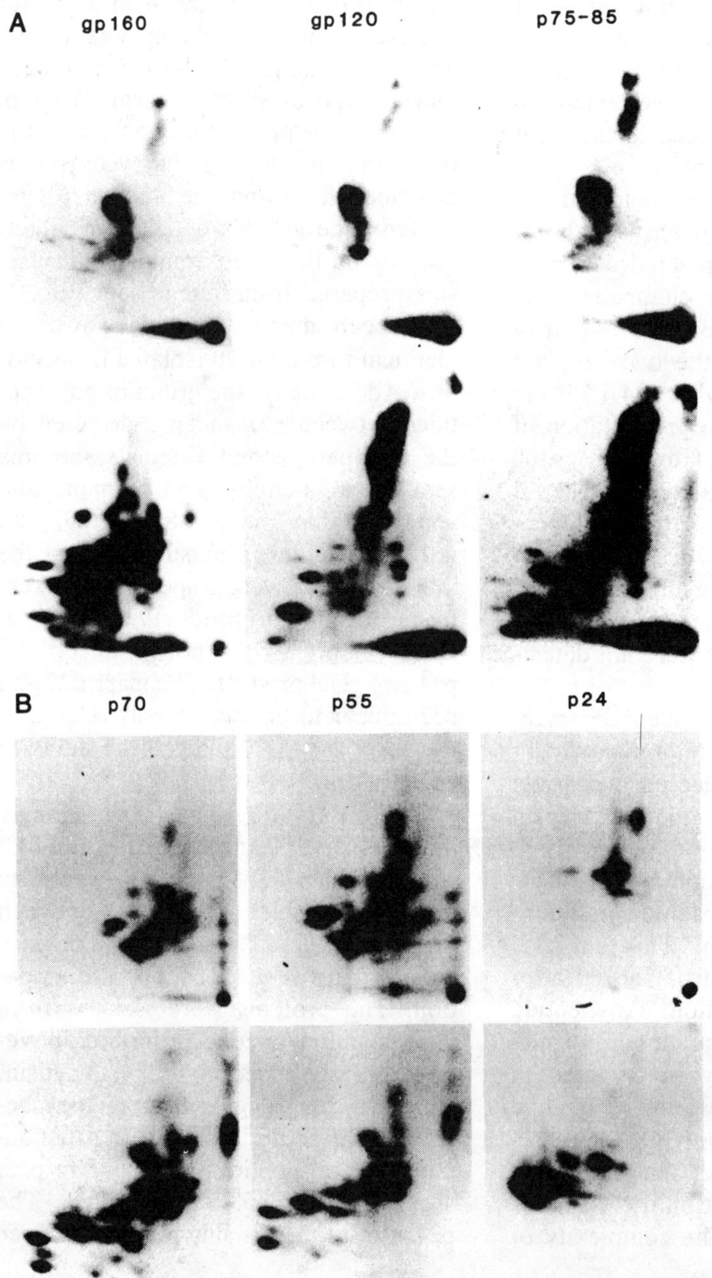

Fig. 2. Two-dimensional oligopeptide maps of HTLV-III envelope gene polypeptides (A) and structural gene polypeptides (B). Trypsin maps (upper row in A and B) and chymotrypsin maps (lower row in A and B) were made as described (*18, 21*). Briefly, polypeptides were isolated from cell culture fluids (gp120, p75-85, p70, p55, and p24) or detergent extracts of HTLV-III–infected cells (gp160) by immunoaffinity chromatography over AIDS IgG–Sepharose, labeled with ^{125}I, concentrated by immunoprecipitation, and localized on 10 percent acrylamide gels by autoradiography. Excised gel bands were digested with TPCK (L - 1 - tosylamide -2 - phenylethyl chloromethyl ketone)–trypsin or α-chymotrypsin, and resulting peptides were subjected to electrophoresis (first dimension) and ascending chromatography (second dimension). The origin for electrophoresis is in the lower right corner of each map.

gene product, p70, may be cleaved to p55 and further processed to p24. Additional experiments will determine the translational control (*16*) and kinetic relation between p70 and p55.

Polypeptide p34 (Fig. 1, lane 1) is a candidate for the other cleavage product resulting from the processing of p55 to p24. Other investigators have speculatively identified a precursor of p24 in the range of 50,000 (50K) to 55K molecular weight (*3, 4, 10*). Polypeptide p70 has previously not been included in the p24 precursor scheme. A likely explanation is that the size of the cellular pool may be small, and indeed p70 is barely detectable in immunoprecipitates of metabolically labeled cell extracts but is readily iodinated. The major p24 precursor in metabolically labeled cytoplasmic extracts was p55, in agreement with other observations (*10*). In any case, our data show that p70 and p55 both contain sequences of p24.

Additional proteins invariably detected included a 46K glycoprotein (gp46) and often a 200K polypeptide (p200). Both were precipitated by various sera from noninfected subjects, such as normal human, normal rabbit, and immune rabbit. Initial peptide map data indicate that gp46 is not related to gp120. The presence of antibodies to gp41 in electrotransfer tests has been considered the most sensitive diagnostic criterion of HTLV-III infection (*4, 5*). Although gp41 has been conspicuously absent in immunoaffinity assays with the above sera, the 149, A3, and A4 sera all strongly react with p41 as determined in Western blot electrotransfers (*17*). We have occasionally detected small quantities of a nonglycosylated polypeptide (p41-43) in immunoaffinity experiments and have usually seen small amounts of it in immunoprecipitates of metabolically labeled cells. This nonglycosylated polypeptide was precipitated only by sera that strongly reacted with p24, suggesting that it is a minor intermediate in the processing of p55 to p24. Either the electrotransfer method must be highly sensitive to detect gp41, or gp41 is refractive to iodination. The identities of both gp41 and gp46 require further investigation.

These results show that the primary HTLV-III envelope gene product is a 160K glycoprotein that is processed to a 120K glycoprotein and something else. Both gp160 and gp120 appear to be subject to proteolytic (*18, 19*) and glycosidic degradation. The data also confirm that a major intermediate in the synthesis of p24 is p55 (*6, 9*) and identify another primary *gag* gene product of p70. That HTLV-III is a partially cytolytic virus in H9 cells (*1*) can account for the virus polypeptide precursors in both cytoplasmic extracts and extracellular virions. Finally, the detection of the relatively large envelope gene products of HTLV-III is consistent with the study by Gonda *et al.* (*9*), which suggested that HTLV-III may be closely related to the cytopathic visna lentivirus whose envelope glycoprotein has been reported to be gp135 with a precursor gp150 (*15*).

The identification of the major glycoprotein of HTLV-III should facilitate studies on the induction of neutralizing antibody and resolve the question of whether a state of protection can be achieved. At present, no individual exposed to HTLV-III is known to be protected. However, HTLV-III antibody-positive individuals in several candidate antibody-positive groups can be considered. These include the AIDS patients with Kaposi's sarcoma who have no opportunistic infections and relatively intact immune systems, ARC patients whose lymphadenopathy has improved, selected partners of AIDS patients who

472

have remained well, and hemophiliacs who recently may have been exposed to inactivated virus in heat-treated factor VIII preparations. The techniques described above should clearly delineate whether patterns of antibody response to *env*, *gag*, or other HTLV-III gene products could indicate protection or antedate shifts in the status of the patient.

If genomic variants of HTLV-III indicate either a large number of subtypes or antigenic drift as seen in the related visna virus, then the number of glycoprotein epitopes required for the induction of immune protection may be extensive. Peptide mapping of the envelope glycoproteins of representative variant HTLV-III's will clarify this situation. The ability to isolate HTLV-III glycoproteins of various sizes could lead to attempts to induce protection against infection and seroconversion by a homologous virus or viruses in animal models such as the chimpanzee. Although extensive variations in the *env* gene restriction endonuclease pattern do not engender optimism for the successful establishment of protective immunity in humans, broadly protective group-specific and interspecies-specific neutralizing antibodies have been induced in model animal retrovirus systems by means of purified *env* gene products (*13, 20*).

References and Notes

1. M. Popovic, M. G. Sarngadharan, E. Read, R. C. Gallo, *Science* **224**, 497 (1984).
2. R. C. Gallo *et al.*, *ibid.*, p. 500.
3. J. Schüpbach *et al.*, *ibid.*, p. 503.
4. M. G. Sarngadharan, M. Popovic, L. Bruch, J. Schüpbach, R. C. Gallo, *ibid.*, p. 506.
5. B. Safai *et al.*, *Lancet* **1984-I**, 1438 (1984).
6. R. C. Gallo *et al.*, Eds., *Human T-Cell Leukemia/Lymphoma Virus* (Cold Spring Harbor Laboratory, Cold Spring Harbor, N.Y., 1984).
7. B. H. Hahn *et al.*, *Nature (London)* **312**, 166 (1984).
8. G. M. Shaw *et al.*, *Science* **226**, 1165 (1984).
9. M. A. Gonda *et al.*, *ibid.* **227**, 173 (1985).
10. L. W. Kitchen *et al.*, *Nature (London)* **312**, 367 (1984).
11. M. Essex *et al.*, *Science* **220**, 859 (1983); F. Barré-Sinoussi *et al.*, *ibid.*, p. 868; M. Essex *et al.*, *ibid.* **221**, 1061 (1983).
12. S. Z. Salahuddin *et al.*, *Lancet* **1984-II**, 1418 (1984).
13. W. Schäfer and D. P. Bolognesi, in *Contemporary Topics in Immunobiology*, M. G. Hannar, Jr., and F. Rapp, Eds. (Plenum, New York, 1977), vol. 6, p. 127.
14. This serum is from one of six chimpanzees inoculated with HTLV-III. All animals have seroconverted, and infectious HTLV-III has been recovered from the peripheral blood leukocytes of all six chimpanzees [D. C. Gajdusek *et al.*, *Lancet* **1985-1**, 8419 (1985)].
15. R. Vigne *et al.*, *J. Virol.* **42**, 1046 (1982).
16. Y. Yoshinaka, I. Katoh, T. D. Copeland, S. Oroszlan, *Proc. Natl. Acad. Sci. U.S.A.*, in press.
17. H. Towbin, T. Staehelin. J. Gordon, *ibid.* **76**, 4350 (1979).
18. J. H. Elder, F. C. Jensen, M. L. Bryant, R. A. Lerner, *Nature (London)* **267**, 23 (1977).
19. L. E. Henderson *et al.*, *Virology* **85**, 319 (1978); M. J. Krantz, M. Strand, J. T. August, *J. Virol.* **22**, 804 (1977).
20. P. J. Fischinger, W. Schäfer, D. P. Bolognesi, *Virology* **71**, 169 (1976); G. Hunnsman, V. Moening, W. Schäfer, *ibid.* **66**, 327 (1975).
21. W. G. Robey, W. J. Kuenzel, G. F. VandeWoude, P. J. Fischinger, *Cancer Res.* **42**, 2523 (1982); W. G. Robey, G. A. Dekaban, J. K. Ball, C. M. Poore, P. J. Fischinger, *Virology* **142**, 183 (1985).
22. We thank C. M. Poore for technical assistance and W. C. Saxinger for serum 149 from an AIDS patient.
23. Supported in part by contract N01-CO-23910 with Program Resources, Inc., and contract N01-CO-23909 with Litton Bionetics.

18 January 1985; accepted 13 March 1985

87. Major Glycoprotein Antigens That Induce Antibodies in AIDS Patients Are Encoded by HTLV-III

J.S. Allan, J.E. Coligan, F. Barin, M.F. McLane, J.G. Sodroski, C.A. Rosen, W.A. Haseltine, T.H. Lee, and M. Essex

Human T-cell lymphotropic viruses (HTLV) are a group of exogenous retroviruses that have been implicated in a variety of clinical syndromes (*1–5*). HTLV-III, which is the probable etiologic agent of the acquired immune deficiency syndrome (AIDS) (*4, 5*) has several characteristics in common with HTLV-I and -II. These characteristics include an apparent tropism for OKT4$^+$T cells (*4, 6*), a reverse transcriptase with Mg^{2+} preference (*4, 7*), an ability to *trans*-activate retroviral transcription in infected cells (*8*), and an association with immunosuppression (*4, 9, 10*). That HTLV-I and HTLV-II are highly related is indicated by their primary nucleotide sequences (*11, 12*) and their serological cross-reactivities (*5, 13*). HTLV-III, which is presumably closely related to the lymphadenopathy-associated virus (*14*), contains limited regions of nucleic acid homology with the HTLV-I (*15–17*), partial serological cross-reactivity for the major *gag* and *env* gene products (*5, 10, 18*), and most recently has been shown to contain regions of homology with lentiviruses (*19*).

According to cell membrane immunofluorescence and immunoprecipitation studies with serum samples from infected individuals, the most immunogenic proteins of HTLV-I and HTLV-II are cell surface–expressed glycoproteins (*12, 18, 20*). These glycoproteins are derived from the *env* gene of HTLV, gp61–68 for type I and gp67 for type II (*12*), and are thought to be precursor envelope proteins that may subsequently be processed to an exterior glycoprotein (gp46–52) and smaller transmembrane protein (gp21 or 22) (*12*). The most immunogenic proteins recognized in HTLV-III–infected cells by the sera of patients with AIDS or AIDS-related complex (ARC), hemophiliacs, and exposed healthy homosexuals are also glycoproteins (*21*) of approximately 160 kD (gp160) and 120 kD (gp120). Using Western blot techniques, investigators at other laboratories have reported an additional protein (p41) which is predominant in virus preparations and is thought to be a glycoprotein (*5*). P41 is only weakly reactive in our cellular preparations when analyzed by radioimmunoprecipitation.

Recently, HTLV-III proviruses were cloned from an HTLV-III–infected H9 cell line (*16*). HTLV-III contains, in addition to *gag* and *pol*, a 2.5-kilobase open reading frame located in the 3' end of the genome corresponding to the *env* and /or gene regions of HTLV I and HTLV-II (*17*). The nucleotide and amino acid sequence for the first 210 nucleotides of this region are given in Table 1. We report that the major glycoproteins gp160 and gp120, recognized by the sera of HTLV-infected individuals, are encoded at least in part by this 2.5-kb open reading frame of HTLV-III.

To determine the HTLV-III–specific coding region for gp160 and gp120, we analyzed the sequence of the NH_2-terminus by Edman degradation of the proteins labeled with [^{3}H]leucine and [^{35}S]cysteine. The proteins were prepared by immunoprecipitation and isolation from sodium dodecyl sulfate (SDS)–polyacrylamide gels. Gp160 and gp120 gave the same sequence of labeled amino acids for the first 40 degradation cycles (Fig. 1). Leucine peaks were observed at positions 4 and 22 and a cysteine peak was observed at position 24. The repetitive yield for these sequences was greater than 93 percent. A number of minor radioactive peaks were evident in the gp160 profile and are believed to be related to contaminating proteins. Gp160 and gp120 were also labeled with [^{3}H]valine and again sequenced from the NH_2-terminus. Valine peaks were evident in both at positions 6, 8, 12, 14, 35, and 38 (Fig. 1C). Comparing this result with the deduced amino acid sequence based on the primary nucleotide sequence of HTLV-III, we conclude that gp160 and gp120 are encoded by the 2.5-kb open reading frame of HTLV-III. When one compares the leucine, cysteine, and valine positions in the first 40 amino acids

Table 1. 5′ Nucleotide sequence and predicted amino acid sequence of the HTLV-III envelope gene region. The HTLV-III sequence is derived from Ratner *et al.* (*17*). The dark arrow indicates the site for cleavage of the leader sequence from the envelope glycoproteins resulting in the protein species gp160 and gp120. Asterisks indicate cysteine, leucine, and valine residues determined by radiolabel sequence analysis. The first nucleotide presented corresponds to nucleotide sequence 5802 of the HTLV genome.

```
ATG AGA GTG AAG GAG AAA TAT CAG CAC TTG TGG AGA TGG GGG TGG AGA TGG GGC ACC ATG
 M   R   V   K   E   K   Y   Q   H   L   W   R   W   G   W   R   W   G   T   M20

CTC CTT GGG ATG TTG ATG ATC TGT AGT GCT ACA GAA AAA TTG TGG GTC AGA GTC TAT TAT
 L   L   G   M   L   M   I   C   S   A ▼ T   E   K   L*  W   V*  T   V*  Y   Y40

GGG GTA CCT GTG  TGG AAG GAA GCA ACC ACC ACT CTA TTT TGT GCA TCA GAT GCT AAA GCA
 G   V*  P   V*  W   K   E   A   T   T   T   L*  F   C*  A   S   D   A   K   A60

TAT GAT ACA GAG GTA CAT AAT GTT TGG GCC
 Y   D   T   E   V*  H   N   V*  W   A
```

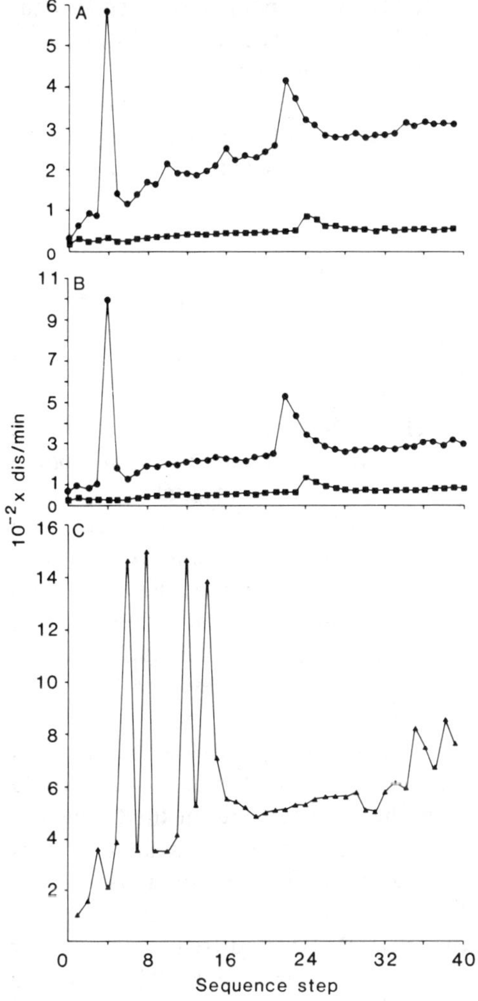

Fig. 1. Amino acid sequence analysis of the NH₂-terminus of the HTLV-III glycoproteins gp160 (A) and gp120 (B) labeled with [³⁵S]cysteine and [³H]leucine and subjected to Edman degradation as described (*18, 24*). Radioactivity is shown for each degradation cycle: ●, [³H]leucine; ■, [³⁵S]cysteine. Leucine peaks were observed at positions 4 and 22, and a cysteine peak was determined at position 24. Gp120 and gp160 were also labeled with [³H]valine as shown in (C) for gp160. Valine peaks were observed at 6, 8, 12, 14, 35, and 38 (▲). Proteins were purified from radioimmunoprecipitated HTLV-infected-cell, lysate by SDS-PAGE as described (*18*). Briefly, approximately 30 × 10⁶ HTLV-III–infected cells (H9) were radiolabeled with 10 mCi of [³H]leucine and 5 mCi of [³⁵S]cysteine or 10 mCi of [³H]valine for 8 hours in appropriate media. Cell lysates were cleared with 200 µl of normal human serum prior to immunoprecipitation with 200 µl of reference HTLV-III–positive serum and the eluted proteins were subjected to electrophoresis on 10 percent SDS–polyacrylamide gels. The protein bands were then cut from the gel, electroeluted, dialyzed, and lyophilized before being sequenced.

of gp120 and gp160 to the predicted sequence (Table 1), one finds a perfect match. The probability of finding such a sequence in any given HTLV-specific protein by chance alone is less than $(1/19)^{1+2+6} \times (17/20)^{40-9}$ or 1.97×10^{-14}. An initation codon is present 30 amino acids upstream from the NH₂-terminus, based on the nucleotide sequence. By analogy with results previously obtained with HTLV-I and HTLV-II (*10*), and because of their relative hydrophobicity,

these 30 residues probably represent the signal sequence which is removed during glycosylation.

To demonstrate a precursor-product relationship for these glycoproteins, we performed pulse-chase studies. HTLV-III–infected cells were starved for 1 hour in cysteine-free medium and then metabolically labeled for 5 minutes with [³⁵S]cysteine (0.2 mCi/ml). The cells were then chased with excess cysteine in complete medium, harvested at 0, 0.2,

0.4, 1, 2, 4, and 8 hours, immunoprecipitated and subjected to SDS-PAGE. Gp160 was initially the most prominent glycoprotein species observed, whereas gp120 became discernible only after 2 hours, with a concurrent loss of gp160. Furthermore, we compared the glycoproteins seen in virus preparations with those of cell lysates. When we immunoprecipitated [^{35}S]cysteine-labeled proteins from virus harvested at 12 hours and concentrated from cell culture supernatants, only gp120 was observed. In contrast, both gp160 and gp120 were seen in the cell lysates which suggests that gp120 is a more mature envelope gene product.

The 2.5-kb open reading frame of HTLV-III is predicted to code for a protein of approximately 90 kD. Tunicamycin treatment of HTLV-III–infected cells was performed to characterize the non-glycosylated forms of the HTLV-III proteins. Tunicamycin is a glycosylation inhibitor and has been used to identify the nascent envelope proteins of many other animal retroviruses, such as Rous sarcoma virus (22). A new protein species of approximately 88 kD was observed when the cell lysate was immunoprecipitated and subjected to SDS-PAGE (Fig. 2A). Although there is a difference of approximately 70 kD between gp160 and p88, this could conceivably be due to glycosylation alone since there are 31 potential glycosylation sites predicted from the gene sequence. The loss of both gp160 and gp120 and the appearence of only one new protein band suggests either that both the unglycosylated forms of gp160 and gp120 are identical or that the inhibition of glycosylation prevents further processing. We therefore isolated gp160 and gp120 by lentil lectin affinity chromatography and subjected them to endoglycosidase H digestion (Fig. 2B). The loss of radioactivity associated with gp160 and gp120 was accompanied by the appearance of two new proteins of approximately 88 kD (p88) and a smaller protein that migrated as a broad band.

Retrovirus biosynthesis typically involves the processing of an *env* gene precursor protein to a mature exterior glycoprotein and a transmembrane protein derived from the carboxyl terminus. Additionally, the glycosylation of the envelope proteins is usually modified from envelope precursors that contain high mannose residues and are sensitive to endoglycosidase H to an exterior glycoprotein containing complex sugar residues. Thus p88 may represent the native unglycosylated form of gp160 which is also seen in tunicamycin studies. The broad protein band between 70 and 80 kD may represent a partially glycosylated form of gp120. On the basis of the nucleotide sequence, one can predict from the cleavage site for the transmembrane protein an unglycosylated exterior glycoprotein of approximately 55 kD. We therefore isolated gp120 by preparative SDS-PAGE and treated the protein with endoglycosidase F, which digests both complex and high mannose sugar moieties. A broad protein band from about 58 to 68 kD was observed, lending further evidence that gp120 may be a cleavage product of gp160, although it is not fully digested as evidenced by the broad band and by the somewhat larger size than that predicted for the exterior glycoprotein.

In general, the *env* genes of animal retroviruses encode glycoproteins that are the most immunogenic proteins as detected by the sera of infected animals (23). In separate studies (21) we found

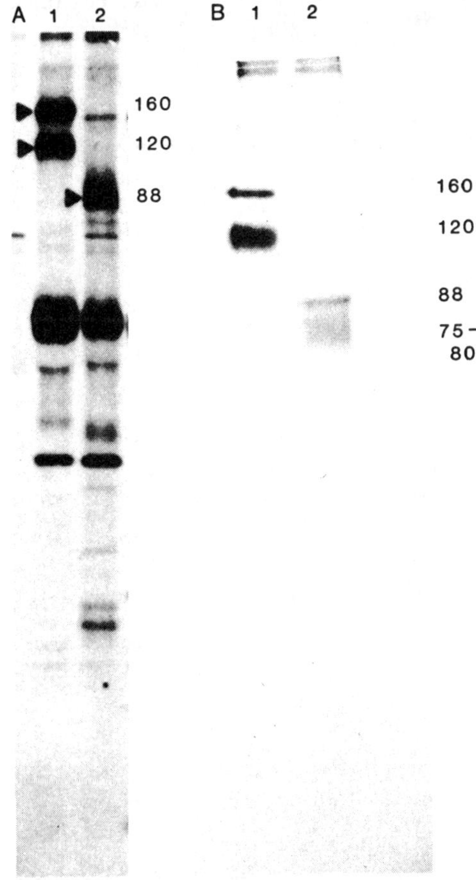

Fig. 2. Analysis of HTLV-III glycoproteins. (A) H9 cells infected with HTLV-III were treated with tunicamycin (*18*) and subjected to radioimmunoprecipitation and SDS-PAGE. Lane 1, proteins immunoprecipitated from untreated [^{35}S]cysteine-labeled infected H9 cells; lane 2, proteins from tunicamycin-treated cells. The infected H9 cells (4 × 10^6 cells) were incubated with tunicamycin (20 μg/ml) for 2 hours and then labeled with [^{35}S]cysteine for an additional 3 hours in the presence of tunicamycin. Cell lysates were prepared, cleared with 20 μl of negative human serum, and immunoprecipitated with 20 μl of known HTLV-III–positive serum. (B) HTLV-III glycoproteins were purified with lentil lectin and digested with endoglycosidase H (*18*). The [^{35}S]cysteine-labeled glycoproteins from HTLV-III–infected cells were immunoprecipitated and incubated (lane 1) in the absence of endoglycosidase H or (lane 2) in the presence of endoglycosidase H and run on 10 percent SDS–polyacrylamide gels. Procedures for endoglycosidase H digestion were described previously (*18*). Briefly, HTLV-III glycoproteins were first incubated with lentil lectin Sepharose 4B for 4 hours and then eluted with 0.2*M* methyl mannoside. The resulting proteins were then immunoprecipitated with HTLV-III reference serum, and the precipitates bound to protein A Sepharose were dissociated from antibody by boiling for 2 minutes in the presence of 0.1 percent SDS and 0.15*M* sodium citrate, *p*H 5.5. Equal portions were then incubated for 3 hours at 37°C in the presence or absence of 0.25 μg of endoglycosidase H. The reaction was terminated by the addition of five volumes of cold 95 percent ethanol, and the proteins were precipitated overnight at −20°C. The samples were then centrifuged at 12,000*g* for 15 minutes and the proteins were reconstituted with electrophoresis sample buffer, boiled for 3 minutes, and subjected to electrophoresis.

that gp120 and gp160 were the HTLV-related species most probably precipitated by the antibodies found in patients with AIDS or AIDS-related complex, healthy homosexual men who had been exposed to HTLV-III, and asymptomatic hemophiliacs. The evidence presented clearly identifies two large glycoproteins that are encoded by the *env* gene of HTLV-III, and we suggest that gp160 represents the envelope gene precursor protein and gp120, a mature envelope glycoprotein. We have not yet identified the transmembrane protein of HTLV-III, although a 41-kD protein has been observed in virus preparations by Western blotting (*5*).

Further characterization of gp160 and gp120 is likely to be important for serodiagnosis of the HTLV-III carrier state as well as for prospective immunoprophylactic approaches to the prevention of

AIDS. The possibility that these glyco-proteins are directly involved in the pathologic consequences of HTLV-III infection on the T helper cell population must also be considered.

References and Notes

1. B. J. Poiesz *et al.*, *Proc. Natl. Acad. Sci. U.S.A.* **77**, 7415 (1980).
2. D. Catovsky *et al.*, *Lancet* **1982-I**, 639 (1982); K. Takatsuki *et al.*, *Jpn. J. Clin. Oncol.* **9**, 317 (1979).
3. V. S. Kalyanaraman *et al.*, *Science* **218**, 571 (1982).
4. M. Popovic *et al.*, *ibid.* **224**, 497 (1984); R. C. Gallo *et al.*, *ibid.*, p. 500; J. Schüpbach *et al.*, *ibid.*, p. 503.
5. M. Sarngadharan *et al.*, *ibid.*, p. 506.
6. M. Popovic *et al.*, *ibid.* **219**, 856 (1983).
7. H. M. Rho *et al.*, *Virology* **112**, 355 (1981).
8. J. G. Sodroski, C. A. Rosen, W. A. Haseltine, *Science* **225**, 381 (1984); J. Sodroski *et al.*, *ibid.* **227**, 171 (1985).
9. M. Essex *et al.*, *ibid.* **221**, 1061 (1983); H. W. Jaffe *et al.*, *ibid.* **223**, 1309 (1984); M. Essex *et al.*, in *Human T-Cell Leukemia Viruses*, R. C. Gallo, M. Essex, L. Gross, Eds. (Cold Spring Harbor Laboratory, Cold Spring Harbor, N.Y., 1984), p. 355; M. Essex, M. F. McLane, T. H. Lee, in *Acquired Immune Defiency Syndrome,* M. S. Gottlieb and J. E. Groopman, Eds. (Liss, New York, 1984), p. 91; M. Popovic *et al.*, *Science* **226**, 459 (1984).
10. M. Essex *et al.*, *Science* **220**, 859 (1983).
11. J. Sodroski *et al.*, *ibid.* **225**, 421 (1984).
12. I. S. Chen *et al.*, *Nature (London)* **305**, 502 (1983).
13. T. H. Lee *et al.*, *Proc. Natl. Acad. Sci. U.S.A.* **81**, 7579 (1984).
14. F. Barré-Sinoussi *et al.*, *Science* **220**, 868 (1983).
15. B. Hahn *et al.*, *Nature (London)* **312**, 166 (1984).
16. G. M. Shaw *et al.*, *Science* **226**, 1165 (1984).
17. L. Ratner *et al.*, *Nature (London)* **313**, 277 (1985).
18. T. H. Lee *et al.*, *Proc. Natl. Acad. Sci. U.S.A.* **81**, 3856 (1984).
19. M. A. Gonda *et al.*, *Science* **227**, 173 (1985).
20. J. Schüpbach, M. G. Sarngadharan, R. C. Gallo, *ibid.* **224**, 607 (1984).
21. L. Kitchen *et al.*, *Nature (London)* **312**, 367 (1984); F. Barin *et al.*, *Science* **228**, 1094 (1985).
22. R. Stohrer and E. Hunter, *J. Virol.* **32**, 412 (1979).
23. T. Taniyama and H. T. Holden, *J. Exp. Med.* **150**, 1367 (1979); D. C. Flyer, S. J. Burakoff, D. V. Faller, *Nature (London)* **305**, 815 (1983).
24. J. E. Coligan *et al.*, *Methods Enzymol.* **91**, 413 (1983); J. E. Coligan and T. J. Kindt, *J. Immunol. Methods* **47**, 1 (1981).
25. Supported by NIH grants CA 37466, CA 13885, and 2T32-CA09031. We thank R. Gallo for reference reagents and P. Fischinger and G. Robey for stimulating discussions.

8 February 1985; accepted 12 April 1985

Report

31 May 1985

88. Virus Envelope Protein of HTLV-III Represents Major Target Antigen for Antibodies in AIDS Patients

F. Barin, M.F. McLane, J.S. Allan, T.H. Lee, J.E. Groopman, and M. Essex

One of the first suggestions that a retrovirus might have a role in the etiology of the acquired immune deficiency syndrome (AIDS) was the finding that a minority of patients with AIDS and AIDS-related complex (ARC) had antibodies that reacted with antigens found in cells infected with human T-cell leuke-mia virus type I (HTLV-I) (*1*). The low titers of these antibodies and the observation that only about 25 percent of the patients had antibodies that would precipitate the HTLV-I encoded gp61 or p24 proteins suggested that cross-reacting antibodies to a related agent could be responsible for the initial observation (*1*,

2). Subsequently, retroviruses that were cytopathic for T-helper lymphocytes were isolated from numerous AIDS and ARC patients. Although these viruses were usually designated HTLV-III (*3*), some were designated lymphadeno-pathy-associated virus (LAV) (*4, 5*) or AIDS-related virus (ARV) (*6*). HTLV-III, LAV, and ARV probably represent the same class of agent (*7, 8*), but on the basis of their antigenic cross-reactivity and several short stretches of amino acid homology they appear to be only distant-ly related to HTLV-I (*2, 7, 9*). However, both HTLV-I and HTLV-III infect T-helper lymphocytes and have a Mg^{2+}-dependent reverse transcriptase (*3*).

The major envelope (*env*) gene prod-ucts of HTLV-III have been identified as glycoproteins of 160 kD (gp160) and 120 kD (gp120 (*10*). These two glycoproteins have the same amino acid sequence at the amino terminus (*10*). We now report that gp120 and gp160 are the HTLV-III proteins detected most readily in ra-dioimmunoprecipitation assays of serum samples from patients with AIDS or ARC. In AIDS patients, the *env* gene encoded proteins are detected about twice as readily as p24, which is the *gag* gene encoded protein of HTLV-III that represents the major antigen found in virus particles.

Serum samples were initially screened for antibodies to HTLV-III by indirect cell membrane immunofluorescence (MIF) using the H9/HTLV-III cell line as described (*11*) (Table 1). Whereas 48 of 50 (96 percent) of the AIDS patients and 43 of 50 (86 percent) of the ARC patients were positive, 34 of 73 (47 percent) of the healthy homosexual males but none of 27 healthy laboratory workers were posi-tive.

All of the samples from the same 190 individuals were also tested by radioim-munoprecipitation and sodium dodecyl sulfate–polyacrylamide gel electrophore-sis (RIP/SDS-PAGE) with [^{35}S]cysteine-labeled H9/HTLV-III and uninfected H9 cells (*11*). As shown in Table 1, samples that were positive by MIF were also positive by RIP/SDS-PAGE, and one sample from an AIDS patient and three

Table 1. Presence of antibodies to membrane antigens (HTLV-III-MA) and to HTLV-III gp120 and p24 proteins in patients with AIDS or ARC and in healthy homosexual controls and healthy laboratory workers. Positivity for HTLV-III-MA was determined by MIF (*11*) and the presence of antibodies to gp120 and p24 was determined by RIP/SDS-PAGE (*11*).

Category*	Number tested	Number and percent positive for			Ratio of number positive for p24 to number positive for gp120
		HTLV-III-MA	gp120	p24	
AIDS	50	48 (96)	49 (98)	22 (44)	0.45
ARC	50	43 (86)	46 (92)	37 (74)	0.80
Healthy homosexual males	73	34 (47)	36 (49)	26 (36)	0.72
Healthy laboratory workers	27	0	0	0	

*Serum samples were taken from subjects who came to a community health clinic in a high-risk area and to area hospitals in 1983–1984. The samples were coded to prevent experimental bias.

samples from ARC patients that were negative by MIF were also positive by RIP/SDS-PAGE.

Figure 1 shows the RIP/SDS-PAGE reactions for 15 representative samples of human serum that were positive by MIF (lanes 2 to 16) and one sample that was negative (lane 1). Whereas all the HTLV-III membrane antigen antibody-positive samples regularly reacted with the *env* gene encoded gp120 and gp160 proteins, only 85 of 131 (62 percent) also detected the p24 protein of HTLV-III. Although some sera from patients with AIDS and ARC patients and some samples from healthy homosexual males have readily detectable antibodies to p24 or to the *gag* gene precursor protein p55 (for example, Fig. 2, lanes 2, 10, 12 to 14, and 16), others lack readily detectable antibodies to these proteins (for example, Fig. 1, lanes 4, 5, 7, 11, and 15). Several other bands were precipitated in various proportions from the sera of AIDS and ARC patients, including proteins of about 41 kD (gp41), 38 kD (p38), 17 kD (p17), and a second band near p24 that migrates close to the 24-kD band precipitated by reference rabbit antisera to whole disrupted HTLV-III (Fig. 2C, lane 7b) or by a reference monoclonal antibody to HTLV-III p24 (Fig. 2C, lane 5b).

To establish the specificity of these sera for HTLV-III proteins, we tested all of them by RIP/SDS-PAGE on uninfected H9 cells. The serum samples from eight highly reactive AIDS patients failed to detect proteins of similar sizes in uninfected control cells (Fig. 2A). The results were similar for five ARC patients (Fig. 2B, lanes 1 to 4, and Fig. 2C, lane 8) and for four antibody-positive healthy homosexual males (Fig. 2B, lanes 5 to 8). No bands of the same sizes were detected on either the HTLV-III infected or the uninfected H9 cells when sera from antibody-negative healthy homosexual males (Fig. 2C, lanes 1 and 2)

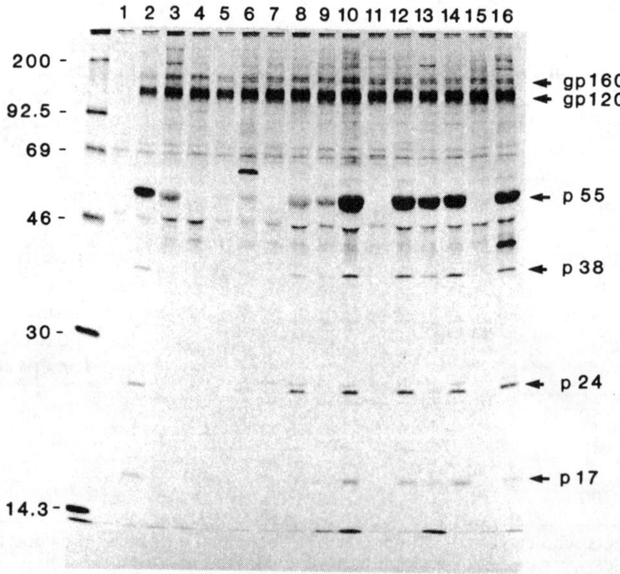

Fig. 1. Reactivity of serum samples for antibody to HTLV-III proteins as determined by RIP/PAGE (*10, 11*). Cell lysates were prepared from [^{35}S]cysteine-labeled HTLV-III–infected H9 cells and immunoprecipitated with sera from the following individuals: a laboratory worker whose serum was negative for antibody to HTLV-III membrane antigens (lane 1); seven ARC patients (lanes 2, 6, 7, 10, 11, 12, and 16); three AIDS patients (lanes 3, 5, and 15); and five healthy homosexuals who were positive for antibody to HTLV-III membrane antigens (lanes 4, 8, 9, 13, 14).

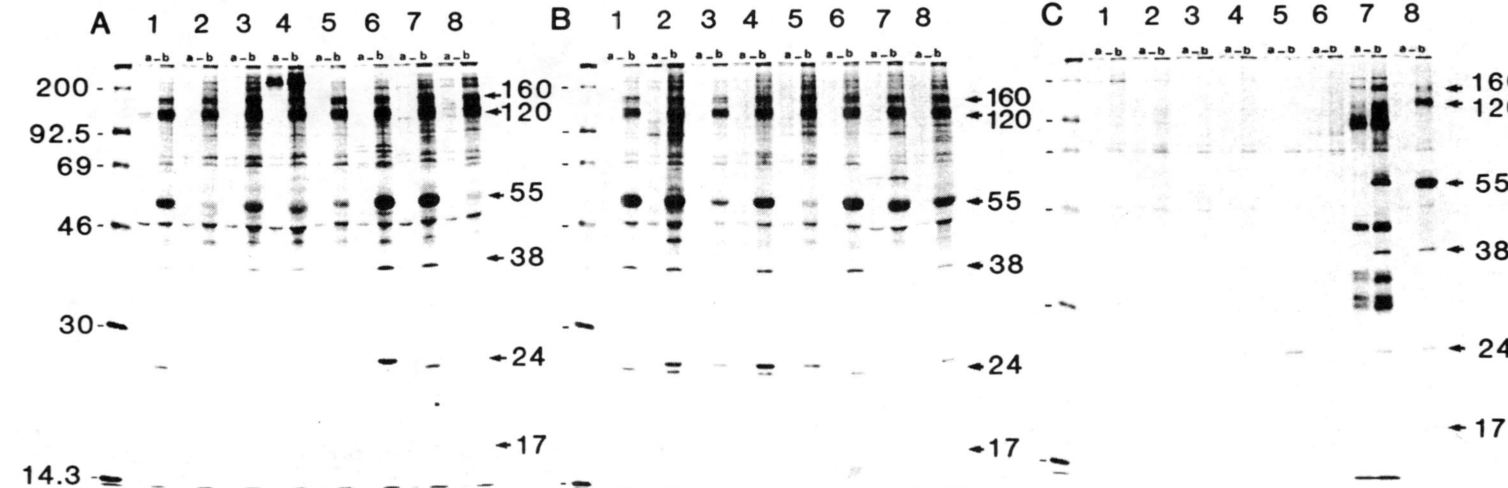

Fig. 2. Analysis of human serum samples for antibodies to HTLV-III proteins. Soluble cell lysates labeled with [^{35}S]cysteine from uninfected H9 cells (a) and infected H9 cells (b) were reacted with (A) sera from eight AIDS patients (lanes 1 to 8); (B) sera from four ARC patients (lanes 1 to 4), and four positive healthy homosexual males (lanes 5 to 8); and (C) sera from two healthy homosexual males (lanes 1 and 2) and two laboratory workers (lanes 3 and 4), all of whom were negative for antibody to HTLV-III membrane antigens; mouse monoclonal antibody to p24 of HTLV-III (lane 5), normal rabbit serum (lane 6), reference rabbit antiserum to disrupted HTLV-III (lane 7), and a positive control from an ARC patient (lane 8).

or healthy laboratory workers (Fig. 1, lane 1, and Fig. 2C, lanes 3 and 4) were checked.

Representative antibody-positive sera were also tested on glycoprotein preparations of H9/HTLV-III cells enriched through the use of a lentil lectin column. Samples from four antibody-positive AIDS patients precipitated proteins of about 120 kD, 160 kD, and 41 kD (Fig. 3, lanes 1 to 4; these are the same sera as in Fig. 2A, lanes 1 to 4). Similar results were obtained with two antibody-positive ARC patients (Fig. 3, lanes 5 and 6; these are the same sera as in Fig. 2B, lanes 1 and 2) and with two antibody positive healthy homosexual males (Fig. 3, lanes 7 and 8; these are the same sera as in Fig. 2B, lanes 5 and 6). No proteins of related sizes were detected in sera from antibody-negative healthy homosexual males (Fig. 3, lanes 9 and 10) or with sera from laboratory workers (Fig. 3, lanes 11 and 12).

None of the human serum samples that we tested contained antibodies to p24 or other *gag*-related HTLV-III antigens without also containing readily detectable antibodies to gp120 and gp160. Conversely, when examined in the same RIP/SDS-PAGE preparation, less than half of the AIDS patients that had antibodies to gp120 also revealed detectable antibodies to p24 (Table 1). Although this ratio was higher for ARC patients and antibody-positive healthy homosexual males, only about three-fourths of the individuals in these categories that had readily detectable antibodies to gp120 and gp160 also had readily detectable antibodies to p24. Other, more sensitive assay systems could conceivably reveal a higher proportion of individuals with antibodies to p24. However, for assays based on equimolar amounts of undenatured antigen, the gp120/160 complex, which has been mapped to the *env* gene of HTLV-III, would presumably be

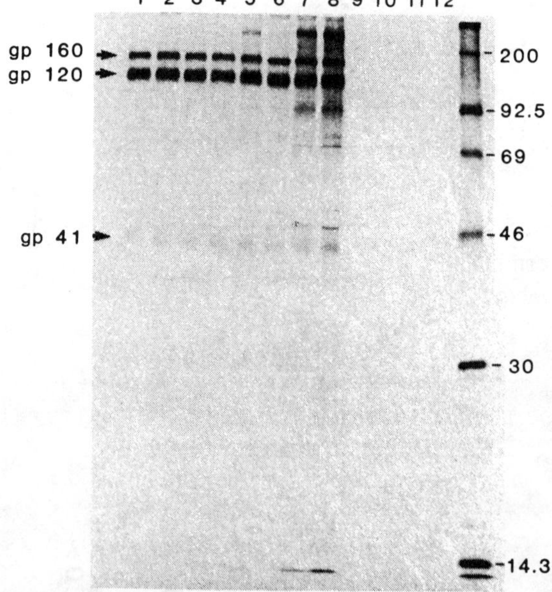

Fig. 3. Analysis of glycoproteins from HTLV-III–infected cells. Cell lysates from [^{35}S]cysteine-labeled H9 cells infected with HTLV-III were enriched for glycoproteins by lentil lectin affinity chromatography as described (*10, 11*). The bound fraction was reacted with antibodies in the sera of four AIDS patients (lanes 1 to 4, same as in Fig. 2A, lanes 1 to 4); two ARC patients (lanes 5 and 6, same as in Fig. 2B, lanes 1 and 2); two healthy homosexual males who were positive for antibodies to HTLV-III membrane antigens (lanes 7 and 8, same as Fig. 2B, lanes 5 and 6); two healthy homosexual males who were negative for antibodies to HTLV-III membrane antigens (lanes 9 and 10, same as Fig. 2C, lanes 1 and 2); and two laboratory workers (lanes 11 and 12, same as Fig. 2C, lanes 3 and 4).

the antigen of choice. This might be particularly important for patients involved in differential diagnoses for AIDS, since such individuals had lower amounts of antibody to p24.

We recently reported that asymptomatic hemophiliacs that tested positive by MIF also regularly had antibodies to gp120/160 (*11*). At that time we had not established that these proteins were encoded by HTLV-III. However, as we now find with AIDS patients, ARC patients, and healthy homosexual males, a significant fraction of the asymptomatic hemophiliacs had antibodies to gp120/gp160 in the absence of antibodies to p24 that could be detected with the same procedure. We also recently reported that four healthy individuals from "high risk" backgrounds carried infectious HTLV-III but had no antibodies detectable by the MIF, ELISA (enzyme-linked immunosorbent assay), or Western blotting procedures (*12*). Three of these individuals were also tested by RIP/SDS-PAGE and were also found to be negative by this procedure.

These results suggest that RIP/SDS-PAGE should be considered as a possible confirmatory test for establishing reactivity of selected serum samples that give uninterpretable results by procedures such as ELISA and Western blotting, especially potential "false positives." Although the ELISA and Western blotting procedures are clearly more adaptable for use in broad-scale screening, to our knowledge the RIP/SDS-PAGE described here is the only assay currently available that regularly reveals a reactivity with a spectrum of the major HTLV-encoded proteins of both the *gag* and *env* genes, virtually eliminating the possibility that false positives would be a problem with this procedure.

References and Notes

1. M. Essex *et al. Science* **220**, 859 (1983).
2. T.-H. Lee *et al.*, *Proc. Natl. Acad. Sci. U.S.A.* **81**, 7579 (1984); M. Essex, M. F. McLane, T. H. Lee, in *Acquired Immune Deficiency Syndrome*, M. S. Gottlieb and J. E. Groopman, Eds. (Liss, New York, 1984), pp. 91–100.
3. M. Popovic *et al.*, *Science* **224**, 497 (1984); R. C. Gallo *et al.*, *ibid.*, p. 500; J. Schüpbach *et al.*, *ibid.*, p. 503; M. Sarngadharan *et al.*, *ibid.*, p. 506; J. Groopman *et al.*, *ibid.* **226**, 447 (1984); D. Zagury *et al.*, *ibid.*, p. 449; D. D. Ho *et al.*, *ibid.*, p. 453; G. M. Shaw *et al.*, *Adv. Intern. Med.* **30**, 1 (1984).
4. F. Barré-Sinoussi *et al.*, *Science* **220**, 868 (1983).
5. L. Montagnier *et al.*, *ibid.* **225**, 63 (1984); P. M. Feorino *et al.*, *ibid.*, p. 69.
6. J. A. Levy *et al.*, *ibid.*, p. 840.
7. L. Ratner *et al.*, *Nature (London)* **313**, 277 (1985).
8. S. Wain-Hobson *et al.*, *Cell* **40**, 9 (1985); R. Sanchez-Pescador *et al.*, *Science* **227**, 484 (1985).
9. S. K. Arya *et al.*, *Science* **223**, 927 (1984).
10. J. S. Allan *et al.*, *ibid.* **228**, 1091 (1985).
11. L. W. Kitchen *et al.*, *Nature (London)* **312**, 367 (1984).
12. S. Z. Salahuddin *et al.*, *Lancet* **1984-II**, 1418 (1984).
13. Supported by NIH grants CA 37466, CA 13885, and 2T32-CA09031. F.B. is a visiting scientist from Université Francois Rabelais in Tours, France and was supported by the Association pour le Development de la Recherche sur le Cancer, the Fondation pour la Recherche Medicale, and the Phillipe Fondation. We thank R. Gallo and M. Sarngadharan for the reference rabbit antisera and mouse monoclonal antibodies to HTLV-III and for the H9/HTLV-III cells.

13 February 1985; accepted 12 April 1985

Report

7 June 1985

89.   Isolation of T-Cell Tropic HTLV-III–Like Retrovirus from Macaques

M.D. Daniel, N.L. Letvin, N.W. King, M. Kannagi, P.K. Sehgal, R.D. Hunt, P.J. Kanki, M. Essex, and R.C. Desrosiers

Converging lines of research strongly suggest that a T-cell tropic retrovirus called HTLV-III or LAV is the cause of the acquired immune deficiency syndrome (AIDS) in humans (1–6). Recent data on the increasing prevalence of infection with HTLV-III indicate that this is a public health problem of major proportions (7). An immune deficiency syndrome of macaque monkeys with many similarities to human AIDS has been described (8–10); affected animals at the New England Regional Primate Research Center (NERPRC) die with opportunistic infections, impaired T-cell function, and lymphoproliferative disorders (8). Because of the need to develop animal systems for the study of HTLV infection and to define the etiological agent (or agents) of the spontaneous immune deficiency syndrome at the NERPRC, we have been studying T-cell tropic retroviruses of macaques.

Serological surveys have indicated that several Old World primate species are extensively infected with an HTLV-I–related virus (11), and HTLV-I seropositivity has been correlated with lymphomas and lymphoproliferative disorders in the NERPRC macaque colony (12). T-cell tropic retroviruses have been isolated from Old World primates, and the biologic, antigenic, and genetic characteristics of these viruses suggest that

they are closely related to HTLV-I (13). Evidence for natural infection of nonhuman primates with a retrovirus that has properties similar to those of HTLV-III has not been presented. Here we describe the isolation of such a virus from four sick macaques of the NERPRC colony.

For virus isolation, peripheral blood lymphocytes, splenic lymphocytes, or cell-free serum samples were cocultivated with the following cell types: (i) HUT-78 cells, a human tumor T-cell line (14), and (ii) human T cells that had been cultured in the presence of T-cell growth factor [interleukin-2 (IL-2)]. Cell cultures were monitored for the appearance of reverse transcriptase activity in cell-free supernatants (Fig. 1). In cultures established with lymphocyte or serum samples from four of the macaques, reverse transcriptase activity was detected 12 to 18 days after initiation of cocultivation and reached maximum levels approximately 10 days later. High levels of reverse transcriptase activity have been maintained for more than 3 months of continuous cultivation of infected HUT-78 cells.

We have found no difference in the sensitivity of the two types of cultured cells for isolation or growth of these macaque retrovirus isolates. However, the use of T-cell tumor lines (15) has several advantages over the use of normal T cells. HUT-78 cells grow continuously in culture and are independent of exogenously added IL-2. Also, infection of HUT-78 cells with these macaque retroviruses resulted in the appearance

Table 1. Isolation of HTLV-III–like virus from macaques.

Animal*	Blood sample used for isolation	Clinical-pathological features
Mm251-79	Frozen splenocytes†	Malignant lymphoma
Mm239-82	Frozen serum	Macrophage infiltrates in brain, oroesophageal candidiasis, cryptosporidiosis, intestinal trichomoniasis
Mm220-82	Frozen serum	Macrophage infiltrates in brain, oroesophageal candidiasis, cryptosporidiosis, intestinal trichomoniasis
Mm142-83‡	Lymphocytes	Diarrhea, facial rash, generalized lymphadenopathy, splenomegaly

*Mm, *Macaca mulatta* (rhesus monkey). †Splenocytes were stored viably frozen in 15 percent dimethyl sulfoxide in liquid nitrogen. ‡The only live animal from which virus was isolated.

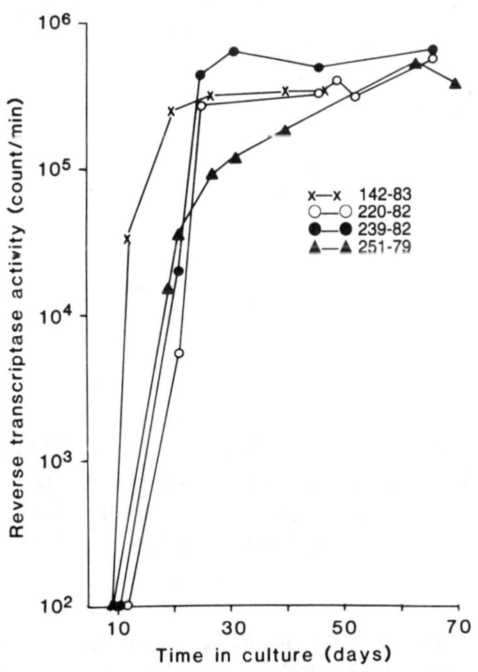

Fig. 1. Appearance of reverse transcriptase activity after cocultivation of macaque samples with HUT-78 cells. The samples indicated in Table 1 were cocultivated with HUT-78 cells (American Type Culture Collection). Lymphocytes and splenocytes were prepared

by banding cells over Ficoll-Hypaque solutions. The four positive samples are a composite of cocultivations started on different dates. At each time point, 2 to 3 ml of cells were centrifuged at 1300g for 10 minutes. The supernatant was removed and centrifuged again at 1300g for 10 minutes to ensure that all cells were removed. Supernatant (1.4 ml) was centrifuged at 12,000g for 90 minutes to pellet virus. The virus pellet was resuspended on ice in 20 μl of dissociation buffer [0.01M tris-HCl, pH 7.3, 0.2 percent Triton X-100, 0.001M EDTA, 0.005M dithiothreitol (DTT), and 0.06M KCl]. To this was added 60 μl of a solution containing 0.05M tris-HCl, pH 8.3, 0.007M MgCl$_2$, 0.06M KCl, 0.08 mg/ml poly-(ribocytidylate)oligo(deoxyguanylate) [(rC)-oligo(dG)]primer, 0.007M DTT, and 3.3 μCi of α-^{32}P-labeled dGTP (3000 Ci/mmol). Samples were incubated at 37°C for 60 minutes and 60 μl of each sample was spotted onto a Whatman No. 3 disk. Radioactivity incorporated in trichloroacetic acid–precipitable material was measured by Cerenkov counting. Backgrounds from uninfected cells varied from 500 to 1000 count/min. Samples from 68 other macaques gave negative results. These 68 samples were of two types: peripheral blood lymphocytes of live, healthy macaques (54 samples) and frozen sera from macaques that had died previously with immune deficiency (14 samples).

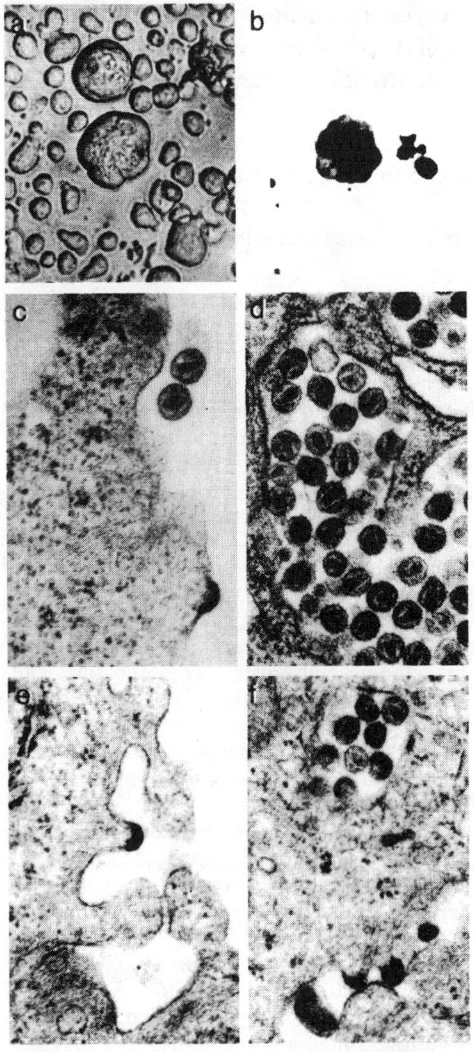

Fig. 2. Photomicrographs of HUT-78 cells infected with STLV-III. (a) Cytopathic effect of STLV-III infection of HUT-78 cells. (b) Large multinucleated cell after hematoxylin and eosin staining. (c) Electron micrograph of a portion of an STLV-III infected HUT-78 cell in which there is a single, budding retrovirus particle and two mature, extracellular particles with dense cylindrical nucleoids. Preformed, cytoplasmic, A-type particles were not observed. (d) Numerous mature, retrovirus particles with dense cylindrical nucleoids resembling HTLV-III. (e) Electron micrograph of a portion of a lymphocyte from a lymph node of Mm 239-82 in which there is a single retrovirus particle budding from the cell membrane. (f) Electron micrograph of a portion of the same cell as in (e) in which there are several tangentially sectioned, budding retrovirus particles and an aggregate of mature extracellular particles with dense, cylindrical nucleoids.

of a characteristic cytopathic effect (Fig. 2, a and b). Infected HUT-78 cells became pleomorphic, and multinucleated giant cells were formed. The multinucleated giant cells appeared quite similar to those previously described for HT cells that had been infected with HTLV-III (*1*). Furthermore, like HTLV-III, but unlike HTLV-I and -II, filtered cell-free supernatants from cells infected with the new macaque virus isolates could infect

T-cell cultures with high efficiency. Unlike type D retroviruses (*16*), these new retrovirus isolates did not replicate detectably in Raji cells, a B-cell line. Conversely, type D retroviruses did not replicate significantly in HUT-78 cells.

Peripheral blood lymphocytes prepared from heparinized human blood, were treated with monoclonal antibody plus complement and cell populations enriched in helper (T4) and suppressor

(T8) cells were isolated. The replication of the macaque virus in fractionated as well as unfractionated cells growing in the presence of IL-2 was determined. The new macaque retrovirus replicated efficiently in T4$^+$ cells but much less efficiently in T8$^+$ cells (Table 2). These results are similar to previous findings with HTLV-III and LAV (*17*).

Cell cultures containing high reverse transcriptase activity (Fig. 1) were processed for electron microscopy as described (*16*). The four macaque T-cell tropic retrovirus isolates displayed a similar morphology. Budding particles with the morphology of type C retroviruses were observed in infected cells (Fig. 2c). Nucleoids were seen only in those viral particles that were in the process of budding from the cell membrane; preformed nucleoids were not observed. Mature, extracellular enveloped viral particles 110 to 130 nm in diameter typically had a cylindrical nucleoid (Fig. 2d). This type of nucleoid is a characteristic of HTLV-III that is not found with HTLV-I or -II. Thus, the formation of budding particles and the morphology of extracellular particles appeared identical to that previously observed for HTLV-III (*3*). Intracytoplasmic type A particles, typically seen in type D retrovirus-infected cells, were not observed.

The histories of the four macaques from which virus was isolated may be relevant to the potential pathogenicity of this virus and are summarized in Table 1. A rhesus monkey (*Macaca mulatta*), designated Mm251-79, died with a lymphoma 26 months after inoculation with minced tissue from a spontaneous *M. mulatta* lymphoma (*18*). Inoculation of seven macaques with minced Mm251-79 lymphoma tissue resulted in the death (range, 47 to 511 days; median, 63 days)

Table 2. STLV-III replication occurs preferentially in T4$^+$ lymphocytes.

Cell population*	Infection†	Reverse transcriptase activity (cpm)‡	
		Day 9	Day 15
Unseparated	STLV-III	34,631	12,141
	None	537	281
T4-enriched	STLV-III	33,905	6,853
	None	574	344
T8-enriched	STLV-III	4,537	237
	None	526	297

*Human peripheral blood lymphocytes (PBL) were treated twice with monoclonal antibody to T4 (19Thy5D7) + complement (C) or monoclonal antibody to T8(7PT3F9) + C, stimulated in vitro with phytohemagglutinin for 3 days, and then similarly treated a third time. Cell staining and fluorescence-activated cell-sorter analysis of these populations after the last treatment demonstrated that the unseparated PBL were comprised of 80 percent T11$^+$, 48 percent T4$^+$, and 29 percent T8$^+$ lymphocytes; the T4-enriched PBL were 72 percent T11$^+$, 72 percent T4$^+$, and 0 percent T8$^+$ lymphocytes; the T8-enriched PBL were 68 percent T11$^+$, 1 percent T4$^+$, and 63 percent T8$^+$ lymphocytes. †Cell populations were incubated for 3 days with aliquots of culture medium containing cell-free virus or control medium, washed, and then maintained in culture with IL-2, the cell number being adjusted to 1 × 10^6/ml every 3 to 4 days. Growth of these cell populations was comparable during the course of this experiment. ‡Assay performed as described (legend to Fig. 1) on supernatants sampled immediately prior to addition of fresh IL-2 and adjustment of cell concentration; cpm, count/min.

of all seven animals with one or more of the following opportunistic infections: candidiasis, generalized cytomegalovirus (CMV), and cryptosporidiosis. Two of these animals were described in more detail previously (*19*). These findings were consistent with an immune deficiency disorder. Pooled blood samples from three of these seven animals were inoculated into an additional six animals with similar results; all six animals died 50 to 65 days after inoculation. Filtered, cell-free plasma from one of these six animals (Mm61-82) was inoculated into Mm220-82 and Mm239-82, both of which died 71 and 85 days later, respectively, with oroesophageal candidiasis, cryptosporidiosis, intestinal trichomoniasis, and multifocal perivascular macrophage infiltrates in the brain. Retrovirus was isolated, not only from viably frozen splenocytes of the original Mm251-79 but also from serum frozen for longer than 1 year from the time of death of Mm220-82 and Mm239-82.

HTLV-III has recently been detected in the brains of AIDS encephalopathy patients (20). Histopathologic features of the brain lesions of Mm220-82 and Mm239-82 appeared similar to brain lesions sometimes seen in AIDS encephalopathy. Extensive electron microscopic examination of thin sections of lymph nodes taken from Mm220-82 and Mm239-82 just prior to death revealed budding and extracellular retrovirus particles indistinguishable in morphology from HTLV-III (Fig. 2, e and f).

Virus was also isolated from a living rhesus monkey Mm142-83. This monkey had lymphadenopathy, splenomegaly, hemoglobin of 6.8 g/dL, and a peripheral blood smear demonstrating atypical lymphocytosis and monocytosis. Peripheral blood lymphocytes from this animal exhibited depressed blastogenic responses after in vitro stimulation with pokeweed mitogen, xenogeneic cells, and *Candida* antigen. The ratio of helper to suppressor T lymphocytes (T4/T8) of this animal was 1.2. Mm142-83 had no connection with the transmission study described above. The retrovirus was isolated from Mm142-83 on two separate occasions, 4 months apart. Mm142-83 died 3 weeks after the second virus isolation.

In a separate study, the antigens of this newly isolated macaque retrovirus have been shown to be closely related to the proteins previously defined for HTLV-III (21). Since the morphology, growth characteristics, and antigenic properties of the new macaque retrovirus clearly indicate that it is similar to HTLV-III, we refer to this virus as simian T-lymphotropic virus type III (STLV-III) of macaques.

The STLV-III isolates described in this report cannot be due to HTLV-III introduced artificially through cell culture contamination or infection by HTLV-III–inoculated animals; HTLV-III has never been present in the laboratories where STLV-III was isolated nor have animals been inoculated with HTLV-III or AIDS material at NERPRC. Thus, these macaques were naturally infected with STLV-III.

We have readily isolated type D retrovirus from NERPRC macaques with an immune deficiency syndrome (16, 22), and type D retroviruses have also been isolated from macaques at other centers where immune deficiency syndromes are endemic (10, 23). However, experimental infection of naive macaques with D/New England isolates did not induce any features suggestive of the immune deficiency syndrome (24). Three of the four samples which yielded STLV-III (Mm251-79, Mm220-82, and Mm239-82) did not yield type D retrovirus upon cocultivation with Raji cells and with canine thymus cells (cell lines which are the most sensitive for type D retrovirus recovery) (10, 16). Cell-free supernatants from the four T-cell lines producing STLV-III did not yield a type D retrovirus when incubated with Raji and canine thymus cells. We were also not able to isolate type D retrovirus from the Mm61-82 filtered plasma used for inoculation of Mm220-82 and Mm239-82 nor from blood samples of Mm220-82 or Mm239-82 themselves on five separate occasions following inoculation, including those taken at the time of death. Continued investigation will be needed to determine the roles of STLV-III and type D retrovirus in spontaneous disease in our colony.

Studies of the pathogenesis of AIDS as well as the development of an effective vaccine would be aided if HTLV-III had the ability to infect and cause disease in a laboratory animal. However, attempts to infect nonhuman primates other than chimpanzees with HTLV-III have generally been unsuccessful (25). Because of the endangered status of chimpanzees, their use for this purpose will probably be limited. If STLV-III is indeed pathogenic in macaques, useful approaches to the development and testing of a vaccine for AIDS may emerge.

References and Notes

1. M. Popovic *et al.*, *Science* **224**, 497 (1984).
2. R. Gallo *et al.*, *ibid.*, p. 500.
3. J. Schüpbach *et al.*, *ibid.*, p. 503.
4. M. Sarngadharan *et al.*, *ibid.*, p. 506.
5. B. Safai *et al.*, *Lancet* **1984-I**, 1438 (1984).
6. F. Brun-Vezinet *et al.*, *Science* **226**, 453 (1984).
7. Center for Disease Control, *Morbid. Mortal. Weekly Rep.* **33**, 661 (1984).
8. N. Letvin *et al.*, *Proc. Natl. Acad. Sci. U.S.A.* **80**, 2718 (1983); N. King *et al.*, *Am. J. Pathol.* **113**, 382 (1983); L. Chalifoux *et al.*, *Lab. Invest.* **51**, 22 (1984).
9. R. Henrickson *et al.*, *Lancet* **1983-I**, 388 (1983); R. Henrickson *et al.*, *Lab. Anim. Sci.* **34**, 140 (1984).
10. K. Stromberg *et al.*, *Science* **224**, 289 (1984).
11. I. Miyoshi *et al.*, *Lancet* **1982-II**, 658 (1982); M. Hayami *et al.*, *ibid.* **1983-II**, 620 (1983); G. Hunsmann *et al.*, *Int. J. Cancer* **32**, 329 (1983); T. Ishida *et al.*, *Microbiol. Immunol.* **27**, 297 (1983); N. Yamamoto *et al.*, *Lancet* **1983-I**, 240 (1983); I. Miyoshi *et al.*, *Int. J. Cancer* **32**, 333 (1983); M. Hayami *et al.*, *ibid.* **33**, 179 (1984).
12. T. Homma *et al.*, *Science* **225**, 716 (1984).
13. I. Miyoshi *et al.*, *Gann* **73**, 848 (1982); *Lancet* **1983-I**, 166 (1983); N. Yamamoto *et al.*, *J. Gen. Virol.* **65**, 2259 (1984); N. Yamamoto *et al.*, *Int. J. Cancer* **34**, 77 (1984); A. Komuro *et al.*, *Virology* **30**, 373 (1984).
14. A. Gazdar *et al.*, *Blood* **55**, 409 (1980); J. Gootenberg *et al.*, *J. Exp. Med.* **154**, 1403 (1981).
15. M. Popovic, E. Read-Connole, R. Gallo, *Lancet* **1984-II**, 1472 (1984).
16. M. Daniel *et al.*, *Science* **223**, 602 (1984).
17. D. Klatzmann *et al.*, *ibid.* **225**, 59 (1984); A. Dalgleish *et al.*, *Nature (London)* **312**, 763 (1984).
18. R. Hunt *et al.*, *Proc. Natl. Acad. Sci. U.S.A.* **80**, 5085 (1983).
19. N. Letvin *et al.*, *Lancet* **1983-II**, 599 (1983).
20. G. Shaw *et al.*, *Science* **227**, 177 (1985).
21. P. Kanki *et al.*, *ibid.* **228**, 1199 (1985).
22. R. Desrosiers *et al.*, *J. Virol.* **54**, 552 (1985).
23. P. Marx *et al.*, *Science* **223**, 1083 (1984).
24. N. Letvin *et al.*, *J. Virol.* **52**, 683 (1984).
25. H. Alter *et al.*, *Science* **226**, 549 (1984); D. Gajdusek *et al.*, *Lancet* **1984-I**, 1415 (1984); D. Gajdusek *et al.*, *ibid.* **1985-I**, 55 (1985); Center for Disease Control, *Morbid. Mortal. Weekly Rep.* **33**, 442 (1984).

26. We thank H. Robinson for suggestions on the reverse transcriptase assay; E. Reinherz and S. Schlossman for providing monoclonal antibodies; D. Schmidt, J. Yetz, J. MacKey, and M. Elliott for technical expertise; and B. Blake for editorial assistance. Supported by NIH grants AI20729, CA38205, CA13885, and CA37466; by a training grant in veterinary and comparative pathology 5T32 RR07000; by the Division of Research Resources RR00168; and by a contract from the Massachusetts Department of Public Health.

19 February 1985; accepted 12 April 1985

Report

7 June 1985

90.   Serologic Identification and Characterization of a Macaque T-Lymphotropic Retrovirus Closely Related to HTLV-III

P.J. Kanki, M.F. McLane, N.W. King, Jr., N.L. Letvin, R.D. Hunt, P. Sehgal, M.D. Daniel, R.C. Desrosiers, and M. Essex

The human T-lymphotropic retroviruses (HTLV) are a group of related exogenous agents that preferentially infect helper T lymphocytes. There are three known types. HTLV-I is characterized by its widespread yet geographically distinct distribution; in endemic regions it has been closely linked with the development of a unique lymphoma of mature T cells designated the adult T-cell leukemia/lymphoma (ATLL) (*1*). HTLV-II is closely related to the type I virus, but its distribution and relation to human disease has not been established (*2*). HTLV-III, also known as LAV and ARV, is the prototype virus isolated from patients with the acquired immune deficiency syndrome (AIDS) (*3, 4*). Thus, it appears that at least two members of this virus family are highly associated with different types of human diseases that include a malignancy and an ablative disorder of the same T4$^+$ lymphocyte population.

The existence of a virus related to HTLV-I in nonhuman primates was first reported by Miyoshi and his colleagues (*5*). Studies with healthy Japanese macaques, *Macaca fuscata*, indicated that various proportions of healthy adults (of this species) had antibodies that reacted with HTLV-I–related antigens. Type C retroviruses that were presumably responsible for this activity were then detected in lymphoid cultures established from seropositive animals (*6*). Subsequent serologic studies have demonstrated the presence of antibodies to HTLV-I in Asian and African Old World primate species, whereas New World primates and prosimians have been uniformly seronegative (*7, 8*). Proviral sequence analyses of viruses derived from seropositive baboons, African green monkeys, and *Macaca* species indicate that the nonhuman primate viruses are closely related to, yet distinct from, HTLV-I (*9*).

We recently reported an association between exposure to an HTLV-I–related virus and the development of spontaneous lymphoma and lymphoproliferative disorders in three species of macaques. Antibodies highly cross-reactive with HTLV-I–related antigens were detected by means of membrane immunofluorescence (MIF) and radioimmunoprecipitation (RIP) techniques (*8*). Macaque sera that were MIF-positive immunoprecipitated the same major HTLV-I proteins encoded by the *gag* and *env* genes that had previously been identified and characterized for the human virus (*8, 10*).

The lymphoma could be transmitted in vivo to other macaques by inoculation of tumor cell suspensions and karyotypic analysis of the tumors so induced confirmed successful transmission by an infectious agent (*11*).

In other studies involving the inoculation of materials from a macaque with lymphoma, the induction of clinical and histopathologic features of macaque immune deficiency syndrome was observed (*11–13*). That this syndrome could be induced so easily prompted us to direct our efforts toward the identification of an HTLV-type virus from macaques with immune deficiency syndromes. We report here on the serologic identification and characterization of a new macaque retrovirus that has striking similarities to the human AIDS virus HTLV-III; we therefore refer to it as the simian T-lymphotropic virus of macaques related to HTLV-III (STLV-III) (*12*).

The viral-related proteins were identified by radioimmunoprecipitation and sodium dodecyl sulfate–polyacrylamide gel electrophoresis (RIP/SDS-PAGE) of [^{35}S]cysteine-labeled whole cell lysates of virus-infected cells. One reference cell line used was HUT-78/STLV-III (HUT-78 cells that were infected with STLV-III), a stable producer of the primate T-lymphotropic virus related to human HTLV-III (*12*). The uninfected HUT-78 cells represent a well-characterized mature human T-cell line (*12, 14*). All sera were similarly reacted with antigens prepared from the HTLV-III–infected human H9 reference cell line (*3, 4*). Human reference positive sera with known reactivity to all HTLV-III type–specific proteins, and monoclonal antibodies directed to p24, the major core protein of HTLV-III, were also subjected to RIP with the same cells (*4, 15*). Serum sam-

ples from representative macaques were included with serum from rhesus macaque Mm251-79, from which the virus was isolated. The four representative human and macaque sera that were positive for precipitation of either HTLV-III proteins or STLV-III proteins, or both, were prescreened for antibodies by MIF as described (*10, 15*) and found to be positive (four of four) on both types of infected cells but negative on the uninfected cells.

The major antigens recognized by antibody-positive human sera from patients with AIDS-related complex (ARC) have previously been described for the H9/HTLV-III cell line (*4, 15*). Monoclonal antibodies to the p24 of HTLV-III recognized a 24-kD species on H9/HTLV-III but not on the uninfected H9 line (Fig. 1A). Human reference positive sera from ARC patients precipitated 160-, 120-, 55-, and 24-kD species and these were not recognized by a human reference negative serum. A representative serum sample from the MIF-antibody–positive macaque Mm251-79, from which STLV-III was isolated, recognized a 55-kD and a 24-kD species upon reaction with H9/HTLV-III cell lysates, but not from lysates prepared from the control H9 cells.

HUT-78/STLV-III and uninfected HUT-78 cell lines were metabolically labeled with S[^{35}S]cysteine according to the same procedure (*10, 15*) and RIP of whole cell lysates was performed with the same sera as described above (Fig. 1B). Monoclonal antibody to p24 of HTLV-III recognized a 24-kD species in the STLV-III–infected antigen preparation. Human ARC reference serum positive for HTLV III proteins immunoprecipitated a 55-kD and 24-kD species on the STLV-III–infected HUT-78 cell line where weak reactivity to the 120- and

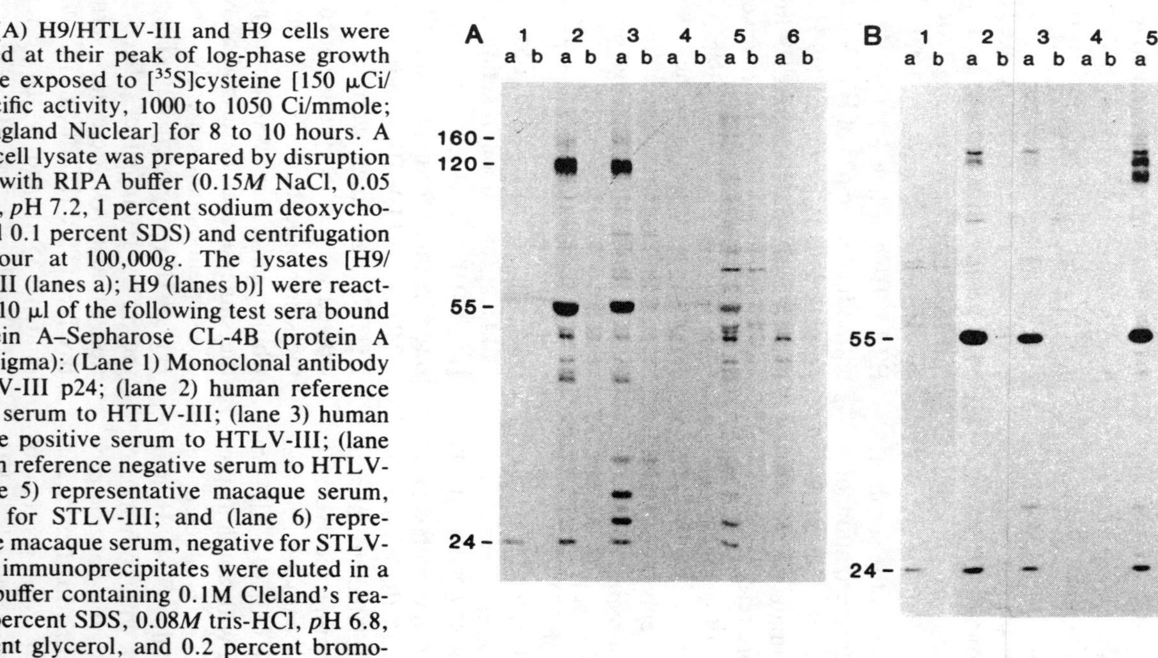

Fig. 1. (A) H9/HTLV-III and H9 cells were harvested at their peak of log-phase growth and were exposed to [^{35}S]cysteine [150 μCi/ml; specific activity, 1000 to 1050 Ci/mmole; New England Nuclear] for 8 to 10 hours. A soluble cell lysate was prepared by disruption of cells with RIPA buffer (0.15M NaCl, 0.05 tris-HCl, pH 7.2, 1 percent sodium deoxycholate, and 0.1 percent SDS) and centrifugation for 1 hour at 100,000g. The lysates [H9/HTLV-III (lanes a); H9 (lanes b)] were reacted with 10 μl of the following test sera bound to protein A–Sepharose CL-4B (protein A beads, Sigma): (Lane 1) Monoclonal antibody to HTLV-III p24; (lane 2) human reference positive serum to HTLV-III; (lane 3) human reference positive serum to HTLV-III; (lane 4) human reference negative serum to HTLV-III; (lane 5) representative macaque serum, positive for STLV-III; and (lane 6) representative macaque serum, negative for STLV-III. The immunoprecipitates were eluted in a sample buffer containing 0.1M Cleland's reagent, 2 percent SDS, 0.08M tris-HCl, pH 6.8, 10 percent glycerol, and 0.2 percent bromophenol blue by boiling at 100°C or 2 minutes. Samples were analyzed in a 10.0 percent acrylamide resolving gel with a 3.5 percent stacking gel according to the discontinuous buffer system of Laemmli (*19*). (B) HUT-78/STLV-III (lanes a) and uninfected HUT-78 (lanes b) cell lysates were prepared as described above. (Lane 1) Monoclonal anti-p24 HTLV-III; (lane 2) human reference positive serum to HTLV-III; (lane 3) human reference positive serum to HTLV-III; (lane 4) human reference negative serum to HTLV-III; (lane 5) representative macaque serum, positive for STLV-III; (lane 4) representative macaque serum, positive for STLV-III; and (lane 7) representative macaque serum, negative for STLV-III.

160-kD species was also observed. Similar species were not detected with uninfected HUT-78 cells. Proteins of the same size were immunoprecipitated by representative macaque sera including MIF antibody-positive sera taken from Mm251-79. The same serum samples reacted positively with the major *gag*-related proteins of HTLV-III. Human reference negative sera and representative negative macaque serum did not react with the STLV-III viral antigen preparation. Human sera with previously determined serologic reactivity to HTLV-I viral proteins failed to recognize STLV-III viral proteins in either MIF or RIP assays. Reference antisera to HTLV-I and macaque sera containing antibodies to the macaque virus that is related to HTLV-I (*8*) were also seronegative with STLV-III.

The same human and macaque serum samples were reacted with glycoproteins prepared from HUT-78/STLV-III cells by using lentil-lectin affinity chromatography (Fig. 2). Human positive reference sera and macaque positive sera similarly recognized two protein species from the eluate fraction that migrated at approximately 160 and 120 kD; these were not recognized by reference negative sera. The high molecular weight HTLV-III proteins gp160 and gp120 are glycosylated and encoded by the *env* region of the HTLV-III genome (*15, 16*). Seroepidemiologic studies indicate that these are the most immunogenic protein species recognized by antibody-positive humans exposed to HTLV-III (*15, 16*).

These data indicate that the viral proteins immunoprecipitated from the STLV-III–infected cell line are of the same molecular sizes as those seen for HTLV-III, and that the larger species (gp120 and gp160) are apparently glyco-

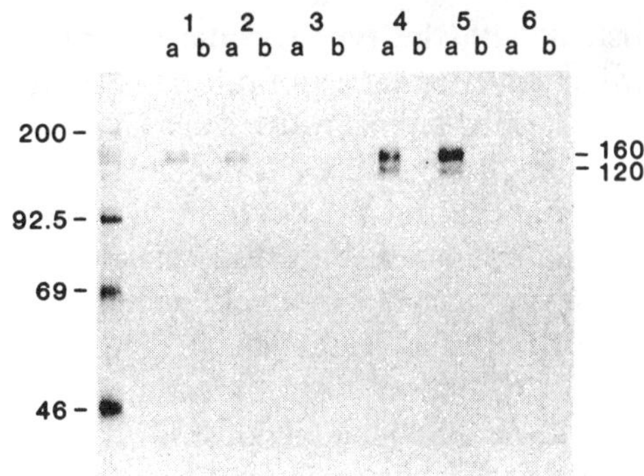

Fig. 2. Reactivity of serum samples with the glycoprotein preparation of HUT-78/STLV-III and uninfected HUT-78 (*10*). The glycoproteins were prepared from soluble cell lysates of HUT-78/STLV-III (lanes a) and HUT-78 (lanes b) made with RIPA buffer lacking sodium deoxycholate. The lysates were passed through a lentil-lectin–Sepharose CL-4B (Pharmacia, Sweden) column at a ratio of 20×10^6 cells to 1 to 2 ml of undiluted lentil-lectin–Sepharose Cl-4B. The glycoproteins were eluted from the column with a buffer consisting of 0.15*M* NaCl, 0.05*M* tris-HCl, *p*H 7.2, 1 percent Triton X-100, and 0.2*M* methyl-α-D-mannoside. The eluted bound fraction was reacted with 10 μl of test sera that had been bound to protein A beads. The same sera was used in lane 1 to 6, respectively, as described for lanes 2 to 7 in Fig. 1B. The immunoprecipitates were eluted from protein A beads and subjected to SDS-PAGE, as described above.

sylated as they are for HTLV-III. Although the high molecular weight glycoproteins of HTLV-III are the most immunogenic antigens in exposed humans, sera from STLV-III antibody–positive macaques showed minimal reactivity to these proteins, indicating an apparent one-way cross-reactivity of antibodies directed to these glycoproteins. STLV-III may thus be distinct from HTLV-III, at least to the degree of the type-specific immunoreactivity to the *env*-encoded glycoproteins. This observation is consistent with the type-specific nature of *env*-encoded antigens of other previously described animal retroviruses.

From Mm251-79 we obtained tumor cells and cell-free preparations that were inoculated into seven rhesus macaques. All seven macaques, which were previously free of disease, succumbed to a variety of opportunistic infections with clinical signs and pathologic lesions similar to those observed in spontaneous immune deficiency disease of macaques (*11–13*). Other STLV-III isolates were obtained from three rhesus macaques with clinical or histopathologic features of an immunosuppressive disorder (*12*). We therefore hypothesize that this virus may be immunosuppressive and etiologically linked to the macaque immune deficiency syndrome. Type D retroviruses have been isolated at the New England Regional Primate Research Center (NERPRC) and at two other primate colonies where spontaneous immune deficiency syndromes in macaques have been described (*17*). Three of the four macaques from which MTLV-III isolates were obtained were apparently free of the type D retrovirus on the basis of repeated unsuccessful isolation attempts (type D retrovirus was recovered from Mm142-83) (*12*). There have been no studies at the NERPRC involving inoculation of HTLV-III or AIDS materials into any primates, nor have HTLV-III–infected cell lines been maintained at this facility. The inadvertent inoculation of multiple macaques or contamination of cell cultures therefore seems highly unlikely.

Serologic studies of macaques at the NERPRC indicate that at least some animals possess antibodies reactive to both HTLV-I and HTLV-III proteins. Three of four macaques that yielded STLV-III isolates were also seropositive for the HTLV-I–related virus of macaques (Mm251-79, Mm239-82, and Mm220-82). There are at least two possible explanations for this observation. The existence of three distinct members of the HTLV family has been established in humans; it is therefore possible that analogous macaque T-lymphotropic virus types could also exist and multiply infect a given animal. Second, cross-reactivity between antibodies directed to different HTLV types has been demonstrated and is presumably due in part to *env* gene conservation between HTLV types (*18*). Therefore, it is conceivable that some of the macaques in our study that had antibodies to an HTLV-I–related agent also had antibodies to STLV-III that were cross-reactive to the same conserved epitopes of the two viruses. Macaques with both HTLV-III– and HTLV-I–related viruses should provide useful models for studies of this family of viruses. The availability of a nonhuman primate naturally infected with a virus related to HTLV-III may facilitate studies of the pathogenesis and treatment or prevention of AIDS.

Noted added in proof: In seroepidemiologic studies of a variety of African primate species we have noted that a significant number of healthy African green monkeys (*Ceropithecus aethiops*) possess antibodies reactive to the STLV-III viral proteins described herein, and that these show significant cross-reactivity with viral proteins of HTLV-III. This observation may be significant with regard to our understanding of the origin of HTLV-III and the pathobiology of AIDS in Africa (*20*).

References and Notes

1. B. Poiesz *et al., Proc. Natl. Acad. Sci. U.S.A.* **77**, 7415 (1980); M. S. Reitz, Jr., *et al., ibid.* **78**, 1887 (1981); H. M. Rho *et al., Virology* **112**, 335

(1981); V. S. Kalyanaraman *et al.*, *J. Virol.* **38**, 906 (1981); B. J. Poiesz *et al.*, *Nature (London)* **294**, 268 (1981); Y. Hinuma *et al.*, *Proc. Natl. Acad. Sci. U.S.A.* **78**, 6476 (1981); I. Miyoshi *et al.*, *Nature (London)* **296**, 770 (1981); M. Yoshida, I. Miyoshi, Y. Hinuma, *Proc. Natl. Acad. Sci. U.S.A.* **79**, 2031 (1982).
2. V. S. Kalyanaraman *et al.*, *Science* **218**, 571 (1982).
3. M. Popovic *et al.*, *Science* **224**, 497 (1984); S. Z. Salahuddin *et al.*, *ibid.*, p. 500.
4. J. Schüpbach *et al.*, *ibid.*, p. 503; M. G. Sarngadharan *et al.*, *ibid.*, p. 506.
5. I. Miyoshi *et al.*, *Gann* **73**, 848 (1982); *Lancet* **1982-II**, 658 (1982).
6. I. Miyoshi *et al.*, *Lancet* **1981-I**, 1016 (1981); *ibid.* **1982-II**, 166 (1982); Y. Ohtsuki *et al.*, *Arch. Virol.* **8**, 329 (1984).
7. M. Hayami *et al.*, *Lancet* **1983-II**, 620 (1983); G. Hunsmann *et al.*, *Int. J. Cancer* **32**, 329 (1983); T. Ishida *et al.*, *Microbiol. Immunol.* **27**, 297 (1983); N. Yamamoto *et al.*, *Lancet* **1983-I**, 240 (1983); I. Miyoshi *et al.*, *Int. J. Cancer* **32**, 333 (1983); M. Hayami *et al.*, *ibid.* **33**, 179 (1984); W. C. Saxinger *et al.*, in *Human T-cell Leukemia Viruses*, R. C. Gallo, M. Essex, L. Gross, Eds. (Cold Spring Harbor Laboratory, Cold Spring Harbor, N.Y., 1984), p. 323.
8. T. Homma *et al.*, *Science* **225**, 716 (1984).
9. H.-G. Guo, F. Wong-Staal, R. C. Gallo, *ibid.* **223**, 1195 (1984); N. Yamamoto *et al.*, *Int. J. Cancer* **34**, 77 (1984); M. Hayami, personal communication; A. Komuro *et al.*, *Virology*, in press.
10. T. H. Lee *et al.*, *Proc. Natl. Acad. Sci. U.S.A.* **81**, 3856 (1984); *Science* **226**, 57 (1984).
11. R. D. Hunt *et al.*, *Proc. Natl. Acad. Sci. U.S.A.* **80**, 5085 (1983).
12. M. D. Daniel *et al.*, *Science* **228**, 1201 (1985).
13. N. L. Letvin *et al.*, *Proc. Natl. Acad. Sci. U.S.A.* **80**, 2718 (1983); N. W. King, R. D. Hunt, N. L. Letvin, *Am. J. Pathol.* **113**, 382 (1983).
14. A. F. Gazdar *et al.*, *Blood* **55**, 409 (1980); B. J. Poiesz *et al.*, *Proc. Natl. Acad. Sci. U.S.A.* **77**, 6815 (1980).
15. L. W. Kitchen *et al.*, *Nature (London)* **312**, 367 (1984); F. Barin *et al.*, *Science* **228**, 1094 (1985).
16. J. Allan *et al.*, *Science* **228**, 1091 (1985).
17. M. D. Daniel *et al.*, *ibid.* **223**, 602 (1984); K. Stromberg *et al.*, *ibid.* **224**, 289 (1984); P. A. Marx, *ibid.* **223**, 1083 (1984).
18. T. H. Lee *et al.*, *Proc. Natl. Acad. Sci. U.S.A.* **81**, 7579 (1984).
19. J. K. Laemmli, *Nature (London)* **227**, 680 (1970).
20. P. J. Kanki *et al.*, in preparation.
21. We thank R. C. Gallo for the reference cell cultures, M. G. Sarngadharan for monoclonal antibody to HTLV-III p24, and J. Groopman for human reference sera from patients with ARC. This research was supported by NIH Institutional Research Service Award 5TRRR07000; NIH grants CA37466, CA18216, AI20729, and CA38205; Division of Research Resources grant RR00168; and a contract from the Massachusetts Department of Public Health.

19 February 1985; accepted 12 April 1985

Report

7 June 1985

91. Naturally Occurring Antibodies Reactive with Sperm Proteins: Apparent Deficiency in AIDS Sera

Toby C. Rodman, Jeffrey Laurence, Fred H. Pruslin, Nicholas Chiorazzi, and Ronald Winston

In the course of our studies on the proteins of mammalian spermatozoa (*1*), we have identified a set of immunoglobulin M (IgM) antibodies in human serum that, although immunologically reactive with defined components of human sperm, appear to be normal constituents of circulating Ig's. This inference is based on the finding that these antibodies are present in more than 99 percent of the sera from healthy males and females ranging in age from 1 day to 40 years and from those hospitalized for other than diseases of the immune system (Table 1).

The possibility that antigens derived from sperm may have a role in the patho-

Table 1. Presence or absence of IgM antibody reactive with acrosomal cap region of human sperm in sera from individuals with and without (control) AIDS or ARC.

Group	Status or type of donor	Sera examined (number)	Sera positive for IgM antibody* (number)	Sera negative for IgM antibody*	
				Number	Percent
	Homosexual males				
AIDS or at risk for AIDS	No symptoms	14	11	3	21
	ARC	45	30	15	33
	AIDS	20	12	8	40
	Others†				
	No symptoms	9	8	1‡	
	ARC	3	3	0	
	AIDS	1	0	1‡	
	Total	92	64	28	
Control	Adult males§	45	44	1	
	Adult females§	35	35	0	
	Hospitalized adults‖	21	21	0	
	Hospitalized children¶	30	30	0	
	Total control	131	130	1	

*IgM antibodies reactive with acrosomal cap region of human sperm (see Fig. 1).   †Intravenous drug users, hemophiliacs, and infants born to women with AIDS.   ‡Female prostitute.   §Sera obtained from routine medical examination (sexual preference not known.)   ‖From miscellaneous hospital admissions (for diseases other than of the immune system).   ¶Ages, 1 day to 2 years; hospitalized for other than immune system diseases.

genesis of the acquired immune deficiency syndrome (AIDS) in homosexual men has been proposed, with the expectation that elevated titers of sperm-specific antibodies would be detectable in the sera of these individuals (2). However, rather than elevated titers, we have detected absence or marked deficiency of the naturally occurring, sperm-reactive IgM antibodies in sera of 40 percent of patients diagnosed with AIDS, 33 percent of patients with AIDS-related complex (ARC), and 21 percent of homosexual men at risk for AIDS but without symptoms of the disease (Table 1).

The relative specificity of the IgM antibody deficiency is indicated by the observation that the total concentration of IgM antibody in these sera is within the normal range. Further, serial specimens of serum from each of two patients showed a distinct correlation between absence of the IgM antibodies and deterioration of the immune system. These data suggest a relation between the immune-suppressive aspect of AIDS and its prodromes and deficiency of antibodies reactive with, but not likely to have been elicited by, sperm.

The more general implication of these observations is that specific subsets of antibodies in human serum may have a role in immune regulation and may be vulnerable to challenge by foreign proteins bearing epitopes with which the antibodies are reactive. Accordingly, we have attempted to characterize the subset of sperm-reactive IgM antibodies present in normal and deficient in AIDS-related sera and of the molecular entities of human sperm with which the antibodies are reactive. A semen specimen from either of two donors with a high count of motile, morphologically normal sperm was used for cytologic study (3), and pooled specimens from eight donors were used for biochemical studies. All control sera (Table 1) were examined for reactivity with human sperm smears by indirect immunofluorescence with heterologous antibodies to the human M, G, and A isotypes (4). When assayed in this manner, the sperm neck and tail were stained nonspecifically and with variable intensity by each Ig antibody. However, the acrosomal cap region of the head was stained only with the IgM antibody; the postacrosomal region of the head did not stain (Fig. 1, A, B, and C). Staining of the acrosomal cap region with this antibody was abolished by treating the sperm with Triton X-100 (Fig. 1D). Staining of the neck and tail regions with any of the Ig antibodies was not abolished by this treatment. The characterization of the set of antibodies reactive with sperm heads as IgM was confirmed by a "double sandwich" immunofluorescence procedure with monoclonal antibodies to human IgM or IgG (5). Thus, human serum appears normally to contain a set of antibodies, specifically characterized as IgM, that bind to moieties in the acrosomal cap region of human spermatozoa. The proteins bearing those reactive epitopes are soluble in Triton X-100.

Sera of AIDS patients and of individuals at risk for AIDS were examined by the immunofluorescence procedure and showed variable staining of the sperm neck and tail regions, but the IgM staining of the acrosomal cap region was absent as noted in Table 1 (see Fig. 1E). Immunoreactivity was estimated on the basis of intensity of fluorescence at serum dilutions of 1:5 to 1:40; a negative designation was made when there was no acrosomal cap staining at a serum dilution of 1:5 (Fig. 1E). Intensity of fluorescence was generally lower in sera from children (see Fig. 1, A and B); however, there was no ambiguity of designation of a serum as negative because any acrosomal cap fluorescence, even at low intensity, was accentuated by the absence of staining in the postacrosomal region. All negative and 10 percent of the positive sera (Table 1) were reexamined in a blind fashion; no discrepancy was observed.

The results of the immunofluorescence procedure were confirmed by immunoblots of electropherograms of sperm head proteins that were soluble in Triton X-100 (6). Sera designated as positive by immunofluorescence were reactive with a series of polypeptides in the molecular weight range of 29 to 95 kilodaltons, representing less than 10 percent of the bands on the stained electropherogram (Fig. 2, lane 2). Reactivity was displayed on the immunoblot with the IgM antibody and not with the IgG antibody. Sera designated as negative by immunofluorescence showed no reactivity on the immunoblots (see Fig. 2, lane f). With the exceptions noted (Fig. 2), the positive sera of all subjects (Table 1) were reactive with the same bands. We conclude, therefore, that a discrete set of IgM antibodies normally present in human serum binds to epitopes on a specific subset of proteins from human sperm.

Total concentrations of circulating IgM in sera from AIDS patients or those at risk for AIDS that were deficient in the specific IgM antibodies reactive with sperm head proteins were within the limits of the normal range (7), which is consistent with previous reports (8) that isohemagglutinin as well as IgM titers are normal or elevated in sera of AIDS or

ARC patients. These observations suggest that the deficiency represents depletion of specific classes of IgM antibodies rather than an overall impairment of IgM production.

The possibility that the presence or absence of the sperm-reactive IgM antibodies may be related to the severity of the immune-deficient state of the patient is supported by two case histories (Fig.

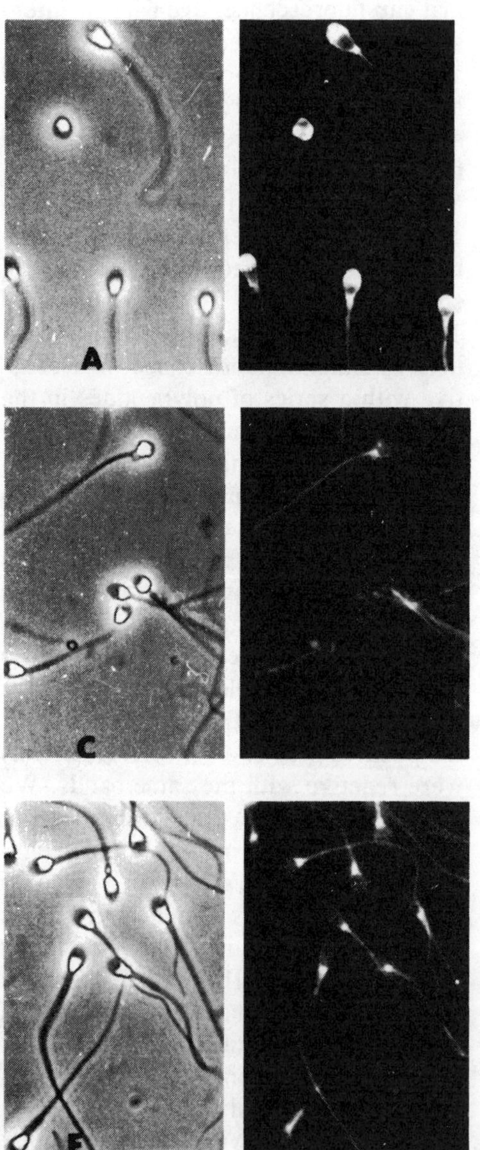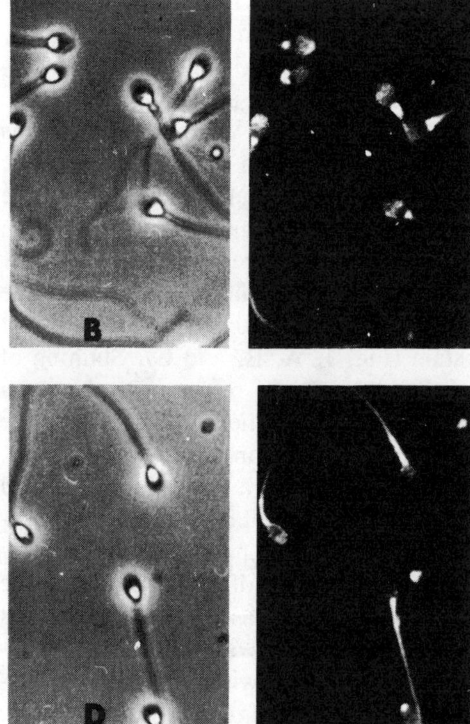

Fig. 1. Indirect immunofluorescence of human sperm with antibodies in human serum. (A) Serum from an adult, heterosexual male developed with FITC-conjugated antiserum to human IgM. (B) Serum from a 10-month-old female (pediatric serum) developed with FITC-conjugated antiserum to human IgM. (C) Same serum as (A) developed with FITC-conjugated antiserum to human IgG. (D) Sperm treated with Triton X-100, same procedure as (A). (E) Serum from a male homosexual with AIDS developed with FITC-conjugated antiserum to human IgM. All sera were used at 1:5 dilution. The acrosomal cap staining indicates a high titer of the specific IgM antibodies in the adult male serum, a lower titer in the pediatric serum, and absence in the AIDS serum.

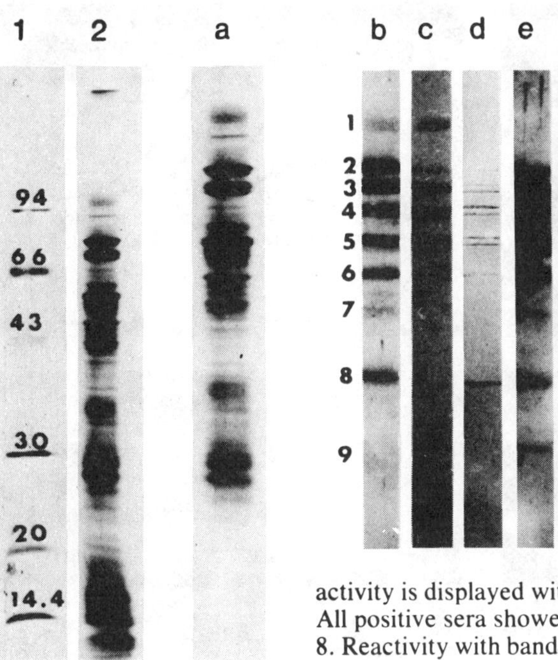

Fig. 2. (Lane 1) Molecular weight markers; (lane 2) SDS–polyacrylamide gel electrophoresis of fraction of sperm head proteins soluble in Triton X-100; (lane a) enlarged excerpt of lane 2. (Lanes b to f) Immunoblots with human sera and peroxidase-conjugated antibody to human IgM. (Lane b) Serum from a normal female; (lane c) serum from a normal heterosexual male; (lane d) pediatric serum; (lane e) serum from a homosexual male with AIDS (antibody-positive; see Table 1); (lane f) serum from a homosexual male with AIDS (antibody-negative; see Fig. 3B). All sera were used at 1:50 dilution. Reactivity is displayed with nine polypeptide bands (or doublets). All positive sera showed reactivity with bands 2, 3, 4, 5, 6, and 8. Reactivity with bands 1, 7, and 9 was detectable in some sera at apparently low titer, suggesting that it may be present at still lower, nondetectable titers in the others.

3). In case 1, the initial serum specimen, taken from a homosexual male with ARC, was positive for the IgM antibodies reactive with the acrosomal cap region of sperm heads (Fig. 3A). The second serum specimen, taken 11 months later when a diagnosis of AIDS with *Pneumocystis carinii* was established 1 month before the death of the patient (*9*), was devoid of those antibodies (Fig. 3B). In case 2, a serum specimen from a homosexual male with ARC contained no IgM antibodies reactive with the acrosomal cap region of sperm heads (Fig. 3C). A specimen taken 1 month later was still negative (Fig. 3D). The clinical and immunologic status of the patient, however, showed progressive improvement (*10*), and a serum sample taken 6 months after the first signs of remission showed that the IgM antibodies reactive with sperm heads were restored (Fig. 3E).

Thus, the decline in the clinical status of patient 1 was correlated with depletion of the antibodies, and clinical improvement in patient 2 was correlated with restoration of the antibodies.

Studies were carried out in vitro to determine whether the sperm proteins recognized by circulating IgM antibodies (Fig. 2) display immunomodulatory properties. A fraction of sperm head proteins soluble in Triton X-100 was chromatographed on a Sephadex G-50 column by elution with phosphate-buffered saline (PBS; *p*H 7.2), and the fractions were tested for effect on phytohemagglutinin (PHA) stimulation of T-cell mitogenesis (Fig. 4). A marked inhibitory effect by fractions 50 to 60 was observed. Repeated experiments with various quantities of the fraction of sperm head proteins soluble in Triton X-100, examined for both PHA- and poke-

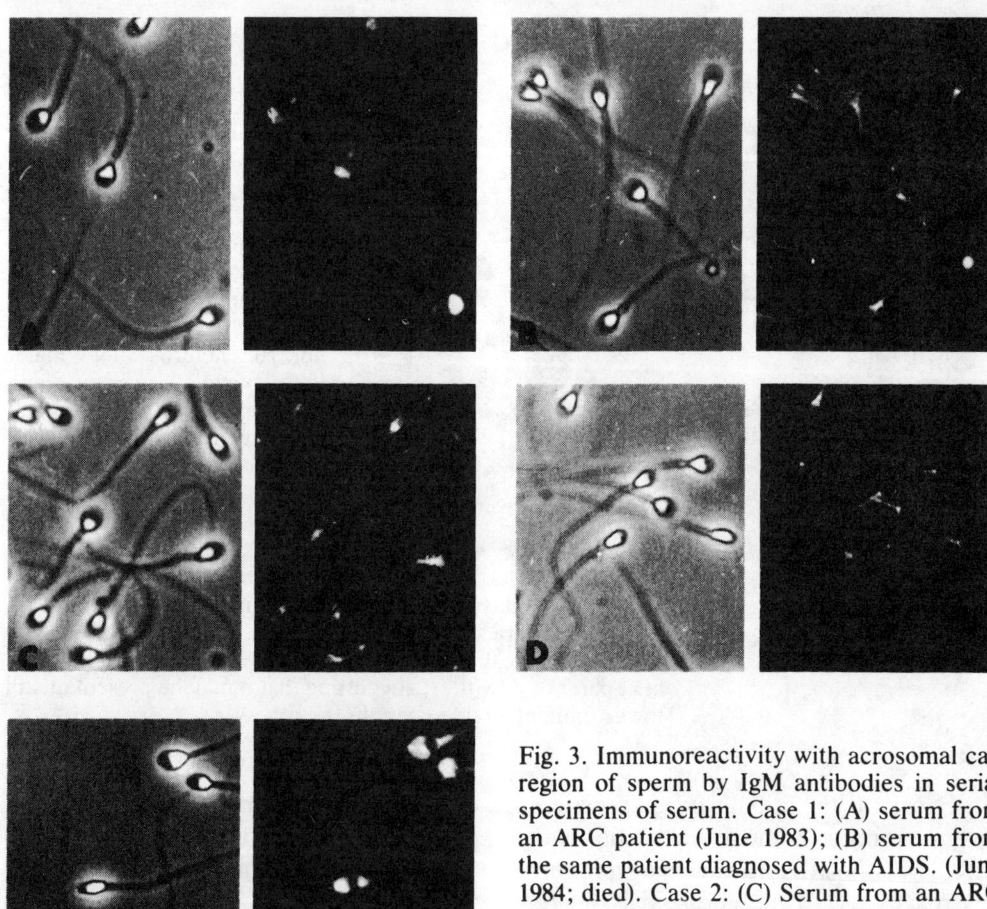

Fig. 3. Immunoreactivity with acrosomal cap region of sperm by IgM antibodies in serial specimens of serum. Case 1: (A) serum from an ARC patient (June 1983); (B) serum from the same patient diagnosed with AIDS. (June 1984; died). Case 2: (C) Serum from an ARC patient (June 1983); (D) serum from the same patient (July 1983); (E) serum from the same patient (November 1983; symptoms and clinical status improved) (*11*).

weed mitogen–induced DNA synthesis confirmed this observation.

Because proteins were also distributed in other fractions of the chromatogram, it was relevant to determine which fractions included the antigenic moieties recognized by the circulating IgM antibodies and whether concordance of antigenicity and inhibition of T-cell mitogenesis could be shown. The fractions were segregated into seven pools (Table 2), the protein content of each pool was

determined, and the immunoreactivity of two normal adult sera with each pool was assayed (Table 2). The major part (~90 percent) of the reactivity between the fraction of sperm head proteins soluble in Triton X-100 and the IgM antibodies of human sera was due to the proteins segregated in fractions 50 to 60 (Fig. 4). Thus, a subset of proteins in the acrosomal cap region of human sperm, which includes a factor (or factors) displaying an immunomodulatory property in vitro, is reactive with a subset of IgM antibodies that appear to be components of the normal set of circulating antibodies.

Considerable evidence has linked a human T-cell leukemia virus–lymphadenopathy-associated virus to the etiolo-

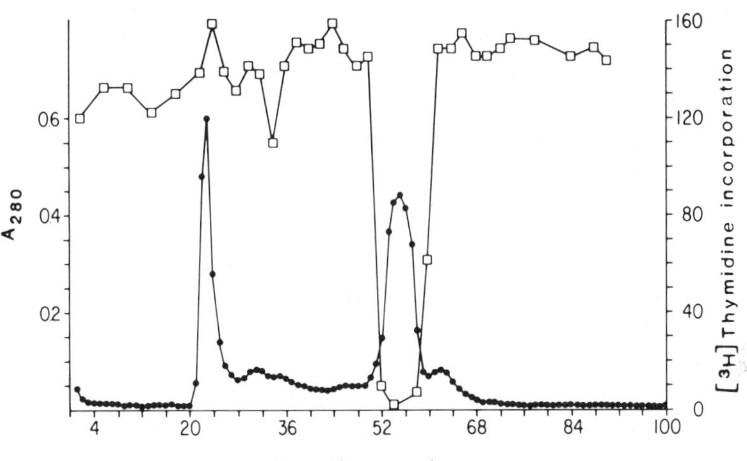

Fig. 4. Proteins of sperm heads soluble in Triton X-100, chromatographed on a Sephadex G-50 column. The 100 fractions were tested for inhibition of PHA-stimulated T-lymphocyte mitogenesis as described (15). Symbols: ($\square$) [^{3}H]thymidine incorporation (with no sperm protein added, specific activity, 140×10^3 count/min); ($\bullet$) protein concentration.

Table 2. Results of radioimmunoassay (2) of the reactivity of subfractions of sperm head proteins soluble in Triton X-100 (see Fig. 4) with IgM antibodies in normal human serum. ^{125}I-labeled goat antibody to human IgM was used as a probe. The total immunoreactivity of each pool was calculated as follows: $A_M \times M = R_t$, where A_M is the activity (in counts per minute) in 5 μg of protein, M is the amount of protein (in micrograms) in the pool, and R_t is the total reactivity. We have assumed a linear relation for the activity in 5 μg of protein, but even if this is not the case, the data show (i) that the immunoreactivity between the IgM antibodies and the fraction of sperm head proteins soluble in Triton X-100 is distributed similarly among the subsets of that fraction of proteins in the two normal human sera and (ii) that the major part of this reactivity (~90 percent) is in the proteins in pool 5. The fractions (see Fig. 4) were grouped as follows: pool 1, fractions 1 to 20; pool 2, fractions 21 to 28; pool 3, fractions 29 to 36; pool 4, fractions 37 to 49; pool 5, fractions 50 to 60; pool 6, fractions 61 to 68; and pool 7, fractions 69 to 100.

Fraction	M	Serum 1		Serum 2	
		A_M	R_t	A_M	R_t
Total		5261		5483	
Pool 1	15	17	50	14	42
2	1875	503	1.9×10^5	470	1.8×10^5
3	270	440	2.4×10^4	388	2.2×10^4
4	225	405	1.8×10^4	379	1.7×10^4
5	2115	5483	2.4×10^6	5568	2.4×10^6
6		14			
7		14			
No protein		18			

gy of AIDS (*11*). However, although antibodies to one or another of the variants of that virus are detectable in sera of more than 30 percent of symptom-free homosexual men and more than 80 percent of those with ARC, only a small proportion of those proceed to AIDS (*12*). Thus, as is frequently stated (*13*), the epidemiological data suggest that the assault by the virus requires a predisposing or cooperative factor.

Because spermatozoa are characterized by a number of specific components, many of which are formed de novo after the individual has attained sexual maturity, sperm-specific moieties are believed to have a high potential for immunogenicity. During anal intercourse, sperm are introduced into milieux where that potential may be maximized (*14*), and some investigators have sought to identify sperm antibodies in the sera of homosexual men at risk for AIDS as evidence of an immunogenic cofactor in the disease (*2*).

In view of our data, a distinction should be made between antibodies elicited by sperm and antibodies immunologically reactive with, but not elicited by, sperm moieties. We have identified a set of IgM antibodies that are clearly of the latter class. Their distribution in the general population (Table 1) suggests that these antibodies are not the result of sperm-induced immunity but are normal constituents of human serum and thus may be components, possibly regulatory, of the immune system.

A relation between deficiency in those IgM antibodies and impairment of the immune system is shown in Table 1 and Fig. 3, and immunologic reactivity between a discrete subset of IgM antibodies and a specific subset of sperm-derived proteins is shown in Fig. 2. A dichotomy is suggested because sperm

moieties may be implicated in the pathogenesis of AIDS. Thus, one hypothesis suggested by these observations is that certain IgM antibodies may have a role in maintaining immunologic homeostasis, and the introduction or an overload of the proteins with which a specific set of IgM antibodies are reactive may result in disruption of an equilibrium. The immunogenic factor in AIDS, therefore, might be depletion of a critical set of IgM antibodies, thereby establishing a medium in which the AIDS-associated retrovirus may be effectively pathogenic. An alternative hypothesis would take into account the demonstrated T-cell mitogenic inhibitory property of the sperm proteins. An overload of these proteins could suppress proliferation of a specific fraction of T cells, leading to an immunodeficient state.

The question then arises as to whether a deficiency of the IgM antibodies identified in this study or of other naturally occurring antibodies can be demonstrated in sera of patients with other immune disorders. A study consisting of a broad survey of such sera is underway.

References and Notes

1. T. C. Rodman *et al.*, *J. Cell Biol.* **80**, 605 (1979); F. H. Pruslin, M. Romani, T. C. Rodman, *Exp. Cell Res.* **128**, 207 (1980); T. C. Rodman, F. H. Pruslin, V. G. Allfrey, *J. Cell Sci.* **53**, 227 (1982); F. H. Pruslin and T. C. Rodman, *Exp. Cell Res.* **144**, 115 (1983); T. C. Rodman, F. H. Pruslin, V. G. Allfrey, *ibid.* **150**, 269 (1984).
2. G. M. Mavligit *et al.*, *J. Am. Med. Assoc.* **251**, 237 (1984); S. S. Witkin and J. Sonnabend, *Fertil. Steril.* **39**, 337 (1983); G. M. Shearer and U. Hurtenbach, *Immunol. Today* **3**, 153 (1982).
3. Sperm was collected by centrifugation and then washed three times in PBS (*pH* 7.2). A drop of sperm suspension, untreated or treated with Triton X-100 [T. C. Rodman *et al.*, *Gamete Res.* **8**, 129 (1983)], was placed on a slide, air-dired, and prepared (unfixed) for indirect immunofluorescence study with human serum.
4. The fluorescein isothiocyanate (FITC)–conjugated antibodies to human Ig's were selected to provide evidence of specific antibody recognition: F(ab')₂ goat antibody to human IgM (μ chain–specific); F(ab')₂ goat antibody to human IgG (Fc fragment–specific); and affinity-purified goat antibody to human serum IgA (α chain–

specific). Use of F(ab')$_2$ fragments as the fluoresceinated probe eliminates the possibility of nonspecific reactivity of the probe with Fc receptors on sperm.

5. D. Posnett, N. Chiorazzi, H. G. Kunkel, *J. Clin. Invest.* **70**, 254 (1982).
6. A fraction of sperm heads, cleanly separated from tails, was treated with Triton X-100 without mechanical disruption of the heads (*1*). The proteins that were soluble in Triton X-100 were recovered in PBS (*p*H 7.2) as described [P. W. Holloway, *Anal. Biochem.* **53**, 304 (1973)] and subjected to electrophoresis on a sodium dodecyl sulfate gel. Blots of the separated proteins were tested with human sera and peroxidase-conjugated (goat) antibody to human IgM or IgG.
7. Total concentrations of IgM in six control sera (Table 1) were 55 to 103 mg per 100 ml and in four antibody-negative sera from patients at risk for AIDS (Table 1) were 39 to 99 mg per 100 ml. The IgM titer for the pediatric serum (Fig. 1B), which showed reactivity with sperm head proteins, was 55 mg per 100 ml; that for the AIDS serum (Fig. 1E), which showed no sperm head immunofluorescence, was 69 mg per 100 ml. Similarly, the IgM titer for the pediatric serum (Fig. 2, lane d) was 83 mg per 100 ml and that for the AIDS serum (Fig. 2, lane f and Fig. 3B) was 88 mg per 100 ml.
8. H. Masur *et al.*, *N. Engl. J. Med.* **305**, 1431 (1981); R. W. Schroff, *et al.*, *Clin. Immunol.* *Immunopathol.* **27**, 300 (1983); A. J. Ammann *et al.*, *ibid.*, p. 315.
9. W. G. Jones, personal communication.
10. The clinical history of case 2 has been reported [J. Laurence and L. Mayer, *Science* **225**, 66 (1984); patient Sel].
11. R. C. Gallo *et al.*, *Science* **224**, 500 (1984); J. Laurence *et al.*, *N. Engl. J. Med.* **311**, 1269 (1984).
12. M. G. Sarngadharan *et al.*, *Science* **224**, 506 (1984); J. J. Goedert *et al.*, *Lancet* **1984-II**, 711 (1984).
13. G. Shearer, *Immunol. Today* **4**, 181 (1983); M. Seligman *et al.*, *N. Engl. J. Med.* **311**, 1286 (1984); R. Weiss, *Nature (London)* **309**, 12 (1984).
14. W. W. Darrow *et al.*, *Lancet* **1982-II**, 160 (1982); G. M. Shearer and A. S. Rabson, *Nature (London)* **308**, 230 (1984), G. M. Mavligit *et al.*, *J. Am. Med. Assoc.* **251**, 237 (1984).
15. J. Laurence, A. B. Gottlieb, H. G. Kunkel, *J. Clin. Invest.* **72**, 2072 (1983).
16. We thank J. Jones for technical assistance and V. G. Allfrey, D. A. Fischman, and G. W. Siskind for critical reading of the manuscript and helpful suggestions. J. L. is supported by a grant from the New York Affiliate of the American Heart Association, the New York Community Trust, and by grant CA 35018-02 from the National Institutes of Health.

25 February 1985; accepted 11 April 1985

Report

7 June 1985

92. Deregulation of Interleukin-2 Receptor Gene Expression in HTLV-I–Induced Adult T-Cell Leukemia

Martin Krönke, Warren J. Leonard, Joel M. Depper, and Warner C. Greene

The type C retrovirus, human T-lymphotropic virus, type I (HTLV-I), has been identified as the etiologic agent in adult T-cell leukemia (ATL) (*1*). HTLV-I infection of human T cells is uniformly associated with expression of large numbers of cellular receptors for interleukin-2 (IL-2) (*2*, *3*). Together, IL-2 and its cellular receptor play an essential role in the control of normal T-cell growth (*4*). The relation of IL-2 receptor expression to HTLV-I infection is still unexplained. However, since most ATL cell lines do not transcribe IL-2 messenger RNA (mRNA) nor secrete IL-2, an autocrine growth model based on the continuous interaction of IL-2 with its receptor is unlikely (*5*). Furthermore, there is evidence that the IL-2 receptor is not the cellular receptor mediating entry of the HTLV-I virus (6). The finding that HTLV-I is not integrated at unique sites within the human genome argues against IL-2 receptor gene activation by adjacent insertion of HTLV-I promoter-enhancer sequences (7). We (8) and others (9) have recently isolated complementary DNA's (cDNA's) encoding the human IL-2 receptor. Using these IL-2 receptor cDNA probes, we have studied the deregulated expression of the IL-2 receptor gene in HTLV-I–infected T lymphocytes.

To investigate the possibility that IL-2 receptor expression reflects constitutive synthesis of IL-2 receptor mRNA, we used ^{32}P-labeled IL-2 receptor cDNA to analyze total cellular RNA from five ATL cell lines by Northern blotting. Each of these ATL lines constitutively expressed IL-2 receptor mRNA species similar in size to those present in mitogen-activated normal T cells (Fig. 1).

In an attempt to detect subtle differences between IL-2 receptor mRNA species from ATL cells and those from normal T cells, which might not have been evident in the Northern blotting analyses, we performed S1 nuclease protection studies with IL-2 receptor mRNA obtained from normal T cells and ATL cells (Fig. 2). As reported earlier (8), the formation of mature IL-2 receptor mRNA involves extensive post-transcriptional processing, including alternate splicing and the use of at least two, and probably three, separate polyadenylation [poly(A)] sites. In a first set of experiments, we used the Eco RI–Nae I cDNA fragment of pIL-2R3, corresponding to 910 base pairs (bp) at the 5′ end of the published sequence of pIL-2R3 (8). This fragment contains an internal 216-bp segment that may be removed by alternate splicing (8, 9). Each of the ATL cell lines, like normal activated T cells, expressed both spliced and unspliced forms of IL-2 receptor mRNA's (Fig. 2). The spliced mRNA was detected in the S1 nuclease protection assay by identifying two fragments of sizes 549 bp and 155 bp, indicating the lack of protection

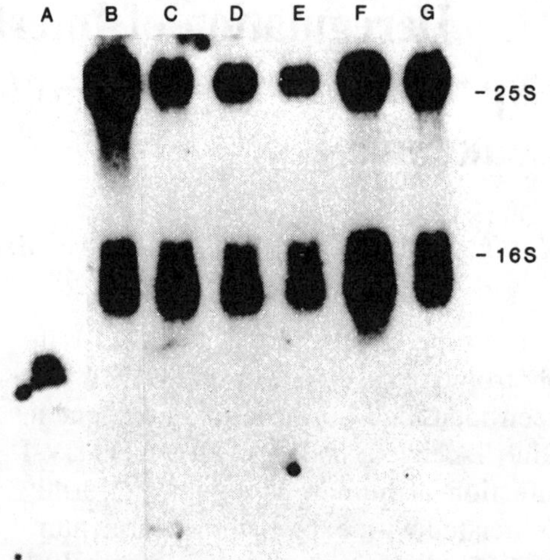

Fig. 1. Northern blot analysis of IL-2 receptor mRNA expression in normal T cells and ATL cell lines. Normal T cells were incubated in RPMI 1640 culture medium and stimulated for 18 hours with PHA (1 μg/ml) and PMA (50 ng/ml). Total cellular RNA (10 μg) from unstimulated T cells (A), T cells stimulated with PHA and PMA (B), and ATL cell lines HUT 102 (C), PL/P6 (D), C91/PL (E), MJ (F), and C5/MJ (G) were size-fractionated on formaldehyde-agarose gels, transferred to nitrocellulose filters, and hybridized to pIL2R2 and pIL2R4 cDNA probes (8) labeled with ^{32}P by nick translation. The origin and cell surface phenotype of these cell ATL lines have been described (3).

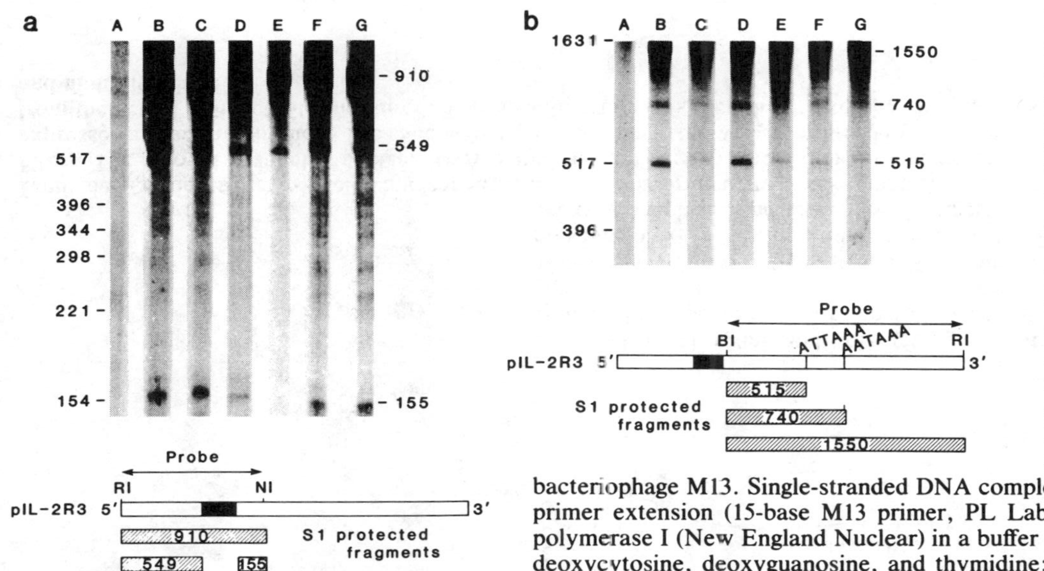

Fig. 2. S1 nuclease protection assay of IL-2 receptor mRNA in normal T cells and ATL cells. Total RNA from resting T cells (A), T cells stimulated with PHA and PMA (B), HUT 102 (C), PL/P6 (D), C91/PL (E), MJ (F), and C5/MJ (G) was hybridized either to the ^{32}P-labeled single-stranded M13 IL-2 receptor "5' probe" (Eco RI–Nae I fragment, base pairs 1 to 910, left panel) or "3' probe" (Bgl I–Eco RI fragment, base pairs 785 to 2335, right panel) and subsequently digested with S1 nuclease. The solid region depicted within the IL-2 receptor cDNA clone pIL-2R3 represents the 216-bp segment that may be removed by alternate splicing (8). Size markers indicate the migration of ^{32}P-phosphorylated pBR322 Hinf I fragments. Each of the respective cDNA probes was subcloned into bacteriophage M13. Single-stranded DNA complementary to mRNA was uniformly labeled by primer extension (15-base M13 primer, PL Laboratories) using the large fragment of DNA polymerase I (New England Nuclear) in a buffer containing 1 mM each of the triphosphates of deoxycytosine, deoxyguanosine, and thymidine; 5μM deoxyadenosine triphosphate (dATP); and 2.5 $\mu M[\alpha^{32}P]$dATP (400 Ci/mmol, Amersham). After digestion with Hind III, the homogeneously labeled DNA was electrophoresed on a gel containing 5 percent polyacrylamide, 8M urea, and single-strength TBE (180 mM tris-borate, 180 mM boric acid, and 2 mM EDTA). The band corresponding in size to the desired probe was excised, electroeluted, and precipitated with ethanol. Total cellular RNA (5 μg) was then hybridized at 50°C for 16 hours to the probe (50,000 cpm) in a buffer containing 0.2M NaCl, 0.2M Pipes (pH 6.8), 5 mM EDTA, and 70 percent formamide. The reactants were then digested with 5000 units of S1 nuclease (Boehringer-Mannheim) in a buffer containing 0.25M NaCl, 30 mM sodium acetate (pH 4.4), and 1 mM ZnCl$_2$ for 30 minutes at 37°C. The samples were then analyzed on a sequencing gel prepared with 5 percent polyacrylamide, 8M urea, and single-strength TBE.

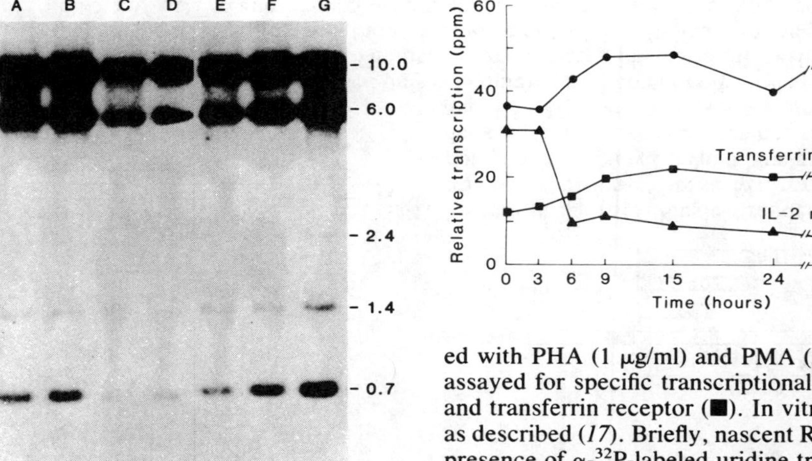

Fig. 3 (left). Southern blot analysis of HTLV-I–infected T cells from ATL patients. DNA from normal T cells (G) and from T-cell lines established from the peripheral blood of six ATL patients [YO (A), TO (B), TA (C), ST (D), SK (E), and HA (F)] was digested with Eco RI, size-fractionated on agarose gels, transferred to nitrocellulose paper, and hybridized with ^{32}P-labeled pIL2R2 and pIL2R4 cDNA probes (8). Size markers indicate migration of lambda DNA–Hind III fragments. Fig. 4 (right). Nuclear transcription assays in HUT 102 cells. HUT 102 cells were stimulated with PHA (1 μg/ml) and PMA (50 ng/ml). At the indicated times, nuclei were isolated and assayed for specific transcriptional activities of genes encoding HLA (●), IL-2 receptor (▲), and transferrin receptor (■). In vitro transcription assays with isolated nuclei were performed as described (17). Briefly, nascent RNA chains were allowed to elongate in isolated nuclei in the presence of α-^{32}P-labeled uridine triphosphate. The labeled nuclear RNA was then purified by deoxyribonuclease and proteinase K digestion, phenol extraction, and ethanol precipitation. Equivalent amounts of ^{32}P-labeled nuclear RNA were then hybridized to excess amounts of specific cDNA probes immobilized on nitrocellulose filters. The amount of labeled nuclear RNA bound to the filters was determined by liquid scintillation counting. The transcriptional activity is expressed as parts per million. The specific parts-per-million value was determined by subtracting the background hybridization to pBR322 DNA from the actual radioactivity measured. This specific value was then divided by the total input radioactive nuclear RNA (in counts per minute) and multiplied by 10^6.

within the 216-bp segment of the labeled Eco RI–Nae I fragment. The unspliced mRNA species is translated into an IL-2 binding receptor (8), but the function and the protein product encoded by the alternately spliced mRNA species are still undefined.

In a second series of S1 nuclease experiments, the 3′ Bgl I–Eco RI fragment of pIL-2R3 corresponding to base pairs 785 to 2335 (8) was used to study the RNA poly(A) signal sequences. These studies revealed three major bands, indicating the use of three different poly(A) signals. We had earlier proposed three potential poly(A) sites, including the sequence ATTAAA (A, adenine; T, thymine) at position 1298, AATAAA at position 1523, and a third site 3′ to the end of the isolated pIL-2R3 clone (8). As shown in the S1 nuclease protection assays (Fig. 2), ATL cells utilize each of these three possible poly(A) signals. Furthermore, the frequency of use does not differ substantially from that occurring in normal activated T cells. Thus, IL-2 receptor mRNA processing appears to be quite similar in normal T cells and ATL cells.

Expression of a full-length IL-2 receptor cDNA isolated from HUT 102 cells in either COS-1 (8) or L cells (10) resulted in the display of IL-2 receptors that recapitulated the abnormal receptor size characteristic of HUT 102 cells (molecular size 50 kD, compared to 55 kD in normal activated T cells). The IL-2 receptor aberrancy in the HUT 102 cell line is secondary to altered post-transcriptional processing but specific for the IL-2 receptor since other cell surface glycoproteins are processed normally (11). These findings suggest the possibility that differences in the primary structure of the normal and HUT 102 IL-2 receptor may exist. However, no unex-

pected fragments were obtained in the S1 nuclease protection assays with either mRNA from normal activated T cells or mRNA from two M13 subclones derived from the HUT 102 cDNA that spanned the entire protein coding region of the IL-2 receptor. These data suggest that the amino acid sequence of the IL-2 receptor in normal T cells and ATL cells are identical. Notwithstanding, it is possible that the S1 nuclease protection assays may fail to detect single base pair mismatches. Final resolution of the question of potential differences in the primary sequence of the IL-2 receptor in HUT 102 and normal T cells must await complete nucleotide sequence analysis of the normal IL-2 receptor gene.

To investigate whether the constitutive high-level expression of IL-2 receptor mRNA was secondary to HTLV-I–induced perturbation of the IL-2 receptor gene structure, we performed Southern blot analyses of restricted DNA extracted from leukemic T-cell lines established from the peripheral blood of six ATL patients (Fig. 3). The five Eco RI restriction fragments for the IL-2 receptor were identical in size in both the ATL and normal T cells. These data suggest that HTLV-I–associated IL-2 receptor expression is probably not due to, or associated with, IL-2 receptor gene rearrangement. Furthermore, these studies provided no evidence for selective IL-2 receptor gene amplification in the ATL cell lines studied. The single-copy IL-2 receptor gene is located on the short arm of chromosome 10 (10p14-15) (12). Karyotype analysis of several ATL cell lines has not revealed consistent translocations involving chromosome 10, suggesting that chromosomal breakage is not involved in the high-level expression of IL-2 receptors characteristic of ATL cells.

508

To further study the deregulation of IL-2 receptor gene expression in ATL cells, we used nuclear transcription assays with isolated HUT 102 nuclei (Fig. 4). In contrast to normal T cells, which must be activated with antigen or mitogen before IL-2 receptors are expressed (*13*), the IL-2 receptor gene was constitutively transcribed in HUT 102 cells. This constitutive expression of the IL-2 receptor gene may reflect direct or indirect *trans*-acting transcriptional activation by the "LOR protein" encoded by the long open reading (LOR) frame associated with the pX region of HTLV-I. Sodroski *et al.* (*14*) showed that the LOR region of HTLV-I encodes a 42-kD protein that can enhance the transcription of genes under the control of the HTLV-I long terminal repeat (LTR) in a *trans*-acting manner. These authors have speculated that the LOR protein enhances HTLV-I replication and also may activate cellular genes involved in neoplastic transformation.

In normal T cells, stimulation with phytohemagglutinin (PHA) and phorbol myristate acetate (PMA) induces transcription of the IL-2 receptor gene within 3 hours (*15*). Paradoxically, stimulation of HUT 102 cells with PHA and PMA resulted in rapid and selective inhibition of IL-2 receptor gene transcription (Fig. 4). This effect was not the result of a generalized nonspecific inhibition of gene expression, since PHA and PMA addition did not alter active transcription of genes encoding histocompatibility antigen (HLA), transferrin receptor (Fig. 4), or c-*myc* (not shown). IL-2 receptor gene transcription is a transient event in normal PHA- and PMA-activated T cells (*15*). After peak transcription at 6 hours, IL-2 receptor gene transcription gradually declines, perhaps secondary to the action of a co-induced repressor mechanism similar to that described for the IL-2 gene (*16*). The constitutive expression of the IL-2 receptor gene in ATL cells may indicate that this putative repressor system is silent. We are intrigued by a model of ATL whereby the LOR protein selectively stimulates IL-2 receptor gene transcription but fails to activate the repressor mechanism. The addition of PHA and PMA, however, may activate the repressor mechanism and result in diminished IL-2 receptor transcription. This hypothesis can be formally tested when the promoter region of the IL-2 receptor gene is isolated. Furthermore, the IL-2 receptor promoter region can be compared with the LTR of HTLV-I for possible sequence homologies and functional LOR protein-binding capacity.

Deregulated expression of genes controlling cell growth and differentiation, including cellular oncogenes, has been associated with the genesis of various neoplasms. Further study of the abnormal regulation of IL-2 receptor gene expression in ATL cells may provide important insights into the molecular mechanisms of HTLV-I–mediated leukemogenesis.

References and Notes

1. B. J. Poiesz *et al.*, *Proc. Natl. Acad. Sci. U.S.A.* **77**, 7415 (1980); V. S. Kalyanaraman *et al.*, *Nature (London)* **294**, 271 (1981).
2. W. J. Leonard *et al.*, *Nature (London)* **300**, 267 (1982); J. M. Depper *et al.*, *J. Immunol.* **133**, 1691 (1984).
3. M. Popovic *et al.*, *Science* **219**, 856 (1983).
4. D. A. Morgan, F. W. Ruscetti, R. C. Gallo, *ibid.* **193**, 1007 (1976); K. A. Smith, *Immunol. Rev.* **51**, 337 (1980).
5. S. K. Arya, R. C. Gallo, F. Wong-Staal, *Science* **223**, 1086 (1984).
6. I. Weissmann, personal communication.
7. M. Seiki, R. Eddy, T. Shows, M. Yoshida, *Nature (London)* **309**, 640 (1984).
8. W. J. Leonard *et al.*, *ibid.* **311**, 626 (1984).
9. T. Nikaido *et al.*, *ibid.*, p. 631; D. Cosman *et al.*, *ibid.* **312**, 768 (1984).
10. W. C. Greene *et al.*, *J. Exp. Med.*, in press.
11. W. J. Leonard *et al.*, *Proc. Natl. Acad. Sci. U.S.A.* **80**, 6957 (1983); Y. Wano *et al.*, *J.*

Immunol. **132**, 3005 (1984); W. J. Leonard *et al.*, *J. Biol. Chem.* **260**, 1872 (1985).
12. W. J. Leonard *et al.*, *Science*, in press.
13. R. J. Robb, A. Munck, K. A. Smith, *J. Exp. Med.* **154**, 1455 (1981).
14. J. G. Sodroski, C. A. Rosen, W. A. Haseltine, *Science* **225**, 381 (1984).
15. W. J. Leonard *et al.*, in preparation.
16. S. Efrat and R. Kaempfer, *Proc. Natl. Acad. Sci. U.S.A.* **81**, 2601 (1984).
17. M. Krönke *et al.*, *ibid.*, p. 5214.
18. We thank M. Popovic and R. C. Gallo for providing the ATL cell lines and A. McClelland for providing the transferrin receptor cDNA clone. M.K. is supported by the Deutsche Forschungsgemeinschaft.

13 February 1985; accepted 1 April 1985

93. Studies of the Putative Transforming Protein of the Type I Human T-Cell Leukemia Virus

Dennis J. Slamon, Michael F. Press, Lawrence M. Souza, Douglas C. Murdock, Martin J. Cline, David W. Golde, Judith C. Gasson, and Irvin S.Y. Chen

The human T-cell leukemia viruses, HTLV-I and HTLV-II, are closely associated with specific malignancies of T cells in humans (*1*) and are capable of transforming normal peripheral blood T lymphocytes in vitro (*2*). The putative transforming gene of these viruses, termed *x*, is located between the *env* gene and the 3′ long terminal repeat (LTR) (*3*). The proteins encoded by this gene in both HTLV-I and HTLV-II have been identified (*4, 5*). A 40-kilodalton (kD) protein called p40^{xI} and a 37-kD protein called p37^{xII} were found in cells infected with HTLV-I and HTLV-II, respectively (*4*). The same proteins have been called p42^{lor} and p38^{lor} (*5*). Attention has been focused on the biology of these proteins because of their possible role in induction of T-cell malignancies. In this report we describe studies on the amount of p40^{xI} in infected cells, the kinetics of intracellular turnover of the protein, and its subcellular localization.

Previously, we used synthetic peptides representing determinants of the predicted translation products of the *x* genes of HTLV-I and HTLV-II to generate antisera to these proteins (*4*). Earlier studies had shown that antibodies to proteins produced in bacteria via expression vectors are useful in detecting the products of viral transforming genes (*6, 7*). Here, we generated antibodies to the COOH-terminus of the p40^{xI} protein. The antiserum was tested in an immunoprecipitation assay with cells that had been infected with HTLV-I (SLB-I) and labeled with [^{35}S]methionine as described (*4*). As with the antisera to the peptides, the antiserum to the COOH-terminus recognized a 40-kD protein in HTLV-I–infected cells (Fig. 1). The antibody titers achieved in rabbits that had been injected with either the synthetic peptides or the bacterially promoted protein (fusion protein) were similar (*8*). However, in experiments with a fixed

510

amount of isotopically labeled cell lysate and an equivalent amount of antiserum, antiserum to the fusion protein was three to five times better at immunoprecipitating the $p40^{x/}$ protein than antiserum to the peptide (Fig. 1, lanes b, c, e, and f). This may have been due to the greater number of potential epitopes in the bacterially promoted 54-amino-acid $x^{/}$ polypeptide compared to the 14- or 17-amino-acid synthetic peptides. The antiserum to the promoted protein, however, did not recognize the $p37^{x//}$ protein in HTLV-II–infected cells (JLB-I). It is known that the proteins encoded by the x genes have less sequence homology at the COOH-termini than at the NH_2-termini (9).

The level of $p40^{x/}$ protein synthesis compared to that of other cellular and viral proteins in HTLV-I–infected cells was estimated by immunoprecipitation. A known amount of isotopically labeled cell lysate was assayed and the radioactivity in the 40-kD protein band was eluted, counted, and compared to the total trichloroacetic acid–precipitable material in the cell lysate (10). Approximately 0.15 percent of the total [^{35}S]methionine incorporation was associated with $p40^{x/}$. The amount of $p40^{x/}$ precipitated was not limited by the amount of antiserum in the experiment, as increasing the amount of antiserum (lane c) did not result in an increased amount of precipitated $p40^{x/}$.

The kinetics of intracellular turnover of the $p40^{x/}$ protein was determined by pulse-chase labeling experiments. HTLV-I–infected cells were labeled with

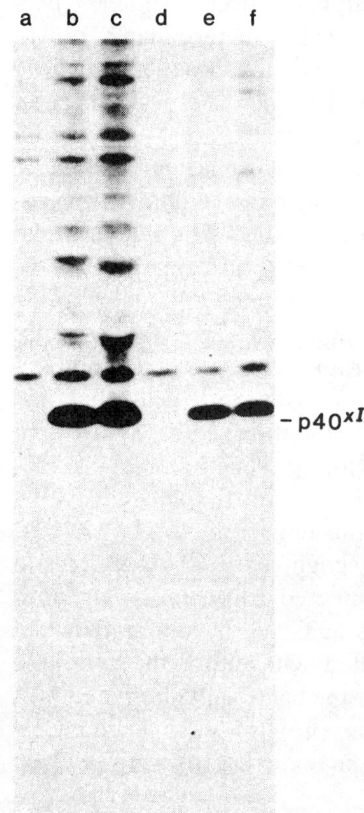

Fig. 1. Immunoprecipitation with antibodies against a $p40^{x/}$ fusion protein. The derivative "runaway" plasmid pCFM516 (25), containing a bacterial tryptophan synthetase promoter and a synthetic bovine growth-hormone (bGH) gene (26), was used to generate a bGH-$p40^{x/}$ fusion protein in *Escherichia coli*. A Sca I–Hinc II DNA fragment coding for the COOH-terminus of the $p40^{x/}$ protein was ligated into M13 mp11 (27). The COOH-terminal $p40^{x/}$ DNA fragment was excised from M13 mp11 with Sst I and Bam HI and placed in the bGH expression vector to form a fusion protein containing the NH_2-terminal 76 amino acids of bGH and the COOH-terminal 54 amino acids of the $p40^{x/}$ protein. The fusion protein was purified from bacterial whole cell lysate by SDS-PAGE (28). The purified bGH-$p40^{x/}$ fusion product was then used to immunize rabbits by the method previously described (4). Antisera were tested in an immunoprecipitation assay with HTLV-I–infected cells (SLB-I) metabolically labeled with [^{35}S]methionine for 4 hours (4). (Lane a) SLB-I cell lysate and sera from unimmunized rabbits; (lane b) SLB-I cell lysate and 5 μl of antiserum to $p40^{x/}$ fusion protein; (lane c) SLB-I cell lysate and 15 μl of antiserum to the $p40^{x/}$ fusion protein; (lane d) SLB-I cell lysate and 5 μl of sera from unimmunized rabbits; (lane e) SLB-I cell lysate and 5 μl of antiserum to the pX IV-6 peptide (4); and (lane f) SLB-I cell lysate and 15 μl of antiserum to the pX IV-6 peptide.

[^{35}S]methionine for 60 minutes, then chased with excess unlabeled methionine (Fig. 2). As a control, the half-life of a protein with known kinetics was studied in the same cells. The transferrin receptor is a 95-kD protein with a half-life of 60 hours (*11*). It is initially seen as a doublet of 95 kD and 90 kD. The smaller protein has a much shorter half-life, being converted into the larger protein within 4 hours (*11*). This pattern was demonstrable in the HTLV-I–infected cells. With the same whole cell lysate, the half-life of the p40^{xI} protein was 120 minutes (Fig. 2).

In cellular fractionation studies, HTLV-I–infected cells were disrupted mechanically in a hypotonic detergent buffer and separated into nuclear, cytoplasmic, and membrane fractions (Fig. 3). The nuclear fraction was monitored microscopically (*12, 13*) to ensure that all intact cells had been eliminated and that only nuclei remained (Fig. 3A). How-

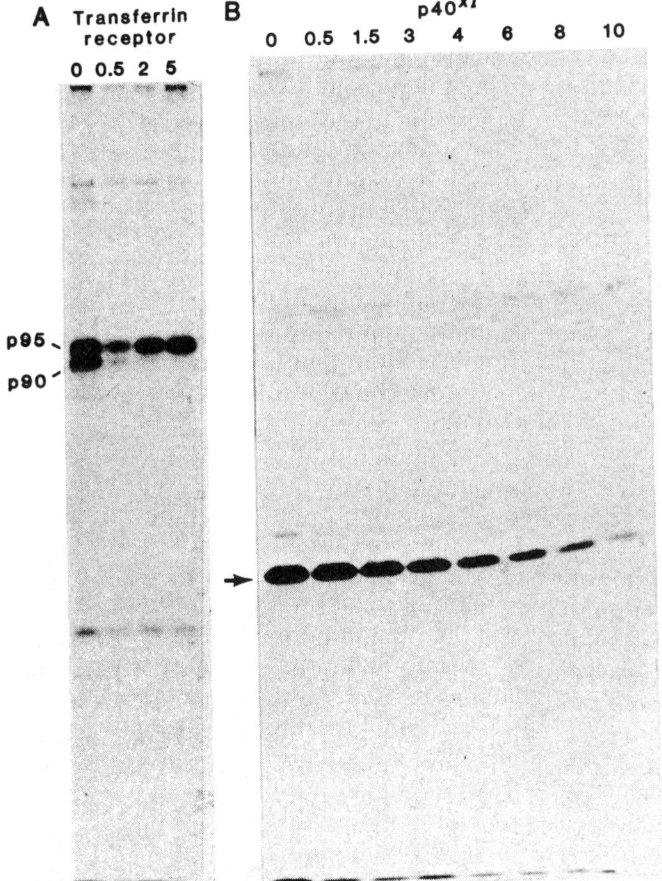

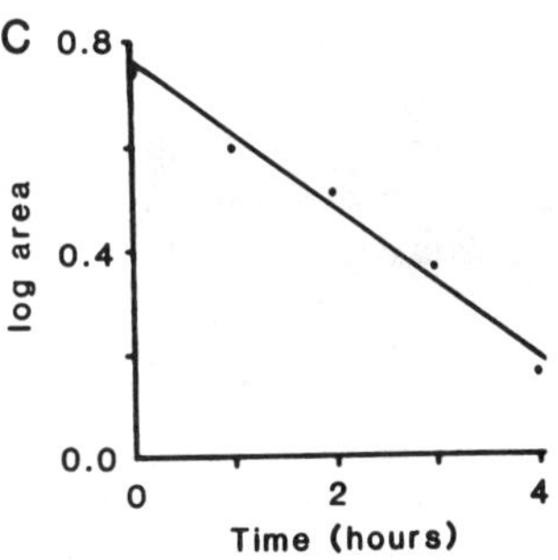

Fig. 2. (A) Kinetics of transferrin receptor turnover in HTLV-I–infected cells (SLB-I). Cells were labeled with [^{35}S]methionine for 60 minutes (*4*) and placed in culture media containing 5×10^4-fold excess of unlabeled methionine for the time periods designated at the top of the gel (in hours). The decrease in intensity in the signal seen at 30 minutes is due to loss of some of the precipitated labeled pellet before it was loaded on the gel; however, the absence of the 90-kD protein in the 2- and 5-hour lanes is still readily apparent. (B) Kinetics of turnover of p40^{xI} in HTLV-I–infected cells (SLB-I). Cells were labeled as above and chased in medium containing unlabeled methionine for the designated periods of time (in hours). Arrow indicates p40^{xI}. The resulting radioautograph was subjected to soft laser densitometry scanning and the rate of disappearance of the p40^{xI} signal corresponded to a half-life of 120 minutes (C).

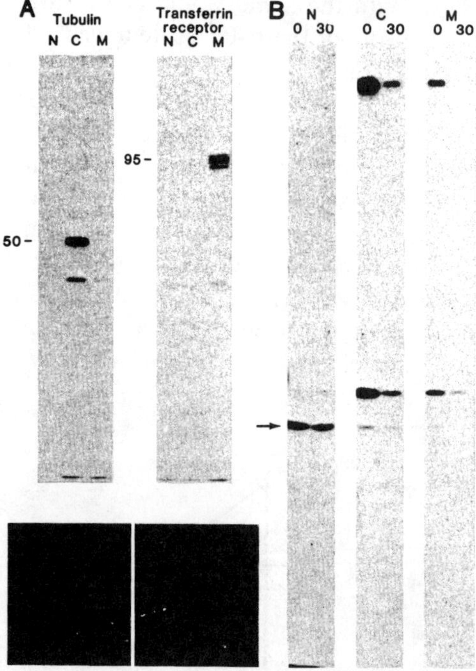

Fig. 3. (A) Subcellular localization of the p40^{xI} protein; N, nucleus; C, cytoplasm; M, membrane. HTLV-I–infected cells were labeled for 2 hours and fractionated with a modification of a previous method (29). In brief, 2×10^7 cells in hypotonic homogenization buffer (5 mM KCl, 1 mM MgCl$_2$, 20 mM Hepes, pH 7.4) were disrupted with 30 strokes in a glass dounce homogenizer (0.002 inches clearance). The lysate was centrifuged at 1000 rev/min for 5 minutes at 4°C and the nuclear pellet was further clarified by centrifugation (1100 rev/min, 6 minutes, 4°C) through 200-μl sucrose cushion (30 percent sucrose, 1 mM EDTA, 25 mM tris, pH 7.5). The pellet was washed once in a Kyro EOB detergent buffer (30) and a sample was examined microscopically to assess purity. (Bottom left) Cells before lysis; (bottom right) nuclei after lysis. The nuclear pellet was then lysed in RIPA buffer (4), passed through a 25-gauge needle, and subjected to immunoprecipitation with either 1 μl of monoclonal antiserum to tubulin or 2 μl of a monoclonal antiserum to the transferrin receptor. The supernatant from the initial dounce homogenization, containing the cytoplasmic and membrane fractions, was centrifuged (40,000 rev/min in a Beckman Ty65 rotor, 1 hour, 4°C) to produce a pellet of the membrane fragments. The resulting supernatant was designated the cytoplasmic fraction. Both the cytoplasmic and membrane fractions were placed in RIPA buffer (4) and analyzed by immunoprecipitation assay. (B) Subcellular localization of the p40^{xI} protein. Lysates described in (A) were also immunoprecipitated with the antiserum to p40^{xI} fusion protein. Most of the p40^{xI} protein (arrow) was found in the nuclear fraction of cell lysates after either 2 hours of metabolic labeling or 2 hours of labeling and 30 minutes of chase with cold methionine.

ever, microscopic evaluation cannot be used to reliably determine the integrity of cytoplasmic and membrane fractions. Immunoprecipitation studies with lysates from all three fractions and an antiserum to a known cytoplasmic protein, tubulin, resulted in detection of a 50-kD protein corresponding to the size of human tubulin (14) in the cytoplasmic fraction, but not in the nuclear or membrane fractions (Fig. 3a). Likewise, immunoprecipitation with antiserum directed against a known membrane protein, the transferrin receptor, resulted in detection of a 90- and 95-kD protein in the membrane, but not in the nuclear or cytoplasmic fractions (Fig. 3a). Immunoprecipitation of lysates with antiserum to p40^{xI} showed that most of this protein in HTLV-I–infected cells is in the nucleus, with smaller amounts of p40^{xI} found in the cytoplasmic and membrane fractions (Fig. 3b). Since we have demonstrated that the nuclear fraction was not appreciably cross-contaminated with cytoplasmic or membrane proteins, this result can be interpreted as true nuclear localization of the p40^{xI} protein.

We confirmed the nuclear localization of p40^{xI} by incubating antiserum to p40^{xI}

with fixed, frozen sections of HTLV-I–infected cells and then subjecting the sections to an indirect immunoperoxidase staining procedure. Examination of the sections by light microscopy revealed specific staining of the p40^{xl} protein in the nuclei of approximately 80 percent of the cells (Fig. 4, a and b). The intensity of staining in individual cells was variable, but all staining was nuclear. Staining did not occur when HTLV-I–infected cells were incubated with preimmune sera (Fig. 4c), nor did it occur when uninfected, transformed human T cells (MOLT-4) were incubated with antiserum to p40^{xl} (Fig. 4d).

The cytoplasmic p40^{xl} could be explained by de novo synthesis of the protein in the cytoplasm. In immunoprecipitation experiments in which we used a lactoperoxidase bead technique (Enzymobead, Bio-Rad) to iodinate outer surface membrane proteins of HTLV-I–infected cells, no p40^{xl} was found. Thus, the small amount of p40^{xl} found in the membrane fraction is not displayed on the extracellular membrane.

Finally, to determine if any of the p40^{xl} protein was a component of the virion itself, we purified extracellular virus from the culture medium of HTLV-I–infected cells, disrupted the viral particles, and labeled the component virion proteins with ^{125}I. These proteins were then subjected to immunoprecipitation either with patient sera that were reactive with *gag* proteins or with antiserum to p40^{xl} and analyzed by sodium dodecyl sulfate–polyacrylamide gel electrophoresis (SDS-PAGE). The p24 *gag* proteins of the virions were easily detected (Fig. 5, lane b). However, p40^{xl} protein was not observed (Fig. 5, lane a), indicating that the p40^{xl} is not packaged in detectable amounts in the HTLV-I virus.

Our data show that an antiserum to the bacterially promoted COOH-terminus of the x^l gene product of HTLV-I recognized the same 40-kD protein that was identified by antisera to potential epitopes from the NH$_2$-terminus (*4*). This confirms that the 40-kD protein is the gene product of the x gene. Because the synthetic peptides used to generate antisera against the NH$_2$-terminus of the protein were from epitopes upstream of the first methionine in the x open reading frame of HTLV-I, we predicted that the 40-kD protein represented the product of a spliced messenger RNA consisting predominantly of x sequences, as well as 5′ viral sequences (*4*). This has been confirmed with data indicating that a methionine initiation codon from *env* and one nucleotide of the next codon is spliced to the x open reading frame (*15, 16*). From this information, the exact size of the protein encoded by the x message is predicted to be 39.89 kD, which is consistent with the 40-kD protein identified previously (*4*) and studied in greater detail here.

By means of cellular fractionation techniques as well as immunocytochemistry, most of the intracellular p40^{xl} protein was found to be in the nucleus of transformed cells (Figs. 3 and 4). The subcellular localization of p40^{xl} to the nucleus places the protein in a cellular compartment consistent with its proposed function as a *trans*-acting enhancer of gene transcription (*17–19*).

The half-life of the p40^{xl} protein is relatively short (120 minutes) (Fig. 2), which is what might be expected for a protein with regulatory function. Proteins encoded by two other transforming viruses, the *myc* protein of the MC-29 virus and the E1A protein of adenovirus are involved in regulation of gene tran-

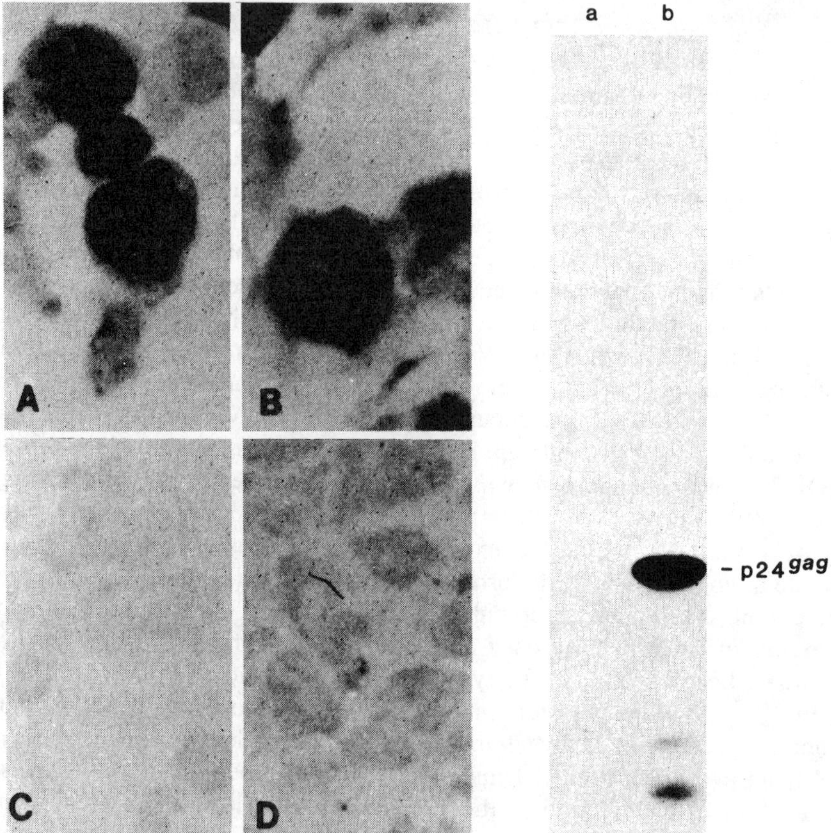

Fig. 4 (left). Immunocytochemical localization of the p40^{x1} protein in HTLV-I–infected cells (SLB-I) with an indirect immunoperoxidase technique (*31*). Antiserum to the p40^{x1} fusion protein was diluted 1:25, 1:50, or 1:100 and absorbed with both rat liver powder and human immunoglobulin G (IgG) and applied to frozen sections of cells that had been fixed with 95 percent alcohol, acetone, picric acid–paraformaldehyde (*32*), or periodate-lysine-paraformaldehyde (*33*). This was followed by treatment with goat antibody to rabbit IgG coupled to peroxidase (Sternberger-Meyer, 1:25 dilution). Each application of antiserum was followed by three 5-minute washes in phosphate-buffered saline (PBS), and treatment with a solution of diaminobenzidine (0.6 mg/ml) and 0.03 percent H_2O_2 in PBS. (A) Specific staining for p40^{x1} in SLB-I cells that had been incubated with antiserum to the bGH-p40^{x1} fusion protein. (B) Occasional cells had large, clear, unstained intranuclear areas which were interpreted as nucleoli. (C) SLB-I cells that were incubated with pre-immune sera and stained. (D) MOLT-4 (a transformed human T-cell line not infected with HTLV-I) were incubated with the antiserum to p40^{x1} and stained.   Fig. 5 (right). Extracellular HTLV-I virus was obtained from 1.5 liters of culture supernatant of SLB-I cells. The media was filtered through gauze and centrifuged (18,000 rev/min, Beckman type 19 rotor 2.5 hours, 4°C). The pellet was collected in cold TEN buffer (10 mM tris, 1 mM EDTA, 100 mM NaCl, pH 7.4) and gently homogenized. The virus was then purified by banding on a 20 to 50 percent sucrose gradient and the viral band was harvested and dialyzed against TEN buffer overnight at 4°C. Virus was pelleted by centrifugation (30,000 rev/min, SW40 rotor, 1 hour, 4°C) and disrupted into individual viral proteins (*34*). Protein concentration was determined with the Bio-Rad protein assay and 1 μg was iodinated by a modification of the chloramine-T method (*35*). The disrupted virion proteins (3 × 10^6 count/min) were immunoprecipitated with (lane a) 10 μl of the antiserum to p40^{x1} fusion protein or (lane b) 10 μl of sera from patients with adult T-cell leukemia which recognize the p24 *gag* proteins.

scription (*20*). Both of these proteins also have short half-lives (*21, 22*), and both are found in the nuclei of infected cells (*12, 23, 24*).

If the $p40^{xI}$ protein is responsible for activation of the viral LTR and for viral gene transcription as postulated (*17–19*), a remaining question is how viral transcription is initially carried out in newly infected cells before the *x* gene is transcribed. At least two possibilities exist: (i) like reverse transcriptase, the $p40^{xI}$ protein may be packaged in the virion, thus facilitating viral gene transcription upon infection, or (ii) low levels of gene transcription occur in the absence of the $p40^{xI}$ protein and subsequently increase as the amount of $p40^{xI}$ increases. We found no detectable levels of $p40^{xI}$ protein in disrupted viral particles (Fig. 5), which argues against the first possibility. Moreover, we have found that low levels of viral transcription do occur in the absence of the x^{II} gene in HTLV-II–infected cells (*18*). A similar mechanism is likely for HTLV-I–infected cells.

It has been postulated that the product of the *x* gene interacts with viral LTR sequences to facilitate viral gene transcription. This function may also activate a cellular gene or genes involved in T-cell proliferation, thus inducing malignancy.

Note added in proof: After submission of this manuscript, Goh *et al.* published results in agreement with Fig. 3b of this study, that is, nuclear localization of the *x* protein (*36*).

References and Notes

1. B. J. Poiesz *et al.*, *Proc. Natl. Acad. Sci. U.S.A.* **77**, 7415 (1980); Y. Hinuma *et al.*, *ibid.* **78**, 6476 (1981); V. S. Kalyanaraman *et al.*, *Science* **218**, 571 (1982); A. Saxon, R. H. Stevens, D. W. Golde, *Ann. Intern. Med.* **88**, 323 (1978).
2. I. Miyoshi *et al.*, *Nature (London)* **294**, 770 (1981); N. Yamamoto *et al.*, *Science* **217**, 737 (1982); M. Popovic *et al.*, *ibid.* **219**, 856 (1983); I. S. Y. Chen, S. G. Quan, D. W. Golde, *Proc. Natl. Acad. Sci. U.S.A.* **80**, 7006 (1983).
3. M. Seiki *et al.*, *ibid.*, p. 3618.
4. D. J. Slamon *et al.*, *Science* **226**, 61 (1984).
5. T. H. Lee *et al.*, *ibid.*, p. 57.
6. J. B. Gibbs, R. W. Ellis, E. M. Scolnick, *Proc. Natl. Acad. Sci. U.S.A.* **81**, 2674 (1984).
7. K. H. Klempnauer *et al.*, *Cell* **33**, 345 (1983).
8. Serial dilutions of the antisera to the peptide or the fusion protein antisera, respectively, were tested by means of enzyme-linked immunoadsorbent assay (ELISA) with either the appropriate synthetic peptides (pX IV-5 or pX IV-6) or the bGH-$p40^{xI}$ fusion protein serving as antigen. All antisera gave a positive reaction at a dilution of 1:100,000 but not at greater dilutions.
9. K. Shimotohno *et al.*, *Proc. Natl. Acad. Sci. U.S.A.*, in press.
10. B. D. Hames, in *Gel Electrophoresis of Proteins: A Practical Approach*, B. D. Hames and D. Rickwood, Eds. (IRL Press, Oxford, England, 1981), pp. 55–59.
11. M. B. Omary and I. S. Trowbridge, *J. Biol. Chem.* **256**, 12888 (1981).
12. H. D. Abrams, L. R. Rohrschneider, R. N. Eisenman, *Cell* **29**, 427 (1982).
13. T. Curran *et al.*, *ibid.* **36**, 259 (1984).
14. J. C. Bulinski and G. G. Borisy, *Proc. Natl. Acad. Sci. U.S.A.* **76**, 293 (1979).
15. W. Wachsman *et al.*, *Science* **226**, 177 (1984).
16. W. Wachsman *et al.*, *ibid.*, in press.
17. J. G. Sodroski, C. A. Rosen, W. A. Haseltine, *ibid.* **225**, 381 (1984).
18. I. S. Y. Chen *et al.*, *Science*, in press.
19. M. Yoshida, personal communication.
20. R. E. Kingston, A. J. Baldwin, P. A. Sharp, *Nature (London)* **312**, 280 (1984); A. J. Berk *et al.*, *Cell* **17**, 935 (1979); J. R. Nevins, *ibid.* **26**, 213 (1981); M. R. Green, R. Treisman, T. Maniatis, *ibid.* **35**, 137 (1983).
21. R. N. Eisenman *et al.*, *Mol. Cell. Biol.* **5**, 114 (1985).
22. K. R. Spindler and A. J. Berk, *J. Virol.* **52**, 706 (1984).
23. L. T. Feldman and J. R. Nevins, *Mol. Cell. Biol.* **3**, 829 (1983).
24. B. Kreppl *et al.*, *Proc. Natl. Acad. Sci. U.S.A.* **81**, 6988 (1984).
25. B. E. Uhlin and K. Mordstrom, *Mol. Genet.* **165**, 167 (1978).
26. I. C. Hart *et al.*, *Biochem. J.* **224**, 93 (1984).
27. J. Messing, *Methods Enzymol.* **101**, 20 (1983).
28. M. W. Hunkapiller *et al.*, *ibid.* **91**, 227 (1983).
29. K. H. Klempnauer *et al.*, *Cell* **37**, 537 (1984).
30. W. J. Boyle *et al.*, *Proc. Natl. Acad. Sci. U.S.A.* **81**, 4265 (1984).
31. L. A. Steinberger, in *Immunocytochemistry*, L. A. Steinberger, Ed. (Wiley, New York, 1979).
32. M. Stefanini, C. De Martino, L. Zamboni, *Nature (London)* **216**, 173 (1967).
33. I. W. McLean and P. W. Nakane, *J. Histochem. Cytochem.* **22**, 1077 (1974). SLB-I cells were more strongly stained when the cells were fixed with acetone or a formaldehyde-containing fixative than when fixed with alcohol.
34. E. Fleissner, *J. Virol.* **8**, 778 (1971).
35. W. M. Hunter and F. C. Greenwood, *Nature (London)* **194**, 495 (1962).
36. W. C. Goh *et al.*, *Science* **227**, 1227 (1985).

37. Supported by grants from Triton Biosciences, Inc., and the U.S. Public Health Service (CA 32737). The antisera against tubulin and against the transferrin receptor were provided by J. Bulinski and O. Witte, respectively, of the University of California at Los Angeles. We thank D. Keith, L. Ramos, S. Quan, A. Healy, N. Nousek-Goebl, B. Koers, and G. Helfand for technical assistance and B. Colby and D. Lindsey for their advice.

26 February 1985; accepted 29 April 1985

94. A Transcriptional Activator Protein Encoded by the x-*lor* Region of the Human T-Cell Leukemia Virus

Joseph Sodroski, Craig Rosen, Wei Chun Goh, and William Haseltine

Human T-cell leukemia viruses (HTLV) comprise a retroviral family associated with lymphoid disorders. HTLV types have been identified on the basis of immunocompetition analysis of *gag* proteins (*1*). HTLV-I is associated with adult T-cell leukemia-lymphoma (ATLL) that is endemic in certain geographic regions (*2*). HTLV-II is a rare isolate associated with a benign form of hairy T-cell leukemia (*1*). HTLV-III has been identified as a probable cause of the acquired immune deficiency syndrome (AIDS) (*3*). Bovine leukemia virus (BLV), the etiological agent of enzootic leukosis in domestic cattle, demonstrates antigenic relatedness to the HTLV viruses in some of the virion proteins (*4*).

HTLV-I, -II, and BLV have been categorized as a separate family (HTLV-BLV) of transforming retroviruses (*5*) because of their characteristic structural and biological properties. The HTLV-BLV viruses can be distinguished from chronic murine leukemia viruses in that the former exhibit *trans*-acting transcriptional activation of the viral long terminal repeat (LTR), which governs viral gene expression, in infected cells (*6, 7*). Cells infected by these viruses contain factors that greatly augment steady-state levels of RNA produced by the viral LTR, without stimulating the replication of the template DNA (*7, 8*). The *trans*-acting factors act most efficiently on the LTR of the infecting virus (*7*), suggesting that a virus-specific rather than host cell-specific factor mediates *trans*-activation.

In addition to the *gag, pol,* and *env* genes typical of chronic leukemia viruses, the HTLV-BLV viruses possess a sequence (called the X region) located between the envelope gene and the 3' LTR (*5, 9*). This region of HTLV-I and HTLV-II contains a gene called x-*lor* that encodes a 42- and 38-kilodalton (kD) protein in HTLV-I and -II, respectively (*10*). These proteins are greater than 90 percent homologous at the amino acid level (*5, 9*) and are located predominately in the nuclei of infected cells (*11*).

Studies correlating the presence of the x-*lor* protein in various nonvirus-producing HTLV transformed cell lines with LTR *trans*-activation provide indirect evidence implicating an x-*lor* product in transcriptional regulation (*12*). Here we examine directly the effects of x-*lor* products on gene expression under the control of the viral LTR's.

The x-*lor* genes of HTLV-I and -II lack initiator methionine codons but have splice acceptor consensus sequences at their 5' ends (*5, 9, 13*). The x-*lor* proteins are made from spliced 2-kilobase (kb) messages that often contain, in addition to regions homologous to LTR and x-*lor*, sequences surrounding the *pol-env* junction (*14*). To gain insight into the composition of the natural x-*lor* protein, we mapped selected splice donors and acceptors in the HTLV-I–immortalized C81-66-45 cell line. Our experience, and that of other investigators (*10, 12*), is that this cell line has only HTLV-related messenger RNA (mRNA) that is 2 kb in size and expresses only the 42-kD x-*lor* product detectable by antiserum from patients with adult T-cell leukemia-lymphoma. A 3' end-labeled probe spanning from 86 base pairs (bp) 5' of the start codon of the *env* gene to the middle of the *env* gene (Fig. 1) was annealed to C81-66-45 RNA and treated with S1 nuclease. The size of the protected fragment was determined by comparison with Maxam-Gilbert sequencing reactions performed on the probe (*15*). The terminus of the protected fragment maps at a splice donor consensus sequence located immediately 3' of the *env* gene start codon. In a similar manner, we mapped the C81-66-45 splice acceptor to a consensus sequence located 172 bp 5' of the Cla I site in the x-*lor* gene, in a position identical to that determined for the HTLV-II x-*lor* message (*13*). Since C81-66-45 RNA does not hybridize to probes derived from the region bounded by these splice donor and acceptor sites, we conclude that these sites are juxtaposed in the C81-66-45 cell line to produce the 2-kb x-*lor* message. A probable scheme for production of the natural x-*lor* message and protein product is presented in Fig. 1. By means of a dual splicing event, the HTLV *env* gene contributes its initiation codon plus a single guanosine residue to the x-*lor* gene, resulting in an in-frame coding sequence.

Knowledge of the splicing pattern for the x-*lor* message suggested that the natural x-*lor* products could be expressed in eukaryotic cells by placing the HTLV-I LTR 5' to the *env*-X regions of the HTLV-I and HTLV-II genomes (plasmids envX$_I$ and envX$_{II}$ in Fig. 2). These plasmids could potentially express envelope proteins, x-*lor* proteins, and other products from the 3' half of the HTLV genome. Another plasmid (pCATLOR$_{II}$) was designed to express only a fusion protein consisting of nine NH$_2$-terminal residues encoded by the bacterial chloramphenicol acetyltransferase (CAT) gene (*16*) and the product of the entire HTLV-II x-*lor* gene extending from the splice acceptor to the termination codon (*5, 9*). This hybrid gene was also placed under the transcriptional control of the HTLV-I LTR. As negative controls, three additional plasmids containing the same sequences as envX$_I$ or pCATLOR$_{II}$ in a configuration not suitable for protein expression were constructed: IenvX$_I$, containing the entire env-X region of HTLV 3' to the HTLV-I LTR, but in an orientation opposite to that of envX$_I$; pTACLOR$_{II}$, containing the HTLV-I LTR and bacterial CAT gene

518

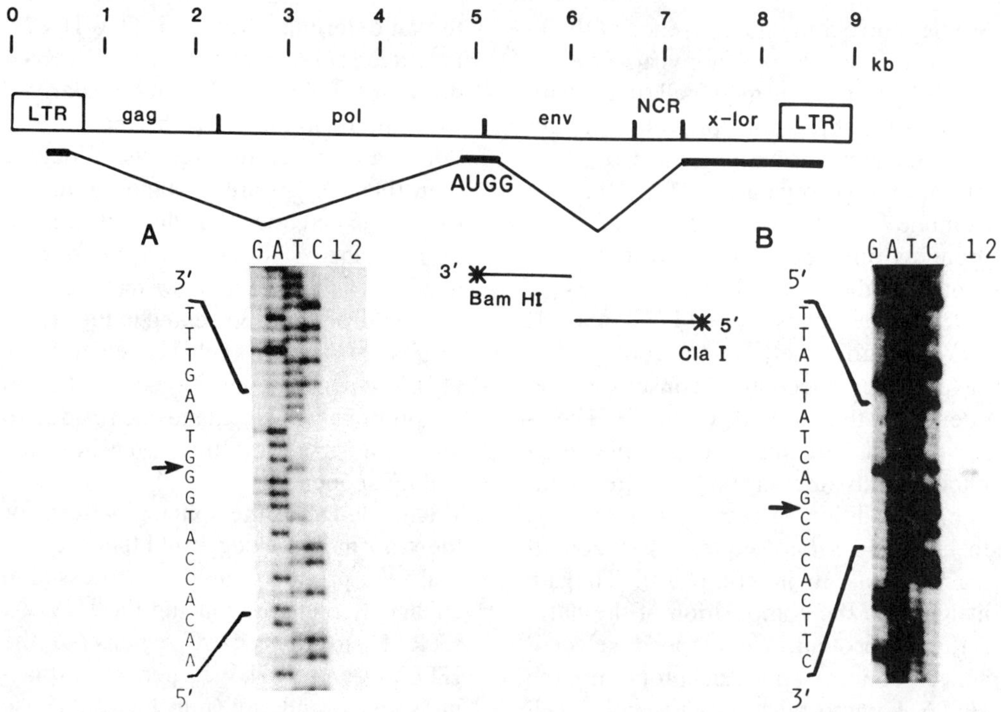

Fig. 1. Mapping of splice sites of the HTLV-related message in the C81-66-45 cell line. NCR represents the region that is not conserved between HTLV-I and HTLV-II (5). A model for generation of the 2-kb x-*lor* message from the HTLV-I genome is shown beneath the genome. Solid horizontal bars represent exons, and thin diagonal lines encompass the regions spliced from the mature message. The C81-66-45 mRNA was characterized for splice donor and acceptor sites relevant to the generation of the x-*lor* open reading frame. A 0.6-kb Bam HI-Sal I fragment [nucleotides 5094 to 5672 of the HTLV-I sequence of Seiki *et al.* (9)], end-labeled at the 3' position of the Bam HI site, was used as a probe for the splice donor (A). A 1.8-kb Sal I-Cla I fragment (nucleotides 5672 to 7474) end-labeled at the 5' position of the Cla I site was used to define the splice acceptor (B). Denatured probes were annealed to total RNA of C81-66-45 (lane 1) or HUT 78 (an HTLV-negative T-lymphocyte line) (lane 2) and treated with S1 nuclease (24). The protected fragments were then analyzed on denaturing acrylamide gels alongside Maxam-Gilbert sequencing reactions (15) performed on the probe fragments. The sequencing gels are oriented so that the sequence of the sense strand can be read directly (G, guanine reaction; A, adenine plus guanine reaction; T, thymine plus cytosine reaction; C, cytosine reaction). Arrows denote the position of the protected fragments. The 5'-most splice donor of the HTLV-I genome was not mapped; thus, the 5'-most splice donor depicted in the figure is based only upon the presence of consensus sequences located in the R region of the LTR. The splice acceptor sequence in the *pol* gene has been mapped approximately to positions 4990 to 5100 of the sequence of Seiki *et al.* (9).

sequences in the opposite orientation to that of pCATLOR$_{II}$; pCATLOR$_{II}$fs, identical to pCATLOR$_{II}$ except for a 2-bp deletion in the CAT gene sequences of pCATLOR$_{II}$, resulting in a +1 frameshift mutation in the x-*lor* reading frame.

The ability of each of these plasmids to affect the rate of gene expression directed by the HTLV-I and -II LTR sequences was examined. Cells were cotransfected with test plasmids and indicator plasmids in which the CAT gene

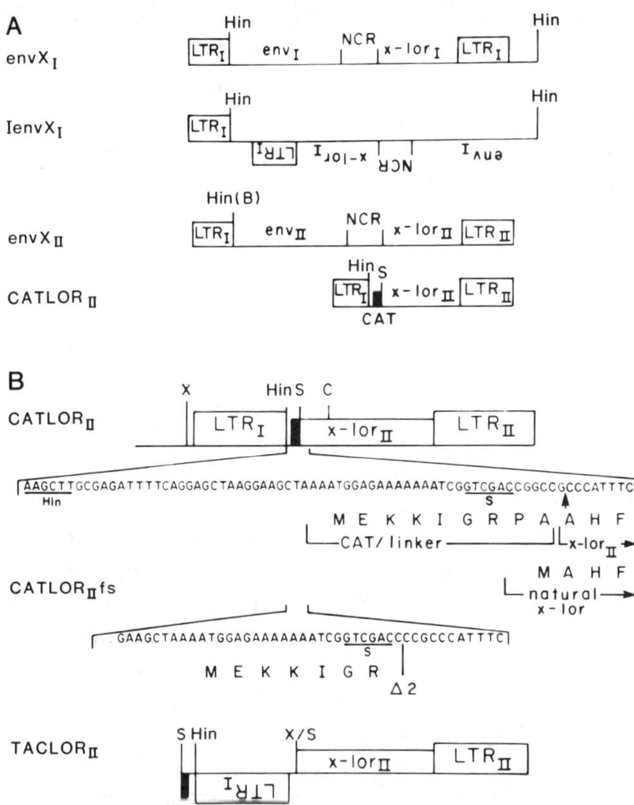

Fig. 2. HTLV x-*lor* expressor and control plasmids. The darkened boxes show sequences derived from the CAT gene. Hin, Hind III site; Hin(B), Hind III adjacent to a Bgl II site via a polylinker; S, Sal I; C, Cla I; X/S, Xho I-Sal I ligation; X, Xho I; NCR, nonconserved region between HTLV-I and HTLV-II. (A) Constructions designed to express the HTLV-I or HTLV-II x-*lor* proteins. The Xho I-Hind III fragment containing the HTLV-I LTR sequences of pU3R-I (7) was used as a promoter element. For envX$_I$ and IenvX$_I$, the Hind III fragment of pCR-1 (25) containing the 3′ end of the HTLV-I genome was inserted in both orientations into the Hind III site of pU3R-Igpt (7) In envX$_I$, the Hind III site of the pU3R-I LTR is located 190-bp 5′ to the *env* gene ATG codon. In envX$_{II}$, the HTLV-I LTR of pU3R-I is located at the Bam HI site 88 bp 5′ to the *env* gene ATG codon of HTLV-II proviral clone MO1A (26). Plasmid pCATLOR$_{II}$ consists of 5′ sequences derived from pU3R-I, including the 5′-most segment of the CAT-gene coding sequence, and a 3′ sequence derived from the HTLV-II provirus in clone MO1A (26). Plasmid pCATLOR$_{II}$ was made by digestion of pU3R-I at a single Pvu II site within the CAT gene and limited digestion of DNA with Bal31 exonuclease. Similarly, a plasmid subclone of MO1A was linearized at the Bgl II site 227 bp 5′ to the x-*lor* splice acceptor and treated with Bal31 exonuclease. Sal I 8-bp linkers (New England Biolabs) were ligated to the exonuclease-treated fragments, which were subsequently digested with Sal I, recircularized, and cloned after transfection of *Escherichia coli*. Fragments from selected clones were then religated to yield constructions with the CAT coding sequence fused in-frame (pCATLOR$_{II}$) and out-of-frame (pCATLOR$_{II}$fs) with the x-*lor* gene. The structure of these plasmids near the Sal I junction was confirmed by DNA sequencing. In addition to the sequences illustrated, all plasmids contain pBR322 sequences (origin of replication and ampicillinase gene) and the SV40 early-region promoter. Plasmid envX$_{II}$ contains enhancer sequences derived from the Moloney murine leukemia virus LTR (27) (from the 5′ limit of the LTR to the Sac I site located upstream of the TATA box) located immediately 5′ to and in the same orientation as the HTLV-I LTR. (B) Details of pCATLOR$_{II}$ and variants. The nucleotide sequences surrounding the junction of the CAT gene and the HTLV-II x-*lor* gene in pCATLOR$_{II}$ are shown. In addition to the methionine of the natural x-*lor* product, the potential pCATLOR$_{II}$-derived product has eight NH$_2$-terminal residues derived from the CAT gene. The vertical arrow designates the position of the known x-*lor*$_{II}$ splice acceptor (13). The plasmid pCATLOR$_{II}$fs is identical to pCATLOR$_{II}$ except for a 2-bp deletion (Δ2) just 5′ to the junction between CAT and x-*lor* resulting in a +1 frameshift in the potential protein product. The plasmid pTACLOR$_{II}$ has the HTLV-I LTR and ATG codon of the CAT gene in an orientation opposite to that of pCATLOR$_{II}$. All plasmids were purified by centrifugation in cesium chloride prior to transfection. Amino acid designations: A, alanine; E, glutamic acid; F, phenylalanine; G, glycine; H, histidine; I, isoleucine; K, lysine; M, methionine; P, proline; R, arginine.

520

was placed under the control of various eukaryotic promoter elements. The CAT-containing plasmids include those previously shown to respond to HTLV-I or -II *trans*-acting factors, pU3R-I (containing HTLV-I LTR sequences) and pU3-II (containing HTLV-II LTR sequences (7). To assess the specificity of any observed effect, CAT-containing plasmids that do not respond to HTLV-I or -II *trans*-acting factors (7) were used. The latter include pSV2CAT (with the SV40 early promoter), pBLVCAT (with the bovine leukemia virus LTR), pU3R-III (with the HTLV-III LTR), and pC55 (with the HTLV-I LTR deleted so as to render it unresponsive to viral *trans*-acting factors) (7, 8, 17, 18). Cell lines used as recipients include uninfected human OKT4+ T lymphocytes (HUT 78), a simian kidney cell line containing a functional SV40 T antigen (COS-1), a feline kidney cell line (CCCS+L−), and a murine fibroblast line (NIH 3T3). Forty-eight hours after transfection, CAT enzymatic activity was determined, a measurement previously shown to correlate with CAT mRNA levels (17, 19).

The results of these experiments are summarized in Table 1 and Fig. 3. In all cell lines examined, cotransfection with the plasmids that contained the x-*lor* gene of either HTLV-I or -II in a configuration suitable for expression led to a marked increase in the level of HTLV-I LTR-directed CAT gene expression as compared to experiments done in parallel with the control plasmids. For example, the level of CAT activity directed by pU3R-I in HUT 78, COS-1, and NIH 3T3 cells transfected with pCATLOR$_{II}$ is 66 times, 30 times, and 7.7 times that observed upon cotransfection of the same cell lines with pU3R-I and pCATLOR-$_{II}$fs. No stimulation of CAT activity was detected upon cotransfection of the test plasmids with CAT plasmids containing the SV40 early promoter or the LTR's of BLV or HTLV-III. Similarly, none of the x-*lor* expressor plasmids stimulated the CAT activity directed by pC55. The plasmid pC55 is identical to pU3R-I except that sequences 5′ to the promoter (TATA box), which are necessary for response to viral *trans*-acting factors, have been deleted (8). This suggests that HTLV-I LTR sequences necessary for *trans*-activation in infected cells are also required for the response to the cotransfected x-*lor* expressor plasmids. Furthermore, the stimulation of pU3R-I CAT activity by the envX$_{II}$ and pCATLOR$_{II}$ constructions is consistent with the ability of the *trans*-acting factors in HTLV-II–infected cells to activate HTLV-I LTR transcription (7). We conclude that products of the HTLV x-*lor* region are able to activate specifically gene expression directed by the HTLV-I LTR.

The *trans*-acting factors in all HTLV-I–infected cells examined to date preferentially activate HTLV-I LTR-mediated gene expression, with detectable, but relatively weak, activation of the HTLV-II LTR (7). To examine the effect of the x-*lor* products on HTLV-II LTR promoter activity, the control plasmids and the x-*lor* expressor plasmids were cotransfected into eukaryotic cells along with the HTLV-II LTR-CAT plasmid, pU3-II. In CCCS+L− feline kidney cells, COS-1 monkey kidney cells, or NIH 3T3 murine fibroblasts, both the x-*lor*$_I$ expressor plasmid (envX$_I$) and the x-*lor*$_{II}$ expressor plasmids (envX$_{II}$ and pCATLOR$_{II}$) stimulated CAT activity directed by the HTLV-II LTR (Fig. 3, Table 1). By contrast, in HUT 78 human T lymphocytes, the x-*lor*$_I$ and x-*lor*$_{II}$ expressor plasmids had only slight stimulatory effects on the HTLV-II LTR, despite the marked stimulation of the HTLV-I LTR by these plasmids in the same cell line. That both x-*lor*$_I$ and x-*lor*$_{II}$ expressor plasmids efficiently activate the HTLV-II LTR in some cell lines only, suggests that the apparent LTR type-selectivity observed in HTLV-I–infected cells (7) is probably not due to structural differences between the HTLV-I and HTLV-

Table 1. CAT activity after cotransfection. Transfections were carried out as described (7), with the DEAE-dextran technique for lymphocytes and CaPO$_4$-DNA coprecipitation for adherent cell lines. For lymphocytes, 8 μg of CAT plasmid DNA and 4 μg of cotransfected test plasmid were used for approximately 10^7 cells. For adherent cell lines, 2 μg CAT plasmid DNA and 2 μg test plasmid DNA were transfected onto 10^6 cells. Forty-eight hours after transfection, equivalent amounts of protein (representing roughly one half of the total cell lysate) were analyzed for CAT activity (7). Percentage conversion of chloramphenicol to acetylated forms per 1-hour reaction time is shown. The pSV2CAT plasmid replicates in COS-1 cells, whereas the other CAT-containing plasmids do not. For this cell line, shorter reaction times and lower amounts of cell lysate were used to remain within the linear scale of the reaction; values obtained were subsequently adjusted to correspond to those obtained with the other cell lines over a 1-hour reaction. All experiments were performed at least twice with a variation of less than 30 percent in CAT activities observed between experiments. ND, not done.

Cotransfected test plasmid	Acetylation of chloramphenicol (%)					
	pU3R-I	pU3-II	pSV2CAT	pC55	pBLVCAT	pU3R-III
HUT 78 (human T lymphocytes)						
pCATLOR$_{II}$	79	0.5	1.0	0.5	0.2	1.0
pCATLOR$_{II}$fs	1.2	0.3	0.9	0.5	ND	ND
pTACLOR$_{II}$	1.1	0.3	0.9	0.5	0.2	0.7
envX$_I$	4.5	1.0	1.0	0.5	0.2	0.7
envX$_{II}$	4.9	0.9	1.0	ND	ND	ND
IenvX$_I$	0.8	0.8	1.0	0.5	0.2	0.9
COS-1 (simian kidney cells)						
pCATLOR$_{II}$	11900	2970	2990			
pCATLOR$_{II}$fs	391	11.4	2980			
pTACLOR$_{II}$	390	14.5	3000			
envX$_I$	900	305	3000			
envX$_{II}$	1402	290	2990			
IenvX$_I$	418	14.9	2990			
NIH 3T3 (murine fibroblasts)						
pCATLOR$_{II}$	18.5	6.6	2.4			
pCATLOR$_{II}$fs	2.4	ND	ND			
pTACLOR$_{II}$	2.8	2.1	3.5			
envX$_I$	52.5	19.6	3.5			
envX$_{II}$	81.6	31.5	2.9			
IenvX$_I$	2.5	1.8	3.6			
CCCS+L− (feline kidney cells)						
pCATLOR$_{II}$		19.9	7.2			
pCATLOR$_{II}$fs		1.1	4.9			
pTACLOR$_{II}$		ND	ND			
envX$_I$		4.3	7.0			
envX$_{II}$		34.1	7.4			
IenvX$_I$		1.9	6.6			

Fig. 3. CAT assays after co-transfection of HUT 78 lymphocytes and CCCS+L− cells with x-*lor* expressor plasmids. Transfection was performed as described in the legend to Table 1. Forty-eight hours after transfection, equivalent amounts of protein from cell

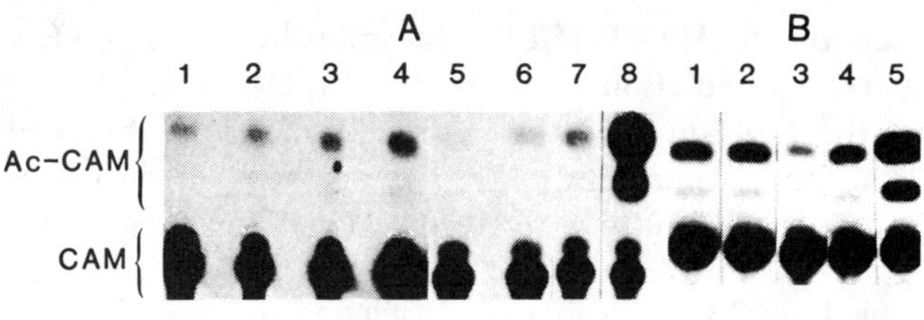

lysates were incubated with ^{14}C-labeled chloramphenicol in the presence of acetyl coenzyme A as described (7, 17). Unacetylated chloramphenicol (CAM) and acetylated forms (Ac-CAM) were determined by thin layer chromatography after a 1-hour reaction. (A) HUT 78 and (B) CCCS+L− cells are the transfected cells. The CAT plasmids used for transfection are: (lanes A1 and A2) pC55 [an HTLV-I LTR-deletion mutant that is unresponsive to viral *trans*-acting factors (8)]; (lanes A3, A4, B1, and B2) pSV2CAT (containing SV40 sequences); (lanes A5 and A6 and B3 to B5) pU3-II (containing HTLV-II LTR sequences); and (lanes A7 and A8) pU3R-I (containing HTLV-I LTR sequences). Cotransfected plasmids used were pCATLOR$_{II}$fs (lanes A1, A3, A5, and A7), pCATLOR$_{II}$ (lanes A2, A4, A6, and A8), IenvX$_I$ (lanes B1 and B3), envX$_I$ (lane B4), and envX$_{II}$ (lanes B2 and B5).

II x-*lor* products. A more tenable explanation is that the HTLV-II LTR is more dependent both upon viral and cellular transcriptional factors than is the HTLV-I LTR. Thus, even in the presence of a functional x-*lor* product, the lack of appropriate cellular factors can prevent efficient HTLV-II LTR-directed gene expression. The ability of the HTLV-II LTR to be *trans*-activated in COS-1, NIH 3T3, and CCCS+L− cells and the poor *trans*-activation in HUT 78 cells suggests that such cellular factors are not necessarily cell type (lymphocyte)-specific.

Our experiments provide direct evidence that products of the HTLV x-*lor* gene are able to act in *trans* to stimulate gene expression directed by the HTLV LTR. The magnitude of LTR *trans*-activation after cotransfection with x-*lor* expressor plasmids approximates that observed in HTLV-infected cell lines (7). In the pCATLOR$_{II}$ construction, only the HTLV-II x-*lor* region is available for expression, suggesting that products of this region are sufficient for *trans*-activa-tion. Disruption of the open reading frame known to encode the 38-kD HTLV-II protein results in a complete loss of *trans*-activating ability. This observation suggests that the known products of the HTLV x-*lor* genes are necessary for *trans*-activation. They are probably sufficient as the x-*lor*$_I$ and x-*lor*$_{II}$ expressor plasmids activate both the HTLV-I and -II LTR in the appropriate cell type, despite the observation that no other potential protein products of the HTLV-I and -II x-*lor* region are structurally related (5, 9).

Consistent with their involvement in the stimulation of gene expression by the LTR, we will refer to the 42- and 38-kD x-*lor* products as the tat$_I$ and tat$_{II}$ proteins, for *trans*-activating transcriptional proteins. We also propose that the HTLV gene encoding this protein be called the *tat* gene, in keeping with the tradition that retroviral genes be named according to function. Viral proteins are likely to mediate the *trans*-acting stimulation of LTR-directed gene expression in cells infected with BLV and HTLV-III

(7, 18) as well. Since retroviral replication is highly dependent on proviral transcription, these products serve critical functions in virion production.

In addition to their role in the virus life cycle, the *tat* products may mediate the pathogenic effects of these retroviral agents. Tumors associated with HTLV-I are monoclonal, yet lack preferred proviral integration sites (20). In addition, HTLV-I and HTLV-II can immortalize primary lymphocytes in vitro despite their lack of a host cell-derived oncogene (9, 21). The HTLV *tat* product is maintained in all in vitro–immortalized cells examined to date, in some cases to the exclusion of all other detectable viral proteins (10, 12). These observations suggest that HTLV might transform lymphocytes by production of this viral product (10, 12). This report directly links the HTLV *tat* product to transcriptional *trans*-activation, whereby host cellular genes involved in T-cell proliferation might be modulated in the absence of adjacent *cis*-acting proviral integrations (7). The HTLV *tat* product may share functional similarities to the immortalizing proteins of adenovirus and SV40, as well as to the cellular *myc* oncogene product. Like the HTLV *tat* product, these proteins are located in the nucleus (22) and can exert regulatory effects on the transcription of viral or cellular genes (23). The expression of a biologically active HTLV *tat* protein in eukaryotic cells should allow a direct examination of the ability of this protein to regulate the transcription of host cell genes and to immortalize primary lymphocytes.

References and Notes

1. V. S. Kalyanaraman *et al.*, *Science* 218, 571 (1982).
2. B. J. Poiesz *et al.*, *Proc. Natl. Acad. Sci. U.S.A.* 77, 7415 (1980); V. S. Kalyanaraman *et al.*, *Nature (London)* 294, 271 (1981); M. Robert-Guroff *et al.*, *J. Exp. Med.* 154, 1857 (1981); M. Yoshida, I. Miyoshi, Y. Hinuma, *Proc. Natl. Acad. Sci. U.S.A.* 79, 2031 (1982); M. Popovic *et al.*, *Nature (London)* 300, 63 (1982); W. A. Blattner *et al.*, *J. Infect. Dis.* 147, 406 (1983).
3. M. Popovic *et al.*, *Science* 224, 497 (1984); R. C. Gallo *et al.*, *ibid.*, p. 500; J. Schüpbach *et al.*, *ibid.*, p. 503; M. Sarngadharan *et al.*, *ibid.*, p. 506.
4. J. F. Ferrer, C. Avila, N. D. Stock, *Cancer Res.* 32, 1864 (1977); S. Oroszlan, in *Human T-Cell Leukemia/Lymphoma Virus*, R. C. Gallo, M. Essex, L. Gross, Eds. (Cold Spring Harbor Laboratory, Cold Spring Harbor, N.Y., 1984).
5. W. A. Haseltine *et al.*, *Science* 225, 419 (1984).
6. D. Celander and W. A. Haseltine, *Nature (London)* 312, 159 (1984).
7. J. G. Sodroski, C. A. Rosen, W. A. Haseltine, *Science* 225, 381 (1984); C. A. Rosen *et al.*, *ibid.* 227, 320 (1985); D. Derse, S. J. Caradonna, J. W. Casey, *ibid.*, p. 317.
8. C. A. Rosen, J. G. Sodroski, W. A. Haseltine, in preparation.
9. M. Seiki *et al.*, *Proc. Natl. Acad. Sci. U.S.A.* 80, 3618 (1983); N. R. Rice *et al.*, *Virology* 138, 82 (1984); K. Shimotohno *et al.*, *Proc. Natl. Acad. Sci. U.S.A.* 81, 6657 (1984).
10. T. H. Lee *et al.*, *Science* 226, 57 (1984); D. J. Slamon *et al.*, *ibid.*, p. 61.
11. W. C. Goh *et al.*, *Science* 227, 1227 (1985).
12. J. G. Sodroski *et al.*, *J. Virol.*, in press.
13. W. Wachsman *et al.*, *Science* 226, 177 (1984).
14. G. Franchini, F. Wong-Staal, R. C. Gallo, *Proc. Natl. Acad. Sci. U.S.A.* 81, 6207 (1984).
15. A. Maxam and W. Gilbert, *ibid.* 74, 560 (1977).
16. N. Alton and D. Vapnek, *Nature (London)* 282, 864 (1979).
17. C. M. Gorman, L. F. Moffat, B. H. Howard, *Mol. Cell. Biol.* 2, 1044 (1982); C. M. Gorman *et al.*, *Proc. Natl. Acad. Sci. U.S.A.* 79, 6777 (1982).
18. J. G. Sodroski *et al.*, *Science* 227, 171 (1985).
19. M. D. Walker *et al.*, *Nature (London)* 306, 557 (1983); J. M. Keller and J. C. Alwine, *Cell* 36, 381 (1984); L. Herrera-Estrella *et al.*, *Nature (London)* 310, 115 (1984).
20. M. Seiki *et al.*, *Nature (London)* 309, 640 (1984); B. Hahn *et al.*, *ibid.* 305, 340 (1983).
21. I. Miyoshi *et al.*, *ibid.* 294, 770 (1981); M. Popovic *et al.*, *Proc. Natl. Acad. Sci. U.S.A.* 80, 5402 (1983); N. Yamamoto *et al.*, *Science* 217, 737 (1982); I. S. Y. Chen, S. G. Quan, D. W. Golde, *Proc. Natl. Acad. Sci. U.S.A.* 80, 7006 (1983).
22. J. H. Pope and W. P. Rowe, *J. Exp. Med.* 120, 121 (1964); D. Kalderon *et al.*, *Nature (London)* 311, 33 (1984); L. T. Feldman and J. R. Nevins, *Mol. Cell. Biol.* 3, 829 (1983); M. Green, K. H. Brackerman, M. A. Cartas, T. Matsuo, *Virology* 42, 30 (1982); L. A. Lucher *et al.*, *ibid.* 52, 136 (1984); P. Donner, I. Greiser-Wilke, K. Moelling, *Nature (London)* 296, 262 (1982); H. D. Abrams, L. R. Rohrschneider, R. N. Eisenman, *Cell* 29, 427 (1982).
23. J. Keller and J. Alwine, *Cell* 36, 381 (1984); J. Brady *et al.*, *Proc. Natl. Acad. Sci. U.S.A.* 81, 2040 (1984); N. Jones and T. Shenk, *ibid.* 76, 3665 (1979); J. R. Nevins, *Cell* 26, 213 (1981); A. Berk *et al.*, *ibid.* 17, 935 (1979); R. B. Gaynor,

524

D. Hillman, A. Berk, *Proc. Natl. Acad. Sci. U.S.A.* **81**, 1193 (1984); R. E. Kingston, A. S. Baldwin, Jr., P. A. Sharp, *Nature (London)* **312**, 280 (1984).
24. A. J. Berk and P. A. Sharp, *Cell* **12**, 721 (1977).
25. V. Manzari *et al.*, *Proc. Natl. Acad. Sci. U.S.A.* **80**, 1574 (1983).
26. E. P. Gelmann *et al.*, *ibid.* **81**, 993 (1984).
27. L. Laimins *et al.*, *J. Virol.* **49**, 183 (1984).
28. We thank R. Gallo, C. Gorman, and F. Wong-Staal for materials; K. Campbell and D. Perkins for expert technical assistance; D. Artz for

expert secretarial assistance; and D. Celander and R. Crowther for helpful discussions. Supported by NIH postdoctoral fellowships CA07580 and CA07094 (J.G.S. and C.A.R), an American Cancer Society grant RD-186, NIH grant CA36974, and a contract from the Massachusetts Department of Public Health.

7 March 1985; accepted 23 April 1985

Report

28 June 1985

95. Expression of the *pX* Gene of HTLV-I: General Splicing Mechanism in the HTLV Family

Motoharu Seiki, Atsuko Hikikoshi, Tadatsugu Taniguchi, and Mitsuaki Yoshida

Human T-cell leukemia virus type I (HTLV-I) was the first isolated member of the HTLV family (*1–3*). It is closely associated with adult T-cell leukemia (ATL) (*2–4*), which is endemic in southwest Japan (*5*), the West Indies (*6*), and Africa (*7*). Infection of a target cell with this virus is a prerequisite for development of ATL (*8*).

Nucleotide sequence analysis of the HTLV-I genome indicated unusual structural features on the basis of which HTLV-I was classified into a new group of retroviruses (*9, 10*). These features include an unusually long R sequence (a repeated sequence that is found at both ends of viral RNA genome) and a potential novel secondary structure in the R region. The large stem and loop structure in the R region may function in the efficient termination of transcription and polyadenylation (*10*). Another unusual

structure is an extra sequence (*pX*) between *env* and the long terminal repeat (LTR) that has the capacity to code for a protein of 40 kilodaltons (kD) (*10*). Other members of the HTLV family, namely HTLV-II (*11*), bovine leukemia virus (BLV) (*12*), and simian T-cell leukemia virus (STLV) (*13*), also have these unusual structural features of the LTR and *pX* regions. This conservation of the R and *pX* regions among distantly related viruses of the HTLV family suggests that these regions have important functions in viral replication or pathogenicity.

Recently, a 40-kD product of the *pX* gene, p40^x, was identified by means of specific antibodies to the COOH-terminal region of the protein predicted from the *pX* nucleotide sequence (*14*). Moreover, p40^x was suggested to enhance transcription initiated at its own LTR in a *trans*-acting manner (*15*). This finding suggested that p40[x] is also involved in leukemogenesis by activating certain cellular genes whose regulation is similar to the LTR. We have previously excluded the possibility of *cis*-function of the LTR of the integrated provirus genome because the site of integration of the provirus in tumor cells varied among different ATL patients (*16*). This *trans*-acting viral protein could be the *pX* gene product, p40[x]. The structure of p40[x] could not be predicted from the genomic sequence, because the open reading frame in the *pX* sequence coding for p40[x] lacks an initiation codon (ATG) at its 5′ end, although the frame has the capacity to encode the 40-kD protein. Therefore, p40[x] was suggested to be encoded by spliced messenger RNA (mRNA) (*14*). Information on the mechanism of mRNA formation and the NH$_2$-terminal structure of p40[x] would be useful for understanding regulation of *pX* expression in infected cells and the function of p40[x]. We now describe cloning of complementary DNA (cDNA) and structural analysis of p40[x] mRNA and propose a general mechanism for viral gene expression in the HTLV family.

A rat T-cell line, TARL-2 (*17*), was used as a source of mRNA, because this cell line has one copy of the intact provirus genome in contrast to other human T-cell lines, which contain multiple copies of the proviruses including defective ones (*3, 18*). Cytoplasmic, polyadenylated RNA was isolated by oligo(dT)-cellulose column chromatography and analyzed by blot-hybridization. Three species of viral RNA were detected with a representative HTLV-I probe (Fig. 1A). They were 8.5, 4.2, and 2.1 kilobases (kb) in size and were concluded to be genomic RNA and subgenomic mRNA's for *env* and *pX*, respectively,

by their sizes and gene-specific hybridization. The RNA's were separated by centrifugation in a sucrose gradient, and fractions containing 2.1-kb mRNA were collected and used as template for complementary DNA (cDNA) synthesis. Oligo(dC)-tailed double stranded cDNA was synthesized by the method of Land *et al.* (*19*) and annealed to oligo(dG)-tailed pBR322 at the Pst I site. The DNA was transfected into the MC 1061 strain of *Escherichia coli* (*20*), and colonies were screened by in situ hybridization with the *pX* region of the HTLV-I as a probe. Five positive colonies were obtained from 4×10^4 transformants and one plasmid, containing the largest insert (1.5 kb), was analyzed further. Initial restriction enzyme analysis showed that this clone contained the 5′ region of mRNA but had lost about 500 bases of the 3′ portion of the coding frame. This defect in the 3′-portion should be due to the incomplete DNA synthesis of the second strand.

To confirm that this cDNA clone is functionally active for the expression of p40[x], the defective 3′ portion of the cDNA was first replaced with the sequence containing a complete 3′ portion isolated from the proviral clone pATK08 (*10*) (Fig. 1B), and then the constructed cDNA was joined in place of the *neo* gene in the pSV2neo (*21*) (Fig. 1B). The resultant plasmid, pSVpX, was transfected into COS-7 cells and the transient expression of the *pX* gene was analyzed (Fig. 1C). A single band of the mRNA containing the *pX* sequence was detected in cells transfected with pSVpX, but not in those infected with pSV2neo. The size of the mRNA (3.1 kb) in the transfectant was different from that in the HTLV-I–infected T-cell line. This was expected as the transcription of the *pX* gene in the plasmid is terminated by the SV40 termination signal instead of the LTR sequence, and so the mRNA should be slightly larger than the original mRNA. The 40-kD protein was also detected in pSVpX transfectants with serum from a patient who had ATL (Fig. 1C) or with rabbit antibodies against synthetic peptide corresponding to the COOH-terminal portion of p40^x. These results indicate that the cDNA clone contained enough information to express p40^x.

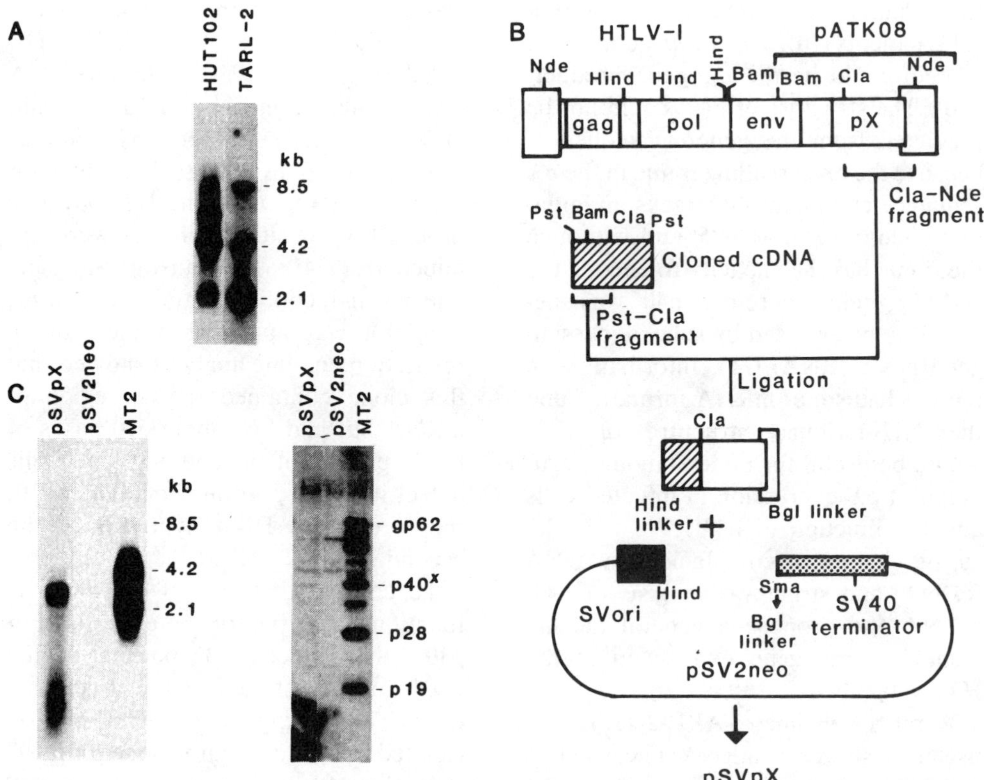

Fig. 1. Construction of plasmid for p40^x expression. (A) Detection of subgenomic *pX* mRNA in HTLV-I–infected cells. Cytoplasmic mRNA was isolated from human T-cell line HUT102 and rat T-cell line TARL-2 and fractionated by formaldehyde-agarose gel electrophoresis. The viral RNA was detected with a ^{32}P-labeled HTLV-I probe. (B) Construction of pSVpX for *pX* gene expression. The complete cDNA clone was reconstructed from a cloned cDNA with defects in the 3′-terminal region, and a provirus clone pATK08 (*10*). The reconstructed cDNA was inserted into the SV40 expression vector. (C) Expression of p40^x. COS-7 cells were transfected (*28*) with 10 μg of pSVpX, or with 10 μg of pSV2neo as a control. After incubation for 48 hours, cells were collected and RNA (left) and proteins (right) were analyzed. (Left) Cytoplasmic RNA was analyzed by the blotting procedure as in (A) but with *pX*-specific probe. (Right) Transfected cells were lysed and sonicated in RIPA buffer (50 m*M* Tris-HCl, *p*H 7.5, 150 m*M* NaCl, 0.1 percent sodium dodecyl-sulfate, 1 percent Triton X-100, and 1 percent sodium deoxycholate) and analyzed by blot-hybridization with sera from ATL patients and ^{125}I-labeled antibody to human immunoglobulin. As control, an HTLV-producing human T-cell line, MT2, was included. Nde, NdeI; Hind, Hind III; Bam, Bam HI; Cla, Cla I; Pst, Pst I; Bgl, Bgl I.

Comparison of the cDNA sequence with that of the provirus genome revealed that the cDNA is composed of three blocks (Fig. 2A). The first block consists of 118 nucleotides derived from the R region (from the cap site at position 354 to position 471) of the LTR. This spliced position at 471 is followed by the consensus sequence (*22*) for the splicing donor site AGGTAAG at positions 470 to 476 in the R region. The second block consists of 191 nucleotides (position 4993 to 5183) in the *pol* region. The junction sites at the two ends of this block correspond to the splicing acceptor sequence TATTTCAAG (4984 to 4992) and donor sequence GGGTAAG (5182 to 5188) in the proviral DNA. The initiation codon ATG (5180 to 5182) for the *env* gene (*10, 23*) is located just 5′ to the donor sequence. The third block consists of all of the *pX* sequence starting from position 7032, which is preceded by the splicing acceptor site TATTATCAG (position 7293 to 7301). Presence of the splicing site at this position was previously demonstrated by S_1 nuclease analysis (*24*). As a result of this second splicing, the *pX* reading frame (7032 to 8356), which can code for 352 amino acids, is joined to the ATGG (5180 to 5183) of the *env* gene so that ATG is aligned in the frame. Thus, the initiation codon ATG for *env* is used for initiation of p40^x translation. The other four cDNA clones showed similar restriction maps although they are also defective, supporting the conclusion that the sequenced cDNA clone represents the majority of the *pX* mRNA population. This conclusion was also consistent with the observation that the 2.1-kb mRNA did not significantly hybridize with the U5 probe. Similar splicing was also found in HTLV-II by Wachsman *et al.* (see *24a*).

The structure of the cDNA clone showed that subgenomic mRNA for p40^x is formed by two-step splicing (Fig. 3A) and that one of the splice donor sites is located in the R region of LTR. This feature is unique to HTLV and might relate to the unusually long R region. We have proposed (*10*) that the ability of the long R sequence to form a secondary structure at the 3′ end of viral mRNA plays a role in transcriptional termination. In addition to this, the R sequence was suggested to regulate mRNA splicing expressing the *env* and *pX* genes, because a complementary sequence to this splicing donor site is found in the R region just after this donor site. Thus the donor site can form a stem structure with 18 bases (Fig. 3B). The secondary structure of the transcript at this splicing donor site would allow this region to compete with U1 RNA in a small nuclear ribonucleoprotein complex; the U1 complex is involved in exact RNA splicing (*25*). Alteration of the pairing ratio of U1 RNA to the stem and loop structure may control the splicing in the R region, eventually affecting the expression of the *env* and *pX* genes. For specific regulation of the *pX* expression, other mechanisms may be required.

One of the splicing acceptor sites is located in the *pol* region, 187 bases upstream from the ATG for the *env* gene. This structure indicates that the subgenomic RNA generated by single splicing is *env* mRNA (Fig. 3A). The calculated size of this spliced product, 3985 bases without the polyadenylated stretch, is consistent with that of one of the subgenomic mRNA's detected in infected cell lines. Probably, the other splicing takes place on the *env* mRNA and produces *pX* mRNA coding for p40^x. In this mRNA, the initiation codon, ATG for

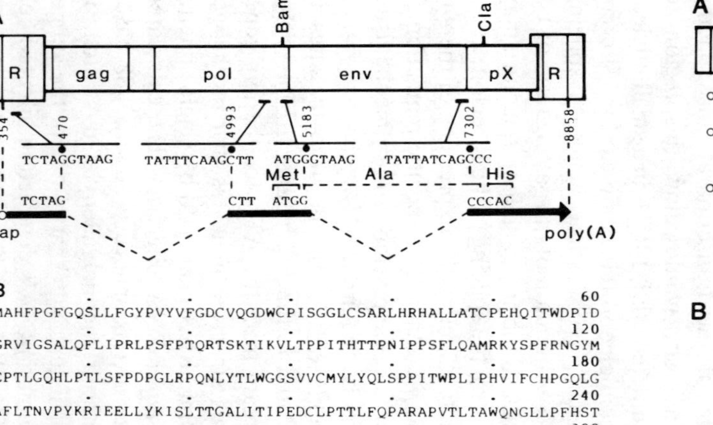

Fig. 2 (left). Summary of nucleotide sequence analysis of the cDNA clone of *pX* mRNA. (A) Splicing sites for mRNA formation. The cDNA, composed of three contiguous segments as shown by thick lines, and its correspondence to the proviral genome are shown. The third domain, the open reading frame from the *pX* region, was sequenced from position 7302 to 7950, which was the 3′ end of the cDNA clone. The sequence determined was identical to that of the provirus genome reported previously except for the following base replacements: T to A at position 5171, G to A at 7374, G to C at 7725, and G to A at 7801. (B) The complete amino acid sequence of p40^x was deduced from the nucleotide sequence of the cDNA clone. The calculated molecular weight of the protein is 39,482 daltons. The following abbreviations were used for amino acids: A, alanine; C, cysteine; D, aspartic acid; E, glutamic acid; F, phenylalanine; G, glycine; H, histidine; I, isoleucine; K, lysine; L, leucine; M, methionine; N, asparagine; P, proline; Q, glutamine; R, arginine; S, serine; T, threonine; V, valine; W, tryptophan; Y, tyrosine.

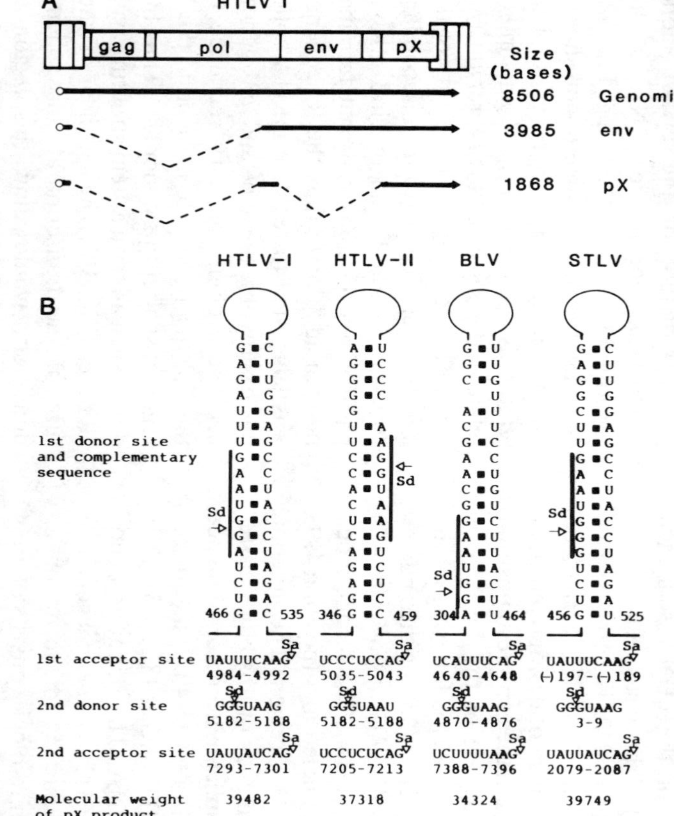

Fig. 3 (right). Conservation of splicing signals in the HTLV family. (A) Splicings to generate the subgenomic mRNA of HTLV. Thick lines represent RNA segments transcribed from the provirus genome and dotted lines indicate portions spliced out from the genomic RNA. (B) Conserved sequences for characteristic splicings in HTLV family members. Possible donor and acceptor sites in HTLV family members, HTLV-I, HTLV-II, BLV, and STLV are compared. For identification of the splicing sites, bases are numbered from the first base of the 5′-LTR except for the second splicing of STLV, where the bases are numbered from the first base of the *env* gene (as the total nucleotide sequence of the genome is not known). Bars beside stems of the stem and loop structure indicate the consensus sequences (*22*) for the splicing donor sites; arrows with Sd and Sa indicate splicing donor and acceptor sites, respectively.

the *env*, is used to initiate the translation of p40^x, and only the first methionine is brought onto p40^x from the *env* domain. Thus the molecular weight of the *pX* gene product was calculated as 39,482.

The key sequences for splicing found in HTLV-I are also present at corresponding positions in HTLV-II (*11, 26*), BLV (*12*), and STLV (*13*) as shown in Fig. 3, suggesting that the unusual splicing mechanisms producing the *env* and *pX* mRNA's are common to all four viruses. A minor exception occurs in BLV; the initiation codon for *pX* translation is located 44 bases downstream from that of the *env* gene, out of the frame. Thus, the *pX* and *env* genes do not share the same initiation codon. However, AIDS-associated viruses (*27*) are different from the other members of HTLV family in the organization of these critical sequences. Thus, a mechanism of the gene expression of AIDS-associated viruses seem to be different from the others.

References and Notes

1. B. J. Poiesz *et al.*, *Proc. Natl. Acad. Sci. U.S.A.* **77**, 7415 (1980); M. R. Reitz *et al.*, *ibid.* **78**, 1887 (1981).
2. Y. Hinuma *et al.*, *ibid.*, p. 6476.
3. M. Yoshida, I. Miyoshi, Y. Hinuma, *ibid.* **79**, 2031 (1982).
4. M. Robert-Guroff *et al.*, *Science* **215**, 975 (1982); V. S. Kalyanaraman *et al.*, *Proc. Natl. Acad. Sci. U.S.A.* **79**, 1653 (1982).
5. Y. Hinuma *et al.*, *Int. J. Cancer* **29**, 631 (1982).
6. W. A. Blattner *et al.*, *ibid.* **30**, 257 (1982); J. D. Schüpback, *et al.*, *Cancer Res.* **43**, 886 (1983).
7. W. Saxinger *et al.*, *Science* **225**, 1473 (1984).
8. M. Yoshida *et al.*, *Proc. Natl. Acad. Sci. U.S.A.* **81**, 2534 (1984).
9. M. Seiki, S. Hattori, M. Yoshida, *ibid.* **79**, 6899 (1982).
10. M. Seiki *et al.*, *ibid.* **80**, 3618 (1983).
11. K. Shimotohno *et al.*, *ibid.* **81**, 6657 (1984); W. A. Haseltine *et al.*, *Science* **225**, 419 (1984).
12. N. R. Rice *et al.*, *Virology* **138**, 82 (1984); N. Sagata *et al.*, *Proc. Natl. Acad. Sci. U.S.A.* **82**, 677 (1985).
13. A. Komuro *et al.*, *Virology* **138**, 373 (1984); T. Watanabe *et al. ibid.* **144**, 59 (1985); H.-G. Guo, F. Wong-Staal, R. C. Gallo, *Science* **223**, 1195 (1984).
14. T. Kiyokawa *et al.*, *GANN* **75**, 747 (1984); M. Miwa *et al.*, *ibid.*, p. 751; T. H. Lee *et al.*, *Science* **226**, 57 (1984); D. J. Slamon *et al.*, *ibid.*, p. 61.
15. J. G. Sodroski, C. A. Rosen, W. A. Haseltine, *Science* **225**, 381 (1984); J. Fujisawa *et al.*, *Proc. Natl. Acad. Sci. U.S.A.* **82**, 2277 (1985).
16. M. Seiki, R. Eddy, T. B. Shows, M. Yoshida, *Nature (London)* **309**, 640 (1984).
17. M. Tateno *et al.*, *J. Exp. Med.* **159**, 1105 (1984).
18. T. Watanabe, M. Seiki, M. Yoshida, *Virology* **133**, 238 (1984).
19. H. Land *et al.*, *Nucleic Acids Res.* **9**, 2251 (1981).
20. M. Casadaban adn S. M. Cohen, *J. Mol. Biol.* **138**, 179 (1980).
21. P. J. Southern and P. Berg, *J. Mol. Appl. Genet.* **1**, 327 (1982).
22. P. A. Sharp, *Cell* **23**, 643 (1984).
23. T. H. Lee *et al.*, *Proc. Natl. Acad. Sci. U.S.A.* **81**, 3856 (1984).
24. W. Wachsman *et al.*, *Science* **226**, 177 (1984).
24a. W. Wachsman *et al.*, *ibid.* **228**, 1534 (1985).
25. M. R. Lerner *et al.*, *Nature (London)* **283**, 220 (1980); J. Rogers and R. Wall, *Proc. Natl. Acad. Sci. U.S.A.* **77**, 1877 (1980).
26. K. Shimotohno *et al.*, *ibid.* **82**, 3101 (1985).
27. L. Ratner *et al.*, *Nature (London)* **313**, 277 (1985); R. Sanchez-Pescador *et al.*, *Science* **227**, 484 (1985); M. A. Muesing *et al.*, *Nature (London)* **313**, 450 (1985); S. Wain-Hobson *et al.*, *Cell* **40**, 9 (1985).
28. P. Mellon *et al.*, *Cell* **27**, 279 (1981).
29. We thank G. Yamada, Institute for Molecular and Cellular Biology, Osaka University, for his useful discussion and help. Supported in part by a Grant-in-Aid for Special Project Research, Cancer-Bioscience; a Grant-in-Aid for Cancer Research, from the Ministry of Education, Science and Culture of Japan; and by a Research Grant of the Princess Takamatsu Cancer Research Fund.

12 February 1985; accepted 29 April 1985

Report

28 June 1985

96.   HTLV *x*-Gene Product: Requirement for the *env* Methionine Initiation Codon

William Wachsman, David W. Golde, Patricia A. Temple, Elizabeth C. Orr, Steven C. Clark, and Irvin S.Y. Chen

The human T-cell leukemia viruses (HTLV-I and HTLV-II) are associated with specific T-cell malignancies in man. HTLV-I-related adult T-cell leukemia is endemic to parts of Japan, the Caribbean, and Africa; HTLV-II is associated with a single case of T-cell–variant hairy-cell leukemia (*1–5*). Both viruses will transform normal, human, peripheral blood T cells in vitro as defined by their continued proliferation in the absence of exogenous interleukin-2 (*6–9*). The mechanism of HTLV-induced T-cell transformation is unknown, although these retroviruses, and bovine leukemia virus (BLV), appear to use a mechanism distinct from that of other animal retroviruses. Molecular studies of the HTLV genome in tumor cells from patients and transformed cell lines indicated that there are no preferential sites of viral integration (*10, 11*). DNA hybridization and nucleic acid sequence analyses of HTLV-I and HTLV-II genomes revealed that the HTLV proviral genome has no homology with known oncogenes or normal cellular sequences (*12, 13*). However, nucleic acid sequence analysis of HTLV-I by Seiki *et al.* identified a region of unknown function (designated X) that is located between *env* and the 3' long terminal repeat (LTR) (*12*). A similar X region was identified in the HTLV-

II and BLV genomes (*14–17*). Recently, we and others demonstrated that this X region of the HTLV genome contains a new gene, *x* (*18, 19*). This gene is transcribed into a 2.1-kilobase (kb) messenger RNA (mRNA) and encodes a protein of 40 or 37 kilodaltons (kD), (designated p40^{xI} or p37^{xII}), in cells infected with HTLV-I or HTLV-II, respectively. Thus, unlike other replication-competent retroviruses, the HTLV class of retrovirus contains four genes: *gag, pol, env*, and *x*. As the *x* gene only occurs in this class of retrovirus, it is hypothesized that its product is responsible for the transforming properties of HTLV.

The exact primary structure of p40^{xI} and p37^{xII} is unknown. Immunoprecipitation of p40^{xI} and p37^{xII} with antisera directed against synthetic peptides (with the peptide sequences deduced from the HTLV-I nucleic acid sequence) demonstrated that the *x* product is encoded primarily from the major open reading frame of the X region (*19*). The size of the *x*-encoded proteins, and the fact that antisera were developed against peptides derived from sequences upstream of the first methionine codon in *x*, led us to predict that the NH$_2$-terminus of these proteins is derived from upstream viral sequences not contiguous with the major open reading frame. We demonstrate here an RNA processing scheme that would generate the complete *x*-encoded product. On the basis of the nucleic acid sequence of the HTLV-I and HTLV-II *x* mRNA, we have deduced the primary structure of p40*xI* and p37*xII* as well as a predicted *x* protein from BLV.

Typically, retroviral subgenomic mRNA's are composed of 5' leader sequences extending from the cap site in the LTR into the *gag* gene, and a downstream exon such as *env* or *src* (*20–22*). Analyses of the HTLV-I and HTLV-II nucleic acid sequences did not reveal any potential initiation codon from the *gag* region that would maintain the *x* open reading frame and contribute less than 0.8 kb to the 2.1-kb *x* mRNA [as at least 1.5 kb of the mRNA would be derived from the downstream exon that contains the *x* gene sequences (*15, 18*)]. Therefore, we postulated the existence of a third exon that contains the initiation codon for the *x* gene and is located between a 5' leader exon and the 3' *x* gene exon. Further analysis of the HTLV-I and HTLV-II nucleic acid sequences in the region of the *pol–env* junction revealed the conservation of potential splice donor signals, located just downstream of the *env* methionine initiation codon, that would maintain the major open reading frame of *x* in a spliced mRNA.

To confirm the existence of these potential splice donor sites, we performed S_1 nuclease analysis on RNA from the HTLV-II–infected cell lines Mo-T and JLB-II, and from the HTLV-I–infected cell lines SLB-I and SLB-II. The hybridization probes (Fig. 1A) were prepared from the pH-6 clone of HTLV-II and the pHT-1 clone of HTLV-I to span the *pol–env* junction. Figure 1B shows the DNA fragments protected by hybridization to the RNA. A band indicative of a 90- and 93-nucleotide long protected fragment was observed for RNA from HTLV-I– and HTLV-II–infected cells, respectively. These coincide exactly with the location of the potential splice donor sequences in *env* at base pair 5183 in both the HTLV-I and HTLV-II proviral genomes (*12, 23*). A second band of 238 nucleotides for HTLV-I and 257 nucleotides for HTLV-II was observed; it corresponds to the protection, presumably by genomic or *env* mRNA, of the full length probe. No protected DNA fragments were observed when uninfected 729-6 cell RNA was hybridized with either probe and then digested with S_1 nuclease. The splice donor site occurs after a single nucleotide 3' of the *env* initiation codon in HTLV-I and HTLV-II. A termination codon is present in the same reading frame, 36 and 24 codons upstream of the *env* initiation codon, in HTLV-I and HTLV-II, respectively. Therefore, the *x* gene uses the *env* initiation codon for its translation and the complete *x* coding sequences are formed by this initiation codon and one additional nucleotide spliced to the downstream major open reading frame of the *x* gene.

We also isolated a complementary DNA (cDNA) clone made from mRNA of HTLV-II–infected Mo-T cells (Fig. 1C), which contains this same sequence at the splice junction of the *x* mRNA. This clone is about 400 nucleotides in size, and part of its sequence (Fig. 1C) verifies that the splicing of HTLV-II *x* mRNA involves the joining of a small segment of *env* with the downstream acceptor site of *x* at sequence locations determined by S_1 mapping.

To obtain further evidence that this splice junction is present in the 2.1-kb *x* subgenomic message, we analyzed RNA

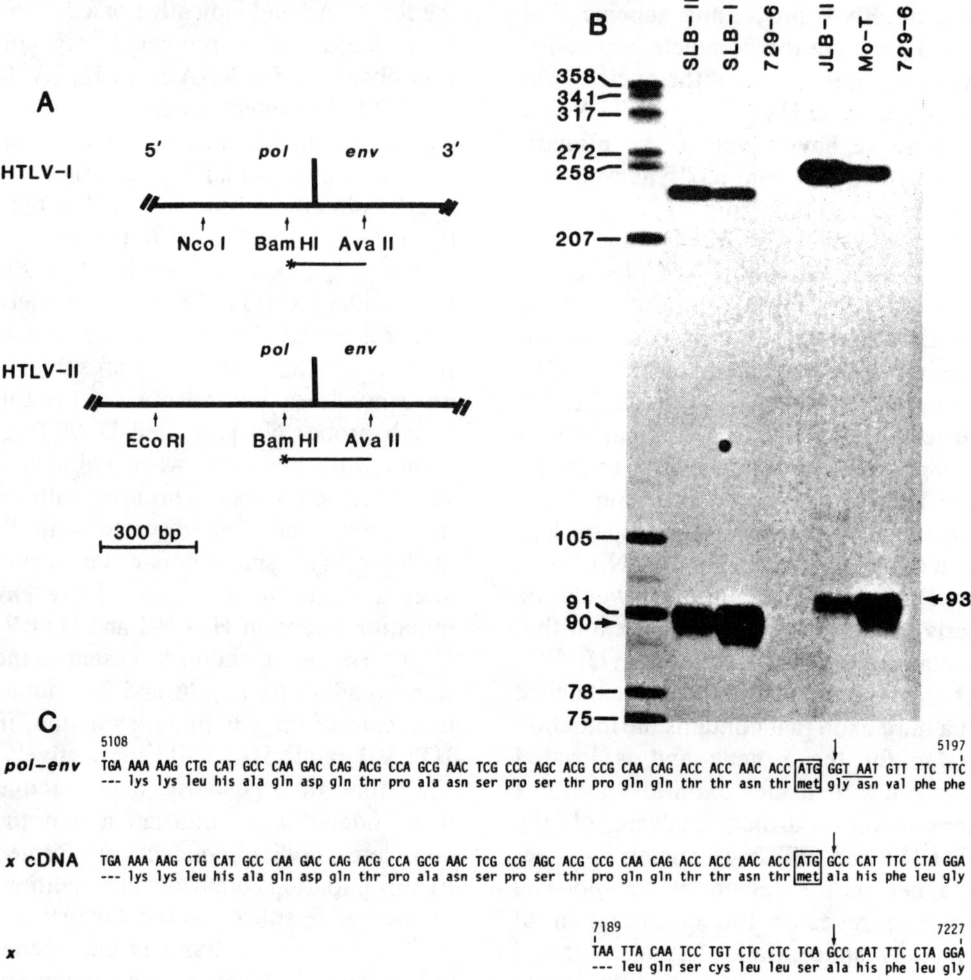

Fig. 1. Localization of the *x* gene splice donor sequences in *env*. (A) Partial restriction enzyme map of the pHT-1 (HTLV-I) and pH-6 (HTLV-II) DNA clones. The junction between *pol* and *env* is indicated as a vertical bar. The Bam HI–Ava II hybridization probe used for S_1 nuclease mapping is shown as a thin line below each map with an asterisk denoting the site at which 3' ^{32}P end-labeling was done by means of the large fragment of DNA polymerase. (B) Hybridization-S_1 nuclease analysis was performed as described (*36, 37*). RNA was extracted from the HTLV-I–infected SLB-I and SLB-II cell lines (*18, 38*), the HTLV-II–infected Mo-T (*4, 39*) and JLB-II (*9*) cell lines, and the uninfected 729-6 B-cell line. The size of the marker DNA fragments is shown in nucleotides. The 90- and 93-nucleotide protected fragment for HTLV-I and HTLV-II, respectively, is denoted by an arrow. No protected fragment was observed after hybridization of control 729-6 RNA to the probe. (C) Nucleic acid and predicted amino acid sequence of a portion of an HTLV-II *x* cDNA clone isolated from a Mo-T cDNA library (*40*). Sequences from the *pol–env* junction and *x* open reading frame of HTLV-II are homologous to the *x* cDNA clone upstream and downstream, respectively, of the *x* cDNA splice junction. Nucleotide positions in the HTLV-II proviral genome are indicated (*23*). The methionine initiation codon of *env* and the *x* gene is denoted by a box. The arrow demarcates the respective sites for the *env* splice donor, *x* gene *env-x* splice junction, and the *x* splice acceptor. In the *pol-env* sequences the underlined TAA shows the position of the *pol* stop codon.

from both HTLV-II–infected and –uninfected cell lines by Northern hybridization (Fig. 2). An oligonucleotide probe was synthesized to correspond with the sequence at the *env-x* splice junction. Under appropriate conditions of hybridization, a single 2.1-kb species of RNA was detected in the HTLV-II–infected cells but not in the uninfected Daudi or CEM cell lines. This mRNA is identical in size to that previously defined as the *x* subgenomic message. Control studies with a probe specific for actin mRNA showed hybridization at a single 2.1-kb band in all three cell lines.

The BLV genome contains sequences, analogous to the HTLV X region, between *env* and the 3′ LTR (*16, 17*). We analyzed the BLV genome for sequences comparable to the HTLV-I and HTLV-II *env* splice donor and *x* splice acceptor sites. At nucleotide position 51, as described by Rice *et al.* (*16*), there is a potential splice donor site (ATGG/GTAA) that is identical in sequence to that in HTLV. In BLV, the ATG in this sequence, although near the start of *env*, does not appear to be the *env* initiation codon. However, like HTLV, the TAA in this potential splice site represents the termination codon of *pol*. A potential splice acceptor site (AG/CAAGT) occurs at the 5′ terminus of the longest open reading frame in the BLV X region [between nucleotides 2487 and 2488 in the pX2 reading frame (*16*)]. This site is preceded by pyrimidines, which is analogous to the splice acceptor site of *x* in HTLV-I and HTLV-II. Because of the similarities in sequence among BLV, HTLV-I, and HTLV-II, we believe that these potential BLV splice sites are used to generate a BLV *x* mRNA. As with HTLV-I and HTLV-II, this predicted *x* coding region would be formed by splic-

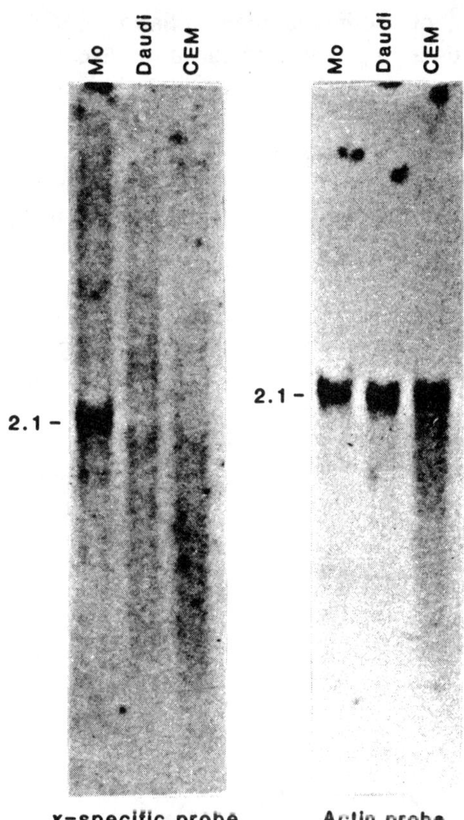

Fig. 2. Confirmation of the spliced junction sequences in *x*-specific mRNA. Polyadenylated RNA was extracted from the indicated cell lines and analyzed by Northern hybridization (*41*). The *x*-specific probe was derived by 5′ end-labeling of an oligonucleotide, 5′ AAATGGGCCATGGTGTTG 3′, which is complementary to the sequence surrounding the splice donor and acceptor junction. Under appropriate conditions of hybridization [4× standard saline citrate (SSC) at 30°C] and washing (2× SSC at 37° to 40°C), this probe hybridized only to sequences that are precisely complementary. This probe did not hybridize to noncontiguous complementary sequences, such as genomic mRNA in which the *env* splice donor and *x* splice acceptor sequences are separated. The actin probe was made from a human cDNA clone that had been isolated from a Mo-T cell cDNA library. Size is shown in kilobases. The Mo-T cells are infected with HTLV-II; the Daudi and CEM cells are uninfected.

534

ing of the methionine initiation codon plus a single base to the downstream x open reading frame. Figure 3 shows the sequences surrounding the HTLV-I and HTLV-II x gene splice junction as well as that predicted for BLV. The consensus sequence for this splice junction is also shown.

The first two amino acids of the translated protein, methionine-alanine, are the same for all three viruses. The predicted size of the primary translation product from HTLV-I and HTLV-II x mRNA is consistent with the respective 40-kD and 37-kD proteins previously demonstrated to be encoded by x (*19*); however, post-translational modification

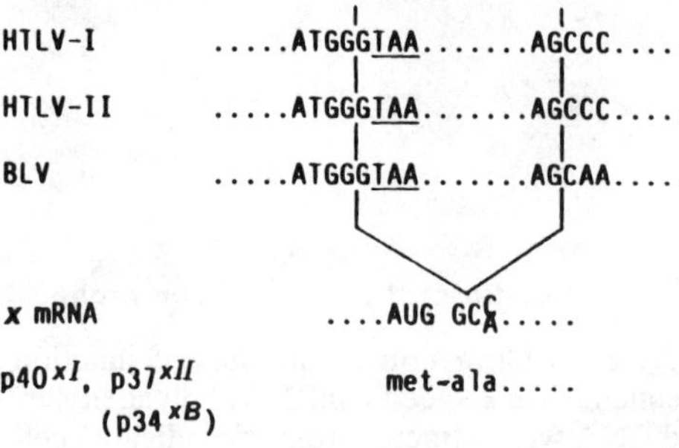

Fig. 3. Schematic representation of mRNA processing to generate the NH$_2$-terminal codons of the x gene. The sequence surrounding the x mRNA splice donor in *env* and the x mRNA splice acceptor in x for HTLV-I and HTLV-II as well as the predicted analogous sequences for BLV x mRNA are shown. The first two codons of the predicted primary translation product formed by mRNA processing are indicated. Although post-translational modifications cannot be excluded we speculate that the met-ala represents the NH$_2$-terminal amino acids of HTLV-I p40^{xI}, HTLV-II p37^{xII}, and p34^{xB} predicted for BLV. The TAA is underlined to indicate the termination codon for *pol*. The nucleotide positions at the *env* splice donor/x splice acceptor junction are: 5183/7302 in HTLV-I (*12*), 5183/7214 in HTLV-II (*23*), and 51/2428 in BLV (*16*).

cannot be excluded. On the basis of the published sequence of BLV, we predict that its x-encoded protein is 34 kD in size. Recombinant constructs of the HTLV-I and HTLV-II x gene synthesized according to the predicted mRNA structure have accurately expressed either p40^{xI} or p37^{xII}.

Retroviral mRNA's start from the cap site at the U3/R junction in the 5' LTR and terminate at the R/U5 junction in the 3' LTR (*24–26*). Further S$_1$ nuclease analysis of RNA from these HTLV-I– and HTLV-II–infected cells identified a potential splice acceptor site upstream of the *env* and x methionine codon at nucleotide 5183 in both HTLV-I and HTLV-II. In addition, there was at least one potential splice donor site located in the HTLV-II 5' LTR at nucleotide 449. Therefore, the HTLV x mRNA consists of at least three exons and has a total size of approximately 1.8 kb if the 3' polyadenylate sequences are excluded. The major open reading frame of the x gene is contained in the 1.5-kb 3' exon of this subgenomic message. Immediately 5' to this exon is a second exon of about 140 nucleotides that spans the *pol–env* junction and provides the initiation codon for the x gene. The 5' exon appears to be a leader sequence of about 135 nucleotides. It extends from the cap site to a splice donor site located in the stem of the potential hairpin loop that has been proposed for the HTLV-I and HTLV-II LTR (*12, 27, 28*). We believe this to be the entire structure of the HTLV-II x subgenomic message. These data are also consistent with the observations of Seiki *et al.* (*29*) regarding the structure of HTLV-I x mRNA.

The functional basis for this precise scheme of mRNA processing to generate the x mRNA is unclear. The only other example of retroviral RNA processing in which the virus contains a gene between *env* and the 3' LTR is Rous sarcoma virus (*30, 31*). In this case, sequences from *env* are not required to generate the *src* gene product (*32, 33*). It is possible that this type of mRNA processing, which adds only four nucleotides of coding sequence to downstream *x* sequences for HTLV, is a primary regulatory mechanism for the production of the *x* product. The function of p40^{xI} and p37^{xII} is unknown. These proteins may be important in viral transcription (*34, 35*). Recent *x* gene mutagenesis studies in our laboratory indicate that the *x* protein increases the efficiency of HTLV transcription (*35a*). Regulation of the expression of the *x* protein may be important for viral transcription and replication as well as for the initiation and maintenance of cellular transformation.

References and Notes

1. B. J. Poiesz *et al.*, *Proc. Natl. Acad. Sci. U.S.A.* **77**, 7415 (1980).
2. Y. Hinuma *et al.*, *ibid.* **78**, 6476 (1981).
3. W. A. Blattner *et al.*, *Int. J. Cancer* **30**, 257 (1982).
4. A. Saxon, R. H. Stevens, D. W. Golde, *Ann. Intern. Med.* **88**, 323 (1978).
5. V. S. Kalyanaraman, M. G. Sarngadharan, M. Robert-Guroff, I. Miyoshi, D. Blayney, D. Golde, R. C. Gallo, *Science* **218**, 571 (1982).
6. I. Miyoshi, I. Kubonishi, S. Yoshimoto, T. Akagi, Y. Ohtsuki, Y. Shiraishi, K. Nagata, Y. Hinuma, *Nature (London)* **294**, 770 (1981).
7. N. Yamamoto *et al.*, *Science* **217**, 737 (1982).
8. M. Popovic *et al.*, *ibid.* **219**, 856 (1983).
9. I. S. Y. Chen, S. G. Quan, D. W. Golde, *Proc. Natl. Acad. Sci. U.S.A.* **80**, 7006 (1983).
10. M. Seiki, R. Eddy, T. B. Show, M. Yoshida, *Nature (London)* **309**, 640 (1984).
11. J. C. Gasson, personal communication.
12. M. Seiki *et al.*, *Proc. Natl. Acad. Sci. U.S.A.* **80**, 3618 (1983).
13. I. S. Y. Chen *et al.*, *Nature (London)* **305**, 502 (1983).
14. W. A. Haseltine *et al.*, *Science* **225**, 419 (1984).
15. K. Shimotohno *et al.*, *Proc. Natl. Acad. Sci. U.S.A.* **81**, 6657 (1984).
16. N. R. Rice *et al.*, *Virology* **138**, 82 (1984).
17. N. Sagata *et al.*, *EMBO J.* **3**, 3231 (1984).
18. W. Wachsman *et al.*, *Science* **226**, 177 (1984).
19. D. J. Slamon *et al.*, *ibid.*, p. 61; T. H. Lee *et al.*, *ibid.*, p. 57.
20. P. Mellon and P. H. Duesberg, *Nature (London)* **270**, 631 (1977).
21. B. Cordell *et al.*, *Cell* **15**, 79 (1978).
22. P. B. Hackett *et al.*, *J. Virol.* **41**, 527 (1982).
23. K. Shimotohno *et al.*, *Proc. Natl. Acad. Sci. U.S.A.*, in press.
24. H. M. Temin, *Cell* **28**, 3 (1982).
25. T. Yamamoto, B. de Crombrugghe, I. Pastan, *ibid.* **22**, 787 (1980).
26. E. W. Benz, Jr., *et al.*, *Nature (London)* **288**, 665 (1980).
27. J. Sodroski *et al.*, *Proc. Natl. Acad. Sci. U.S.A.* **81**, 4617 (1984).
28. N. Sagata *et al.*, *ibid.*, p. 4741.
29. M. Seiki *et al.*, *Science* **228**, 1532 (1985).
30. S. R. Weiss, H. E. Varmus, J. M. Bishop, *Cell* **12**, 983 (1977).
31. N. Quintrell *et al.*, *J. Mol. Biol.* **143**, 363 (1980).
32. A. F. Purchio *et al.*, *Proc. Natl. Acad. Sci. U.S.A.* **75**, 1567 (1978).
33. K. Beemon and T. Hunter, *J. Virol.* **28**, 551 (1978).
34. J. G. Sodroski, C. A. Rosen, W. A. Haseltine, *Science* **225**, 381 (1984).
35. C. A. Rosen, J. G. Sodroski, R. Kettman, A. Burny, W. A. Haseltine, *ibid.* **227**, 320 (1985).
35a. I. S. Y. Chen *et al.*, *ibid.*, in press.
36. A. J. Berk and P. A. Sharp, *Cell* **12**, 721 (1977).
37. R. Weaver and C. Weissman, *Nucleic Acids Res.* **7**, 1175 (1979).
38. SLB-I and SLB-II are cell lines derived by infection of normal human leukocytes with HTLV-I in vitro.
39. A. Saxon *et al.*, *J. Immunol.* **120**, 777 (1978).
40. The cDNA clone was selected by hybridization to an oligonucleotide probe, 5'-CAAATCCTAGGAAATGG-3' (complementary to nucleotides 7215–7231) (*23*), which is downstream of the *x* splice-acceptor site, and by the lack of hybridization to an oligonucleotide probe, 5'-CTCCTCTCAGCCCATTTCC 3', which spans the *x* splice acceptor sequences (nucleotides 7204–7222) (*23*). A third hybridization probe was an HTLV-II cDNA clone previously described and located within the *x* gene (*13*). Nucleic acid sequencing of this portion of the *x* cDNA clone was performed by the standard dideoxy technique.
41. H. Lehrach *et al.*, *Biochemistry* **16**, 4743 (1977).
42. We thank J. Gasson for helpful comments on the manuscript, S. G. Quan for artwork, C. Nishikubo, S. G. Quan, A. Healy, and J. Fujii for technical assistance, and H. Merriman, B. Koers and W. Aft for editorial assistance. Supported by NCI grants CA 30388, CA 32737, CA 38597, CA 09297, and CA 16042; by grants PF-2182 and JFRA-99 from the American Cancer Society, and by a Bank of America-Giannini Foundation Fellowship (W.W.).

14 February 1985; accepted 2 May 1985

Report

28 June 1985

97. Localization of the Gene Encoding the Human Interleukin-2 Receptor on Chromosome 10

Warren J. Leonard, Tim A. Donlon, Roger V. Lebo, and Warner C. Greene

Interleukin-2 (IL-2, also referred to as T-cell growth factor) is a lymphokine synthesized and secreted by T cells after they are activated with an antigen or mitogen that permits long-term growth of human lymphoid cells in vitro (*1*). Interleukin-2 has been biochemically characterized (*2*), molecularly cloned (*3*), and identified as being encoded by a single gene on human chromosome 4 (*4*). The entire DNA sequence of the IL-2 gene has been determined (*5*).

Interleukin-2 acts by binding to specific high-affinity membrane receptors present on the surface of activated T cells (*6*) and may also in some circumstances have biological effects on B cells (*7*). Receptors for IL-2, which are absent on resting T cells, are expressed after cellular stimulation with antigen or lectin. Under appropriate conditions, IL-2 itself can upregulate the expression of IL-2 receptors (*8*). These receptors have been biochemically characterized (*9*) and are present in large numbers on leukemic cells infected with type I human T-cell lymphotrophic virus (HTLV-I) (*10*). Complementary DNA's (cDNA's) for this receptor have been isolated and sequenced (*11, 12*), and both alternate polyadenylation and messenger RNA splicing events have been described (*11*). The finding of relatively simple hybridization patterns on genomic Southern blots sug-

gested that the human IL-2 receptor was encoded by a single structural gene (*11*). We have now localized this gene to chromosome 10p14 → 15.

The 24 human chromosome types were sorted into 21 fractions according to the complementary Hoechst and chromomycin fluorescent emission (*13*). Filter-bound chromosomal DNA was denatured and hybridized to ^{32}P-labeled IL-2 receptor cDNA's prepared by the random priming method (*14*). We used IL-2 receptor cDNA's pIL2R2 and pIL2R4 in these studies. The pIL2R2 cDNA contains an insert corresponding to bases 1 to 937 of the published sequence for pIL2R3 (*11*); pIL2R4 is a full-length cDNA except that it lacks a 216–base pair segment in the middle of the protein-coding region (*11*). A gene-specific hybridization signal was obtained with the filter-bound DNA from chromosomes 9, 10, 11, and 12, indicating that the IL-2 receptor gene was on one of these chromosomes (Fig. 1). Fluorescent sorting technology does not separate these four Hoechst-chromomycin–stained chromosomes.

In situ hybridization studies (conducted by T.A.D.) with ^{3}H-labeled IL-2 receptor cDNA's were used to determine the specific location of the receptor gene. When these studies were performed, the results of the DNA spot-blot

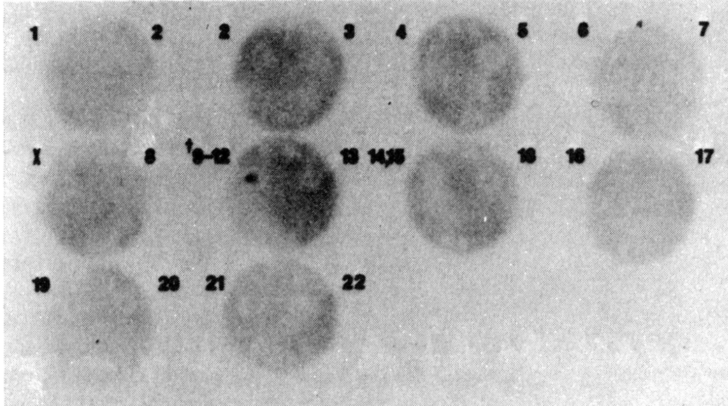

Fig. 1. Chromosome suspensions were prepared from a lymphocyte cell line in trisspermine buffer and stained with the Hoechst - chromomycin A3 stain pair (*13*). A dual-laser custom FACS IV chromosome sorter (*24*) was used to sort 30,000 chromosomes of each type directly onto a single spot of a nitrocellulose filter paper. The filter-bound chromosomal DNA was denatured, neutralized, prehybridized, and hybridized in 10 percent dextran sulfate (*13*) for 18 hours to IL-2 receptor cDNA's labeled with ^{32}P by the "random priming" method (*14*). After excess probe was removed by washing, a specific hybridization signal was detected autoradiographically over the area of the nitrocellulose filter onto which DNA from chromosomes 9 to 12 was spotted (denoted by dagger).

analysis had not yet been obtained. The pIL2R2 and pIL2R4 cDNA's were labeled by nick translation to specific activities of 1.9×10^7 and 2.0×10^7 cpm/μg, respectively, with the ^{3}H-labeled nucleotides deoxyadenosine triphosphate (51.9 Ci/mmol), deoxycytidine triphosphate (61.1 Ci/mmol), and thymidine triphosphate (103.3 Ci/mmol) (all from New England Nuclear). Peripheral blood lymphocytes from normal males were cultured in RPMI 1640 medium (Gibco) supplemented with 10 percent fetal bovine serum and synchronized in the cell cycle by the method of Yunis and Chandler (*15*). The hybridization technique was as described by Harper and Saunders (*16*), except that a fluorescent R-band procedure was used to stain the hybridized chromosome preparations after autoradiography (*17*). This modification permitted consistent, unequivocal chromosome identification through the use of simultaneous fluorescent and transmitted illumination. The hybridizations were performed at 42°C for 14 hours, with nick-translated IL-2 receptor

DNA at a final concentration of 0.02 ng/μl. The autoradiographs were exposed at 4°C for 9 days and developed in Kodak Dektol. The preparations were analyzed, then destained in methanol and G-band–stained with Wright's stain (*15*) to show the location of the silver grains.

The IL-2 receptor cDNA's pIL2R2 and pIL2R4 contain overlapping sequences and gave virtually identical results when used as probes. The major site of hybridization was to chromosome 10 at bands p14 and p15. In 56 of 300 cells, the label was associated with 10p14 → 15, and 57 of the 520 grains were found at 10p14 → 15. In Fig. 2, both chromosomes 10 were labeled over this region, which was the strongest site of hybridization.

Figure 3 shows the intensity of hybridization to 10p14 → 15 relative to the rest of the karyotype. These data permit assignment of the IL-2 receptor to this locus. Five other loci (3p24 → pter, 12q24 → qter, 7p15 → p21, 7q32 → q34, 11p15 → pter) showed lower but statistically significant degrees of hybridization

538

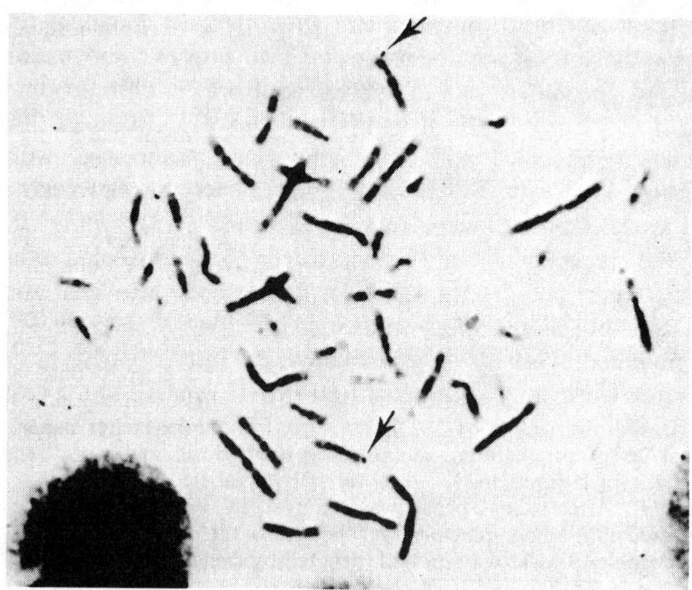

Fig. 2. Peripheral blood lymphocytes from normal males were activated with phytohemagglutinin. The chromosomes were prepared, hybridized to nick-translated pIL2R4, and autoradiographed for 9 days. Both chromosome 10's are labeled at band p15 (indicated by arrows).

to the IL-2 receptor cDNA. These secondary sites of hybridization include three regions to which oncogenes have been mapped (*RAF1* at 3p25, Harvey *ras* at 11p15, and Kirsten *ras* at 12q24 → ter) (*18*). The enhanced autoradiographic signal in these chromosomal regions may be due at least in part to (i) possible active transcription of these regions in stimulated lymphocytes, which would result in greater accessibility of the probe and therefore greater nonspecific in situ hybridization or (ii) the possible occurrence of DNA sequences homologous to the IL-2 receptor cDNA in these regions in addition to the oncogene sequences, which are not homologous to the IL-2 receptor.

No oncogenes, growth factors, or growth factor receptors have previously been localized to chromosome 10. Other key T-lymphocyte membrane proteins such as the β chain of the antigen receptor and proteins of the major histocompatibility complex are located on different chromosomes [chromosomes 7 and 6, respectively (*19, 20*)] and thus are not linked to the IL-2 receptor gene. Chromosome 10 contains the hexokinase locus, which when absent leads to a hemolytic anemia (*21*). Thus, a polymorphism for the IL-2 receptor locus, when identified, might be useful to test for segregation frequency in families with hexokinase deficiency. A polymorphic IL-2 receptor can also serve as a known mapped marker to test for segregation with other unmapped disease genes in studies analogous to those of the Huntington's disease locus, which was subsequently mapped to chromosome 4 (*22*). Polymorphic sites of the IL-2 receptor gene that exhibit tight linkage with genetic disease loci could be useful in prenatal diagnosis.

The short arm of chromosome 10, although apparently not involved in translocations in T-cell lymphomas, was identified in a translocation t(10:11) (p15;q23.3) in an acute nonlymphocytic lymphoma (*23*). Whether these neoplastic cells displayed IL-2 receptors is un-

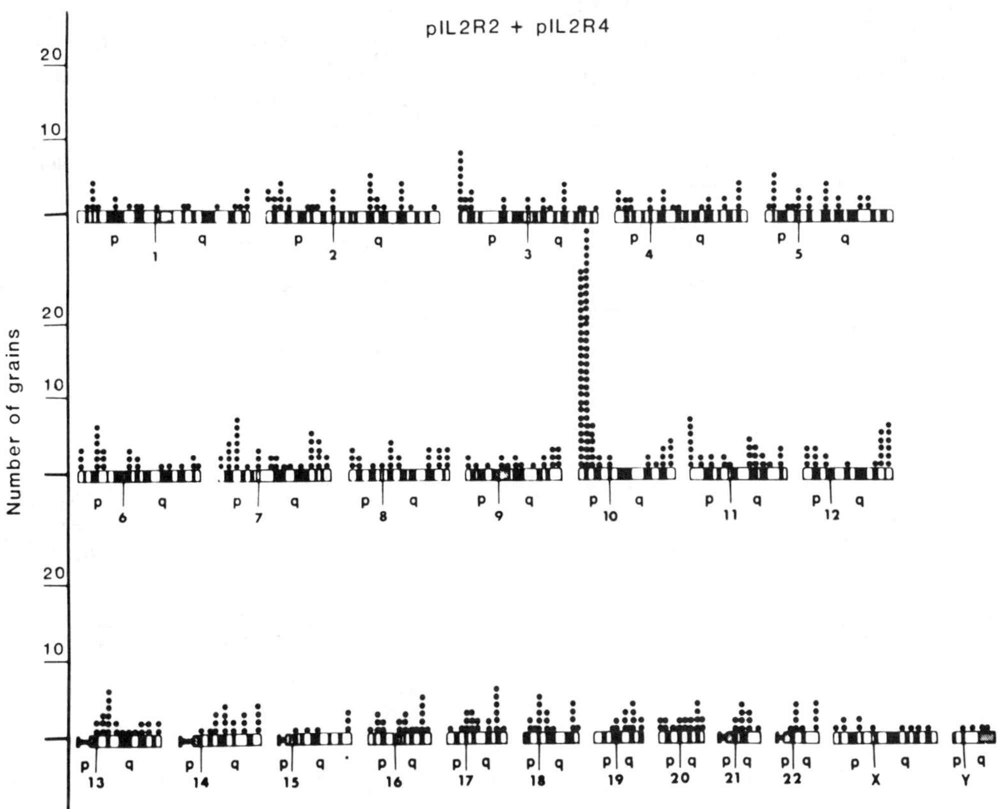

Fig. 3. Histogram indicating the location and number of grains from experiments with either pIL2R2 or pIL2R4. The distributions observed with the two probes were identical and therefore the data have been combined. Of 300 cells, 18.7 percent had label over 10p14 → 15. Of 520 total grains, 11 percent were found at this site.

known. However, augmented IL-2 receptor expression is a hallmark of HTLV-I–induced adult T-cell leukemia (*10*). Since no uniform karyotypic abnormality of chromosome 10 has been found in this leukemia, the deregulated IL-2 receptor expression does not appear to be due to a chromosomal translocation involving the IL-2 receptor gene.

References and Notes

1. D. A. Morgan, F. W. Ruscetti, R. C. Gallo, *Science* **193**, 1007 (1976); K. A. Smith, *Immunol. Rev.* **51**, 337 (1980).
2. R. J. Robb, R. M. Kutny, V. Chowdhry, *Proc. Natl. Acad. Sci. U.S.A.* **80**, 5990 (1983).
3. T. Taniguchi *et al.*, *Nature (London)* **302**, 305 (1983); R. Devos *et al.*, *Nucleic Acids Res.* **11**, 4307 (1983).
4. L. J. Seigel *et al.*, *Science* **223**, 175 (1984).
5. T. Fujita *et al.*, *Proc. Natl. Acad. Sci. U.S.A.* **80**, 7437 (1983); N. Holbrook *et al.*, *ibid.* **81**, 1634, 1984.
6. R. J. Robb, A. Munck, K. A. Smith, *J. Exp. Med.* **154**, 1455 (1981).
7. M. Tsudo, T. Uchiyama, H. Uchino, *ibid.* **160**, 612 (1984); T. A. Waldmann *et al.*, *ibid.*, p. 1450; M. C. Mingari *et al.*, *Nature (London)* **312**, 641 (1984).
8. G. Reem and N.-H. Yeh, *Science* **225**, 429 (1984); K. Welte *et al.*, *J. Exp. Med.* **160**, 1390 (1984); J. M. Depper *et al.*, *Proc. Natl. Acad. Sci. U.S.A.*, in press.
9. W. J. Leonard *et al.*, *Nature (London)* **300**, 267 (1982); W. J. Leonard *et al.*, *Proc. Natl. Acad. Sci. U.S.A.* **80**, 6957 (1983); W. J. Leonard *et al.*, in *Receptors and Recognitions*, M. Greaves, Ed. (Chapman and Hall, London, 1984), series B, vol. 17, p. 145; Y. Wano *et al.*, *J. Immunol.* **132**, 3005 (1984); W. J. Leonard *et al.*, *J. Biol.*

Chem. **260**, 1872 (1985).
10. J. M. Depper *et al.*, *J. Immunol.* **133**, 1691 (1984).
11. W. J. Leonard *et al.*, *Nature (London)* **311**, 626 (1984).
12. T. Nikaido *et al.*, *ibid.*, p. 631; D. Cosman *et al.*, *ibid.*, **312**, 768 (1984).
13. R. V. Lebo *et al.*, *Science* **225**, 57 (1984).
14. A. P. Feinberg and B. Vogelstein, *Anal. Biochem.* **132**, 6 (1983).
15. J. J. Yunis and M. E. Chandler, in *Progress in Clinical Pathology*, M. Steffanini, A. A. Hossaini, and H. D. Isenberg, Eds. (Grune & Stratton, New York, 1977), pp. 267–288.
16. M. E. Harper and G. F. Saunders, *Chromosoma* **83**, 431 (1981).
17. T. A. Donlon *et al.*, *Am. J. Hum. Genet.* **35**, 1097 (1983).
18. Human Gene Mapping 7, *Cytogenet. Cell. Genet.* **37**, 1 (1984).
19. P. E. Barker *et al.*, *Science* **226**, 348 (1984).
20. C. C. Morton *et al.*, *Am. J. Hum. Genet.* **34**, 136A (1982).
21. V. A. McKusick, *Clin. Genet.* **25**, 88 (1984).
22. J. F. Guzella *et al.*, *Nature (London)* **306**, 234 (1983).
23. J. J. Yunis and A. L. Soreng, *Science* **226**, 1199 (1984).
24. R. V. Lebo and A. M. Bastian. *Cytometry* **3**, 213 (1982).
25. We thank Meichi Cheung for help with spot blot analysis.

20 February 1985; accepted 1 May 1985

98.   More About the HTLV's and How They Act

Jean L. Marx

The human T-lymphotropic viruses (HTLV's) have been closely linked to two serious human diseases—adult T-cell leukemia and acquired immune deficiency syndrome (AIDS). That alone would be sufficient to make them the subjects of an intense research effort. But, like other viruses that infect mammalian cells, they are also interesting because of what they may reveal about the innermost secrets of those cells.

All three HTLV's infect T lymphocytes, which are needed for many immune responses. Infection by HTLV-I or -II, the viruses that have been associated with leukemias and lymphomas, leads to uncontrolled cell proliferation. In contrast, HTLV-III, the AIDS virus which is also called lymphadenopathy/AIDS virus (LAV) and AIDS-associated retrovirus (ARV), kills the cells it infects.

Finding out how the viruses produce these opposite effects could therefore give an improved understanding of cellular growth control. As William Haseltine of Harvard's Dana-Farber Cancer Institute has said, "These viruses may have put their fingers on the pulse of the replicative cycle of the T4 cell." The possibility that the information might also provide the means of interrupting the often fatal progression of the diseases caused by the viruses does not diminish interest in the research.

A recent profusion of reports, most of them appearing in *Science* over the past 3 or 4 weeks, has yielded new clues to the ways in which the HTLV's act. Earlier research had indicated that all three of the viruses produce *trans*-activating proteins that stimulate the expression of viral genes. The proteins might also alter cellular gene expression, thus disrupting growth control in infected cells.

It will now be easier to test this hypothesis. The viral genes coding for the *trans*-activating proteins have been definitively identified in all three viruses, thus confirming that HTLV-III, like HTLV-I and -II, does have such a gene. "It reinforces the notion that these retroviruses are unique in having this function," says Flossie Wong-Staal of the National Cancer Institute (NCI).

HTLV-III provided a surprise, however. Its *trans*-activating gene is in an unexpected location and is distinctly different in structure from those of HTLV-I and -II. The difference may help explain the diametrically opposed effects of HTLV-I and -II on the one hand and of HTLV-III on the other. It may also be new grist for the mills of those who already think that the AIDS virus is too unlike HTLV-I and -II to carry the same family name (*Science*, 22 March 1985).

Nevertheless, despite the differences in the *trans*-activating genes, the new work shows that transcription of all three into the corresponding messenger RNA's (mRNA's), which is the first step in the synthesis of the proteins, follows the same unusual pattern. Finally, investigators are defining the control sequences on the target genes that respond to *trans*-activation. These are also unusual and may be representatives of a new class of genetic regulatory elements.

When the original evidence for *trans*-activation by HTLV-I and -II was obtained about a year ago, the prediction was that the protein causing this activity would be encoded in a region of the viral genomes that had been designated "pX"

because its function was unknown. The right-hand half of the pX region, which is sometimes designated the *lor* (for long open reading frame) region, codes for a protein with a molecular weight of about 40,000 and is very similar in the two viruses, a finding which may mean that it has an essential function.

Two groups, using different approaches, have now confirmed that the *x-lor* region codes for the *trans*-activating proteins of HTLV-I and -II. Haseltine, Joseph Sodroski, and their Dana-Farber colleagues have shown that the *x-lor* region of either virus is all that is needed to stimulate the expression of genes under the control of the viral regulatory sequences (*1*).

In addition, in a report in the 5 July 1985 issue of *Science*, Irvin Chen, Dennis Slamon, and their colleagues at the University of California School of Medicine in Los Angeles describe HTLV-II mutants in which the *x-lor* region can no longer make its protein product. Transcription of the viral genes is greatly reduced in the mutants, which fail to replicate. "This is direct evidence that the *x-lor* gene is necessary for replication because it is necessary for transcriptional activation," Chen says. Both the Haseltine (*2*) and the Chen (*3*) groups have found that the *x-lor* proteins are largely located in the cell nucleus, the appropriate site for proteins that alter gene transcription.

Chen and his colleagues could not detect the *trans*-activating protein in the HTLV-I particle. Apparently the virus does not carry it into newly infected cells but must make it after arrival there. The results with the *x-lor* mutant suggest that a low level of transcription occurs even in the absence of the *trans*-activating protein. If the same is true for

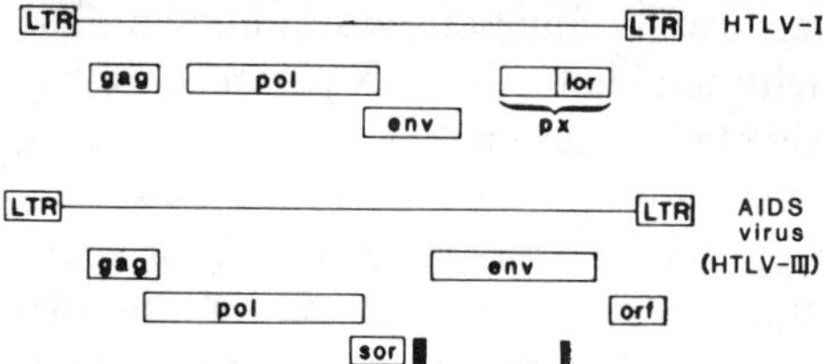

Organization of the HTLV-I and -III genomes. The black bars indicate the regions coding for the *trans*-activating protein of the AIDS virus.

the normal, wild-type virus, then it may initially produce a small amount of the protein, thus stimulating more transcription and producing a positive feedback that allows efficient virus replication.

In any event, now that the function of the *x-lor* region has been established, Haseltine proposes that it be given the designation *tat*—for *trans*-activating transcriptional gene—with the subscripts I or II to indicate the specific virus.

If the HTLV-III genome followed the same organizational pattern as HTLV-I and -II, then its *trans*-activating protein ought to have been encoded in the open reading frame that is located to the right of the viral envelope (*env*) gene and extends into the right-hand long terminal repeat (LTR). That is not what has been found, however.

In the 5 July 1985 issue of *Science*, Wong-Staal and her NCI colleagues and Sodroski, Haseltine, and their colleagues report that they have identified the HTLV-III *tat* gene. It consists of three exons, the first of which does not code for protein structure. The second and third exons encode a total of 86 amino acids, which makes the protein about one-fourth the size of the HTLV-I and -II *trans*-activating proteins. The second exon, which codes for 72 amino acids, is

located approximately in the middle of the viral genome between a short open reading frame, designated *sor*, and the start of the *env* gene. That region had not previously been thought to have protein-coding capabilities. The remaining 14 amino acids are encoded by a small exon located within the *env* gene. Only the second exon is absolutely required for *trans*-activation.

The sequence of the HTLV-III protein does not resemble those of any other protein, including the HTLV-I and -II *tat* proteins. It is rich in basic amino acids, a finding that is consistent with its proposed role in altering gene expression.

Investigators who favor the inclusion of the AIDS virus in the HTLV family and those who oppose it can both find support in these results. The gene encoding the AIDS virus *trans*-activating protein is clearly different from those of HTLV-I and -II. Nevertheless, the identification of such a gene in the AIDS virus buttresses the arguments of those who think that it is truly an HTLV. "At a minimum the viruses have all evolved a *trans*-activating mechanism for speeding up their own replication," Haseltine explains. "It is a new property these viruses have and they have new genes to go along with it."

Among the RNA-containing viruses, only the three HTLV's and the related bovine leukemia virus have definitively been shown to have *trans*-activating capabilities. Although there has been a report of *trans*-activation by Rous sarcoma virus, other investigators, including Haseltine, have had trouble confirming the result and this situation awaits further clarification. The HTLV's and BLV may in fact more closely resemble certain DNA-containing viruses in their mode of action than other retroviruses. For example, the DNA viruses SV40 and adenovirus, both of which can transform appropriate cell types, make *trans*-activating proteins.

Synthesis of the *trans*-activating gene messengers provides another point of similarity between HTLV-III and the other two HTLV's. The Haseltine and Chen groups (*4*) and also that of Mitsuaki Yoshida at the Tokyo Cancer Institute (*5*) have found that the *tat* genes of HTLV-I and -II consist of three exons separated by two introns, an organization similar to that of the HTLV-III gene, despite its other differences. Formation of the corresponding mRNA's thus requires two splicing steps to remove the introns and join the exons. This is a very unusual mode of synthesis for a retroviral mRNA. Two exons and a single splicing event is more typical.

In addition, the first four nucleotides coding for the *trans*-activating proteins of HTLV-I and -II are located not in *x-lor* region, which forms the third exon, but come from the start of the *env* gene, which is some distance away in the second exon. "There is a completely novel pattern for generating the *x-lor* mRNA," Chen points out. The unusual splicing pattern may provide a means by which the HTLV's can control the synthesis of their *trans*-activating proteins.

The supposition is that the *trans*-activating proteins of HTLV-I and -II are the transforming proteins of the viruses. In addition to stimulating transcription of viral genes, they may perhaps increase the transcription of cellular genes that stimulate cell division, thus producing the uncontrolled growth characteristic of transformed cells. Although the potential cellular targets of the HTLV-I and -II *trans*-activating proteins are still unknown, the gene for the interleukin-2 receptor remains a good candidate. Transformed cells have greatly increased

numbers of this receptor, which mediates the growth stimulating effects of the lymphokine interleukin-2.

However, the *trans*-activating proteins by themselves may not be sufficient to generate a cancerous tumor, Chen points out. Although cultured cells that have been transformed by HTLV-I or -II make the corresponding mRNA's, tumor cells that have been isolated from leukemic patients do not. The *trans*-activating proteins may be needed early in oncogenesis to give the cells the ability to divide continuously. This would be consistent with the role proposed for the *trans*-activating proteins of such DNA viruses as SV40 and adenovirus. Other, additional steps may then be required to complete the cancerous transformation.

In contrast to the role proposed for the HTLV-I and -II *trans*-activating proteins, the *trans*-activating protein of HTLV-III may turn off a gene needed for cell division or stimulate one that suppresses cell division. "Now that we have the proteins isolated we can test this hypothesis," Haseltine says.

A complete understanding of *trans*-activation requires identification of the regulatory sequences on the target genes that respond to the *tat* proteins. Haseltine and his colleagues have identified these sequences for the HTLV-I genome and have found that they, like so many other HTLV features, are unusual (*6*).

Most genes have at least two regulatory elements, a promoter that helps to determine accurately the start site for transcription and an enhancer that governs the rate of transcription from the promoter. In retroviruses these regulatory regions are in the LTR's at the ends of the genome.

The Haseltine group has found that the regulatory sequence for HTLV-I *trans*-activation, which they call the *tar* (for *trans*-acting responsive) sequence, lies between nucleotide -159 and nucleotide $+315$ (counting from the transcription start site). It includes part of the enhancer, which extends from nucleotide -350 to nucleotide -55, plus the promoter, which is located about 35 nucleotides before the start site. But neither the enhancer nor the promoter is by itself sufficient for *trans*-activation.

Also unusual, Haseltine stresses, is the efficacy with which this regulatory region seems to work. *Trans*-activation by the HTLV's gives greater increases in transcription than other systems, including the SV40 system, usually do. "We think that it may be a new kind of regulatory sequence that will be found in other genes that need to be turned on in a hurry," Haseltine says. He suggests that it may be similar to another regulatory sequence that was recently found by Nam-Hai Chua of Rockefeller University and his colleagues in a totally unrelated gene coding for a plant photosynthetic protein. All in all, the HTLV's are proving to be estimable guides to the molecular biology of the mammalian cell.

References

1. J. Sodroski, C. Rosen, W. C. Goh, W. Haseltine, *Science* **228**, 1430 (1985).
2. W. C. Goh *et al.*, *ibid.* **227**, 1227 (1985).
3. D. J. Slamon *et al.*, *ibid.* **228**, 1427 (1985).
4. W. Wachsman *et al.*, *ibid.*, p. 1534 (1985).
5. M. Seiki, A. Hikikoshi, T. Taniguchi, M. Yoshida, *ibid.*, p. 1532 (1985).
6. C. A. Rosen, J. G. Sodroski, W. A. Haseltine, *Proc. Natl. Acad. Sci. U.S.A.*, in press.

Letter to the Editor

5 July 1985

99. AIDS Repository

Richard A. Kaslow

The National Institute of Allergy and Infectious Diseases and the National Cancer Institute have developed a repository of biological specimens from homosexual men. The specimens were collected through contracts with five major U.S. universities for studies of the natural history of acquired immune deficiency syndrome (AIDS). Information about applying for collaborative use of these specimens and pertinent epidemiological data is now available from the Project Officer, AIDS Repository, Epidemiology and Biometry Section, National Institute of Allergy and Infectious Diseases, Westwood Building, Room 739, National Institutes of Health, Bethesda, Maryland 20205.

100. The *x* Gene is Essential for HTLV Replication

Irvin S.Y. Chen, Dennis J. Slamon, Joseph D. Rosenblatt, Neil P. Shah, Shirley G. Quan, and William Wachsman

The human T-cell leukemia viruses (HTLV) are associated with specific T-cell malignancies (*1–3*). Human T-cell leukemia virus type I (HTLV-I) is the likely etiologic agent for adult T-cell leukemia (ATL), which is endemic to parts of Japan, the Caribbean, and Africa (*1, 2*). Human T-cell leukemia virus type II (HTLV-II) was associated with a neoplasm in a single patient with a relatively benign T-cell variant of hairy cell leukemia (*4*). Despite the difference in associated diseases, both viruses will infect normal human T cells in vitro, causing their continued proliferation in the absence of exogenous interleukin-2 (*5–8*). The mechanism by which HTLV induces T-cell malignancies in vivo and T-cell transformation in vitro is unknown. Nucleic acid hybridization to cellular DNA (*9–11*) and nucleic acid sequencing (*12–14*) of the complete HTLV-I and HTLV-II proviral genomes have not revealed sequences in HTLV that are related to classical viral oncogenes. Unlike such replication-competent retroviruses as the lymphoid leukosis viruses (*15–17*), Moloney murine leukemia viruses (*18–20*), and mouse mammary tumor viruses (*21*), the HTLV proviral genome does not integrate near specific cellular sequences in tumors (*22*). This finding argues against the theory of transformation by insertional mutagenesis. Therefore, malignant transformation by HTLV appears to involve a novel mechanism.

The genomic structure of HTLV-I and HTLV-II is different from that of other retroviruses. In addition to the *gag, pol,* and *env* genes, HTLV has a fourth gene between *env* and the 3′ long terminal repeat (LTR), termed *x* (*12*) [also referred to as *lor* (*14*)]. RNA processing generates a subgenomic messenger RNA (mRNA) (*23*) that encodes a protein of 40 kilodaltons (kD) in HTLV-I–infected cells and 37 kD in HTLV-II–infected cells (*24–26*). The function of these proteins is unknown; however, the conservation of the *x* gene in the genomes of both HTLV-I (*12*) and HTLV-II (*14, 27*) suggests a role for the *x*-encoded protein in cellular transformation. It has been proposed that these proteins have a role in the enhancement of transcription by the HTLV LTR's (*28*), which would be analogous to the immediate early gene functions of the adenoviruses (*29, 30*), the papovaviruses (*31*), and some herpesviruses (*32*). We have used a clone of infectious, proviral HTLV-II DNA (*11, 27, 33*) to study the role of the *x* gene of HTLV in viral replication. The results demonstrate that the *x* gene is essential for high levels of HTLV-II transcription. In the absence of a functional *x* gene, approximately 100-fold lower levels of viral mRNA are transcribed.

As with T cells, B cells will also support a productive HTLV infection although HTLV does not transform B cells. Some Epstein-Barr virus (EBV)–transformed B-cell lines infected with HTLV-I have been isolated from ATL patients (*34*) and an EBV-transformed B-cell line infected with HTLV-II was obtained from peripheral blood of the patient Mo (*8*). The kinetics of productive infection by HTLV-II in B-cell lines in vitro is similar to in vitro infection of peripheral blood T cells. Therefore, infection of B-cell lines by HTLV provided a model system in which to study HTLV replication. We have previously described a transfection system for HTLV-II in B-cell lines (*27, 33*).

An activity in HTLV-infected cells has been found which enhances the transcription of HTLV LTR's introduced into the cells by DNA transfection (*28*). It was hypothesized that this transcriptional regulatory function was the product of the *x* gene. To examine these findings with respect to HTLV-II, we made a recombinant construct in which the expression of the gene for chloramphenicol acetyltransferase (CAT) (*35*) was dependent on the function of the HTLV-II LTR. We used an HTLV-II LTR derived from a proviral DNA clone of HTLV-II that had been isolated from HTLV-II–transformed T cells. The clone is infectious in DNA transfection assays (*27, 33*) and results in replication-competent HTLV-II capable of transforming normal human peripheral blood T cells. Thereby we ensured that the LTR was representative of the wild-type HTLV-II genome. The LTR-CAT recombinant constructs were transfected into uninfected and HTLV-II–infected EBV-transformed B-cell lines, termed 729 and 729pH6neo, respectively. Cell line 729pH6neo produces HTLV-II after sta-

ble transfection with cloned HTLV-II proviral DNA. Expression of the CAT gene by the LTR's was not detectable in the uninfected cells. In cells infected with HTLV-II, more CAT was expressed under the control of the LTR than by the SV40 early promoter (Fig. 1). Similar results were obtained with a second LTR from another infectious clone of HTLV-II and with a second pair of B cells, one uninfected and the other infected with HTLV-II. Although it is possible that selection for cells competent to transcribe HTLV RNA occurred during the course of infection of cells, it is unlikely to have occurred in the cell line transfected stably by cloned HTLV-II; the only selection was for maintenance of the neo^R marker in the vector. Thus, HTLV-II LTR function is enhanced in the HTLV-II–infected cells. These results are consistent with the demonstration of enhanced function of the HTLV-I LTR in the infected cells of a pair of HTLV-I–infected and –uninfected fibroblast cell lines (*28*). A *trans*-acting viral function in HTLV-II–infected cell lines appears to be necessary for efficient LTR function.

A possible candidate for a virally encoded *trans*-acting protein is the product of the *x* gene, p37^{xII}. We constructed mutants of HTLV-II by means of a plasmid (pH6neo) that contains a complete HTLV-II provirus and was previously demonstrated to be infectious (*13, 27, 33*). A unique Cla I site located within the *x* gene (approximately 50 codons from the NH$_2$ terminus) was cleaved and subjected to Bal 3l exonuclease digestion to generate a series of deletions of varying size within the *x* gene (Fig. 2). The activity of these mutant proviruses was analyzed by DNA transfection into B-cell lines.

The complete wild-type proviral ge-

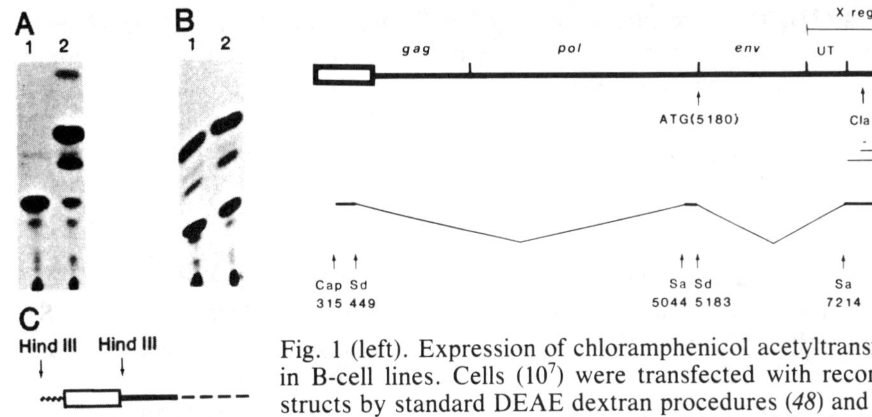

Fig. 1 (left). Expression of chloramphenicol acetyltransferase (CAT) in B-cell lines. Cells (10^7) were transfected with recombinant constructs by standard DEAE dextran procedures (*48*) and harvested 42 hours after transfection. Assays for CAT activity in disrupted cells were as previously described (*35*). Migration of [^{14}C]chloramphenicol in thin-layer chromatography plates is from bottom to top. The acetylated form of chloramphenicol, indicating presence of CAT activity, is the furthest migrating form. (A) The LTR and flanking cell sequences of an infectious HTLV-II proviral clone (pH6) were isolated by digestion with Hind III (within cell sequences) and Eco RI (nucleotide position 786, 23 nucleotides from the 3′ end of the 5′ LTR) and substituted for the SV40 early promotor of pSVCAT by ligation with Hind III synthetic linkers. (Lane 1) 729-6; (lane 2) 729pH6neo. (B) pSVCAT, containing the SV40 early promoter, was modified from a previously described construction (*49*). (C) The LTR CAT and SV CAT constructs. Symbols are wavy line, human DNA sequences; open box, LTR sequences; dotted line, SV40 sequences—early promoter and termination sequences; solid bar, CAT gene.   Fig. 2 (right). Schematic representation of the HTLV-II proviral genome and position of the deletions in constructed mutant genomes. The HTLV-II proviral genome is shown schematically at the top with the relative position of the four genes indicated. The X region is as defined by Seiki *et al.* (*12*) and includes an untranslated region (UT) and the *x* gene. The position of the initiation methionine used for both *env* and *x* is indicated. The position of deletions in the X region are indicated beneath the HTLV-II genome as thin solid lines. The number to the right of the deletion designates specific proviral mutants. The structure of the processed HTLV-II mRNA which encodes the *x* gene is shown beneath the HTLV-II genome. The position of the three exons is shown. The numbers beneath the mRNA indicate the nucleotide position of the cap site, splice donors (Sd), splice acceptors (Sa), and polyadenylation sites of the *x* mRNA (*13*). Deletions were generated in the proviral clone of HTLV-II, pH6neo, by cleavage with Cla I followed by Bal 31 exonuclease digestion. Sal I linkers were introduced at the point of deletion to facilitate screening and nucleic acid sequence analysis of mutant proviral DNA.

nomes of HTLV subcloned into pSV2neo (*11, 36*) were transfected into a B-cell line, 729-6, and transfected cells were selected for Geneticin (G418) resistance (*33*). About 15 to 20 percent of the G418-resistant clones transfected with the wild-type HTLV-II provirus expressed infectious, transforming HTLV-II. In contrast, the transfection of cells by three mutants containing *x* gene dele-

tions of various sizes did not result in stable G418-resistant clones capable of producing infectious transforming HTLV-II. This is despite the fact that more than 90 independent G418-resistant clones of this type were tested for expression of one of the viral core antigens (p19) by indirect immunofluorescence (*8*) and for viral RNA expression by "dot blot" analysis with HTLV-II–

specific probes (33). These results were confirmed in separate experiments by pooling clones of cells stably transfected with either wild-type provirus or each of the three deletion mutants and testing for production of transforming virus by a cocultivation assay with peripheral blood T cells (8). The pooled group of control cells transfected with wild-type HTLV-II was capable of transforming normal human peripheral blood T cells, whereas the pooled cells transfected with mutant HTLV-II did not produce transforming virus. This assay is capable of detecting as few as 50 HTLV-II–infected donor cells. Therefore, deletion mutations in the x gene appear to abrogate viral replication.

We further analyzed individual clones of 729 cells stably transfected with mutant HTLV-II to study the genetic basis for the restriction in transcriptional activity. DNA was extracted from several of the cell lines and analyzed by Southern hybridization for the presence of the complete HTLV-II mutant genome. An example of three clones in which the mutant HTLV-II genomes are integrated is shown in Fig. 3. None of these clones expressed detectable viral RNA by dot-blot analysis over a period of 8 months in culture, although the complete mutant genome is present. Furthermore, these clones did not produce transforming virus as assayed by cocultivation with peripheral blood T cells.

The nucleotide sequence surrounding the point of deletion in clone 729ΔCla35-8 was determined (Fig. 4). This clone has a deletion of 187 nucleotides and an insertion of two Sal I synthetic linkers. If p37^{xII} is required for efficient HTLV-II transcription, then superinfection with wild-type HTLV-II should provide wild-type p37^{xII} in *trans* and "rescue" the inactive provirus. We tested this predic-

tion by infecting the 729ΔCla35-8 cells with HTLV-II. Four independent HTLV-II–infected cultures expressed the HTLV-II x gene product p37^{xII} (Fig. 5A). As expected, the parent cell line containing the mutant HTLV-II did not express detectable levels of p37^{xII}.

We determined whether the resident mutant HTLV-II provirus was transcribed in these infected cells by S1 nuclease analysis. An S1 nuclease hybridization probe that includes the deleted region will distinguish between expression of wild-type and mutant RNA. Wild-type RNA would be expected to protect the entire length of the probe (201 nucleotides), whereas the mutant RNA would protect only a part of the hybridization probe (52 nucleotides). S1 nuclease analysis of RNA from the parent cell line prior to superinfection revealed a low level of HTLV-II ΔCla35 RNA that was detectable only in long autoradiographic exposures (Fig. 5B). This RNA is transcribed beginning at the cap site of the mutant provirus LTR. By contrast, the superinfected cell lines expressed high levels of both wild-type and mutant RNA. The amount of mutant RNA expressed in the superinfected cells is comparable to wild-type RNA and about 100 to 200 times the amount expressed in the parent cells. Only the 201-nucleotide band, representative of wild-type RNA, was detected when RNA from a cell line that had been transfected only with wild-type HTLV-II was analyzed (Fig. 5B, 729pH6neo). To further confirm the "rescue" of the defective genome, we investigated the ability of the mutant genome in the infected cells to be packaged as virions and form unintegrated viral DNA after infection of uninfected 729-6 B cells. Analysis by Southern hybridization of cytoplasmic, linear, unintegrated viral DNA demon-

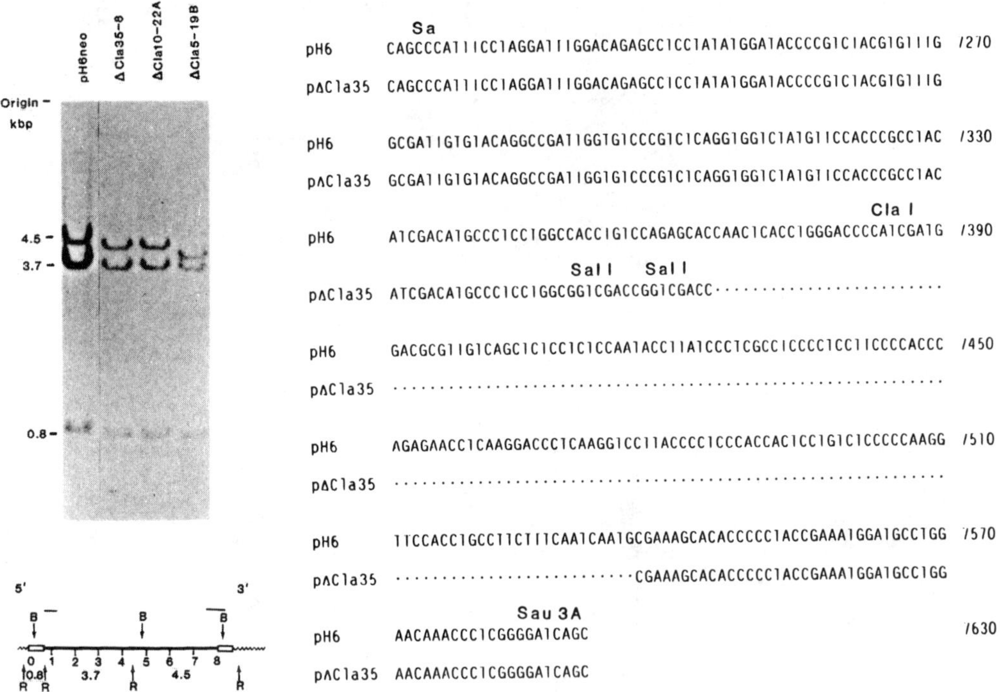

Fig. 3 (left). Presence of mutant HTLV-II proviral genomes in 729-6 B cells. Cells were transfected with wild-type HTLV-II, pH6neo, and derivative mutant genomes pΔCla5, pΔCla10, and pΔCla35 by spheroplast fusion as described (*33*). G418-resistant clones of cells were propagated, DNA-extracted, and analyzed by Southern hybridization after digestion with Eco RI. The location of the hybridization probe (thin, straight horizontal line) indicated above the HTLV-II genome and fragments of the cloned wild-type provirus predicted after Eco RI digestion are shown below the autoradiogram. B, Bam HI; R, Eco RI; open box, LTR; wavy line, human DNA sequences.   Fig. 4 (right). Nucleic acid sequence of the *x* gene in deletion-mutant clone pΔCla35. The clone was sequenced about the point of deletion in the *x* gene (*50*). The sequence of the wild-type HTLV-II genome (pH6) (*13, 27*) is aligned for comparison. The position of the splice acceptor at the 5' end of the *x* open reading frame (*23*) is indicated. Only relevant restriction enzyme sites are shown. The nucleotide positions with respect to the entire HTLV-II genome (*13*) are shown to the right of the sequence.

strated the presence of mutant viral DNA, distinguished from wild-type by the presence of a Sal I restriction enzyme site. Similar results were also obtained with the virus that had been rescued from the cell line 729ΔCla10-22A (see Fig. 3).

Thus, the *x* gene of HTLV-II is necessary for efficient transcription of the HTLV genome. A mutant that lacks a functional *x* gene transcribes viral RNA at levels 1/100 to 1/200 as efficiently as the wild-type provirus. These results, considered with the activation of LTR function as assayed by transfection of LTR recombinant constructs into virus-infected cells, indicate that the *x* gene product enhances viral transcription by acting on the initiation of transcription by the HTLV LTR. The recent demonstration of nuclear localization of p40^*xl* is consistent with this function (*26*).

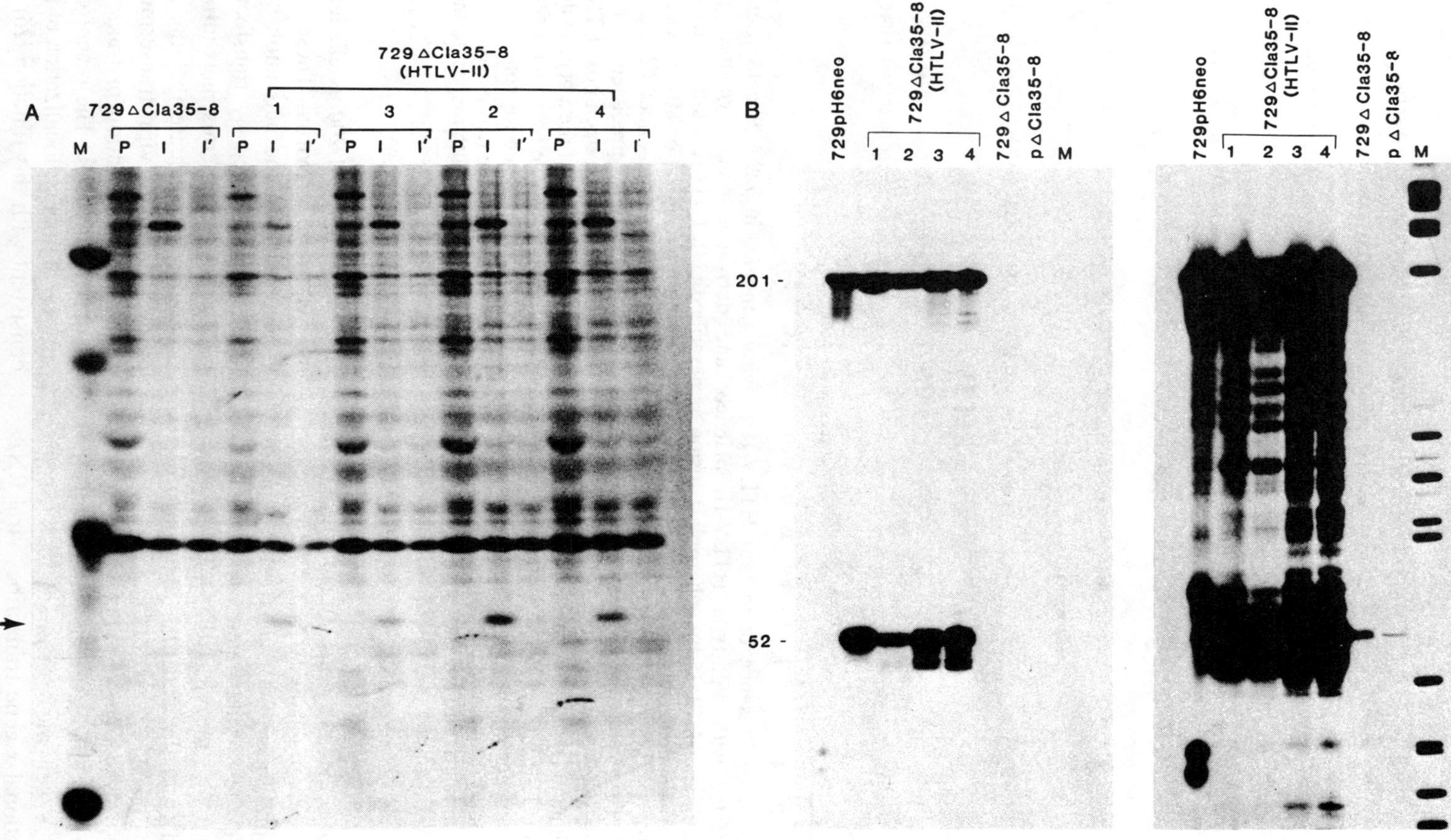

A
729△Cla35-8
729△Cla35-8
(HTLV-II)
1   3   2   4
M   P I I'   P I I'   P I I'   P I I'   P I I'
B
729pH6neo
729△Cla35-8
(HTLV-II)
1 2 3 4
729△Cla35-8
p△Cla35-8
M
201 -
52 -
729pH6neo
729△Cla35-8
(HTLV-II)
1 2 3 4
729△Cla35-8
p△Cla35-8
M

A low level of viral transcription occurs in the absence of x gene function. In the mutant provirus of pΔCla35-8 the deletion of sequences and insertion of synthetic oligonucleotide linkers has fortuitously maintained the reading frame (see Fig. 4). Therefore, although unlikely, we cannot exclude the possibility that a weakly functional x gene product is present. The deletion results in a loss of a substantial number of amino acids from within the NH_2-terminal region of the protein and adds irrelevant amino acids by the introduction of the two synthetic oligonucleotide linkers. Also, loss of this part of the protein would be expected to be deleterious, because this region is the most highly conserved between HTLV-I and HTLV-II x proteins and also has some conserved sequences with bovine leukemia virus (36).

The low level of transcription seen in cells transfected with mutant HTLV-II could explain how the wild-type virus replicates. After integration into the genome of the host cell, low levels of x mRNA are transcribed, resulting in some p37^{xII}. This x protein would activate LTR function, in turn producing higher levels of x protein to further activate the LTR to transcribe RNA at greater levels. This proposed process is consistent with the kinetics of HTLV infection in B cells (37). Unlike a typical retrovirus infection, in which stable RNA expression is dependent solely upon passage of the newly infected cell through the S phase, stable HTLV expression is a much slower process. Multiple cell generations are required to generate high levels of virus expression, consistent with the hypothesis that expression of HTLV occurs via a positive regulatory mechanism.

An x gene is also found in bovine leukemia virus (36), which shares many molecular, biological, and pathological

Fig. 5. (facing page) (A) Radioimmunoprecipitation of ^{35}S methionine-labeled cell lysates with antibodies reactive to HTLV-II p37^{xII} (24). Preimmune serum (10 μl), a mixture of two immune antibodies α pXIV-5 and α pXIV-6 (5 μl each) or a mixture of the same antibodies plus the synthetic peptides against which the antibodies are directed (I′), was used to immunoprecipitate p37^{xII} from 10^7 count/min of labeled lysate from 729ΔCla35-8 or from each of four independent HTLV-II–infected lines. Competition with the synthetic peptides was performed as previously described (24). P, preimmune sera; I, immune sera; I′, immune sera plus synthetic peptides. Arrow indicates the position of p37^{XII}. The protein standards (M) are 92.6, 68, 43, and 25.7 kD in size. (B) Expression of mutant HTLV-II RNA in 729 ΔCla35-8 cells infected with wild-type HTLV-II. For each infection 5 × 10^6 729ΔCla35-8 cells were infected with HTLV-II by cocultivation with an equal number of HTLV-II–infected B cells, termed J-WIL. Following 2 days of cocultivation, the J-WIL cells were killed by addition of G418 (1.5 mg/ml) to the culture medium. The infected cells were propagated for an additional 6 weeks, at which time approximately 80 percent of the cells expressed HTLV-II p19 antigen as assayed by indirect immunofluorescence. Total RNA was extracted from four independently infected cell populations and analyzed by S1 nuclease analysis (51) in parallel with RNA from the parent cell line, 729ΔCla35-8, and a cell line transfected with the wild-type HTLV-II genome, 729pH6neo. The hybridization probe is a DNA fragment of wild-type HTLV-II from the Cla I site (nucleotide 7385) to the Sau 3A site (nucleotide 7584) (see Fig. 4). The Sau 3A site was labeled with γ^{32}P ATP and T4 polynucleotide kinase. S1 nuclease assays were performed as previously described with 50 μg of total RNA for all samples, except in the case of 729pH6neo, where 20 μg of RNA was used. The pΔCla35-8 refers to the fragment of the clone from the Sal I site in the linker inserted at the point of deletion in pΔCla35-8 to the Sau 3A site present in the same position as the Sau 3A site of the wild-type genome (see Fig. 4). This fragment was 5′ end-labeled at the Sau 3A site and, therefore, serves as a marker for the distance from the labeled end to the point of deletion. The marker is Sau 3A–digested pBR322 DNA. Sizes are indicated in nucleotides. (Left) Five-hour exposure of gel; (right) 48-hour exposure.

552

features with HTLV (*38–40*). The telio-logic basis for the evolution of the *x* gene in HTLV/BLV is unknown. Its product may regulate viral expression under some circumstances. A unique mRNA-processing mechanism operates in this retrovirus family whereby the *env* methionine initiation codon and one nucleotide of the next codon are joined to the major open reading frame of the *x* gene to generate the complete coding region (*41, 42*). This processing scheme may be a means of modulating *x* gene expression, thereby allowing further regulation of overall viral expression.

The *x* gene is functionally analogous to *trans*-acting transcriptional regulatory genes of some DNA viruses, the best studied example of which is the EIA gene of adenoviruses. The product of this immediate early gene is required for efficient expression of the other adenovirus genes (*43, 44*); however, a complete replication cycle can occur in the absence of EIA functions, although with delayed kinetics (*45*). The functional analogies between EIA and *x* are relevant to potential mechanisms of HTLV transformation since adenoviruses will transform rodent cells, and EIA has been demonstrated to be capable of transforming cells (*46, 47*). Therefore, the functions of the *x* gene in transcriptional activation are likely to be important in understanding the ability of HTLV to cause T-lymphoid malignancies.

Note added in proof: The low level of viral transcription in the absence of a functional *x* gene is also observed in cell line 729ΔCla5-19B (Figs. 2 and 3) which contains a mutant provirus deleted for more than 500 nucleotides in *x*.

References and Notes

1. R. C. Gallo *et al.*, *Cancer Res.* **43**, 3892 (1983).
2. Y. Hinuma *et al.*, *Proc. Natl. Acad. Sci. U.S.A.* **78**, 6476 (1981).
3. V. S. Kalyanaraman *et al.*, *Science* **218**, 571 (1982).
4. A. Saxon, R. H. Stevens, D. W. Golde, *Ann. Intern. Med.* **88**, 323 (1978).
5. I. Miyoshi, *Nature (London)* **294**, 770 (1981).
6. N. Yamamoto *et al.*, *Science* **217**, 737 (1982).
7. M. Popovic *et al.*, *Proc. Natl. Acad. Sci. U.S.A.* **80**, 5402 (1983).
8. I. S. Y. Chen, S. G. Quan, D. W. Golde, *ibid.*, p. 7006.
9. F. Wong-Staal *et al.*, *Nature (London)* **302**, 626 (1983).
10. M. Yoshida *et al.*, *Proc. Natl. Acad. Sci. U.S.A.* **81**, 2534 (1984).
11. I. S. Y. Chen, J. McLaughlin, D. W. Golde, *Nature (London)* **309**, 276 (1984).
12. M. Seiki *et al.*, *Proc. Natl. Acad. Sci. U.S.A.* **80**, 3618 (1983).
13. K. Shimotohno *et al.*, *ibid.* **82**, 3101 (1985).
14. W. A. Haseltine *et al.*, *Science* **225**, 419 (1984).
15. W. S. Hayward, B. G. Neel, S. M. Astrin, *Nature (London)* **290**, 475 (1981).
16. G. S. Payne, J. M. Bishop, H. E. Varmus, *ibid.* **295**, 209 (1982).
17. M. R. Noori-Daloii *et al.*, *ibid.* **294**, 574 (1981).
18. P. N. Tsichlis, P. G. Strauss, L. F. Hu, *ibid.* **302**, 445 (1983).
19. G. Lemay, P. Jolicoeur, *Proc. Natl. Acad. Sci. U.S.A.* **81**, 38 (1984).
20. D. Steffen, *ibid.*, p. 2097.
21. R. Nusse *et al.*, *Nature (London)* **307**, 131 (1984).
22. M. Seiki *et al.*, *ibid.* **309**, 640 (1984).
23. W. Wachsman *et al.*, *Science* **226**, 177 (1984).
24. D. J. Slamon *et al.*, *ibid.*, p. 61.
25. T. H. Lee *et al.*, *ibid.*, p. 57.
26. W. C. Goh *et al.*, *ibid.* **227**, 1227 (1985); D. J. Slamon *et al.*, *ibid.* **228**, 1427 (1985).
27. K. Shimotohno *et al.*, *Proc. Natl. Acad. Sci. U.S.A.* **81**, 6657 (1984).
28. J. Sodroski *et al.*, *Science* **225**, 421 (1984).
29. R. B. Gaynor, D. Hillman, A. J. Berk, *Proc. Natl. Acad. Sci. U.S.A.* **81**, 1193 (1984).
30. R. Treisman, M. R. Green, T. Maniatis, *ibid.* **80**, 7428 (1983).
31. J. Brady *et al.*, *ibid.* **81**, 2040 (1984).
32. R. J. Watson and J. B. Clements, *Nature (London)* **285**, 329 (1980).
33. I. S. Y. Chen, J. McLaughlin, D. W. Golde, *ibid.* **309**, 276 (1984).
34. N. Yamamoto *et al.*, *ibid.* **299**, 367 (1982).
35. C. M. Gorman, L. F. Moffat, B. H. Howard, *Mol. Cell. Biol.* **2**, 1044 (1982).
36. N. Sagata *et al.*, *EMBO J.* **3**, 3231 (1984).
37. J. Rosenblatt, unpublished observations.
38. N. Sagata *et al.*, *Proc. Natl. Acad. Sci. U.S.A.* **81**, 4741 (1984).
39. N. Sagata *et al.*, *ibid.* **82**, 677 (1985).
40. A. Burny *et al.*, *Mechanisms of Viral Leukaemogenesis* (Churchill Livingstone, London, 1984), p. 229.
41. W. Wachsman *et al.*, *Science* **228**, 1534 (1985).
42. M. Seiki *et al.*, *ibid.*, p. 1532.
43. N. Jones and T. Shenk, *Proc. Natl. Acad. Sci. U.S.A.* **76**, 3665 (1979).
44. A. J. Berk *et al.*, *Cell* **17**, 935 (1979).
45. R. B. Gaynor and A. J. Berk, *ibid.* **33**, 683 (1983).
46. H. E. Ruley, *Nature (London)* **304**, 602 (1983).
47. A. Houweling, P. van den Elsen, A. van der Eb, *Virology* **105**, 537 (1980).

48. J. Banerji, L. Olson, W. Schaffner, *Cell* **33**, 729 (1983).
49. J. Banerji, personal communication.
50. A. M. Maxam and W. Gilbert, *Proc. Natl. Acad. Sci. U.S.A.* **74**, 560 (1977).
51. A. J. Berk and P. A. Sharp, *Cell* **12**, 721 (1977).
52. We thank D. Golde for continued assistance and support; J. Gasson and A. Cann for helpful comments on the manuscript; and M. Ahdieh, C. Nishikubo, A. Healy, J. Fujii, H. Merriman, B. Koers, and W. Aft for technical assistance. Supported by NCI grants CA 32737, CA 38597, CA 09297, and CA 16042; by grants PF-2182 and JFRA-99 from the American Cancer Society; and by a Bank of America–Giannini Foundation Fellowship (W.W.).

12 March 1985; accepted 14 May 1985

Report

5 July 1985

101. *Trans*-Activator Gene of Human T-Lymphotropic Virus Type III (HTLV-III)

Suresh K. Arya, Chan Guo, Steven F. Josephs, and Flossie Wong-Staal

Human T-lymphotropic virus type-III (HTLV-III) is etiologically associated with the acquired immune deficiency syndrome (AIDS) (*1, 2*). It belongs to the group of exogenous retroviruses called HTLV whose other members include HTLV-I and HTLV-II. HTLV-I has been etiologically linked to human adult T-cell leukemia-lymphoma (ATLL) (*3, 4*), and HTLV-II, isolated originally from a patient with hairy cell leukemia (*5*), has not yet been linked to any human disease. These viruses share a number of biological and structural properties which include a tropism for OKT4$^+$ lymphocytes (*2, 6*), the ability to induce giant multinucleated cells in vivo and in vitro (*2, 7*), weak immunologic cross-reactivity of some virally encoded proteins (*8*), and distant nucleic acid sequence homologies (*9, 10*). Despite these similarities, HTLV-III differs from HTLV-I and HTLV-II in many aspects of its structure and biology. For exam-ple, while infection of human T lymphocytes with HTLV-I or HTLV-II often results in transformation and immortal-ization (*3, 4*), infection with HTLV-III generally leads to cell death (*1, 2*).

The genomes of HTLV-III and related viruses have been molecularly cloned and sequenced (*10–14*), and five open reading frames (ORF's) have been iden-tified (*11–15*) (Fig. 1). On the basis of the predicted amino acid sequence and align-ment with known proteins of other retro-viruses, it was postulated that the first, second, and fourth reading frames from the 5' end of the genome constituted the *gag*, *pol*, and *env* genes of HTLV-III. The third open reading frame, termed *sor*, has no correspondence in the HTLV-I or HTLV-II genome and its function is unknown. The fifth open reading frame (3'-*orf*) extends into the 3' long terminal repeat (3'-LTR) and is truncated in some HTLV-III clones. HTLV-III–infected cells contain a *trans-*

acting factor which activates the expression of LTR-linked genes (*16*). Similar factors in HTLV-I, HTLV-II, and bovine leukemia virus (BLV) are the products of a unique viral gene termed *tat* (also called *x-lor*) (*17*). On the basis of structural similarities of the predicted protein of 3′-portion of the unusually long *env* gene of HTLV-III with that of *tat* gene products, it was suggested that the *trans*-acting factor of HTLV-III is encoded by the 3′-portion of *env* gene. However, we show here that the major functional domain of the *trans*-activator gene of HTLV-III is located in what was previously thought to be a noncoding region between the *sor* and *env* genes. This gene consists of three exons and its transcription into a functional messenger RNA (mRNA) involves double splicing. We also describe the characteristics of the putative 3′-*orf* gene, which also consists of three exons, and identify putative mRNA's for *env* and *gag-pol* genes.

To identify *trans*-activator and other genes of HTLV-III, we took the direct approach of obtaining functional complementary DNA (cDNA) clones. In HTLV-III–infected cells there are at least four abundant virus-specific RNA's of 9.4, 4.2, 2.0, and 1.8 kilobases (kb) (*18*). To assess the genetic composition of the individual mRNA's and thus design strategies for obtaining specific cDNA clones, virus-specific RNA's were characterized further by Northern blotting with subgenomic viral DNA probes. As shown in Fig. 1, a 9.4-kb virus-specific RNA was detected by all the subgenomic probes. The ease of detection of other virus-specific RNA's was dependent on the probe used. All RNA species were scored by the probe designated C1, which was a cDNA clone containing leader sequences and a small

5′-part of the *gag* gene. The 4.2-kb RNA was detected by all the probes used in this study except H8, which gave a signal of only marginal relative intensity.

The 2.0-kb and 1.8-kb RNA's were easily scored by the probes representing the 3′-half of the viral genome (probes B8 and H5), and also but faintly by the probe B2. Additional hybridization of these RNA's with a leader sequence probe suggested that their synthesis involved at least one, probably two, splicing events. These results also suggested that the 4.2-kb mRNA was probably the *env* message and that the 9.4-kb RNA could be the genomic RNA as well as the viral readthrough message encoding *gag* proteins. Since the *pol* gene of HTLV-III is in a different reading frame from the *gag* gene, a spliced mRNA involving a frameshift must be synthesized to encode *pol*, but this may not be resolved from the unspliced genomic mRNA. If one assumes that the 3′-*orf* gene transcribes abundant message or messages, either the 2.0-kb or 1.8-kb RNA, or both, are candidates for its transcripts. Similar observations were reported by Muesing *et al.* (*15*). By analogy to the mRNA of the *trans*-activating gene of HTLV-I and HTLV-II, which is also 2.0 kb in size, we speculated that one of the smaller mRNA's of HTLV-III encodes the *trans*-activating function.

We, therefore, screened cDNA libraries of RNA from HTLV-III–infected cells with probes C1 and B8, searching for clones with viral inserts of 2.0 kb or less. Two cDNA libraries were constructed for this purpose. One library was constructed in a mammalian expression vector (here termed pPL) containing SV40 regulatory sequences (*19*). The second library was constructed in a high-efficiency cloning vector lacking mam-

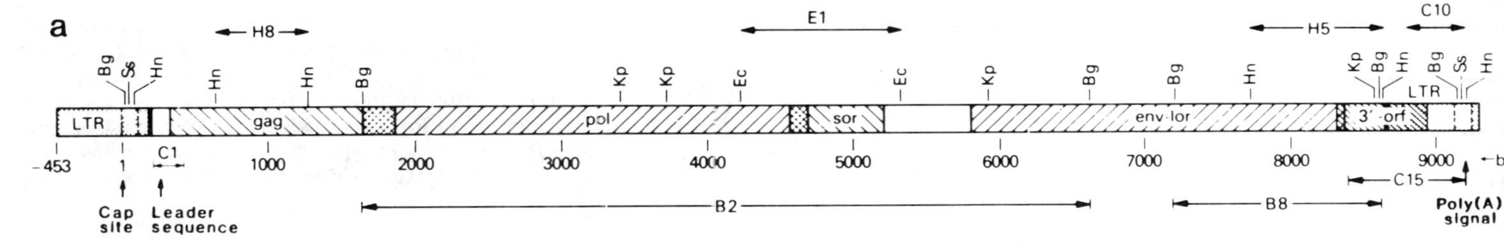

Fig. 1. Analysis of HTLV-III transcripts in virus-infected cells. Poly(A)-selected cellular RNA was hybridized with HTLV-III subgenomic probes by the Northern blot procedure (28). The derivation of the subgenomic probes, designated C1, H8, B2, E1, B8, and H5, along with a physical map of HTLV-III, is shown at the top. Lanes 1 and 2 in each panel are for uninfected and HTLV-III–infected H4 cells, respectively. Subgenomic probes were obtained by subcloning in plasmid vectors the fragments of HTLV-III genome generated by cleavage with specific restriction enzymes. The subclones were selected and characterized by restriction mapping, hybridization, and DNA sequencing. The restriction enzyme designations are Bg, Bg1 II; Ss, Sst I; Hn, Hind III; Kp, Kpn I; and Ec, Eco RI.

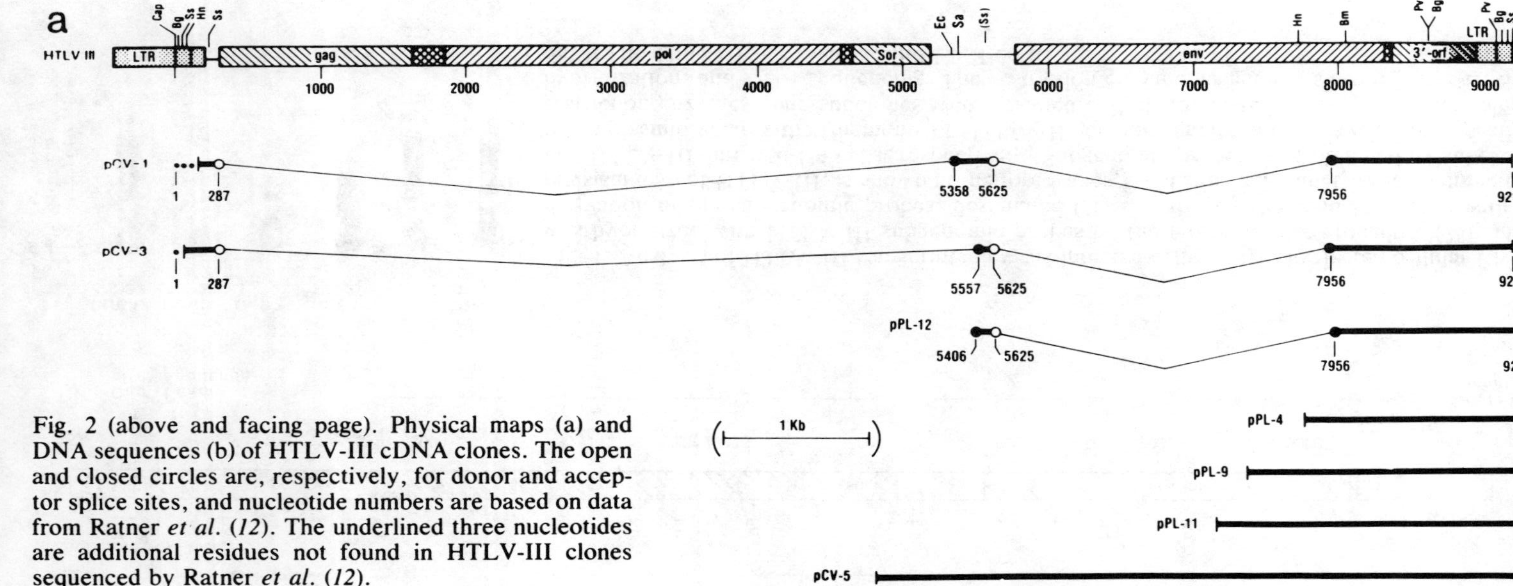

Fig. 2 (above and facing page). Physical maps (a) and DNA sequences (b) of HTLV-III cDNA clones. The open and closed circles are, respectively, for donor and acceptor splice sites, and nucleotide numbers are based on data from Ratner *et al.* (*12*). The underlined three nucleotides are additional residues not found in HTLV-III clones sequenced by Ratner *et al.* (*12*).

b

```
                                             .            .         Hind III
                                 pCV3 aacccactgcttaagcctcaataaagct  82

         .            .             .             .             .             .
pCV3 tgccttgagtgcttcaagtagtgtgtgcccgtctgttgtgtgactctggtaactagagatccctcagacc  152

         .            .       U5--|-tRNA lysine PBS-|             .             .
pCV1 CTTTTAGTCAGTGTGGAAAATCTCTAGCAGTGGCGCCCGAACAGGGACTTGAAAGCGAAAGGGAAACCAG  221
pCV3 ------------------------------------------------------------------------

                                                          pCV1 splice  287 5358
     Sst I                                                                   \/
pCV1 AGGAGCTCTCTCGACGCAGGACTCGGCTTGCTGAAGCGCGCACGGCAAGAGGCGAGGGGCGGCGACTGAA  5359
pCV3 --------------------------------------------------------a--------(
                                                   ***
pCV1 TTGGGTGTCGACATAGCAGAATAGGCGTTACTCGACAGAGGAGAGCAAGAAATGGAGCCAGTAGATCCTA  5429
                                   pPL12 ------------------->

pCV1 GACTAGAGCCCTGGAAGCATCCAGGAAGTCAGCCTAAAACTGCTTGTACCAATTGCTATTGTAAAAAGTG  5499
                                         pCV3 splice  287 5557
                                                         \/
pCV1 TTGCTTTCATTGCCAAGTTTGTTTCATAACAAAAGCCTTAGGCATCTCCTATGGCAGGAAGAAGCGGAGA  5569
                                         pCV3   )-------------
                         pCV1, pCV3 common splice 5625 7956
                                                     \/
pCV1 CAGCGACGAAGACCTCCTCAAGGCAGTCAGACTCATCAAGTTTCTCTATCAAAGCAACCCACCTCCCAAT  7969
pCV3 ------------g---a---gaa------------------------------------------------
                         ***
pCV1 CCCGAGGGGACCCGACAGGCCCGAAGGAATAGAAGAAGAAGGTGGAGAGAGAGACAGAGACAGATCCATT  8039
pCV3 ----------------------------------------------------------------------
                  Bam HI
pCV1 CGATTAGTGAACGGATCCTTAGCACTTATCTGGGACGATCTGCGGAGCCTGTGCCTCTTCAGCTACCACC  8109
pCV3 ----------------------------------------------------------------------

pCV1 GCTTGAGAGACTTACTCTTGATTGTAACGAGGATTGTGGAACTTCTGGGACGCAGGGGGTGGGAAGCCCT  8179
pCV3 ----------------------------------------------------------------------

pCV1 CAAATATTGGTGGAATCTCCTACAATATTGGAGTCAGGAGCTAAAGAATAGTGCTGTTAGCTTGCTCAAT  8249
pCV3 ----------------------------------------------------------------------

pCV1 GCCACAGCTATAGCAGTAGCTGAGGGGACAGATAGGGTTATAGAAGTAGTACAAGAAGCTTATAGAGCTA  8319
pCV3 --------c--------------------------------------------g-----g---------

pCV1 TTCGCCACATACCTAGAAGAATAAGACAGGGCTTGGAAAGGATTTTGCTATAAGATGGGTGGCAAGTGGT  8389
pCV3 ----------------------------------------------------------------------

pCV1 CAAAAAGTAGTGTGGTTGGATGGCCTGCTGTAAGGGAAAGAATGAGACGAGCTGAGCCAGCAGCAGATGG  8459
pCV3 ----------------------------------------------------------------------
                     Xho I
pCV1 GGTGGGAGCAGCATCTCGAGACCTAGAAAAACATGGAGCAATCACAAGTAGCAACACAGCAGCTAACAAT  8529
pCV3 ----------------------------------------------------------------------
                                                                     Kpn I
pCV1 GCTGCTTGTGCCTGGCTAGAAGCACAAGAGGAGGAGAAGGTGGGTTTTCCAGTCACACCTCAGGTACCTT  8599
pCV3 ----------------------------------------------------------------------
                       Pvu II Bgl II                              |--U3
pCV1 TAAGACCAATGACTTACAAGGCAGCTGTAGATCTTAGCCACTTTTTAAAAGAAAAGGGGGGACTGGAAGG  8669
pCV3 ----------------------------------------------------------------------

pCV1 GCTAATTCACTCCCAACGAAGACAAGATATCCTTGATCTGTGGATCTACCACACACAAGGCTACTTCCCT  8739
pCV3 ----------------------------------------------------------------------

pCV1 GATTGGCAGAACTACACACCAGGACCAGGGATCAGATATCCACTGACCTTTGGATGGTGCTACAAGCTAG  8809
pCV3 ----------------------------------------------------------------------

pCV1 TACCAGTTGAGCCAGAGAAGTTAGAAGAAGCCAACAAAGGAGAGAACACCAGCTTGTTACACCCTGTGAG  8879
pCV3 -------------->

pCV1 CCTGCATGGAATGGATGACCCGGAGAGAGAAGTGTTAGAGTGGAGGTTTGACAGCCGCCTAGCATTTCAT  8949

pCV1 CACGTGGCCCGAGAGCTGCATCCGGAGTACTTCAAGAACTGCTGATATCGAGCTTGCTACAAGGGACTTT  9019

pCV1 CCGCTGGGGACTTTCCAGGGAGGCGTGGCCTGGGCGGGACTGGGGAGTGGCGAGCCCTCAGATCCTGCAT  9089
        Pvu II             U3--|--R                              Sst I
pCV1 ATAAGCAGCTGCTTTTTGCCTGTACTGGGTCTCTCTGGTTAGACCAGATCTGAGCCTGGGAGCTCTCTGG  9159
pCV3                                                             <---------
                         poly A (sig.)                    poly A
pCV1 CTAACTAAGGAACCCACTGCTTAAGCCTCAATAAAGCTTGCCTTGAGTGCTGTC                  9213
pCV3 -------g---------------------------------------------- --
```

malian regulatory sequences (*20*), and the cDNA inserts of selected clones from this library were transferred to a second mammalian expression vector (*21, 22*), here termed pCV, which contained hybrid regulatory sequences (Fig. 3). Several selected cDNA clones from these libraries were characterized by restriction mapping and complete or partial DNA sequencing (Fig. 2).

It was clear that clones pCV-1 and pCV-3, each with about 1.8-kb inserts of viral sequences, corresponded to mRNA's whose synthesis involved two splicing events, consistent with our hybridization results. The pCV-1 message was apparently transcribed with the use of a donor splice site at nucleotide 287 and an acceptor splice site at nucleotide 5358, with the second donor and acceptor splice sites located at nucleotides 5625 and 7956, respectively (Fig. 2). Synthesis of the pCV-3 message used the same first donor and second acceptor and donor splice sites, but the first acceptor splice site was located at nucleotide 5557 (Fig. 2). In each case, the donor and acceptor splice site sequences were GT and CAG, respectively. The viral insert in clone pPL-12 contained sequences in common with clone pCV-1, utilizing the same second splice junction (Fig. 2), and appeared to be a partial transcript of the message similar or identical to that contained in clone pCV-1. The other cDNA clones shown in Fig. 2 were partial transcripts of viral genomic or subgenomic mRNA's as determined by restriction mapping and confirmed in some cases (for example, pCV-5) by direct DNA sequencing.

To ascertain which of these cDNA clones contained sequences with *trans*-activating function, we constructed a plasmid containing HTLV-III LTR sequences 5′ to the bacterial chloramphenicol acetyltransferase (CAT) gene (pC15CAT) (Fig. 3). It was shown previously that the LTR of HTLV-III can function as a promoter for the CAT gene in human lymphoid and other cells (*16*). The activity of the CAT gene in transfected cells can be conveniently measured and is correlated with steady-state CAT messenger levels (*23*). The cloned cDNA's were then cotransfected with pC15CAT DNA into human lymphoid H9 and JM cells by the DEAE-dextran protocol, and the CAT activity in the cytoplasm was measured. For representative results of such assays see Fig. 3; the data are compiled in Table 1. The results were reproducible within the experimental errors indicated (Table 1). Clones pCV-1 and pPL-12 clearly enhanced the CAT gene activity promoted by HTLV-III LTR as did the clone pCV-5. The other clones were consistently negative. The lack of enhancement by clones pCV-3 and pPL-11 compared with clones pCV-1 and pPL-12 could not be attributed to differing transfection efficiencies, because the cells transfected with these DNA's contained equivalent levels of plasmid DNA's when analyzed by the Southern blot procedure. We also cotransfected cDNA clones with pRSV-CAT DNA, which contains Rous sarcoma virus LTR linked to CAT gene (*23*). None of the clones enhanced the CAT gene activity promoted by RSV LTR.

The structure-function analysis of cDNA clones used here allowed us to define the HTLV-III sequences responsible for its *trans*-activating function. Each of the clones pCV-1, pCV-3, and probably also clone pPL-12, consists of three exons (Fig. 2). Functional mRNA's of HTLV-III are synthesized by using two splicing events [see herein and (*16*)].

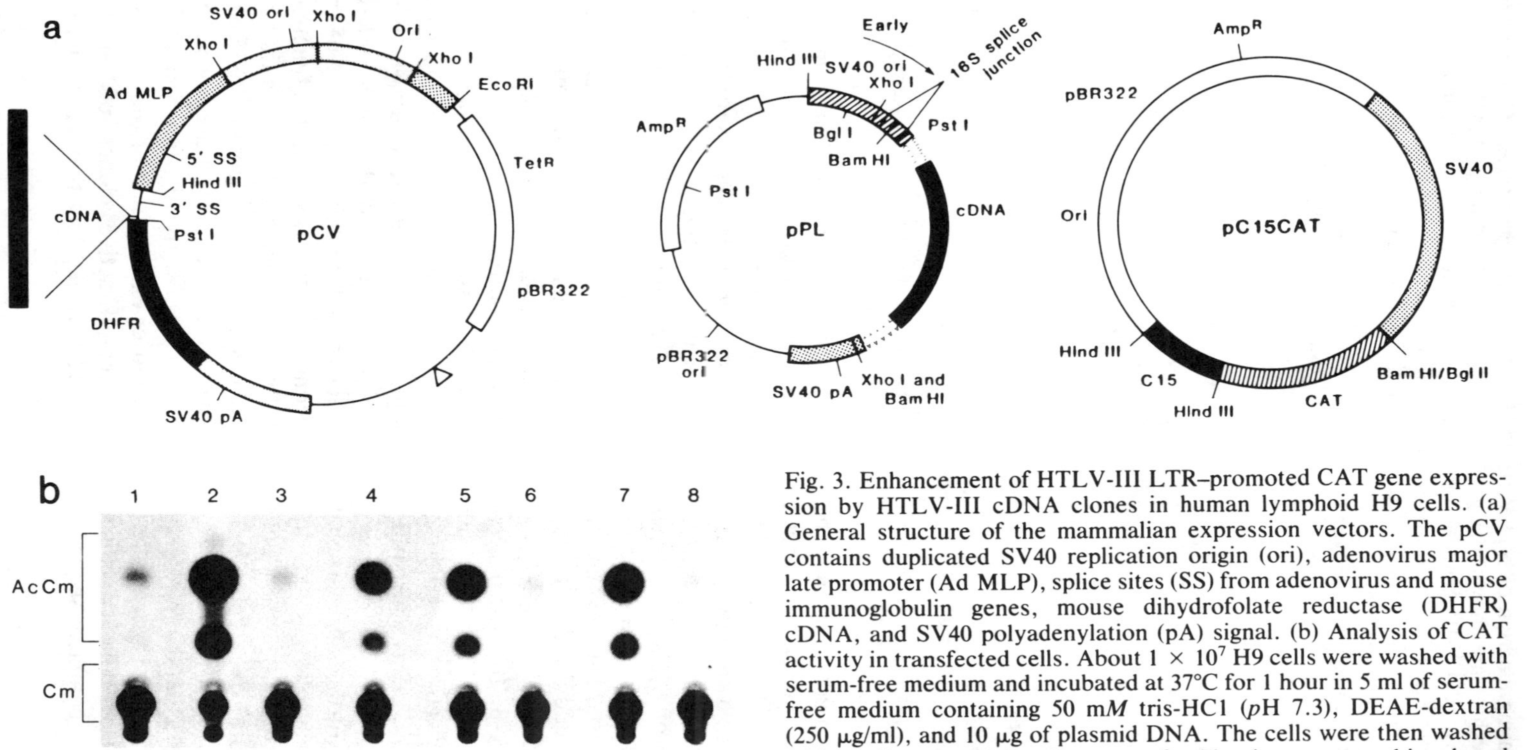

Fig. 3. Enhancement of HTLV-III LTR–promoted CAT gene expression by HTLV-III cDNA clones in human lymphoid H9 cells. (a) General structure of the mammalian expression vectors. The pCV contains duplicated SV40 replication origin (ori), adenovirus major late promoter (Ad MLP), splice sites (SS) from adenovirus and mouse immunoglobulin genes, mouse dihydrofolate reductase (DHFR) cDNA, and SV40 polyadenylation (pA) signal. (b) Analysis of CAT activity in transfected cells. About 1×10^7 H9 cells were washed with serum-free medium and incubated at 37°C for 1 hour in 5 ml of serum-free medium containing 50 mM tris-HC1 (pH 7.3), DEAE-dextran (250 µg/ml), and 10 µg of plasmid DNA. The cells were then washed with medium containing 20 percent fetal bovine serum and incubated in 20 ml of serum-containing medium at 37°C. Forty-eight hours after transfection, cells were washed with phosphate-buffered saline and suspended in 100 µl of 0.25M tris-HCl (pH 7.4), and cellular extracts were prepared by three cycles of freezing (in ethanol and dry ice) and thawing (37°C). CAT activity was measured by incubating 20-µl aliquots of extracts with ^{14}C-labeled chloramphenicol (Cm) and 2.5 mM acetyl coenzyme A at 37°C overnight, and separating the acetylated chloramphenicol (AcCm) from the unacetylated form by ascending thin-layer chromatography. The chromatogram was autoradiographed and spots cut from the plate were then quantitated by scintillation counting. Lanes 1 to 8 are, respectively, for cells transfected with DNA's of (1) pSV$_0$CAT, (2) pRSVCAT, (3) pC15CAT, (4) pC15CAT plus pCVHXb3, (5) pC15CAT plus pCV-1, (6) pC15CAT plus pCV-3, (7) pC15CAT plus pPL-12, and (8) pC15CAT plus pPL-11.

Table 1. *Trans*-activating function of HTLV-III cDNA clones. The structures of many of the plasmid DNA's listed here are shown in Fig. 2. Others are pCV-0, vector pCV DNA without any insert; pCVHXb3, HTLV-III genomic clone HXb3 with cellular flanking sequences (*10*) inserted into the unique Xba I site of a derivative of the pCV vector (*22*); pSV$_0$-CAT, SV40CAT plasmid from which viral promoter has been deleted (*23*). Experiments were performed as described in the legend for Fig. 3.

Plasmid DNA	Relative activity of CAT gene	
	H9 cells	JM cells
pC15CAT	1	1
pC15CAT + pCV-0	0.9 ± 0.1*	
pC15CAT + pCV-1	23.6 ± 5.6†	90.4
pC15CAT + pCV-3	0.82 ± 0.12†	3.1
pC15CAT + pCV-5	7.3 ± 2.7*	16.8
pC15CAT + pPL-12	33.0 ± 6.5†	52.5
pC15CAT + pPL-4	1.0 ± 0.2*	0.6
pC15CAT + pPL-9	1.0 ± 0.2*	
pC15CAT + pPL-11	0.82 ± 0.26†	1.2
pC15CAT + pCVHXb3	16.7 ± 7.6†	48.9
pSV$_0$-CAT	1.10 ± 0.36†	0.6

*Average of two transfection assays.   †Mean and standard deviation of four transfection assays.

A double splicing mechanism for the synthesis of the *tat* mRNA has been suggested for HTLV-I (*17, 24*) as well as BLV (*25*) and may be a common property of the HTLV-BLV group of retroviruses. Comparison of the active clones pCV-1 and pPL-12 with the inactive clone pCV-3 suggests that the critical *trans*-activating functional domain is located in the second exon, which is truncated in clone pCV-3. It also suggests that the first and third exons are not sufficient for *trans*-activating function. The fact that clone pCV-5, and also pPL-12, both of which lack the first exon, are functionally active further suggests that the first exon is not necessary for gene activity. The lack of activity of clones that contain the third exon completely and exclusively, or nearly so (for example, pPL-4), suggests that the third exon by itself is not sufficient for *trans*-activating function. Further, all of the clones tested contained the complete sequence of the gene designated 3'-*orf*, which is located within the third exon; many of these clones were inactive. This suggests that the 3'-*orf* gene is not likely to be the *trans*-activator gene of HTLV-III. This is further supported by the fact that pCV-3, which contains a single ORF corresponding to 3'-*orf* and which probably represents the functional mRNA of this gene, is functionally inactive. The work of Sodroski *et al.* (*26*) confirms these observations and further demonstrates that entire deletion of the 3'-*orf* sequences does not affect *trans*-activating function. The fact that clone pPL-12 is active and contains only part of the second exon narrows down the functional domain further and indicates that sequences between nucleotides 5357 and 5405 of the second exon are not necessary for *trans*-activating function.

A closer examination of the DNA sequences of active clones pCV-1 and pPL-12 revealed that they contained, in

a

```
pCV1                                                    ATGGAGCCAGTAGATCCTA   5429
                                                       MetGluProValAspProArg  (7)


pCV1  GACTAGAGCCCTGGAAGCATCCAGGAAGTCAGCCTAAAACTGCTTGTACCAATTGCTATTGTAAAAAGTG  5499
      LeuGluProTrpLysHisProGlySerGlnProLysThrAlaCysThrAsnCysTyrCysLysLysCys   (30)


pCV1  TTGCTTTCATTGCCAAGTTTGTTTCATAACAAAAGCCTTAGGCATCTCCTATGGCAGGAAGAAGCGGAGA  5569
      CysPheHisCysGlnValCysPheIleThrLysAlaLeuGlyIleSerTyrGlyArgLysLysArgArg   (53)
                                              5625 7956
                                                \/
pCV1  CAGCGACGAAGACCTCCTCAAGGCAGTCAGACTCATCAAGTTTCTCTATCAAAGCAACCCACCTCCCAAT  7969
      GlnArgArgArgProProGlnGlySerGlnThrHisGlnValSerLeuSerLysGlnProThrSerGlnSer (77)


pCV1  CCCGAGGGGACCCGACAGGCCCGAAGGAATAG  8001
      ArgGlyAspProThrGlyProLysGlu      (86)
```

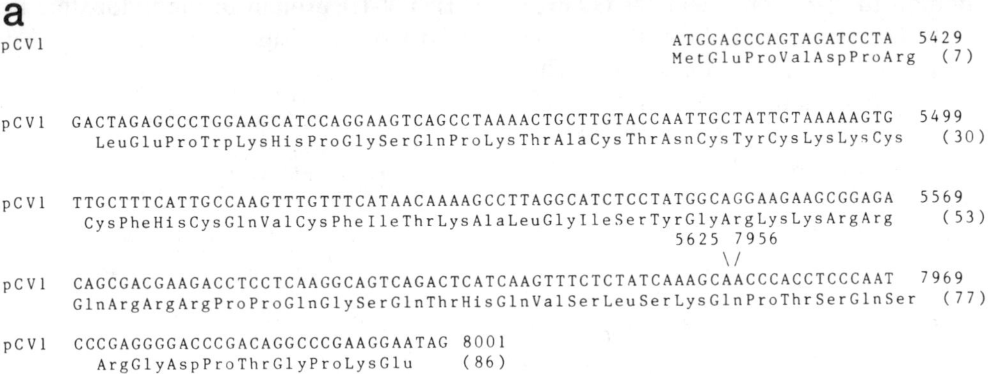

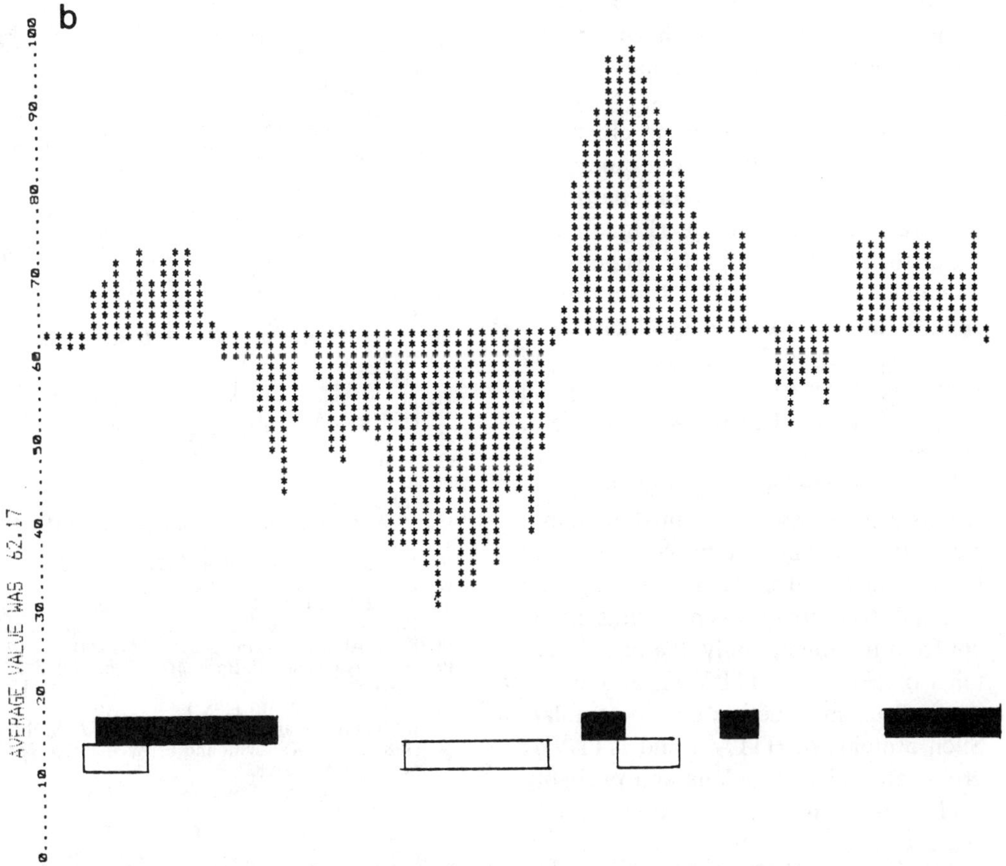

Fig. 4. Open reading frame found in cDNA clones pCV-1 and pPL-12. (a) Nucleotide and predicted amino acid sequence. (b) Hydrophilicity profile and predicted secondary structure of the putative polypeptide analyzed according to Kyte and Doolittle (29) and Chou and Fasman (30). Open and closed boxes represent α-helical structures and β-turns, respectively.

562

addition to 3'-*orf*, an identical ORF of 258 bp consisting of 215 bp of the second exon and 43 bp of the third exon. This ORF starts with the initiator codon ATG located at position 5411 in the second exon and ends with the termination codon at position 7999 in the third exon (Fig. 4). It is absent in the inactive clone pCV-3, as this clone lacks the first 145 bp, including ATG. It is interesting that this ORF is well conserved among divergent HTLV-III isolates, suggesting the functional importance of this region. This ORF predicts a polypeptide of 86 amino acid residues (9 to 10 kD) rich in basic amino acids and with an uncommonly large number of prolines and arginines, and with no potential glycosylation sites. There is a striking cluster of lysine-arginine residues from amino acids 49 to 57. The hydrophilic nature of the predicted polypeptide (Fig. 4) and the absence of a hydrophobic signal peptide–like sequence at the NH_2-terminus suggest an intracellular localization of this protein. Its highly basic composition would be consistent with its being an intranuclear and DNA-binding protein. If the *trans*-activating function of HTLV-III is mediated by a protein, the results provide strong circumstantial evidence that the putative polypeptide may be the functional protein. Although the size and structure of this protein is different from the functionally analogous proteins of HTLV-I, HTLV-II, and BLV, its mechanism of action may be similar. Such proteins of HTLV-I and HTLV-II are located in the nucleus and probably act by direct binding to viral and possibly some cellular regulatory nucleotide sequences (*17, 27*). Since these proteins play a critical role in the transforming activity of HTLV-I and HTLV-II, it will be of interest to determine the role of this

HTLV-III protein in the cytopathic activity of the virus.

References and Notes

1. F. Barré-Sinoussi *et al.*, *Science* **220**, 868 (1983).
2. M. Popovic, M. G. Sarngadharan, E. Read, R. C. Gallo, *ibid.* **224**, 497 (1984); R. C. Gallo *et al.*, *ibid.*, p. 500.
3. B. J. Poiesz *et al.*, *Proc. Natl. Acad. Sci. U.S.A.* **77**, 7415 (1980); B. J. Poiesz *et al.*, *Nature (London)* **294**, 268 (1981); M. Popovic *et al.*, *Science* **219**, 856 (1983); V. Manzari *et al.*, *Proc. Natl. Acad. Sci. U.S.A.* **80**, 1574 (1983); R. C. Gallo, in *Cancer Surveys*, L. M. Franks, J. Wyke, R. A. Weiss, Eds. (Oxford Univ. Press, Oxford, 1984), pp. 113–159.
4. I. Miyoshi *et al.*, *Nature (London)* **294**, 770 (1981); M. Yoshida *et al.*, *Proc. Natl. Acad. Sci. U.S.A.* **79**, 2031 (1982); F. A. Vyth-Drees and J. E. de Vries, *Lancet* **1982-II**, 993 (1982); B. F. Haynes *et al.*, *Proc. Natl. Acad. Sci. U.S.A.* **80**, 2054 (1983); D. Catovsky *et al.*, *Lancet* **1982-I**, 639 (1982).
5. V. S. Kalyanaraman *et al.*, *Science* **218**, 571 (1982).
6. D. Klatzmann *et al.*, *ibid.* **225**, 59 (1984).
7. H. Hoshino *et al.*, *Proc. Natl. Acad. Sci. U.S.A.* **80**, 6061 (1983); P. Clapham, K. Nagy, R. A. Weiss, *ibid.* **81**, 2886 (1984).
8. J. Schüpbach *et al.*, *Science* **224**, 503 (1984); M. G. Sarngadharan *et al.*, *ibid.*, p. 506.
9. I. S. Y. Chen *et al.*, *Nature (London)* **305**, 502 (1983); E. P. Gelmann *et al.*, *Proc. Natl. Acad. Sci. U.S.A.* **81**, 993 (1984); G. M. Shaw *et al.*, *ibid.*, p. 4544.
10. B. H. Hahn *et al.*, *Nature (London)* **312**, 166 (1984); G. M. Shaw *et al.*, *Science* **226**, 1165 (1984).
11. M. Alizon *et al.*, *Nature (London)* **312**, 757 (1984); P. A. Luciw *et al.*, *ibid.*, p. 760.
12. L. Ratner *et al.*, *ibid.* **313**, 277 (1985).
13. S. Wain-Hobson *et al.*, *Cell* **40**, 9 (1985).
14. R. Sanchez-Pescador *et al.*, *Science* **227**, 484 (1985).
15. M. A. Muesing *et al.*, *Nature (London)* **313**, 450 (1985).
16. J. Sodroski *et al.*, *Science* **227**, 171 (1985).
17. J. G. Sodroski, C. A. Rosen, W. A. Haseltine, *ibid.* **225**, 381 (1984); J. Sodroski *et al.*, *ibid.* **228**, 1430 (1985); B. Felber *et al.*, *ibid.*, in press.
18. S. K. Arya *et al.*, *ibid.* **225**, 927 (1984).
19. H. Okayama and P. Berg, *Mol. Cell. Biol.* **3**, 280 (1983).
20. ———, *ibid.* **2**, 161 (1982).
21. R. Kaufman and P. A. Sharp, *ibid.* **2**, 1304 (1982); R. J. Kaufman and P. A. Sharp, *J. Mol. Biol.* **159**, 601 (1982).
22. S. C. Clark *et al.*, *Proc. Natl. Acad. Sci. U.S.A.* **81**, 2543 (1984).
23. C. M. Gorman *et al.*, *Mol. Cell. Biol.* **2**, 1044 (1982); C. M. Gorman *et al.*, *Proc. Natl. Acad. Sci. U.S.A.* **79**, 6777 (1982); M. D. Walker *et al.*, *Nature (London)* **306**, 577 (1983).
24. A. Aldovini *et al.*, in preparation.
25. R. Mamoun *et al.*, *J. Virol.*, in press.
26. J. Sodroski *et al.*, *Science* **229**, 74 (1985).
27. W. C. Goh *et al.*, *ibid.* **227**, 1227 (1985).

28. S. K. Arya, F. Wong-Staal, R. C. Gallo, *ibid.*
    223, 1086 (1984); S. K. Arya and R. C. Gallo,
    Biochemistry **23**, 6690 (1984).
29. J. Kyte and R. F. Doolittle, *J. Mol. Biol.* **157**,
    105 (1981).
30. P. Y. Chou and G. D. Fasman, *Biochemistry* **13**,
    222 (1974).

31. We thank L. Jagodzinski and R. Lieu and their
    colleagues for assistance with the DNA se-
    quencing, L. Seigal and R. Kaufman for the
    pCIS-CAT plasmid and pCV vector, respective-
    ly, and R. C. Gallo for encouragement.

23 May 1985; accepted 6 June 1985

Report

5 July 1985

102.   Location of the *Trans*-Activating Region on the Genome of Human T-Cell Lymphotropic Virus Type III

Joseph Sodroski, Roberto Patarca, Craig Rosen, Flossie Wong-Staal, and William Haseltine

Human T-cell lymphotropic virus type III (HTLV-III/LAV) is the etiological agent of the acquired immune deficiency syndrome (AIDS) and associated diseases (*1*). Like HTLV types I and II and the related bovine leukemia virus (*2*), gene expression directed by the long terminal repeat (LTR) of HTLV-III is stimulated in *trans* in infected cells (*3*). The virus-associated *trans*-acting factors are specific for the infecting virus and have been postulated to play critical roles in increasing viral gene expression and possibly in pathogenesis (*2, 3*).

Trans-activation of the HTLV-I and HTLV-II LTR's is mediated by a novel gene product (*4*). In addition to the virion structural proteins and reverse transcriptase, the genomes of HTLV-I and -II encode 42- and 38-kilodalton (kD) proteins, respectively (*5*). These nuclear proteins (*6*) are encoded by a gene called

tat, for *trans*-activating transcriptional regulation, located within the pX region between the envelope glycoprotein gene and the 3' LTR (*7*).

Identification of the region in HTLV-III that is responsible for *trans*-activation was not possible by direct analogy with HTLV-I or HTLV-II since the organization of the HTLV-III genome differs from that of the other HTLV's. Five long open reading frames have been identified in HTLV-III (Fig. 1) (*8*). In addition to the *gag, pol,* and *env* genes, there are two open reading frames, one located immediately 3' to the *pol* gene (*sor*) and one 3' to the *env* gene (3' *orf*) (*8*). Numerous other open reading frames that could encode polypeptides of 10 kD or smaller also exist (*8*).

Recently, a complete clone of HTLV-III proviral DNA was shown to produce infectious virions upon transfection into

Fig. 1. Structure and *trans*-activation ability of the HTLV-III deletion mutants. The restriction map of the complete HTLV-III provirus in plasmid pHXBc2 is shown (H, Hind III; K, Kpn I; E, Eco RI; S, Sal I; T, Sst I; Bg, Bgl II; B, Bam HI; X, Xho I). The LTR's are indicated by boxes at either end of the provirus with the U3, R, and U5 regions depicted. Numbers correspond to the nucleotide numbers of the deletion endpoints and are based on the sequence of Ratner *et al.* (*8*), where the RNA cap site is designated +1. All deletion mutants were made with available restriction endonuclease cleavage sites (shown above the deletion endpoints), in some cases in the presence of ethidium bromide to promote partial digestion. All deletion mutants utilize HTLV-III LTR sequences responsive to *trans*-activating factors as promoters. The promoter for plasmid pΔ(83-5365/8053-9296) and derivatives consists of HTLV-III LTR sequences from −167 to +83. All 3′ *orf*-related sequences are deleted from this promoter, which retains the ability to respond to *trans*-activating factors (*14*). The zig-zag lines mark the position of polyadenylation and splice signals derived from the SV40 small t–antigen coding region. Transfections were carried out as described in the legend to Table 1. The percentage conversion of chloramphenicol to its acetylated forms was measured after transfection of HeLa (human epithelial) or H9 (human T lymphocyte) cells with the test plasmid and the pU3R-III CAT plasmid; a 1-hour time point and equivalent amounts of protein lysate were used for each reaction. ND, not determined.

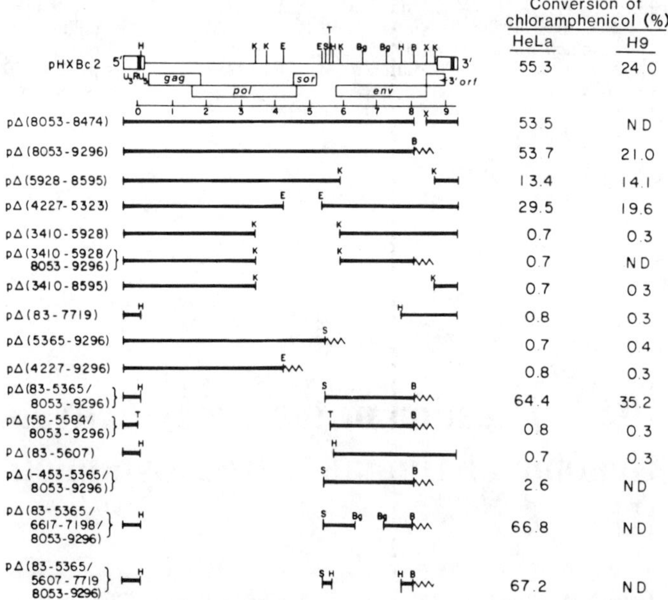

lymphocytes (*9*). Initially, we determined whether *trans*-activating factors specific for the HTLV-III LTR could be expressed by this complete proviral clone. Lymphoid and nonlymphoid cells were cotransfected with a plasmid that contained the complete HTLV-III provirus (pHXBc2) and an indicator plasmid that contained the HTLV-III LTR 5′ to the gene for chloramphenicol acetyltransferase (CAT) of *Escherichia coli* (pU3R-III CAT) (*3, 10*). Cotransfections were also done with the pSV2CAT plasmid, which contains the SV40 early promoter 5′ to the CAT gene (*10*). Cells of lymphoid and nonlymphoid lineage were used as recipients. At 48 hours after transfection, CAT enzyme activity, which correlates with CAT messenger RNA (mRNA) levels (*11*), was assayed, providing a measurement of promoter strength for the sequences 5′ to the CAT gene. All experiments to be described were performed at least twice with a range of values of not more than ±30 percent of the reported value. The effect of plasmid pHXBc2 on CAT activity directed by pSV2CAT was the same as that of a control plasmid that contained only the HTLV-III LTR sequences (pIII) (Table 1). By contrast, a marked stimulation of LTR-directed CAT activity was observed in pU3R-III CAT after cotransfection with pHXBc2 but not with the negative control DNA. We conclude that the entire HTLV-III provirus in plasmid pHXBc2 encodes *trans*-acting factors that stimulate HTLV-III LTR-directed gene expression.

The stimulation of LTR-directed CAT activity by the HTLV-III provirus in clone pHXBc2 was seen in all cell lines examined (Table 1). These included feline epithelial cells as well as human lymphoid and epithelial cell lines. Thus, neither efficient promoter activity nor *trans*-activation of the HTLV-III LTR is restricted to cells that normally serve as targets for viral infection. This observation demonstrates that, unlike the murine leukemia viruses (*12*), cell type–specific restriction of LTR-directed gene expression is not a major determinant of the tropism of these viruses.

The stimulation of HTLV-III LTR-directed CAT activity in the cotransfec-

Table 1. Cotransfection in different eukaryotic cell lines. Cotransfection of CAT plasmids and plasmids to be tested for *trans*-activating ability were carried out with 2 μg CAT plasmid DNA and approximately 2 μg test plasmid DNA, the latter adjusted so that molar equivalents of DNA were used. For adherent cells, 1×10^6 cells were transfected overnight by calcium phosphate-DNA coprecipitation (*2*). For cells grown in suspension, the DEAE-dextran technique (*19*) was employed, with 1×10^7 cells per transfection. Forty-eight hours after transfection, CAT lysates were prepared by freeze-thawing (*2*). CAT assays were done with equivalent amounts of protein from each lysate (approximately 200–300 μg protein per assay) as described (*10*), except that the final acetyl coenzyme A concentration in the reaction mix was 3 m*M*. At 10-, 30-, and 60-minute time points, reaction mixes were evaluated by thin-layer chromatography for percentage conversion of chloramphenicol to acetylated forms. The time points for the values shown in the table were chosen so that values fall within the linear range of the assay.

Cell line	Description	CAT plasmid	Cotransfected DNA	Conversion of chloramphenicol (%)
HeLa	Human cervical carcinoma epithelial cells	pSV2CAT	pIII	6.3
			pHXBc2	4.3
		pU3R-III	pIII	0.8
			pHXBc2	55.3
H9	Human T lymphocytes	pU3R-III	pIII	0.2
			pHXBc2	21.7
HUT78	Human T lymphocytes	pU3R-III	pIII	0.33
			pHXBc2	12.0
Raji	Human B lymphocytes	pU3R-III	pIII	0.66
			pHXBc2	76.0
CCCS+L−	Feline kidney epithelial cells	pU3R-III	pIII	0.5
			pHXBc2	52.0

tion experiments was less than that observed in the same cell lines infected with HTLV-III (*3*). This difference may be due to the lower levels of viral protein expressed transiently in transfected cells as compared with those produced in infected cells (*13*). To determine if the effect observed in the cotransfection experiments was qualitatively the same as that in infected cells, the response of CAT plasmids that carried alterations in the HTLV-III LTR sequences affecting

in vivo *trans*-activation (*14*) was analyzed in cotransfection experiments with the pHXBc2 plasmid. The LTR mutants that could respond to *trans*-activating factors in virus-infected cells also responded to factors produced upon cotransfection with the pHXBc2 plasmid (Table 2). Those LTR mutants that had lost the ability to respond to the factors present in infected cells were not activated by cotransfection with the pHXBc2 plasmid. We conclude that the stimula-

Table 2. Effect of cotransfected DNA on CAT plasmids. Transfections and CAT assays were carried out as described in the legend to Table 1, with 1×10^6 HeLa cells as recipients. The construction of the CAT plasmids and an evaluation of their responsiveness to *trans*-activating factors present in cells infected with HTLV-III are as described (*14*). Relative CAT activity is the ratio of chloramphenicol conversion to acetylated forms obtained in H9 cells infected with HTLV-III to that obtained with an equivalent amount of transfected DNA, protein lysate, and reaction conditions in uninfected H9 cells (*14*).

CAT plasmid	Promoter	Relative CAT activity	Cotransfected DNA	Conversion of chloramphenicol (%)*
pSV2CAT	SV40 early region promoter	1.0	pIII	6.3
			pHXBc2	4.3
			pΔ(83-5365/8053-9296)	5.1
pU3R-III	HTLV-III LTR (−453 to +83)	400–800	pIII	0.8
			pHXBc2	55.3
			pΔ(83-5365/8053-9296)	65.2
p-167	HTLV-III LTR deleted to −167 from the cap site	400–800	pIII	2.9
			pHXBc2	95.7
			pΔ(83-5365/8053-9296)	98.2
p-167/+21	Same as above but R region deleted to +21	1.0	pIII	0.7
			pHXBc2	0.6
			pΔ(83-5365/8053-9296)	0.7
pRSV/−44	Rous sarcoma virus enhancers at −44 of HTLV-III LTR	170	pIII	0.7
			pHXBc2	55.8
			pΔ(83-5365/8053-9296)	61.2
pSV2/−17	SV40 enhancer and promoter at −17 of HTLV-III LTR	40	pIII	0.9
			pHXBc2	31.6
			pΔ(83-5365/8053-9296)	42.6
pHEP/−17	HTLV-I enhancer and promoter at −17 of HTLV-III	1.0	pIII	0.6
			pHXBc2	1.5
			pΔ(83-5365/8053-9296)	1.3

*Measured after a 1-hour reaction period.

tion of HTLV-III LTR-directed CAT activity observed upon cotransfection with pHXBc2 DNA is qualitatively the same as the effect observed in cells infected with HTLV-III virions.

To understand what regions of the HTLV-III genome are necessary for determining *trans*-activation, deletions were introduced into the pHXBc2 plasmid. All deleted plasmids retained an LTR capable of *trans*-activation as a promoter element. Because the HTLV-I and HTLV-II *trans*-activating proteins are encoded by the 3′ end of the genome (*4*), our initial effort focused on testing deletions in this part of the HTLV-III genome (Figs. 1 and 2). Plasmids with deletions of major portions [pΔ(8053-8474)] or all [pΔ(8053-9296)] of the 3′ long open reading frame (3′ *orf*) had nearly the same *trans*-activating activity as the wild-type pHXBc2 plasmid. Plasmid pΔ(5928-8595), in which almost the entire *env* gene and the 3′ open reading frame are deleted, retained *trans*-activating ability, albeit at a reduced level compared to the pHXBc2 plasmid. In plasmid pΔ(83-5365/8053-9296), all of the 3′ long open reading frame sequences in the 5′ LTR were also deleted, yet the plasmid retained the ability to stimulate HTLV-III LTR-directed CAT expression (see below). These experiments exclude the 3′-*orf* and the complete *env* gene as sequences required for *trans*-activation.

Plasmid pΔ(4227-5323) has the entire potential coding region designated *sor* deleted. This plasmid retained most of the *trans*-activating ability of the wild-type plasmid. Thus, *sor* is not necessary for *trans*-activation.

Deletion of the region from nucleotides 3410 to 5928 in the plasmids capable of *trans*-activating HTLV-III LTR gene expression consistently resulted in

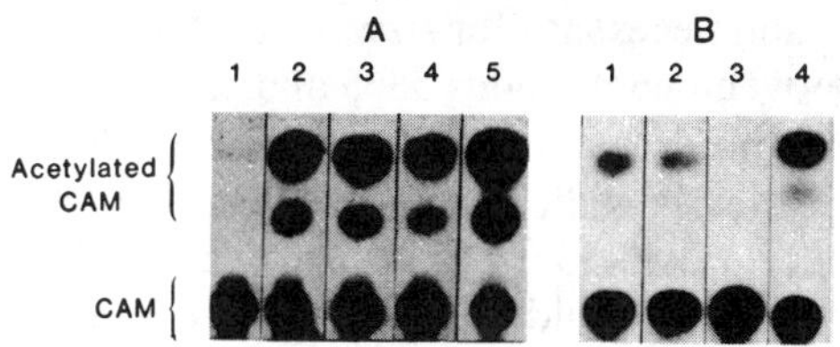

Fig. 2. Typical CAT assays after cotransfection into H9 (A) or HeLa (B) cells. Conversion of chloramphenicol (CAM) to its acetylated form after a 60-minute reaction is shown. CAT plasmids utilized for transfection were pU3R-III (lanes A1–A5), pSV2CAT (lanes B1 and B2), or pSV2/-17 (lanes B3 and B4). Cotransfected plasmids used were pIII (lanes A1, B1, and B3), pHXBc2 (lane A2), pΔ(8053-9296) (lane A3), pΔ(5928-8595) (lane A4), and pΔ(83-5365/8053-9296) (lanes A5, B2, and B4).

a loss of activity (Fig. 1). For example, although pΔ(4227-5323) was competent for *trans*-activation, plasmid pΔ(3410-5928) exhibited no *trans*-activating ability. The 3′ boundary of the necessary region was determined by placing SV40 polyadenylation signals at nucleotide positions 4227, 5365, and 8053. While pΔ(8053-9296) retained *trans*-activating ability, plasmids pΔ(4227-9296) and pΔ(5365-9296) were inactive. We conclude that the 3′ boundary of the region necessary for *trans*-activation lies between 5365 and 8053. The actual 3′ boundary is likely to be between 5365 and 5928 since plasmid pΔ(5928-8595) also showed *trans*-activating ability.

To define the 5′ border of the region necessary for *trans*-activation, the HTLV-III LTR was placed at nucleotides 5365, 5584, and 5607. Plasmid pΔ(83-5365/8053-9296) *trans*-activates the CAT plasmid containing the HTLV-III LTR, but plasmids pΔ(58-5584/8053-9296) and pΔ(83-5607) do not (Fig. 1). This indicates that the 5′ boundary of the region necessary for *trans*-activation lies between nucleotides 5365 and 5584. Furthermore, sequences from 5365 to 8053 are clearly sufficient for *trans*-activation, since pΔ(83-5365/8053-9296) was as active as the wild-type pHXBc2 clone in the cotransfection assay. The pΔ(83-5365/8053-9296) plasmid *trans*-activated the same HTLV-III LTR mutants as did the wild-type plasmid (Table 2). Thus, *trans*-activation by pΔ(83-5365/8053-9296) is both quantitatively and qualitatively similar to that observed for the complete proviral clone.

These studies define a region from positions 5365 to 5928 that is necessary for the ability to *trans*-activate the HTLV-III LTR. Expression of this region is a prerequisite for efficient *trans*-activation, as a plasmid that contains this region without 5′ promoter sequences [pΔ(-453-5365/8053-9296)] was almost inactive in the cotransfection assay.

Knowledge of the HTLV-III splicing patterns provides insight into how this genomic region might be expressed. Multiple double-spliced messages with exons including this region have been identified in infected cells (*8, 15*). The nucleotide sequence contains a splice acceptor followed by a methionine codon. This codon initiates an open reading frame that could encode a protein 72 amino acids long (Fig. 3). Immediately 5′ to the stop codon is a splice donor (*8, 15*). The corresponding splice acceptor at position 7955 precedes an in-phase open reading frame capable of encoding an additional 14 amino acids. The potential protein product of the two exons is 86 amino acids long. Deletion of sequences contained within the intron did not affect the *trans*-activating ability of plasmids. For example, plasmids pΔ(83-5365/8053-9296) and pΔ(83-5365/6617-

7198/8053-9296) exhibited comparable activities in stimulating HTLV-III LTR-directed CAT expression in the cotransfection assay (Fig. 1).

When the putative downstream exon is deleted, as in plasmid pΔ(5928-8595), a truncated protein of 72 amino acids encoded by the upstream exon can be made. Since plasmid pΔ(5928-8595) still showed *trans*-activating ability, the residues encoded by the second exon must not be essential to the activity of the putative protein product. In plasmid pΔ(83-5365/5607-7719/8053-9296), a stop codon has been placed at position 5612, precluding use of the second exon and prematurely terminating translation from the first exon. This plasmid still *trans*-activated, even though its potential protein product lacks 19 carboxyl terminal amino acids compared to the wild-type protein. The open reading frames are well conserved among the different HTLV-III/LAV isolates. However, the ARV-2 strain of HTLV-III is altered such that the second putative exon could encode 28 rather than 14 amino acids. These observations suggest that some heterogeneity in the carboxyl terminus of the putative *trans*-activating protein is permissible without compromising function.

Amino acid residues 49 through 57 in the potential product of this region comprise a strongly basic domain (Fig. 3). Such arginine- or lysine-rich regions have been found in several nuclear proteins that bind to nucleic acids (*16*). This basic stretch is invariant among the HTLV-III isolates examined (*8*). No homology exists between the potential product of this region and other sequenced proteins, including the *tat* products of HTLV-I, HTLV-II, and BLV.

The conserved nature of this open reading frame among different AIDS virus isolates, the inclusion in spliced mRNA, and the dramatic reduction in *trans*-activating ability of proviruses with this reading frame deleted suggest that the potential protein product is involved in *trans*-activation. Since some of the deletion mutants containing this open reading frame exhibit slightly decreased *trans*-activating ability compared to the wild-type provirus, these data do not exclude the possibility that additional viral products play auxiliary roles in

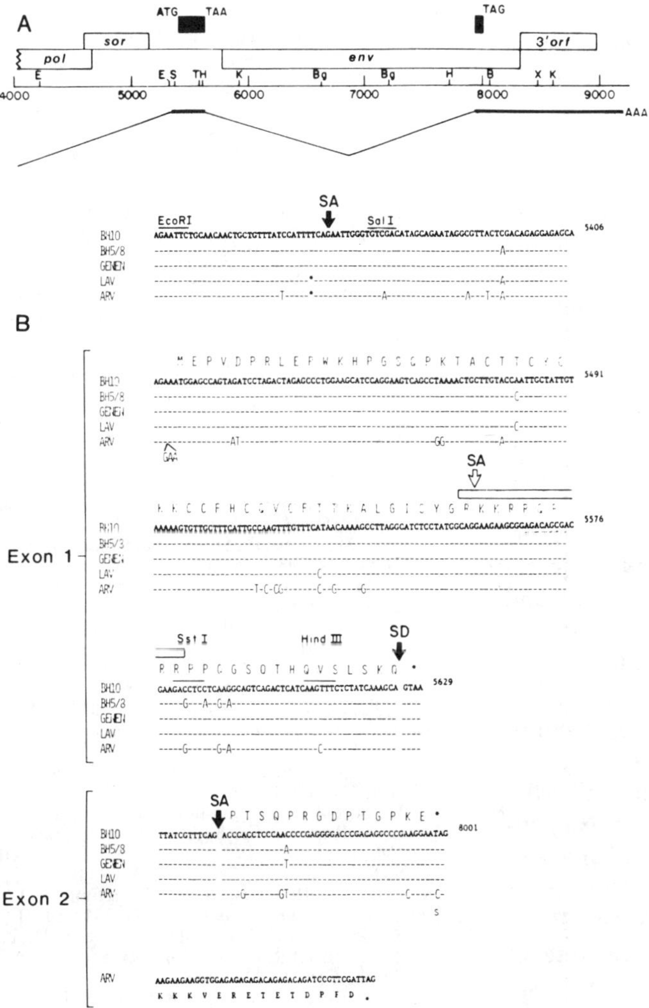

Fig. 3. The HTLV-III/LAV genome and potential protein product. The 3' half of the HTLV-III/LAV genome is shown in the upper figure. The restriction endonuclease map is depicted, with enzyme abbreviations as in Fig. 1, and nucleotide positions corresponding to those of Ratner *et al.* (*8*). The two exons potentially encoding the *trans*-activating protein are shown as black boxes above the restriction map. The splicing pattern of the message for this potential coding region, based on the sequence of cDNA's cloned from HTLV-III–infected cells (*8*, *15*), is shown beneath the genome. Dark horizontal bars represent exons and thin diagonal lines introns (AAA, polyadenylation site). The nucleotide sequence of this region (*8*) is shown in the lower figure. Viral isolate designations are at the left. Restriction endonuclease cleavage sites and splice donors (SD) and acceptors (SA) are noted (*8*, *15*). The splice donors and acceptors depicted with dark arrows are those probably used for production of the *trans*-activating protein. The splice acceptor depicted with the open arrow is also used (*8*, *15*), probably for mRNA encoding the 3' open reading frame. The translated amino acid sequence of the open reading frame in this region is shown above the nucleotide sequence. The open bar above the amino acid sequence delimits a highly conserved stretch of basic residues typical of nucleic acid–binding proteins located in the nucleus (*16*). The asterisks indicate stop codons.

trans-activation. These results are consistent with studies of the HTLV-III *trans*-activating factor by means of complementary DNA (cDNA) expression vectors (*15*).

Characterization of the genomic regions of HTLV-I and HTLV-III encoding *trans*-activating factors, as well as their target sequences in the LTR, allows a comparison between *trans*-activation in these two viruses. In both viruses, *trans*-activation is accompanied by an increase in steady-state levels of LTR-directed RNA, with no replication of the template DNA (*14, 17*). Both the HTLV-I and HTLV-III target sequences in the LTR are located near the promoter element (TATA box) and include sequences 3' to the mRNA start site (*14, 17*). *Trans*-activating factors do not stimulate the enhancers of either HTLV-I or HTLV-III (*14, 17, 18*). Both *trans*-activating factors can be made from multiply spliced mRNA's, which is unusual for retroviral messages (*4, 8, 15*). However, the location of the *trans*-activating regions on the genome and the sizes and characteristics of the potential protein products differ. Another difference is that sequences 5' to the promoter of HTLV-I are necessary for the response to *trans*-activating factors (*17*). This is not the case for HTLV-III, in which the LTR sequences responsive to *trans*-activation are located between −17 and +80 (*14*). Thus, while the mechanism of *trans*-activation of the HTLV-I LTR appears to be an increase in the rate of transcription initiation, the mechanism whereby HTLV-III LTR-directed gene expression is increased in infected cells remains an open question.

The expression of host cellular genes might also be regulated by the *trans*-activating factors synthesized by the HTLV's. The expression of the HTLV-III *trans*-activating factor in specific T-lymphocyte subpopulations may result in the inappropriate expression of lethal or growth-suppressive genes. The availability of plasmids exclusively expressing the *trans*-activating factor should allow a direct test of this hypothesis.

References and Notes

1. M. Popovic *et al.*, *Science* **224**, 497 (1984); R. C. Gallo *et al.*, *ibid.*, p. 500; J. Schüpbach *et al.*, *ibid.*, p. 503; M. G. Sarngadharan *et al.*, *ibid.*, p. 506; F. Barré-Sinoussi *et al.*, *ibid.* **220**, 868 (1983); D. Klatzmann *et al.*, *Nature (London)* **313**, 767 (1984); J. A. Levy *et al.*, *Science* **225**, 840 (1984).
2. J. G. Sodroski, C. A. Rosen, W. A. Haseltine, *Science* **225**, 381 (1984); C. A. Rosen *et al.*, *ibid.* **227**, 320 (1985); J. Fujisawa *et al.*, *Proc. Natl. Acad. Sci. U.S.A.* **82**, 2277 (1985).
3. J. G. Sodroski *et al.*, *Science* **227**, 171 (1985).
4. J. G. Sodroski *et al.*, *ibid.* **228**, 1430 (1985).
5. T. H. Lee *et al.*, *ibid.* **226**, 57 (1984); D. J. Slamon *et al.*, *ibid.*, p. 61.
6. W. C. Goh *et al.*, *ibid.* **227**, 1227 (1985).
7. M. Seiki *et al.*, *Proc. Natl. Acad. Sci. U.S.A.* **80**, 2618 (1983); W. A. Haseltine *et al.*, *Science* **225**, 419 (1984); K. Shimotohno *et al.*, *Proc. Natl. Acad. Sci. U.S.A.* **81**, 6657 (1984).
8. L. Ratner *et al.*, *Nature (London)* **313**, 227 (1985); R. Sanchez-Pescador *et al.*, *Science* **227**, 484 (1985); M. A. Muesing *et al.*, *Nature (London)* **313**, 450 (1985); S. Wain-Hobson *et al.*, *Cell* **40**, 9 (1985).
9. M. Fisher *et al.*, *Nature (London)*, in press.
10. C. M. Gorman, L. F. Moffat, B. H. Howard, *Mol. Cell. Biol.* **2**, 1044 (1982).
11. C. M. Gorman *et al.*, *Proc. Natl. Acad. Sci. U.S.A.* **79**, 6777 (1982); M. D. Walker *et al.*, *Nature (London)* **306**, 557 (1983); J. M. Keller and J. C. Alwine, *Cell* **36**, 381 (1984); L. Herrera-Estrella *et al.*, *Nature (London)* **310**, 115 (1984).
12. D. Celander and W. A. Haseltine, *Nature (London)* **312**, 159 (1984).
13. J. Sodroski *et al.*, unpublished observations.
14. C. A. Rosen, J. G. Sodroski, W. A. Haseltine, *Cell*, in press.
15. S. K. Arya *et al.*, *Science* **229**, 69 (1985).
16. E. M. DeRobertis, R. F. Longthorne, J. B. Guron, *Nature (London)* **272**, 254 (1978); D. Kalderon *et al.*, *ibid.* **311**, 33 (1984); D. Kalderon, B. L. Roberts, W. D. Richardson, A. E. Smith, *Cell* **39**, 499 (1984).
17. C. A. Rosen, J. G. Sodroski, W. A. Haseltine, *Proc. Natl. Acad. Sci. U.S.A*, in press.
18. ______, in preparation.
19. C. Queen and D. Baltimore, *Cell* **33**, 741 (1983).
20. We thank K. Campbell and J. Potz for their invaluable help with these experiments, S. Arya for communication of results prior to publication, D. Celander, W. C. Goh and R. Crowther for helpful discussions, and D. Artz and L. DeFurio for help in preparation of this manu-

script. This work was supported by grants from the State of Massachusetts (W.H.) and the National Institutes of Health CAA07580 (C.R.) and CA07094 (J.S.), and a scholarship from Consejo Nacional de Investigaciones Científicas of Venezuela (R.P.).

23 May 1985; accepted 6 June 1985

Report

2 August 1985

103. *Cis*- and *Trans*-Acting Transcriptional Regulation of Visna Virus

Jay L. Hess, Janice E. Clements, and Opendra Narayan

The lentiviruses are a group of non-oncogenic retroviruses that produce a variety of chronic progressive diseases with unusually long incubation periods. Visna virus, the prototype of this group of so-called "slow" viruses, causes chronic pneumonitis and a progressive demyelinating disease in sheep months to years after the initial infection (*1*). Interest in visna virus has increased considerably with the discovery by Gonda *et al.* (*2*) that the virus is morphologically similar to and shares sequence homology with human T-cell lymphotropic virus type III (HTLV-III), the presumptive etiologic agent of the acquired immune deficiency syndrome (AIDS) (*3*).

Visna virus replicates to high titers in tissue culture, eventually killing its host cell, a feature that distinguishes it from most other retroviruses. This high level of expression suggests that the visna virus promoter sequence has a high transcriptional rate in infected cells. Regulation of such transcription may depend on the promoter containing strong enhancer sequences—segments of DNA that in-

crease the transcriptional rate of proximal promoters in a manner relatively independent of position and orientation (*4*). In addition, regulation may be achieved through the production of *trans*-acting transcriptional activators (*5–8*). Studies on HTLV-I, a virus associated with adult T-cell leukemia (*5*), HTLV-II, which is associated with hairy cell leukemia (*5*), HTLV-III (*6*), and bovine leukemia virus (BLV), which is associated with B-cell leukemia of cattle (*7, 8*), indicate that transcription from the long terminal repeats (LTR's) of all of these viruses is much greater in infected than uninfected cells. Recently, transcription from the Rous sarcoma virus (RSV) promoter was shown to be increased by a product of the *gag* gene, providing further evidence for *trans*-acting factors playing a role in the regulation of retroviral transcription (*9*).

Here we report the nucleotide sequence of the U3 region of visna virus, and present evidence that both *cis*-acting enhancer sequences and *trans*-acting transcriptional activating factors contrib-

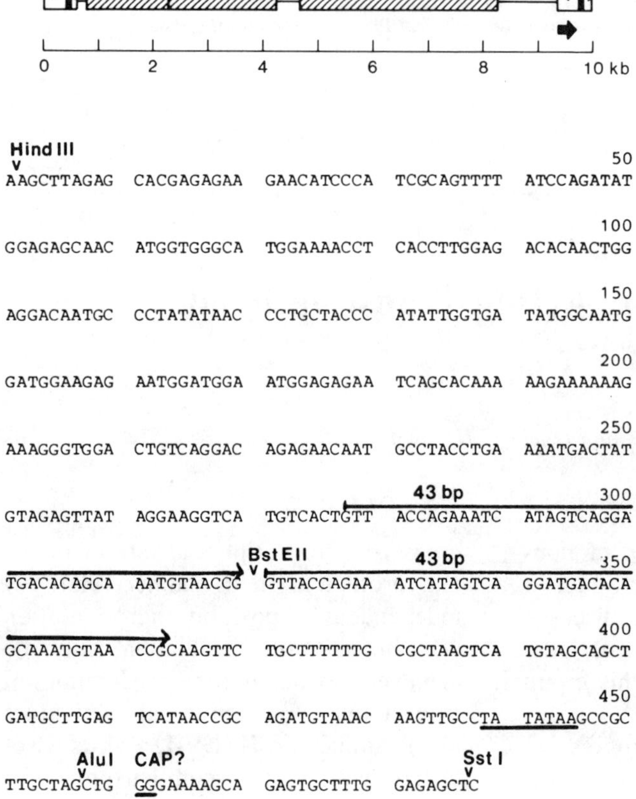

Fig. 1. (Top) Organization of the proviral form of visna virus DNA. Positions of the *gag*, *pol*, and *env* coding regions are approximate. The arrow indicates the position of the Hind III–Sst I fragment used for sequencing, and for construction of recombinant plasmids. The cloning of visna virus from unintegrated DNA has been described (*26*). (Bottom) Nucleotide sequence of the Hind III–Sst I DNA fragment spanning the U3 region of the visna virus 3′ LTR. This fragment was subcloned into bacteriophage M13 (*27*) and sequenced by the method of Sanger *et al.* (*28*). The 43-bp tandem repeats are indicated with arrows, and the TATA box and possible RNA transcription initiation sites are underlined. Restriction sites used for constructing recombinant plasmids are also labeled.

ute to the high rate of visna virus transcription in infected cells.

Promoter and enhancer sequences that govern the initiation and rate of retroviral RNA transcription are located within the U3 region of the retroviral LTR (*4, 10*) (Fig. 1, top). The nucleotide sequence of this region of visna virus (Fig. 1, bottom) shares little homology with other retroviruses, including BLV, HTLV-I, HTLV-II, or HTLV-III, or other retroviruses isolated from AIDS patients (*11*). Eukaryotic and viral promoters often contain the sequence CCAAT 70 to 90 base pairs (bp) 5′ to the cap site (the start site for RNA transcrip-

tion) (*12*), and the sequence TATA^A_TA^T_A (the TATA box) 20 to 30 bp 5′ to the cap site (*13*). Sequences similar to the CCAAT consensus sequence appear in the visna LTR beginning with bases 352 (CAAAT) and 364 (CAAGT). A well-defined TATA box (TATATAA) begins with base 438. On the basis of the position of these promoter elements we place the cap site on a guanine residue somewhere between bases 460 to 480. There is no polyadenylation signal in this sequence.

Enhancer sequences of retroviruses often appear as short (40 to 80 bp) tandemly repeated sequences located 100 to

250 bp upstream from the RNA cap site. The U3 region of visna virus contains a pair of 43-bp perfect tandem repeats spanning the region approximately 100 to 180 bp upstream from the putative cap site. These repeats do not contain a good example of the "core" sequence $GTGG^{AAA}_{TTT}G$ which is found in many viral and eukaryotic enhancers (4), but the juxtaposition of the tandem repeats with classical promoter elements strongly suggests that they function as enhancer sequences.

We tested the ability of visna virus sequences to function as a promoter by constructing plasmids in which portions of the U3 region of the virus containing either one (pVIS1CAT) or both (pVIS-2CAT) 43-bp tandem repeats, including the region containing the TATA box, were inserted 5' to the bacterial gene chloramphenicol acetyltransferase (CAT) (Fig. 2) (14, 15). These plasmids were transfected into a variety of eukaryotic cells by the DEAE-dextran method (16) coupled with an osmotic shock (10 percent dimethyl sulfoxide) (17, 18). The CAT activity of cell extracts was measured by an enzyme assay 48 hours later (19). CAT activity is closely correlated with CAT-related messenger RNA at this time (14, 15), providing a sensitive way to quantitate the transcriptional rate of transfected plasmids.

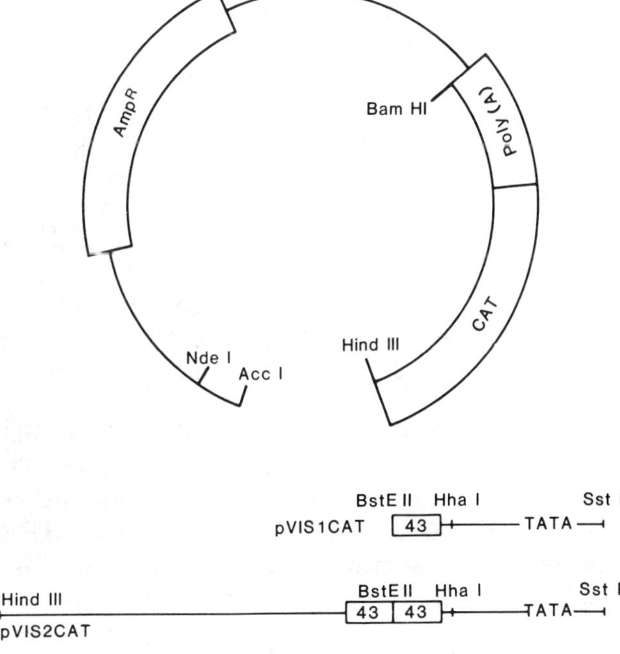

Fig. 2. Construction of plasmids that express the bacterial CAT gene under the transcriptional control of visna promoter sequences. pSV2CAT contains the CAT gene 3' to the SV40 early region promoter (14). pVIS2CAT is derived from pSV2CAT by replacing the SV40 promoter and pBR322 sequences between the Acc I and Hind III sites with a 488-bp Hind III–Sst I fragment of visna DNA containing promoter sequences and both tandem repeats. The ends of both the vector and insert were made blunt ended by using Klenow enzyme and T4 DNA polymerase, and were joined so the Hind III end of the viral insert was ligated to the Acc I site of the plasmid; the Sst I end of the insert was ligated to the Hind III end of the insert. pVIS1CAT was derived from pVIS2CAT by cleaving with Nde I and Bst EII, deleting 50 bp of pBR322 sequence and 170 bp of 5' visna virus DNA. The endonuclease-cut plasmid was treated with Klenow enzyme and religated. This plasmid contains 170 bp of visna DNA which includes one 43-bp repeat and the downstream viral promoter elements. All plasmids were gradient-purified prior to use in transfections.

The plasmids pSV2CAT and RSVCAT, containing the SV40 early region promoter and RSV promoters, respectively, 5' to the CAT gene (*14, 15*), were included in the assays along with plasmids containing visna viral sequences for comparison (Table 1). The percentage conversion of ^{14}C-labeled chloramphenicol to its acetylated derivatives per hour of incubation was normalized to the percentage conversion by pRSVCAT. The results (Table 1) indicate that the visna promoter, with either one (pVIS1CAT) or both (pVIS2CAT) 43-bp tandem repeats, directed high and equivalent levels of transcriptional activity in a variety of cell types. In mouse L cells, the CAT activity directed by pVIS-1CAT and pVIS2CAT was comparable to that directed by pSV2CAT. The results were similar in H9 cells, a human T-lymphocyte cell line in which HTLV-III replicates to high titers. In sheep choroid plexus (SCP) cells and SV40-transformed sheep macrophages (both being cells in which visna virus replicates) the levels of CAT activity directed by pVIS-1CAT or pVIS2CAT were more than tenfold higher than pSV2CAT.

The presence of 43-bp tandem repeats upstream from classical promoter elements suggested that these repeats might function as enhancer sequences. We next examined the ability of these sequences to enhance transcription from an SV40 promoter from which its own enhancer sequences had been deleted. Plasmids were constructed with the visna U3 region inserted both 3' and 5' to the SV40 promoter in both sense and antisense orientations (Fig. 3). These plasmids were transfected into mouse L cells, and CAT activity was measured 48 hours later. The results are expressed as the ratio of the percentage acetylation of

[14]C-labeled chloramphenicol by a given plasmid divided by the percentage acetylation by pSV1CAT, a plasmid containing the "enhancer-less" SV40 promoter without any visna virus DNA insert (Table 2). These data show that the visna insert, which contains both 43-bp repeats, functions as a strong enhancer. As has been found in other viruses (*20*), the enhancer sequences showed an orientation preference, working three to four times better in the sense as opposed to the antisense orientation. The visna virus enhancer sequences are unusual in that they appear to function better when positioned downstream rather than 5' to the SV40 promoter.

The *trans*-acting transcriptional activation recently described in the human T-cell lymphotropic viruses, BLV, and Rous sarcoma virus (RSV) prompted us to look for a similar activation of the visna promoter in infected cells. We introduced the plasmids already described into SCP cells and alveolar macrophages 24 hours after they were infected with visna virus. In SCP cells, the CAT activity directed by pVIS1CAT (containing the visna promoter and one 43-bp repeat) was substantially higher in infected than uninfected cells (Table 1). In infected SCP cells, the ratio of the activity directed by pVIS1CAT to that directed by pRSVCAT was approximately sevenfold greater than the ratio in uninfected SCP cells. The amount of CAT activity in infected macrophages was roughly three times higher than that in uninfected cells. Results for SCP cells and macrophages are the average of three separate transfections. Variation among values was less than 40 percent in infected cells and less than 30 percent in uninfected cells. To ensure that these effects were not due to differences in DNA uptake between

Table 1. Transient expression of the CAT gene in uninfected and visna virus–infected cells. The results represent the average of a minimum of three separate transfections and are expressed as the ratio of the percentage conversion of chloramphenicol to its acetylated forms by a given plasmid, compared to the percentage conversion directed by pRSVCAT in cells transfected in parallel. Results were highly reproducible with variation between values less than 40 percent in most cases. For the methods used for transfections and CAT assays, see (18, 19).

Cell type	pVIS1CAT Visna/visna*	pVIS2CAT Visna/visna*	pSV1-3 CATs Visna/SV40*	pSV1-3′CATa Visna/SV40*	pSV1CAT SV40†	pSV2CAT SV40/SV40*	pRSVCAT RSV/RSV*
Mouse L cells	10.1	9.4	9.7	2.9	0.1	12.6	1.0
Human H9 cells	0.6					0.5	1.0
Goat synovial membrane (GSM)	2.6	2.8				1.3	1.0
Sheep alveolar macrophages							
Uninfected	11.2	12.0				0.5	1.0
Infected	40.0	33.9				1.0	1.0
SCP cells							
Uninfected	12.0	10.0	0.7	0.6	0.4	1.8	1.0
Infected	83.7	69.9	5.2	2.2	0.6	5.0	1.0

*Enhancer/promoter.   †Promoter.

Table 2. Expression of the CAT gene directed by plasmids with an SV40 promoter and visna enhancer sequences. The L cells were transfected as described in the text with the plasmids described in Fig. 3. The results represent the average of three separate transfections and are expressed as the ratio of the percentage conversion of chloramphenicol to its acetylated forms by a given plasmid compared to the percentage conversion by pSV1CAT. The range of values observed for each plasmid is indicated in parentheses.

	pSV1-5′CATs Visna/SV40*	pSV1-5′CATa Visna/SV40*	pSV1-3′CATs Visna/SV40*	pSV1-3′CATa Visna/SV40*	pSV1CAT SV40†	pSV2CAT SV40/SV40*
CAT activity related to pSV1CAT	21.9	6.8	68.7	20.7	1.0	89.1
Range of values	(15.8–26.3)	(6.0–7.6)	(57.7–81.7)	(17.6–25.0)		(70.6–110.5)

*Enhancer/promoter.   †Promoter.

Fig. 3. Construction of plasmids for testing the ability of visna virus sequences to enhance transcription from the SV40 promoter. pSV1CAT has an SV40 promoter deleted of enhancer sequences and was derived from pSV2CAT by deleting sequences from Acc I to the distal Sph I site. A 457-bp Hind III to Alu I visna fragment containing both 43-bp tandem repeats (in addition to viral promoter sequences) was inserted into pSV1CAT at the Nde I site in either the sense (pSV1-5′s) or antisense (pSV1-5′a) orientation; this fragment was also inserted into the Bam HI site in either the sense (pSV1-3′s) or antisense (pSV1-3′a) orientation. Plasmids were constructed by treating both the vector and viral DNA insert with Klenow enzyme, followed by blunt end ligation as described (29). Plasmids were gradient-purified prior to use in transfections.

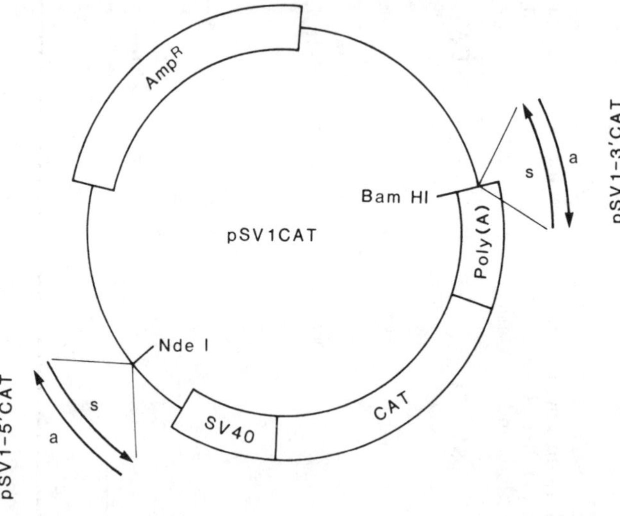

infected and uninfected cells, DNA dot blots were done to quantitate the amount of plasmid DNA in infected and uninfected cells 3, 24, and 48 hours after transfection. These dot blots confirmed that DNA uptake in infected and uninfected cells was equivalent, and also showed that the plasmids did not replicate in either group of cells.

The results of the CAT assays indicate that the visna virus promoter is not dependent on virally encoded or induced *trans*-acting factors for activity. The high transcriptional activity of the visna LTR can be explained in part by the presence of strong enhancer sequences, probably contained within the 43-bp tandem repeats of the viral promoter. That the visna LTR can direct high levels of CAT activity in both fibroblastic and lymphoid cells suggests that the visna enhancer sequences show relatively little tissue specificity and in this respect are similar to those of SV40.

In addition to increasing transcription from the visna promoter, cells infected with visna virus also activate transcription from the promoter of caprine arthritis-encephalitis virus (CAEV) (21), another macrophage-tropic lentivirus, to the same extent as the visna promoter. Since the sequences of the U3 regions of the two viruses are somewhat divergent, but their tandem repeats are closely homologous, it seems likely that the *trans*-acting factor interacts with these putative enhancer sequences. In SCP cells infected with visna, transcription from the SV40 promoter was consistently increased (typically two- to threefold), whereas transcription from pRSVCAT was unaffected. This indicates that there is some latitude in the ability of the *trans*-acting factor to activate transcription from promoters other than the viral LTR. The result is similar to that for the RSV encoded *trans*-acting factor, which activates transcription of the rat preproinsulin II gene in addition to the RSV LTR (9).

The magnitude of transcriptional activation by visna virus infection is not as large as observed for HTLV-I, HTLV-II, HTLV-III, and BLV (5–8). We believe that the degree of activation observed in visna-infected SCP cells is limited in part by the cytopathic effects of virus replication. The absence of the R region in the visna viral DNA used to transcribe the CAT gene in our experiments may also have limited the extent of *trans*-activation we observed. Work by Derse *et al*. has shown that *trans*-acting transcriptional activation of the BLV promoter is reduced by almost 90 percent when most of the R region of the viral LTR is deleted (8).

The phenomenon of *trans*-acting transcriptional activation occurs in several DNA viruses. Transcription from the adenovirus early transcriptional units is increased by the Ela gene product (22), and similar transcriptional enhancement occurs with the immediate early gene of herpes simplex virus type I (23). There is also evidence that the SV40 T antigen activates transcription of late region genes of SV40 (24). The recent discovery of *trans*-acting transcriptional activation in several retroviral systems has prompted speculation that these viruses, like some DNA viruses, code for their own *trans*-acting enhancer proteins (5–7). In support of this theory, spliced RNA transcripts and protein products encoded by additional open reading frames have been detected in some infected cells (25). In the case of RSV, a region of the viral genome has been identified which activates transcription in *trans* from a plasmid containing the viral LTR (9). Our experiments suggest that cells infected with visna virus also produce a *trans*-

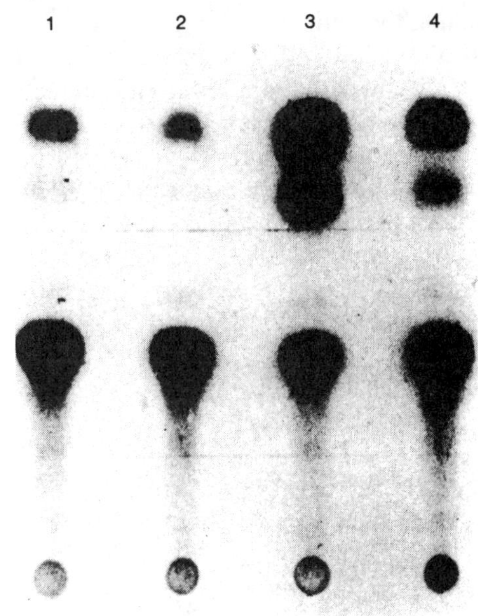

Fig. 4. A representative CAT assay on infected and uninfected SCP cells. SCP cells were either infected or "mock" infected with visna virus strain 1514 at a multiplicity of 0.1 infectious unit per cell. The cells were transfected 24 hours later, and collected for CAT assay 72 hours after infection. Infected and uninfected cell extracts contained equivalent amounts of protein and equal amounts of plasmid DNA as determined by DNA dot blots. Lane 1, pVIS-1CAT (uninfected); lane 2, pSV2CAT (uninfected); lane 3, pVIS1CAT (infected with visna virus); and lane 4, pSV2CAT (infected with visna virus).

acting factor. However, we have not identified a viral gene product responsible for transcriptional activation of the visna LTR, and we cannot exclude the possibility that the *trans*-acting transcriptional activator is a cellular protein that is induced by viral infection.

Addendum: Recent experiments indicate the magnitude of *trans*-activation of the visna virus promoter is considerably increased when the R-U5 region is included in the plasmids. Plasmids con-

578

taining the entire visna virus LTR located 5' to the CAT gene show a 40-fold increase in activity in visna virus-infected SCP cells, giving levels of CAT activity more than 430 times that directed by the RSV promoter. To date we have no evidence that HTLV-III infection can *trans*-activate the visna virus promoter, or that visna virus infection can *trans*-activate the HTLV-III promoter.

References and Notes

1. B. Sigurdsson, P. Palsson, H. Grimsson, *J. Neuropathol. Exp. Neurol.* **16**, 389 (1957); B. Sigurdsson and P. A. Paulsson, *J. Exp. Neurol.* **39**, 519 (1958); A. T. Haase, *Curr. Top. Microbiol. Immunol.* **72**, 101 (1975).
2. M. A. Gonda *et al.*, *Science* **227**, 173 (1985).
3. M. Popovic *et al.*, *ibid.* **224**, 497 (1984); R. C. Gallo *et al.*, *ibid.*, p. 500; J. E. Groopman *et al.*, *ibid.* **226**, 447 (1984); D. Zagury *et al.*, *ibid.*, p. 449; D. D. Ho *et al.*, *ibid.*, p. 451; B. Safai *et al.*, *Lancet* **1984-I**, 1438 (1984); J. Groopman *et al.*, *N. Engl. J. Med.* **311**, 1419 (1984).
4. Y. Gluzman and T. Shenk, Eds., *Enhancers and Eukaryotic Gene Expression* (Cold Spring Harbor Laboratory, Cold Spring Harbor, N.Y., 1983); G. Khoury and P. Gruss, *Cell* **33**, 313 (1983).
5. J. G. Sodroski, C. A. Rosen, W. A. Haseltine, *Science* **225**, 381 (1984).
6. J. G. Sodroski *et al.*, *ibid.* **227**, 171 (1985).
7. C. A. Rosen *et al.*, *ibid.*, p. 320.
8. D. Derse *et al.*, *ibid.*, p. 317.
9. S. Broome and W. Gilbert, *Cell* **40**, 537 (1985).
10. H. M. Temin, *ibid.* **28**, 3 (1982).
11. L. Ratner *et al.*, *Nature (London)* **313**, 277 (1985); M. A. Muesing *et al.*, *ibid.*, p. 450; B. Starcich *et al.*, *Science* **227**, 538 (1985); R. Sanchez-Pescador *et al.*, *ibid.*, p. 484; S. Wain-Hobson *et al.*, *Cell* **40**, 9 (1985).
12. A. Efstratiadis *et al.*, *Cell* **21**, 653 (1980).
13. E. Gilboa *et al.*, *ibid.* **16**, 863 (1979); F. Gannon *et al.*, *Nature (London)* **278**, 428 (1979).
14. C. M. Gorman, L. F. Moffat, B. H. Howard, *Mol. Cell. Biol.* **2**, 1044 (1982).
15. C. M. Gorman *et al.*, *Proc. Natl. Acad. Sci. U.S.A.* **79**, 6777 (1982).
16. J. H. McCutchan and J. S. Pagano, *J. Natl. Cancer Inst.* **41**, 351 (1968).
17. M. A. Lopata, D. W. Cleveland, B. Sollner-Webb, *Nucleic Acids Res.* **12**, 5707 (1984).
18. Nearly confluent monolayers of L cells, SCP cells (*30*), sheep alveolar macrophages (*31*), and goat synovial membrane cells (*32*) grown in 35-mm dishes were transfected by using the DEAE-dextran technique coupled with a dimethyl sulfoxide shock (*16, 17*). The SCP cells or sheep macrophages were infected by adding visna virus (strain 1514) 24 hours prior to transfection at multiplicities of 0.1 (SCP) or 1.0 (macrophages). Cells to be transfected were washed with serum-free medium and then DNA was added (3 μg/ml in 1 ml of serum-free medium containing DEAE-dextran, 200 μg/ml). After 4 hours at 37°C the cells were treated with 1 ml of Hepes buffered saline, *pH* 7.1 (*31*) containing 10 percent dimethyl sulfoxide for 2 minutes at room temperature. The cells were washed once with phosphate-buffered saline (PBS), then modified Eagle's medium containing 10 percent fetal bovine serum (Dulbecco's modified Eagle's medium containing 2 percent lamb serum was used for the sheep macrophages) was added and the cells were incubated for 48 hours at 37°C. The H-9 cells were transfected as described elsewhere (*6*).
19. Cells grown in monolayers were harvested for CAT assay by trypsinization. The cells were washed twice with cold PBS (*pH* 7.4), then lysed by freeze-thawing three times in 60 μl of 250 mM tris-HCl (*pH* 7.8). Cell debris was pelleted by centrifugation, and 30 μl of the cellular supernatant was assayed for CAT activity as described (*14, 15*). The percentage acetylation of ^{14}C-labeled chloramphenicol (New England Nuclear) after 1 or 2 hours was measured by separating the acetylated and unacetylated forms by thin-layer chromatography, then counting spots cut from the plate by liquid scintillation. The results are expressed as the percentage conversion of ^{14}C-labeled chloramphenicol to its acetylated derivatives per hour normalized to the percentage conversion by either pRSVCAT (Table 1) or pSV1CAT (Table 2).
20. N. Rosenthal *et al.*, *Science* **222**, 749 (1983); S. Kenney *et al.*, *ibid.* **226**, 1337 (1984); L. Laimons *et al.*, *Virology* **49**, 183 (1984).
21. L. C. Cork *et al.*, *Infect. Disease* **129**, 134 (1974); T. B. Crawford *et al.*, *Science* **207**, 997 (1980); J. M. Pyper *et al.*, *J. Virol.* **51**, 713 (1984).
22. A. J. Berk *et al.*, *Cell* **17**, 935 (1979); J. R. Nevins, *ibid.* **26**, 213 (1981); N. Jones and T. Shenk, *Proc. Natl. Acad. Sci. U.S.A.* **76**, 3665 (1979).
23. C. M. Preston, *J. Virol.* **29**, 275 (1979); R. A. F. Dixon and P. A. Schaffer, *ibid.* **36**, 189 (1980); R. J. Watson and J. B. Clements, *Nature (London)* **285**, 329 (1980).
24. J. Brady *et al.*, *Proc. Natl. Acad. Sci. U.S.A.* **81**, 2040 (1984); J. M. Keller and J. C. Alwine, *Cell* **36**, 381 (1984).
25. T. H. Lee *et al.*, *Science* **226**, 57 (1984); D. J. Slamon *et al.*, *ibid.*, p. 61.
26. S. Molineaux and J. E. Clements, *Gene* **23**, 137 (1983).
27. J. Messing, R. Crea, P. H. Seeburg, *Nucleic Acids Res.* **9**, 309 (1981).
28. F. Sanger, S. Nickelen, R. Coulson, *Proc. Natl. Acad. Sci. U.S.A.* **74**, 5463 (1977).
29. T. Maniatis *et al.*, in *Molecular Cloning: A Laboratory Manual* (Cold Spring Harbor Laboratory, Cold Spring Harbor, N.Y., 1982).
30. O. Narayan, D. E. Griffin, A. M. Silverstein, *J. Infect. Dis.* **135**, 800 (1977).
31. H. E. Gendelman *et al.*, *Lab. Invest.* **51**, 547 (1984).
32. O. Narayan *et al.*, *J. Gen. Virol.* **41**, 343 (1980).
33. We thank D. Garrett, D. Sheffer, and S. Parnell for technical assistance, K. Beemon for pSV1CAT and B. Howard for pSV2CAT and pRSVCAT, M. Gonda for H-9 cells, L. Kelly for

typing the manuscript, and K. Beemon, G. Ketner, and H. Smith for critical review of the manuscript. Supported by NIH grants NS-16145 and NS-15721.

19 February 1985; accepted 29 May 1985

104. Hepatitis B Virus DNA Sequences in Lymphoid Cells from Patients with AIDS and AIDS-Related Complex

F. Laure, D. Zagury, A.G. Saimot, R.C. Gallo, B.H. Hahn, and C. Brechot

A human T-lymphotropic retrovirus (HTLV-III, LAV) (*1–5*) has been isolated from patients with the acquired immune deficiency syndrome (AIDS) or AIDS-related complex (ARC) and from clinically asymptomatic individuals (*3, 6*). This virus has been causally related to AIDS and ARC, and it appears to be a necessary etiologic agent of these syndromes (*7*). However, infection by HTLV-III/LAV induces different responses depending on the individuals, suggesting that one or more other factors, such as hepatitis B virus (HBV), cytomegalovirus (CMV), or Epstein-Barr virus (EBV) (*8*), might also have a role in the pathogenic mechanism that leads to immune deficiency or might enhance the likelihood of disease manifestations of HTLV-III/LAV infection. Indeed, on the basis of epidemiological and biological considerations, several authors have proposed an etiologic role for HBV (*9*). Serological markers of HBV have frequently been detected in patients with AIDS and in people at high risk for AIDS (for example, homosexual men, hemophiliacs, and intravenous drug abusers), and HBV DNA sequences have been identified in bone marrow cells (*10*) and mononuclear blood cells of such subjects (*11, 12*). These data prompted us to investigate concomitant hepatitis B infections in patients with AIDS and ARC. We report here that HBV DNA sequences were present in lymphocytes derived from AIDS patients who were serologically HBV-positive or HBV-negative. In the lymphocyte populations assayed, we also detected a common pattern consistent with the integration of the HBV DNA and with free monomeric viral forms.

Lymphoid cell DNA from four patients, two with AIDS (one of them with Kaposi's sarcoma) and two with ARC, were assessed. That each of the patients was infected with HTLV-III/LAV was demonstrated by (i) the presence of antibodies to HTLV-III in the serum samples detected by indirect immunofluorescence as described (*13*), (ii) the identification of reverse transcriptase activity (RT) in the supernatant of primary mononuclear cell cultures and H9 cocultures, and (iii) the detection of HTLV-III antigens p15 and p24 in acetone-fixed cultured lymphocytes by indirect immunofluorescence in the presence of specific monoclonal antibodies (*1, 14*).

Serological markers for HBV were identified by commercial solid-phase radioimmunoassay (Abbott). One patient was positive for hepatitis B surface antigen (HBsAg) and positive for antibodies to the core (HBc) protein. Two other patients were negative for HBsAg but positive for antibodies to HBs and HBc. The last patient and five normal individuals (control group) were negative for all HBV serological markers.

Fresh mononuclear cells from peripheral blood lymphocytes (PBL) or lymph nodes derived from patients with AIDS or ARC and from normal donors were obtained by separation through a Ficoll-Hypaque gradient. Primary cultures of 5×10^5 to 6×10^5 PBL were seeded in medium (RPMI 1640 with 20 percent fetal calf serum) containing phytohemagglutinin (PHA). After 2 to 3 days, T-cell growth-factor interleukin-2 (IL-2), antibody to human α-interferon (α-IFN) (neutralizing titer 6 IU at a dilution of 10^5), and hydrocortisone (5 μg) were added.

Long-term T-cell cultures were obtained as described (*15*). Briefly, 10^3 to 10^4 fresh PBL were cultured with a feeder cell layer consisting of irradiated (4000 rads) lymphoid cells in a medium containing PHA and, after 2 to 3 days, IL-2, antibody to α-IFN, and hydrocortisone. When maintained at a density of 0.3×10^6 to 1×10^6 cells per milliliter, the PBL proliferated in the presence of IL-2 for up to 2 months.

When RT activity was found (day 6 to 10), in the primary cultures from AIDS patients, portions of cells were cocultivated with uninfected H9 cells as described (*1, 14*). These cocultures, which proliferated in a medium deprived of IL-2 for long periods, were found to contain cells morphologically similar to H9 cells as well as multinuclear giant cells. The presence of retrovirus in the cocultures was demonstrated by finding RT activity in the culture fluids and HTLV-III p15 and p24 antigens in acetone-fixed cells by indirect immunofluorescence in the presence of specific monoclonal antibody (*14*).

Fresh mononuclear cells, long-term cultures of lymphocytes, and H9 cocultures were examined for the presence of HBV DNA sequences by Southern blotting (*16*). The purified viral HBV DNA probe was obtained from a recombinant plasmid after digestion with Eco RI, electrophoresis, and electroelution (*17*). The cellular DNA was studied before and after digestion (Fig. 1) with the following restriction enzymes: Eco RI and Xba I, which generally cut the HBV genome at one and two sites, respectively, and Hind III and Sac I, which usually do not cut the HBV DNA (*18*).

As shown in Table 1, HBV DNA sequences were detected in the long-term cultures of T lymphocytes from all four patients tested. We also tested cellular DNA from fresh mononuclear cells of three of these patients and identified viral DNA in cells from two of them. The samples of cellular DNA, both before and after digestion with Eco RI, showed a single band at the 3.2-kb position. After digestion with Hind III and Sac I, discrete bands corresponding to high molecular weight DNA (at the 12- and 23-kb positions, respectively) were associated with the 3.2-kb band.

Taken together, these results are consistent with the integration of the viral genome with a dimeric or multimeric

Fig. 1. Representative restriction pattern of HBV DNA hybridization in mononuclear cells from patient No. 1 (Fig. 1). Southern blot analysis of cellular DNA from fresh mononuclear cells (lanes A and D), long-term cultures of T lymphocytes (lanes B, E, G, and J), and T lymphocytes cocultivated with H9 cells (lanes C, F, H, I, and K). Samples (5 μg) of undigested or digested DNA's were separated through an 0.8 percent agarose gel and transferred to a nitrocellulose membrane. The filters were hybridized with a nick-translated HBV DNA (1.5×10^7 count/min) insert from pcP10 (3×10^8 count/min per microgram of DNA) in 15 ml of 50 percent formamide, $5\times$ SSC (standard saline citrate), $1\times$ Denhardt's solution, 10 percent of dextran sulfate, 20 mM Na$_2$HOP$_4$, pH 6.5, and sonicated salmon sperm DNA. After overnight incubation at 42°C, the filters were washed under stringent conditions in $2\times$ SSC with 0.1 percent sodium dodecyl sulfate (SDS) for 5 minutes at room temperature and then in $0.1\times$ SSC with SDS at 65°C for 3 hours. The specificity of these results was supported by the negativity of the H9 cells and the control samples. Bacterial DNA contamination was eliminated by the absence of hybridization with the ^{32}P-labeled PBR$_{322}$ probe.

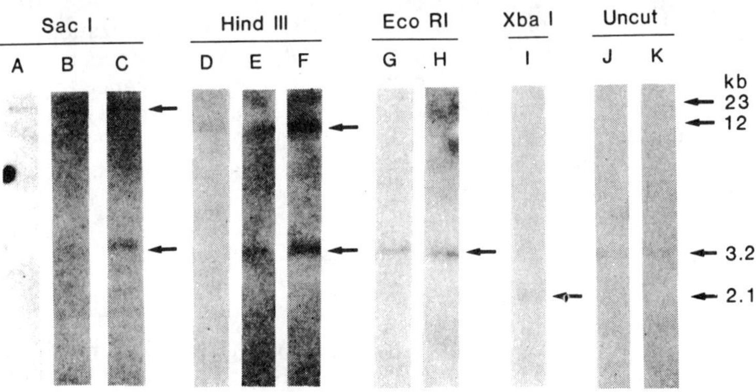

organization of HBV DNA. Since HBV DNA sequences were detected at the 3.2-kb DNA position both before digestion with restriction enzymes and after digestion with Hind III and Sac I, the results also suggest the presence of free monomeric viral DNA forms. However, the presence of discrete bands after digestion with Hind III and Sac I that were absent from the undigested DNA pattern is consistent with clonal proliferation of infected cells. These bands were observed at the same positions in the genomic DNA from different patients. When more cellular DNA becomes available it will be possible to clone the viral DNA sequences and determine the integration sites for the HBV DNA. It will also be possible to compare restriction patterns for such sequences with patterns from liver DNA (*19*). Free monomeric HBV DNA but no viral DNA replicative forms were identified in samples of the long-term cultures. It is interesting that HBV DNA, although absent from the reference H9 cell line, was detected in the cocultures of H9 cells with mononuclear cells from the AIDS patients. If one assumes that the primary PBL had died after 3 weeks in coculture, which was when we detected the HBV DNA, this result implies that the H9 cells acquired the HBV from the patients' mononuclear blood cells.

Studies with five additional AIDS patients, two of whom were negative for conventional HBV markers, showed that HBV DNA sequences were present in cell populations derived from different lymphoid sources: bone marrow, semen, lymph node, as well as PBL. The concomitant infections of HBV-HTLV-III/LAV found in all of these patients, even in the absence of conventional serological HBV markers, are consistent with the possibility that HBV may be a cofactor in the development of AIDS, as previously suggested for CMV and EBV (*8*).

Table 1. Results of serological and HBV DNA hybridization studies. HTLV-III/LAV was identified in mononuclear cells from AIDS or ARC patients by antibodies to HTLV-III in the serum samples revealed by an indirect immunofluorescence test, HTLV-III antigens detected by fixed-cell indirect immunofluorescence, and RT activity in the supernatant of primary mononuclear cells culture and H9 coculture (1, 13, 14). The HBV serological markers were identified by a commercial solid-phase radioimmunoassay (Abbott) and the HBV DNA sequences were detected as described in Fig. 1.

Patient number	HTLV III	Serological markers for HBV			Hepatitis B virus DNA sequences		
		HBsAg	Anti-HBc	Anti-HBs	Fresh PBL	Long-term cultures of T cells	Cocultured T cells with H9 cells
1 (AIDS)	+	−	−	−	NT*	+	+
2 (AIDS)	+	+	+	−	+	+	+
3 (ARC)	+	−	+	+	+	+	+
4 (ARC)	+	−	+	+	−	+	+
Control subjects (n = 5)	−	−	−	−	−	−	−

*NT, not tested.

Further studies are needed to assess this hypothesis, and it will be necessary to conduct similar studies with DNA probes for other viruses, such as EBV and CMV, and to determine the role of all of these viruses in the pathogenesis of AIDS.

References and Notes

1. M. Popovic et al., Science 224, 497 (1984); R. Gallo et al., ibid., p. 500.
2. B. H. Hahn et al., Nature (London) 312, 166 (1984).
3. F. Barre-Sinoussi et al., Science 220, 868 (1983).
4. M. Alizon et al., Nature (London) 312, 757 (1984).
5. P. A. Luciw et al., ibid., p. 760.
6. Centers for Disease Control, Morbid. Mortal. Week. Rpt. 32, 688 (1984); J. W. Curran et al., N. Engl. J. Med. 310, 69 (1984); G. B. Scott et al., ibid., p. 76; J. Oleske et al., J. Am. Med. Assoc. 249, 2345 (1983).
7. S. Broder and R. C. Gallo, N. Engl. J. Med. 311, 1292 (1984); F. Wong-Staal and R. C. Gallo, Blood 62, 253 (1985).
8. M. S. Hirsch et al., Rev. Infectious Dis. 6, 726 (1984).
9. R. T. Ravenholt, Lancet 1983-II, 885 (1983); M. I. McDonald, J. D. Hamilton, D. T. Durack, ibid., p. 882; T. Wright, S. Freidman, D. Alt-man, Gastroenterology 84, 1402 (1983); R. E. Anderson et al., in Viral Hepatitis and Liver Disease, G. N. Vyas, Ed. (Grune & Stratton, New York, 1984), p. 339.
10. E. Elfassi et al., Proc. Natl. Acad. Sci. U.S.A. 81, 3526 (1984).
11. P. Pontisso et al., Br. Med. J. 288, 1563 (1984).
12. L. E. Lie-Injo et al., DNA 2, 301 (1983).
13. D. Matez et al., Lancet 1984-I, 799 (1984).
14. M. D. Sarngadharan et al., Science 224, 506 (1984); D. Zagury et al., ibid. 226, 439 (1984).
15. D. Zagury et al., J. Immunol. Methods 43, 67 (1981).
16. E. M. Southern, J. Mol. Biol. 93, 503 (1975).
17. M. F. Dubois et al., Proc. Natl. Acad. Sci. U.S.A. 77, 4549 (1980).
18. P. Valenzuala et al., Nature (London) 280, 815 (1979); P. Charnay, C. Pourcel, A. Louise, A. Fritsch, P. Tiollais, Proc. Natl. Acad. Sci. U.S.A. 76, 2222 (1979).
19. C. Brèchot et al., Proc. Natl. Acad. Sci. U.S.A. 78, 3906 (1981); C. Brèchot et al., in Viral Hepatitis and Liver Disease, G. N. Vyas, Ed. (Grune & Stratton, New York, 1984), p. 395.
20. The work of F. Laure on DNA sequences was performed at the Pasteur Institute (Unité de Recombinaison et Expression Génétique). Supported by grants from the Association pour la Recherche Contre le Cancer (Villejuif), Ligue Nationale Française contre le Cancer, Federation André Maginot and Delegation de la Recherche et des Equipements Techniques. We thank V. Thiers and C. Pasquinelli and thank A. Cova for typing the manuscript.

27 March 1985; accepted 4 June 1985

Report

9 August 1985

105. Infection of HTLV-III/LAV in HTLV-I–Carrying Cells MT-2 and MT-4 and Application in a Plaque Assay

Shinji Harada, Yoshio Koyanagi, and Naoki Yamamoto

In 1984, retroviruses termed HTLV-III and AIDS-related virus (ARV) were isolated in the United States from the peripheral blood lymphocytes of patients with AIDS or pre-AIDS (*1*). A similar virus, LAV_1, had been isolated in France from patients with lymphadenopathy syndrome (*2*). Determination of the complete nucleotide sequences of the genome of these viruses revealed that they were variants of the same virus (*3*). That this virus is the causative agent of AIDS is indicated by studies showing that patients with AIDS or AIDS-related complex (ARC) frequently possess serum antibodies against this virus (*4*) and that the virus is found with high frequency in AIDS and ARC patients (*5*), causes specific cytopathogenic changes in $OKT4^+$ cells (*6*), is transmissible through blood transfusions (*7*), and causes a similar disease in chimpanzees (*8*).

Transmission of HTLV-III to an established T-cell line, H9, was first achieved by Popovic *et al.* (*1*). The same group of investigators subsequently showed that several $OKT4^+$ cell lines were susceptible to HTLV-III infection (*9*). The discovery of cell lines that continuously grow and produce the virus after infection greatly facilitated further studies of this virus. It was also reported that LAV could be adapted to grow in Epstein-Barr virus–transformed B lymphoblastoid cell lines or in the CCRF-CEM T-cell line (*10*). However, viral replication in all of these cell lines, and in primary human lymphocytes, requires a considerable time lag after infection. (Growth of the virus in primary human lymphocytes usually results in cell lysis.) In H9 cells infected with concentrated HTLV-III, viral activity is detectable 6 days after infection by the appearance of immunofluorescent antigens or the presence of reverse transcriptase (RT) (*1*).

We undertook these studies to find other cell culture systems that allow the efficient replication of HTLV-III. Sodroski *et al.* (*11*) had already shown that chloramphenicol acetyltransferase (CAT) expression from recombinants of the HTLV-I long terminal repeat (LTR) and the CAT gene is more enhanced in HOS cells infected with HTLV-I than in uninfected HOS cells. In this system, HTLV-I produced a transregulatory protein that influenced LTR-directed CAT expression. Chen *et al.* (*12*) obtained an analogous result with the HTLV-II–neo^R gene system. Moreover, Dalgleish *et al.* and Klatzmann *et al.* had shown that the OKT4 molecule is an essential com-

584

ponent of the receiver for HTLV-III/ LAV (*13*). On the basis of these observations we selected the MT-2 and MT-4 cell lines as the target for HTLV-III/ LAV infection since both cell lines strongly express HTLV-I antigens and are positive for OKT4 surface antigens. We report here the efficient replication of HTLV-III/LAV in these cell lines and the use of these lines in a plaque assay.

Lines MT-2 and MT-4 were established from cord blood lymphocytes that had been cocultured with leukemic cells from patients with adult T-cell leukemia (ATL) (*14*). The cells in these T-cell lines resemble leukemic T cells of ATL in terms of cell surface markers. After infection with HTLV-III derived from H9/ HTLV-III cells, the MT-2 and MT-4 cells showed differences in morphology, viability, and growth characteristics (Fig. 1 and 2A). MT-2 cells usually be-

came attached to the plastic surface of the culture dish (Fig. 1A) after subculture in the fresh medium. Three days after exposure to a 1:10 dilution of culture fluid from H9/HTLV-III cells, the MT-2 cells showed cytopathic changes with the appearance of multinuclear giant cells (Fig. 1B), apparently due to cell fusion, that attached to the surface of the culture dish. Floating cells started to show swelling and the features of ghost cells. These cells, and many others that did not change in size, degenerated very rapidly. Cell multiplication was impaired and viability started to decrease rapidly 3 days after infection (Fig. 2A).

The cytopathic changes in MT-4 cells infected with HTLV-III were somewhat weaker than those in the MT-2 cells. MT-4 cells are smaller than MT-2 cells and do not attach to the surface of the culture dish when placed in fresh medi-

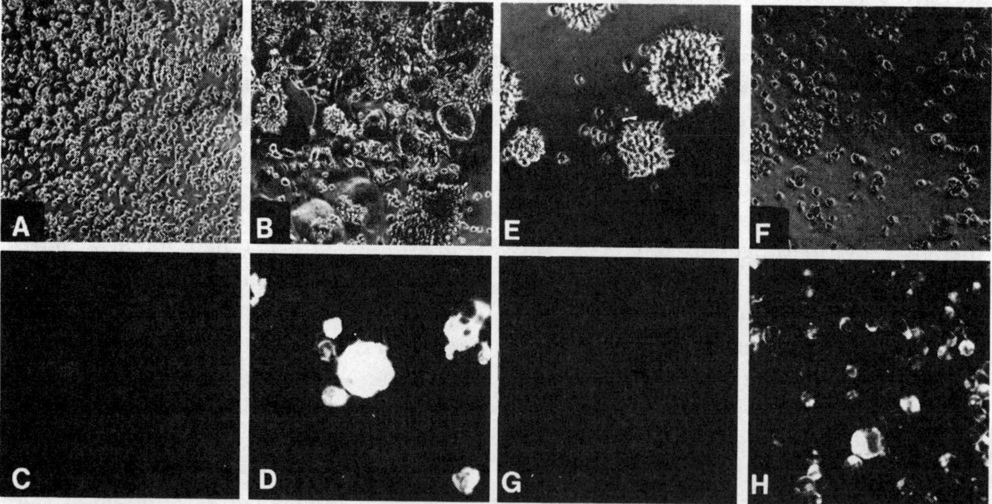

Fig. 1. HTLV-III–infected MT-2 (B and D) and MT-4 (F and H) cells and uninfected MT-2 (A and C) and MT-4 (E and G) cells. Virus was obtained from H9/HTLV-III culture medium after incubation for 4 days at 37°C. After removal of cells by centrifugation at 900*g* for 10 minutes, the supernatant was passed through a 0.22-μm Millipore membrane and stored at −80°C. Cells were infected with tenfold diluted virus preparation and photographed 3 days later by phase-contrast microscopy (A and B, ×60; E and F, ×120) or by immunofluorescent microscopy (C, D, G, and H, ×240) after staining.

585

um (Fig. 1E). Three days after infection with tenfold dilutions of culture fluid from H9/HTLV-III cells, the MT-4 cells became rounded and lost their surface characteristics. Then they became dark and showed shrinkage of the nucleus but usually no swelling (Fig. 1F). When control H9 cells were exposed to tenfold dilutions of H9/HTLV-III culture fluids, multinuclear giant cells appeared after about 5 days; an additional 5 days were required for all the cells to become infected. In MT-2 and MT-4 cells, the time course of the appearance of these cytopathic effects depended on the viral dose.

The MT-2 and MT-4 cell cultures inoculated with the tenfold dilutions of virus culture fluids were examined by immunofluorescence (IF) with a standard antibody (A-1) to HTLV-III from a patient with AIDS (IF titer; 1:1280) as described (1) (Figs. 1 and 2B). The first antigen-positive cells appeared as early as 1 day after infection in both cell lines (Fig. 1, D and H) and increased with time. However, the proportion of cells with detectable antigen increased more rapidly in MT-4 cells than in MT-2 cells: about 5 percent at 1 day, 33 percent at 2 days, and nearly 100 percent after 3 days of culture (Fig. 2B). When the cells were infected with the undiluted culture fluid of H9/HTLV-III cells, the first antigen-positive cells appeared within 16 hours and almost all the cells became antigen-positive within 24 hours. In the MT-2 cultures, almost all the cells became antigen-positive 6 days after inoculation. Under the same conditions, H9 cells started to show antigen positivity at 4 days, and the frequency of antigen-positive cells reached 100 percent about 10 days after infection. If the HTLV-III preparations were treated with human antibodies to HTLV-III obtained from

an AIDS patient (A-1) or a hemophiliac boy (He-1; IF titer, 1:4096), the frequency of antigen-positive cells was greatly

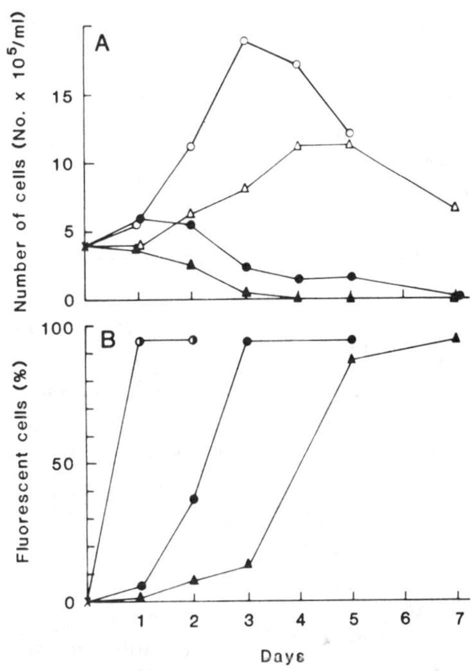

Fig. 2. Effect of HTLV-III infection on growth of cells and induction of HTLV-III–specific immunofluorescent antigens in MT-2 and MT-4 cells. MT-2 and MT-4 cells were infected with the various concentrations of HTLV-III. Virus suspension (0.5 ml, appropriately diluted) was added to the pellet of 2×10^6 cells of the target cells. The mixture was then incubated for 1 hour at 37°C for virus adsorption. Then, 4.5 ml of complete medium (RPMI 1640 with 10 percent fetal calf serum) was added to each tube, and the cells (1 ml per well) were inoculated into a 24-well plastic tray. After incubation at 37°C in a humidified atmosphere with CO_2, the cells were investigated for growth by the trypan blue dye exclusion method under the low-power microscope (A) and for HTLV-III antigen synthesis by indirect immunofluorescence (B) at the indicated times after infection. Symbols: △, uninfected MT-2 cells; ▲, MT-2 cells infected with HTLV-III (1:10); ○, uninfected MT-4 cells; ●, MT-4 cells infected with HTLV-III (1:10); and ◑, MT-4 cells infected with the undiluted HTLV-III.

reduced and the cytopathogenic changes were blocked at lower dilutions of the sera.

When these experiments were repeated with LAV prepared from cultures of CEM/LAV$_1$ cells (15), we obtained essentially the same results. To ensure that the cytopathic effects and the appearance of immunofluorescent antigens were indeed caused by HTLV-III, we performed immunoprecipitation experiments (16). In MT-4 cells infected with the virus, eight dominant polypeptide bands were specifically precipitated with antisera to HTLV-III. The molecular weights of these polypeptides were approximately 120,000, 55,000, 46,000, 40,000, 36,000, 33,000, 24,000, and 17,000. In none of the experiments were HTLV-I antigens observed when the two HTLV-III antibodies were used.

We then tested whether MT-4 cells could be used as target cells for an HTLV-III–induced plaque assay (17). Since MT-4 cells were not adherent to the culture vessel, we used plates coated with poly-L-lysin (PLL) (molecular weight 90,000; Sigma) to make a monolayer of cells (18). The dilution experiment data (Fig. 3C) suggest that a single infectious virus particle is sufficient for infection and plaque formation (17, 19), but this test does not prove that every virion present is able to create a plaque. To determine whether plaques are formed by HTLV-III, we incubated portions [40 plaque-forming units (PFU)] of the virus preparation with various dilutions of sera from two seronegative controls and two patients with hemophilia A who were both seropositive to HTLV-III. Serum from patient 1, who had a high titer (1:4096) of antibody detected by IF (1), completely inhibited plaque at 1:10 and 1:20 dilutions (Table 1). The

titer of neutralizing antibody to HTLV-III in the sera from both patients was almost 1:160, judged by the 50 percent reduction in plaque formation. In contrast, sera from two healthy donors (negative IF) did not remarkably reduce plaque formation, although some reduction in the number of plaques was observed. This result may reflect experimental variation due to the small number of PFU used as virus controls or the sensitivity of the assay. It may be necessary to improve the technique to minimize the standard deviation of the number of plaques. To confirm that plaque formation was specific to HTLV-III infection, we compared PFU, median tissue culture infectious doses (TCID$_{50}$), and the activity of RT from different preparations of virus (Table 2). There was a parallel relation between PFU titer and RT activity, suggesting that PFU reflected the amount of the retrovirus. Also, PFU was well correlated with TCID$_{50}$, as determined by the CPE of infected MT-4 cell cultures. Thus the values obtained were the same within the range of experimental error. Plaque formation was also observed when HTLV-III/LAV–infected cells were used instead of cell-free virus (22).

Sodroski et al. reported that gene expression directed by the LTR sequence of HTLV-III is stimulated only in cell lines infected with HTLV-III and not with HTLV-I or -II (23). Gallo and his colleagues showed that an HTLV-I–positive cell line, C91/PL, was susceptible to HTLV-III infection although H9 cells were more efficient in terms of viral replication (9). Using a large panel of HTLV-I–positive cell lines of human and monkey origin, we determined whether the efficient replication of HTLV-III observed in MT-2 and MT-4 cells is a

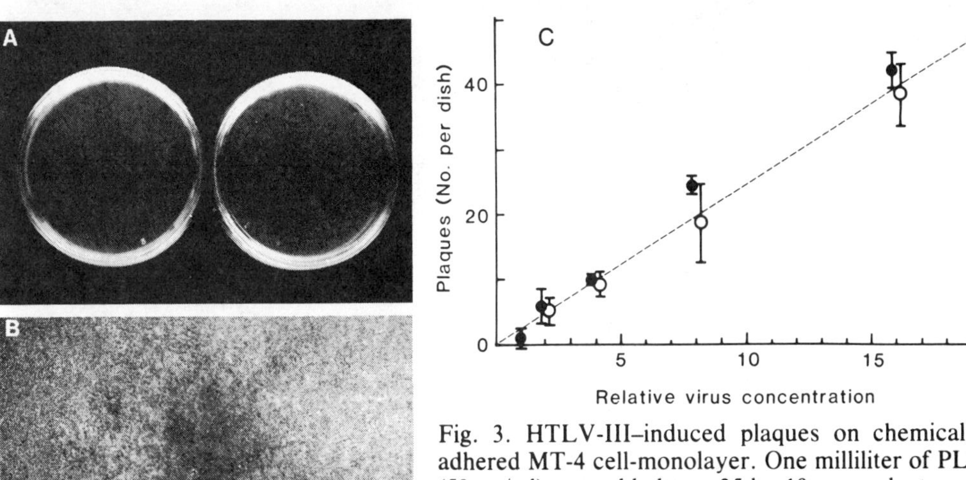

Fig. 3. HTLV-III–induced plaques on chemically adhered MT-4 cell-monolayer. One milliliter of PLL (50 μg/ml) was added to a 35 by 10 mm polystyrene tissue culture dish (Falcon). The coated plates were incubated for 60 minutes at room temperature and rinsed three times in phosphate-buffered saline (PBS). Portions (1.5 ml) of MT-4 cells (150×10^4 per milliliter) were washed three times in PBS and added to each PLL-coated plate. After incubation for another 30 minutes the unbound cells were removed by gently washing the plates three times with PBS. The MT-4 cell-monolayer was prepared, and 100 μl of diluted virus was slowly dropped onto cells. The plates were then incubated for 60 minutes at 4°C. After adsorption of the virus, 1 ml of the agarose medium was overlayed [Sea Plaque Agarose, Marine Colloid Corporation: RPMI 1640 medium supplemented with 10 percent fetal calf serum, penicillin (100 IU/ml), streptomycin (100 μg/ml), and 0.6 percent agarose]. The plates were incubated (CO_2 atmosphere) at 37°C for 3 days; 1 ml of agarose overlay medium containing neutral red (1:50,000) was added; and incubation was continued for another 3 days in the dark. On day 6, plaque production was observed (A) with the naked eye (right, infected; left, uninfected) and (B) microscopically. At this time, plaque diameter was 1 to 2 mm. HTLV-III–specific antigen detected by IF was expressed in the cells picked from the plaques. (C) Linear relation between number of plaques and virus concentration. Values for the relative virus concentration were chosen arbitrarily; however, a concentration of 16 corresponds to a 1:100 dilution of filtrated supernatant (4×10^3 PFU/ml) from H9/HTLV-III cell culture. Then, a twofold dilution of the virus was made. The dashed line represents the theoretical dose response of plaque formation according to the one-particle hypothesis (*19*). Open and solid circles display two independent experiments. The number of plaques per dish was expressed as the mean value of three dishes. The bars reveal the standard deviations ($n = 3$).

general phenomenon in HTLV-I–positive cell lines. Thirteen of 21 cell lines showed more rapid appearance and increase of viral antigens after HTLV-III infection than the H9 cells used as a control. However, HTLV-III replication efficiency did not appear to be correlated with the frequency of the cells positive for the HTLV-I antigens detectable by IF (*24*). Thus it is not known whether HTLV-III replication after infection is correlated with LOR gene expression in these HTLV-I–carrying cells.

It is also not known whether the virus produced from HTLV-I–positive cell lines after HTLV-III infection are phenotypically altered [an interaction has been observed between HTLV-I and vesicular stomatitis virus (VSV) (*25*)]. Cell-free HTLV-I usually fails to infect and

Table 1. Inhibition of HTLV-III–induced plaque formation by the treatment of the virus with sera from two seropositive patients with hemophilia and two seronegative controls. Aliquots of HTLV-III (200 μl of 800 PFU/ml) derived from H9/HTLV-III cultures were incubated with 200 μl of twofold diluted sera from two patients and two controls for 2 hours at 4°C. Then 100 μl of each mixture was inoculated onto MT-4 monolayers. Triplicate plaque assays were performed (average $\pm$ standard error of the mean are given). When PBS was used instead of sera, 41.0 $\pm$ 12.2 plaques per plate were counted as the virus control. No plaque was observed without inoculation of the virus. The percentage reduction of the plaque is shown in parentheses and was calculated as follows: $[(P_c - P_t)/P_c] \times 100$, where P_c is the number of plaques in the virus control and P_t the number in the test. N.T., not tested.

Donor	Antibody titer* against HTLV-III	Dilution of serum				
		1:10	1:20	1:40	1:80	1:160
Patient 1 (He-1)	1:4096	0 (100)	1.3 ±2.3 (96.8)	2.0 ± 1.0 (95.1)	9.0 ± 6.6 (78.0)	17.7 ± 10.5 (56.8)
Patient 2	1:512	7.3 ± 1.5 (82.2)	6.7 ± 1.5 (83.7)	9.0 ± 2.6 (78.0)	13.0 ± 6.6 (68.3)	18.0 ± 5.2 (56.1)
Healthy 1	<1:5	37.0 ± 7.9 (9.8)	37.0 ± 17.0 (9.8)	30.3 ± 6.7 (26.1)	N.T.	N.T.
Healthy 2	<1:5	36.7 ± 12.9 (10.5)	29.5 ± 4.9 (28.0)	29.0 ± 9.9 (29.3)	N.T.	N.T.

*Antibody titers were determined by indirect immunofluorescence of fixed H9/HTLV-III cells (*1*).

Table 2. Plaque-forming units (PFU), $TCID_{50}$, and RT activity of virus preparations from various sources. Portions (15 ml) of filtrated supernatants from MT-2 cell, H9/HTLV-III cells, HTLV-III–infected MT-4 cells, and MT-4 cell cultures were tested for PFU, $TCID_{50}$, and RT activity. Plaque formation was performed as described in Fig. 3. In order to determine the $TCID_{50}$, 100 μl of 60×10^4 per milliliter of MT-4 cells was plated into each flat well of microtiter plate (Terumo, Tokyo). The same volume of tenfold diluted supernatants was then inoculated into each well. Quadruplicate experiments were performed for each dilution. Half of the medium (RPMI 1640 with 10 percent fetal calf serum and antibiotics) was changed twice a week. Plates were incubated at 37°C for 4 weeks. Remarkable pH change of the medium and cytopathic effects of infected cells were counted. The Reed and Muench method (*20*) was used for calculation of the 50 percent end point. RT activity was detected as described by Poiesz *et al.* (*21*).

Viral source	Time in culture (days)	Quantitation of the virus		
		PFU/ml	$TCID_{50}$/ml	RT (count/min)
Medium		0	0	1.5×10^3
MT-2 cells	4	0	0	2.3×10^3
H9/HTLV-III cells	1	2.7×10	$10^{1.2}$	6.3×10^3
H9/HTLV-III cells	4	4.0×10^3	$10^{3.3}$	2.3×10^4
HTLV-III–infected MT-4 cells	4	2.2×10^5	$10^{5.5}$	1.7×10^6
MT-4 cells	4	0	0	3.8×10^3

transform normal lymphocytes, although there are some exceptions ascribed to the labile envelope of the virus (*26*). We found no biological activity of HTLV-I in filtrates of the culture medium of MT-2 and MT-4 cells after HTLV-III infection; however, the biological activity of HTLV-III seemed to be enhanced (*27*).

The establishment of a system that permits rapid and efficient replication of HTLV-III and cell death opens the way to the routine detection and isolation of HTLV-III from the infected patients and may facilitate studies of the AIDS virus.

References and Notes

1. M. Popovic *et al.*, *Science* **224**, 497 (1984); J. A. Levy *et al.*, *ibid.* **225**, 840 (1984).
2. F. Barré-Sinoussi *et al.*, *ibid.* **220**, 868 (1983).
3. L. Ratner *et al.*, *Nature (London)* **313**, 277 (1985); R. Sanchez-Pescador *et al.*, *Science* **227**, 484 (1985); S. Wain-Hobson *et al.*, *Cell* **40**, 9 (1985).
4. M. G. Sarngadharan *et al.*, *Science* **224**, 506 (1984); V. S. Kalyanaraman *et al.*, *ibid.* **225**, 321 (1984).
5. R. C. Gallo *et al.*, *ibid.* **224**, 500 (1984).
6. D. Klatzmann *et al.*, *ibid.* **225**, 59 (1984).
7. P. M. Feorino *et al.*, *ibid.*, p. 69; L. W. Kitchen *et al.*, *Nature (London)* **312**, 367 (1984).
8. H. J. Alter *et al.*, *Science* **226**, 549 (1984); D. P. Francis *et al.*, *Lancet* **1984-II**, 1275 (1984).
9. M. Popovic, E. Read, R. C. Gallo, *ibid.*, p. 1472.
10. L. Montagnier *et al.*, *Science* **225**, 63 (1984).
11. J. G. Sodroski, C. A. Rosen, W. A. Haseltine, *ibid.*, p. 381.
12. I. Chen *et al.*, *Nature (London)* **309**, 276 (1984).
13. A. G. Dalgleish *et al.*, *ibid.* **312**, 763 (1984); D. Klatzmann *et al.*, *ibid.*, p. 767.
14. I. Miyoshi *et al.*, *ibid.* **296**, 770 (1981); I. Miyoshi *et al.*, *Gann Monogr.* **28**, 219 (1982); Y. Koyanagi *et al.*, *Med. Microbiol. Immunol.* **173**, 127 (1984).
15. R. Cheingson-Popov *et al.*, *Lancet* **1984–II**, 477 (1984).
16. N. Yamamoto *et al.*, *Int. J. Cancer* **32**, 281 (1983); J. Schneider *et al.*, *Virology* **132**, 1 (1984).
17. The plaque assay was originally developed by R. Dulbecco [*Proc. Natl. Acad. Sci. U.S.A.* **38**, 747 (1952)].
18. R. D. Stulting and G. Berke, *J. Exp. Med.* **137**, 932 (1973).
19. R. Dulbecco and M. Vogt, *ibid.* **99**, 167 (1954).
20. L. J. Reed and H. Muench, *Am. J. Hyg.* **27**, 493 (1983).
21. B. J. Poiesz *et al.*, *Proc. Natl. Acad. Sci. U.S.A.* **77**, 7415 (1980).
22. S. Harada and N. Yamamoto, *Jpn. J. Cancer Res. (Gann)* **76**, 432 (1985).
23. J. Sodroski *et al.*, *Science* **227**, 171 (1985).

24. Y. Koyanagi *et al.*, in preparation.
25. K. Nagy *et al.*, in *Human T-Cell Leukemia Viruses*, R. C. Gallo, M. Essex, L. Gross, Eds. (Cold Spring Harbor Press, Cold Spring Harbor, N.Y., 1984), p. 121.
26. N. Yamamoto *et al.*, *Science* **217**, 737 (1982); T. Chosa *et al.*, *Gann* **73**, 844 (1982); P. Clapham *et al.*, *Science* **222**, 1125 (1983); N. Yamamoto *et al.*, *Z. Naturforsch.* **37**, 731 (1982).
27. S. Harada *et al.*, in preparation.
28. We thank R. C. Gallo and J. C. Chermann for supplying H9 and H9/HTLV-III and CEM/LAV cells, respectively, and Y. Koyanagi for typing the manuscript. Supported by Grants-in-Aid for Cancer Research from the Ministry of Education, Science, and Culture, Japan.

25 March 1985; accepted 6 June 1985

Report

16 August 1985

106.   The pX Protein of HTLV-I Is a Transcriptional Activator of Its Long Terminal Repeats

Barbara K. Felber, Harry Paskalis, Carol Kleinman-Ewing, Flossie Wong-Staal, and George N. Pavlakis

The exogenous retrovirus human T-cell leukemia virus type I (HTLV-I) appears to be the etiologic agent of adult T-cell leukemia-lymphoma (*1, 2*). HTLV-I is a member of a family of human retroviruses that display some structural and functional similarities, including the tropism for a restricted cell type, the OKT4 helper T lymphocyte. HTLV-I resembles a chronic leukemia virus in that it is replication competent, causes a monoclonal malignancy after a long latency period, and does not contain any recognizable cell-derived oncogene. However, HTLV-I can efficiently immortalize normal human lymphocytes in vitro, a property previously associated with acute transforming viruses containing oncogenes (*3*). In spite of the monoclonality of HTLV-I associated malignancies, no specific chromosomal sites have been detected for the integration of the provirus (*4*). There is evidence that the

HTLV viruses, HTLV-I, HTLV-II, and HTLV-III, together with bovine leukemia virus (BLV), may constitute a group of retroviruses that can be characterized by the way in which they interact with the infected cell. There is a great increase in the level of steady-state messenger RNA (mRNA) directed from the promoter in the long terminal repeats (LTR's) in cell lines infected with HTLV-I compared to uninfected parent cells (*5–7*). It has been postulated that this is a transcriptional activation caused directly or indirectly by a viral product (*5, 8*). In addition to the typical retroviral genes *gag*, *pol*, and *env*, the HTLV-I genome contains four overlapping open reading frames at the 3' end of the genome (*9*). One of these, the extended X_{IV} (*9*) or LOR (*8*) reading frame (here referred to as the X-LOR) is highly conserved between HTLV-I and HTLV-II (*10*). A splice acceptor at the beginning of this reading frame is also conserved among HTLV-I, HTLV-II (*11*), and probably BLV (*12*). Furthermore, a protein of the expected molecular weight was identified in cells infected with HTLV-I or HTLV-II by immunoprecipitation and partial radiosequencing (*13*). It was proposed that this viral product (here referred to as pX) may be responsible for the observed *trans*-activation. Alternatively, virus-permissive cell lines may constitutively produce specific factors that, upon infection with virus, allow the increased transcription from the LTR (*6, 7*). To distinguish between these explanations, and to understand the role of pX in the life cycle of the virus and its relation to leukemogenesis, we have expressed the pX protein in animal cells and studied its structural and functional properties.

The strategy we used is depicted in Fig. 1A. The promoter and the first structural exon of the mouse metallothionein I (MT) gene were ligated to HTLV-I upstream of the mapped splice acceptor within the X-LOR reading frame (*11*). If the MT splice donor can splice to the HTLV-I splice acceptor, a protein should be produced that would contain seven amino acids from the NH_2 terminal end of MT and the entire pX reading frame from the splice acceptor to the terminator within the LTR. A frameshift mutation within the X-LOR reading frame was constructed by inserting a dinucleotide at the Cla I site at position 7472 of HTLV-I. These two constructs were inserted into vector pJYM that contains a part of the plasmid pBR322 and the entire SV40 genome linearized at the Bam HI site (*14*). This resulted in plasmids pMXL and pMXfL, containing the X-LOR and the frameshift mutant, respectively.

Plasmids pMXL and pMXfL were introduced into CV1 cells, a monkey kidney cell line, by using the calcium phosphate coprecipitation technique (*15*). Total RNA was isolated and analyzed by S1 mapping (*16*) with the use of probes a and b (Fig. 1A). S1 mapping with probe a revealed that most of the stable mRNA was correctly spliced (Fig. 2A). Two bands of 174 and 192 nucleotides were specifically protected in the transfected cells. The lower band is derived from hybridization to correctly spliced mRNA and the upper band from hybridization to unspliced mRNA. No bands were protected after S1 mapping of RNA from cells transfected with salmon sperm DNA or with vector pJYMMT(L) (*17*), a JYM plasmid (*14*) with a 4-kilobase (kb) MT gene insert. S1 mapping experiments with probe b, which spans the entire HTLV-I part of the intervening sequence, gave a band at 174 nucleotides corresponding to spliced mRNA, and a substantial amount of full-length probe, indicating the presence of unspliced mRNA (Fig. 2B). There appeared to be no other major splice donors or acceptors within this region. Therefore, most (>90 percent) of the mRNA is correctly spliced, and both plasmids pMXL and pMXfL direct the synthesis of similar amounts of mRNA after transfection.

Cells transfected with plasmid pMXL were also examined by indirect immunofluorescense with the use of patient sera containing high titers of antibody to HTLV-I (*18*). Approximately 10 percent of the CV1 cells were positive in this assay. All positive cells contained strongly fluorescing nuclei, indicating that most of the HTLV-I protein encoded by plasmid pMXL was localized in the nucleus (Fig. 3A). Identical results were obtained after transfection with

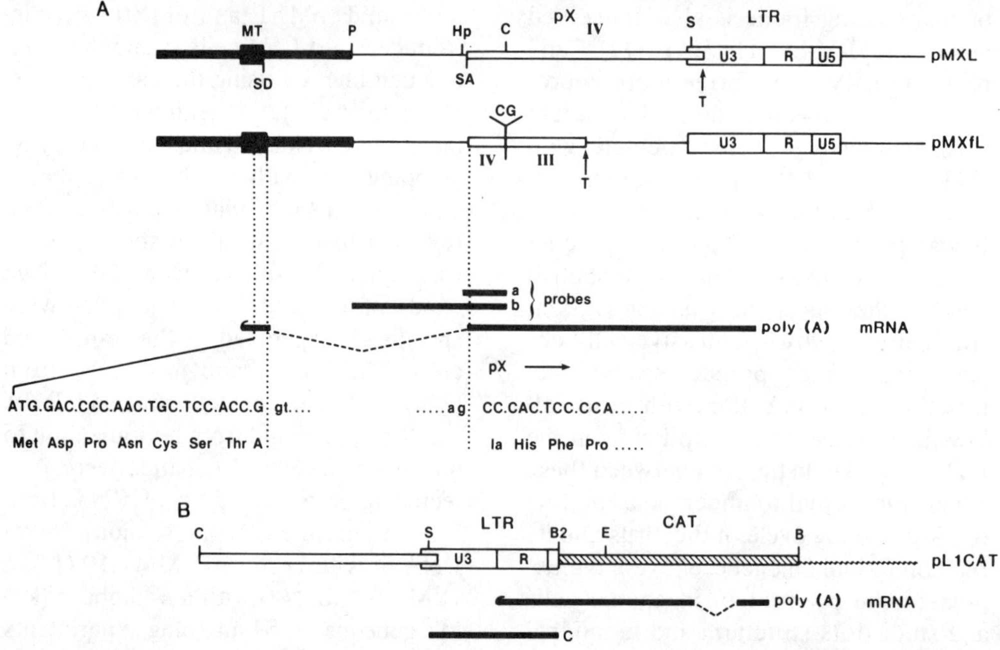

Fig. 1. (A) Structure of the recombinant plasmids for the expression of pX of HTLV-I. A 2.3-kb piece of the mouse MT gene (solid rectangles) containing the promoter, the first exon, and part of the first intervening sequence was ligated upstream from the splice acceptor (SA) of HTLV-I. This construct was inserted into vector pJYM that contains the complete SV40 linearized at the Bam HI site (plasmid pMXL). The SV40 genome is adjacent to the LTR. The direction of transcription of the MT promoter is the same as that of the late region of SV40. The expected protein contains seven amino acids from the NH_2 terminus of metallothionein and the complete X-LOR reading frame from the splice acceptor [position 7301; the sequence is numbered as in (9)]. The HTLV-I clone used (31) was partially sequenced. Only three differences were found between this clone and that of Seiki et al. (9) within the sequenced region. These were G to A at position 5195 T to C at position 5234, and C to T at position 7271, which destroys a Pst I site. A frameshift was constructed in the X-LOR reading frame by inserting a CG dinucleotide in the Cla I site by filling in with the Klenow fragment of DNA polymerase I and converting it into a Nru I site (plasmid pMXfL). The expected protein contains seven amino acids of metallothionein, 58 amino acids of the X-LOR reading frame, and 111 amino acids of the X_{111} reading frame from position 7464 to 7809. The structures of the expected mRNA and protein are indicated. The bars labeled a and b are the S1 mapping probes used in Fig. 2: a, Hpa I–Cla I probe; b, Pst I–Cla I probe. For the S1 mapping experiments, uniformly ^{32}P-labeled single-stranded probes were generated by primer extension from appropriate restriction fragments subcloned into M13 vectors. (B) Structure of plasmid pL1CAT. A Cla I–Sau 3AI fragment containing the U3, R, and part of the U5 region of the LTR of HTLV-I was ligated upstream of the CAT coding sequences in plasmid CAT3M (32). The bar labeled c represents the Sma I–Sau 3AI S1 mapping probe used in Fig. 4F. Symbols: MT, metallothionein; SD, splice donor; SA, splice acceptor; T, terminator; LTR, long terminal repeat; P, Pst I; Hp, Hpa I; C, Cla I; S, Sma I; B2, Bgl II; E, Eco RI; B, Bam HI.

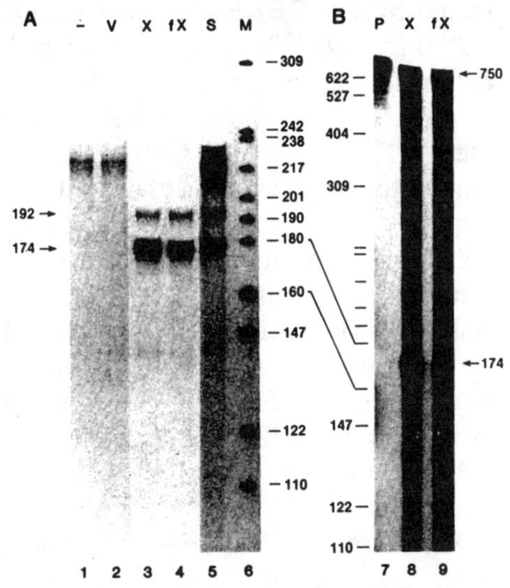

Fig. 2. (A) S1 mapping analysis of mRNA with the use of probe a. At 48 hours after transfection, total RNA was prepared by the guanidinium isothiocyanate–cesium chloride method. Ten micrograms of RNA were hybridized at 40°C overnight and treated with S1 nuclease (16). We expected a band of 192 nucleotides from the unspliced mRNA and a band of 174 nt from the spliced mRNA. CV1 cells were transfected with lane 1, salmon sperm DNA; lane 2, pJYMMT(L) vector DNA; lane 3, pMXL DNA; lane 4, pMXfL DNA. Lane 5, S1 mapping of total RNA isolated from the stable producer cell line BXL40 with probe a. Lane 6, end-labeled Hpa II digest of pBR322 DNA as molecular weight markers. (B) S1 mapping of the same RNA preparations using probe b. Lane 7, probe b. Lanes 8 and 9, CV1 cells transfected with pMXL DNA and pMXfL DNA, respectively. The same 174-nucleotide band is protected by the spliced mRNA.

plasmid pMXfL. The numbers of cells positive in transfections with pMXL and with pMXfL were about equal. Untransfected cells or cells transfected with vector pJYMMT(L) DNA were not stained by the antibody (Fig. 3B). Recently Goh et al. (19) reported that pX is present in both the nuclear and the cytoplasmic fractions of HTLV-I–infected transformed lymphocytes.

We have also established permanent cell lines that overexpress pX protein by inserting the constructs shown in Fig. 1A into bovine papilloma virus vectors as described (20). These cell lines, which will be described elsewhere, contain correctly spliced pX mRNA (Fig. 2A, lane 5). They also express the pX protein as determined by indirect immunofluorescence as well as by immunoprecipitations and immunoblots of cell lysates.

The effect of the pX protein on the transcription of the LTR of HTLV-I was next tested by cotransfection experiments. First, plasmid pL1CAT (Fig. 1B)

was constructed by ligating the LTR of HTLV-I 5′ to the body of the gene for chloramphenicol acetyltransferase (CAT). Transcription from the promoter in the LTR is expected to produce CAT, which was monitored by the acetylation of ^{14}C-labeled chloramphenicol as described (21). Plasmid pL1CAT was introduced into CV1 cells in the presence or absence of plasmid pMXL or plasmid pMXfL. Cell lysates were assayed for CAT activity, or total RNA was isolated and used for quantitative S1 mapping (Fig. 4A). pL1CAT alone directed the synthesis of low levels of CAT in CV1 cells [Fig. 4A, lane (−)]. When a coprecipitate of pMXL and pL1CAT was applied on the cells, a 50-fold increase of the CAT activity was observed (lane X). Cotransfection of pL1CAT with pMXfL (lane fX) resulted in a small increase in CAT activity, approximately fourfold greater than that seen with pL1CAT alone. Mixing plasmid pMXL and pMXfL increased the CAT activity to

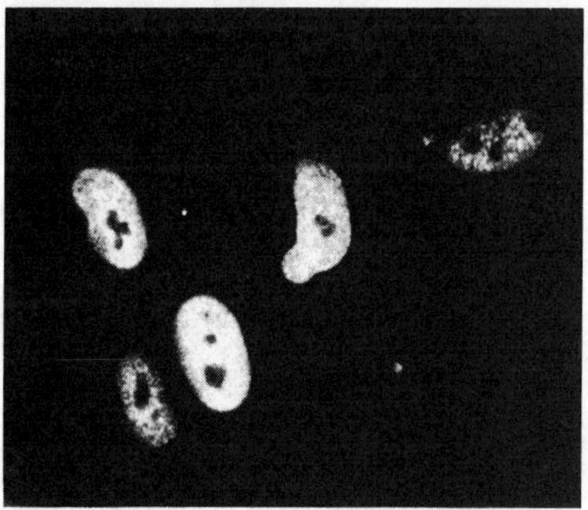

Fig. 3. Localization of pX by indirect immunofluorescence in CV1 cells transfected with plasmid pMXL. At 48 hours after transfection, the cells were fixed in 3.7 percent formaldehyde, made permeable with 0.1 percent NP-40 in phosphate-buffered saline (PBS), treated with serum from a human patient and then with FITC-conjugated goat anti–human immunoglobulin G (Cappel) to identify the pX protein.

the same extent as pMXL alone (lane X + fX). These results indicate that the activation is caused by the gene product of the X-LOR reading frame acting in *trans*, and not by competition of the incoming plasmid DNA for cellular factors. To verify this conclusion, we cotransfected increasing amounts of pMXL into CV1 cells with 10 μg of pL1CAT (Fig. 4B). The CAT activity was significantly stimulated by 0.1 μg of pMXL (1:200 molar ratio, pMXL:pL1CAT). As a control, the same experiment was repeated with a number of other promoters linked to the CAT gene, such as pSV2CAT and pRSVCAT (21). The presence of various amounts of pMXL did not affect the promoter activity of the SV40 early promoter (Fig. 4C), the Rous sarcoma virus LTR promoter, or the mouse metallothionein promoter.

The extent of HTLV-I LTR activation in a lymphoid cell line was also tested. The human T-cell line H9 (22) was transfected by the DEAE-dextran technique (23) (Fig. 4D). The results obtained by cotransfection of pL1CAT with pMXL or pMXfL were similar to the results in the CV1 cell line. No factors that are unique to lymphoid cells appeared to be required for the activation of the LTR by pX. Similar results were obtained after transfection of plasmid pL1CAT into the stable pX-producing cell lines BXL14 and BXL40. The CAT activity was 20-fold higher in BXL40 cells (Fig. 4E) than in control 7-4 cells containing a similar BPV vector without any HTLV-I sequences.

The increased CAT levels observed in these assays could, in principle, be due to a transcriptional activation of the LTR promoter, an increase in CAT mRNA accumulation, a change in translational efficiency of the hybrid mRNA or in protein stability, or some combination of the above. To distinguish among these possibilities and to examine whether the same promoter is used in the presence of pX, we transfected CV1 cells with pL1CAT in the presence or absence of pX. Total RNA was isolated and mapped by S1 nuclease for the presence of correctly initiated LTR mRNA with the use of probe c (Fig. 1B). Because plasmid pMXL contains a copy of the HTLV-I LTR, a different plasmid, pMX ΔL, was used in these experiments. pMX ΔL has the entire LTR deleted 3′ to the Sma I site (Fig. 1A); therefore, it produces a pX protein that lacks 16 amino acids from the carboxy terminus. This protein was found to be functional in the pL1CAT transactivation assay.

Correctly initiated mRNA was detected in the cells cotransfected with pL1CAT and pMX ΔL (Fig. 4F, lanes 2 and 3). No mRNA starting at the correct initiation site was detected in cells trans-

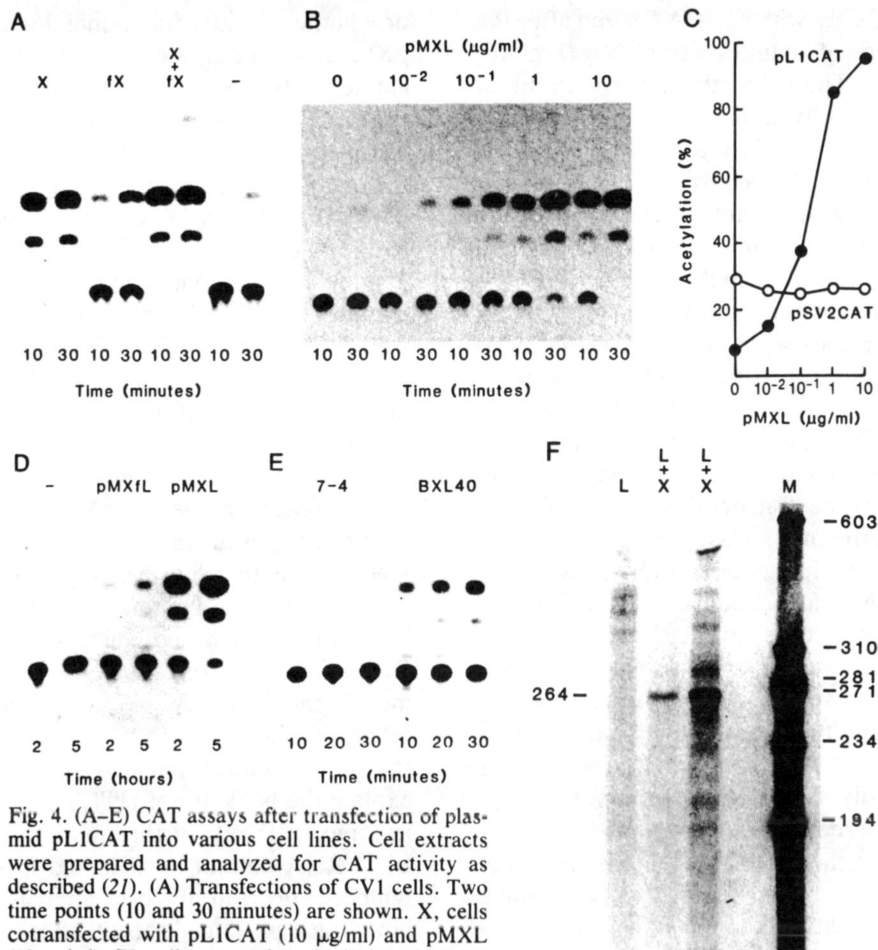

Fig. 4. (A–E) CAT assays after transfection of plasmid pL1CAT into various cell lines. Cell extracts were prepared and analyzed for CAT activity as described (*21*). (A) Transfections of CV1 cells. Two time points (10 and 30 minutes) are shown. X, cells cotransfected with pL1CAT (10 μg/ml) and pMXL (10 μg/ml); fX, cells cotransfected with pL1CAT (10 μg/ml) and pMXfL (10 μg/ml); X+fX, cells cotransfected with pL1CAT (10 μg/ml), pMXL (10 μg/ml) and pMXfL (10 μg/ml); (−), cells transfected only with pL1CAT (10 μg/ml). (B) Cotransfection of pL1CAT (10 μg/ml) in CV1 cells with different amounts of pMXL (0 to 10 μg) as indicated. Two time points for each concentration are shown (10 and 30 minutes). In all cases, the final DNA concentration in the precipitate was adjusted to 35 μg/ml by the addition of JYMMT(L) vector DNA. (C) Plot of data in (B). The 10-minute time points were quantitated by liquid scintillation counting. Under the same conditions, the expression of pSV2CAT is not affected by pMXL. (D) Cotransfections of plasmids pL1CAT with pMXL or pMXfL in H9 cells, a lymphoid cell line permissive for HTLV-I. Two time points (2 and 5 hours) of the CAT assay are shown. −, Cells transfected with pL1CAT (1 μg/ml); pMXfL, cells transfected with pL1CAT (1 μg/ml) and pMXfL (1 μg/ml); pMXL, cells transfected with pL1CAT (1 μg/ml) and pMXL (1 μg/ml). (E) Transfections of pL1CAT (10 μg/ml) into a stable cell line producing pX. Three time points of the CAT assay are shown (10, 20, and 30 minutes). 7-4 is a control cell line transformed with a BPV vector not containing HTLV-I sequences. BXL40 produces high quantities of pX. (F) S1 mapping of the LTR promoter of HTLV-I in the presence and absence of pX, using probe c. Lane 1, 50 μg of total RNA from cells transfected with pL1CAT. Lane 2, 1 μg of total RNA from cells cotransfected with pL1CAT and pMX ΔL. Lane 3, 5 μg of total RNA as in lane 2. Lane 4, molecular weight markers (end-labeled φX Hae III digest).

fected only with pL1CAT, even after the addition of 50 times more RNA (Fig. 4F, lane 1). Therefore, the induction ratio of the correctly initiated mRNA from the LTR promoter in the presence of pX is approximately 500-fold. This is almost one order of magnitude greater than the estimate based on the CAT assay. There appears to be a high basal level in the CAT assay due to transcripts initiated in other places within the transfected plasmid. Such possible aberrant initiation sites can explain the protected bands in Fig. 4F, lane 1. When we included a plasmid containing a human α-globin gene in the transfection coprecipitates, no difference was detected in the amounts of α-globin mRNA, indicating that the transfection efficiencies of the different coprecipitates were similar. Nuclear runoff experiments, deletion mutagenesis of the pL1CAT plasmid (24), and the data presented above indicated that the activation of LTR by pX is primarily, if not exclusively, a transcriptional event.

Since the product of pMXL in animal cells is a mutant pX protein containing seven additional amino acids at the NH_2-end, the question arises whether the properties of this mutant are similar to those of pX. The authentic pX protein is generated by a double-spliced mRNA that brings the envelope AUG next to the X-LOR reading frame. Using a similar approach, we have expressed the authentic pX protein in animal cells by splicing of the viral RNA and have shown that the two proteins give qualitatively similar results in the *trans*-activation assays (24). The observed fourfold induction of CAT with the frameshift mutant pfX indicates that pfX protein is partially active. We did not determine whether the 111 amino acids of the X_{111} reading frame contribute to this activity,

or whether a major functional domain of pX exists within the 58 NH_2-terminal amino acids that are identical in pX and pfX. The low induction by pMXfL could also be due to a frameshift suppression that generates a small amount of pX from pMXfL. Our *trans*-activation experiments were done in the presence of SV40 T antigen, a known modulator of gene expression (25). We obtained similar results with another set of pX-producing vectors that do not contain SV40 sequences (24). Therefore, *trans*-activation of the LTR by pX is not dependent on the presence of T antigen.

Two general models of pX action may now be proposed. In the first, pX would bind directly to a specific site in the LTR and influence the binding of other cellular factors or RNA polymerase with the DNA. In the second model, pX would modify the expression or the activity of other cellular factors that interact with the LTR. Neither model is sufficient to explain the behavior of HTLV-I or BLV in vivo without further assumptions. BLV RNA cannot be detected in fresh lymphocytes from infected animals (26), but virus is produced shortly after culturing the cells (27). Fresh leukemic cells from four of five ATL patients do not express detectable quantities of HTLV-I mRNA (28). Therefore, at least the majority of peripheral blood cells containing the provirus appear to counteract the activation of the LTR promoter by pX. This could be caused either by an inhibition of pX production or by an inhibition of transcription by cellular repressors. The existence of additional regulatory circuits is supported by the observation that after cultivation of leukemic cells, the provirus is actively transcribed and transmissible virus can be detected. The production of pX may be linked to cell cycle. Therefore, nondividing peripheral blood lymphocytes of leukemic patients would not contain substantial quantities of pX mRNA.

These data demonstrate that HTLV-I carries its own transcriptional activator that functions well in other cell types as well as in lymphoid cells. HTLV-I, HTLV-II, and BLV appear to have properties that justify their classification in the same class of retroviruses. To our knowledge this is the first identification of a group of retroviruses (29) that can code for a protein that has some properties characteristic of the transforming proteins of DNA tumor viruses, such as nuclear localization, ability to activate a homologous viral promoter (or promoters), and ability to modulate the expression of certain cellular promoters (24). It will therefore be interesting to examine whether pX is a transforming protein of HTLV-I, perhaps analogous to adenovirus E1A products or SV40 and polyoma T antigens (25, 30). The ability of pX to modulate the activity of other promoters may be important for triggering the sequence of events that lead to leukemogenesis. Since little or no pX protein occurs in fresh leukemic cells from patients, it could be involved in the initiation but not the maintenance of transformation. Alternatively, low levels of pX acting during inappropriate stages in the cell cycle may be enough to maintain the transformed phenotype in the leukemic cell. Availability of vectors producing authentic and mutant pX proteins in animal cells may help answer these questions. Since the name pX implies an unknown function of the gene product, it is no longer adequate. We propose to call this the Ta I protein, for transcriptional activator of the LTR.

References and Notes

1. B. J. Poiesz *et al.*, *Proc. Natl. Acad. Sci. U.S.A.* **77**, 7415 (1980); V. S. Kalyanaraman *et al.*, *Nature (London)* **294**, 271 (1981); M. Robert-Guroff *et al.*, *J. Exp. Med.* **154**, 1957 (1981); M. Yoshida *et al.*, *Proc. Natl. Acad. Sci. U.S.A.* **79**, 2031 (1982).
2. For recent reviews, see R. C. Gallo, M. Essex, L. Gross, Eds., *Human T-Cell Leukemia Viruses* (Cold Spring Harbor Laboratory, Cold Spring Harbor, N.Y., 1984); F. Wong-Staal and R. C. Gallo, *Blood* **65**, 253 (1985).
3. I. Miyoshi *et al.*, *Nature (London)* **294**, 770 (1981); M. Popovic *et al.*, *Proc. Natl. Acad. Sci. U.S.A.* **80**, 5402 (1983); S. Merl *et al.*, *Blood* **64**, 967 (1984).
4. M. Seiki *et al.*, *Nature (London)* **309**, 640 (1984).
5. J. Sodroski *et al.*, *Science* **225**, 381 (1984); J. Sodroski *et al.*, *ibid.* **227**, 171 (1985).
6. I. S. Y. Chen *et al.*, *Nature (London)* **309**, 276 (1984).
7. D. Derse *et al.*, *Science* **227**, 317 (1984).
8. W. A. Haseltine *et al.*, *ibid.* **225**, 419 (1984).
9. M. Seiki *et al.*, *Proc. Natl. Acad. Sci. U.S.A.* **80**, 3618 (1983).
10. K. Shimotono *et al.*, *ibid.* **81**, 6657 (1984).
11. W. R. Wachsman *et al.*, *Science* **226**, 177 (1984); T. Okamoto *et al.*, *Virology*, in press.
12. N. R. Rice *et al.*, *Virology* **138**, 82 (1984); N. R. Rice, *ibid.* **142**, 357 (1985); N. Sagata *et al.*, *Proc. Natl. Acad. Sci. U.S.A.* **82**, 677 (1985).
13. T. H. Lee *et al.*, *Science* **226**, 57 (1984); D. J. Slamon *et al.*, *ibid.*, p. 61; T. Kiyokawa *et al.*, *Gann* **75**, 747 (1984).
14. M. Lusky and M. Botchan, *Nature (London)* **293**, 79 (1981).
15. F. J. Graham and A. J. Van der Eb, *J. Virol.* **52**, 456 (1973).
16. A. J. Berk and P. A. Sharp, *Cell* **12**, 721 (1977); R. F. Weaver and C. Weissmann, *Nucleic Acids Res.* **7**, 1175 (1979).
17. D. H. Hamer and M. J. Walling, *J. Mol. Appl. Genet.* **1**, 273 (1982).
18. J. Schüpbach *et al.*, *Cancer Res.* **43**, 886 (1983).
19. W. C. Goh, J. Sodroski, C. Rosen, M. Essex, W. A. Haseltine, *Science* **227**, 1227 (1985).
20. N. Sarver *et al.*, *Mol. Cell. Biol.* **1**, 486 (1981); G. N. Pavlakis and D. H. Hamer, *Proc. Natl. Acad. Sci. U.S.A.* **80**, 397 (1983); *Recent Prog. Horm. Res.* **39**, 353 (1983); unpublished results.
21. C. M. Gorman *et al.*, *Mol. Cell Biol.* **2**, 1044 (1982); C. M. Gorman, G. T. Merlino, M. C. Willingham, I. Pastan, B. H. Howard, *Proc. Natl. Acad. Sci. U.S.A.* **79**, 6777 (1982).
22. M. Popovic *et al.*, *Science* **224**, 497 (1984).
23. J. J. McCutchan and J. S. Pagano, *J. Natl. Cancer Inst.* **41**, 351 (1968).
24. G. N. Pavlakis and B. K. Felber, in preparation.
25. J. Tooze, Ed., *DNA Tumor Viruses: Molecular Biology of Tumor Viruses* (Cold Spring Harbor Laboratory, Cold Spring Harbor, N.Y., 1981); S. I. Reed *et al.*, *Proc. Natl. Acad. Sci. U.S.A.* **73**, 3083 (1976); D. Rio *et al.*, *ibid.* **77**, 5706 (1980); R. Tjian, *Cell* **13**, 165 (1981); J. Brady, F. Wong-Staal, R. C. Gallo, *Proc. Natl. Acad. Sci. U.S.A.* **81**, 2040 (1984).
26. R. Kettmann *et al.*, *Leuk. Res.* **4**, 509 (1980).
27. V. Baliga and J. F. Ferrer, *Proc. Soc. Exp. Biol. Med.* **156**, 388 (1977).
28. G. Franchini *et al.*, *Proc. Natl. Acad. Sci. U.S.A.* **81**, 6207 (1984).
29. A potential addition is Rous sarcoma virus; see S. Broome in *Eucaryotic Viral Vectors*, Y. Gluzman, Ed. (Cold Spring Harbor Laboratory, Cold Spring Harbor, N.Y., 1982); S. Broome and W.

Gilbert, *Cell* **40**, 538 (1985).
30. N. Jones and T. Shenk, *Proc. Natl. Acad. Sci. U.S.A.* **76**, 3665 (1979); J. R. Nevins, *Cell* **26**, 213 (1981); C. T. Feldman, M. J. Imperiale, J. R. Nevins, *Proc. Natl. Acad. Sci. U.S.A.* **79**, 4952 (1982); A. Berk *et al.*, *Cell* **17**, 935 (1979).
31. V. Manzari *et al.*, *Proc. Natl. Acad. Sci. U.S.A.* **80**, 1574 (1983).
32. L. A. Laimins *et al.*, *J. Virol.* **49**, 183 (1984).
33. We thank M. Satake for help with the immuno-fluorescence, M. G. Sarngadharan and R. C.

Gallo for human patient sera and for discussions, B. Howard and L. Laimonis for CAT vectors, H.-U. Affolter for advice, S. Hughes, D. Hamer, and Y. Ito for discussions and comments, and H. Marusiodis and V. Koogle for editorial assistance. Research sponsored by NCI, DHHS, under contract No. N01-C0-23909 with Litton Bionetics, Inc.

4 April 1985; accepted 1 July 1985

107. Genomic Diversity of Human T-Lymphotropic Virus Type III (HTLV-III)

Flossie Wong-Staal, George M. Shaw, Beatrice H. Hahn, S. Zaki Salahuddin, Mikulas Popovic, Phillip Markham, Robert Redfield, and Robert C. Gallo

Human T-lymphotropic virus type-III (HTLV-III), also referred to as lymphadenopathy-associated virus (LAV) and AIDS-related virus (ARV), is the etiologic agent of the acquired immune deficiency syndrome (AIDS) and related immunological disorders (*1, 2*). Diversity, or heterogeneity, in the genomes of different isolates of HTLV-III was first noted by our laboratory in the course of our initial characterization of the virus (*3*) and subsequently by the comparison of the nucleotide sequences of four different AIDS virus isolates (*4–6*). The latter studies also suggested that the extent of divergence between isolates could be minor (1 to 2 percent among BH-10, BH-5/8, and LAV-1A) or more extensive (7 percent between BH-10 and ARV-2) but, because so few isolates had been examined, the extent of variation among AIDS viruses was unclear. Thus, to gain

more information on the extent and nature of genomic variation in the HTLV-III group of viruses, we analyzed by Southern hybridization the viral DNA from 17 consecutively studied patients with either AIDS or AIDS-related complex (ARC) and one subject at risk for AIDS but with no apparent clinical disease.

Virus from nine patients with AIDS or ARC and one healthy subject was transmitted to established neoplastic T-cell lines (H4, H9, or JM) or to normal peripheral blood lymphocytes (PBL) (*1, 7*). Primary tissues (lymph node or brain) from the eight AIDS or ARC patients were examined directly (Table 1). DNA from cultured cells or primary tissues was digested with a panel of restriction enzymes and analyzed by Southern hybridization to 9-kb cloned HTLV-III probe (BH-10) (*3*). DNA bands constitut-

Table 1. Patients evaluated for HTLV-III DNA.

Isolate	DNA source	Patient diagnosis	Risk factor	Geographic location	Year of isolation
H9/HTLV-III$_B$	PBL/H9*	AIDS and ARC	Homosexuals	New York and New Jersey	1983
RF	PBL/H4*	AIDS	Haitian	Haiti and Philadelphia	1983
RH	PBL†	Healthy	Homosexual	Washington, D.C.	1984
TM	PBL/N-PBL*	AIDS	Homosexual	Boston	1984
HW	PBL/N-PBL*	AIDS	Heterosexual promiscuity	Europe and Africa	1984
MN	PBL/JM*	ARC	Child whose mother used intravenous drugs	New York and New Jersey	1984
SL	PBL/N-PBL*	ARC	Homosexual	New York and New Jersey	1984
SC	PBL/N-PBL*	ARC	Homosexual	California	1984
JS	PBL/N-PBL*	ARC	Homosexual	California	1984
MJ	PBL/H9*	AIDS	Child of Haitian mother	Haiti and Miami	1985
RJ	PBL/N-PBL*	AIDS	Homosexual	Boston	1985
FO	Lymph node‡	AIDS	Homosexual	New York and New Jersey	1984
KC	Lymph node‡	ARC	Intravenous drug user	New York and New Jersey	1984
JR 1	Brain‡	AIDS	Child whose mother used intravenous drugs	New York and New Jersey	1984
JR 2	Brain‡	AIDS	Homosexual	New York and New Jersey	1984
LS	Brain‡	AIDS	Child whose mother had ARC	New York and New Jersey	1984
JT	Brain‡	AIDS	Homosexual	New York and New Jersey	1984
RC	Brain‡	AIDS	Homosexual	New York and New Jersey	1984
RR	Brain‡	AIDS	Homosexual	New York and New Jersey	1984

*Virus transmitted from patients' PBL into H9, H4, or JM cell lines, or into normal allogeneic PBL. †Virus grown directly in patient's own PBL without transmission. ‡Viral DNA detected and analyzed in uncultured tissue.

ing an entire genomic complement were detected by this probe for each of the viruses under high stringency hybridization and wash conditions indicating that a high degree of homology exists among all of the isolates (Fig. 1). Despite this overall conservation in sequence homology, a striking degree of restriction enzyme site polymorphism was found among the isolates. For example, Sst I generated three predominant genotypic patterns: a 9.0-kb fragment (isolates RH, RF, and TM), 5.5- and 3.5-kb fragments (isolates HW, JS, and SC), and 5.5-, 1.8-, and 1.7-kb fragments (isolates MN and SL). The cell line H9/HTLV-III$_B$ (Fig. 1, lane IIIB), which was derived from the HT line that was infected by virus from several different patients (8), contains both the 9.0-kb and (5.5 + 3.5)-kb Sst I genotypes. Although all 18 isolates that we examined contained one of the three Sst I patterns described above, digestion of these isolates with three other enzymes (Bgl II, Hind III, and Pst I) yielded overall restriction patterns different for each of the viruses. It should be noted that the interpretation of restriction site differences between HTLV-III isolates is complicated by the simultaneous presence of unintegrated linear and circular DNA as well as integrated proviral DNA (3); we avoided this problem by using enzymes (Sst I, Bgl II, and

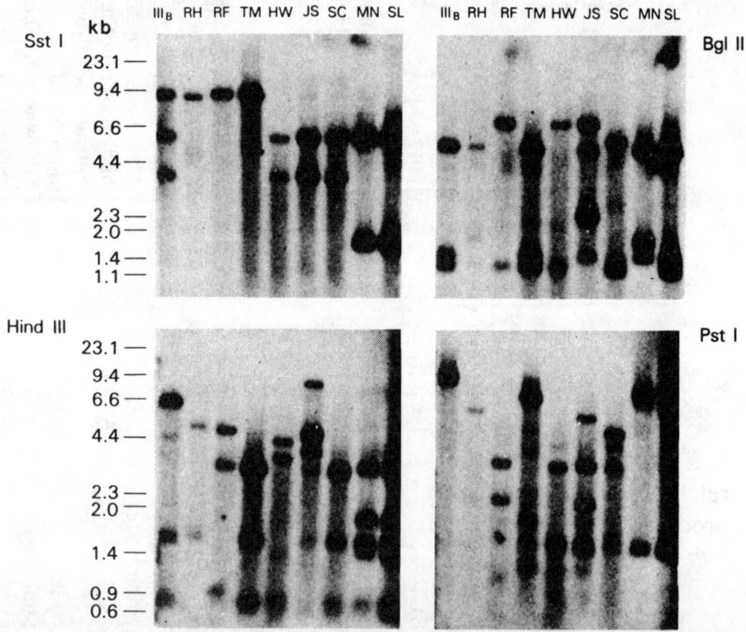

Fig. 1. Heterogeneity of HTLV-III genomes. High-molecular-weight DNA was extracted from virus infected cells (see Table 1) as (3). The DNA (5 to 15 μg) was digested with the indicated restriction enzymes according to the manufacturers' recommendations. The DNA was then subjected to electrophoresis through 0.6 cm thick 0.8 percent agarose slab gels and blotted in 10× SSC (standard saline citrate) onto 0.1 μm nitrocellulose filters (Schleicher and Schuell). Hybridizations were performed at 37°C for 18 hours in 2.4× SSC, 40 percent formamide, 10 percent dextran sulfate, 1 mg each, per milliliter, of bovine serum albumin, polyvinylpyrrollidone, and Ficoll, and 20 μg of transfer RNA per milliliter. Filters were washed for 2 hours at 65°C in 1× SSC. The probe used was the 9 kb Sst I-Sst I insert from BH-10 (3) which contains the entire HTLV-III genome less 180 basepairs of LTR sequences, 3 × 10^6 dpm/ml (specific activity approximately 2 × 10^8 dpm/g). Blots were exposed to Kodak XAR-5 film for 2 days.

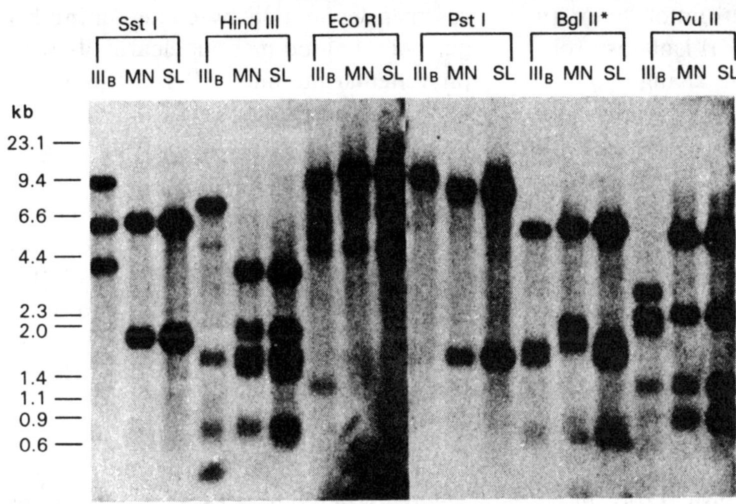

Fig. 2. Comparison of two closely related HTLV-III isolates. DNA from MN and SL (Table 1) was analyzed with six enzymes, with HTLV-III$_B$ used for comparison. Methods were as described in the legend to Fig. 1. As shown, MN and SL differ only in the size of one Bgl II fragment.

Hind III) whose site in the viral LTR is well conserved (9) and by identifying internal restriction fragments. In sum, each of the 18 viral genomes could be distinguished from the others by at least one, and usually many, restriction site differences and no genotypic pattern was evident that correlated with a particular disease state such as AIDS, ARC, or asymptomatic carrier.

The results in Fig. 1 suggested that different isolates of HTLV-III represent a spectrum of related viruses. To evaluate further this spectrum of diversity, we compared two closely related isolates, MN and SL, with the more distantly related isolates in the H9/HTLV-III$_B$ producer cell line (Fig. 2). This blot-hybridization shows that MN and SL differ from each other in only 1 of 23 restriction sites (see Bgl II digestion), yet they differ from HTLV-III$_B$ in more than half of the sites tested.

To determine how the differences in restriction patterns of the isolates shown in Figs. 1 and 2 correlate with differences in nucleotide sequence, we have, in oth-er studies, determined the nucleotide sequence of a full-length clone of the isolate RF. This RF clone (HAT-3) differs from the BH-10 clone of the H9/HTLV-III$_B$ line in 14 of 31 restriction sites and in 8.5 percent of base pairs over the entire length of the viral genome (10). Similarly, ARV-2 differs from BH-10 in approximately half of its restriction sites and in 6.5 percent of its base pairs, while LAV-1A is very similar to BH-10 in restriction pattern and differs in 1.9 percent of its base pairs. Thus, as expected, the extent of restriction site differences between AIDS virus isolates correlates with their degree of nucleotide sequence divergence, and comparison of restriction patterns provides an important estimate of their overall relatedness. It should be noted, however, that while genomic restriction mapping is useful in evaluating overall similarities between viral isolates, it does not adequately reflect the clustering of nucleotide sequence changes that have been identified in certain regions of the viral genome, especially the envelope (6, 11).

The finding of a spectrum of diversity among different HTLV-III isolates probably reflects progressive changes in the viral genome over time. Isolates MN and SL were both isolated at approximately the same time (1984) from patients in the New York–New Jersey area and they are quite similar in restriction pattern. Similarly, HTLV-III$_B$ and LAV were both isolated from patients with contacts in the New York–New Jersey area in 1983 and their nucleotide sequences are also quite similar (5). Conversely, isolates ARV and RF were obtained from patients from California and Haiti, respectively, and they are considerably more divergent (5, 6, 10).

Characterization of viral DNA in cultured and primary cells has allowed us to determine whether more than one viral genotype could be present in a given patient at any one point in time. Of the 18 patients evaluated, two (JS and RJ) had evidence of infection with more than one viral genotype. This is shown for patient JS in Fig. 1, where enzymes that cut in the viral LTR (Bgl II and Hind III) generated bands adding up to more than one 10-kb genomic complement. This finding was confirmed by using other enzymes including double digestions with Sst I, which also cuts within the LTR. Although more than one viral genotype was not found in the other 16 patients, it is possible that they were present in the uncultured tissues but not in amounts sufficient for detection by blot-hybridization [fresh tissue specimens generally contain only very small amounts of viral DNA; see (3, 11)]. At the same time, propagation of virus in vitro could provide a selective growth advantage for one form of the virus and that other forms present in vivo could go unrecognized. However, we cultured virus from patient JS by cocultivating his peripheral blood mononuclear cells with phytohemagglutinin (PHA)-stimulated allogeneic lymphocytes (7) on four separate occasions over a period of 1 year, and on each occasion two similar viral forms were identified by restriction analysis. This suggests that the virus which grows in culture is representative of predominant forms in vivo but still does not rule out the possibility that some viral forms may not grow readily in vitro.

We have also analyzed the effects of long-term propagation of the virus in vitro on its genomic restriction pattern. Figure 3 demonstrates that the major internal restriction fragments for Sst I, Pvu II, and Hind III (as well as for Bgl II, Eco RI, and Pst I, not shown) were unchanged for H9/HTLV-III$_B$ after 9 months in culture. This cell line has served as the principal source of reagents for characterizing the HTLV-III virus and for detecting antibodies in patient sera directed specifically against it (1). In studies of two other viral isolates (RF and MOV), we have observed similar genomic stability after cultivation of infected cell lines in vitro for 3 to 9 months (6). In other studies (3), we have shown that infection of allogeneic lymphocytes and two different T-cell lines by the same virus isolate does not lead to changes in its genomic restriction pattern. These results thus indicate that the genomic differences described here for the ten cultured isolates are not due to changes introduced by cultivation of these viruses in vitro.

Although the HTLV-III$_B$ restriction patterns did not change noticeably in vitro, what did change in this virus-producing permanent cell line was the number of different viral genotypes present and their state of integration. The

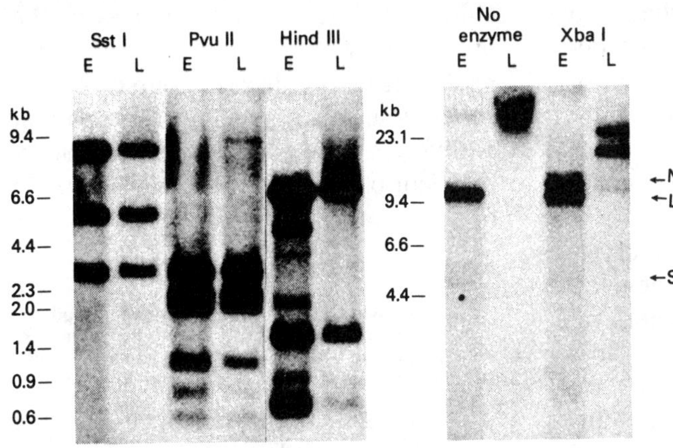

Fig. 3. Comparison of viral DNA in early and late passage H9/HTLV-III$_B$ cells. These cells were harvested on two occasions: 2 months after infection (early, E) and after continuous propagation in culture for an additional 9 months (late, L). Arrows indicate positions of different forms of unintegrated DNA; S. supercoiled; L, linear; N, nicked circular; Sst I, Pvu II, and Hind III cut in the viral LTR and internally. Xba I does not cut within the virus genome. Hybridization conditions were those described in Fig. 1.

disappearance of a subset of Hind III bands (Fig. 3) corresponds to the loss of a specific viral genotype. The appearance of two discrete high-molecular-weight bands in Xba I–digested DNA of late-passage cells, and the disappearance of bands migrating as linear, superhelical, and nicked-circular DNA in the same DNA, reflect a change from predominantly unintegrated viral DNA to predominantly integrated viral DNA. That two discrete high-molecular-weight bands are generated by Xba I, an enzyme that does not cut within the HTLV-III$_B$ genomes, suggests that the cells containing these sequences are proliferating in a clonal fashion. It should be noted that these studies in vitro, involving propagation of a virally infected cell line such as H9/HTLV-III$_B$, do not address the question of the rate and extent of genomic divergence of AIDS viruses since the viral progeny in these lines probably do not progress through a complete life cycle including reverse transcription. It is in this step catalyzed by the RNA-dependent DNA polymerase that changes in the viral genome would

be expected to occur most frequently. Studies of viral changes occurring in vivo and after repeated reinfection in vitro will be necessary to examine these issues.

Our results indicate that genomic diversity is a characteristic and prominent feature of the AIDS viruses, that the variation between isolates ranges from slight to rather extensive, and that most patients appear to be infected with only one or two predominant forms of the virus at any one time. Other studies indicate that it is the envelope gene that varies most among different viral isolates (5, 6, 10). These findings, along with the demonstration that HTLV-III and visna virus are related in their nucleotide sequence, morphology, cytopathic effects, and propensity to infect brain cells (11, 12), point to genomic diversity of HTLV-III as a property likely to be fundamentally important to its biologic activity and pathogenicity. Both visna virus and equine infectious anemia virus (EIAV) are believed to avoid elimination by host immune defense mechanisms by undergoing progressive changes in their enve-

604

lope proteins during the course of infection (*13*). It is not yet known whether a similar type of immunologic escape occurs with HTLV-III, but the existence of neutralizing antibodies in infected individuals (*14*) and the relatedness of HTLV-III to visna virus and EIAV make this a serious consideration.

Another question is why some individuals infected with HTLV-III develop AIDS, others ARC, and still others no disease at all (*15*). Viral genotype, host immune response, and other factors are likely to be determinants of clinical outcome. From our analysis of the 18 HTLV-III isolates, we were unable to identify any disease-specific restriction pattern. In fact, each of the 18 viral isolates was different from the next and none were identical to HTLV-III$_B$, LAV, or ARV. Further nucleotide sequence analyses and deletion mutant studies (*16*) will be needed to identify regions of the HTLV-III genome responsible for the virus's biologic effects and for correlating viral genotype with clinical outcome.

Finally, it is of interest that in most patients only one predominant form of the AIDS virus was identified. If this is not the result of selective pressures introduced by cultivation in vitro, it suggests that some sort of interference process may occur, since these patients, especially the hemophiliacs, homosexuals, and intravenous drug addicts, are subject to repeated exposures to genotypically diverse viruses. The data would also then suggest that if genotypic variation is being generated in vivo as occurs

with visna virus and EIAV (*13*), then either it is a rather slow process or the preexisting viral strains are largely eliminated during the disease course. Analyses of viral isolates from the same patient at different time points and from donor-recipient pairs of individuals would help to address these questions.

References and Notes

1. M. Popovic, M. G. Sarngadharan, E. Read, R. C. Gallo, *Science* **224**, 497 (1984); R. C. Gallo *et al.*, *ibid.*, p. 500; M. G. Sarngadharan *et al.*, *ibid.*, p. 506; F. Wong-Staal and R. C. Gallo, *Blood* **65**, 253 (1985).
2. F. Barré-Sinoussi *et al.*, *Science* **220**, 868 (1983); F. Brun-Vezinet, *et al.*, *Lancet* **1984-I**, 1253 (1984); L. Montagnier *et al.*, in *Human T-Cell Leukemia/Lymphoma Viruses*, R. C. Gallo, M. Essex, L. Gross, Eds. (Cold Spring Harbor Press, Cold Spring Harbor, N.Y., 1984), pp. 363–370; J. Levy *et al.*, *Science* **225**, 840 (1984).
3. B. H. Hahn *et al.*, *Nature (London)* **312**, 166 (1984); G. M. Shaw *et al.*, *Science* **226**, 1165 (1984).
4. L. Ratner *et al.*, *Nature (London)* **313**, 277 (1985); S. Wain-Hobson *et al.*, *Cell* **40**, 9 (1985); R. Sanchez-Pescador *et al.*, *Science* **227**, 484 (1985).
5. L. Ratner, R. C. Gallo, F. Wong-Staal, *Nature (London)* **313**, 636 (1985).
6. B. H. Hahn *et al.*, *Proc. Natl. Acad. Sci. U.S.A.*, in press.
7. S. Z. Salahuddin *et al.*, *ibid.*, in press.
8. See M. Popovic *et al.* in (*1*), p. 498.
9. L. Ratner *et al.*, in preparation.
10. B. Starcich *et al.*, in preparation.
11. G. M. Shaw *et al.*, *Science* **227**, 177 (1985).
12. M. A. Gonda *et al.*, *ibid.*, p. 173.
13. J. E. Clements, F. S. Pederson, O. Narayan, W. A. Haseltine, *Proc. Natl. Acad. Sci. U.S.A.* **77**, 4454 (1980); R. C. Montelaro, B. Parekh, A. Orrego, C. J. Issel, *J. Biol. Chem.* **259**, 10539 (1984).
14. M. Robert-Guroff, M. Brown, R. C. Gallo, *Nature (London)*, in press; D. Ho *et al.*, *ibid.*, in press; R. A. Weiss *et al.*, *ibid.*, in press.
15. H. W. Jaffe *et al.*, *Ann. Intern. Med.* **102**, 627 (1985).
16. A. G. Fisher *et al.*, *Nature (London)*, in press.
17. We thank J. Oleske, J. Hoxie, S. Broder, J. Groopman, L. Epstein and R. Price for supplying clinical specimens, W. Parks for providing viral isolate MJ, and A. Mazzuca for editorial assistance.

3 April 1985; accepted 3 July 1985

108.   The Epidemiology of AIDS: Current Status and Future Prospects

James W. Curran, W. Meade Morgan, Ann M. Hardy, Harold W. Jaffe, William W. Darrow, and Walter R. Dowdle

The first cases of acquired immune deficiency syndrome (AIDS) were reported in mid-1981 (*1*). The initial occurrence of the syndrome among homosexual men and users of intravenous drugs suggested a transmissible agent as the cause. The transmissible agent hypothesis became more widely accepted by early 1983, with the well-documented occurrence of the syndrome in persons with hemophilia and recipients of blood transfusions (*2*). During the next year, a retrovirus variously termed lymphadenopathy-associated virus (LAV), human T-lymphotropic virus type III (HTLV-III), or AIDS-associated retrovirus (ARV) was isolated and shown to be the cause of AIDS (*3*).

Magnitude of the Problem

Cases in the United States. By 30 August 1985, 12,932 cases of AIDS had been reported to the Centers for Disease Control (CDC); more than half had been reported during the preceding 12 months. Over 6,480 (50 percent) persons were known to have died; the case fatality rate was over 75 percent for patients diagnosed before January 1983. Of the 12,767 adult cases, more than 73 percent were in homosexual or bisexual men (12

percent who also used intravenous drugs); 17 percent occurred in heterosexual men or women who used intravenous drugs. An additional 195 (1.5 percent) patients with no other risk factors had received a transfusion of whole blood or one of its components within 5 years of diagnosis, and 86 (0.7 percent) were persons with hemophilia who had received clotting factor concentrates. There were 129 (1.0 percent) heterosexual partners of AIDS patients or persons at increased risk for AIDS. The remaining 814 (6.4 percent) could not be classified by recognized risk factors for AIDS; this group included 341 persons born outside the United States, in countries where most AIDS cases have not been associated with known risk factors. Most of these cases in the United States were among Haitians. Of the 165 cases diagnosed among infants and children, 116 (70 percent) were born to a parent who had AIDS or belonged to an identified risk group for AIDS, 25 (15 percent) had received transfusions, 9 (5 percent) had hemophilia, and the remaining 15 had no identified risk factor or incomplete epidemiologic investigations.

Cases have been reported from 46 states, the District of Columbia, and three U.S. territories. Most cases have been reported from New York, Califor-

606

nia, New Jersey, and Florida, but proportionately greater increases have been noted recently from other states. The geographic distribution of AIDS cases in children with parents in high-risk groups is similar to that seen in heterosexual adult patients with AIDS.

The ad hoc model described in Fig. 1 predicts that over 12,000 additional cases will be diagnosed between July 1985 and June 1986 inclusive (4). Over half of these cases are predicted to be from states other than New York and California.

Cases outside the United States. By March 1985, 940 cases of AIDS had been reported from Europe to the World Health Organization Collaborating Center on AIDS (5). The largest number of cases were reported from France (307) and the Federal Republic of Germany (162). Seventy-two percent of cases re-

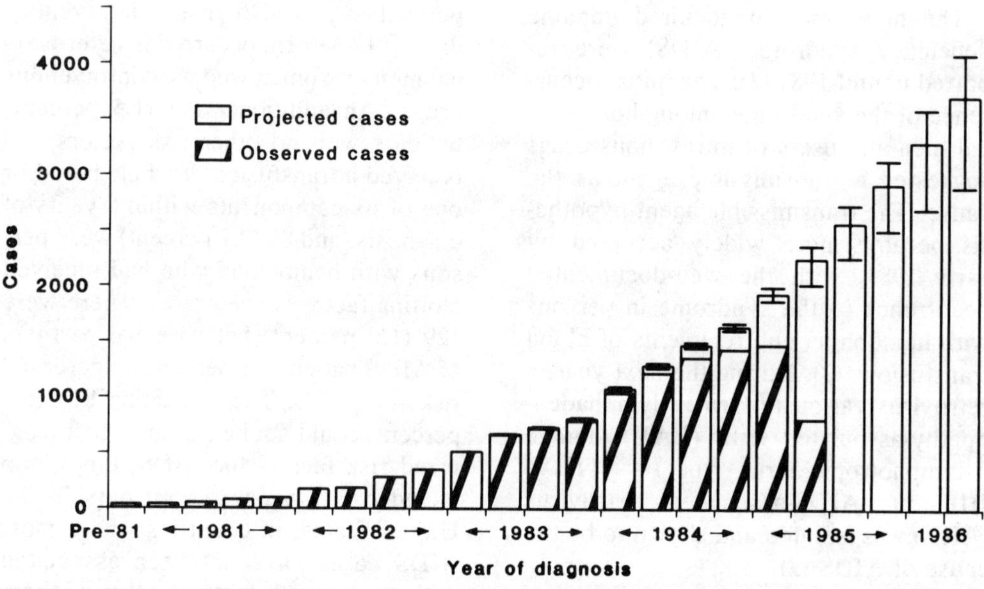

Fig. 1. Incidence of AIDS in the United States, by quarter of diagnosis projected from cases reported as of 30 June 1985. The AIDS cases in the United States reported to CDC as of 30 June 1985 (shaded bars) were used to project the number of cases expected to be diagnosed through the second quarter of 1986 (open bars). The projections were made in two stages. First, with the assumption that the distribution of delays between the actual diagnosis of AIDS and the report of these cases to CDC will remain constant over time, the cases reported each month were adjusted to obtain estimates of the cases actually diagnosed. The adjustment indicates that approximately 13,600 cases of AIDS were diagnosed as of 30 April 1985. Second, to project future cases to be diagnosed, a polynomial model was fitted to the adjusted case counts as transformed by the Box-Cox method (4). The transformation was used to obtain homoscedastic residuals suitable for calculating prediction intervals. The 95 percent confidence intervals for the first quarter of 1985 and before account for the expected variation in adjusting for reporting delays; the prediction intervals for the second quarter of 1985 and beyond account for the usual residual variance as well as that introduced by adjusting the case counts and applying the Box-Cox transformation. The model indicates that approximately 12,500 new AIDS cases will be diagnosed between 1 July 1985 and 30 June 1986, with a 95 percent prediction interval ranging from 10,000 to 14,000.

ported were in homosexual men, but only 1.5 percent were in heterosexual men and women who used intravenous drugs. As of December 1984, 111 (15 percent) of the European patients were born in one of 18 African countries. Twenty-four (3 percent) of the European patients were born in Caribbean countries, with the majority from Haiti.

In the Americas, 778 cases had been reported from 14 countries other than the United States, the largest numbers being from Haiti (340), Canada (190), and Brazil (182) (6). Outside Europe and the Americas, the only country with a large number of reported cases is Australia (95).

Cases have been reported in residents of nearly 20 countries in Africa, but studies of AIDS have been conducted primarily in Zaire and Rwanda (7). In Zaire, the male to female ratio was approximately 1.1 to 1, and the annual incidence was estimated to be between 17 and 40 per hundred thousand population.

Incidence rates and mortality. Estimates of population-specific annual incidence rates of AIDS place the magnitude of the AIDS problem in the United States in perspective (Fig. 2) (8). Single men in Manhattan and San Francisco, intravenous drug users in New York City and New Jersey, and hemophilia A patients had high rates of disease (>250 per 100,000). For these groups, 1984 incidence rates of AIDS were similar to U.S. population incidence rates of all cancers (1973–1977 average annual incidence rate of 331.5 per 100,000) and mortality rate of heart disease (1982 mortality rate of 191 per 100,000) (9).

Recent Haitian entrants had estimated incidence rates much higher than Haitians who had entered the United States prior to 1978. This finding is consistent with the observation that AIDS is also a fairly new disease in Haiti.

Female partners of men who use intravenous drugs and recipients of blood transfusions had much lower estimated rates of AIDS. The estimated rate for transfusion-associated AIDS in children was nearly five times that in adults. Most pediatric patients had received their transfusions at the time of birth. Whether this observed increased risk is related to an increased susceptibility due to an immature immune system, to coexisting diseases, to a shorter latency period, or to other factors is unknown. The incidence rate of AIDS for those not in any of the groups listed is extremely low, about 0.1 per 100,000.

The high case fatality rate and the relative youth of those affected by AIDS leads to a dramatic effect on life expectancy in groups with a high incidence of disease. One way to examine this is with "years of potential life lost" (YPLL) before age 65, a measure of premature mortality (Table 1). In single (never-married) men aged 25 to 44 years in the United States, YPLL due to AIDS in 1984 was only slightly less than YPLL attributable to all cancers. In Manhattan and San Francisco, AIDS-related YPLL ranked above the other individual causes examined. In the United States in 1984, AIDS increased YPLL due to all causes among single men aged 25 to 44 years by at least 5 percent. In Manhattan and San Francisco this increase will be 43 and 74 percent, respectively.

Natural History of HTLV-III/LAV Infection

Prevalence of infection by risk group. Of homosexual men tested in large cities in the United States or Europe, 17 to 67

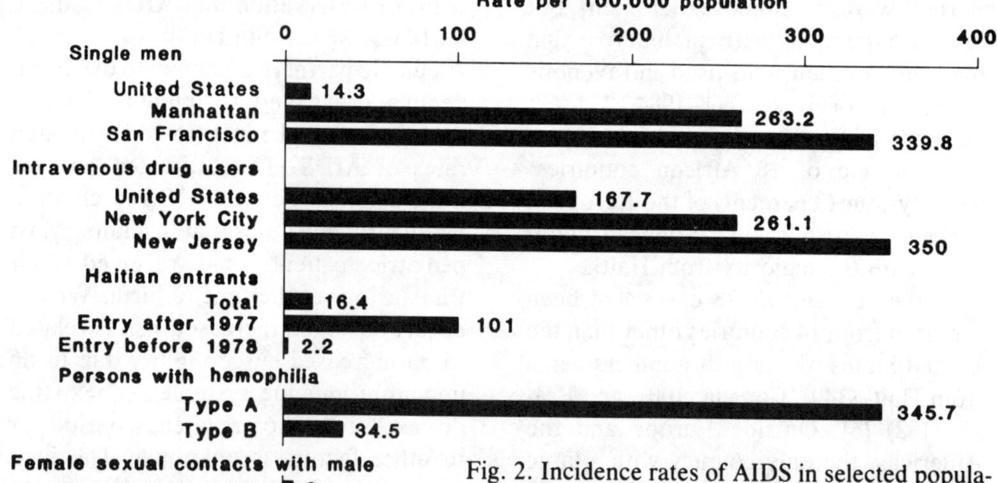

Fig. 2. Incidence rates of AIDS in selected population groups in the United States in 1984. Rates were calculated by dividing AIDS cases diagnosed in 1984 and reported to CDC by 13 May 1985 by estimates of the number in the various population groups and adjusting these to rates per 100,000 population. These denominator estimates were obtained as follows: for single men, 1980 census figures for single (never-married) men aged 15 years or older were used; estimates of intravenous drug users were provided by the National Institute on Drug Abuse, the New Jersey State Health Department, and the New York State Division of Substance Abuse Services; the figure for Haitian entrants includes legal immigrants, apprehended illegal entrants, and an estimate of undetected illegal entrants through 1984 as determined by the Immigration and Naturalization Services; an estimate of the number of persons with hemophilia was available from a survey done in 1976; the number of female partners of male intravenous drug users was assumed to be 80 percent of the total number of male intravenous drug users; for blood transfusion recipients, figures obtained from the American Blood Commission of blood recipients from 1978 to 1983 were adjusted to include only recipients who would survive long enough to develop clinically apparent AIDS (8).

percent have been reported to have antibody to HTLV-III/LAV, depending on the characteristics of the population (10). Antibody prevalence estimates in intravenous drug users in New York and New Jersey ranged from 50 to 87 percent, while prevalence in Europe is reported to be lower, 1.5 to 36 percent (10, 11). Persons with hemophilia A who had received clotting factor concentrates had 72 to 85 percent seropositively rates, and exposure to HTLV-III/LAV through use of cryoprecipitate has also been documented (12). Hemophiliacs in Europe also demonstrated serologic evidence of infection (10, 13).

In some developing countries such as Haiti and Zaire, the prevalence of HTLV-III/LAV antibody in adults ranged from 4 to 8 percent (3, 14). HTLV-III/LAV antibody was reported to have been found in 50 of 75 serum samples collected from healthy children in Uganda as early as 1972 and 1973 (15). Since AIDS has not been reported from Uganda, the interpretation of this finding is unclear.

In high-risk populations, infection with HTLV-III/LAV is considerably more common than AIDS. A retrospective analysis of 6,875 members of a hepatitis B study cohort in San Francisco

Table 1. Years of potential life lost (YPLL) by cause of death and geographic area for single men aged 25 to 44 years. YPLL before age 65 can be used as a measure of premature mortality and are derived by multiplying the cause-specific number of deaths in each age category by the difference between 65 years and the midpoint age of each category. YPLL due to AIDS are for 1984; all other causes are for 1980 and were calculated from data provided by the National Center for Health Statistics.

Cause of death	United States	Manhattan	San Francisco
All	642,400	16,100	5,800
Accidents	188,000	1,400	1,500
Homicide, suicide	174,600	4,800	2,000
Cancer	39,500	800	400
AIDS	32,300	7,000	4,300

showed that, by the time the first two cases of AIDS were diagnosed, 24 percent had antibody to HTLV-III/LAV (Table 2). In 1980, the ratio of seropositive persons to persons with AIDS was 825:1. In 1984, 68 percent of the men had antibody to HTLV-III/LAV, and over 2.4 percent had been diagnosed with AIDS, indicating that serologic evidence of infection was then 28 times more common than AIDS. The lag between virus infection and the occurrence of AIDS has prevented the community or high-risk population from recognizing the severity of the AIDS problem until a large number of individuals have been infected. We assume that the infection in most areas of the United States lags behind the 1984 HTLV-III infection-to-AIDS rates of the San Francisco cohort. If the infection-to-AIDS ratio is currently between 50:1 and 100:1, then it can be estimated that between 500,000 to 1,000,000 Americans have been infected with HTLV-III/LAV to date. The number of cases of AIDS projected to be diagnosed next year (Fig. 1) would then represent an annual attack rate of from 1 to 2 percent of those currently infected with the virus.

Persistence of infection with HTLV-III/LAV. Retrovirus infections in animals persist for prolonged periods, usu-

ally for life. HTLV-III/LAV infection in humans can also persist, at least for several years. The virus has been isolated months to years after the onset of symptoms from 85 percent or more of seropositive individuals with AIDS, lymphadenopathy, or other associated conditions (*3*). In investigations of cases of transfusion-associated AIDS, HTLV-III/LAV was isolated from specimens obtained from 22 of 23 seropositive blood donors an average of 28 months after the implicated donation (*16*). All but one of the high-risk blood donors were asymptomatic at the time of donation, and 15 of 22 remained asymptomatic when virus was isolated from 1 to 4 years later. In another study, HTLV-III/LAV was isolated from the blood of 8 of 12 homosexual men who had been asymptomatic and seropositive for 4 to 69 months. Low T-helper to T-suppressor ratios were most frequent in men who had been seropositive the longest (*17*). Because persistent infection with HTLV-III/LAV can be readily demonstrated in asymptomatic persons, the presence of specific antibody should be considered presumptive evidence of current infection and infectibility.

The spectrum of HTLV-III/LAV infection and AIDS. An acute mononucleosis-like illness characterized by fever, mal-

Table 2. Estimate of number of individuals with HTLV-III/LAV antibody and AIDS, 1978–1984 (from San Francisco CDC cohort study (n = 6875).

Variable	1978	1979	1980	1981	1982	1983	1984
Seropositive (%)	4	12	24	35*	46*	57*	68
Estimated number seropositive	275	825	1650	2406	3162	3919	4675
Cumulative number reported with AIDS	0	0	2	14	41	84	166

*Estimated.

aise, gastrointestinal symptoms, myalgia, sore throat, diarrhea, and generalized lymphadenopathy described in 11 homosexual men within days to weeks after exposure provides evidence of an acute clinical and immunologic response to infection with HTLV-III/LAV (18). In three of these individuals, seroconversion to HTLV-III/LAV occurred after onset of clinical and immunologic findings. These findings support the concept of an acute, transient, and generally nonspecific HTLV-III/LAV syndrome, but the time interval from infection to diagnosis of AIDS may be quite long. The median interval between receipt of blood transfusion and diagnosis of AIDS among cases reported to date is 29 months in adults and 14 months in infants (2, 19). However, this estimate is probably low since only cases with the shortest incubation times have been diagnosed. A recent study estimates the mean incubation period for transfusion-associated AIDS to be 4.5 years (20). In another study, among homosexual men developing AIDS, the average interval between seroconversion and diagnosis of AIDS exceeded 3 years (21).

In a representative sample of 474 homosexual men in the San Francisco cohort study, initially seen between 1978 and 1980 and enrolled in a follow-up study in 1984, AIDS had been diagnosed and reported in 2.7 percent. Another 25.8 percent had clinical signs or symptoms or laboratory evidence of AIDS-related conditions, particularly generalized lymphadenopathy (Table 3). Over 57 percent of those with no signs of illness were seropositive for HTLV-III/LAV (21). The estimated mean follow-up after seroconversion was just over 3 years, and approximately 3.6 percent of those with antibody have been diagnosed with AIDS.

The short-term prognosis is reported to be worse in persons who have AIDS-related conditions severe enough to require medical care. In these studies', from 6 to 20 percent of patients were diagnosed with AIDS during 2 years of follow-up (22). In one prospective study of generalized lymphadenopathy, patients were more likely to be subsequently diagnosed with AIDS if they initially had low T-helper cell counts, anemia, lymphopenia, and other symptoms in addition to the generalized lymphadenopathy (22).

Modes of Transmission

HTLV-III/LAV has been isolated from peripheral blood, semen, saliva, and tears (23). In most cases of AIDS in the United States, the virus appears to have been transmitted through one or more of four routes: sexual contact, intravenous drug administration with contaminated needles, administration of blood and blood products, and passage of the virus from infected mothers to their newborns. Several epidemiologic studies have identified specific behavioral risk factors for AIDS and HTLV-III/LAV infection in homosexual men (22, 24). An increased number of sexual partners was the most consistent risk factor associated with acquisition of infection or AIDS in homosexual men. In addition, receptive anal intercourse and other practices associated with rectal trauma often differentiated cases from controls in these studies. Heterosexual transmission of HTLV-III/LAV infection appeared to be most closely associated with being a steady heterosexual partner of a person with AIDS or of a seropositive individual in a risk group (25). Studies in Central Africa and the United States have also shown that sexual contact with prostitutes and large numbers of heterosexual partners are risk factors for AIDS in heterosexual men (7, 26).

Among intravenous drug users, the sharing of needles, presumably contaminated with infectious blood, has been implicated as a risk factor for AIDS and HTLV-III/LAV infection (11).

Transfusion-associated AIDS has been caused by receipt of a unit of whole blood or blood component from a donor infected with HTLV-III/LAV. Frequently the donor is asymptomatic. Patients who received blood components from large numbers of donors were more likely to be exposed. Blood components implicated in transmission include red cells, platelets, plasma, and whole blood (2, 19). HTLV-III/LAV infection has been transmitted to persons with hemophilia through pooled plasma products, specifically clotting factor concentrates. HTLV-III seroprevalence increases with severity of hemophilia and increased use of clotting factor (12). Recently, the use of cryoprecipitate has also been implicated in the transmission of HTLV-III/LAV (2, 12).

Most infants with AIDS were born to mothers with AIDS or in high-risk groups. The occurrence of symptoms shortly after birth and the absence of cases in older children suggests transmission in utero, or during or shortly

Table 3. Prevalence of AIDS, related conditions, and HTLV-III/LAV antibody in homosexual men, San Francisco Health Department/CDC cohort study, 1984 [adapted from Jaffe *et al.* (17)].

Condition*	Number of men (%)		Number of antibody-positive/ number tested (%)	
AIDS	13	(2.7)	10/10	(100.0)
Generalized lymphadenopathy	98	(20.7)	82/89	(92.1)
Other signs or symptoms suggesting AIDS prodrome	14	(3.0)	11/14	(78.6)
Hematologic abnormalities	10	(2.1)	10/10	(100.0)
None of the above	339	(71.5)	180/312	(57.7)
Total	474	(100.0)	293/435	(67.4)

*If more than one condition was present, the participant was included only in the group listed first. Definitions for AIDS-related conditions were as follows. Generalized lymphadenopathy: palpable nodes of at least 1.0 cm diameter in two or more extrainguinal sites, not more than one of which was cervical. Other signs or symptoms suggesting AIDS prodrome: fever or diarrhea lasting at least 2 weeks or weight loss of at least 10 lbs in last 4 months; oral candidiasis on examination. Hematologic abnormalities: hematocrit <40.0, absolute lymphocyte count <1500 per cubic millimeter, or absolute neutrophil count <1200 per cubic millimeter.

after birth (*27*). Recently, HTLV-III/LAV seroconversion was described in an infant of a mother who had acquired HTLV-III/LAV infection postnatally from a blood transfusion. It has been hypothesized that transmission occurred from the mother to the infant as a result of breast-feeding or other close mother-to-infant contact (*28*).

Epidemiologic studies of AIDS suggest that heterosexual transmission accounts for a larger proportion of cases in developing countries, although homosexual transmission, transmission through blood transfusion, and from infected mothers to newborns have also been reported. The association of HTLV-III/LAV infection with the number of injections received for therapeutic and nontherapeutic purposes in some developing countries suggests that reuse of nonsterile needles may contribute to transmission (*14, 29*).

Of the 10,533 cases of AIDS reported by 24 May 1985, 371 (3.5 percent) were in health-care workers. All but 31 (8.4 percent) of these health-care workers belonged to known AIDS risk groups. In the completed investigations of cases outside risk groups, no specific occupational exposures could be documented. Five hundred and twelve health-care workers have been enrolled in a prospective evaluation of persons exposed by a parenteral or mucous membrane route to blood or body fluids from patients with AIDS or symptoms suggestive of AIDS. Serologic testing for HTLV-III/LAV has been completed for 105, 82 percent of whom had parenteral exposure from needlesticks or cuts from sharp instruments. None of the 105 participants demonstrated seroconversion to HTLV-III/LAV after an average 8-month follow-up

(*30*). In another study, none of 85 employees with nosocomial exposure seroconverted to HTLV-III/LAV, including 32 individuals who encountered needlestick accidents or other parenteral exposures to blood (*31*). A recent report, however, describes a nurse in England who developed confirmed HTLV-III/LAV antibody following a needlestick injury and exposure to the blood of an AIDS patient. This seroconversion occurred 27 to 45 days after exposure and was accompanied by lymphadenopathy and fever, consistent with the acute symptoms described with HTLV-III/LAV (*32*). From the data available, the risk of HTLV-III/LAV infection to health-care and laboratory workers appears to be small, even following parenteral exposure to blood from patients with AIDS. However, these workers should continue to follow precautions when caring for persons with definite or suspected AIDS or with serologic or epidemiologic evidence of infection and when handling specimens from these patients. Summaries of these precautions have been published (*33*). There is no evidence of transmission of HTLV-III/LAV infection from health-care workers to individuals under their care.

Although concern has been expressed that HTLV-III/LAV might be present in hepatitis B vaccine, there is now considerable evidence concerning the safety of this vaccine in regard to HTLV-III/LAV transmission. Epidemiologic studies have not detected an association between vaccine and AIDS in cases of AIDS reported to the Centers for Disease Control and in members of AIDS risk groups who received hepatitis B vaccine. Further, several of the inactivation steps used in the manufacture of the

U.S.-licensed hepatitis B vaccine have been shown to reduce HTLV-III/LAV virus to undetectable levels in vitro (*34*).

Similarly, no cases of AIDS or HTLV-III/LAV infection have been attributed to the use of immunoglobulins. These pooled products undergo fractionation with ethyl alcohol, which has been shown to inactive HTLV-III/LAV in vitro (*35*). Although high levels of antibody to HTLV-III/LAV were detected in commercial hepatitis B immunoglobulin, there was no evidence of HTLV-III/LAV transmission from this product. In 19 recipients of 31 doses of HBIG containing antibody to HTLV-III/LAV, low levels of passively acquired antibody were detected shortly after injection, but the reactivity did not persist. Six months after the immunoglobulin injection, all patients were seronegative to HTLV-III/LAV and remained clinically well (*36*).

After 4 years of close observation of AIDS in the United States, there has been no evidence of transmission of HTLV-III/LAV infection or AIDS through food, by arthropods, or from casual contact.

Determinants of Outcome Among Individuals with HTLV-III/LAV

Most individuals infected with HTLV-III/LAV do not develop AIDS within the first few years. Whether or how cofactors or host susceptibility factors increase the risk of AIDS in infected persons is unknown. The higher rate of transfusion-associated AIDS in infants suggests that infection in the perinatal period may be especially virulent, perhaps because of the immaturity of the neonatal immune system. Whether other factors that suppress the immune system, such as medical use of steroids or antineoplastic agents, other coexisting immunosuppressant diseases, severe protein-calorie malnutrition, or even old age, may increase the risk of AIDS in persons infected with HTLV-III/LAV is unknown. The occurrence of AIDS in previously healthy young persons from all risk groups, however, suggests that, while such cofactors may modify the course of infection, they are not likely to be essential for AIDS to develop in an individual infected with HTLV-III/LAV.

The rates of individual opportunistic diseases occurring in AIDS patients vary by risk groups. Tuberculosis has been reported more frequently in users of intravenous drugs and patients from developing countries, cryptococcal meningitis is more common in Africans with AIDS, and disseminated toxoplasmosis occurs in proportionately more cases among persons born in Haiti (*29, 37*).

More puzzling are the differential rates of Kaposi's sarcoma (KS). In the United States, KS has been reported in over 34 percent of homosexual men with AIDS, but only 6 percent of patients in all other groups. Both classic KS as well as KS in AIDS have been associated with the presence of the HLA DR5 haplotype (*38*), but this association cannot explain the excess occurrence in homosexual men compared with other groups with AIDS. An increased frequency of use of nitrite inhalants has been reported in homosexual men with KS compared to homosexual men with other manifestations of AIDS or with asymptomatic HTLV-III/LAV infection (*39*). In addition, cytomegalovirus (CMV) infection has been associated with classic KS, and there is a high frequency of CMV infection in homosexual men with and without AIDS (*40, 41*). Both CMV and the use of nitrite inhalants deserve further attention as possible cofactors for KS in persons with HTLV-III/LAV infection.

Prospects for Prevention and Control

Substantial progress has been made in prevention of HTLV-III/LAV transmission through blood and blood products. In March 1983, the U.S. Public Health Service advised that members of high risk groups for AIDS voluntarily refrain from donating blood (*41*). The Food and Drug Administration (FDA) also published guidelines to that effect for blood and plasma centers in the United States. Serologic tests for antibody to HTLV-III/LAV were licensed in March 1985 and are currently being used to screen blood and plasma donations in virtually every center in the United States. Preliminary results reported by the FDA show repeatable enzyme-linked immunosorbent assay (ELISA) reactivity in 0.25 percent of the first 1,100,000 units of donated blood tested (*42*). The low prevalence of repeatable ELISA reactivity is consistent with a low level of infectivity among current blood and plasma donors and indicates that discarding these units will decrease the risk of virus transmission and have minimal effect on blood supplies. The interpretation of positivity in the ELISA and the effect of notification of blood donors are currently under study.

HTLV-III/LAV is sensitive to heat in vitro (*35, 43*). Heat-treated clotting factor concentrates have been developed and are commercially available. The National Hemophilia Foundation has recommended that all patients with hemophilia be treated with these products. Preliminary follow-up studies of seronegative hemophiliacs suggest that these products do not transmit HTLV-III/LAV infection. Screening donated blood and plasma for HTLV-III/LAV and using safer clotting factor concentrates should greatly reduce transmission of HTLV-III/LAV through blood and blood products in the future. Because of the long incubation period of AIDS, however, cases in hemophiliacs and recipients of blood transfusions will continue to be reported in those who have been already infected.

In March 1983, the Public Health Service recommended that members of high-risk groups reduce the number of their sexual partners to avoid acquiring or transmitting the infection causing AIDS (*41*). Surveys confirm a substantial reduction in the average number of reported sexual partners in homosexual men during the past 2 years. During this time the number of reported sexually transmitted infections in homosexual men was greatly reduced (*44*). Cases of rectal gonorrhea in men attending the San Francisco city health department clinics declined 73 percent between 1980 and 1984. Undoubtedly this trend reflects a major change in behavior leading to transmission of sexually transmitted infections. While cases of rectal gonorrhea declined by 73 percent, the prevalence of antibody to HTLV-III/LAV in homosexual men increased 280 percent in the hepatitis B study cohort previously described. Thus, the risk of exposure to HTLV-III/LAV for homosexual men may be greater now than it was in the early 1980's despite substantial behavior changes. To be safe from risk of exposure to HTLV-III/LAV infection, persons should avoid any sexual activity that involves the exchange of body fluids, such as semen, with an individual who is known or suspected to be infected. When the prevalence of any sexually transmitted infection is high in a population, as is true with HTLV-III/LAV in homosexual men, any sexual contact with an individual whose infection status is unknown should be considered high risk. For uninfected individuals likely to continue sexual exposure to HTLV-III/LAV, such preventive measures as condoms, diaphragms, or spermicides offer some theoretical protection, but their efficacy is unproved. With other sexually transmitted infections, these measures reduce but do not eliminate the risk of infection.

The risk of HTLV-III/LAV infection and of AIDS in infants born to infected mothers is substantial but has not yet been quantified. The Public Health Service has recommended that women with clinical, epidemiologic, or serologic evidence of infection with HTLV-III/LAV should postpone or avoid pregnancy to prevent transmission to the fetus or newborn (45). Women who may have been exposed should have a serologic test for HTLV-III/LAV before considering pregnancy. Premarital and prenatal screening for antibody to HTLV-III/LAV should be seriously considered by physicians or clinics providing care for women in populations with increased risk of infection, such as intravenous drug users.

Individuals with clinical, epidemiologic, or serologic evidence of infection with HTLV-III/LAV should avoid transmission to others through sexual intercourse and sharing needles and should refrain from donating blood, plasma, body organs, other tissues, or sperm (45). In addition, donors of organs, tissue, or sperm should be serologically tested for HTLV-III/LAV to prevent transmission (46).

The Future

Future strategies for preventing HTLV-III/LAV infection will involve vaccine or specific antiviral therapy, should either or both become available. Currently, preventing HTLV-III/LAV infections depends upon education and counselling to prevent sexual transmission and transmission among intravenous drug users and from infected mothers to newborns. Prevention efforts begin with providing up-to-date, accurate information and sound recommendations to individuals on how to prevent transmission. Community prevention programs must proceed now, before definitive evidence of their effectiveness is available. They should be evaluated according to their ability to prevent HTLV-III/LAV infection as well as to influence behavior. To maximize efficiency and chance for success, prevention efforts of public health agencies and community groups should be coordinated.

In the absence of vaccine or therapy, the incidence of AIDS in the United States is likely to increase during the next few years. Since HTLV-III/LAV infection has wide-ranging effects on the immune system, infection may affect the course and prognosis of other diseases; knowledge of HTLV-III/LAV infection status will become increasingly important for the management of many medical disorders. More widespread use of the serologic test will make apparent the

616

need for carefully considered policies for safe and equitable handling of infected persons in day-care centers, schools, prisons, and chronic care institutions (*47*). Concerns about confidentiality will threaten to jeopardize research and public health control efforts unless they are adequately and credibly addressed.

It is unlikely that casual contact will play a significant role in transmission of HTLV-III/LAV infection. Current modes of transmission will remain stable, and sexual transmission of the virus will account for the vast majority of cases in the United States for many years to come. Homosexual men and persons who abuse intravenously administered drugs will remain at extraordinary risk for AIDS; the disease will probably become the major cause of death in these populations.

During the past 4 years, research has resulted in an understanding of the etiology and pathogenesis of AIDS and the modes of transmission of the virus causing it. A continued commitment to research is needed to develop a vaccine and therapy and to further understand the natural history of HTLV-III/LAV infection. Control of AIDS and HTLV-III/LAV infection cannot await the benefits of future research. There is an urgent need for community groups and health professionals to work together and utilize the tools available to prevent AIDS and care for its victims.

References and Notes

1. Centers for Disease Control (CDC), *Morbid. Mortal. Weekly Rep.* **30**, 250 (1981); *ibid.*, p. 305.
2. CDC, *ibid.* **31**, 365 (1982); *ibid.*, p. 652; J. W. Curran *et al.*, *N. Engl. J. Med.* **310**, 69 (1984).
3. F. Barré-Sinoussi *et al.*, *Science* **220**, 868 (1983); R. C. Gallo *et al.*, *ibid.* **224**, 500 (1984); J. A. Levy *et al.*, *ibid.* **225**, 840 (1984).
4. G. E. P. Box and D. R. Cox, *J. R. Statist. Soc. Ser. B* **26**, 211 (1964).
5. CDC, *Morbid. Mortal. Weekly Rep.* **34**, 471 (1985).
6. R. K. St. John, Pan American Health Organization, unpublished data.
7. P. Piot *et al.*, *Lancet* **1984-II**, 65 (1984); P. Vande Perre *et al.*, *ibid.*, p. 62; J. M. Mann *et al.*, paper presented at International Conference on AIDS, Atlanta, Georgia, April 1985.
8. A. M. Hardy, J. R. Allen, W. M. Morgan, J. W. Curran, *J. Am. Med. Assoc.* **253**, 215 (1985).
9. J. L. Young and E. S. Pollack, in *Cancer Epidemiology and Prevention*, D. Schottenfeld and J. F. Fraumeni, Eds. (Saunders, Philadelphia, 1982), pp. 138–165; *Health, United States, 1983* (PHS Pub. No. 84-1232, Department of Health and Human Services, Washington, D.C., 1983).
10. CDC, *Morbid. Mortal. Weekly Rep.* **33**, 377 (1984); B. Safai *et al.*, *Lancet* **1984-I**, 1438 (1984); J. Schüpbach *et al.*, *N. Engl. J. Med.* **312**, 265 (1985); R. Cheingsong-Popov *et al.*, *Lancet* **1984-II**, 477 (1984); H. W. Jaffe *et al.*, *Ann. Intern. Med.*, in press.
11. S. H. Weiss *et al.*, paper presented at International Conference on AIDS, Atlanta, Georgia, April 1985; H. Cohen, *et al.*, *ibid.*
12. CDC, *Morbid. Mortal. Weekly Rep.* **34**, 241 (1985); G. McGrady *et al.*, paper presented at International Conference on AIDS, Atlanta, Georgia, April 1985; M. E. Eyster *et al.*, *J. Am. Med. Assoc.* **253**, 2219 (1985); B. L. Evatt *et al.*, *N. Engl. J. Med.* **312**, 483 (1985).
13. M. Melbye *et al.*, *Lancet* **1984-II**, 1444 (1984).
14. J. M. Mann *et al.*, paper presented at International Conference on AIDS, Atlanta, Georgia, April 1985; J. W. Pape *et al.*, *ibid.*
15. W. C. Saxinger *et al.*, *Science* **227**, 1036 (1985).
16. P. M. Feorino *et al.*, *N. Engl. J. Med.* **312**, 1293 (1985).
17. H. W. Jaffe *et al.*, *Ann. Intern. Med.* **102**, 627 (1985).
18. D. A. Cooper *et al.*, *Lancet* **1985-I**, 537 (1985).
19. T. A. Peterman *et al.*, paper presented at International Conference on AIDS, Atlanta, Georgia, April 1985.
20. K.-J. Lui *et al.*, unpublished data.
21. H. W. Jaffe *et al.*, *Ann. Intern. Med.*, in press.
22. D. B. Fishbein *et al.*, *J. Am. Med. Assoc.*, in press; J. J. Goedert *et al.*, *Lancet* **1984-II**, 711 (1984); U. Mathur-Wagh *et al.*, *ibid.* **1984-I**, 1033 (1984); D. I. Abrams, B. J. Lewis, J. H. Beckstead, C. A. Casavant, L. Drew, *Ann. Intern. Med.* **100**, 801 (1984).
23. J. E. Groopman, S. Z. Salahuddin, M. G. Sarngadharan, P. D. Markham, M. Gonda, A. Sliski, R. C. Gallo, *Science* **226**, 447 (1984); D. Zagury *et al.*, *ibid.*, p. 449; L. S. Fujikawa *et al.*, *Lancet*, **1985-II**, 529 (1985).
24. H. W. Jaffe *et al.*, *Ann. Intern. Med.* **99**, 145 (1983); M. Marmor *et al.*, *ibid.* **100**, 809 (1984); M. Melbye *et al.*, *Br. Med. J.* **289**, 573 (1984).
25. J. K. Kreiss *et al.*, *Ann. Intern. Med.* **102**, 623 (1985); J. M. Mann *et al.*, paper presented at International Conference on AIDS, Atlanta, Georgia, April 1985; C. A. Harris *et al.*, *ibid.*
26. N. Clumeck *et al.*, paper presented at International Conference on AIDS, Atlanta, Georgia, April 1985; C. Rabkin *et al.*, *ibid.*; CDC, *Morbid. Mortal. Weekly Rep.* **33**, 661 (1984).
27. J. Oleske *et al.*, *J. Am. Med. Assoc.* **249**, 2345 (1983); A. Rubinstein *et al.*, *ibid.* p. 2350; P. A. Thomas *et al.*, *ibid.* **252**, 639 (1984); G. B. Scott *et al.*, *ibid.* **253**, 363 (1985); N. LaPointe *et al.*, *N. Engl. J. Med.* **312**, 1325 (1985).

28. J. B. Ziegler *et al.*, *Lancet* **1985-I**, 896 (1985).
29. J. W. Pape *et al.*, *N. Engl. J. Med.* **309**, 945 (1983); B. M. Kapita *et al.*, paper presented at International Conference on AIDS, Atlanta, Georgia, April 1985.
30. E. McCray *et al.*, paper presented at International Conference on AIDS, Atlanta, Georgia, April 1985; CDC, *Morbid. Mortal. Weekly Rep.* **34**, 101 (1985).
31. M. S. Hirsch *et al.*, *N. Engl. J. Med.* **312**, 1 (1985).
32. Anonymous, *Lancet* **1984-I**, 1376 (1984).
33. CDC, *Morbid. Mortal. Weekly Rep.* **31**, 577 (1982); ______, *ibid.* **32**, 450 (1983); J. E. Conte, W. K. Hadley, M. Sande., *N. Engl. J. Med.* **309**, 740 (1983).
34. CDC, *Morbid. Mortal. Weekly Rep.* **33**, 685 (1984); I. M. Jacobson *et al.*, *N. Engl. J. Med.* **311**, 1030 (1984).
35. L. S. Martin *et al.*, paper presented at International Conference on AIDS, Atlanta, Georgia, April 1985; B. Spire, F. Barré-Sinoussi, L. Montagnier, J. C. Chermann, *Lancet* **1984-II**, 899 (1984).
36. R. S. Tedder, A. Uttley, R. Cheingsong-Popov, *Lancet* **1985-I**, 815 (1985).
37. J. Vierra, E. Frank, T. J. Spira, S. H. Landesman, *N. Engl. J. Med.* **308**, 129 (1983); N. Clumeck *et al.*, *ibid.* **310**, 492 (1984); A. E. Pitchenik *et al.*, *Ann. Intern. Med.* **98**, 277 (1983).
38. A. E. Friedman-Kien *et al.*, *Ann. Intern. Med.* **96**, 693 (1982); M. S. Pollack, B. Safai, B. DuPont, *Disease Markers* **1**, 135 (1983).
39. H. W. Haverkos *et al.*, paper presented at International Conference on AIDS, Atlanta, Georgia, April 1985; A. R. Moss *et al.*, *ibid.*
40. M. F. Rogers *et al.*, *Ann. Intern. Med.* **99**, 151 (1983); G. Giraldo *et al.*, *Int. J. Cancer* **15**, 839 (1975); G. Giraldo *et al.*, *ibid.* **22**, 126 (1978); G. Giraldo *et al.*, *ibid.* **26**, 23 (1980); W. L. Drew *et al.*, *J. Infect. Dis.* **143**, 188 (1981); W. L. Drew *et al.*, *Lancet* **1982-II**, 125 (1982).
41. CDC, *Morbid. Mortal. Weekly Rep.* **32**, 101 (1983).
42. CDC, *ibid.* **34**, 477 (1985).
43. CDC, *ibid.* **33**, 589 (1984); J. S. McDougal *et al.*, *J. Clin. Invest.*, in press.
44. CDC, *Morbid. Mortal. Weekly Rep.* **33**, 295 (1984); F. N. Judson, *Lancet* **1983-II**, 159 (1983); M. T. Schechter *et al.*, *ibid.* **1984-I**, 1293 (1984).
45. CDC, *Morbid. Mortal. Weekly Rep.* **34**, 1 (1985).
46. CDC, *ibid.*, p. 294.
47. CDC, *ibid.*, p. 517.
48. We thank R. Byers, R. Selik, D. Echenberg, and E. McCray for sharing data and Q. V. Harris and A. Navin for technical assistance.

List of Authors

J.S. Allan, *Department of Cancer Biology, Harvard School of Public Health, Boston, Massachusetts 02115.*

Harvey J. Alter, *Blood Bank Department, Clinical Center, National Institutes of Health, Bethesda, Maryland 20205.*

A.A. Ansari, *Navy Medical Research Unit No. 3, Cairo, Egypt, FPO New York, New York 09527.*

D. Armstrong, *Department of Medicine, Memorial Sloan-Kettering Cancer Center, New York, New York 10021.*

Larry O. Arthur, *Biological Products Laboratory, Program Resources, Inc., NCI—Frederick Cancer Research Facility, Frederick, Maryland 21701.*

Suresh K. Arya, *Laboratory of Tumor Cell Biology, National Cancer Institute, Bethesda, Maryland 20205.*

C. Axler-Blin, *Institut Pasteur, Département de Virologie, 75724 Paris Cédex 15, France.*

F. Barin, *Department of Cancer Biology, Harvard School of Public Health, Boston, Massachusetts 02115.*

A.D. Barone, *Centocor, Inc., 244 Great Valley Parkway, Malvern, Pennsylvania 19355.*

Philip J. Barr, *Chiron Research Laboratories, Chiron Corporation, 4560 Horton St., Emeryville, California 94608.*

Françoise Barré-Sinoussi, *Institut Pasteur, Département de Virologie, 75724 Paris Cédex 15, France.*

J. Michael Bedford, *Department of Obstetrics and Gynecology, Cornell University Medical College, New York, New York 10021.*

Raoul E. Benveniste, *Laboratory of Viral Carcinogenesis, NCI—Frederick Cancer Research Facility, Frederick, Maryland 21701.*

J. Bernard, *Institut Jean Godinot, Reims, 75005 Paris, France.*

R. Biggar, *National Cancer Institute, Bethesda, Maryland 20205.*

J. Edwin Blalock, *Department of Microbiology, University of Texas Medical Branch, Galveston, Texas 77550.*

W.A. Blattner, *National Cancer Institute, Bethesda, Maryland 20205.*

Douglas Blayney, *Epidemiology Branch, National Cancer Institute, Bethesda, Maryland 20205.*

Madeleine Boncy, *Haitian Study Group on Kaposi's Sarcoma and Opportunistic Infections (GHESKIO), Post Office Box 15267, Pétion-ville, Haiti.*

E.H. Braff, *San Francisco City Clinic, 356 7th St., San Francisco, California 94103.*

C. Brechot, *Unité de Recombinaison et Expression Génétique, INSERM Unit 163, CNRS-LA-271 Institut Pasteur, Paris, France.*

C. Bridts, *University of Antwerp, Antwerp, Belgium.*

Debra Briggs, *Dana-Farber Cancer Institute, Department of Pathology, Harvard Medical School, Boston, Massachusetts 02115.*

Samuel Broder, *Laboratory of Tumor Cell Biology, National Cancer Institute, Bethesda, Maryland 20205.*

Sheryl L. Brown-Shimer, *Chiron Research Laboratories, Chiron Corporation, 4560 Horton St., Emeryville, California 94608.*

Lilian Bruch, *Department of Cell Biology, Litton Bionetics, Inc., 5516 Nicholson Lane, Kensington, Maryland 20895.*

620

C. Bruck, *Department of Molecular Biology, University of Brussels, 1640 Rhode St., Genèse, Belgium.*

Françoise Brun-Vézinet, *Hôpital Claude Bernard, Laboratoire Central—Virologie, 10 avenue de la Porte d'Aubervilliers, 75019 Paris, France.*

J.B. Brunet, *Direction Générale de la Santé, Paris, France.*

Arsene Burny, *Department of Molecular Biology, University of Brussels, 1640 Rhode St., Genèse, Belgium.*

C.D. Cabradilla, *Center for Infectious Diseases, Centers for Disease Control, Atlanta, Georgia 30333.*

Doreen A. Cantrell, *Department of Medicine, Dartmouth Medical School, Hanover, New Hampshire 03756.*

Salvatore J. Caradonna, *Department of Pharmacology, Louisiana State University Medical Center, New Orleans, Louisiana 70112.*

James W. Casey, *Section of Genetics, Laboratory of Viral Carcinogenesis, NCI—Frederick Cancer Research Facility, Frederick, Maryland 21701.*

S. Chamaret, *Institut Pasteur, Département de Virologie, 75724 Paris Cédex 15, France.*

P.K. Chanda, *Centocor, Inc., 244 Great Valley Parkway, Malvern, Pennsylvania 19355.*

N.T. Chang, *Centocor, Inc., 244 Great Valley Parkway, Malvern, Pennsylvania 19355.*

T.W. Chang, *Centocor, Inc., 244 Great Valley Parkway, Malvern, Pennsylvania 19355.*

R. Cheingsong-Popov, *Institute of Cancer Research, Chester Beatty Laboratories, Fulham Road, London SW3 6JB, England.*

Irvin S.Y. Chen, *Division of Hematology-Oncology, Department of Medicine, UCLA School of Medicine, Los Angeles, California 90024.*

Jean-Claude Chermann, *Institut Pasteur, Département de Virologie, 75724 Paris Cédex 15, France.*

Nicholas Chiorazzi, *Department of Immunology, Rockefeller University, New York, New York 10021.*

Eun-Sook Cho, *Department of Pathology, University of Medicine and Dentistry of New Jersey, Newark, New Jersey 07103.*

P. Clapham, *Institute of Cancer Research, Chester Beatty Laboratories, Fulham Road, London SW3 6JB, England.*

J. Clark, *National Cancer Institute, Bethesda, Maryland 20205.*

Steven C. Clark, *Genetics Institute, 87 Cambridge Park Drive, Cambridge, Massachusetts 02140.*

Janice E. Clements, *Department of Neurology, Johns Hopkins University School of Medicine, Baltimore, Maryland 21205.*

Martin J. Cline, *Division of Hematology-Oncology, Department of Medicine, UCLA School of Medicine, Los Angeles, California 90024.*

N. Clumeck, *Saint-Pierre Hospital, University of Brussels, 1000 Brussels, Belgium.*

J. Cogniaux, *Institut Pasteur du Branbant, 1180 Brussels, Belgium.*

John E. Coligan, *Laboratory of Immunogenetics, National Institute of Allergy and Infectious Diseases, Bethesda, Maryland 20205.*

Jeffrey Cossman, *Laboratory of Tumor Cell Biology, National Cancer Institute, Bethesda, Maryland 20205.*

S. Cran, *Saint-Pierre Hospital, University of Brussels, 1000 Brussels, Belgium.*

R. Crookes, *South African Blood Transfusion Service, Johannesburg, South Africa.*

Barbara J. Culliton, *SCIENCE, 1333 H St., N.W., Washington, D.C. 20005.*

James W. Curran, *Center for Infectious Diseases, Centers for Disease Control, Atlanta, Georgia 30333.*

Marinos C. Dalakas, *Infectious Diseases Branch, National Institute of Neurological and Communicative Disorders and Stroke, Bethesda, Maryland 20205.*

Muthiah D. Daniel, *New England Regional Primate Research Center, Harvard Medical School, Southborough, Massachusetts 01772.*

William W. Darrow, *AIDS Branch, Division of Viral Diseases, Center for Infectious Diseases, Centers for Disease Control, Atlanta, Georgia 30333.*

Charles Dauguet, *Institut Pasteur, Département de Virologie, 75724 Paris Cédex 15, France.*

N.K. Day, *Cancer Research Program, Oklahoma Medical Research Foundation, Oklahoma City, Oklahoma 73104.*

Guy de Thé, *Laboratoire d'Épidémiologie et Immunovirologie des Tumeurs, Lyon, France.*

A.G. Dean, *International Agency for Research in Cancer, Lyon, France.*

Joel M. Depper, *Metabolism Branch, National Cancer Institute, Bethesda, Maryland 20205.*

David Derse, *Section of Genetics, Laboratory of Viral Carcinogenesis, NCI—Frederick Cancer Research Facility, Frederick, Maryland 21701.*

J. Desmyter, *Rega Institute, University of Leuven, Leuven, Belgium.*

Ronald C. Desrosiers, *New England Regional Primate Research Center, Harvard Medical School, Southborough, Massachusetts 01772.*

David Dickson, *SCIENCE, 1333 H St., N.W., Washington, D.C. 20005.*

Dino Dina, *Chiron Research Laboratories, Chiron Corporation, 4560 Horton St., Emeryville, California 94608.*

R.Y. Dodd, *American Red Cross Blood Services Laboratories, Bethesda, Maryland 20814.*

Tim A. Donlon, *Department of Genetics, Children's Hospital Medical Center, Boston, Massachusetts 02115.*

Walter R. Dowdle, *AIDS Branch, Division of Viral Diseases, Center for Infectious Diseases, Centers for Disease Control, Atlanta, Georgia 30333.*

B. Dupont, *Department of Human Immunogenetics, Memorial Sloan-Kettering Cancer Center, New York, New York 10021.*

Jorg W. Eichberg, *Virology and Immunology Department, Southwest Foundation for Biomedical Research, San Antonio, Texas 78284.*

R.W. Engelman, *Cancer Research Program, Oklahoma Medical Research Foundation, Oklahoma City, Oklahoma 73104.*

Leon G. Epstein, *Laboratory of Central Nervous System Studies, National Institute of Neurological and Communicative Disorders and Stroke, Bethesda, Maryland 20205.*

M. Essex, *Department of Cancer Biology, Harvard School of Public Health, Boston, Massachusetts 02115.*

B.L. Evatt, *Center for Infectious Diseases, Centers for Disease Control, Atlanta, Georgia 30333.*

M. Exley, *Institute of Cancer Research, Chester Beatty Laboratories, Fulham Road, London SW3 6JB, England.*

L. Falk, *Department of Cancer Biology, Harvard School of Public Health, Boston, Massachusetts 02115.*

Anthony S. Fauci, *Laboratory of Immunoregulation, National Institute of Allergy and Infectious Diseases, Bethesda, Maryland 20205.*

F.M. Feinsod, *National Institute of Allergy and Infectious Disease, Bethesda, Maryland 20205.*

Barbara K. Felber, *LBI-Basic Research Program, NCI—Frederick Cancer Research Facility, Frederick, Maryland 21701.*

M. Feldman, *Weizmann Institute, Rehovot, Israel.*

P.M. Feorino, *Center for Infectious Diseases, Centers for Disease Control, Atlanta, Georgia 30333.*

Peter J. Fischinger, *NCI—Frederick Cancer Research Facility, Frederick, Maryland 21701.*

D. Fishbein, *Center for Infectious Diseases, Centers for Disease Control, Atlanta, Georgia 30333.*

N. Flomenberg, *Department of Human Immunogenetics, Memorial Sloan-Kettering Cancer Center, New York, New York 10211.*

Theresa Flynn, *Infectious Disease Unit, Massachusetts General Hospital, Harvard Medical School, Boston, Massachusetts 02114.*

Paul Foster, *Department of Medicine, University of North Carolina, Chapel Hill, North Carolina 27514.*

D.P. Francis, *Center for Infectious Diseases, Centers for Disease Control, Atlanta, Georgia 30333.*

R.W. Fulton, *Department of Microbiology, College of Veterinary Medicine, Oklahoma State University, Stillwater, Oklahoma 74078.*

D. Carleton Gajdusek, *Laboratory of Central Nervous System Studies, National Institute of Neurological and Communicative Disorders and Stroke, Bethesda, Maryland 20205.*

Robert C. Gallo, *Laboratory of Tumor Cell Biology, National Cancer Institute, Bethesda, Maryland 20205.*

Murray B. Gardner, *Department of Pathology, School of Medicine, University of California, Davis, California 95616.*

Judith C. Gasson, *Division of Hematology-Oncology, Department of Medicine, UCLA School of Medicine, Los Angeles, California 90024.*

Wendy W. Gee, *Chiron Research Laboratories, Chiron Corporation, 4560 Horton St., Emeryville, California 94608.*

Edward P. Gelmann, *Laboratory of Tumor Cell Biology, National Cancer Institute, Bethesda, Maryland 20205.*

D. Geroldi, *Institut Pasteur, Départment de Virologie, 75724 Paris Cédex 15, France.*

J.P. Getchell, *Center for Infectious Diseases, Centers for Disease Control, Atlanta, Georgia 30333.*

W. Ellis Giddens, Jr., *Department of Pathology, School of Medicine, University of Washington, Seattle, Washington 98195.*

Raymond V. Gilden, *Program Resources, Inc., NCI—Frederick Cancer Research Facility, Frederick, Maryland 21701.*

Jean Claude Gluckman, *Laboratoire d'Immunologie Nephrologique et de Transplantation, UER Pitié-Salpétrière, 75634 Paris Cédex 13, France.*

Wei Chun Goh, *Dana-Farber Cancer Institute, Department of Pathology, Harvard Medical School, Boston, Massachusetts 02115.*

J. Gold, *Department of Medicine, Memorial Sloan-Kettering Cancer Center, New York, New York 10021.*

David W. Golde, *Division of Hematology-Oncology, Department of Medicine, UCLA School of Medicine, Los Angeles, California 90024.*

D. Goldfinger, *Cedars-Sinai Medical Center, Los Angeles, California 90048.*

Matthew A. Gonda, *Laboratory of Cell and Molecular Structure, Program Resources, Inc., NCI—Frederick Cancer Research Facility, Frederick, Maryland 21701.*

R.A. Good, *Cancer Research Program, Oklahoma Medical Research Foundation, Oklahoma City, Oklahoma 73104.*

J. Gootenberg, *Laboratory of Tumor Cell Biology, National Cancer Institute, Bethesda, Maryland 20205.*

M.S. Gottlieb, *Department of Medicine, UCLA School of Medicine, Los Angeles, California 90024.*

Maneth Gravell, *Infectious Diseases Branch, National Institute of Neurological and Communicative Disorders and Stroke, Bethesda, Maryland 20205.*

Warner C. Greene, *Metabolism Branch, National Cancer Institute, Bethesda, Maryland 20205.*

Claude Griscelli, *Département de Pédiatrie, Hôpital des Enfant Malades, Paris, France.*

Jerome E. Groopman, *Department of Medicine, New England Deaconess Hospital, Boston, Massachusetts 02215.*

J. Gruest, *Institut Pasteur, Départment de Virologie, 75724 Paris Cédex 15, France.*

D. Guétard, *Unité d'Oncologie Virale, Institut Pasteur, 75724 Paris Cédex 15, France.*

Chan Guo, *Laboratory of Tumor Cell Biology, National Cancer Institute, Bethesda, Maryland 20205.*

Hong-Guang Guo, *Laboratory of Tumor Cell Biology, National Cancer Institute, Bethesda, Maryland 20205.*

Beatrice H. Hahn, *Laboratory of Tumor Cell Biology, National Cancer Institute, Bethesda, Maryland 20205.*

Shinji Harada, *Department of Virology and Parasitology, Yamaguchi University School of Medicine, Ube, Yamaguchi, 755 Japan.*

Ann M. Hardy, *AIDS Branch, Division of Viral Diseases, Center for Infectious Diseases, Centers for Disease Control, Atlanta, Georgia 30333.*

Mary E. Harper, *Laboratory of Tumor Cell Biology, National Cancer Institute, Bethesda, Maryland.*

A.K. Harrison, *Center for Infectious Diseases, Centers for Disease Control, Atlanta, Georgia 30333.*

William A. Haseltine, *Dana-Farber Cancer Institute, Department of Pathology, Harvard Medical School, Boston, Massachusetts 02115.*

H.W. Haverkos, *Center for Infectious Diseases, Centers for Disease Control, Atlanta, Georgia 30333.*

Barton F. Haynes, *Department of Medicine, Duke University School of Medicine, Durham, North Carolina 27710.*

H. Hemmi, *Laboratory of Tumor Cell Biology, National Cancer Institute, Bethesda, Maryland 20205.*

Roy V. Henrickson, *California Primate Research Center, University of California, Davis, California 95616.*

Jay L. Hess, *Department of Neurology, Johns Hopkins University School of Medicine, Baltimore, Maryland 21205.*

Atsuko Hikikoshi, *Department of Viral Oncology, Cancer Institute, Kami-Ikebukuro, Toshima-ku, Tokyo 170, Japan.*

Martin S. Hirsch, *Infectious Disease Unit, Massachusetts General Hospital, Harvard Medical School, Boston, Massachusetts 02114.*

David D. Ho, *Infectious Disease Unit, Massachusetts General Hospital, Harvard Medical School, Boston, Massachusetts 02114.*

Anthony D. Hoffman, *Cancer Research Institute, Department of Medicine, University of California School of Medicine, San Francisco, California 94143.*

Mei Hoh, *Laboratory of Tumor Cell Biology, National Cancer Institute, Bethesda, Maryland 20205.*

Constance Holden, *SCIENCE, 1333 H St., N.W., Washington, D.C. 20005.*

T. Homma, *Department of Cancer Biology, Harvard School of Public Health, Boston, Massachusetts 02115.*

Sidney A. Houff, *Infectious Diseases Branch, National Institute of Neurological and Communicative Disorders and Stroke, Bethesda, Maryland 20205.*

C.W.S. Howe, *Department of Cancer Biology, Harvard School of Public Health, Boston, Massachusetts 02115.*

J. Huang, *Centocor, Inc., 244 Great Valley Parkway, Malvern, Pennsylvania 19355.*

Ronald D. Hunt, *New England Regional Primate Research Center, Harvard Medical School, Southborough, Massachusetts 01772.*

P. Jacobs, *University of Cape Town Medical School, Cape Town, South Africa.*

R. Jacobson, *Georgetown University Hospital, Washington, D.C. 20007.*

P. Jacquemin, *Institut Pasteur du Branbant, 1180 Brussels, Belgium.*

Harold W. Jaffe, *Center for Infectious Diseases, Centers for Disease Control, Atlanta, Georgia 30333.*

624

Warren D. Johnson, Jr., *Division of International Medicine, Cornell University Medical College, New York, New York 10021.*

Cheryl L. Jorcyk, *Laboratory of Molecular Oncology, NCI—Frederick Cancer Research Facility, Frederick, Maryland 21701.*

Steven F. Josephs, *Laboratory of Tumor Cell Biology, National Cancer Institute, Bethesda, Maryland 20205.*

Kayembe Kalambayi, *University Hospital, University of Kinshasa, Zaire.*

V.S. Kalyanaraman, *Center for Infectious Diseases, Centers for Disease Control, Atlanta, Georgia 30333.*

P.J. Kanki, *Department of Cancer Biology, Harvard School of Public Health, Boston, Massachusetts 02115.*

M. Kannagi, *New England Regional Primate Research Center, Harvard Medical School, Southborough, Massachusetts 01772.*

J. Kaplan, *Center for Infectious Diseases, Centers for Disease Control, Atlanta, Georgia 30333.*

Joan C. Kaplan, *Infectious Disease Unit, Massachusetts General Hospital, Harvard Medical School, Boston, Massachusetts 02114.*

Mark Kaplan, *Division of Infectious Diseases, North Shore University Hospital, Manhusset, New York 11030.*

Richard A. Kaslow, *Epidemiology and Biometry Section, National Institute of Allergy and Infectious Diseases, National Institutes of Health, Bethesda, Maryland 20205.*

C.K. Kasper, *Department of Medicine, University of Southern California Orthopedic Hospital, Los Angeles, California 90007.*

Richard Kettman, *Department of Molecular Biology, University of Brussels, 1640 Rhode St., Genèse, Belgium.*

B.W. Kilbourne, *Center for Infectious Diseases, Centers for Disease Control, Atlanta, Georgia 30333.*

Norval W. King, Jr., *New England Regional Primate Research Center, Harvard Medical School, Southborough, Massachusetts 01772.*

David Klatzmann, *Laboratoire d'Immunologie Néphrologique et de Transplantation, UER Pitié-Salpétrière, 75634 Paris Cédex 13, France.*

Carol Kleinman-Ewing, *LBI-Basic Research Program, NCI—Frederick Cancer Research Facility, Frederick, Maryland 21701.*

Gina Kolata, *SCIENCE, 1333 H St., N.W., Washington, D.C. 20005.*

Yoshio Koyanagi, *Department of Virology and Parasitology, Yamaguchi University School of Medicine, Ube, Yamaguchi, 755 Japan.*

Susan M. Kramer, *Cancer Research Institute, Department of Medicine, University of California School of Medicine, San Francisco, California 94143.*

J. Kreiss, *Wadsworth Veterans Administration Hospital, Los Angeles, California 90073.*

Martin Krönke, *Metabolism Branch, National Cancer Institute, Bethesda, Maryland 20205.*

Ruth Kulstad, *SCIENCE, 1333 H St., N.W., Washington, D.C. 20005.*

A. Claude LaRoche, *Haitian Study Group on Kaposi's Sarcoma and Opportunistic Infections (GHESKIO), Post Office Box 15267, Pétion-ville, Haiti.*

A. Landay, *Cellular Immunobiology Unit of the Tumor Institute, University of Alabama, Birmingham, Alabama 35294.*

Jill A. Landis, *Cancer Research Institute, Department of Medicine, University of California School of Medicine, San Francisco, California 94143.*

H. Clifford Lane, *Laboratory of Immunoregulation, National Institute of Allergy and Infectious Diseases, Bethesda, Maryland 20205.*

Gunhild Lange-Wantzin, *Bispebjerg Hospital, Copenhagen, Denmark.*

F. Laure, *Laboratoire de Physiologie Cellulaire, Université Pierre et Marie Curie, Paris, France.*

Jeffrey Laurence, *Department of Medicine, New York Hospital—Cornell Medical Center, New York, New York 10021.*

Francine Laurent, *Laboratory of Tumor Cell Biology, National Cancer Institute, Bethesda, Maryland 20205.*

James A. Lautenberger, *Laboratory of Molecular Oncology, NCI—Frederick Cancer Research Facility, Frederick, Maryland 21701.*

D.N. Lawrence, *Center for Infectious Diseases, Centers for Disease Control, Atlanta, Georgia 30333.*

Roger V. Lebo, *Department of Medicine, University of California, San Francisco, California 94143.*

Tun-Hou Lee, *Department of Cancer Biology, Harvard School of Public Health, Boston, Massachusetts 02115.*

Jacque Leibowitch, *Department of Immunologie, Hôpital Raymond Poincaré, 92380 Garches, France.*

Warren J. Leonard, *Metabolism Branch, National Cancer Institute, Bethesda, Maryland 20205.*

Nicholas W. Lerche, *California Primate Research Center, University of California, Davis, California 95616.*

Norman L. Letvin, *New England Regional Primate Research Center, Harvard Medical School, Southborough, Massachusetts 01772.*

Paul H. Levine, *Clinical Epidemiology Branch, National Cancer Institute, Bethesda, Maryland 20205.*

Jay A. Levy, *Cancer Research Institute, Department of Medicine, University of California School of Medicine, San Francisco, California 94143.*

A. Ley, *Department of Medicine, Memorial Sloan-Kettering Cancer Center, New York, New York 10021.*

Bernard Liautaud, *Haitian Study Group on Kaposi's Sarcoma and Opportunistic Infections (GHESKIO), Post Office Box 15267, Pétion-ville, Haiti.*

S.G. Lindner, *Laboratory of Tumor Cell Biology, National Cancer Institute, Bethesda, Maryland 20205.*

Richard E. Lloyd, *Department of Microbiology, University of Texas Medical Branch, Galveston, Texas 77550.*

William T. London, *Infectious Diseases Branch, National Institute of Neurological and Communicative Disorders and Stroke, Bethesda, Maryland 20205.*

Linda J. Lowenstine, *California Primate Research Center, University of California, Davis, California 95616.*

Paul A. Luciw, *Chiron Research Laboratories, Chiron Corporation, 4560 Horton St., Emeryville, California 94608.*

Abe M. Macher, *Laboratory of Pathology, National Cancer Institute, Bethesda, Maryland 20205.*

David L. Madden, *Infectious Diseases Branch, National Institute of Neurological and Communicative Disorders and Stroke, Bethesda, Maryland 20205.*

Dean Mann, *Laboratory of Human Carcinogenesis, National Cancer Institute, Bethesda, Maryland 20205.*

Phillip D. Markham, *Department of Cell Biology, Litton Bionetics, Inc., 5516 Nicholson Lane, Kensington, Maryland 20895.*

Jean L. Marx, *SCIENCE, 1333 H St., N.W., Washington, D.C. 20005.*

Preston A. Marx, *California Primate Research Center, University of California, Davis, California 95616.*

Henry Masur, *Critical Care Medicine Department, Clinical Center, National Institutes of Health, Bethesda, Maryland 20205.*

626

Jean-Robert Mathurin, *Haitian Study Group on Kaposi's Sarcoma and Opportunistic Infections (GHESKIO), Post Office Box 15267 Pétion-ville, Haiti.*

Shuzo Matsushita, *Clinical Oncology Program, National Cancer Institute, Bethesda, Maryland 20205.*

Donald H. Maul, *California Primate Research Center, University of California, Davis, California 95616.*

Lloyd Mayer, *Department of Immunology, Rockefeller University, New York, New York 10021.*

Mbendi N. Mazebo P., *University Hospital, University of Kinshasa, Zaire.*

J. McCormick, *Centers for Disease Control, Atlanta, Georgia 30333.*

J.S. McDougal, *Center for Infectious Diseases, Centers for Disease Control, Atlanta, Georgia 30333.*

S. McKinney, *Centocor, Inc., 244 Great Valley Parkway, Malvern, Pennsylvania 19355.*

M.F. McLane, *Department of Cancer Biology, Harvard School of Public Health, Boston, Massachusetts 02115.*

Mary Megson, *Laboratory of Tumor Cell Biology, National Cancer Institute, Bethesda, Maryland 20205.*

Kapita Bila Mirlangu, *Mama Yemo Hospital, Kinshasa, Zaire.*

S. Mitchell, *Centers for Disease Control, Atlanta, Georgia 30333.*

Hiroaki Mitsuya, *Laboratory of Tumor Cell Biology, National Cancer Institute, Bethesda, Maryland 20205.*

Jasmine Moghissi, *Laboratory of Tumor Cell Biology, National Cancer Institute, Bethesda, Maryland 20205.*

Luc Montagnier, *Institut Pasteur, Département de Virologie, 75724 Paris Cédex 15, France.*

Peggy Moody, *California Primate Research Center, University of California, Davis, California 95616.*

W. Meade Morgan, *AIDS Branch, Division of Viral Diseases, Center for Infectious Diseases, Centers for Disease Control, Atlanta, Georgia 30333.*

William R. Morton, *Regional Primate Research Center, University of Washington, Seattle, Washington 98195.*

N. Mourali, *Institute Salah Azaiz, Bab Saadoun, Tunis, Tunisia.*

J.I. Mullins, *Department of Cancer Biology, Harvard School of Public Health, Boston, Massachusetts 02115.*

Robert J. Munn, *Department of Pathology, School of Medicine, University of California, Davis, California 95616.*

Douglas C. Murdock, *Amgen, 1900 Oak Terrace Lane, Thousand Oaks, California 91320-1789.*

F.A. Murphy, *Center for Infectious Diseases, Centers for Disease Control, Atlanta, Georgia 30333.*

K. Nagy, *Institute of Cancer Research, Chester Beatty Laboratories, Fulham Road, London SW3 6JB, England.*

Opendra Narayan, *Department of Neurology, Johns Hopkins University School of Medicine, Baltimore, Maryland 21205.*

R. Narayanan, *Center for Infectious Diseases, Centers for Disease Control, Atlanta, Georgia 30333.*

William G. Nash, *Section of Genetics, NCI—Frederick Cancer Research Facility, Frederick, Maryland 21701.*

Bradford A. Navia, *Department of Neurology, Cornell University Medical College, New York, New York 10021.*

F.K. Nkrumah, *University of Ghana, Medical School, Accra, Ghana.*

Marie Thérèse Nugeyre, *Département de Virologie, Institut Pasteur, 75724 Paris Cédex 15, France.*

Stephen J. O'Brien, *Section of Genetics, NCI—Frederick Cancer Research Facility, Frederick, Maryland 21701.*

M.J. O'Connell, *New England Regional Primate Research Center, Harvard Medical School, Southborough, Massachusetts 01772.*

Carl J. O'Hara, *Department of Medicine, New England Deaconess Hospital, Boston, Massachusetts 02215.*

Hans D. Ochs, *Department of Pediatrics, Division of Immunology and Rheumatology, School of Medicine, University of Washington, Seattle, Washington 98195.*

Takashi Okamoto, *Laboratory of Tumor Cell Biology, National Cancer Institute, Bethesda, Maryland 20205.*

James M. Oleske, *Division of Allergy, Immunology, and Infectious Disease, University of Medicine and Dentistry of New Jersey, Newark, New Jersey 07103.*

Stephen Oroszlan, *Laboratory of Molecular Virology, Litton Bionetics, Inc., NCI— Frederick Cancer Research Facility, Frederick, Maryland 21701.*

Elizabeth C. Orr, *Genetics Institute, Inc., 87 Cambridge Park Drive, Cambridge, Massachusetts 02140.*

Kent G. Osborn, *California Primate Research Center, University of California, Davis, California 95616.*

Lyndon S. Oshiro, *Viral and Rickettsial Disease Laboratory, California Department of Health Services, Berkeley, California 94704.*

Thomas J. Palker, *Department of Medicine, Duke University School of Medicine, Durham, North Carolina 27710.*

Molière Pamphile, *Haitian Study Group on Kaposi's Sarcoma and Opportunistic Infections (GHESKIO), Post Office Box 15267, Pétion-ville, Haiti.*

Takis S. Papas, *Laboratory of Molecular Oncology, NCI—Frederick Cancer Research Facility, Frederick, Maryland 21701.*

Jean W. Pape, *Haitian Study Group on Kaposi's Sarcoma and Opportunistic Infections (GHESKIO), Post Office Box 15267, Pétion-ville, Haiti.*

Harry Paskalis, *LBI-Basic Research Program, NCI—Frederick Cancer Research Facility, Frederick, Maryland 21701.*

Roberto Patarca, *Dana-Farber Cancer Institute, Department of Pathology, Harvard Medical School, Boston, Massachusetts 02115.*

George N. Pavlakis, *LBI-Basic Research Program, NCI—Frederick Cancer Research Facility, Frederick, Maryland 21701.*

Vergniaud Pean, *Haitian Study Group on Kaposi's Sarcoma and Opportunistic Infections (GHESKIO), Post Office Box 15267, Pétion-ville, Haiti.*

Dennis Perkins, *Dana-Farber Cancer Institute, Department of Pathology, Harvard Medical School, Boston, Massachusetts 02115.*

Carol K. Petito, *Department of Neurology, Cornell University Medical College, New York, New York 10021.*

P. Piot, *Institute of Tropical Medicine, Antwerp, Belgium.*

M.-C. Poon, *Cellular Immunobiology Unit of the Tumor Institute, University of Alabama, Birmingham, Alabama 35294.*

Mikulas Popovic, *Laboratory of Tumor Cell Biology, National Cancer Institute, Bethesda, Maryland 20205.*

D. Portetelle, *Department of Molecular Biology, University of Brussels, 1640 Rhode St., Genèse, Belgium.*

Michael D. Power, *Chiron Research Laboratories, Chiron Corporation, 4560 Horton St., Emeryville, California 94608.*

Srinivasa Prahalada, *California Primate Research Center, University of California, Davis, California 95616.*

Michael F. Press, *Department of Pathology, University of Chicago School of Medicine, Chicago, Illinois 60637.*

Richard W. Price, *Department of Neurology, Cornell University Medical College, New York, New York 10021.*

628

Fred H. Pruslin, *Department of Cell Biology, Rockefeller University, New York, New York 10021.*

Shirley G. Quan, *Division of Hematology-Oncology, Department of Medicine, UCLA School of Medicine, Los Angeles, California 90024.*

T.C. Quinn, *National Institute of Allergy and Infectious Disease, Bethesda, Maryland 20205.*

Harvey Rabin, *LBI-Basic Research Program, NCI—Frederick Cancer Research Facility, Frederick, Maryland 21701.*

Anne Randolph, *Chiron Research Laboratories, Chiron Corporation, 4560 Horton St., Emeryville, California 94608.*

Lee Ratner, *Laboratory of Tumor Cell Biology, National Cancer Institute, Bethesda, Maryland 20205.*

Elizabeth Read, *Laboratory of Tumor Cell Biology, National Cancer Institute, Bethesda, Maryland 20205.*

Robert Redfield, *Department of Virus Diseases, Walter Reed Army Institute of Research, Washington, D.C. 20012.*

Gabrielle H. Reem, *Department of Pharmacology, New York University Medical Center, New York, New York 10016.*

Marvin S. Reitz, Jr., *Laboratory of Tumor Cell Biology, National Cancer Institute, Bethesda, Maryland 20205.*

Andre Renard, *Chiron Research Laboratories, Chiron Corporaton, 4560 Horton St., Emeryville, California 94608.*

F. Rey, *Institut Pasteur, Département de Virologie, 75724 Paris Cédex 15, France.*

D.P. Rhodes, *Centocor, Inc., 244 Great Valley Parkway, Malvern, Pennsylvania 19355.*

Jon M. Richards, *Department of Obstetrics and Gynecology, Cornell University Medical College, New York, New York 10021.*

Ersell Richardson, *Laboratory of Tumor Cell Biology, National Cancer Institute, Bethesda, Maryland 20205.*

Marjorie Robert-Guroff, *Laboratory of Tumor Cell Biology, National Cancer Institute, Bethesda, Maryland 20205.*

W. Gerard Robey, *NCI—Frederick Cancer Research Facility, Frederick, Maryland 21701.*

Toby C. Rodman, *Department of Cell Biology and Anatomy, Cornell University Medical College, New York, New York 10021.*

Craig A. Rosen, *Dana-Farber Cancer Institute, Department of Pathology, Harvard Medical School, Boston, Massachusetts 02115.*

Joseph D. Rosenblatt, *Division of Hematology-Oncology, Department of Medicine, UCLA School of Medicine, Los Angeles, California 90024.*

Teresa R. Rota, *Infectious Disease Unit, Massachusetts General Hospital, Harvard Medical School, Boston, Massachusetts 02114.*

Christine Rouzioux, *Hôpital Claude Bernard, Laboratoire Central—Virologie, 10 avenue de la Porte d'Aubervilliers, 75019 Paris, France.*

W. Rozenbaum, *Hôpital La Pitié-Salpétrière, Département de Santé Publique et Médecine Tropicale, 97 Boulevard de l'Hôpital 75013 Paris, France.*

Bijan Safai, *Dermatology Service, Memorial Sloan-Kettering Cancer Center, New York, New York 10021.*

A.G. Saimot, *Pathologie Infectieuse et Tropicale, Hôpital Claude Bernard, Paris, France.*

S. Zaki Salahuddin, *Laboratory of Tumor Cell Biology, National Cancer Institute, Bethesda, Maryland 20205.*

Kenneth P. Samuel, *Laboratory of Molecular Oncology, NCI—Frederick Cancer Research Facility, Frederick, Maryland 21701.*

Ray Sanchez-Pescador, *Chiron Research Laboratories, Chiron Corporation, 4560 Horton St., Emeryville, California 94608.*

Prem S. Sarin, *Laboratory of Tumor Cell Biology, National Cancer Institute, Bethesda, Maryland 20205.*

M.G. Sarngadharan, *Laboratory of Tumor Cell Biology, National Cancer Institute, Bethesda, Maryland 20205.*

W. Carl Saxinger, *Laboratory of Tumor Cell Biology, National Cancer Institute, Bethesda, Maryland 20205.*

Robert T. Schooley, *Infectious Disease Unit, Massachusetts General Hospital, Harvard Medical School, Boston, Massachusetts 02114.*

Jörg Schüpbach, *Laboratory of Tumor Cell Biology, National Cancer Institute, Bethesda, Maryland 20205.*

Prabhat K. Sehgal, *New England Regional Primate Research Center, Harvard Medical School, Southborough, Massachusetts 01772.*

Leonard J. Seigel, *Laboratory of Tumor Cell Biology, National Cancer Institute, Bethesda, Maryland 20205.*

Motoharu Seiki, *Department of Viral Oncology, Cancer Institute, Kami-Ikebukuro, Toshima-ku, Tokyo 170, Japan.*

John L. Sever, *Infectious Diseases Branch, National Institute of Neurological and Communicative Disorders and Stroke, Bethesda, Maryland 20205.*

Neil P. Shah, *Division of Hematology-Oncology, Department of Medicine, UCLA School of Medicine, Los Angeles, California 90024.*

George M. Shaw, *Laboratory of Tumor Cell Biology, National Cancer Institute, Bethesda, Maryland 20205.*

Gene M. Shearer, *Immunology Branch, National Cancer Institute, Bethesda, Maryland 20205.*

C.W. Shearman, *Centocor, Inc. 244 Great Valley Parkway, Malvern, Pennsylvania 19355.*

Joni M. Shimabukuro, *Cancer Research Institute, Department of Medicine, University of California School of Medicine, San Francisco, California 94143.*

Kunitada Shimotohno, *National Cancer Center Research Institute, Chuo-ku, Tokyo 104, Japan.*

Gurdip D. Sidhu, *Department of Pathology, New York University Medical Center, New York, New York 10010.*

Dennis J. Slamon, *Division of Hematology-Oncology, Department of Medicine, UCLA School of Medicine, Los Angeles, California 90024.*

Ann Sliski, *Laboratory of Tumor Cell Biology, National Cancer Institute, Bethesda, Maryland 20205.*

Kendall A. Smith, *Department of Medicine, Dartmouth Medical School, Hanover, New Hampshire 03756.*

Joseph G. Sodroski, *Dana-Farber Cancer Institute, Department of Pathology, Harvard Medical School, Boston, Massachusetts 02115.*

Lawrence M. Souza, *Amgen, 1900 Oak Terrace Lane, Thousand Oaks, California 91320-1789.*

T.J. Spira, *Center for Infectious Diseases, Centers for Disease Control, Atlanta, Georgia 30333.*

S. Sprecher-Goldberger, *Institut Pasteur du Branbant, 1180 Brussels, Belgium.*

Marie-Myrtha A. St. Amand, *Haitian Study Group on Kaposi's Sarcoma and Opportunistic Infections (GHESKIO), Post Office Box 15267, Pétion-ville, Haiti.*

Rosalyn E. Stahl, *Department of Pathology, New York Veterans Administration Hospital, New York, New York 10010.*

G. John Stanton, *Department of Microbiology, University of Texas Medical Branch, Galveston, Texas 77550.*

Bruno Starcich, *Laboratory of Tumor Cell Biology, National Cancer Institute, Bethesda, Maryland 20205.*

Kathelyn S. Steimer, *Chiron Research Laboratories, Chiron Corporation, 4560 Horton St., Emeryville, California 94608.*

S.F. Stein, *Department of Medicine, Emory University School of Medicine, Atlanta, Georgia 30322.*

Michelle M. Stempien, *Chiron Research Laboratories, Chiron Corporation, 4560 Horton St., Emeryville, California 94608.*

Kurt Stromberg, *Laboratory of Viral Carcinogenesis, NCI—Frederick Cancer Research Facility, Frederick, Maryland 21701.*

630

M. Strong, *Naval Medical Research Institute, Bethesda, Maryland 20014.*

N. Tachibana, *Department of Cancer Biology, Harvard School of Public Health, Boston, Massachusetts 02115.*

H. Taelman, *Institute of Tropical Medicine, Antwerp, Belgium.*

S.H. Tam, *Centocor, Inc., 244 Great Valley Parkway, Malvern, Pennsylvania 19355.*

Tadatsugu Taniguchi, *Institute for Molecular and Cellular Biology, Osaka University, Suita-shi, Osaka 565, Japan.*

Patricia A. Temple, *Genetics Institute, Inc., 87 Cambridge Park Drive, Cambridge, Massachusetts 02140.*

L. Thiry, *Institut Pasteur du Branbant, 1180 Brussels, Belgium.*

Franck Thomas, *Haitian Study Group on Kaposi's Sarcoma and Opportunistic Infections (GHESKIO), Post Office Box 15267, Pétion-ville, Haiti.*

Ze'ev Trainin, *Department of Cancer Biology, Harvard School of Public Health, Boston, Massachusetts 02115.*

Cecelia Trainor, *Laboratory of Tumor Cell Biology, National Cancer Institute, Bethesda, Maryland 20205.*

Che-Chung Tsai, *Regional Primate Research Center, University of Washington, Seattle, Washington 98195.*

Hannah Ungar-Waron, *Department of Immunology, Kimron Veterinary Institute, Bet-Dagan, Israel.*

Etienne Vilmer, *Département de Pédiatrie, Hôpital des Enfant Malades, Paris, France.*

D.J. Volkman, *Laboratory of Immunoregulation, National Institute of Allergy and Infectious Disease, Bethesda, Maryland 20205.*

William Wachsman, *Division of Hematology-Oncology, Department of Medicine, UCLA School of Medicine, Los Angeles, California 90024.*

D.T. Warfield, *Center for Infectious Diseases, Centers for Disease Control, Atlanta, Georgia 30333.*

Toshiki Watanabe, *Department of Viral Oncology, Cancer Institute, Kami-Ikebukuro, Toshima-ku, Tokyo 170, Japan.*

R.A. Weiss, *Institute of Cancer Research, Chester Beatty Laboratories, Fulham Road, London SW3 6JB, England.*

Dorothee Wernicke, *Department of Cancer Biology, Harvard School of Public Health, Boston, Massachusetts 02115.*

Gilbert White, *Department of Medicine, University of North Carolina, Chapel Hill, North Carolina 27514.*

L. Wilson, *University of Cape Town Medical School, Cape Town, South Africa.*

Ronald Winston, *Harry Winston Research Foundation, New York, New York 10019.*

Steven S. Witkin, *Department of Obstetrics and Gynecology, Cornell University Medical College, New York, New York 10021.*

Odio Wobin, *University Hospital, University of Kinshasa, Zaire.*

Flossie Wong-Staal, *Laboratory of Tumor Cell Biology, National Cancer Institute, Bethesda, Maryland 20205.*

Naoki Yamamoto, *Department of Virology and Parasitology, Yamaguchi University School of Medicine, Ube, Yamaguchi, 755 Japan.*

C.S. Yang, *College of Medicine, National Taiwan University, Taipei, Taiwan.*

Robert Yarchoan, *Clinical Oncology Program, National Cancer Institute, Bethesda, Maryland 20205.*

Ning-Hsing Yeh, *Department of Pharmacology, New York University Medical Center, New York, New York 10016.*

Mitsuaki Yoshida, *Department of Viral Oncology, Cancer Institute, Kami-Ikebukuro, Toshima-ku, Tokyo 170, Japan.*

D. Zagury, *Institut Jean Godinot, Reims, 75005 Paris, France.*

Susan Zolla-Pazner, *Department of Pathology, New York Veterans Administration Hospital, New York, New York 10010.*

Research News, News and Comment, and Letters to the Editor

Subject Index